MOSBY'S COMPREHENSIVE REVIEW OF DENTAL HYGIENE

MOSBY'S

Comprehensive Review of Dental Hygiene

Edited by

Michele Leonardi Darby, R.D.H., M.S.

Professor and Chairman,
Department of Dental Hygiene and Dental Assisting,
Old Dominion University,
Norfolk, Virginia

Eleanor J. Bushee, B.S., D.D.S., F.A.C.D.

Professor and Assistant Dean for Administration,
Southern Illinois University,
School of Dental Medicine,
Alton, Illinois

Illustrated

THE C. V. MOSBY COMPANY

ST. LOUIS • TORONTO • PRINCETON   1986

MOSBY

A TRADITION OF PUBLISHING EXCELLENCE

Editor: Alison Miller
Assistant editor: Susan R. Epstein
Manuscript editors: Judith Bange, Marybeth Engelhardt, Jean Babrick
Book designer: Nancy Steinmeyer
Production: Teresa Breckwoldt, Kathleen L. Teal

Printed in the United States of America

Library of Congress Cataloging in Publication Data

Main entry under title:

Mosby's comprehensive review of dental hygiene.

   Includes bibliographies and index.
   1. Dental hygiene. 2. Dental hygiene—Examinations, questions, etc. I. Darby, Michele Leonardi.
II. Bushee, Eleanor J. III. Title: Comprehensive review of dental hygiene. [DNLM: 1. Dental Prophylaxis—outlines. WU 18 M894]
RK60.7.M67 1986   617.6'01   85-15483
ISBN 0-8016-1237-3

AC/VH/VH 9 8 7 6 5 4   01/C/031

Contributors

Stephen C. Bayne, M.S., Ph.D., F.A.D.M.

Associate Professor, Section Head of Biomaterials, Department of Operative Dentistry, School of Dentistry, University of North Carolina at Chapel Hill, Chapel Hill, North Carolina

Marcia K. Brand, R.D.H., M.S.

Associate Professor, Department of Dental Hygiene, College of Allied Health Sciences, Thomas Jefferson University, Philadelphia, Pennsylvania

Catherine C. Davis, R.D.H., M.S.D.

Formerly Assistant Professor, Department of Dental Hygiene, University of Iowa, College of Dentistry, Iowa City, Iowa

Beverly Entwistle, R.D.H., M.P.H.

Assistant Professor, Department of Applied Dentistry, University of Colorado School of Dentistry, Denver, Colorado

Dianne M. Frazier, Ph.D., M.P.H., R.D.

Assistant Professor, Department of Biochemistry and Nutrition, School of Medicine, University of North Carolina at Chapel Hill, Chapel Hill, North Carolina

Jan Shaner Greenlee, R.D.H., M.S.

Penns Commons Dental Group, Ltd., Private Practice, Reading, Pennsylvania

Charlotte Hangorsky, R.D.H., M.S.

Formerly Chairman and Assistant Professor, Department of Dental Hygiene, School of Dental Medicine, University of Pennsylvania, Philadelphia, Pennsylvania

Olga A. C. Ibsen, R.D.H., M.S.

Associate Clinical Professor, Columbia University School of Dental and Oral Surgery, New York, New York

Donald E. Isselhard, B.S., D.D.S., F.A.G.D.

Creve Coeur, Missouri

Marlene Klyvert, R.D.H., M.S., M.Ed., Ed.D.

Associate Professor, Columbia University, Divisions of Dental Hygiene and Orofacial Growth and Development, School of Dental and Oral Surgery, New York, New York

Sandra Kramer, R.D.H., M.A.

Oakland, California

Mary M. Lee, R.D., Dr. P.H.

Assistant Professor, Department of Oral Diagnosis, School of Dentistry, University of North Carolina at Chapel Hill, Chapel Hill, North Carolina

Susan Schwartz Miller, R.D.H., M.S.

Formerly Assistant Professor and Graduate Program Director, Department of Dental Hygiene, Baltimore College of Dental Surgery, Dental School, University of Maryland at Baltimore, Baltimore, Maryland

John M. Powers, Ph.D.

Professor, Department of Dental Materials, University of Michigan School of Dentistry, Ann Arbor, Michigan

Lynn Ray, R.D.H., B.S.

Test Development Administrator, Central Regional Dental Testing Service, Inc., Tulsa, Oklahoma

Barbara Requa-Clark, Pharm. D.

Professor, School of Dentistry, University of Missouri–Kansas City, Kansas City, Missouri

Lindsay L. Rettie, R.D.H., M.S., Ed.D.

Associate Vice-President for Academic and Financial Affairs and Associate Professor, Department of Dental Hygiene and Dental Assisting, Old Dominion University, Norfolk, Virginia

Hazel O. Torres, C.D.A., R.D.A., M.A.

Director Emeritus, Registered Dental Assisting Program, College of Marin, Kentfield, California

Nancy B. Webb, R.D.H., M.S.

Assistant Professor, Department of Dental Hygiene and Dental Assisting, Old Dominion University, Norfolk, Virginia

K. Cy Whaley, Ed.D.

Adjunct Associate Professor, School of Allied Health Sciences, University of North Carolina at Chapel Hill, Chapel Hill, North Carolina

Esther M. Wilkins, B.S., R.D.H., D.M.D.

Associate Clinical Professor, Department of Periodontology, Tufts University School of Dental Medicine, Boston, Massachusetts

Pamela Zarkowski, R.D.H., B.S., M.P.H.

Associate Professor, Department of Dental Hygiene, University of Detroit School of Dentistry, Detroit, Michigan

To my husband, Dennis, and our daughter, Devan —
for the joy and peace they bring me

M.L.D.

To the memory of my brothers, Ralph and Ray,
whose support and encouragement were so helpful at
the beginning of this venture and so sadly
missed at its completion

E.J.B.

Preface

Developing a book that comprehensively reviews the current body of dental hygiene knowledge is a challenge. This book meets that challenge with several key purposes in mind: first, to assist the dental hygiene student in reviewing the knowledge, skills, and judgments required on national, regional, and state dental hygiene board examinations; second, to prepare the individual for reentry into the field by updating knowledge required for contemporary dental hygiene practice; and third, to provide dental hygiene educators with salient information that can be used for developing relevant course materials.

Mosby's Comprehensive Review of Dental Hygiene is divided into 19 independent, yet interrelated, chapters. Fifteen of the chapters cover the subject areas traditionally found on the National Board Dental Hygiene Examination. The remaining four chapters focus on preparing for board examinations; concepts and practice of four-handed, six-handed, and TEAM dentistry; practice management and career development strategies; and historical, professional, ethical, and legal issues facing dental hygienists.

Chapter 1 contains detailed information and practical suggestions for anyone preparing for a board examination. Chapters 2 through 19 contain subject information in an outline format, review questions, and answers with rationales explaining why the correct answer is correct, as well as the reason why each incorrect choice is wrong. This information should enable the reviewer to truly learn from each mistake.

A comprehensive index enables the user to locate information quickly and easily. Illustrations throughout the text and the appendices included separately should minimize the need to refer back to a textbook. Reference lists are provided for those who desire a more indepth review.

We would like to express our sincere appreciation to those who helped make *Mosby's Comprehensive Review of Dental Hygiene* a reality. The outlined materials, questions, and rationales used in this book were submitted by educators and practitioners who are recognized experts. The exemplary work of these contributors is certain to make *Mosby's Comprehensive Review of Dental Hygiene* a classic in the field.

A very special thanks is extended to the faculty and staff of the Department of Dental Hygiene and Dental Assisting at Old Dominion University and to the administration of Southern Illinois University School of Dental Medicine who made it possible for us to complete the text despite the demands of continuing responsibilities. From Old Dominion University we would especially like to thank instructors Constance Lady, Barbara McGrady, and Linda Wilson; assistant professors Deborah Bauman, Lynn Tolle, and Nancy Webb; associate professors Pamela Brangan, Patricia Damon-Johnson, and Cameron Lowe; professor James Luton; and staff members Toni Barks, Vanessa Beck, John Donahue, and Deborah Muth; and from Southern Illinois University, Dr. Herbert C. Butts, Dean of the School of Dental Medicine.

Our recognition and appreciation go to Deborah Miller-Carson and B. Yvonne Wilson, graphic illustrators from the Old Dominion University Center for Instructional Development, for some of the illustrations provided. We also acknowledge the authors and publishers who granted permission to use quotes, concepts, photographs, figures, and tables.

Without all these generous and talented people, the book would not have been possible.

Michele Leonardi Darby
Eleanor J. Bushee

Contents

MOSBY'S COMPREHENSIVE REVIEW OF DENTAL HYGIENE

CHAPTER 1

Preparing for National, Regional, and State Dental Hygiene Board Examinations

LYNN RAY

Preparing for board examinations requires careful planning, study and review, time management, organization of information and schedules for applications, and a positive attitude. Conscientious dental hygienists will organize a plan for success well in advance and be prepared to satisfy board requirements with confidence in their professional knowledge and skills. This book is a guide through a comprehensive body of knowledge that constitutes the basis of dental hygiene practice. Systematic use of this book can enable one to reinforce professional education, benefit from exposure to concepts and ideas from a variety of dental hygiene educators, and identify those areas where additional study is needed.

This introductory chapter outlines suggestions on how a dental hygienist—whether a new graduate, a practicing dental hygienist who is moving to another licensing jurisdiction, or a dental hygienist who wishes to begin practicing again after an extended period of inactivity— can prepare for board examinations. The chapter takes into consideration preparation for both theoretic and clinical examinations. A dental hygienist must master the basic subject matter and skills necessary for practice; therefore each chapter of this book focuses on different aspects of such knowledge and skills. However, there have been instances where highly knowledgeable and skillful dental hygienists have failed to successfully complete board examinations. It is just as essential that the dental hygienist be psychologically, emotionally, and physically prepared to demonstrate competence, and be thoroughly familiar with the format, logistics, and requirements of any examination preparatory to licensure.

This chapter provides basic information about how the credentialing system is organized and how it functions with the interaction of many different agencies and organizations. A more detailed discussion is included on the Joint Commission on National Dental Examinations, its testing program, and the development of test items.

Further discussion is devoted to regional testing services and clinical board examinations in general. The chapter concludes with an overview of this review book, including its purposes and organization, as well as instructions on how to use it effectively.

STRUCTURE OF CREDENTIALING AGENCIES

In preparing for board examinations, one should understand the credentialing system. Many dental hygienists, particularly new graduates who have never been licensed, often have only a vague understanding of the system with which they are interacting. Such lack of awareness has even resulted in a few dental hygienists' assuming that receiving a certificate for successful completion of an examination is authorization to practice, and they have begun practicing illegally without a license. Passing board examinations satisfies the major requirements for licensure, but there are usually other prerequisites as well. There is often a complex interrelationship of agencies involved in the board examination process. It behooves the examination candidate to have a clear understanding of which agency is administering an examination, how that agency functions, and by what authority the agency administers examinations and issues credentials.

State Boards of Dentistry/Dental Hygiene

The basic authority to recognize any credential for licensure lies with the state board of dentistry. Each state or licensing jurisdiction has a *state practice act* or some statutes that regulates the practice of dentistry/dental hygiene within that jurisdiction. Such statutes also establish a regulatory agency to enforce the law, conduct examinations for competence, and regulate the practice of dentistry/dental hygiene. There are features that virtually all state practice acts have in common; however, even a cursory review of state practice acts will alert one to the fact that they are inconsistent in defining the legal practice of dentistry/dental hygiene. Great variations exist from state to state in the way regulatory boards are organized, the power or authority they have, and even in the names with which they are entitled. For the purpose of clarity in this text, the term *state board* or *state board of dentistry* is used to refer to the regulatory agency in a respective state that is empowered to determine prerequisites for licensure and issue licenses to practice dental hygiene. One of the first things a candidate for licensure should know is the correct title of the state board for the state(s) in which licensure is sought.

It is far too common for licensure candidates, and even licensed practitioners in a state, to have a fuzzy conception of what the state board actually is. Many professionals confuse the board with the local state dental association. While there are usually strong ties between a state board and the state dental association, legally there are distinct differences in their organization and purpose. The state board of dentistry is a *government agency,* established by law, that functions as an arm of the state legislature to regulate the practice of dentistry. Its sole purpose is to protect the public from incompetent or unethical practitioners. In contrast, a state dental or dental hygiene association is a *voluntary organization* of practitioners who join together to promote the oral health of the public and advance the profession. As one studies the credentialing system, it becomes evident that dental/dental hygiene associations are integrally involved in activities that impact on the legal requirements for licensure. However, it is important to understand the distinction between state boards and professional associations. Professional associations *do not* determine requirements for licensure or regulate practice; that is determined by law and implemented through state boards. Professional associations *do,* however, initiate programs and research projects, studies, and legislative changes that are ultimately incorporated into the legal requirements for practice. Specific examples of the interrelationship between state boards and professional associations are provided with further explanation of the credentialing system.

Since state boards of dentistry are charged with the responsibility of conducting examinations for competence to practice, the candidate for licensure should be aware of how board members are identified. It is of particular interest to candidates for clinical examinations, because state board members are very likely to be the clinical examiners. In the vast majority of states, state board members are appointed by the governor; in only two states (North Carolina and Oklahoma) are board members selected by an elective process within the profession. Despite the fact that gubernatorial appoint-

ments are the prevailing method, professional associations have an impact on this process as well. It is general practice in most states for the state association to submit a list of nominees from which the governor appoints. While the governor is often not limited to such a list, in most instances appointments are made from the nominees designated by the association. Most states have few if any formal criteria for qualifications of board members.

Dental hygienists may be interested in activities of their professional associations that have changed the face of the credentialing system. In the early 1970s state boards consisted almost universally of dentists, with a few boards having public members. As a result of the legislative initiatives of many state dental hygiene associations, within 10 years about 40 state boards included one or more dental hygienists in their membership. The 1980s have brought a thrust in some states to establish separate dental hygiene state boards. Since the 1960s another area of activity in many states has been to expand the functions that constitute the legal practice of dental hygiene. Changes in these functions and in the structure of state boards has had, and will continue to have, an impact on the content and format of board examinations. One should understand that the legislative and political arenas in health professions are fluid and constantly changing, as are technologic advancements. This dictates an ongoing necessity for the dental hygienist to continually update professional skills and knowledge, and it requires constant revision of examinations and redefining of standards of competence. While this places demands on the individual practitioner, on the educational system, and on those agencies that are responsible for evaluating competence, it is the means by which the profession is able to advance its standards of care.

Having briefly reviewed the structure and nature of state boards and how they may interact with professional associations, it is appropriate to refocus attention on the responsibilities of the state boards with respect to board examinations. It is typical of state practice acts to charge the state board with conducting both theoretic and practical examinations to determine competence to practice. Some state laws even define the content of such examinations and specify the passing score. Most practice acts authorize the state board to recognize other examinations equivalent to their own. The act may even specify recognition of certain examinations, such as national or regional boards. This is the basis on which other agencies become a part of the credentialing process, but it must be recognized that the fundamental authorization to recognize credentials for licensure lies with the state board of dentistry.

Dental/Dental Hygiene Professional Associations

Any review of the credentialing system would be incomplete without reference to an essential licensure requirement (i.e., graduation from a program accredited by the Commission on Dental Accreditation of the American Dental Association [ADA]). Since it is implied that dental hygienists preparing for board examinations will have satisfied this requirement, it is not relevant to dwell on a lengthy discussion of accreditation standards. Suffice it to say that accreditation for dental hygiene education programs was instituted in 1951 with the encouragement and extensive involvement of the American Dental Hygienists' Association (ADHA). Graduation from an accredited school has become a basic licensure requirement in most state practice acts. Those states that provide for licensure of a dentist or dental hygienist from a nonaccredited school generally require evidence of an educational program that is equivalent to an accredited program. The diploma or certificate of graduation is an essential credential for licensure that is based on an accreditation program carried out under the auspices of the ADA.

Joint Commission on National Dental Examinations

The National Board Examination Program is another prime example of how the concerns of dental practitioners and educators, expressed through their professional associations, influence the legal requirements for licensure. In the early part of this century, each individual state board prepared and administered its own theoretic and clinical examinations. Obviously, there were extreme variations in the difficulty, content, and format of such exams. Any practitioner wishing to move from one state to another had to take more examinations. While it is reasonably feasible for a practitioner to remain current in clinical procedures and be able to demonstrate competence at any point professionally, it is much more difficult to remain current in all the didactic material included in theoretic examinations. It was equally difficult for state boards to keep their examinations up-to-date and secure the resources to ensure the comprehensiveness and reliability of the exams. Interest grew in developing a national, comprehensive, theoretic examination that would satisfy state board requirements for licensure and reduce barriers to the mobility of dental practitioners. The logical source for organizing such a collaborative effort was the ADA.

In 1928 the ADA established the Council of National Board of Dental Examiners, composed of three ADA members, three members of the American Association of Dental Schools (AADS), and three members of the American Association of Dental Examiners (AADE). The first National Board Dental Examination was administered in 1933. The program gradually gained acceptance, and over a period of years most state practice acts were revised to recognize successful completion of National Board Dental Examinations as satisfying the theoretic examination requirement.

Interest in a dental hygiene national board examination program emerged in the 1950s during the period when national accreditation standards were established for dental hygiene educational programs. In 1959 the ADHA instituted an achievement testing program and also formed a liaison committee with the American Association of Dental Examiners. Working with this liaison committee, and also through its involvement with the ADA's Council on Dental Education accreditation program, the ADHA gained support for a dental hygiene national board examination. In 1960 the ADHA requested that the ADA Board of Trustees consider assigning the development of a dental hygiene national board to an appropriate ADA agency. In 1961 the ADA Council of National Board of Dental Examiners was charged with this responsibility; the ADA agreed to underwrite the developmental costs for the examination, and the ADHA agreed to provide the test-item files and information from the ADHA achievement testing program. This brief history is the basis for the ADA and ADHA involvement in the National Board Dental Hygiene Examination, which was first administered in the spring of 1962.

The original ADA Council of National Board of Dental Examiners has evolved through its own history of structural and political changes up until 1980 when it became the Joint Commission on National Dental Examinations. Its membership is composed of three ADA members, three AADS members, six AADE members, one ADHA member, one public member, and one member from the American Student Dental Association. Dental hygiene involvement has historically been broadened by the Committee on Dental Hygiene, which was established in 1962. This committee has five dental hygienists—two educators and two practitioners appointed by the ADHA (one of whom is the ADHA Commissioner) and a dental hygiene student representative—plus one commissioner from each of the respective parent organizations: the ADA, AADE, and AADS. The Committee on Dental Hygiene assumes fundamental responsibility for guiding the development and administrative policies of the dental hygiene examinations. The committee reviews examinations, considers problems that arise, and recommends policy and regulations for the examination program. The commission has final authority to act on all recommendations of the committee, but historically the

Committee on Dental Hygiene has been the guiding force of the dental hygiene examination program.

Having reviewed the basic structure of the credentialing system and how it is influenced by other professional organizations, it is appropriate to review the actual National Board Dental Hygiene Examination Program in more detail.

NATIONAL BOARD DENTAL HYGIENE EXAMINATION PROGRAM

Examination Format

When the National Board Dental Hygiene Examination was first administered in 1962, the test was organized according to subject matter. That is, 12 subjects were organized into groups of 3 to make a 4-part examination. Special test construction committees were formed to develop test items related to community dental health, dental health education, and clinical dental hygiene. Other subjects, such as microbiology, pathology, and histology, were assigned to appropriate dental test construction committees. The subject-oriented examination format was used from 1962 through 1972.

In 1969 the Committee on Dental Hygiene recommended the development of a comprehensive, function-oriented examination that would be organized according to the services that a dental hygienist may be expected to provide in practice. The purposes were to emphasize the more practical application of knowledge to clinical situations and to eliminate some of the overlapping of test items between subjects. The Committee on Dental Hygiene, in conjunction with the ADHA Education Committee, spent almost 2 years developing a function-oriented examination outline, which was widely circulated throughout the profession for input. The first function-oriented examination was developed and administered in March 1973, and this basic format has remained in effect to date.

Examination Outline

The examination outline should be carefully reviewed by all examination candidates; it is the blueprint from which all editions of the test are constructed. Each major heading is broken down into specific functions that are included in the examination content, and an itemization is provided of the number of questions that are devoted to each function. The outline also breaks the number of questions down into three major categories:

Category A. Background information (recognizing why and when the function is performed, including clinical application of basic sciences)

Category B. Method or technique (how the function is performed)

Category C. Armamentarium (design, care, and use of equipment and materials)

This breakdown allows the examination candidate to perceive where the emphasis is placed in each content area. The examination outline is circulated constantly for review and comment and is routinely refined and modified by the Committee on Dental Hygiene in order to keep the examination current. The examination content includes only those functions that are legal in the majority of states. Functions such as the administration of local anesthesia are covered only to the extent of background information that a dental hygienist is expected to know in relation to such basic sciences as pharmacology or anatomy. Questions regarding functions such as the technique for injection of anesthetic agents are not included unless that function is legal in the majority of states.

It is not appropriate to print the examination outline within this text, since ongoing revisions may render such a duplication inaccurate or misleading. Any dental hygienist preparing for the examination should secure a current copy of the examination outline and use it as a guide for study and review.

Test Construction Committees

National Board Dental Hygiene Examinations are developed through an extensive structure of test construction committees. Test constructors are selected by the Joint Commission on National Dental Examinations from applications solicited from schools, state boards, and professional associations and generally serve a term of 5 years. The membership of test construction committees is balanced according to the content of the examinations being developed and the disciplines that are covered. The commission maintains criteria for the selection of test constructors, and in addition to the qualifications of experience and expertise, geographic distribution is an important consideration.

The function-oriented examination format necessitates the use of interdisciplinary committees to construct the examination. In addition, a special committee is used to develop all test items relating to community dental health. Each interdisciplinary committee is composed of a periodontist, a dentist or dental hygienist with an advanced degree in one of the basic sciences, a dentist or dental hygienist with expertise in radiography, a clinical dental hygienist, a dental hygienist with a strong curriculum background, and a member of the community dental health committee. Each edition of the examination is reviewed by at least two interdisciplinary committees: the first committee drafts the examination, and the second committee reviews and finalizes it. In addition, every examination edition is reviewed after it has been administered and statistics have been generated for each question. Items that are statistically unsatisfactory are reviewed, revised, or discarded. Therefore test construction committees have three routine responsibilities: drafting new examinations, reviewing examination drafts prepared by another committee, and reviewing unsatisfactory test items after an examination has been administered. The test construction committees work with test-item files containing thousands of questions that are classified according to the content area of the examination outline. The committees also develop new items, and questions are constantly solicited from throughout the profession.

Examination Scoring System

A norm-referenced scoring system is used for all National Board Dental Hygiene Examinations to ensure uniform meaning of scores from edition to edition of the tests. The converted score that is reported is known as a standard score, which indicates how an individual's score relates to the average. Standard scores can be averaged and correlated, and the results are generally proportional to differences in raw scores. The examinations maintain a degree of difficulty high enough to spread candidates out over a broad range of performance. Therefore there tend to be distinct differences in the performances of those who pass and those who fail, and guessing correctly on a few test items has minimal effect on an individual's score in relation to the other candidates. The average raw score on an examination is usually around 65%, which would convert to a standard score of approximately 85.

A candidate's examination score depends on two factors. The first, of course, is the raw score or number of correct answers the candidate selects. The second is the distribution of raw scores of the norming group. The norming group used for National Board Dental Hygiene Examinations consists of all candidates taking the examination for the first time who are students in fully accredited dental hygiene programs. The mean raw score of the norming group is always assigned the standard score of 85. Next, the raw score 1.5 standard deviations below the mean raw score is assigned the standard score of 75. All other standard scores are computed using the relationship between these two. There is no fixed failure rate, but the results have remained stable for many years, and the failure rate is typically around 5%. A standard score of 75 is required to pass. It is obvious that as new editions of the examination are drafted, some may be more difficult than others; it is impossible to predict the difficulty level of new questions that are introduced. The norm-referenced scoring system eliminates inconsistencies in the results that may be caused by differences in difficulty between editions of the examination. Another potential inconsistency exists, however, in the possible differences among norming groups. If there is any possibility that the overall performance of new graduates in 1 year was less than that of graduates 5 years previously,

then a norm-referenced score would not mean the same thing from year to year. To measure any significant differences in norming groups from year to year, the commission uses anchor items. Anchor items are selected questions that are used in repeated editions of the examination. The statistics on these anchor items are monitored and compared to see if there is any difference in the performance of the norming groups.

Examination Irregularities

The commission maintains a program to identify any irregularities or cheating on the examinations. For many years this has been done during the scoring process by computer comparison of answers to detect improbable similarities. The commission began implementing a plan in 1984 to use alternate forms of the examination so that different test booklets have the same questions in scrambled order. The commission is committed to maintaining the integrity of each candidate's individual results and can be expected to use as effective a system as possible to control irregularities.

Released Examinations

The commission has traditionally released examinations almost every year and has maintained that policy with the dental examinations. Since the implementation of the function-oriented examination in 1973, National Board Dental Hygiene Examinations have been released far less frequently, at intervals of 3 to 5 years. This is primarily because it is much more difficult to develop questions that require the application of knowledge to specific clinical functions. Test constructors must not only have knowledge in their area of expertise, but they must also understand how that knowledge is relevant to the practice of dental hygiene. The bank of test items must be large enough that the release of questions does not jeopardize the integrity and security of the examination program. The commission recognizes the desirability of releasing examinations frequently and circulating ample information so that misconceptions do not develop about the testing program. They are guided in their decisions by both the need to provide information and the necessity of maintaining a secure bank of reliable test items. Certainly, released examinations are an invaluable study guide for dental hygienists preparing for the National Board Dental Hygiene Examination. However, their greatest value is simply as a study guide; it is not constructive for a candidate to attempt to memorize questions. Changing one or two words in a question can alter the entire item, and the candidate who has memorized questions by rote will be utterly confused. It is far more constructive to invest one's energy in building a solid knowledge base that allows one to respond to many questions.

Release of Examination Results

It takes approximately 7 weeks to process and report examination scores. The candidate receives an individual score report, the school of graduation receives a report, and scores are sent to those state boards that have been specified by the candidate to receive a report. There is no limit on the number of times a candidate may retake the examination; however, a dental hygienist who fails the examination twice within a 25-month period must wait at least 11 months to retake the examination. Some jurisdictions require successful completion of the National Board Dental Hygiene Examination before a candidate is eligible for a clinical examination. The prerequisites of each jurisdiction in which a candidate is interested in obtaining licensure should be researched well in advance so that the necessary preparations to satisfy such requirements can be effectively scheduled.

Examination Availability

The National Board Dental Hygiene Examination is offered three times a year: usually in March, July, and December. Any graduate of an accredited dental hygiene program is eligible to take the examination; students who are certified by their program director as being within four months of graduation are also eligible. The results are accepted in all states except Delaware and Alabama; they are also accepted in the District of Columbia, Puerto Rico, and the Virgin Islands. Some states, such as Arizona, Colorado, Florida, and Hawaii, as well as Puerto Rico and the Virgin Islands, have time restrictions for accepting examination results. These jurisdictions require that examination scores be current within a certain number of years for licensure to be granted.

CHARACTERISTICS OF MULTIPLE-CHOICE TEST ITEMS

National Board Dental Hygiene Examinations are composed of approximately 360 questions, all of which are multiple-choice items. There are several different approved formats for the structure of these items. A multiple-choice item consists of a stem, which poses a problem, and a set of possible answers or options. All questions in this examination must have at least three and not more than eight possible answers. Only one choice should be correct or clearly the best answer. Other possible options are termed distractors, because they are designed to distract the candidate from the correct answer.

Item Stems

The stem of an item either poses a question or forms an incomplete statement. The candidate should be able to determine what is being asked on the basis of the stem alone. The stem should contain all the information necessary to present the question, but there should be no extraneous information. The purpose of the stem is to test, not to teach.

Distractors

The quality of the distractors determines the effectiveness of a question. A good distractor is plausible enough to attract the attention of candidates who lack the knowledge or skill being tested. Common misconceptions are frequently included as distractors, as well as responses that meet some, but not all, of the conditions posed in the stem. Possible answers are usually ordered according to length, and good distractors are of relatively uniform length. A well-constructed question also has distractors that are gramatically consistent with the stem (i.e., all options are nouns or verbs or whatever is appropriate grammar to complete the stem).

Correct Answer

Each test item should have only one option that is correct or clearly the best answer. Every effort is made to use only those items where there is national agreement that an answer is correct or best. Answers that reflect regional philosophies are avoided.

FORMATS OF NATIONAL BOARD MULTIPLE-CHOICE ITEMS

A variety of item formats are approved for use in National Board Dental Hygiene Examinations. Familiarity with these formats and knowing how to respond to each of them will help the candidate avoid confusion. A description of the types of approved formats follows, along with examples of questions that have been extracted from the released March 1983 National Board Dental Hygiene Examination.

Completion-type Items

The stem of a completion-type item contains a statement that is completed by the addition of the selected answer. These items are generally easy to read and understand. For example:

The proper method of clinically prolonging the setting time of alginate hydrocolloids is to
1. Use less water
2. Decrease water temperature
3. Increase water temperature
4. Reduce the amount of retarder in the powder

It should be noted that the options in the above question all contain a verbal phrase that completes the statement in the stem in the proper grammatical context. The options are ordered according to length.

Question-type Items

The stem of a question-type item contains a complete question. These items are generally simple, straightforward, and easily understood. An example follows:

Which of the following incisors is most likely to have a carious lingual pit?
1. Maxillary lateral
2. Maxillary central
3. Mandibular lateral
4. Mandibular central

Negative Items

A negative test item is characterized by a word such as *except, not,* or *least* in the stem of the question. The key negative word is always italicized to call the candidates' attention to it. Negative items can be either completion-type or question-type items. All the options for a negative item are generally stated in the positive form. Negative items are useful for testing exceptions to general principles. Examples are shown below:

Which of the following is *least* significant in the initiation and progression of periodontitis?
1. Plaque
2. Calculus
3. Food impaction
4. Poorly contoured restoration
5. Insufficient zone of attached gingiva

The above item is a negative question-type item. The question below is a negative completion-type item:

Relative sensitivities of cells and tissues to radiation depend on all of the following *except*
1. Age
2. Dose rate
3. Blood type
4. Type of radiation
5. Specific area involved
6. Variability among species and individuals

Intermediate Answer or Combination Multiple-Choice Items

Some questions have more than one correct answer or a series of responses that are correct. These items lend themselves to a format of intermediate answers. Typically, the item contains a stem followed by a series of responses. To answer the question, the candidate must choose from options containing combinations of the responses. Such items tend to be more complex, require more careful reading, and demand more complete knowledge from the candidate. That is, the candidate may readily know three out of five essential steps in a process, but to answer a question correctly, it may be necessary to recognize all five steps. Combination mul-

tiple-choice items are used fairly extensively in National Board Dental Hygiene Examinations; they may also appear in the negative-item format. Examples of such items appear below:

Avoidance of cross contamination during routine patient treatment requires
(a) Wearing sterilized gloves
(b) Properly sterilizing instruments
(c) Not touching anything unsanitized
(d) Careful handwashing before, during, and after appointments
(e) Adequately sanitizing all equipment that cannot be sterilized
1. a, b, c, and e
2. a, c, and e
3. b, c, and d
4. b, c, d, and e
5. b, d, and e

Salicylates are *not* the drug of choice for patients
(a) With gastric ulceration
(b) With hemorrhagic disorders
(c) With rheumatoid arthritis
(d) Receiving anticoagulant therapy
1. a, b, and c
2. a, b, and d
3. a, c, and d
4. a and d
5. b and d

Paired True-False Items

In a paired true-false item, the stem is the only portion of the question that varies. The stem consists of two statements on the same topic. The options always provide all possible true-false combinations. An example appears below:

In health, bone is constantly undergoing resorption and formation. In periodontitis, only bone resorption occurs.
1. Both statements are true
2. Both statements are false
3. The first statement is true; the second is false
4. The first statement is false; the second is true

Paired true-false items do not occur frequently in National Board Dental Hygiene Examinations.

Cause-and-Effect Items

A cause-and-effect item is very similar to a paired true-false item in that the only portion of the question that varies is the stem. The stem contains a statement and a reason, which are written as a single sentence and connected by *because*. The possible answers are always the same, as in the example below:

Protection from radiation may be aided by the use of aluminum filters and a lead diaphragm *because* the filters reduce the

amount of soft radiation reaching the patient's face and the diaphragm reduces the area exposed.
1. Both statement and reason are correct and related
2. Both statement and reason are correct but *not* related
3. The statement is correct, but the reason is *not*
4. The statement is *not* correct, but the reason is an accurate statement
5. *Neither* statement nor reason is correct

This type of item requires the candidate to judge both the accuracy and the relationship of two statements. Such items should be read very carefully to avoid confusion. Cause-and-effect items generally appear with limited frequency in National Board Dental Hygiene Examinations.

Matching Items

The most recently approved item format for National Board Dental Hygiene Examination questions is the matching item. There are currently no released examples of such items. A matching question groups several test items together; for instance, test items 52 to 57 may consist of matching a list of premises with a list of responses. In responding to each item, the candidate must select an answer from the list of responses that matches an item on the list of premises. Instructions for marking answers should appear with the question. In actuality, matching items merely group together several questions about the same subject matter.

Case Problems

It is typical for several case problems to be presented in an edition of the National Board Dental Hygiene Examination. These items describe a patient's condition or clinical situation and are followed by several test items related to the case problem. The case problem may include only written material or may be supplemented with charts, line drawings, or radiographs. Questions that relate to the case problem may be presented in any of the test-item formats that have been described.

TIPS FOR TAKING MULTIPLE-CHOICE TESTS

There are general stategies that alert candidates will use in taking any multiple-choice examination. A poorly constructed examination will contain many clues for a test-wise candidate. The careful construction process and editing to which National Board Dental Hygiene Examination items are subjected minimizes many of these typical clues. However, developing a system for reading and responding to questions will facilitate a candidate's performance.
1. Read the stem of the question carefully and completely before looking at the answers.
   a. Clearly determine what the question is asking;

identify key words; try to formulate the answer in your mind before looking at the answers.
   b. Read each answer carefully and determine whether it is an appropriate response to the question and gives as complete an answer as possible.
   c. Immediately eliminate any answers that are obviously incorrect, and attempt to narrow the choices to not more than two.
   d. For combination multiple-choice items, narrow the choices by eliminating any answer that contains an incorrect response, and consider only those answers that contain responses that you confidently know are correct.
   e. When the choices have been narrowed as much as possible and the correct answer is still not clear, make an educated guess. There is no penalty for guessing.
2. Avoid selecting any answer that contains such words as *always, never, none, all,* or *every.* There are seldom any conditions that are absolute in the health field, and unconditional responses are usually incorrect answers.
3. Look for the answer that *best* applies to the conditions presented in the question. An option may be partially true or may apply under certain conditions. Select the *best* answer that will generally apply under most conditions and specifically is applicable to the question. If several options might be true but one option would incorporate all possibilities, that option should clearly be the *best* answer.
   a. Avoid selecting answers that are based on isolated rules, are applicable only to certain locales or regions, or refer to procedures and techniques that are not broadly practiced.
   b. If the question asks for an immediate action, such as what is the *first* thing one would do, all of the options may be correct. The *best* answer would have to be based on identified priorities and on the conditions stipulated in the question.
4. Be alert for grammatical clues. A well-edited question will offer options that are all grammatically correct with the stem. If the question indicates a plural response, all the options should be in plural form. Any response that is inconsistent with the flow of the question may be an indication of an incorrect answer.
5. Watch for the words *not, least,* or *except* in the stem of the question. If an item does not make sense, reread it carefully to be sure a key word has not been overlooked.
6. Carefully review questions that include as a response, "all of the above" or "none of the above." These responses impose broadly inclusive and exclusive

conditions. ''None of the above'' has limited usefulness as a response, because it entirely negates the premise of the question.

7. The pattern of numbers for correct answers should be fairly random. Do not be overly concerned if the same-numbered answer is selected repeatedly, and it is not advisable to base answer selections on a pattern of numbers.

8. Be careful to mark the correct space on the answer sheet that relates to the item. Periodically review the answer sheet to make sure you have not inadvertently marked in the wrong space.

9. The spaces on the answer sheet should be completely marked with a dark line, but no marks should extend outside the lines. Listen carefully when instructions are given for marking the answer sheet. Do not assume it is just like others you may have used.

GUIDELINES FOR PREPARING FOR NATIONAL BOARD DENTAL HYGIENE EXAMINATIONS

1. Organize a study plan 4 to 6 months in advance that will allow an orderly, progressive review without undue pressure.

2. Obtain an examination outline and application materials, including a brochure or any information about the examination provided by the Joint Commission on National Dental Examinations. Study the information carefully to understand clearly the format and design of the examination and the protocol for its administration.

3. Obtain a copy of the most recently released National Board Dental Hygiene Examination. Released examinations are usually available through a dental or dental hygiene school library or from the commission itself. Set aside a day without interruptions; take the examination without advance preparation, using the same time limitations that are prescribed in the examination. As you take the test, mark all questions about which you are unsure.

4. Grade yourself with the key that is included in the released examination.

5. Prepare an outline of the areas in which you have identified weaknesses. Be guided by your experience in school as indicated by grades or difficulty in certain subjects, and by the items from the released examination that you missed or marked as questionable. Dental hygienists who have been out of school or practice for some period of time should focus on basic science material and any developments in dental technology or services that may have expanded the knowledge base since their graduation.

6. Gather a personal resource library for ready reference throughout the review process. Properly used, this book should be the mainstay of your study guides; directions for its use are included further on in this chapter. This book is designed to direct you through a comprehensive review of dental hygiene, provide questions by which you can assess your mastery of the subject material, and offer documentation for correct and incorrect answers. This review book should be supplemented with textbooks and appropriate reference material from a professional library when further study is needed in particular areas. Dental hygienists whose textbooks and reference material may be substantially outdated should make it an immediate priority to obtain adequate resources. They might contact recent graduates, requesting an extended loan of textbooks, and visit the nearest dental library to review current publications. Those references that are particularly helpful should be ordered and purchased.

7. If possible, organize a study club of several candidates who are preparing for the examination. The group should be small, perhaps three to five colleagues. It is best to collaborate only with those individuals whose study habits, personal habits, and self-discipline will contribute to the group's efforts; otherwise, it would be better to study alone. Never rely on someone else to do your preparation; however, several heads can be better than one if the group is intentional in its purpose.

8. If a study group is formed, organize a schedule and procedures for it to operate. Content areas can be assigned to individuals for specific study and research; then the members of the group can pool their information and notes to be shared by all. Open discussion of questions or content areas that are confusing can contribute to the review process of each candidate.

9. Outline an orderly system to guide your review, and establish target dates to complete each area. It would be logical to set deadlines for the review of each chapter in this book. You may wish to organize your review around the functions specified in the examination outline, although you should be aware that each function will probably require the review of several different disciplines. Another option would be to assess and prioritize your own needs as you perceive them, and be guided by the priorities you have established. The important point is to plan a system for your review, with goals and deadlines to monitor your progress.

10. When you have formulated a plan, get going and stick with it. If the plan bogs down, reassess the obstacles and modify your goals so you can continue through a comprehensive review.

11. Plan to complete your review at least 3 to 5 days

before the examination date. Having prepared yourself intellectually, you should prepare yourself physically. As an educated health professional, you would be wise to adhere to principles of good health. Eat well-balanced meals, get plenty of sleep, avoid any chemical stimulants, and set aside time for exercise such as brisk daily walks or any form of physical activity to which you are routinely accustomed. Last-minute cramming all night before the examination is not advisable. A good night's sleep is far more likely to enable you to access your knowledge during the test.

12. Prepare yourself psychologically to set aside all distractions or immediate concerns on the day of the test. Focus on whatever enhances your powers of concentration. Above all, read the instructions for the examination thoroughly, and read each question carefully so you are sure you understand exactly what is being asked.

13. Take a watch or accurate timepiece and keep it in front of you during the examination. The time allowed for each section of the examination should be clearly stated, and you should pace yourself accordingly. Do not dwell on difficult items about which you are unsure. Move along and come back to those items as time permits. If time is available when you have completed all items, briefly review all your answers; be sure you have recorded the answer you intended.

14. As breaks are available during the day of the examination, seek out brief activities that are refreshing and help to restore your energy and concentration for the remaining portions of the test.

REGIONAL TESTING AGENCIES ■■■■■■■

Having reviewed some of the structural intricacies of the credentialing system and the National Board Dental Hygiene Examination Program in particular, it is appropriate to devote some discussion to regional testing agencies. The thrust toward regional board examinations began in the late 1960s and gained momentum throughout the 1970s. Because of the barriers to mobility that are created by having to take repeated state board examinations to qualify for licensure in another state, interest grew in consolidating standards so that one examination might qualify a practitioner for licensure in multiple states. There was some impetus for a national clinical examination and licensure at the federal level. However, because of the historical advantages of licensure at the state level, regional examinations were perceived as a viable alternative to usurping those state rights and imposing national requirements. The basic rationale for the formation of regional testing services has been the standardization of requirements among states and the pooling of resources to develop and administer reliable clinical examinations.

There has been a similar pattern in the development of each of the regional boards. Typically, each region began with a core group of states that initiated discussions about joining forces with one another. Usually this was followed by the states' giving simultaneous examinations at a common testing site, then working to consolidate their respective state examinations into one test that they could all accept. As the regions have matured, more states have joined, and the combined examinations have gradually been revised and replaced with a regional test developed with the consensus of the member states. The important feature to be remembered about regional boards, which is often misunderstood by members of the profession, is that they are voluntary organizations made up of individual state boards of dentistry. The regional boards have no authority to supersede state boards or implement policy that goes beyond the statutory authorization of the member state boards. Only the individual state board can make the determination to accept the results of the regional board as satisfying its requirements for licensure. It is typical to find numerous inconsistencies in the policies and procedures of states within the same region. A regional board only standardizes the examination that is offered by the member states; it does not standardize all other aspects of state board responsibilities.

The Northeast Regional Board (NERB) was the first of all the regions and has remained the largest, with 14 member states. NERB began in the late 1960s. The Central Regional Dental Testing Service (CRDTS) followed in 1972, taking in 11 states between the Rocky Mountains and the Mississippi River; the withdrawal of a state in 1984 reduced their membership to 10. In the mid-1970s the Southern Regional Testing Agency (SRTA) was formed, taking in four of the middle southern states. In the late 1970s the Western Regional Examining Board (WREB) was established; it began with three member states, grew to five, and then returned to three with the withdrawal of two states. The concept of regional board examinations has been supported by both the ADA and the ADHA, although these associations have no actual involvement in any of the regional testing services. The political environment of the 1980s, deemphasizing federal involvement in health services and returning control to the states, appears to have diminished the momentum for growth of regional testing services. Nevertheless, the advent of regional testing agencies has had notable impact on the content and format of clinical board examinations in both dentistry and dental hygiene.

The four regional testing agencies, comprising a total of 31 member state boards, are very similar in their organization and structure. Typically, there is a steering committee or board of directors that is responsible for determining policies of the agency and financial management. Generally, each member state board is represented on the steering committee. A second key part of the organizations is usually the examination committee, on which each member state board is also represented. In addition, the examination committee generally has several faculty members representing regional educational institutions. The examination committee is charged with reviewing and revising the examinations and developing new examinations. Most regions have some sort of mechanism to review complaints or appeals of results, and they all maintain their own office and staff separate from that of the member state boards.

While national boards satisfy the state requirements for theoretic examinations, the regional boards' emphasis is on evaluating clinical knowledge and skills. The methodology for testing clinical competence generally involves clinical treatment of patients, but it should not be assumed that hands-on patient procedures are the only mechanisms for assessing clinical ability. It is quite common for clinical examinations to include some written exercises and some clinical simulations using typodonts, radiographs, photographs, models, and so on. There is no general statement that can be made about the distinctions between regional board examinations and state board examinations. Their content and format often appear quite similar on the surface. Obviously, regional board examinations have the advantage of qualifying a candidate for licensure in more than one state and are often offered more frequently than individual state board examinations. They also offer the advantage of bringing collective resources to bear on developing and maintaining reliable examinations. Examiners and educators have a forum in which they can cooperatively determine appropriate standards of competence and concentrate on technical aspects of testing without the distractions of the many other responsibilities that burden state boards. Some candidates believe that regional boards are better organized and present more specific documentation of candidate requirements, scoring systems, and performance criteria. Certainly, the circumstances will vary depending on which jurisdictions and examinations are being compared.

Examiner Selection and Training

The pool of examiners for regional agencies comes from the member state boards. Usually each state has the right to be represented at any or all regional examinations. All active board members of each state board are eligible to serve as examiners. In addition, many states are authorized to designate deputy examiners to represent them; such deputy examiners are generally practi-

tioners who are not board members but are certified to serve as examiners for their state and help carry out the board's examining responsibilities. Testing dates and sites are scheduled well in advance by the region and the schools. The number of candidates at each test determines the number of examiners that is necessary, and each state is asked to assign examiners to represent them. From the pool of examiners assigned to a particular test, further assignments are made to administer the dental hygiene examination or different portions of the dental examination.

Training programs for the examiners vary according to the region, but it is becoming increasingly common for the regions to place heavy emphasis on standardization and grading exercises for examiners, training them to apply the examination criteria. The result of this is a more thorough and specific evaluation for dental hygienists, in comparison with a cursory inspection and flash of the mirror around the mouth, as may have been the practice in some jurisdictions in the past.

STATE AND REGIONAL CLINICAL EXAMINATIONS

Only general statements can be made about the content of clinical dental hygiene board examinations, because it varies from jurisdiction to jurisdiction and is continually being revised. There are three basic categories of clinical skills that are commonly included in regional and state clinical examinations. These are charting or data-gathering skills, the oral prophylaxis, and radiographic skills. Data gathering may include such functions as dental and periodontal charting, head and neck examination, health history taking, and charting the location of subgingival deposits. An oral prophylaxis on at least one patient is a universal requirement. However, requirements for the difficulty of the case may vary, and some jurisdictions demand a complete prophylaxis, whereas others may require a more difficult patient and assign only a portion of the mouth for the purposes of the examination. Some jurisdictions may require treatment of more than one patient as well.

The radiographic evaluation may include an assessment of the ability to interpret or recognize radiographic features and/or an assessment of technical ability. Some jurisdictions require a full-mouth survey of radiographs; others require only selected films. In some instances radiographs may be exposed in advance, whereas other agencies require all radiographic exercises to be completed during the examination.

The time schedule is another factor that may vary considerably in different jurisdictions. Some board examinations place specific time limits for the completion of assignments, whereas others allow such an ample amount of time that it is not a matter of concern for most candidates. It is essential for a candidate to be thoroughly familiar with examination requirements, not only concerning *what* one is expected to do, but *how* and *when* it must be done.

Anonymous Examinations

In recent years there has been a growing trend toward administering clinical board examinations anonymously. This means that the candidates are identified only by number, and the examiners are usually segregated from the candidates. Patients are brought to a clinical area reserved for the examiners, and the candidates are not present while the examiners conduct their evaluations. Candidates often have mixed responses to this arrangement. Some candidates feel it is extremely stressful to be present during the examiners' evaluation and are relieved to avoid it. Others are enormously curious to perceive any clue from the examiners about their performance. Many candidates interrogate their patients about every comment or facial expression they observed among the examiners. Making assumptions based on the reports of patients, who generally understand little about the examination process, invites misinformation and erroneous conclusions. In any case, anonymous evaluations have a definite impact on the logistics of the examination process. The purpose, of course, is to eliminate any potential bias of the examiners based on personality, race, sex, or personal background, so that the candidate's clinical performance is the only basis for the evaluation.

Examination Scoring

There is no uniform scoring system for regional or state board clinical examinations. Such scoring tends to be highly specific to the content, design, and format of each individual examination. However, some generalities can be reviewed. Clinical examinations are ordinarily criterion referenced, as opposed to the norm-referenced scoring system described for National Board Dental Hygiene Examinations. That is, a candidate's clinical performance is measured against a specific standard of competence rather than against the performance of another candidate or group of candidates. The best and most objective clinical examinations are generally considered to be those that set forth specific performance criteria and define the cutoff point that separates acceptable from unacceptable performance.

The emphasis on determining acceptable versus unacceptable performance is a distinctive feature of clinical board examinations. It is not relevant to the purposes of board examinations to rank candidates as good, better, or best; nor is it important whether a candidate scores 85 or 95 on an examination. The essential question is whether or not the candidate has demonstrated adequate competence to be licensed to practice. The critical decisions, then, in clinical board examinations lend themselves to pass/fail or acceptable/unacceptable determinations. Numerical values are almost always assigned to the examiners' determinations of acceptability, but such numerical scores often do not have the same meaning as test scores in school or on other standardized tests. For example, a test score of 100 on a 100-item pathology final would very likely mean that a student answered every question correctly. In contrast, a score of 100 on a criterion-referenced, pass/fail examination would not necessarily indicate that a candidate performed perfectly; it could mean only that the candidate consistently demonstrated minimal competence in all aspects of the examination.

Clinical board examinations generally use raw scores without any kind of conversion system; even written sections of the examination are scored strictly on the basis of the number of correct answers. However, it is common in board examinations to use a system of weighting. Weighting in examinations is simply a method of emphasizing the importance or recognizing the difficulty of certain skills and treatment procedures. For instance, most dental hygienists would acknowledge that subgingival scaling is a more difficult task, and more important to the practice of dental hygiene, than the charting of restorations. Consequently, one would expect to see subgingival scaling weighted with more point value in an examination than dental charting. If dental charting is included in the examination, examiners will carefully evaluate the candidate's ability to chart correctly; however, acceptable performance in dental charting may be worth only 10 points in the overall test as opposed to a weight of 30 points assigned to subgingival scaling. A candidate should strive to demonstrate competence in all skills that are evaluated in an examination. The candidate should study the weighting system before the examination and may wish to concentrate time and attention on each skill in proportion to the weighted importance that is built into the examination.

There undoubtedly is much variation in the amount of information that different testing agencies release about their scoring systems. An examination scoring system is of concern to the candidate to the extent that it appears to be fair and reasonable, and it may offer guidance in preparing the candidate to take the examination. It is unwise, however, for a candidate to become too absorbed in analyzing the grading system. Indeed, some candidates have tended to become more interested in how to *give* the examination than in how to *take* it. The grading system is the testing agency's concern, and demonstrating competence in performing dental hygiene procedures is the candidate's concern. Successful candidates are those who do not allow themselves to be distracted from their primary task.

Clinical Facilities

Most jurisdictions today have access to modern clinical facilities in which to administer board examinations. Fortunately, it is a thing of the past to hear stories of board examinations given in poorly equipped prison clinics or with portable equipment set up in the basement of a courthouse. Today most candidates have the benefit of adequate lighting, water, evacuation systems, and functional equipment. For many states without any educational institutions, gaining access to adequate clinical facilities was a primary reason for joining a regional testing service. There is no state or regional board that owns or operates its own clinical facility. Boards must elicit the cooperation of schools or large clinics to make their facilities available for board examinations. It is no small concession on the part of schools to release their facilities for several days for board examinations. It requires scheduling adjustments and substantial loss of clinic income, and it places heavy demands on faculty and staff to accommodate examination requirements and personnel.

Candidates are often oblivious to clinical facilities as long as they have equipment that is functional, reasonably comfortable, and efficient, and they are able to find what they need when they need it. This poses no problem to candidates who take an examination at their school of graduation or at a familiar site. Problems may arise, however, for those who are operating in an unfamiliar facility. Candidates should be aware that the clinical facility is *not* under the management and control of the board examiners. In fact, the examiners may be scarcely more familiar with the facilities and equipment than are the candidates. The testing site may charge a separate fee to candidates for the use of the facilities and supplies, and may have its own institutional requirements or record keeping for which the candidate is responsible. Rental of equipment or instruments is typically handled through the testing site, as well as obtaining information about the compatibility of handpieces, and so on. An equipment breakdown during the examination can create stress for the candidate and result in the loss of time. Maintenance is also usually managed by the testing site, and many schools are accommodating enough to keep maintenance personnel on call during the examination.

The purpose of this discussion is simply to point out that candidates should not assume that all aspects of the examination process are totally under the control of the testing agency. The candidate will be involved with the testing site, the testing agency, and the state board(s) of the jurisdiction(s) in which licensure is sought. When problems or questions arise, the candidate should be aware of which agency can respond to his or her concerns. The testing site addresses concerns about the facilities; the testing agency addresses questions about the test itself, and the state board deals with actually issuing a license to practice. For those jurisdictions that are not part of a regional testing service, the state board and the testing agency are one and the same.

Patient Selection and Classification

All dental hygiene clinical board examinations place the greatest weight on patient treatment procedures, particularly the oral prophylaxis. Therefore selection of a board patient is undoubtedly the single most important factor in preparation for an examination. Most testing agencies provide some criteria for patient acceptability. Some agencies may be quite specific, to the point of defining exactly how many teeth must have subgingival calculus and how many millimeters wide a band of calculus must be. Other agencies set forth more general descriptions. Experience has shown that no matter how detailed the criteria may be, candidates still worry desperately about whether their patient is acceptable.

One of the difficulties in defining patient criteria is that there is no standardized definition of patient classification that is universally accepted, and, of course, judgments differ among individuals when it comes to placing a patient in a particular category. Most jurisdictions require a patient with moderate to heavy subgingival deposits. Patients exhibiting only plaque or soft deposits are probably not difficult enough to present a valid test of the candidate's skills. A patient with grossly heavy calculus or any patient demonstrating significant periodontal involvement is too difficult for the purposes of a board examination. Many experienced board examiners have observed that educators tend to classify patients as being more difficult than examiners would. Perhaps this is because for most board examinations the baseline for minimally acceptable patients begins with moderate deposits of calculus, and the degree of difficulty escalates from that point.

Many testing agencies classify the difficulty of patients and vary the examination criteria according to such classification. The most common factors that determine the patient's classification are the amounts of subgingival calculus and supragingival stain. The classification of difficulty may be used to determine how well the candidate is expected to perform and/or how much work the candidate is assigned. For example, a candidate who presents a patient with minimal deposits of subgingival calculus and light stain obviously has a much easier task than the candidate whose patient is a pipe smoker and has heavy deposits of subgingival and supragingival calculus. One method of compensating for such variabilities in patient conditions is to assign the first candidate three or four quadrants for the oral prophylaxis and expect at least 85% of the deposits to be completely removed. In contrast, the second candidate may be assigned to treat only one quadrant and be expected to remove at least 75% of the deposits. Such compensation designed into the examination criteria tends to equalize the difficulty of the candidates' tasks and make the examination more equitable for all.

Recruitment of Patients

Most testing agencies cannot and do not provide patients for candidates. The burden of that responsibility falls on the candidate. Candidates frequently turn to the testing site for assistance in recruiting patients, but there is considerable variation in the amount of assistance that may be provided. Schools often assist their students in patient recruitment and selection but are unable to provide patients to other candidates. Some schools will make operatories available for patient screening shortly before a board examination or may screen and make lists of potential board patients through the oral diagnosis department. Ultimately, however, it is the responsibility of the candidate to present a suitable patient, and the examiners make the final decision regarding acceptability. It is not helpful for a candidate to challenge an examiner's decision by pointing out that an instructor or family dentist said the patient would be acceptable. It is the candidate's responsibility to know how a patient may or may not satisfy the examination criteria. It is not advisable to present a marginally acceptable patient and hope to ''squeak by'' the criteria. Having a patient dismissed places enormous stress on the candidate, may penalize the grade or reduce the operating time, and delays the entire examination process.

Candidates often exhibit incredible resourcefulness in recruiting patients. Family and friends are a primary source. One's school, family dentist, or dental hygienist may also be sources for contacts. Students or staff at hospitals or health science centers are frequently recruited. Many candidates have contacted local police and fire stations, studied the shift schedule to determine who would be off duty on the day of the examination, and then visited the station when that shift was on duty in order to screen and recruit patients. Sometimes graduating classes develop plans of action and organize themselves to recruit patients for the entire class. Candidates have been known to advertise in local newspapers or post notices on bulletin boards to obtain patients; some candidates have even accosted people on the streets. Bizarre and unprofessional methods of patient recruitment are obviously directly proportional to the desperation of the candidate. Such desperation can be avoided if the candidate begins a search for patients well in advance and maintains an attitude of professionalism in all contacts with potential patients. The pressure of board examinations can often influence candidates to perceive patients as walking typodonts instead of relating to them as hu-

man beings whose oral health needs certainly extend beyond the day of the examination.

Patient selection is primarily dictated by the criteria that are defined by the testing agency. Such criteria may stipulate requirements for systemic health conditions, calculus deposits, stain, gingival conditions, a minimal number of teeth and items to be charted, and periodontal pockets. There may also be requirements for legal consent from the patient for treatment and requirements for radiation hygiene. Candidates should carefully review all prerequisites before recruiting patients. The wise candidate will also take into consideration the attitude and cooperativeness of the patient and ascertain the patient's pain threshold or tolerance of treatment. Part of the candidate's preparation for the examination should include careful preparation of the patient.

Clinical examinations usually require long treatment sessions and periods of waiting for examiners. It is a difficult day for the patients, who are subjected not only to the necessary treatment by the candidate, but also to inspection and instrumentation by the examiners. Examiners usually do not have the time or opportunity to build rapport with the patient or provide the same kind of support that they would in a practice setting. Moreover, patients frequently ask examiners questions about the candidate's performance that the examiners are not at liberty to answer. The examiners' lack of response to patients and/or candidates may make them appear abrupt, when in actuality they are only doing their job. Candidates are in a stressful situation during the examination, which often makes it more difficult for them to maintain good patient rapport. If patients are poorly prepared for the demands of the examination setting, or if they have not been informed of the amount of time they will be detained, they can cause great difficulty for the candidate by refusing to cooperate, threatening to leave, or actually leaving the examination. Therefore the candidate should advise the patient of the purposes of the examination, its importance to the candidate's career, the treatment that will be provided, what the examiners will be doing, the time schedule, and delays that may be encountered. Certainly, the patient should be made aware of additional treatment that may be necessary but will not be provided during the examination. Some patients are so eager for the candidate to succeed that they may regard the examiners as adversaries. However, when they are made to understand the purpose and format of board examinations, most patients are supportive and appreciative of the efforts of the dental profession to ensure the competence of practitioners.

It is obvious that not all candidates are going to be fortunate enough to find the perfect patient who satisfies all criteria. However, some candidates are able to secure several patients who are potentially suitable. It is highly advisable to recruit more than one patient and have a backup patient available. These patients should be informed that they may not be needed for the examination; however, it is often likely that if the candidate who recruited them does not need them, another candidate will. The candidate should stay in frequent contact with any patients who have been recruited, confirm the time and date, and make sure that transportation is arranged and that the patient has clear directions about where to appear, how to get there, and where to park.

Instrument Requirements

In recent years there has been an increasing tendency for testing agencies to specify certain instruments that are required for the examination. Some testing agencies supply or sell them, and others merely specify what the candidate is responsible for providing. While such requirements may impose some inconvenience on the candidate, it tends to serve the best interests of the candidate by standardizing the examination process. Ordinarily, it is only the examining instruments that are standardized, such as the mirror, explorer, and periodontal probe. Handpieces, scalers, and curettes are usually selected at the candidate's discretion.

Every clinician has certain instruments that are most effective for that individual. Certainly, the candidate should use those instruments that are familiar and provide the best tactile sensitivity. If the examination requires instruments with which the candidate is not familiar, it is advisable to begin practicing with those instruments well in advance. For instance, it may be that a testing agency requires the candidate to have a No. 2 explorer, which the examiners use for detection of calculus. Perhaps the candidate has the greatest tactile sensitivity with a No. 13/14 curette. In preparing for the examination, the candidate should practice with both instruments, double-checking first with the curette and then with the explorer, until the explorer becomes as familiar as an extension of the candidate's operating hand. During the examination the same procedure should be followed, with the candidate exploring delicately and thoroughly for any remaining deposits, before the patient is presented for evaluation.

Candidates should be sure that their instruments are in excellent condition and *very sharp*. It would be poor strategy to provide examiners with a dull curette or scaler with the hope that they could not find or remove any calculus. Very likely, this would only serve to convince examiners that anyone who operates with such dull instruments is a poor practitioner and has only burnished calculus instead of removing it. It is advisable to have extra sterile sets of instruments on hand in case a patient is not acceptable or an instrument is dropped.

The air syringe is an examining instrument that is frequently overlooked or forgotten by candidates. Careful candidates will take the time to thoroughly inspect their work with good light and a dry field before presenting the patient for evaluation.

Examination Forms

For whatever charting, record keeping, or documentation that is necessary during the examination, forms are an important consideration. There are innumerable systems for charting and for taking patient histories, and most individuals are familiar with only those few they have used. If it is possible to obtain examination forms or facsimiles thereof in advance, candidates should study them carefully and practice using them. If examination forms are not available before the test, time should be taken to read and review them at the examination site; candidates should be sure they understand and are properly oriented to the use of the forms before beginning any charting procedures. Most testing agencies will provide adequate orientation to their forms before any clinical exercises begin; however, candidates should not expect the testing agency to tell them how to record every specific oral condition that may occur with a patient. The purpose of a charting examination is to measure a candidate's ability to recognize and record oral conditions; it is not intended to be a copying exercise. Therefore familiarity with the examination forms will allow the candidate to avoid confusion and exercise good clinical judgment in the gathering of data.

Release of Examination Results

Regional board examination results are often reported more slowly than those of state boards; some are released within a few days. Generally speaking, the larger the testing agency, the longer it takes to receive results, and in some instances it may be 8 weeks. Candidates should investigate when they might anticipate receiving results and schedule their practice plans accordingly.

HOW TO PREPARE FOR STATE OR REGIONAL CLINICAL BOARD EXAMINATIONS

1. Obtain application forms, a candidate's guide or brochure, and any information pertaining to the examination that is published by the testing agency. This should be done several months before the examination.
2. Carefully review the application materials and highlight or make a list of all the requirements for the examination, including forms or documentation you must provide, patient requirements, instruments, supplies, etc.
3. Make a note of the application deadline and schedule on your calendar all pertinent dates for completing examination and licensure requirements.

4. If you are taking a regional examination, contact the individual state board offices for the states in which you are seeking licensure. Obtain licensure applications from each state, along with all pertinent information and deadlines for fulfilling licensure prerequisites. It is also advisable to obtain copies of the state dental practice act and rules and regulations for any jurisdiction in which licensure is sought.

5. If you are taking a regional examination, ascertain what additional requirements the state board may have for the jurisdiction(s) in which you are applying for licensure. On successful completion of the regional examination, it is common for a state board to require an examination over its state practice act—perhaps an oral interview or other forms of examination. You should plan your preparation and schedule deadlines for these requirements as well.

6. Begin gathering whatever credentials are necessary to complete the examination and licensure applications. These credentials may include such items as your school transcript, National Board Dental Hygiene Examination score, a copy of your diploma, evidence of malpractice/liability insurance, and a passport-type photograph.

7. It may be helpful to talk with several dental hygienists who have taken the same examination within the past year and ask them for helpful hints in preparing for the examination. Keep the conversation constructive to your concerns. Board examinations create stress for virtually all candidates, and everyone has "war stories" about difficulties they may have encountered or how nervous they were. It is in your best interest to manage such stress constructively, pursue factual information, and employ a positive attitude in your preparations.

8. With the patient-selection criteria firmly in mind, begin searching for suitable patients. Be prepared to present a prospective patient with a clear and professional explanation of both the patient's and your role in the examination. Refer to the section on "Recruitment of Patients" for a more comprehensive discussion of patient selection.

9. Candidates who are enrolled in school should attempt to arrange clinical sessions that duplicate board requirements as much as possible. Many schools conduct "mock boards" for just this purpose; however, additional practice sessions can also be helpful. Seek out those instructors who provide critical, constructive feedback on clinical skills. Make an effort to obtain additional experience with patients whose difficulty level is commensurate with board requirements. Try to sharpen your clinical skills in any area in which you perceive weaknesses.

10. Dental hygienists who are in practice should also set up clinical simulations of board requirements. Begin a period of critical self-assessment; allow time to carefully evaluate your treatment before releasing a patient. Make arrangements with your employer-dentist or with a fellow dental hygienst to occasionally evaluate your performance and give you specific feedback. Many testing agencies do not permit the use of ultrasonic instruments on board examinations. If it is your practice to use ultrasonic scalers routinely for patients with substantial deposits, make a point to limit yourself to hand scalers and curettes until you are sure the strength of your hand and tactile sensitivity with these instruments is at its peak.

11. It is particularly important for dental hygienists who have been out of practice for some period of time to arrange to sharpen their clinical skills. There are a number of dental and dental hygiene schools that periodically offer refresher and update courses for dental hygienists. Such courses should be investigated and pursued well before the examination date, particularly those courses that emphasize clinical skills. A hygienist who is not employed but who is licensed in the jurisdiction might seek the cooperation of a local dentist and/or dental hygienist to treat selected patients in the office and obtain feedback. A nonpracticing hygienist who is not licensed in the jurisdiction might contact a few local hygienists and request assistance through a few practice sessions in the evening—not involving any patient treatment.

12. Ascertain whether there are any specific instruments required for the examination. If so, obtain such instruments and practice using them until they are completely comfortable and familiar. Refer to the previous discussion in this chapter on standardized instruments.

13. If it is possible to obtain examination forms before the test, practice using them. If not, carefully study the examination manual for information about forms and materials to be used during the test.

14. Some examinations require the use of a particular tooth numbering system for the purposes of the test. If a standardized numbering system is used, be sure you are familiar with it and can apply it accurately. Confusion with an unfamiliar system can cause unnecessary charting errors or result in a candidate's failing to comprehend which teeth are assigned by examiners.

15. In addition to your attention to clinical skills, preparation should be ongoing for any written sections of the board examination. The examination manual or guide should contain some information about writ-

ten portions of the test. Many clinical board examinations include written slide examinations covering radiographic recognition or interpretation. In such instances a review of Chapter 5 of this book and a radiographic textbook would be appropriate. Projected slides of common pathologic conditions are also frequently included in board examinations. Your study should be guided by the content of the examination for which you are preparing.

16. A few days before the test, prepare uniforms or clinic attire and organize your instruments and supplies. Be *sure* your instruments are *sharp* and in excellent condition. Confirm arrangements with your patient(s) and make sure the time, date, location, and relevant directions are clearly understood. For safety's sake, it is advisable to check with the patient again the night before the examination.

17. If you are taking the examination at an unfamiliar testing site, try to arrange a brief tour of the clinical facilities before taking the test. Sometimes such a tour is provided in conjunction with a candidate's orientation session that is conducted at the beginning of the examination. Check among your fellow candidates to identify those who are familiar with the facility and request any assistance you may need in locating supplies or in operating equipment.

18. Maintain especially good health habits the final days before the examination so you will be at your best physically, emotionally, and psychologically. This includes a nutritious diet, plenty of rest, and mild, routine exercise. Plan your arrival at the testing site to allow plenty of time for mishaps, traffic, parking problems, locating your operatory, setting up, and orienting yourself. Avoid starting the day feeling rushed, harried, and distracted.

19. At the examination, *listen* carefully to instructions and *read* thoroughly all material that is provided. Above all, follow instructions. Failure to read and follow instructions is undoubtedly the single most important factor in problems encountered by candidates.

20. *Relax* and concentrate on providing the treatment that your entire professional education and experience has prepared you to skillfully deliver. Try to plan appropriate breaks and rest periods during the examination for both yourself and your patient. Eat and drink sensibly during the day to maintain your physical well-being.

CONTENT AND ORGANIZATION OF THIS REVIEW BOOK

This text presents a review in outline form of basic, dental, and clinical sciences. Each review outline is fol-

lowed by related questions that test the candidate's knowledge of concepts, principles, and theories underlying the practice of dental hygiene.

Following the review questions covering the subject matter, each chapter contains a section that provides justification for the correct answer and every distractor. The rationale supporting the correct answer is specified, as well as an explanation of why each distractor is inappropriate as a response to the question. By reviewing these rationales, the candidate should be able to confirm facts and reinforce knowledge.

HOW TO USE THIS BOOK IN STUDYING

1. Review one section of content material at a time. Study the material outlined in the section. Refer to other textbooks and references to research additional details if you encounter any areas that are unclear to you.

2. When you have reviewed the content material, answer the review questions that immediately follow. As you answer each question, write a few words about why you think that answer is correct; in other words, simply justify why you selected that answer. If you guess at an answer to a question, you should make a special mark to identify the answer you selected as a guess. This will enable you to readily identify areas that need further review and clarification of facts. It will also provide a measure of how correct your guessing may be. Remember that analyzing a question, narrowing the choices, and then making an educated guess, if necessary, can improve your performance. On board examinations, guessing is preferable to leaving any blank spaces.

3. Compare your answers with the answers at the end of each chapter. If you answered the item correctly, check the reason you noted for selecting the answer with the rationale that is presented. If you answered the item incorrectly, read the rationale to determine why the distractor you selected is incorrect. In addition, for each item you answered incorrectly, you should review the correct answer and its rationale. If your mistake on that item is still not clear to you, review the theory in the chapter pertaining to that question and research information in your reference material. You should carefully review all questions and rationales for items you identified as guesses, since you did not have mastery of the material covered by the questions.

4. After an interval of several days or weeks, review the chapter again and reanswer the review questions. If you miss the same questions, it should be a clear sign that further study of the material is necessary.

COMPLETION OF THE REVIEW PROCESSES

When a candidate has completed the comprehensive review presented in this book, assessed areas of strength and weakness with the aid of the chapter review questions, reinforced concentrated study of particular material pinpointed by the review, become familiar with the board examination process, protocol, and purpose, and followed instructions for preparation, board examinations can be successfully completed with confidence and composure. Preparation for board examinations actually begins with the first class in dental hygiene school and continues throughout the educational process. This book is designed to present a cohesive, comprehensive review of that professional educational base, reinforce existing knowledge, and guide the candidate toward areas requiring concentrated study.

CHAPTER 2

Histology and Embryology

MARLENE KLYVERT

The dental hygienist's ability to recognize clinical deviations from normal is one essential characteristic of the competent practitioner. However, the competent practitioner also should comprehend the histologic dimension of health and disease and the histologic effects of dental hygiene interventions. A basic knowledge of histology and embryology provides the practicing dental hygienist with the conceptual framework necessary for understanding the complexities of normal growth and development, deviations from the norm, the disease and healing processes, and the histologic changes that occur as a result of dental hygiene intervention. This chapter focuses on the basic concepts relative to general histology and embryology with special emphasis on oral histology and oral and facial development.

General Histology

CELLS (Fig. 2-1)

A. Smallest structures and functionally self-contained units in the body; vary in size, shape, and surface, depending on functional specialization
B. Possess similar common physiologic properties that permit
   1. Growth and reproduction
   2. Response to external stimuli
   3. Assimilation and synthesizing of materials
C. Are the building blocks of tissues in the body attached to each other via cell junctions; there are various types of cell junctions, whose structure is dependent on location and function; types of junctions are
   1. Desmosomes
   2. Tight junctions
   3. Gap junctions
D. Are surrounded by a cell membrane that separates them from the extracellular environment; cell membrane encloses all components of the cell
   1. Cytoplasm
   2. Organelles
   3. Inclusions
   4. Nucleus

Cell Membrane

A. Referred to as plasma membrane or plasmalemma; usually too thin to be seen with a light microscope; average width is approximately 7 nm; is considered selectively permeable, since it controls passage of materials in and out of the cell
B. Trilaminar structure composed of two layers of lipid molecules facing each other into which large globular proteins are inserted (Fig. 2-2)
   1. Lipid bilayers consist mainly of phospholipid molecules; are oriented with hydrophilic ends facing outer and inner surfaces of the cell; hydrophobic ends attract and face each other
   2. Globular proteins are of two types
      a. Integral proteins that extend through the full width of the cell membrane and protrude; may have carbohydrate units attached to them
      b. Peripheral proteins linked or attached to the cell membrane surface

Cytoplasm

A. Translucent homogenous gel enclosed in the cell by the cell membrane; organelles and inclusions are suspended in the cytoplasmic gel
B. All metabolic activities of the cell occur in the cytoplasm
   1. Assimilation (digestion)
   2. Synthesizing of substances such as proteins, proteoglycans, and glycoproteins

Nucleus

A. Controls the two major functions of the cell
   1. Chemical reactions of the cell; synthetic activities
   2. Stores genetic information of the cell
B. Genetic information is stored in chromosomes—chromosomal deoxyribonucleic acid (DNA); human nucleus contains 46 chromosomes
C. Chromosomes are visible only during cell division when they become long, coiled strands; other times chromosomal material is dispersed in granular clumps of material called chromatin

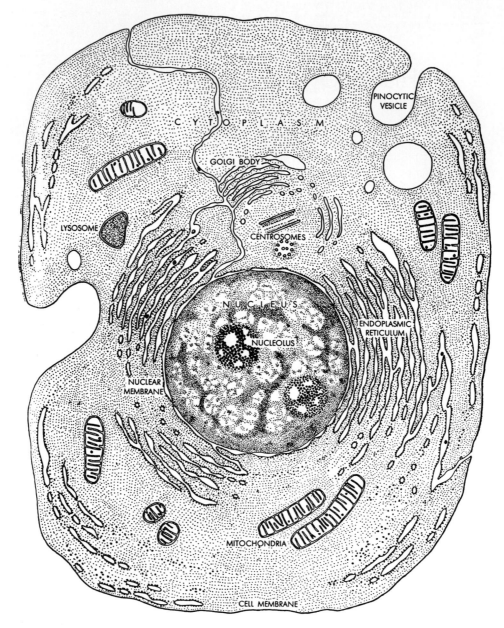

Fig. 2-1 Typical cell. (From Brachet, J.: The living cell, Sci. Am. **205**:50, 1961. Copyright ©
1961 by Scientific American, Inc. All rights reserved.)

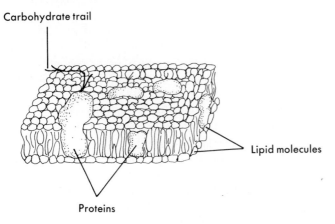

Carbohydrate trail

Lipid molecules

Proteins

Fig. 2-2 Proposed model for structure of cell membrane — two layers of lipid molecules facing each other, into which large globular proteins are inserted (trilaminar membrane).

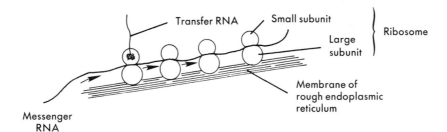

Fig. 2-3 Ribosomes showing protein synthesis on rough endoplasmic reticulum; messenger RNA is being passed through ribosomes on endoplasmic reticulum where transfer RNA becomes incorporated in protein (being formed) that is assembled in ribosome.

D. Each nucleus contains one or more round dense structures referred to as nucleoli; these produce ribosomal ribonucleic acid (RNA) (protein plus RNA)

Synthetic Activities

A. Three types of RNA are necessary for protein synthesis
  1. Messenger RNA—copies of short segments of DNA, the genetic code
    a. Messenger RNA can be compared to a type that contains all the genetic information of proteins but must pass through the ribosomes attached to the endoplasmic reticulum
    b. As the type passes through the ribosomes, transfer RNA adds the exact amino acid to the newly forming proteins (Fig. 2-3)
  2. Transfer RNA—carriers of specific amino acids (building blocks of proteins)
  3. Ribosomal RNA—found floating free in the cytoplasm (polyribosomes) or attached to the endoplasmic reticulum
B. Protein synthesis can also occur on polyribosomes floating free in the cytoplasm; proteins synthesized on the free polyribosomes are used by the cell; proteins synthesized on the ribosomes attached to the endoplasmic reticulum are transported out of the cell

Inclusions

A. Transitory, nonliving metabolic by-products found in the cytoplasm of the cell
B. May appear as lipid droplets, carbohydrate accumulations, or engulfed foreign substances

Lysosomes

A. Membrane-bound organelles responsible for the breakdown of foreign substances engulfed by the cell by the process of phagocytosis or pinocytosis
B. Produced by the golgi complex; they bud off as spherical vesicles containing digestive enzymes; enzymes are first produced by endoplasmic reticulum and then transported to the golgi complex
C. Fuse with engulfed substances, forming a secondary vesicle; vesicle with digestive materials may remain in the cell as a residual body or be discharged outside of the cell

Golgi Complex

A. Stacks of closely spaced membranous sacs where newly formed proteins are concentrated and prepared for export out of the cell (Fig. 2-4)
  1. Small membrane-bound vesicles pinch off from the golgi complex and form secretory granules (newly formed proteins)
  2. Granules attach to the inside of the cell membrane and are then discharged outside of the cell
B. Also involved in production of large carbohydrate molecules and lysosomes

Mitochondria (Fig. 2-5)

A. Membranous structures bounded by a double, inner and outer cell membrane; inner part is thrown into folds (cristae) that extend like shelves inside the mitochondria, providing an additional work surface for the organelle; usually more than one mitochondrion is present in a cell; number tends to be dependent on amount of energy required by the cell
B. Provide the chief source of energy for the cell (oxidation of nutrients) by enzymatic breakdown of fats, amino acids, and carbohydrates

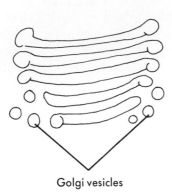

Fig. 2-4 Golgi complex, which consists of a series of flat membranous sacs filled with newly formed proteins; small vesicles pinch off and form secretory granules.

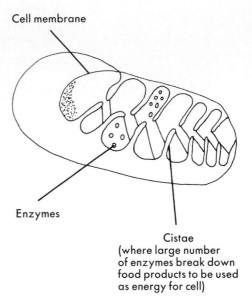

Cell membrane

Enzymes

Cistae (where large number of enzymes break down food products to be used as energy for cell)

Fig. 2-5 Mitochondria.

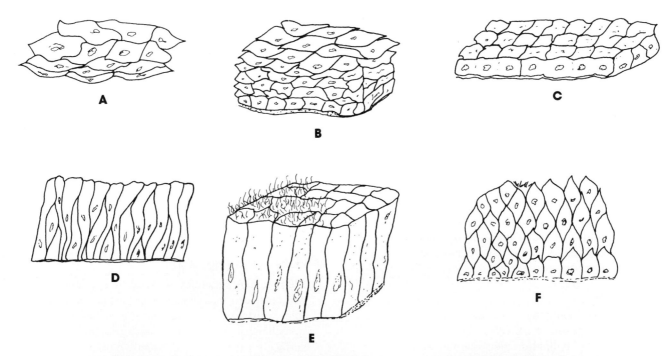

Fig. 2-6 Classification of epithelia according to morphologic shape and number of cell layers. **A,** Simple squamous. **B,** Stratified squamous. **C,** Simple cuboidal. **D,** Pseudostratified columnar. **E,** Simple columnar. **F,** Stratified columnar.

Endoplasmic Reticulum

A. Extensive membranous system found throughout the cytoplasm of the cell; composed of lipoprotein membranes existing in the form of connecting tubules and broad, flattened sacs (cisternea); outer membrane may or may not be covered with ribosomes
  1. Rough-surfaced endoplasmic reticulum (RER)
     or
  2. Smooth-surfaced endoplasmic reticulum (SER), which is minus the ribosomes; agranular
B. Proteins are synthesized on ribosomes attached to the endoplasmic reticulum and are transported to the golgi complex for packaging
C. Smooth endoplasmic reticulum has a number of diverse rolls and is found in a variety of cell types

Filaments and Tubules

A. Threadlike structures about 7 to 10 nm thick; thicker filaments are the same as those seen in muscle (actin strands) and have been associated with contractility in cells
B. Microfilaments act as a support system for the cell cytoskeleton
C. Bundles of microfilaments form tonofibrils and become part of the attachment apparatus (desmosomes) between cells

Microtubules

A. Delicate tubes 20 to 27 nm wide found in cells that are undergoing mitosis and alterations in cell shape
B. Have a support function, particularly in long cellular processes such as neurites or odontoblastic processes

CONCEPTS RELATING TO DENTAL TISSUES

A. All calcified dental tissues are produced by secretory cells that require a great amount of energy in producing their organic matrix, which becomes calcified; organelles such as mitochondria play an important role in helping to provide energy
B. Mitochondria have been associated with the calcification (mineralization) process that occurs in dental tissues
C. Cell organelles help maintain tissues after initial formation by the cell

BASIC TISSUES

A. At the beginning of human development, individual cells multiply and differentiate to perform specialized functions; groups of cells with similar morphologic characteristics and functions come together and form tissues
B. Tissues in the human body can be classified into four types
  1. Epithelial tissue
  2. Connective tissue
  3. Nerve tissue
  4. Muscle tissue
C. Each of the four basic tissues may be further subdivided into several variations

EPITHELIAL TISSUE

A. Consists exclusively of cells held together by specialized junctions (very little intercellular material between the cells); cells rest on an extracellular matrix, the basement membrane
B. Epithelial cells form continuous sheets (tissues) and perform the following functions
  1. Protection—covers all outer surfaces of the body (e.g., skin)
  2. Absorption—lines all inner surfaces of the body (e.g., digestive tract)
  3. Secretion—forms glands (glandular tissue)
C. Epithelial tissue varies depending on its function—may have surface specializations on its free surfaces
  1. Microvilli—for absorption
  2. Cilia—for surface transportation

Types

A. Epithelium is classified according to
  1. Shape of the most superficial cells
     a. Squamous (flat)
     b. Cuboidal
     c. Columnar
  2. Number of cell layers present
     a. One cell layer—simple
     b. Several cell layers—stratified
B. Combination characteristics allow for six different types of epithelium (Fig. 2-6)
  1. Simple squamous
  2. Simple cuboidal
  3. Simple columnar
  4. Stratified squamous
  5. Stratified cuboidal
  6. Stratified columnar

C. Other intermediate forms of epithelium
   1. Pseudostratified columnar (e.g., trachea)
   2. Transitional (e.g., urinary tract)
D. Other cell types found in epithelium
   1. Melanocytes—produce melanin (pigmentation)
   2. Inflammatory cells—transient cells usually associated with inflammation
E. Epithelium lining the oral cavity (oral mucosa) and the skin (dermis) are examples of stratified squamous epithelium

CONNECTIVE TISSUE

Connective Tissue Proper

A. All connective tissue proper develops from embryonic tissue and mesenchyme; has two main functions
   1. Provides mechanical and biologic support
   2. Provides pathways for metabolic substances
B. Other types of connective tissue
   1. Bone
   2. Cartilage
   3. Bone marrow
   4. Lymphoid tissue (tonsils and lymph nodes)
   5. Fat (special type of connective tissue—composed of fat cells)
   6. Dental tissues
      a. Pulp
      b. Dentin
      c. Cementum
C. Types of connective tissues differ in composition of cell products and proportions of products present
   1. Dense connective tissue—consist predominantly of heavy, tightly packed collagen fibers; main function is to resist tension
   2. Loose connective tissue—collagen and reticulin fibers extending in all directions; main function is to provide biologic support and fill spaces between organs and tissues

Connective Tissue Components

A. Cells
   1. Types of cells normally present
      a. Fibroblasts—produce the fibrous matrix and ground substance of connective tissue
      b. Histiocytes—capable of digestive activity
      c. Mast cells—contain vesicles filled with heparin and histamine
   2. Cells that are normally in the bloodstream but that move in and out of the blood vessels into surrounding connective tissue when needed (wandering cells) are
      a. Monocytes
      b. Polymorphonuclear leukocytes
      c. Lymphocytes
      d. Plasma cells
B. Fibrous matrix
   1. Collagen matrix of connective tissue composed of some or all of the following fibers
      a. Collagen fibers—consist of three long protein strands coiled in a left-handed helix to form a tropocollagen unit, which is assembled in a "quarter-stagger" model outside of the cell; are highly resistant to tension; most abundant fibers found in connective tissue (Fig. 2-7)
      b. Reticulin fibers—comparable to collagen fibers in their protein composition; usually found in border areas between connective tissue and other tissues
      c. Elastic fibers—consist of long fibrous proteins different in composition from collagen; are the branching fibers responsible for recoil in tissues when stretched
      d. Oxytalan fibers—resemble elastic fibers in morphology and chemical composition; are thought to be immature elastic fibers

A 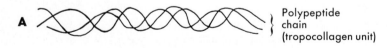 } Polypeptide chain (tropocollagen unit)

B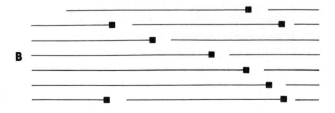

Fig. 2-7 Structural arrangement of polypeptide units forming collagen molecule, **A,** and orderly arrangement of tropocollagen forming collagen fiber—quarter-stagger model, **B.**

C. Ground substance
1. Amorphous substance that consists of many large, highly organized carbohydrate chains attached to long protein cores—proteoglycans
2. Molecular structure and the composition are responsible for the ground substances resistance to compression—compressive loading from any direction

Types (Cartilage and Bone)

Cartilage

A. Cartilage and bone are sister tissues, both highly specialized forms of connective tissues whose intercellular substances have assumed particular properties that allow them to perform support functions
1. Very "bouncy" resilient tissue that is specialized to resist compression; has a gel-like matrix where the ground substance predominates over the intercellular matrix
2. Relatively avascular tissue
3. In humans most of the embryonic skeleton is preformed as hyaline cartilage but is eventually replaced by bone (endochondral ossification); depending on the location and loading pattern imposed on the cartilage, it may specialize and form fibrous or elastic cartilage
4. All mature cartilage is surrounded by a fibrous connective tissue, perichondrium, which serves a biomechanical function; it acts as an attachment site for muscles and tendons
B. Cartilage, like all connective tissues, is composed of three components
1. Cells—chondroblasts and chondrocytes
2. Fibrous matrix—collagen fibers and in some cases elastic fibers
3. Ground substance—proteoglycans, which have a protein core with side chains of chondroitin sulfate and keratin sulfate; because of the chemical nature and organization of the proteoglycans, the ground substance can readily bind and hold water, which allows the tissue to assume a gelatinous nature that can resist compression and also permit some degree of diffusion through the matrix
C. Types
1. Hyaline cartilage
a. Found in the adult human
(1) Covering articular surfaces of movable bones
(2) Forming skeletal support parts of
(a) Trachea
(b) Larynx

(c) External ear
(d) Nasal septum
(e) Ends of ribs
b. Most abundant type of cartilage; forms the human embryonic skeleton in humans; is best suited to resist compression; appears as a homogeneous, translucent tissue because its intercellular matrix dominates its collaginous fibers; major type of fiber in collagen
2. Fibrous cartilage (fibrocartilage)
a. Has a very sparce amount of intercellular substance dominated by collagen fibers, which are in such proportions that they are visible with a light microscope and are seen running between the chondrocytic cells in the cartilage
b. Resembles tendons except for the presence of the chondrocytes enclosed in lacunae
c. Usually found in areas that are subjected to both compression and tension, as in
(1) Intervertebral disk
(2) Temporomandibular joint of older adults
(3) Pubic symphysis
3. Elastic cartilage
a. In areas that are in need of elastic recoil, hyaline cartilage becomes highly specialized and elastic fibers are added to its intercellular matrix, as in
(1) External ear
(2) Epiglottis
b. Elastic fibers are highly branched and form a delicate fibrous matrix, often obscuring the intercellular substance; fibers can be seen only with a light microscope when stained with a specific elastic stain

Bone

A. Very rigid tissue; calcified connective tissue capable of resisting tension; has a calcified matrix that contains the mineral salt hydroxyapatite; very vascular tissue
B. Two main functions
1. Provides skeletal support and protection of soft tissues
2. Acts as a reservoir for calcium and phosphorous ions—when these two ions drop below a critical level in the blood (100 mg Ca/ 100 ml blood and 600 mg P/100 ml blood), they can be withdrawn from the bone

C. Can be identified on two levels
 1. Macroscopic (gross) level—compact (dense) and spongy (cancellous)
  a. Compact (dense) bone appears as a continuous solid mass
  b. Spongy (cancellous) bone appears as branching bony spicules (trabeculae with large intervening marrow spaces between them)
 2. Microscopic level—woven, spongy (cancellous), and lamellar bone
D. Bone morphology
 1. Woven bone—earliest formed embryonic bone; fibers in the matrix have no distinct preferential orientation
 2. Lamellar bone—mature bone has become functionally loaded and can withstand a variety of loading patterns (Fig. 2-8)
  a. Concentric lamellae—form around blood vessels, forming osteons (primary or secondary)
  b. Circumferential lamellae—form on the outer and inner layers of compact bone
  c. Trabecular bone—reflects loading patterns; trabeculae are oriented in two main directions: one parallel with the principle loading direction, the other at right angles with the first; if the loading pattern changes, bone remodeling follows, adjusting the size/shape and direction of the trabeculae to new conditions

  d. Primary osteons—form initially around blood vessels in embryonic woven bone when bone is remodeled and resorbed; are replaced by mature secondary osteons; secondary osteons differ from primary osteons in that their outer surfaces have a scalloped border, rather than a smooth one, as with primary osteons; scalloping reflects the areas of resorbed lacunae by the osteoclasts before the secondary osteon was built
  e. Thickness of any bone (compact lamellar, spongy lamellar) is limited by the nutritional needs of its cells (osteocytes); furthest distance any osteocyte can be from any blood vessel is about 200 μm
E. Bone tissue
 1. Bone, like all connective tissues, has three main components
  a. Cells
   (1) Osteoblasts—bone-forming cells
   (2) Osteoclasts—bone-resorbing cells
   (3) Osteocytes—osteoblasts that are embedded in lacunae of bone matrix and that maintain the bone tissue
  b. Fibrous matrix—collagen fibers (type I) are the dominant component of the bone matrix
  c. Ground substance—proteoglycans containing chonroitin sulfates and seeded with the mineral salt hydroxyapatite
 2. Bone is formed by osteoblasts developed in one of two ways
  a. Intramembranous ossification—mesenchymal cells move closer together (condensation); differentiate into osteoblasts and begin to deposit bone matrix
  b. Endochondral ossification—future bone is preformed in a cartilage model that is eventually resorbed and replaced by new bone formed by osteoblasts (Fig. 2-9)

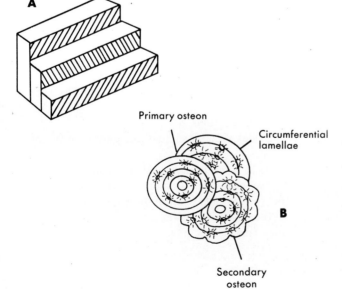

A

Primary osteon

Circumferential lamellae

B

Secondary osteon

Fig. 2-8 Microscopic morphology of bone tissue. **A,** Compact lamellar bone where collagen fibers in each lamella run in opposite direction from adjacent lamella. **B,** Osteons, primary and secondary, that form as result of bone resorption and remodeling; note scalloped edge of secondary osteon. (Modified from Salentijn-Moss, L., and Klyvert, M.: Dental and oral tissues: an introduction for paraprofessionals in dentistry, Philadelphia, 1980, Lea & Febiger.)

(1) Cartilage must undergo two important changes before being resorbed and replaced by new bone
   (a) Chondrocytic hypertrophy
   (b) Calcification of the cartilage model
(2) Endochondral ossification is the process by which all long bones in the human body are formed
   (a) Bone growth in length—occurs in the cartilaginous epiphyseal growth plate
   (b) Bone growth in diameter—occurs in the cellular layer of the fibrous covering connective tissue periosteum, which produces a periosteal bone collar on the outer bone surface

F. Structure of long bones (macroscopic)
   1. Typical long bone is composed of
      a. Diaphysis (shaft)—thick compact bone forming a hollow cylinder with a central marrow cavity; is the primary center of ossification in a long bone
      b. Epiphyses (ends)—spongy bone covered by a thin layer of compact bone; is the secondary growth center
      c. Metaphysis—transitional region between the epiphyses and the diaphysis where the cartilage growth plate is located
      d. All articular surfaces of long bones are covered by articular cartilage
   2. While active, the epiphyseal growth plate usually has four zones, proceeding from first to last
      a. Primary spongiosa with resorption
      b. Hypertrophy and provisional calcification
      c. Proliferation
      d. Resting zone (Fig. 2-9)

BLOOD AND LYMPH

A. Vascular system
   1. Develops embryonically from mesenchymal cells that come together and form delicate tubular structures composed of endothelial cells
   2. Consists of the heart, blood vessels, and lymphatics
      a. Is a closed system that runs from the heart to the organs of the body and back to the heart
      b. Between the heart and the organs, the blood vessels branch progressively into finer and finer vessels and finally enter organs
         (1) Here a delicate network of capillaries form, called the capillary bed—the most essential part of the vascular system
         (2) Exchanges of gases and substances occur in this capillary bed
      c. Blood is then carried back to the heart via larger vessels, the veins
   3. Functions
      a. Carries nutrients, oxygen, and hormones to all parts of the body
      b. Carries metabolic waste products to the kidneys
      c. Transports inflammatory cells and antibodies
      d. Maintains a constant body temperature
B. Lymph vessels empty into filtering organs (nodes); generally flow toward larger lymph vessels, the thoracic duct, and the right lymphatic duct; lymph enters venous branches of the circulatory system

Blood Vessels

A. Arteries—the largest of the blood vessels; walls are composed of
   1. Thick layer of smooth muscle cells
   2. Elastic tissue—the largest amount found in large arteries close to the heart

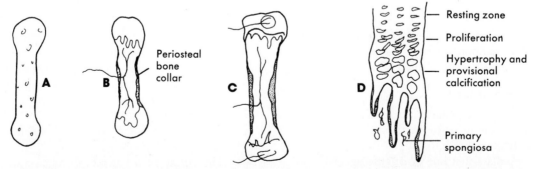

Fig. 2-9 Stages of endochondral bone formation in long bone growth. **A,** Preformed cartilage model of bone. **B,** Primary center of ossification in diaphysis and periosteal collar. **C,** Secondary center of ossification starting in diaphysis. **D,** Growth plate with four zones.

B. Veins—usually accompany arteries but carry blood in the opposite direction
　1. Walls are composed of
　　a. Layer of endothelial cells
　　b. Connective tissue layer
　　c. Occasionally a few smooth muscle cells
　2. Veins contain about 70% of the total blood volume of the body at any given time
C. Capillaries—the simplest of the blood vessels in their structure
　1. Walls consist of a simple layer of endothelial cells and a basal lamina
　2. Usually the diameter of a capillary lumen is so small that only one blood cell at a time can pass through the vessel
　3. Form a barrier between the blood and the tissues
　4. Transport of substances occurs at the capillary level via
　　a. Pores in the endothelial wall of the capillary
　　b. Openings between adjacent endothelial cells
　　c. Pinocytotic vesicles formed by the wall of the capillary

Microvasculature

A. Composed of the smallest arteries and veins located in the capillary bed
　1. At the end of the arterioles is a preferential channel, which has several side branches entering into the capillary bed
　2. Blood passes through the capillary bed from the arterial side to the venous side
B. Selective openings and closings of the capillary bed occur in the microvasculature to ensure regulation of the amount of blood throughout the body at any given time

Blood Components

A. Cells
　1. Red blood cells—erythrocytes; most numerous
　2. White blood cells—leukocytes (granular and nongranular)
　3. Platelets—cell fragments of a specific cell type found in red bone marrow; have no nuclei
B. Plasma—liquid portion of blood

Functions of Blood Cells

A. Red blood cells—contain hemoglobin, which carries oxygen from the lungs to the tissues
B. Granular leukocytes
　1. Neutrophils—first line of defense against bacterial invasion
　2. Eosinophils—involvement in allergy reactions
　3. Basophils—antigen involvement

C. Nongranular leukocytes
　1. Monocytes—can become macrophages in connective tissue
　2. Lymphocytes—produce antibodies
D. Platelets—promote blood clotting

Lymphatic System

A. Made up of a series of vessels that carry excess tissue fluid from the capillaries to filtering organs such as lymph nodes on the way back to the bloodstream
B. Lymph nodes are found along the lymphatic pathway
　1. Consist of masses of lymph tissue that serve as a filtering system for the body
　2. Tonsils and the spleen are both filtering organs for the body
　3. Swollen and palpable lymph nodes can indicate that there may be an infection somewhere in the body
C. Function of lymph is to help protect and maintain the internal fluid environment of the body

NERVE TISSUE ▬▬▬▬▬▬▬

A. Main functions of the nervous system
　1. Directs and helps maintain the complex internal environment of the body
　2. Integrates and interprets incoming stimuli, and directs appropriate responses at a conscious or unconscious level
B. Nervous system can be classified accordingly
　1. Central nervous system (CNS)
　2. Peripheral nervous system (PNS)
　3. Autonomic nervous system (ANS)
C. Afferent nerves transmit impulses (sensations) from the periphery to the CNS (sensory input); efferent nerves transmit impulses (commands) from the CNS to muscles and other organs (motor output) (Fig. 2-10)
D. Divisions of the nervous system
　1. Central nervous system
　　a. Includes the brain and the spinal cord
　　b. Main functions
　　　(1) Receives incoming information at a conscious or unconscious level (sensory)
　　　(2) Integrates outgoing responses (motor) that are transmitted to various parts of the brain and the spinal cord
　2. Peripheral nervous system
　　a. Composed of 31 pairs of spinal nerves and 12 pairs of cranial nerves
　　b. All nerves transmit information to and from the CNS
　　c. Contains both sensory and motor nerves (neurons)

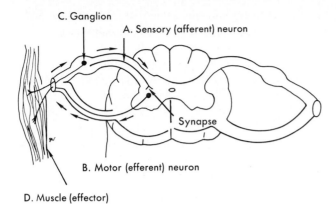

Fig. 2-10 Cross section of spinal cord and pathways used to transmit nerve impulses from periphery to central nervous system (see also Figs. 3-13 to 3-15). *A*, Sensory neuron sending impulses from periphery to central nervous system; *B*, motor neuron leaving spinal cord, transmitting commands to effector; *C*, nerve cell bodies located in dorsal root ganglia; *D*, Effector.

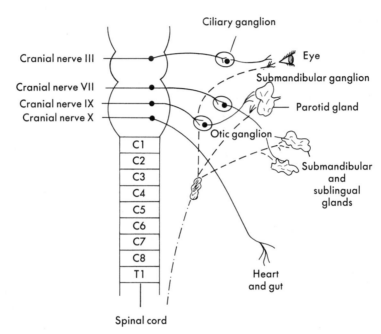

Fig. 2-11 Autonomic pathways for cranial nerves and synapses in their respective ganglia outside central nervous system (see also Fig. 3-17).

3. Autonomic nervous system (Fig. 2-11)
   a. Controls, regulates, and coordinates visceral activities (digestion, body temperature, blood pressure, and glandular secretions) on an unconscious level
   b. Is further subdivided into
      (1) Parasympathetic division—acts to regulate and mobilize activities during emergency and/or stress (flight activities); activities that require large outputs of energy produce an accelerated heart rate and increase in blood pressure
      (2) Sympathetic division—works the opposite of the parasympathetic division; stimulates those activities that restore or conserve energy

Structural Components

A. Neurons (Fig. 2-12)
   1. Structural components of nerve tissue
   2. Receive and transmit information
   3. Highly specialized cells consisting of
      a. Cell body—contains the nucleus and the organelles; located in the ganglia in the CNS and PNS
      b. One or more cytoplasmic extensions
         (1) Dendrites—conduct impulses toward the cell body
         (2) Axons—conduct impulses away from the cell body

4. Classified according to the number of cell processes (Fig. 2-13)
   a. Multipolar neurons—located in the CNS and autonomic ganglia; usually one process is the axon, and the other processes are the dendrites
   b. Unipolar neurons—have a short cell process that leaves the cell body and divides into two long branches; one branch goes to the CNS, and the other goes toward the PNS (sensory neurons)

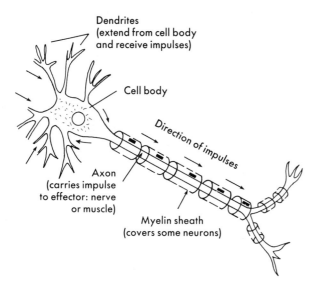

Fig. 2-12 Basic neuron.

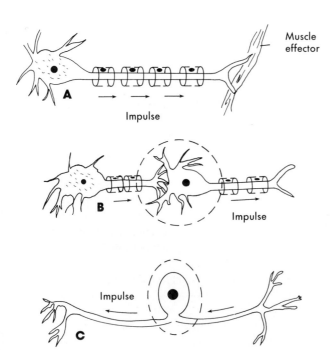

5. Interneurons—lie within the CNS; receive and link sensory and motor impulses to bring about appropriate responses in the body

B. Glial cells—provide structural support and nourishment for the neurons; Schwann cells in the PNS and satellite cells in the ganglia

Definitions

A. Synapse—area that occurs between two neurons or between a neuron and its effector (muscle or gland); between the cell surfaces are
   1. Synaptic cleft—intercellular space separating a presynaptic and postsynaptic membrane
   2. Presynaptic membrane—situated before the synapse
   3. Postsynaptic membrane—situated after the synapse

B. Neurotransmitters—chemicals released from the neuron as electrical impulses travel along the axon and reach the terminal end
   1. They increase the permeability of the cell membranes; impulses are relayed to the effector (impulses can be excitatory or inhibitory)
   2. Two membrane junctions
   3. Kinds of neurotransmitters
      a. Acetylcholine
      b. Norepinephrine

C. Myelin sheath—fatty layer surrounding the axon of the nerve
   1. Myelinated—contains a fatty sheath
   2. Unmyelinated—no fatty sheath is present

D. Free nerve endings—end portions of afferent (sensory) axons that are no longer covered by a supportive Schwann cell; are found in
   1. Dental pulp
   2. Oral epithelium

Fig. 2-13 Classification of neurons based on number of cell processes on neuron. **A,** Multipolar motor neuron with one of its axons going to effector (skeletal muscle). **B,** Two automatic multipolar neurons; axon of one neuron in central nervous system communicates with cell body of neuron outside central nervous system (in ganglion). **C,** Sensory (afferent) neuron; cell process leaves cell body and divides into two processes; one process goes toward central nervous system, and one goes to periphery (e.g., skin, oral mucosa). (Modified from Salentijn-Moss, L., and Klyvert, M.: Dental and oral tissues: an introduction for paraprofessionals in dentistry, Philadelphia, 1980, Lea & Febiger.)

E. Encapsulated nerve endings—are composed of several portions of afferent axons surrounded by a capsule of several Schwann cells without a myelin sheath and some connective tissue; are associated with
   1. Touch perception (Meissner's corpuscles) found in the lamina propria of the oral mucosa
   2. Periodontal ligament

Cranial Nerves

A. Twelve pairs of cranial nerves originate from the brain
   1. Transmit information to the brain from the special sensory receptors, regulating the functions of
      a. Smell
      b. Sight
      c. Hearing
      d. Taste
   2. Bring impulses from the CNS to voluntary muscles of
      a. Eyes
      b. Mouth (masticatory muscles)
      c. Face (facial expression)
      d. Tongue (swallowing and speech)
      e. Larynx
B. Local anesthetic used in the dental profession is injected into a sensory peripheral nerve; it diffuses through the nerve fibers and blocks transmission of impulses to the brain in an area of several teeth or in a localized area of soft tissue

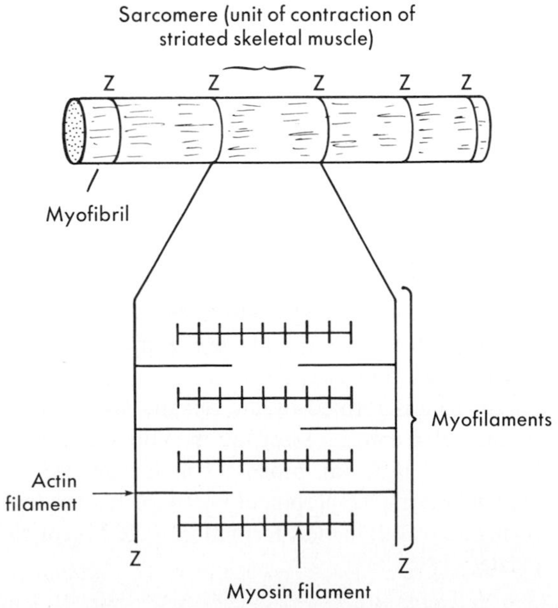

Fig. 2-14 Enlarged segment of myofibril showing arrangement of actin and myosin filaments and their attachment to Z bands (see also Fig. 3-10).

MUSCLE TISSUE

A. Composed mainly of cells called muscle fibers that have differentiated from embryonic mesenchyme and become highly specialized in contracting (shortening)
B. Contracting ability of muscle fibers is a result of large amounts of intracellular, contractile protein filaments: actin and myosin
C. Three muscle tissue types
   1. Skeletal (striated) muscle
      a. Under conscious control; referred to as voluntary musle
      b. Has rapid, short, strong contractions; requires a great deal of energy
      c. Innervated by motor nerves
      d. Skeletal muscles of the head region
         (1) Muscles of mastication
         (2) Muscles of facial expression
      e. Muscle attachments are made possible because of the connective tissues surrounding the muscle, bone, or cartilage; connecting tissues of muscles run directly into the periosteum, covering bone, or the perichondrium, covering cartilage; there may be intermediate structures such as
         (1) Tendons
         (2) Ligaments
         (3) Aponeurosis
   2. Smooth muscle
      a. Under the control of the ANS and not under conscious control
      b. Contractions are slow and can be maintained over a long period of time without the use of much energy
   3. Cardiac muscle
      a. Has some of both skeletal and smooth muscle characteristics
      b. Is involuntary; has fast, powerful contractions

Muscle Contraction

A. Muscle can be stimulated to contract by one or many nerves
B. Each striated muscle contains bundles of highly organized contractile proteins called myofibrils; each myofibril consists of regularly arranged protein filaments: actin and myosin (Fig. 2-14)
C. Protein filaments are attached to a Z band; section of a myofibril between two Z bands is called a sarcomere, which is the contractile unit
D. As a muscle unit contracts, the actin and myosin filaments slide past each other, shortening the length of the individual sarcomere (sliding mechanism) and causing the total shortening of the muscle fiber

Embryology

GENERAL EMBRYOLOGY

A. All human development begins by the uniting of a female germ cell (ovum) with a male germ cell (sperm), called fertilization

B. Each germ cell contains 23 chromosomes (haploid number); during the process of fertilization the number of chromosomes is restored to 46 (diploid number)

C. The developing organism, called the zygote, goes through a series of mitotic divisions, producing
1. Morula—16 to 32 cells having the appearance of a mulberry
2. Blastocele—central cavity develops with an embryonic pole
3. Blastocysts—become attached to and embedded in the uterine wall
   a. Two distinct layers become visible
      (1) Epiblast (ectoderm) layer
      (2) Hypoblast (endoderm) layer
   b. These two layers constitute the embryonic disk, which will give rise to the future embryo

D. Three distinct periods in human development
1. Period of the ovum (first week)—fertilized ovum develops an embryonic disk
2. Embryonic period (second through eighth week)—most of the organs and organ systems develop
   a. Period of differentiation
   b. At the end of this period a recognizable individual has developed
   c. Most congenital malformations occur during this time
3. Fetal period (third through ninth month)—growth of the existing structures takes place

E. Development of some facial and oral structures is dependent on a group of cells (neural crest cells) derived from ectoderm as the neural tube is forming; these cells migrate cephalically and interact with the cephalic ectoderm and mesoderm, resulting in development of
1. Facial skeleton—Meckel's cartilage
2. Neck skeleton—hyoid bone
3. Connective tissue components
4. Tooth development

F. Neural crest cells migrate into each of the branchial arches and surround the existing mesoderm; in each arch the following components develop
1. Cartilage rod—skeleton of each arch—first branchial arch, Meckel's cartilage
2. Muscular component—second branchial arch, facial musculature
3. Vasculature component
4. Nerve component—first branchial arch, trigeminal nerve

G. On the internal aspect of the branchial arches are corresponding pharyngeal pouches that give rise to
1. External auditory meatus
2. Pharyngotympanic tube
3. Palatine tonsils
4. Parathyroid glands

FACIAL DEVELOPMENT

A. Begins in the fourth week of prenatal life (embryonic period) and is complete in the twelfth week

B. Future facial region is located between the bulging forebrain, frontal nasal process, and developing heart

C. At the beginning of the fourth week, five facial swellings appear on the embryo, called branchial arches
1. Located between the first branchial arch and the forebrain is the oral stomadeum (primitive oral cavity) (Fig. 2-15, A and B)
2. Maxilla and mandible develop from the first branchial arch
3. Second through fifth branchial arches are involved with development of the neck

D. Frontal nasal process develops the forehead and nose
1. On the surface of the frontal nasal process two bilateral thickened areas of specialized ectoderm arise—nasal placodes (Fig. 2-15, C), which produce
   a. Two lateral nasal processes—will form the sides of the nose
   b. Two medial nasal processes—will form the bridge of the nose, the nostrils, and the philtrum of the upper lip
2. Face grows downward and forward around the developing nasal and oral cavities

E. Midface is formed by the bilateral processes of the maxillary process, which grow forward and make contact with the mandibular processes and the medial nasal processes

F. Lower face is formed by the bilateral swellings (mandibular processes) of the mandibular arch

G. Several facial or oral processes merge or fuse together during development; incomplete merging or fusing can result in cleft formation—cleft lip or cleft palate

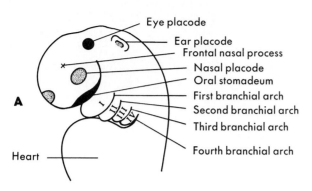
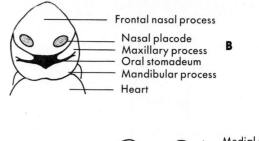
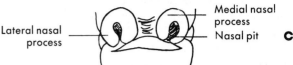

Fig. 2-15 Facial development in fourth week in embryo. **A** and **B,** Facial development beginning with outgrowth of branchial arches; note relationship of oral stomadeum to heart and developing face. **C,** Nasal placodes develop from frontal nasal process and grow to become nostrils and form bridge of nose and philtrum.

PALATAL DEVELOPMENT

A. Primary palate (primitive palate) develops as a result of the merging of the two medial nasal processes and gives rise to
   1. Philtrum of upper lip
   2. Primary palate, which carries the incisor teeth
B. During the sixth week of embryonic life, two palatal shelves develop from each side of the maxilla, lying vertically on each side of the tongue (secondary palate)
C. During the seventh week of embryonic life, the vertical palatal shelves flip up, assume a horizontal position, and fuse with the primary palate
D. Where the two palatal processes (shelves) fuse in midline, trapped epithelium between the two processes may result in epithelium remnants, which may result in cysts

TONGUE DEVELOPMENT

During the fourth week of embryonic life, the tongue develops from several swellings arising on the internal aspect of branchial arches 1 through 4 (pouches); these swellings eventually merge and form the body and root of the tongue

A. Branchial arch 1—two lateral swellings and one medial swelling
B. Branchial arches, 2, 3, and part of 4—corpula
C. Branchial arch 4—epiglottis

Oral Histology

TOOTH DEVELOPMENT

A. Begins in the seventh week of embryonic life with the 20 primary (deciduous) teeth; continues until the late teens with sequential exfoliation of the primary teeth and development and eruption of the secondary dentition—the 32 permanent teeth
B. Tissues of the tooth
   1. Each tooth consists of four tissues (Fig. 2-16)
      a. Enamel—calcified
      b. Cementum—calcified
      c. Dentin—calcified
      d. Pulp—uncalcified
   2. All tissues of the tooth are specialized forms of connective tissue, except enamel
   3. Each tooth is the product of two tissues that interact during tooth development
      a. Mesenchyme—derived from neural crest cells
      b. Epithelium—oral epithelium derived from ectoderm
C. Involves two major events
   1. Morphodifferentiation—shaping of the tooth
   2. Cytodifferentiation—cells differentiate into specific tissue-forming cells
      a. Ameloblasts—enamel-forming cells
      b. Cementoblasts—cementum-forming cells
      c. Odontoblasts—dentin-forming cells
      d. Fibroblasts—pulp-forming cells

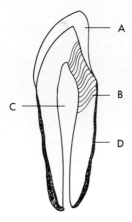

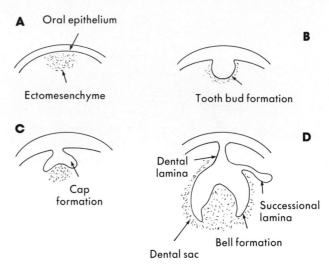

Fig. 2-16 Longitudinal cross section showing tissues of tooth. *A,* Enamel covering crown of tooth; *B,* dentin forming bulk of tooth in crown and root; *C,* pulp tissue centrally located in crown and root; *D,* cementum covering root.

Fig. 2-17 Sequential stages of tooth development. **A,** Initial interaction between oral epithelium and ectomesenchyme. **B,** Bud stage. **C,** Cap stage. **D,** Bell stage.

Morphodifferentiation

A. Oral epithelium and underlying mesenchyme are responsible for shaping the tooth
   1. Both primary and permanent tooth germs go through the same stages of development
   2. Oral epithelium grows down into underlying mesenchyme; small areas of condensed mesenchyme will form future tooth germs
B. Stages (Fig. 2-17)
   1. Bud stage—condensed areas of ectomesenchymal cells that are continuous with oral epithelium; connection between the two is referred to as the dental lamina
   2. Cap stage—future shape of the tooth becomes evident; cells specialize to form the enamel organ
   3. Bell stage—final stage of morphodifferentiation; in the later part of stage, cytodifferentiation begins in the enamel organ
   4. Apposition stage—cells have differentiated into tissue-forming cells; begin to deposit the dental tissues

Cytodifferentiation

A. Stages of cytodifferentiation and morphodifferentiation overlap; both the epithelial and mesenchymal components of the tooth germ become organized
   1. Epithelial components become the enamel organ, which is organized into four distinct cell layers

   a. Outer enamel epithelium (OEE)—outlines the shape of the future developing enamel organ on the outer surface; composed of small cuboidal cells, one cell layer thick
   b. Inner enamel epithelium (IEE)—innermost layer of enamel organ on the concave side of the developing tooth germ; will become the future enamel-producing cells, the ameloblasts; composed of cuboidal-type cells, one cell layer thick
   c. Stratum intermedium (STI)—flat, supporting squamous-type cells; two cell layers thick, lying on top of the inner enamel epithelial cells
   d. Stellate reticulum (STR)—mechanically and nutritionally supporting cells that fill the bulk of the developing enamel organ; are star shaped with large amounts of intercellular space between them (Fig. 2-18)
   2. Mesenchymal components—become subdivided into
   a. Dental sac (follicle)—surrounds the developing tooth germ and provides cells that will form the cementum, periodontal ligament, and the alveolar bone proper
   b. Dental papilla—condensed mesenchyme located on the concavity side of the enamel organ; periphery cells will differentiate into dentin-forming cells, the odontoblasts
   c. Center of the dental papilla will become the dental pulp

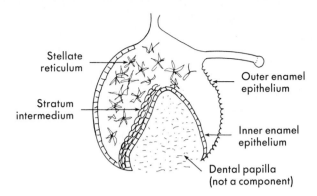

Fig. 2-18 Four distinct components of enamel organ.

B. Is dependent on a series of sequential cellular interactions between epithelial and mesenchymal components of the tooth germ
1. First interaction—between oral epithelium and the mesenchyme; mesenchyme instructs the epithelium to grow down into the mesenchyme and shape the tooth
2. Second interaction—given by cells of inner enamel epithelium (preameloblasts) to mesenchymal cells on the periphery of the dental papilla to differentiate into odontoblasts and begin deposition of dentin
3. Third interaction—as soon as odontoblasts begin to deposit dentin, preameloblasts become true secreting ameloblasts and begin deposition of enamel
4. Fourth interaction—occurs with development of root dentin and cementum

Dentin and Enamel Formation

A. Both enamel- and dentin-forming cells are polarized, tall, columnar secreting cells; just before ameloblasts and odontoblasts begin to deposit enamel and dentin, there is an increase in the number of organelles, especially the mitochondria; organelles move to the basal nonsecretory end of the cell; both cells require tremendous amounts of energy for production of their calcified tissues
B. All dentin and enamel formation begins at the dentoenamel junction of the cup or incisal edge of the tooth and continues in an apical direction
C. Permanent tooth germ grows off the primary (deciduous) tooth germ via an epithelial attachment similar to dental lamina, called successional lamina; true for all of the developing permanent teeth except first, second, and third molars, which develop from the dental lamina, which continues to grow back in oral arches

D. Dentin formation
1. Odontoblasts produce a fibrous connective tissue matrix of predominantly collagen fibers with a rich proteoglycan ground substance; dentinal tissue is calcified by deposition of the calcium salt, hydroxyapatite crystals, into the matrix
2. Each odontoblast has a long cell-extension, odontoblastic process, left behind in the calcified dentin and enclosed in a dentinal tubule (Fig. 2-19, *A*)
3. Dentin remains a vital tissue throughout the life of the tooth; cells continue to produce dentin when needed
E. Enamel formation
1. Ameloblasts produce an enamel matrix with protein components; precise nature of proteins is not yet known; matrix is calcified immediately by deposition of the calcium salt, hydroxyapatite crystals
2. Each ameloblast has a secretory process, Tomes' process; (Fig. 2-19, *B*); ameloblasts deposit enamel; Tomes' process is responsible for the pattern seen microscopically in mature enamel, the enamel prism; processes are not left behind embedded in the calcified enamel
3. When the tooth emerges into the oral cavity, the enamel has no vital cells associated with the tissue; enamel is not a true tissue as the other dental tissues are; is incapable of tissue growth or repair
F. Dentogingival junction formation
1. After enamel formation is completed, remains of the enamel organ (OEE, IEE, STI, and STR) come together
2. These form the reduced enamel epithelium, which plays an important role in formation of the dentogingival junction as the tooth emerges into the oral cavity
G. Cementum formation
1. Formation of root dentin and cementum follows after the crown of the tooth is completed
2. Hertwig's root sheath is formed by the joining of the outer enamel epithelium and the inner enamel epithelium, which continues to grow down; shapes the root of the tooth and formation of root dentin; is followed by differentiation of cells from the dental sac, which produce
a. Cementum
b. Periodontal ligament
c. Alveolar bone proper

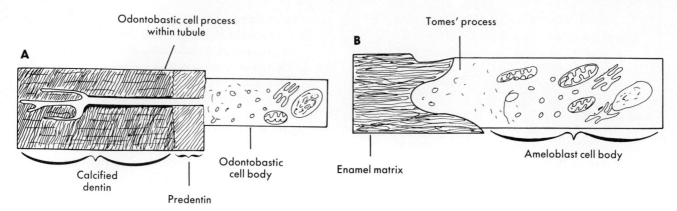

Fig. 2-19 Odontoblast and ameloblast with their cell extensions. **A,** Tall secretory odontoblast with its cell extension (odontoblastic process). **B,** Tall secretory ameloblast with its cell extension (Tomes' process).

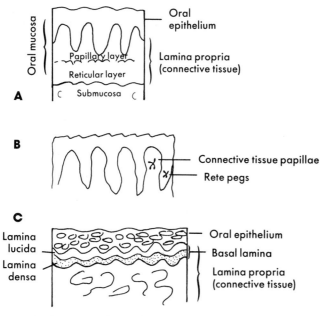

Fig. 2-20 Basic structure of oral epithelium. **A,** Two basic tissue types of oral mucosa: oral epithelium and connective tissue; connective tissue is composed of papillary layer and reticular layer; submucosal layer may or may not be present, depending on location of oral mucosa. **B,** Arrangement of rete pegs and connective tissue. **C,** Basal lamina interface between oral epithelium and connective tissue.

SOFT TISSUE OF THE ORAL CAVITY ▬▬
Oral Mucosa

A. Oral epithelium (Fig. 2-20)
   1. Covered by a layer of stratified squamous epithelium, which
      a. Acts as a mechanical barrier
      b. Protects the underlying tissues
   2. Three types of stratified squamous epithelium are found in the oral cavity
      a. Orthokeratinized
         (1) Effective as a mechanical protector and barrier against fluids
         (2) Least frequently present of the three types
         (3) Layers
            (a) Basal cell layer—deepest layer
            (b) Prickle cell layer
            (c) Granular layer—contains the keratohyaline granules, the precursor to keratin
            (d) Keratinized layer—contains degenerative cells with no nuclei or organelles; cells are filled with keratin; become hard (cornified) and are eventually lost from the surface epithelium
      b. Nonkeratinized
         (1) Functions as a selective barrier, acting as a cushion and as protection against mechanical stress and wear
         (2) Layers
            (a) Basal cell layer
            (b) Prickle cell layer

(c) Outer surface of nonkeratinized cells (squamae); no distinctly recognizable layer above the prickle cell layer; superficial cells in the outermost layer undergo a gradual increase in size; look empty but are filled with fluid sacs; cells act as a cushion and are firmly attached to each other
   c. Parakeratinized
      (1) Intermediate form of epithelium located between the orthokeratinized and nonkeratinized oral mucosa
      (2) Layers
         (a) Basal cell layer
         (b) Prickle cell layer
         (c) Keratinized layer—no distinct granular layer present; gradually becomes filled with keratin; nuclei and other cell organelles remain present until the cell becomes cornified and are eventually lost
   3. Stratified squamous epithelium is constantly being renewed by mitosis at the basal cell layer; turnover rate time ranges from 5 to 16 days
B. Connective tissue—referred to as lamina propria
   1. Subdivided into two layers
      a. Papillary layer—directly under the epithelial layer
      b. Reticular layer—dense fibrous layer located under the papillary layer
   2. Forms a mechanical support system and carries
      a. Blood vessels
      b. Nerves
C. Submucosa
   1. Layer of loosely organized connective tissue
   2. Present only in areas that require a high degree of compressibility and flexibility (e.g., cheeks, soft palate)
   3. When present, is located between the lamina propria and areas where muscle tissue is present
D. Interface
   1. Area of interdigitation between oral epithelium and the connective tissue
   2. Epithelial extensions into the connective tissue (lamina propria) are called rete pegs
   3. Connective tissue extensions into overlying epithelium are called connective tissue papillae
   4. Corrugated arrangement
      a. Increases the surface area between the two tissues

      b. Increases the strength of the junction between the two tissues
      c. Decreases the distance between the blood supply and epithelium, which does not have its own blood supply; blood vessels are carried to epithelium in connective tissue via the connective tissue papillae
E. Basement membrane
   1. Located between oral epithelium and the connective tissue
   2. Noncellular
   3. Produced in part by epithelial cells

Specialized Mucosa of the Tongue

A. Specialized covering found only on the top of the tongue
B. Epithelial layer—statified squamous epithelium that varies in thickness and degree of keratinization
C. Connective tissue papillae form specialized lingual papillae
   1. Fungiform papillae—located on the dorsal aspect of the tongue; mushroom shape; a single taste bud may be present on the top surface
   2. Filiform papillae—most abundant on the papillae; found covering the entire top surface of the tongue; have no taste buds
   3. Vallate papillae—large papillae located in a V-shaped groove at the base of the tongue; encircled by a deep groove; mushroom shaped; taste buds are located on their sides; small salivary glands (von Ebner glands) empty into surrounding grooves of taste buds
   4. Foliate papillae—located along the sides of the tongue, near the base of the tongue; taste buds may be located only on one of the sides
D. No submucosa is present

TISSUES OF THE TOOTH ▰▰▰▰▰▰▰▰
Dentin

A. Mature dentin composition
   1. Chemical composition
      a. Organic matter   18%
      b. Inorganic materials 70%
      c. Water   12%
   2. Tissue composition
      a. Cells—odontoblasts
      b. Fibrous material—collagen fibers
      c. Ground substance—proteoglycans
   3. Calcification—deposition of the calcium salt, hydroxyapatite crystals, in dentin organic matrix

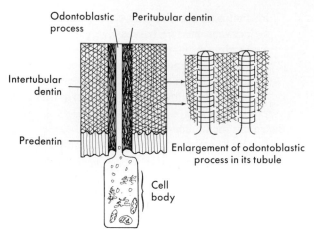

Fig. 2-21 Odontoblastic process with its cell process enclosed in dentinal tubule.

B. Process of dentogenesis
1. Dentin begins to form in the late bell stage of the developing tooth germ
2. Newly differentiated odontoblasts deposit the dentin matrix; odontoblastic processes become surrounded by predentin (a newly deposited uncalcified dentin matrix); predentin becomes calcified as cells deposit more dentin
3. Each cell process in mature calcified dentin is enclosed in a dentinal tubule (Fig. 2-21)
   a. Dentinal tubules can run from the dentoenamel junction to the periphery of the dental pulp, where cell bodies of odontoblasts are located
   b. Tubules follow a primary S-shaped curve (pathway) and secondary S-shaped curves along the length of the tubules
      (1) Primary S-shaped curves are caused by movement of odontoblasts from a wider area to a narrower area, which produces crowding of the odontoblasts; S-shaped curved movement is how odontoblasts adjust to the new crowding while moving back toward the dental pulp
      (2) Secondary S-shaped curves are seen along the length of the dentinal tubule as small waves in the tubules, about 4 μm apart; may possibly be reflecting changes in the movement of the odontoblasts during the night and day
   c. Tubules tend to have more branching at their terminal ends in the crown of the tooth than in the root dentin; root dentin has more lateral branching, with fewer primary S-shaped curves

d. Diameter of tubules changes during the process of dentin formation; widest dentinal tubules are found in children and are about 4 μm wide
4. First layer of dentin immediately adjacent to the dentoenamel junction is called mantle dentin; remainder of the deposited dentin is called circumpulpal dentin (around the pulp)
   a. Mantle dentin
      (1) Layer of dentin about 10 to 30 μm thick
      (2) Differs from circumpulpal dentin because, in addition to collagen fibers normally found in dentin, it contains a second group of thicker and heavier collagen fibers
         (a) These fibers are deposited perpendicular to the dentoenamel junction
         (b) Are referred to as von Korff's fibers
      (3) Is less calcified than circumpulpal dentin
   b. Circumpulpal dentin
      (1) Contains finer collagen fibers than mantle dentin
      (2) Fibers are deposited parallel to the dentoenamel junction
5. Dentin that forms immediately around the odontoblastic process is called peritubular dentin
   a. Forms a sheath around each odontoblastic process about 1 μm thick
   b. Consists of a matrix of delicate collagen fibers
   c. Is highly calcified
   d. First dentin to be decalcified by the bacterial enzymes when exposed to caries is the peritubular dentin
6. Remainder of dentin is called intertubular dentin
   a. Consists of large, coarse collagen fibers
   b. Matrix is less calcified than that of the peritubular dentin
   c. Produced first by the odontoblast, then the odontoblast produces its peritubular dentin
7. Once the dentin is deposited, it does not undergo any remodeling
C. Types
1. Primary dentin—refers to dentin deposited *before* the completion of the apical foramen
2. Secondary dentin—refers to dentin formed *after* the completion of the apical foramen; tends to be more calcified than the primary dentin; forms at a slower rate

3. Reactive dentin—forms rapidly in localized areas where dental tubules have been exposed to external traumas such as
   a. Caries preparations
   b. Attrition or bruxism (enamel has been worn away)
   c. Thermal water sprays

D. Sensory conduction
   1. Nerves associated with dentin are located in the dental pulp, but it is believed that they monitor changes in the environment of odontoblasts, allowing for perceptions of pain
   2. When dentinal tubules become exposed to the outside environment, a direct contact is made with pulp; fluid in open, exposed tubules begins to evaporate, and the movement of fluid caused by evaporation may stimulate nerves nearest odontoblasts to produce pain

Pulp Tissue

A. Structure
   1. Most centrally located tissue in the tooth
   2. Loose connective tissue
   3. Cells
      a. Fibroblasts—undifferentiated mesenchymal cells
      b. Histiocytes—found along blood vessels; sometimes referred to as macrophages when filled with ingested materials
      c. Lymphocytes—when present, tend to be near the odontoblastic layer
      d. Cells present in diseased pulp include monocytes, polymorphonuclear leukocytes, eosinophils, and plasma cells
      e. No fat cells are present
   4. Structural arrangement
      a. Outer periphery of the pulp gives rise to the odontoblastic cell layer
      b. Subjacent layer to the odontoblastic layer is called the cell-free zone or zone of Weil
      c. Next to the cell-free zone is a relatively cell-rich zone
      d. Core of the pulp is centrally located

B. Functions
   1. Nutritive functions—very rich blood supply that forms a capillary plexus that surrounds the odontoblasts
   2. Formative function—peripheral layer of pulp cells give rise to the odontoblasts
   3. Sensory function—naked nerve fibers travel as free nerve endings and make contact with odontoblasts

4. Protective function—pulp can respond to stimuli that occur outside of the tooth; response may trigger the formation of reactive dentin

C. Blood supply and nerves
   1. Blood vessels enter pulp via the apical foramen; one or more small arterioles form a rich capillary plexus under the odontoblastic layer; exchange of nutrients occurs across the capillary wall
   2. Two types of nerve fibers enter the pulp
      a. Autonomic nerve fibers—only the sympathetic autonomic nerve fibers are found; regulate the flow of blood in the vessels
      b. Afferent nerve fibers—come from the second and third branches of the trigeminal nerve; lose their myelin sheath and terminate as free nerve endings in close association with odontoblasts

D. Pulp changes
   1. Changes resulting from age
      a. As the tooth ages, there is an increase in the amount of collagen fibers and a decrease in the number of reticulin fibers; ground substance loses considerable water
      b. Pulp becomes less cellular and more fibrous
      c. Size of the pulp decreases because of the continued deposition of dentin
   2. Small calcified bodies called denticles may be present
      a. Three types of denticles
         (1) True denticles—form during tooth development in the root; have dentinal tubules present in their structure; odontoblasts are present on their periphery
         (2) False denticles—form when components of the pulp start to degenerate; calcify and grow into irregular calcified bodies; dentinal tubules are not usually present
         (3) Diffuse calcifications—occur in sick pulps in many locations; are likely to grow and cause problems
      b. Both true and false denticles may be loose in the dental pulp, attached to the dentin wall, or embedded in the dentin tissue
      c. Calcified structures in pulp appear radiopaque on radiographs

Comparison of Pulp and Dentin

A. Dentin and pulp are closely related functionally and developmentally; both are products of the dental papilla (derived from neural crest cells)

B. Two major differences between the tissues
1. Pulp is a loose, noncalcified connective tissue; dentin is a highly specialized calcified connective tissue
2. Pulp is a very vascular tissue; dentin is avascular
C. Dentin and pulp form the bulk of the fully developed tooth
D. During tooth development the peripheral cells of the dental papilla differentiate into odontoblasts, forming dentin, while the core of the dental papilla becomes the pulp

Enamel

A. Composition
1. Most highly calcified of the dental tissues
2. Composed mainly of inorganic calcium salt, hydroxyapatite, with a small amount of protein material and water in the matrix
   a. Inorganic component   95%
   b. Organic component   1%
   c. Water   4%
B. Process of amelogenesis
1. Enamel formation, like dentin formation, begins in the late bell stage of tooth development
2. Shortly after the deposition of dentin, the inner enamel epithelial cells of enamel organ become secretory ameloblasts
   a. Begin to deposit enamel matrix, which is mineralized almost immediately
   b. Have tall columnar cell bodies that are hexagonal in cross section
   c. Secretory process is shovel shaped and called Tomes' process; shape of the process is closely related to the form of the structural units that make up the fully developed enamel tissue
3. Ameloblasts pass through two main stages while depositing enamel
   a. Secretory stage—ameloblasts deposit enamel matrix, which contains both organic and inorganic components
   b. Resorbing stage—ameloblasts remove most of the water and organic components from the matrix
4. Enamel maturation begins before completion of enamel formation
   a. First, hydroxyapatite crystals deposited in matrix are very thin and needlelike
   b. During process of enamel maturation, crystals increase in all dimensions, which is made possible by continual removal of water and organic components from the matrix

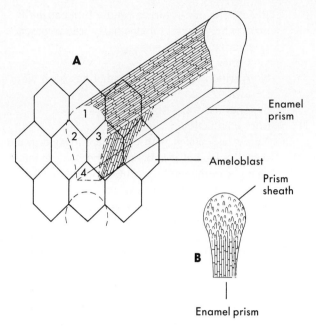

Fig. 2-22 Formation of enamel prism. **A,** Cross-sectional, hexagonal outline of ameloblast is superimposed over cross-sectional, keyhole outline of enamel prism; note that it takes four ameloblasts to form one enamel prism. **B,** Outline of prism with prism sheath surrounding prism head. (Modified from Salentijn-Moss, L., and Klyvert, M.: Dental and oral tissues: an introduction for paraprofessionals in dentistry, Philadelphia, 1980, Lea & Febiger.)

   c. Hydroxyapatite crystals in enamel are four times larger than those in bone, dentin, and cementum
C. Enamel prisms—structural units of enamel
1. Enamel is composed of tightly packed masses of hydroxyapatite crystals called enamel prisms
2. Prism formation is related to the shape of Tomes' process and orientation of crystals as they are deposited by ameloblasts
3. Are rod-shaped structures that run from the dentoenamel junction to the outer edge of the enamel surface
4. Are stacked in rows, one row on top of the other, in an interlocking fashion; stacking arrangement causes prisms to appear keyhole shaped when viewed in cross section, with the top of the keyhole facing the occlusal or incisal edge of the tooth and the tail facing the cervical portion; four ameloblasts contribute to form one keyhole (Fig. 2-22)
5. Average width of an enamel prism is approximately 4 μm; prisms are narrower near the dentoenamel junction and wider near the outer surface of the enamel

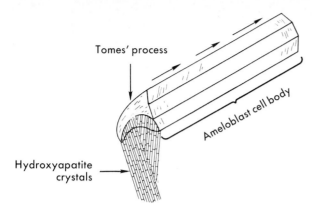

Tomes' process

Ameloblast cell body

Hydroxyapatite
crystals

Fig. 2-23 Ameloblast depositing hydroxyapatite crystals from Tomes' process; note angular change in orientation of crystals being deposited, which accounts for prism sheath around head of prism.

6. Crystals in the prism head region are oriented with their long axis parallel to the long axis of the prism; in the tail region crystals are perpendicular to the long axis of the prism
7. Adjacent prisms are separated from each other by a prism sheath approximately 0.1 to 2.0 μm wide; can be observed in the head region of the prism but are not so clearly defined in the tail region; are produced by an abrupt change in angulation (orientation) of the crystals as they are deposited by the moving ameloblast (Fig. 2-23)
8. Prismless enamel may be found near the dentoenamel junction and outer surface of enamel
9. Are perpendicular to the outer surface of enamel; near the cervix of the tooth they tend to be oriented apically; toward the inner third of the enamel, groups of prisms curve but then straighten out to form right angles with the enamel surface
D. Clinical importance
   1. Dental procedures performed on enamel
      a. Application of fluoride—because enamel is semipermeable, fluoride ions are absorbed on the hydroxyapatite crystals; tooth becomes more resistant to bacteria-produced acids
      b. Acid etching of enamel—structure of enamel (prisms and prism sheaths) allows acid to penetrate enamel for a limited distance (30 μm), attacking the mineral at the periphery of the sheaths; leaves a rough enamel surface so bonding materials adhere more readily; acid may attack the prism core, producing same effect

c. Cavity preparations—all prisms are supported by dentin; margins of cavity will fail if enamel is left unsupported
   2. Tetracycline stains
      a. Appear clinically as dark bands through the enamel, especially near the cervix of the tooth where enamel is thin
      b. Caused by the administration of tetracycline (antibiotic) while teeth were forming
      c. Tetracycline binds chemically to organic and inorganic components of bone and dentin
      d. Resulting darkened area shows through enamel with fully developed tooth becoming esthetically unattractive
      e. Are difficult to bleach out; affected teeth may need crowns for esthetic purposes only
   3. Pits and fissures in enamel
      a. Are often less-calcified areas
      b. Form where ameloblasts become crowded between adjacent areas (cusps), causing incomplete maturation of enamel

Cementum

A. General properties and functions
   1. Calcified connective tissue that covers the roots of the teeth; in conjunction with the alveolar bone proper and the periodontal ligament forms the attachment apparatus of the teeth, allowing the teeth to become suspended in the jaw
   2. Derived from the dental sac (dental follicle)
   3. Resembles bone in structure and composition; major differences are
      a. Bone is a vascularized tissue
      b. Cementum is avascular
   4. Least mineralized of the calcified tissues of the tooth
B. Mature cementum composition
   1. Chemical composition
      a. Organic components   23%
      b. Inorganic components   65%
      c. Water   12%
   2. Tissue composition
      a. Cells—cementoblasts, cementocytes
      b. Fibrous matrix—collagen fibers (type I); dominant component of the tissue, 90%
      c. Ground substance—proteoglycans
C. Process of cementogenesis (Fig. 2-24)
   1. After crown formation is complete, the epithelial root sheath (Hertwig's root sheath) begins to grow down
      a. Shapes the root of the tooth
      b. Induces formation of root dentin

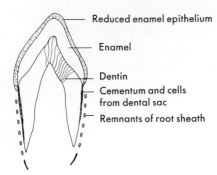

Fig. 2-24 Relationship of epithelial root sheath to the forming root and formation of cementum.

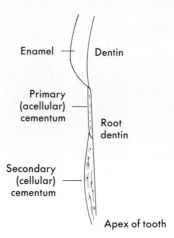

Fig. 2-25 Relationship of primary (acellular) cementum to secondary (cellular) cementum or root of tooth; note thickness of cellular cementum near tooth apex.

2. After the first root dentin is deposited, the root sheath breaks down; cells from the dental sac migrate onto newly deposited dentin; differentiate into cementoblasts

D. Mature cementum (fibrous matrix)
   1. Very little cementum is deposited on the developing root until the tooth reaches functional occlusion (only about two thirds of the root has been formed when the tooth erupts)
   2. Two groups of fibers found in cementum
      a. Group I
         (1) Collagen fibers produced by the cementoblasts
         (2) Form in the fibrous component of cementum
         (3) Run parallel to the long axis of the root (internal fibers)
      b. Group II
         (1) Fibers produced by cells from the dental sac
         (2) Form fibers of the periodontal ligament (external fibers)
         (3) Insert into cementum at right angles to the dentoenamel junction or at right angles to the internal fibers of cementum
   3. Group II fibers (external fibers) are coarser than internal fibers; cores of fibers remain uncalcified in the calcified cementum; referred to as Sharpey's fibers

E. Cellular and acellular cementum (Fig. 2-25)
   1. Acellular cementum
      a. Cervical half of the tooth is covered with a thin layer of cementum, approximately 10 μm thick
      b. Does not contain any embedded cementocytes (cementoblasts) in the lacunae
      c. Forms at a slower rate than cellular cementum
      d. Does not increase during the life of the tooth

      e. Appears to be involved more in maintenance of the tissue than in production
      f. Contains less inorganic matrix than cellular cementum
      g. Better calcified than cellular cementum
   2. Cellular cementum
      a. Apical portion of the tooth is covered with cellular cementum, reaching a thickness of 100 to 150 μm
      b. Contains cementocytes trapped in the lacunae of the tissue
      c. Deposited throughout the life of the tooth
      d. Deposited at intervals (pauses), producing arrest lines—highly calcified lines similar to those seen in bone tissue

F. Abnormalities
   1. Reversal lines
      a. May be present in cementum as in bone tissue
      b. Reflect resorption of the tissue (remodeling)
      c. Resorption of cementum does not occur as frequently as in bone tissue; when it does occur, is usually associated with
         (1) Extreme orthodontic movement of the teeth
         (2) Trauma to the teeth
   2. Cementicles
      a. Small abnormal calcified bodies occasionally found in the periodontal ligament
      b. Result of cellular debris (i.e., degenerating remnants of the epithelial root sheath)
      c. May be found
         (1) Attached to the cementum surface
         (2) Free in the periodontal ligament
         (3) Embedded in the cementum of the root

3. Hypercementosis
   a. Local abnormal thickening of parts of the cementum
   b. Usually found in the apical region, occurring on one or all of the teeth
   c. May be seen in cases of
      (1) Chronic inflammation of the tooth
      (2) Loss of an antagonist tooth (no opposing tooth in the jaw)
      (3) Additional eruption occurs; compensatory cementosis takes place
      (b) Tooth may become fused to surrounding alveolar bone proper

Cementoenamel Junction

A. Three types of cementoenamel relationships can occur during the development of the tooth
   1. Cementum *meets* the enamel edge to edge—occurs in approximately 30% of all teeth
   2. Cementum *overlaps* a small part of the enamel—occurs in approximately 60% of all teeth
   3. Cementum and enamel *do not meet,* exposing dentin—occurs in approximately 10% of all teeth
B. Cementoenamel relationships occur when root-cementum development begins; related to the timing of the disruption (breakdown) of the epithelial root sheath; allow cells from the dental sac to differentiate and begin depositing cementum
C. Differentiation of root dental papilla into odontoblasts is mediated by a cell-to-matrix type of inductive interaction (between the basal lamina of Hertwig's root sheath and undifferentiated root dental papilla)
D. Differentiation of dental sac cells into cementoblasts is mediated by a cell-substrate type of inductive interaction between sac cells and newly deposited dentin
E. Practicing dental hygienists should use caution during instrumentation in areas where cementum is thin or absent
F. Recession of gingiva may also leave exposed cementum or dentin, creating root sensitivity or root caries

SUPPORTING TISSUES ▄▄▄▄▄▄
Alveolar Bone

A. That part of the bony maxilla and mandible, the alveolar process, in which teeth are suspended in alveoli (bony sockets)
B. Existence or presence of alveolar bone is totally dependent on the presence of dental roots; when teeth do not develop and erupt, alveolar bone will

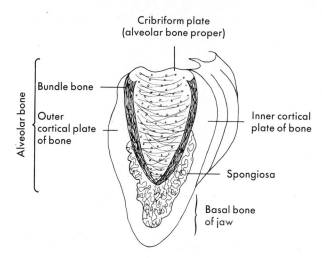

Fig. 2-26 Components of alveolar bone proper. (Modified from Schroeder, H.E.: Orale Strukturbiologie: Entwicklungsgeschichte, Struktur und Funktion Normaler Hart-und Weichgewebeder Mundhohle, Stuttgart, 1976, Georg Thieme Verlag.)

not develop; when teeth are extracted, alveolar bone resorbs
C. Formed during development and eruption of teeth; developing teeth, primary or permanent, are located in bony crypts in bone of the maxilla or mandible
D. Has the same biophysical and chemical properties as other bone tissue in the body; has the same basic components as other connective tissues
   1. Cells—osteoblasts, osteocytes, osteoclasts
   2. Fibrous matrix—collagen fibers dominant component; calcified by deposition of calcium salt, hydroxyapatite, into the matrix
   3. Ground substance—proteoglycans
E. Gross anatomy of a mature bone socket
   1. Each tooth is suspended in its own alveolus (socket), with each alveolus having the same structure and anatomy (Fig. 2-26)
      a. Outer cortical (compact lamellar) plate bone—faces the cheek and lips—buccal
      b. Inner cortical (compact lamellar) plate of bone—faces the tongue and palate—lingual
      c. Spongiosa—cancellous bone sandwiched between cortical plates of bone
   2. Alveolar bone proper—that part of the alveolus directly facing the root of the tooth; follows the general outline of the root; sometimes referred to as the cribriform plate or lamina dura
      a. Cribriform plate
         (1) Contains small numerous openings, allows blood vessels and nerves in the periodontal ligament and bone to communicate

(2) Consists of two layers of bone
(a) Compact lamellar bone
(b) Layer of bundle bone into which the periodontal fibers insert; cores of the fibers remain uncalcified in the calcified tissues of bone or cementum—called Sharpey's fibers
b. *Lamina dura* is purely a radiographic term based on the fact that this area appears more radiopaque on radiographs; is not more calcified than the rest of the bone socket; rather, opaqueness is caused by geometry in the area
c. Alveolar bone proper that forms sockets around multirooted teeth consists of the cribriform plates of both roots and some spongy bone, called interradicular alveolar bone
d. Alveolar bone proper between teeth consists of the cribriform plates of both teeth and some spongy bone, called interdental alveolar bone
e. Spongiosa is composed of small trabeculae of bone with large marrow spaces between the trabeculae
3. Alveolar bone proper/cribriform plate is the only essential part of the bone socket; spongiosa and outer and inner cortical plates of bone are not always present; spongiosa may be absent, and outer and inner cortical cortical plates may be fused together
4. Trabeculae of the spongiosa reflect functional forces or loading patterns imposed on teeth; pattern will change when forces are altered; two principal directions of the trabeculae are parallel and perpendicular to the direction of the imposed forces; trabecular bone orientation can be observed on radiographs
5. Orthodontic movement of teeth always causes remodeling of the alveolar bone proper to accommodate movement of the teeth; affects the insertion of periodontal ligament fibers in the bundle bone, but is a localized type of resorption; when the bundle bone is redeposited, fibers become firmly attached again
6. Radiographs of teeth may be used to show the height and/or slope of the interdental bone septum, which may reflect periodontal or other disease

Periodontal Ligament

A. Specialized form of connective tissue, derived from the dental sac that contributes to attachment of the tooth
B. Made up of groups of fiber bundles called gingival fibers and principal fiber bundles; between the principal fiber bundles are areas of loose connective tissue, blood vessels, and nerves; areas of loose connective tissue are called interstitial spaces
C. Tissue components
1. Fibroblasts of the periodontal ligament (PDL) are responsible for production of fibrous matrix and ground substance; are continually engaged in synthetic activities, rebuilding and producing new fibers to be incorporated into existing fibers, which are constantly being remodeled; PDL has a very fast turnover rate
2. Ground substance—proteoglycans
3. Fibrous matrix is dominant component of the PDL
a. Fibers are collagen and oxytalan with a few elastic fibers associated with blood vessels
b. Fibers are arranged in dense bundles inserted into the alveolar bone proper and the cementum
c. Fibers are arranged into two groups
(1) Gingival fiber bundles (Figs. 2-27 and 2-28; see also Chapter 11, Fig. 11-2)
(a) Dentogingival fibers—extend from the cervical cementum to the free gingiva and from the cervical cementum to the lamina propria of the gingiva, over the alveolar crest
(b) Dentoperiosteal fibers—extend from the cervical cementum over the alveolar crest to the periosteum of the cortical plates of bone
(c) Transseptal fibers—extend from the cementum of the tooth to the adjacent tooth, over the alveolar crest
(d) Circumferential fibers—extend horizontally around the most cervical part of the root, inserting into the cementum and lamina propria of the gingiva and the alveolar crest
(2) Principal fiber bundles (Fig. 2-27; see also Chapter 11, Fig. 11-3)
(a) Alveolar crest fibers—extend from the cervical cementum and insert into the alveolar crest

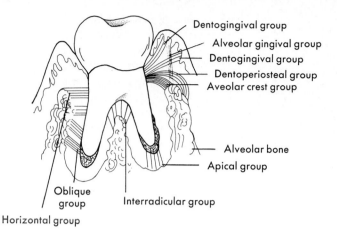

Dentogingival group
Alveolar gingival group
Dentogingival group
Dentoperiosteal group
Aveolar crest group

Alveolar bone
Apical group

Oblique group
Interradicular group

Horizontal group

Fig. 2-27 Connective tissue fibers of gingiva and principal fiber bundles of periodontal ligament (transeptal and circular fibers shown in Fig. 2-28; see also Figs. 11-2 and 11-3).

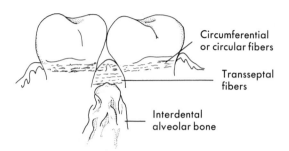

Circumferential or circular fibers

Transseptal fibers

Interdental alveolar bone

Fig. 2-28 Transseptal fibers are shown between two teeth passing over alveolar crest; circumferential fibers are around teeth within free gingiva.

    (b) Horizontal fibers—extend at right angles to the long axis of the root of the tooth in a horizontal plane from the alveolar bone to the cementum; found in the cervical third of the root
    (c) Oblique fibers—slant occlusally from the cementum to the alveolar bone; most abundant of the fiber bundles; start at the apical two thirds of the root
    (d) Apical fibers—radiate from the apical cementum into the alveolar bone
    (e) Interradicular fibers (seen only in multirooted teeth)—extend from the cementum in the furcation area of the tooth to the interradicular alveolar bone
  d. Fiber bundles are oriented to give the tooth optimal resistance to all kinds of functional loading patterns
    (1) Circumferential fibers resist rotational movements of the tooth
    (2) Alveolar crest and apical fibers resist pull of the tooth from its socket
    (3) Transseptal fibers connect all teeth and maintain integrity of the dental arches
  e. Elastic fibers in the PDL do not contribute to support of the tooth; role of the oxytalan fibers is not clear

D. Blood vessels
  1. Blood supply of the PDL is very rich and highly developed, more than in any other connective tissues; vessels are found in the interstitial spaces of the ligament
  2. Each tooth, with its PDL and alveolar bone, has a common blood supply; a small artery will branch off of the main artery that supplies the jaw and enter
    a. Apical foramen of the tooth—supplies pulp of the tooth
    b. Periodontal ligament—supplies areas all around the tooth
    c. Alveolar bone of the tooth
  3. Once blood vessels enter pulp chambers, they are isolated from surrounding tissues, but vessels supplying the PDL and alveolar bone are richly interconnected via openings in the cribriform plate
E. Nerves
  1. PDL contains two types of nerves
    a. Autonomic—sympathetic fibers that travel with blood vessels; regulate flow of blood to the tissues
    b. Afferent sensory fibers—mostly myelinated nerves from branches of the second and third divisions of the trigeminal nerve (cranial nerve V)
  2. Two types of nerve endings are found in the PDL
    a. Free, unmyelinated nerve endings—responsible for pain sensation
    b. Encapsulated nerve endings—responsible for registering pressure changes
F. Width of the PDL varies with functional forces placed on the tooth and at different levels of the root (apex and cervix)
  1. Width is greater in young adults (0.21 mm) than in older adults (0.15 mm)

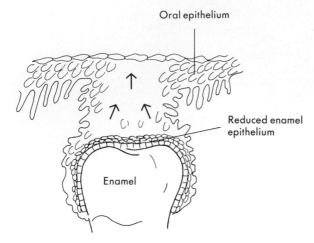

Fig. 2-29 Tooth emerging into oral cavity; note reduced enamel epithelium covering tooth and joining of oral epithelium and reduced enamel epithelium, which will form initial junctional epithelium.

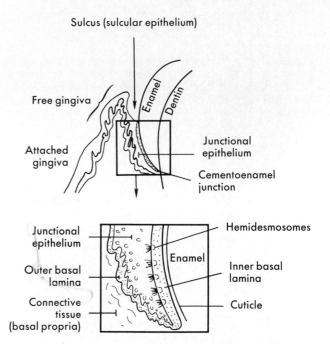

Fig. 2-30 Junctional epithelium and its relationship to clinical and histologic structures; note enlarged section of junctional epithelium showing outer and inner basal lamina that is continuous around junctional epithelium and cuticle that is seen intervening between junctional epithelium and tooth surface.

2. Width is greater near cervical and apical areas than in the middle of the root
3. Minimal movements (rotations) of any tooth occur around the axis in the middle of the root; greatest movements occur near the apex and cervix, accounting for difference in width of the PDL along the root
4. Width is related to the amount of function; actively functioning tooth will have a slightly wider PDL than a nonfunctioning tooth

G. Abnormalities
   1. Cementicles
   2. Epithelial rests (cell rests of Malassez)
      a. Remnants of epithelium from the root sheath that did not disintegrate; formed a cluster of epithelial cells surrounded by a basement membrane
      b. In most cases are harmless, but they have the potential to become cystic
   3. Untreated periodontal disease can result in damage to the supporting apparatus of the tooth, causing eventual loss of the tooth

Dentogingival Junction

A. Area on the tooth where enamel and epithelium form a junction; with age, the junction is displaced more apically between cementum and epithelium
B. First established as the tooth emerges into the oral cavity (Fig. 2-29)
   1. Developing tooth is covered with the reduced enamel epithelium (REE), consisting of
      a. Layer of outer enamel epithelial cells

   b. Remnants of the stratum intermedium cell layers
   c. Stellate reticulum
   d. Postsecretory ameloblasts
   2. Basal cells of oral epithelium covering the emerging tooth and outer layer of cells of the REE begin to proliferate; soon grow together and form one continuous unit; as tooth emerges through the combined epithelia, it forms the initial dentogingival junction on the enamel of the tooth
C. Dentojunctional epithelium
   1. Gingival epithelium that faces the tooth
   2. Composed of nonkeratinized stratified squamous epithelium and divided into
      a. Sulcular epithelium
         (1) Found occlusally at the same height as the free gingiva
         (2) Sulcus forms a shallow pocket around the tooth, about 0.5 mm deep
      b. Junctional epithelium
         (1) Begins at the base of the sulcus
         (2) Is firmly attached to the tooth, enamel, and/or cementum by hemidesmosomes

(3) Located between two basal laminae
    (a) One basal lamina faces the enamel surface
    (b) Second basal lamina faces the connective tissue of the gingiva
    (c) Basal laminae are continuous at the base of the junctional epithelium (Fig. 2-30)
3. A membrane intervenes between the basal lamina of the junctional epithelium and tooth surface, called the primary cuticle
    a. Formed during the late stages of eruption of the tooth
    b. Composition of the cuticle is not known but thickens with age
4. Newly erupted tooth is covered with a thin, delicate membrane called Nasmyth's membrane
    a. Will float off of the tooth surface if placed in a 10% solution of hydrochloric acid
    b. Contains some of cells of the REE and the dental cuticle
5. In the area of the dentogingival junction the junctional epithelium has the capacity to repair itself
6. Site of the dentogingival junction is easily invaded by microorganisms and is where periodontal disease often begins

SUGGESTED READINGS

Guyton, A.C.: A textbook of medical physiology, ed. 6, Philadelphia, 1981, W.B. Saunders Co.

Kelly, D.E., Wood, B.L., and Enders, A.C.: Bailey's textbook of microscopic anatomy, ed. 18, Baltimore, 1984, Williams & Wilkins.

Menaker, L.: The biological basis of dental caries: an oral biology textbook, New York, 1980, Harper & Row, Publishers, Inc.

Osborne, J.W., and Ten Cate, A.R.: Advanced dental histology; dental practitioner's handbook No. 6, ed. 4, London, 1983, Wright PSG

Salentijn-Moss, L., and Klyvert, M.: Dental and oral tissues: an introduction for paraprofessionals in dentistry, Philadelphia, 1980, Lea & Febiger.

Shroeder, H.E.: Orale Strukturbiologie: Entwicklungsgeschichte, Struktur und Funktion Normaler Hart-und Weichgewebeder Mundhohle, Stuttgart, 1976, George Thieme Verlag.

Sperber, G.H.: Craniofacial embryology: dental practitioner's handbook No. 16, ed. 3, Bristol, 1981, John Wright & Sons, Ltd.

Ten Cate, A.R.: Oral histology: development, structure, and funtion, St. Louis, 1980, The C.V. Mosby Co.

Weiss, L.: Histology: cell and tissue biology, ed. 5, New York, 1983, Elsevier Biomedical.

Review Questions

1 Proteins are manufactured in the cell
1. Chromosomes
2. Desmosomes
3. Ribosomes and polyribosomes
4. Lysosomes
5. Mitochondria

2 The cells of the outer layer of keratinized stratified squamous epithelium
1. Constantly go through mitosis
2. Contain fluid-filled vacuoles
3. Contain large amounts of glycogen
4. Contain large amounts of keratin
5. Contain large amounts of melanin

3 While performing a dental oral examination on a Hispanic patient, a dental hygienist notices dark brown spots on the gingival mucosa. These areas of discoloration of the gingiva could be attributed to
1. Melanocytes being present in the tissue
2. Langerhans' cells being present in the tissue
3. Lymphocytes being present in the tissue
4. Keratohyaline granules being present in the tissue
5. Merkel's cells being present in the tissue

4 What kind of tissue makes up the bulk of the lamina propria of the oral mucosa?
1. Connective tissue
2. Muscle tissue
3. Epithelium
4. Nerve tissue
5. Bone tissue

5 To examine the oral mucosa, the mucosa is rolled and compressed between the fingers. This is possible because
1. It is nonkeratinized lining mucosa
2. It is keratinized masticatory mucosa
3. It is oral epithelium that is thicker than anywhere else in the oral cavity
4. Of the deep rete pegs and the deep connective tissue papilla between the epithelium and the lamina propria
5. Of the basal lamina at the interface between the lamina propria and the epithelium

6 Muscle tissue is a highly specialized tissue having the ability to contract because the muscle cells
1. Contain large amounts of sarcoplasm
2. Contain the two proteins actin and myosin filaments
3. Are in close relationship to presynaptic and postsynaptic junctions
4. Contain large numbers of lysosomes in their sarcoplasm
5. Can respond to stimuli via the nervous system

7 During an oral clinical examination, an inspection is made of the lateral borders of the tongue near the base; what structures would one expect to see?
1. Lymph nodes
2. Filiform papillae
3. Rete pegs
4. Taste buds
5. Foliate papillae

8 Connective tissue proper is highly resistant to compressive forces, loading in all directions because of the
1. Orientation of the fibers in the ground substance
2. Proteoglycans in the ground substance
3. Large number of fibroblasts in the tissue
4. Large number of histiocytes in the tissue
5. Arrangement of the oxytalan fibers in the tissue

9 It is important to understand the course of direction of the enamel prisms from the dentinoenamel junction to the outer surface of the enamel because
1. It will help in understanding how the walls of a cavity preparation should be finished off
2. It will help in knowing where to apply topical fluoride to the tooth surface
3. It will provide a better understanding of the caries process
4. It will provide a better understanding of the formation of enamel prisms
5. It will influence the treatment plan when it includes acid etching the enamel surface

10 What process occurs during enamel formation that allows for increased growth in the hydroxyapatite crystals?
1. The crystals reorient themselves at the end of enamel formation, allowing more space for additional growth
2. The enamel-producing cells at the end of enamel formation begin to produce a substance that causes the crystals to increase in size
3. The crystals start to grow because of an inductive interaction between the crystals and the oral mucosa
4. The ameloblast alternates between being a secretory and a resorbing cell while depositing the enamel matrix
5. The crystals do not increase in size after they are initially deposited

11 The peritubular dentin that is found surrounding the odontoblastic process
1. Is more calcified than the intertubular dentin
2. Is less calcified than the intertubular dentin
3. Has no difference in the calcification of the peritubular and the intertubular dentin
4. Is not true dentin
5. Has different type of proteoglycan in its ground substance

12 The main difference between secondary and reactive dentin is
1. Secondary dentin forms only in response to dental trauma such as an insult to the tissue by carries; by

abrasion of the enamel, exposing the dentinal tubules; or by mechanical or thermal overstimulation of the tubules
2. Secondary dentin is all the dentin that is formed after the completion of the apical foramen
3. Secondary dentin will reflect a change in the orientation of the S-shaped pathways of the tubules when seen histologically
4. Secondary dentin has far fewer tubules than reactive dentin
5. Secondary dentin resembles bone in its morphology when seen histologically

13 The first dentin to be deposited by the odontoblasts is mantle dentin, which is different from the rest of the dentin in the tooth because
1. It is not true dentin
2. It does not contain collagen fibers
3. It contains a second group of collagen fibers
4. It does not become fully calcified like the rest of the dentin in the tooth
5. It is deposited only at the start of dentin formation

14 The dentinal tubules follow an S-shaped pathway as they move away from the dentinoenamel junction because of an
1. Adjustment caused by crowding
2. Increase in the number of dentinal tubules
3. Increase in the amount of branching of the tubules
4. Adjustment in the amount of dentin matrix being deposited
5. Increase in the surface area that they are moving to

15 True denticles found in the dental pulp differ from false denticles in that true denticles
1. Contain dentinal tubules
2. Are not calcified like false denticles
3. Are found only attached to the wall of the dentin
4. Are lamellated structures
5. Are more highly calcified than false denticles

16 The following events occur during the formation of cementum on the root of the tooth
1. The reduced enamel epithelium begins to disintegrate after tooth formation
2. The cells of the enamel organ, the stratum intermedium, and the stellate reticulum remain after the completion of the crown
3. The outer enamel epithelial cells remain and induce the formation of cementoblasts
4. The inner enamel epithelial cells remain and induce the formation of cementoblasts
5. The formation of Hertwig's root sheath, followed by its disintegration as the root forms

17 In the mature erupted tooth the dentogingival junction is composed of
1. Junctional epithelium
2. Junctional epithelium, basal lamina with hemidesmosomes, and a primary cuticle

3. Functional epithelium with a cuticle
4. A cuticle with hemidesmosomes
5. Junctional epithelium with desmosomes

18 The blood supply of the periodontal ligament and the alveolar bone proper anastomose and communicate because of the
1. Compact structure of the alveolar bone proper
2. Structure of the cribriform plate of the alveolar bone proper
3. Lamina dura of the alveolar bone proper
4. Bundle bone of the alveolar bone proper
5. Arrangement of Sharpey's fibers in the alveolar bone proper

19 Which of the periodontal fiber groups help to maintain the integrity of the dental arch?
1. Oblique fiber group
2. Apical fiber group
3. Circumferential fiber group
4. Transseptal fiber group
5. Interradicular fiber group

20 The canaliculi or the cell processes of the cementocytes are usually oriented toward the periodontal ligament because
1. The cell processes are forced in this direction when the cementocytes become enclosed in their lacunae
2. The cell processes of the cementocytes project off of the cell only in the direction of the periodontal ligament
3. It is easier for the cementocytes to deposit more cementum
4. They must face a blood supply
5. They can provide nourishment for the periodontal ligament

21 Bone is able to act as a reservoir for calcium and phosphorous ions when the two ions drop below a critical level in the blood. This is because
1. Bone is always supersaturated with these two ions at all times
2. These two ions are major components of bone tissue, and when they are needed for body use, the bone can supply them
3. The osteoblasts, bone-forming cells, can store the two ions and release them when necessary
4. These two ions are always located in the osteocytic lacunae of bone tissue, waiting to be used
5. The arrangement of the collagen fibers in the tissue permits the two ions to be available when needed

22 Histologically, how can one tell that bone has been remodeled?
1. Because of the many arrest lines seen in the tissue
2. Because of the small size of the lamella
3. Because of the change in the orientation of the fibers in each adjacent lamella
4. Because of the reversal lines seen in the tissue
5. Because the periosteum covering the bone tissue looks thinner than in some of the other areas of bone

23 An orthodontist is waiting for an 18-year-old patient to complete most of his growth before scheduling a mandibular resection. Which of the following diagnostic aids could assist the orthodontist in determining if the patient had attained most of his growth?
1. Study models
2. Full-mouth radiographs
3. A radiograph of the hand or leg
4. A clinical examination
5. An occlusal film

24 When bone begins to resorb in localized areas, it could be a result of
1. Osteocytes in their lacunae depositing too much calcium
2. The need for more calcium and phosphorus in the blood
3. The need to resorb and remodel bone in a particular area because the osteocytes are too far from their source of nourishment
4. The need of the cells of the periosteum to be closer to their blood supply
5. Too much calcium and phosphorus in the bone tissue

25 An infant born without a primary palate is presented for consultation. What teeth will never be present, even after a surgical repair of the existing condition?
1. Both the deciduous and the permanent incisors in the maxilla
2. Both the first deciduous and the permanent premolars in the maxilla
3. Both 6-year molars in the maxilla
4. Both the deciduous and the permanent canines in the maxilla
5. Only the deciduous incisors in the maxilla

26 In a person born without teeth, what part of the bone of the maxilla and the mandible would be absent?
1. The cribriform plate of the alveolar bone proper
2. The alveolar bone
3. The basal bone of the maxilla and the mandible
4. The bundle bone of the alveolar bone proper
5. The interradicular bone of the alveolar process

27 A mother brings her newborn infant into a pediatric clinic for a physical examination. It is noted that the infant has a midline cleft of the hard palate. What structures did not fuse during the embryonic stage of facial development?
1. The two medial nasal processes
2. The medial and lateral nasal processes
3. The two palatal shelves
4. The maxillary and lateral nasal processes
5. The primary and secondary palates

28 An occlusal film shows a radiolucent area in the midline of the hard palate. This radiolucent area could be
1. The nasal fossa
2. The maxillary sinus
3. A midline palatal cyst
4. The greater palatine foramen
5. A mucoperiosteal cyst

Answers and Rationales

1. (3) Proteins are manufactured on the ribosomes of the rough endoplasmic reticulum and on the polyribosomes that are floating free in the cytoplasm of the cell. It is where messenger and transfer RNA meet.
   (1) The genetic information of the cell is contained in the chromosomes.
   (2) The desmosomes are attachment plaques that are seen between cells.
   (4) The lysosomes are the organelles that contain digestive enzymes for the cells.
   (5) The mitochondria are the organelles that provide the main source of energy for the cell.
2. (4) The outer cells of keratinized epithelium contain large amounts of keratin, the protein substance that is responsible for the cornification of the cells.
   (1) Keratinized cells are dead cells and do not contain viable nuclei or other organelles.
   (2) There is no fluid contained in the keratinized layer, only keratin plus other broken-down, dying organelles.
   (3) There is no glycogen contained in the keratinized layer.
   (5) Melanin is produced by melanocytes and is the substance responsible for pigmentation, not keratinization.
3. (1) Melanocytes, the cells that produce melanin, are responsible for the pigmentation of a tissue. It is not unusual to find dark brown areas of the gingiva in dark-complexioned people.
   (2) Langerhans' cells are dendritic cells found in the oral epithelium, but they are not associated with pigmentation.
   (3) Lymphocytes are cells associated with inflammation, not pigmentation.
   (4) Keratohyaline granules are the precursors of keratin.
   (5) Merkel's cells, found in the oral mucosa, have been associated with touch sensation.
4. (1) The lamina propria of the oral mucosa is composed of connective tissue, which is a support tissue for the overlying epithelium and which also acts as padding.
   (2) Muscle tissue is a highly specialized tissue having the power of contraction; it is not a support tissue.
   (3) Epithelium is not a form of connective tissue.
   (4) Nerve tissue is a highly specialized tissue whose main function is communication; it is not a support tissue.
   (5) Bone is a calcified skeletal tissue that provides support for organ systems.
5. (1) The oral mucosa is a lining mucosa, with a submucosa present that ties the tissue to muscle, allowing the tissue a great deal of flexibility.
   (2) Keratinized masticatory mucosa does not usually have a submucosa, except on the hard palate, where it is tied to underlying bone tissue with no flexibility.
   (3) The thickness of the epithelium is not related to the flexibility of the mucosa.
   (4) The length of the rete pegs and the connective tissue papilla is not a function of flexibility.
   (5) The basal lamina is a component of the basement membrane and is unrelated to the flexibility of the tissue.
6. (2) The muscle cells contain the proteins actin and myosin, which are the contractile elements of muscle cells.
   (1) The amount of sarcoplasm in the muscle cells is completely unrelated to the ability of the cells to contract.
   (3) The terms *presynaptic junction* and *postsynaptic junction* are part of the neural junction nomenclature but are *not* structures that make coordination possible.
   (4) Lysosomes are organelles found in the sarcoplasm of cells; they contain digestive enzymes and act as macrophages.
   (5) Ability to respond to stimuli is not related to the cell's ability to contract.
7. (5) Foliate papillae are the only lingual papillae located on the lateral borders of the tongue.
   (1) Lymph nodes are found in the underlying connective tissue and cannot be seen clinically.
   (2) Filiform papillae are located on the dorsal aspect of the tongue.
   (3) Pete pegs are epithelial projections seen at the interface between the epithelium and the connective tissue of the oral mucosa.
   (4) Taste buds are located on the lateral sides of the foliate, vallate, and filiform papillae, but they can be seen only with the aid of a microscope.
8. (2) Connective tissue is highly resistant to compressive loading because of the molecular structure and composition of the proteoglycans in the ground substance.
   (1) The orientation of the fibers in the tissue is not the main reason for the tissue to resist compressive loading.
   (3) The fibroblasts in the tissue are the major cells of connective tissue but do not play any role in making the tissue resistant to compression.
   (4) When histiocytes are present in connective tissue, they are associated near blood vessels and act like marcophages.
   (5) Oxytalan fibers are very special fibers that have never been associated with connective tissue proper but have been identified in the periodontal ligament.

For each question the correct answer and rationale are listed first. The other choices are presented in order with the reasons why they are not correct.

9. (1) Knowing the course of the enamel prisms will help in finishing off the walls of a cavity preparation to prevent leaving unsupported rods (prisms), which would lead to leaky cavity margins and fractured restorations.
   (2) The application of topical fluorides has no bearing on the orientation of the enamel rods.
   (3) The course of the prisms is totally unrelated to understanding the caries process.
   (4) Formation of the prism sheath is not related to the course of the prisms but is related to the orientation of the hydroxyapatite crystals as they are deposited by the ameloblast.
   (5) Knowing how to acid etch a tooth relates to understanding the composition of the sheath and the prism core, not to the direction of the enamel prisms.

10. (4) The ameloblast, acting as a secretory and a resorbing cell while depositing its matrix, allows the cell to constantly remove all excess organic matrix and water, thus providing room for crystal growth.
    (1) No reorientation of the crystals occurs in the enamel prisms after they are initially deposited.
    (2) At the end of enamel formation, the enamel-producing cells are more involved in resorbing than in secretory actions.
    (3) The crystals are covered in the tissue by the reduced enamel epithelium following the completion of enamel formation; therefore they could not interact with the oral epithelium.
    (5) The crystals do increase in size during maturation.

11. (1) The peritubular dentin is more calcified than the intertubular dentin because it contains less organic matrix than the intertubular dentin.
    (2) The intertubular dentin contains more organic matrix than the peritubular dentin; therefore it is less calcified.
    (3) There is a definite difference in the degree of calcification between the peritubular and the intertubular dentin based on the differences in amounts of organic and inorganic matrix.
    (4) Peritubular dentin *is* a true type of dentin having the same organic and inorganic components as the intertubular dentin.
    (5) Both types of dentin have the same type of proteoglycans present in their ground substance.

12. (2) Secondary dentin is called secondary dentin because it forms only after the completion of the apical foramen and throughout the life of vital teeth.
    (1) Secondary dentin does not form in response to trauma the way reactive dentin does.
    (3) Secondary dentin does reflect a change in the orientation of the S-shaped pathway of the tubules, but this change is not as extreme as that seen in reactive dentin.

    (4) Secondary dentin does have fewer tubules than primary dentin, but the difference is not as extreme as that seen in reactive dentin.
    (5) Secondary dentin does not resemble bone histologically.

13. (3) Mantle dentin contains a second group of collagen fibers called von Korff's fibers, which are deposited at right angles to the dentinoenamel junction.
    (1) Mantle dentin is a true dentin, since it contains the same components as the rest of the dentin, but it has the addition of von Korff's fibers.
    (2) Mantle dentin does contain collagen fibers.
    (4) Mantle dentin calcifies the same as the rest of the dentin in the tooth.
    (5) The difference between mantle dentin and the rest of the dentin is related to the presence of von Korff's fibers, *not* that it is deposited only at the start of dentin formation.

14. (1) The S-shaped pathway that the dentinal tubules follow as they move away from the dentinoenamel junction is related to crowding of the odontoblasts as they move from a larger surface to a smaller surface.
    (2) The number of tubules does not increase as the odontoblasts move away from the dentinoenamel junction.
    (3) The tubules do branch more in the root dentin, but this has no bearing on the S-shaped pathway that they follow.
    (4) The amount of dentin matrix does not affect the movement of the odontoblasts.
    (5) If the odontoblasts were moving to a larger area, they would follow a straight pathway, since there would be no crowding.

15. (1) True denticles contain dentinal tubules because their formation is related more to an inductive interaction between epithelial remnants from the root sheath, becoming odontoblasts, which form the denticles. False denticles form on a nidus of dead cells, and calcification begins.
    (2) Both types of denticles are calcified bodies.
    (3) Both true and false denticles can become attached to the dentin wall.
    (4) False denticles are the lamellated type.
    (5) There is no evidence to suggest that true denticles and false denticles differ in their degree of calcification.

16. (5) The formation of Hertwig's root sheath and its disintegration is essential to the formation of cementum. As the sheath breaks down, cells from the dental sac make contact with the dentin in the root and differentiate into cementoblasts.
    (1) The reduced enamel epithelium does not play a role in the formation of cementum.
    (2) The cells of the stratum intermedium and the stellate reticulum must collapse first in order for Hertwig's root sheath to form.

(3) The cells of the outer enamel epithelium do not play a role in the formation of cementum unless they are combined with the inner epithelial cells to form the root sheath.

(4) Same answer as given for 3.

17. (2) The dentogingival attachment is composed of junctional epithelium (stratified squamous epithelium), which produces its own epithelium. Like most epithelium, it will also form junctional complexes to attach to other cells or tissues. In this instance the junctional epithelium forms hemidesmosomes to attach to the tooth surface.

(1) Junctional epithelium, such as a junctional complex, would not allow the epithelium to become attached to the tooth surface.

(3) Epithelium will always produce a basal lamina in healthy tissue.

(4) A cuticle with hemidesmosomes is unlikely to form, because the cuticle is structureless and composed of dead blood cells and other unidentified materials.

(5) Desmosomes are seen between cells as a form of cell-to-cell contact but not between cells and other tissue types.

18. (2) The cribriform plate of the alveolar bone proper has minute small openings in it to allow for the passage of blood vessels, which communicate with the blood vesels in the periodontal ligament.

(1) The compact bone of the alveolar bone proper does not have the morphology to permit the blood vessels to pass through and communicate with those in the periodontal ligament.

(3) *Lamina dura* is a radiographic term used to describe an opaque line seen on radiographs outlining the alveolar bone proper.

(4) The bundle bone proper is that part of the bone into which the periodontal ligament is inserted.

(5) Sharpey's fibers are not related to the blood supply of the periodontal ligament or alveolar bone; they are uncalcified cores of the ligament found in cementum and alveolar bone.

19. (4) The transseptal fiber group helps to maintain the integrity of the dental arch by passing over the alveolar crest and attaching adjacent teeth to each other.

(1) The oblique fibers belong to the principal fibers and support the tooth in its alveolus.

(2) The periapical fibers belong to the principal fibers and support and help to resist pull from the bone socket.

(3) The circumferential fibers belong to the principal fibers and resist rotation of the tooth in the bone socket.

(5) The interradicular fibers are support fibers that belong to the principal fibers.

20. (4) Cementum is an avascular tissue and needs to be near a blood supply that is located in the periodontal ligament. Nutrients from the blood reach the cementocytes via their cell processes, which face the periodontal ligament.

(1) There is no histologic evidence to date that the cementocytes are forced in a particular direction once they are in their lacunae.

(2) The cell processes project off of the cell in all directions, but for the most part, the majority face the periodontal ligament for nourishment for the cell.

(3) The direction of the cell processes from the cementocytes is not related to the deposition of cementum.

(5) The cell processes are oriented toward the periodontal ligament for nourishment, not because they can nourish the ligament.

21. (2) Calcium and phosphorous ions are major components of bone, and because of a biofeedback system in the body involving the parathyroid glands, when the two ions are needed by the body, bone will be resorbed.

(1) Supersaturation is not related to the process of bone acting as a reservoir for the two ions.

(3) Osteoblasts are the bone-forming cells and are not the cells that resorb the tissue; nor are they responsible for storage of the two ions.

(4) Osteocytes are trapped in the calcified matrix of bone and are not the cells responsible for the resorption of bone.

(5) Collagen fibers are the major components of the fibrous matrix of bone tissue but have no role in the resorption of bone or in the releasing of the two ions when they are needed.

22. (4) When bone is remodeled, there are reversal lines in the tissue, reflecting where the osteoclasts resorbed the bone tissue, causing a scalloping, and then bone is redeposited in the opposite direction from the resorption.

(1) The arrest lines seen in bone tissue are related to deposition of bone—a phasic deposition, not remodeling.

(2) The size of the lamella is not related to the remodeling process.

(3) The orientation of the fibers in each lamella is always different from that of each adjacent lamella.

(5) The thickness or the thinness of the periosteum is not related to the remodeling process in bone tissue.

23. (3) The fingers and the legs both have epiphyseal growth plates, which can be used to ascertain the degree of growth that the patient may still attain.
    (1) Study models would best be used to give information related to the patient's occlusion.
    (2) A full-mouth radiographic series could exhibit soft or hard tissue pathology and the status of unerupted teeth, if any, but not the degree of growth.
    (4) A clinical examination would best be used to determine the condition of the soft and hard tissues of the oral cavity.
    (5) An occlusal film would provide a panoramic view of the maxilla and the floor of the maxillary sinuses.

24. (3) Bone will resorb in a localized area if the bone becomes so thick that the osteocytes become too distant to allow for the passage of blood through their canaliculi.
    (1) The role of the osteocytes is to maintain the tissue, not deposit bone tissue.
    (2) When there is a need for more calcium and phosphorus in the blood, they are released from the bone, not in a localized area, but by a general resorption of bone.
    (4) Blood vessels that nourish bone tissue are located in the periosteum.
    (5) An overabundance of calcium and phosphorus in bone tissue is not related to localized bone resorption.

25. (1) Incisors develop in the primary palate; if the primary palate is absent, neither deciduous nor permanent incisors will ever be present.
    (2) Premolars would not be affected, because they do not develop in the primary palate.
    (3) First permanent molars do not develop in the primary palate.
    (4) Deciduous and permanent canines do not develop in the primary palate.
    (5) Both the deciduous and the permanent incisors would be affected because the permanent incisors develop from the successional lamina.

26. (2) Alveolar bone will develop in the oral cavity only if teeth develop and erupt into the mouth.
    (1) The cribriform plate could not be present, because it is part of the alveolar bone proper.
    (3) Basal bone would be present because it is that part of the maxilla and mandible below the alveolar bone and is unrelated to tooth formation.
    (4) Bundle bone is part of the alveolar bone proper and would not be present; it houses Sharpey's fibers of the periodontal ligament.
    (5) The interradicular alveolar bone is that part of the alveolar bone located between the roots of multirooted teeth and would not be present.

27. (3) Two palatal shelves develop from both sides of the maxilla and grow down in a vertical position on either side of the tongue. These palatal shelves flip up into a horizontal position and fuse to form the hard palate.
    (1) The two medial nasal processes fuse to form the bridge of the nose and the primary palate.
    (2) The medial and lateral nasal processes fuse to form the nasal passages.
    (4) The maxillary and lateral nasal processes fuse; the entrapped epithelium eventually becomes canalized to form the nasolacrimal duct.
    (5) The fusion of the primary and secondary palates gives rise to the complete anterior portion of the hard palate.

28. (3) When the palatal shelves fuse to form the hard palate, epithelium is sometimes entrapped, becoming epithelial remnants. These remnants have the potential to become cystic.
    (1) The nasal fossa would show a midline structure separating the nasal cavities.
    (2) The maxillary sinuses are not located in the midline of the palate.
    (4) The greater palatine foramen is not located in the middle of the palate.
    (5) A mucoperiosteal cyst is associated with the gingiva and is related to periodontal problems.

CHAPTER 3

Human Anatomy and Physiology

CATHERINE C. DAVIS

Anatomy and physiology are sciences that describe the organization, structure, and function of the human body. The dental hygienist uses basic concepts of anatomy and physiology most often during patient assessment and evaluation. Knowledge of these concepts allows the dental hygienist to determine the location of normal structures and to determine if structures are within normal limits, deviate from normal, or are ectopic. Anatomic landmarks also are important in oral radiologic

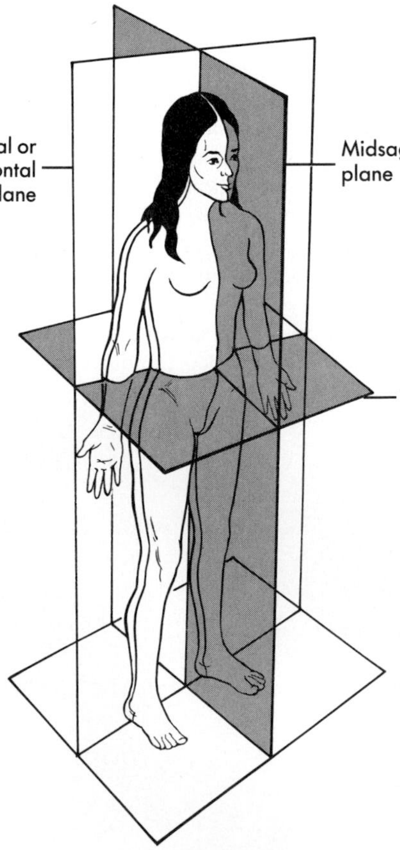

Fig. 3-1 Directions and planes of section. (From McClintic, J.R.: Human anatomy, St. Louis, 1983, The C.V. Mosby Co.)

and pathologic examinations and for the administration of a local anesthetic. The anatomic and physiologic review covers basic concepts, definitions of terms, cell structure and function, and the systems of the body, including the skeletal, muscular, nervous, circulatory, digestive, endocrine, and reproductive systems.

Sciences of Anatomy and Physiology

BASIC CONCEPTS

Anatomy

A. Definition—the science that describes the structure of the body; word is derived from the Greek roots that translate into ''the act of cutting up'' (i.e., dissection)
B. Branches of anatomy
   1. Gross anatomy—study of structures that can be identified with the naked eye; usually involves the use of cadavers (corpses)
   2. Microscopic anatomy (histology)—study of cells that compose tissues and organs; involves the use of a microscope to study the details of the specimens
   3. Developmental anatomy (embryology)—study of an individual from beginning as a single cell to birth
   4. Comparative anatomy—comparative study of the animal structure in regard to similar organs or regions

Descriptive Terms

A. Anatomic position—erect body position with the arms at the sides and the palms upward
B. Plane or section
   1. Definition—imaginary flat surface formed by an extension through an axis
   2. Median plane—a vertical plane that divides a body into right and left halves (Fig. 3-1)

3. Sagittal plane
   a. Any plane parallel to the median plane
   b. Divides the body into right and left portions
4. Frontal plane
   a. Vertical plane that forms at right angles to the sagittal plane
   b. Divides the body into anterior and posterior sections
   c. Synonymous with the term *coronal plane*
5. Transverse plane
   a. Horizontal plane that forms at right angles to the sagittal and frontal planes
   b. Divides the body into upper and lower portions
   c. Synonymous with the term *horizontal plane*

C. Relative positions
1. Anterior
   a. Nearest the abdominal surface and the front of the body
   b. Synonymous with the term *ventral*
   c. In referring to hands and forearms, the terms *palmar* and *volar* are used
2. Posterior
   a. Back of the body
   b. Synonymous with the term *dorsal*
3. Superior
   a. Upper or higher
   b. Synonymous with the term *cranial* (head)
4. Inferior
   a. Below or lower
   b. Synonymous with the term *caudal* (tail)
   c. In refering to the top of the foot and the sole of the foot, the terms *dorsal* and *plantar* are used respectively
5. Medial—near to the median plane
6. Lateral—farther away from the median plane
7. Proximal—near the source or attachment
8. Distal—away from the source or attachment
9. Superficial—near the surface
10. Deep—away from the surface
11. Afferent—conducting toward a structure
12. Efferent—conducting away from a structure

Physiology

A. Definition—study of mechanisms by which the body performs various functions; attempts to explain vital processes by using principles outlined in the biologic, chemical, and physical sciences; roots of the word are derived from the Greek words that translate into ''the study of nature''

B. Branches of physiology
1. Comparative physiology—study of comparing and contrasting the vital processes in different organisms
2. Developmental physiology—study of the vital processes related to embryonic development
3. General physiology—study of the functions of the vital processes
4. Human physiology—study of the functions within the human body
5. Pathologic physiology—study of disease that relates to an imbalance in function

BODY CAVITIES – FORMATION AND CONTENTS (Fig. 3-2)

A. Dorsal cavity—contains the brain and spinal cord
1. Cranial cavity—formed by bones of the skull
2. Vertebral cavity—formed by the vertebrae
B. Ventral cavity
1. Thoracic cavity
   a. Pericardial cavity contains the heart
   b. Pleural cavity contains the lungs
   c. Trachea, bronchi, esophagus, and thymus lie between these subdivisions
2. Abdominopelvic cavity
   a. Upper cavity contains the liver, small and large intestines, stomach, spleen, pancreas, and gallbladder
   b. Lower cavity contains the bladder, rectum, sigmoid colon, and reproductive organs

CELLS

Common Functions

See also Chapter 2, section on general histology and Fig. 2-1
A. Excitability
1. Change in the environment stimulates the cell to bring about a response to adapt to the change in the environment
2. Example—nerve cells conduct impulses
B. Synthesis
1. Cells must be able to form substances to produce products that aid in the body's function
2. Example—glands synthesize and secrete products to aid body function
C. Membrane transport
1. Fluids, chemical elements, and compounds must be able to move both in and out of the cells
2. Example—nutrients are transported across the epithelial lining of the gastrointestinal tract

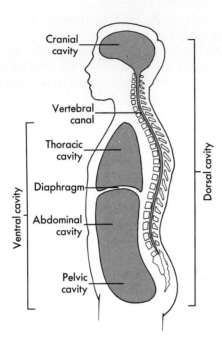

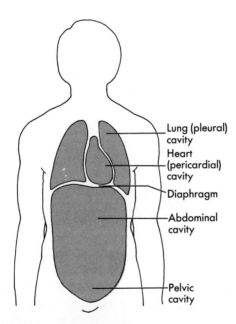

Fig. 3-2 Lateral and anterior views of human figure, identifying body cavities. (From McClintic, J.R.: Human anatomy, St. Louis, 1983, The C.V. Mosby Co.)

D. Reproduction
  1. Cells must be able to preserve the species by giving rise to offspring
  2. Example—union of a sperm and an ovum can lead to the formation of an offspring

Specialization

A. Differentiation
  1. Cells that recognize one another will group together
  2. Cancer cells do not recognize each other
B. Organize chemicals
  1. Chemicals appear early in the development of the embryo
  2. Endocrine substances are produced by one type of cell and can affect other types of cells
C. Cells → tissues → organs → organ systems

Cellular Structures—Organelles

See also Chapter 2, section on general histology, and Chapter 7, sections on procaryotic (bacterial) cell structure and function and on eucaryotic cell structure and function

A. Cell membrane
  1. Surrounds the cell; is semipermeable, allowing some substances to pass though it and others to be excluded
  2. Its permeability may be varied
  3. Selective permeability characteristics
     a. Protects cell from external environment
     b. Permits entrance and exit of selected substrates
     c. Uses active transport, passive transport, or facilitated diffusion
  4. Has a 3:2 ratio of proteins to lipids; lipids and proteins are the major components
  5. Consists of a bipolar membrane with a central core of lipids between two layers of protein
  6. The 8 Å pores in the surface allow diffusion of small lipid insoluble substances
B. Endoplasmic reticulum
  1. A complex series of tubules in the cytoplasm of the cell
  2. Membraneous system of channels that can permeate the entire cytoplasm, sometimes leading from the plasma membrane to the nuclear membrane
  3. Synthesizes, circulates, and packages intracellular and extracellular materials
  4. Contains enzymes and is involved in a variety of metabolic activities (e.g., lipogenesis and glycogenesis)
  5. Granular
     a. Contains ribosomes, which are attached to the cytoplasmic side of the membrane
     b. Site of protein synthesis
  6. Agranular
     a. No ribosomes present
     b. Site of steroid synthesis

C. Golgi apparatus or body
1. Network of flattened smooth membrane and vesicles
2. Responsible for secreting to the external environment a variety of proteins synthesized on the endoplasmic reticulum
3. Major site of membrane formation and recycling
4. Storage site for newly synthesized proteins
5. Site for packaging and transporting many cell products (e.g., polysaccharides, proteins, and lipids)
6. Synthesis site for lysosomes

D. Mitochondria
1. Ellipsoid bodies that consist of an outer and inner membrane that contain enzyme complexes in a particular array (e.g., tricarboxylic acid cycle enzymes)
2. Function as the powerhouse of the cell by transforming the chemical energy bond of nutrients into the high-energy phosphate bonds of adenosine triphosphate (ATP)
3. There may be 50 to 2500 of these organelles in a single cell, depending on the cell's energy needs

E. Lysosomes
1. Tiny closed vesicles with a single limiting membrane containing powerful degradative or hydrolytic enzymes
2. Involved in the normal degradation of both intracellular and extracellular substances that must be removed by the cell
3. Vitamins A and E and zinc are important stabilizers for the membrane

F. Cytoplasm
1. Aqueous environment that surrounds and supports all of the organelles within a cell
2. Transport medium in which all nutrients and metabolites are carried from one organelle to another
3. Contains enzymes and electrolytes in which specific metabolic reactions take place (e.g., glycolysis)

G. Ribosomes
1. Ribonucleoprotein particles usually attached to the endoplasmic reticulum
2. Synthesis site for protein molecules

H. Nucleus
1. Consists of a nuclear membrane, nucleolus, and nuclear matrix with chromosomes
2. Ultimately controls cellular function; determines cellular nutrient needs

3. Genetic code for cell duplication and construction of the cell's proteins is found in the deoxyribonucleic acid (DNA) portion of the chromosome
4. Mitosis—process of cell replication (Fig. 3-3)
   a. Interphase
      (1) Genetic material of each chromosome replicates
      (2) Chromosomes are dispersed as chromatin material in the nucleus
   b. Prophase
      (1) Nuclear envelope disappears
      (2) Two centrioles separate and move to opposite poles of the cell
      (3) Spindle fibers develop
   c. Metaphase
      (1) Chromatids line up at the center
      (2) Spindle fibers attach at the centromere
      (3) Centromere replicates, allowing separation of the chromatids
   d. Anaphase
      (1) Spindle fibers pull the new chromosomes to opposite poles of the cell
   e. Telophase
      (1) Nuclear membrane forms around each set of chromosomes
      (2) Centrioles replicate in each cell

Internal Environment and Homeostasis

A. Extracellular fluid
1. The mass of fluid that circulates on the outside of the cells and in between them
2. Composition must be regulated exactly

$$[Na+] = 142 \text{ mEq/L}$$
$$[K+] = 5 \text{ mEq/L}$$
$$[Cl^-] = 103 \text{ mEq/L}$$
$$[Ca+^2] = 5 \text{ mEq/L}$$
$$pH = 7.4$$

3. Claude Bernarde called it the "milieu interne"

B. Intracellular fluid
1. The fluid located inside the cells of the body
2. Composition must be regulated exactly

$$[Na+] = 10 \text{ mEq/L}$$
$$[K+] = 141 \text{ mEq/L}$$
$$[Cl^-] = 4 \text{ mEq/L}$$
$$[Ca+^2] = <1 \text{ mEq/L}$$
$$pH = 7.0$$

C. Homeostasis
1. The delicate balance that must be maintained between the two fluid compositions
2. Phrase coined by William Cannon

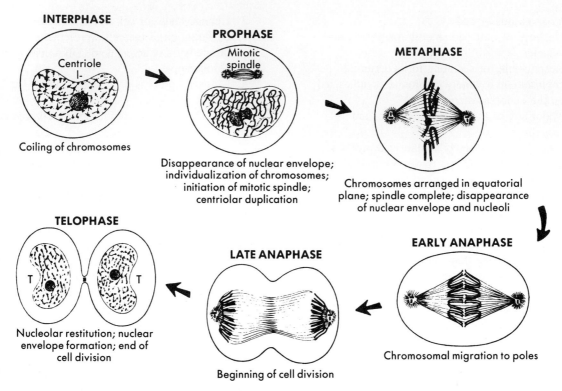

Fig. 3-3 Phases of mitosis. (From Junqueira, L.C., and Carneiro, J.: Basic histology, ed. 4; copyright 1983 by Lange Medical Publications, Los Altos, Calif.)

Transport through the Cell Membrane

A. Diffusion
   1. Definition—continuous movement of molecules among each other in liquids or in gases
   2. Molecules may move across a membrane
   3. Direction of diffusion of a substance is from a region of high concentration to a region of low concentration, which is the diffusion gradient
   4. If equal amounts of a substance are placed at either ends of the chamber, they diffuse toward each other and the net rate of diffusion equals zero
   5. Factors that affect the rate of diffusion
      a. The higher the concentration difference, the greater the rate of diffusion
      b. The greater the cross-sectional area of the chamber, the greater the rate of diffusion
      c. The greater the temperature, the greater the rate of reaction
      d. The lesser the square root of the molecular weight, the greater the rate of reaction
      e. The shorter the distance, the greater the rate of reaction

Diffusion rate $\propto$
$$\frac{\text{Concentration difference} \times \text{Cross-sectional diameter} \times \text{Temperature}}{\sqrt{\text{Molecular weight}} \times \text{Distance}}$$

   6. How rapidly a substance can diffuse through the lipid matrix of the cell membrane is determined by its solubility in lipids
      a. Oxygen, carbon dioxide, and alcohol can diffuse through the membrane rapidly, since they are lipid soluble
      b. Water is not lipid soluble and therefore must depend on another mechanism to diffuse through the cell membrane
   7. Facilitated diffusion involves the use of a carrier substance to transport a nonlipid-soluble substance across the cell membrane
      a. Once the substance reaches the opposite side of the membrane, it breaks away from the carrier
      b. This system does not involve the use of energy
   8. Diffusion through pores
      a. Substance must be less than 8 Å in diameter to move through the pore
      b. Calcium ions line the pores; therefore positive elements such as potassium are repelled
      c. Antidiuretic hormone (ADH) from the hypothalmus can cause the pores in kidney tubule cells to decrease in diameter

B. Osmosis
   1. Definition—process of net diffusion of water through a semipermeable membrane caused by a concentration difference
   2. Osmotic pressure—pressure that develops in a solution as a result of net osmosis into that solution; is affected by the number of dissolved particles per unit volume of fluid
   3. Isotonic solution—when placed on the outside of a cell, will not cause osmosis (e.g., 0.9% sodium chloride)
   4. Hypertonic solution—when placed on the outside of a cell, will cause osmosis out of the cell (e.g., greater than 0.9% sodium chloride) and lead to crenation of the cell
   5. Hypotonic solution—when placed on the outside of a cell, will cause osmosis into the cell (e.g., less than 0.9% sodium chloride) and lead to lysis of the cell)
C. Active transport
   1. Used by a cell when large quantities of a substance are needed inside of the cell and only a small amount is present in the extracellular fluid
   2. Involves pumping the substance against its concentration gradient
   3. Uses a carrier system and energy (ATP)
   4. Keeps sodium extracellularly (sodium pump) and potassium intracellularly; important for transmission of impulses
   5. Almost all monosaccharides are actively transported to the body
D. Phagocytosis—movement of a solid particle into the cell
   1. Cell wall invaginates around the particle
   2. Pinches off from the rest of the membrane and floats inward
E. Pinocytosis—movement of fluid into a cell; similar to phagocytosis, except cell invaginates around fluid

TISSUES

A. Definition—an aggregate of cells that have nonliving intracellular substances between the cells
   1. Classifications
      a. Epithelial
      b. Connective
      c. Nerve
      d. Muscle
   2. Differ in structure because each tissue can differ in function
B. Types
   1. Epithelial tissue
      a. Contains little intercellular substance; therefore is composed mainly of cells
      b. Does not contain blood vessels
      c. Cells composing this tissue undergo mitosis
      d. Subtypes
         (1) Simple squamous
            (a) One layer of flat cells
            (b) Example—lining of blood vessels
         (2) Stratified squamous
            (a) Several layers thick
            (b) Example—mucous membranes
         (3) Simple columnar
            (a) Two types of cells—columnar and goblet
            (b) Example—lining of the intestines
   2. Connective tissue
      a. Contains large amounts and various types of intercellular material and few cells
      b. Is usually highly vascular
      c. Functions
         (1) Supports structures
         (2) Aids in distribution of nutrients
      d. Classifications
         (1) Reticular—network of branching fibers; acts as a filter; loose and stretchable; serves as a connection between structures
         (2) Adipose—located under the skin; insulates
         (3) Dense fibrous—flexible; serves as a connection between structures
         (4) Bone—hard and calcified; serves a supportive, protective function
         (5) Cartilage—firm but flexible; serves a supportive function
         (6) Blood—large amount of fluid within the various cells; carries on vital functions of the body
   3. Nervous tissue
      a. Neurons—nerve cells that are irritable and are the conducting units
      b. Neuroglia—supporting framework
   4. Muscle tissue
      a. Function—contraction
      b. Types
         (1) Skeletal—voluntary, striated
         (2) Cardiac—involuntary, striated
         (3) Visceral—involuntary, smooth

MEMBRANES AND GLANDS
Membranes

A. Function—to cover or line parts of the body
B. Types
   1. Mucous

a. Line cavities of the body that communicate with the exterior
b. Protect, secrete, and absorb
2. Serous
   a. Line cavities that do not communicate with the exterior
   b. Visceral layer covers organs
   c. Parietal layer lines cavities
   d. Synovial membranes line joint cavities
3. Cutaneous
   a. Skin functions in protection, excretion, and sensation
   b. Skin consists of epidermis and dermis
   c. Skin contains hair follicles and glands

Glands

A. Function—synthesizes compounds
B. Types
   1. Endocrine—secrete product directly into the blood system
   2. Exocrine—secrete product directly into ducts
      a. Simple—nonbranching duct
      b. Compound—branching duct

Systems of the Body and Their Components

SKELETAL SYSTEM

A. Functions
   1. Provides a rigid support system
   2. Protect delicate structures (e.g., the protection provided by the bones of the vertebral column to the spinal cord)
   3. Bones supply calcium to the blood; are involved in the formation of blood cells (hemopoesis)
   4. Bones serve as the basis of attachment of muscles; form levers in the joint areas, allowing movement
B. Formation
   1. Bones begin to form during the eighth week of embryonic life in the fibrous membranes (intramembranous ossification) and hyaline cartilage (endochondral ossification)
   2. Ossification
      a. Intramembranous—found in the flat bones of the face
         (1) Mesenchymal cells cluster and form strands
         (2) Strands are cemented in a uniform network, which is known as osteoid

(3) Calcium salts are deposited; osteoid is converted to bone
(4) Trabeculae are formed and make cancellous bone with open spaces known as marrow cavities
(5) Periosteum forms on the inner and outer surfaces of the ossification centers
(6) Surface bone becomes compact bone
   b. Endochondral—primary type of ossification in the human
      (1) Cartilage model is covered with perichondrium that is converted to periosteum
         (a) Diaphysis—central shaft
         (b) Epiphysis—located at either end of the diaphysis
         (c) Growth in length of the bone is provided by the metaphyseal plate located between the epiphyseal cartilage and the diaphysis
      (2) Blood capillaries and the mesenchymal cells infiltrate the spaces left by the destroyed chondrocytes
         (a) Osteoblasts are derived from the undifferentiated cells; form an osseous matrix in the cartilage
         (b) Bone appears at the site where there was cartilage
      (3) Ossification is completed as the proximal epiphysis joins with the diaphysis between the twentieth and twenty-fifth year
C. Microscopic structure
   1. Compact bone is found on the exterior of all bones; cancellous bone is found in the interior
   2. Surface of compact bone is covered by periosteum that is attached by Sharpey's fibers
   3. Blood vessels enter the periosteum via Volkmann's canals and then enter the haversian canals that are formed by the canaliculi and lacunae
   4. Marrow
      a. Fills spaces of spongy bone
      b. Contains blood vessels and blood cells in various stages of development
      c. Types
         (1) Red bone marrow
            (a) Formation of red blood cells (RBCs) and some white blood cells (WBCs) in this location

(b) Predominate type of marrow in the newborn

(c) Found in spongy bone of adults (sternum, ribs, vertebrae, and proximal epiphyses of long bones)

(2) Yellow bone marrow

(a) Fatty marrow

(b) Generally replaces red bone marrow in the adult, except in areas mentioned above

D. Types
1. Long bones (e.g., femur and humerus)
2. Short bones (e.g., wrist and ankle bones)
3. Flat bones (e.g., ribs)
4. Irregular bones (e.g., vertebrae)

E. Descriptive terminology
1. Projections
   a. Process—prominence
   b. Spine—sharp prominence
   c. Tubercle—rounded projection
   d. Tuberosity—larger rounded projection
   e. Trochanter—very large bony prominence
   f. Crest—ridge
   g. Condyle—round process for articulation
   h. Head—enlargement at end of a bone
2. Depression
   a. Fossa—pit
   b. Groove—furrow
   c. Sulcus—synonymous with groove
   d. Sinus—cavity within a bone
   e. Foramen—opening
   f. Meatus—tubelike

F. Divisions of the skeleton (Figs. 3-4 and 3-5)
1. Axial skeleton (74 total)
   a. Upright axis of the skeleton
   b. Consists of the skull, hyoid, vertebral column, sternum, and ribs
2. Appendicular skeleton (126 total)
   a. Bones attached to the axial skeleton
   b. Upper and lower extremities
3. Auditory ossicles (6 total)

G. Articulations
1. Classified according to their structure, composition, and movability
   a. Fibrous joints—surfaces of bones almost in direct contact with limited movement
      (1) Syndesmosis—two bones united by interosseous ligaments
      (2) Sutures—serrated margins of bones united by a thin layer of fibrous tissue
      (3) Gomphosis—insertion of a cone-shaped process into a socket

b. Cartilaginous joints—no joint cavity and contiguous bones united by cartilage
   (1) Synchondrosis—ends of two bones approximated by hyaline cartilage
   (2) Symphyses—approximating bone surfaces connected by fibrocartilage

c. Synovial joints—approximating bone surfaces covered with cartilage; may be separated by a disk; attached by ligaments
   (1) Hinge—permits motion in one plane only
   (2) Pivot—permits rotary movement in which a ring rotates around a central axis
   (3) Saddle—opposing surfaces are convex-concave, allowing great freedom of motion
   (4) Ball and socket—capable of movement in an infinite number of axes; rounded head of one bone moves in a cuplike cavity of the approximating bone

2. Bursae
   a. Sacs filled with synovial fluid that are present where tendons rub against bone or where skin rubs across bone
   b. Some bursae communicate with a joint cavity
   c. Prominent bursae found at the elbow, hip, and knee

3. Movements
   a. Gliding
      (1) Simplest kind of motion in a joint
      (2) Movement on a joint that does *not* involve any angular or rotary motions
   b. Flexion—decreases the angle formed by the union of two bones
   c. Extension—increases the angle formed by the union of two bones
   d. Abduction—occurs by moving part of the appendicular skeleton away from the median plane of the body
   e. Adduction—occurs by moving part of the appendicular skeleton toward the median plane of the body
   f. Circumduction
      (1) Occurs in ball-and-socket joints
      (2) Circumscribes the conic space of one bone by the other bone
   g. Rotation—turning on an axis without being displaced from that axis

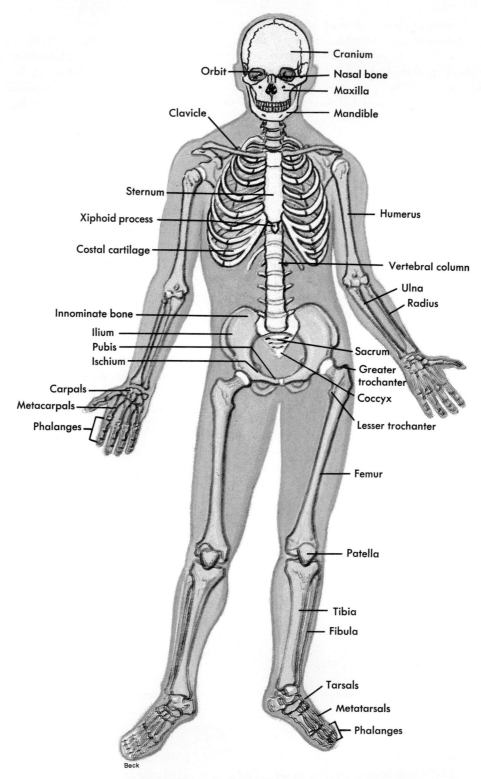

Fig. 3-4 Skeleton, anterior view. (From Anthony, C.P., and Thibodeau, G.A.: Textbook of anatomy and physiology, ed. 11, St. Louis, 1983, The C.V. Mosby Co.)

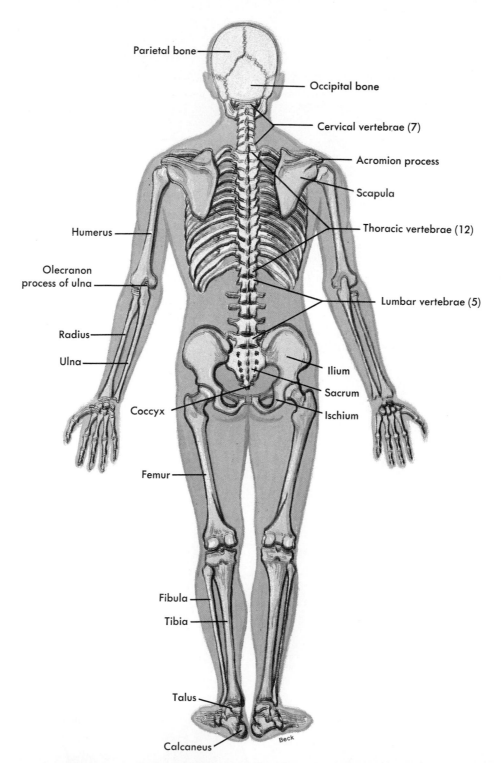

Parietal bone

Occipital bone

Cervical vertebrae (7)

Acromion process

Scapula

Humerus

Thoracic vertebrae (12)

Olecranon
process of ulna

Lumbar vertebrae (5)

Radius

Ulna

Ilium

Sacrum

Coccyx

Ischium

Femur

Fibula

Tibia

Talus

Calcaneus

Beck

Fig. 3-5 Skeleton, posterior view. (From Anthony, C.P., and Thibodeau, G.A.: Textbook of anatomy and physiology, ed. 11, St. louis, 1983, The C.V. Mosby Co.)

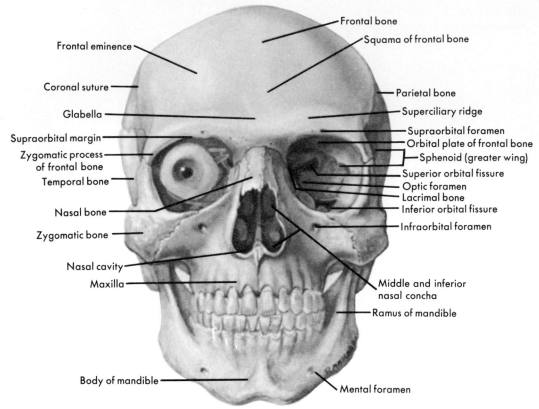

Fig. 3-6 Skull viewed from front. (From McClintic, J.R.: Human anatomy, St. Louis, 1983, The C.V. Mosby Co.)

Frontal bone
Squama of frontal bone
Frontal eminence
Coronal suture
Parietal bone
Glabella
Superciliary ridge
Supraorbital margin
Supraorbital foramen
Orbital plate of frontal bone
Zygomatic process of frontal bone
Sphenoid (greater wing)
Superior orbital fissure
Temporal bone
Optic foramen
Lacrimal bone
Nasal bone
Inferior orbital fissure
Infraorbital foramen
Zygomatic bone
Nasal cavity
Maxilla
Middle and inferior nasal concha
Ramus of mandible
Body of mandible
Mental foramen

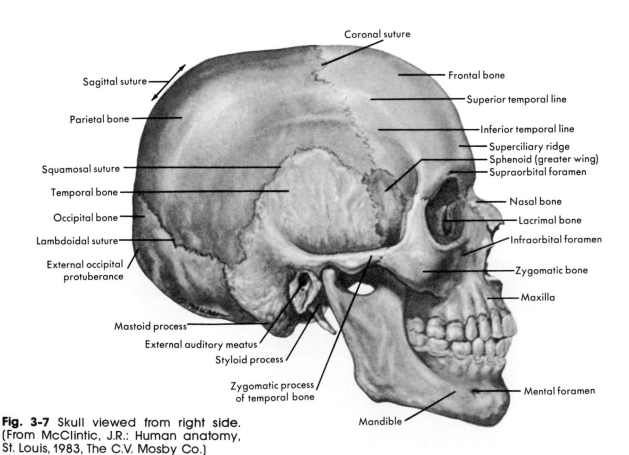

Coronal suture
Sagittal suture
Frontal bone
Superior temporal line
Parietal bone
Inferior temporal line
Superciliary ridge
Sphenoid (greater wing)
Squamosal suture
Supraorbital foramen
Temporal bone
Nasal bone
Occipital bone
Lacrimal bone
Lambdoidal suture
Infraorbital foramen
External occipital protuberance
Zygomatic bone
Maxilla
Mastoid process
External auditory meatus
Styloid process
Zygomatic process of temporal bone
Mental foramen
Mandible

Fig. 3-7 Skull viewed from right side. (From McClintic, J.R.: Human anatomy, St. Louis, 1983, The C.V. Mosby Co.)

Table 3-1 Bones of the skull

Bones	No.
BONES OF THE CRANIUM	
Occipital	1
Frontal	1
Sphenoid	1
Ethmoid	1
Parietal	2
Temporal	2
BONES OF THE FACE	
Mandible	1
Vomer	1
Maxillae	2
Zygomae	2
Lacrimal	2
Nasal	2
Inferior nasal conchae	2
Palatine	2

Axial Skeleton

A. Skull (Figs. 3-6 and 3-7 and Table 3-1)
   1. Cranium
      a. Superior portion formed by the frontal, parietal, and occipital bones
      b. Lateral portions formed by the temporal and sphenoid bones
      c. Cranial base formed by the temporal, sphenoid, and ethmoid bones
      d. Fontanels—soft spots in which ossification is incomplete at birth
   2. Frontal bone
      a. Forms the forehead
      b. Contains the frontal sinuses
      c. Forms the roof of the orbits
      d. Union with the parietal bones forms the coronal suture
   3. Parietal bones
      a. Union with the occipital bone forms the lambdoid suture
      b. Union with the temporal bone forms the squamous suture
      c. Union with the sphenoid bone forms the coronal suture
   4. Temporal bones
      a. Contains the external auditory meatus and middle and inner ear structures
      b. Squamous portion—above the meatus; zygomatic process—articulates with the zygoma to form the zygomatic arch
      c. Petrous portion

         (1) Contains organs of hearing and equilibrium
         (2) Prominent elevation on the floor of the cranium
      d. Mastoid portion
         (1) Protuberance behind the ear
         (2) Mastoid process
      e. Glenoid fossa—articulates with the condyle on the mandible
      f. Styloid process—anterior to the mastoid process; several neck muscles attach here
      g. Stylomastoid foramen—located between the styloid and mastoid processes; facial nerve emerges through this opening
      h. Jugular foramen—located between the petrous portion and the occipital bone; cranial nerves IX, X, and XI exit
   5. Sphenoid bone (Fig. 3-8)
      a. Bounded by the ethmoid and frontal bones anteriorly and the temporal and occipital bones posteriorly
      b. Greater wings—lateral projections
         (1) Form outer wall and floor of the orbits
         (2) Foramen rotundum—maxillary division of cranial nerve V exits
         (3) Foramen ovale—mandibular division of cranial nerve V exits
         (4) Foramen spinosum—transmits an artery to the meninges
         (5) Foramen lacerum—contains the internal carotid artery
         (6) Superior orbital fissure—transmits cranial nerves III and IV and part of cranial nerve V
      c. Lesser wings
         (1) Posterior part of the roof of the orbits
         (2) Optic foramen—cranial nerve II exits
      d. Body
         (1) Sella turcica—holds the pituitary gland
         (2) Contains the sphenoid sinuses
         (3) Medial and lateral pterygoid processes located here
   6. Ethmoid bone
      a. Contributes to the formation of the base of the cranium, the orbits, and the roof of the nose
      b. Perpendicular plate—forms the superior part of the nasal septum
      c. Horizontal plate (cribriform plate)
         (1) Located at right angles to the perpendicular plate
         (2) Olfactory nerves pass through
         (3) Contains the crista galli—meninges of the brain attach to this process

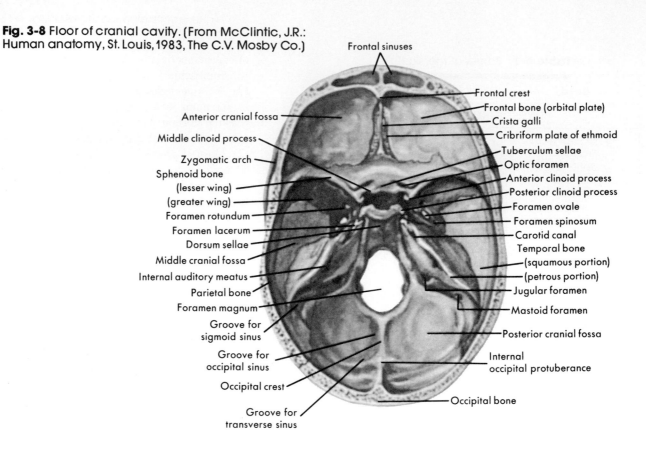

Fig. 3-8 Floor of cranial cavity. (From McClintic, J.R.: Human anatomy, St. Louis, 1983, The C.V. Mosby Co.)

Frontal sinuses

Frontal crest
Frontal bone (orbital plate)
Crista galli
Cribriform plate of ethmoid
Tuberculum sellae
Optic foramen
Anterior clinoid process
Posterior clinoid process
Foramen ovale
Foramen spinosum
Carotid canal
Temporal bone
(squamous portion)
(petrous portion)
Jugular foramen
Mastoid foramen
Posterior cranial fossa
Internal occipital protuberance
Occipital bone

Anterior cranial fossa
Middle clinoid process
Zygomatic arch
Sphenoid bone
(lesser wing)
(greater wing)
Foramen rotundum
Foramen lacerum
Dorsum sellae
Middle cranial fossa
Internal auditory meatus
Parietal bone
Foramen magnum
Groove for sigmoid sinus
Groove for occipital sinus
Occipital crest
Groove for transverse sinus

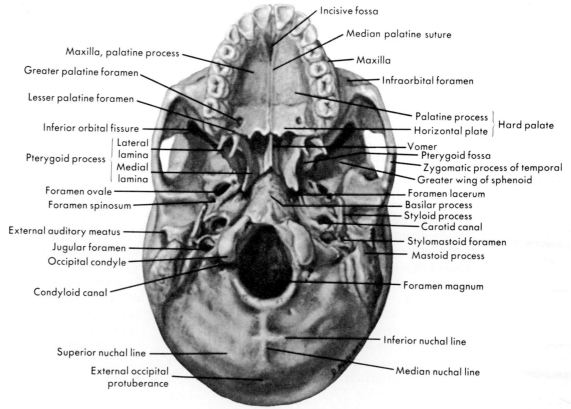

Fig. 3-9 Skull viewed from below. (From McClintic, J.R.: Human anatomy, St. Louis, 1983, The C.V. Mosby Co.)

Incisive fossa
Median palatine suture
Maxilla
Infraorbital foramen
Palatine process
Horizontal plate
Vomer
Pterygoid fossa
Zygomatic process of temporal
Greater wing of sphenoid
Foramen lacerum
Basilar process
Styloid process
Carotid canal
Stylomastoid foramen
Mastoid process
Foramen magnum
Inferior nuchal line
Median nuchal line

Hard palate

Maxilla, palatine process
Greater palatine foramen
Lesser palatine foramen
Inferior orbital fissure
Pterygoid process
Lateral lamina
Medial lamina
Foramen ovale
Foramen spinosum
External auditory meatus
Jugular foramen
Occipital condyle
Condyloid canal
Superior nuchal line
External occipital protuberance

  d. Lateral masses
   (1) Form the orbital plates
   (2) Contain the superior and middle conchae
    (lateral walls of the nose)
   (3) Contain the ethmoid sinuses
 7. Occipital bone (Fig. 3-9)
  a. Forms the posterior part of the cranium
  b. Foramen magnum—spinal cord enters to
   attach to the brainstem
  c. Condyles (two) on either side of the
   foramen magnum—articulate with
   depressions on the C1 vertebra
  d. External occipital protuberance—located on
   the posterior surface
   (1) Superior nuchal lines—curved ridges
    extending laterally
   (2) Inferior nuchal lines—parallels superior
    nuchal lines
  e. Transverse sinuses—located on the inner
   surface
B. Facial bones
 1. Appear suspended from the middle and
  anterior parts of the cranium
 2. Ethmoid and frontal bones also contribute to
  the framework of the face
 3. All the facial bones except the mandible touch
  the maxilla
  a. Alveolar process—forms the upper jaw
   containing the maxillary teeth
  b. Forms the floor of the orbit; infraorbital
   foramen is inferior from the orbit
  c. Forms the walls of the nasal cavities and
   the hard palate (palatine process)
  d. Maxillary sinus—large air space
 4. Mandible
  a. Body—central horizontal portion
   (1) Chin—symphysis in midline
   (2) Alveolar process—contains the
    mandibular teeth
   (3) Mental foramen
    (a) Below the first bicuspid on the
     outer surface
    (b) Transmits nerves and blood
     vessels; frequent site of injections
     of local anesthetics
  b. Ramus—upward process on either side of
   the posterior body of the mandible
   (1) Condyle—articulates with the glenoid
    fossa (neck—constriction located
    inferior to the condyle)
   (2) Coronoid process—attachment site for
    the temporalis muscle
   (3) Mandibular foramen—located on the
    inner surface

 5. Zygomatic bone
  a. Prominence of cheek—attaches to the
   zygomatic process of the temporal bone to
   form the zygomatic arch
  b. Other margin of the orbit
 6. Lacrimal—medial part of the wall of the orbit
 7. Nasal bones—upper bridge of the nose
 8. Inferior nasal concha
  a. Horizontally placed along the lateral wall
   of the nasal fossa
  b. Inferior to the middle and superior conchae
   of the ethmoid
 9. Palatine bones
  a. Horizontal plates—form the posterior part
   of the hard palate
  b. Perpendicular plates—form the
   sphenopalatine foramen
 10. Vomer
  a. Plowshare-shaped
  b. Forms the lower part of the nasal septum
C. Hyoid
 1. U-shaped bone
  a. Body
  b. Greater horn
  c. Lesser horn
 2. Suspended by ligaments from the styloid
  process
D. Vertebral column
 1. Part of the axial skeleton; strong, flexible rod
  a. Supports the head
  b. Gives base to the ribs
  c. Encloses the spinal cord
 2. Vertebrae
  a. Consists of 34 bones composing the spinal
   column
   (1) Cervical—7 bones
   (2) Thoracic—12 bones
   (3) Lumbar—5 bones
   (4) Sacral—5 bones
   (5) Coccygeal—4 to 5 bones
  b. In the adult the vertebrae of the sacral and
   coccygeal regions are united into two bones,
   the sacrum and the coccyx
 3. Curvatures—from a lateral view there are four
  curves, alternately convex and concave
  ventrally
  a. Two convex curves are the cervical and
   lumbar
  b. Two concave curves are the thoracic and
   sacral
 4. Vertebra morphology
  a. Each vertebra differs in size and shape but
   has similar components

b. Body—central mass of bone
   (1) Weight bearing
   (2) Forms anterior part of the vertebra
   (3) Encloses the vertebral foramen
c. Pedicles of the arch—two thick columns that extend backward from the body to meet with the laminae of the neural arch
d. Processes (7)
   (1) One spinous, two transverse, two superior articular, and two inferior articular
      (a) Spinous process extends backward from the point of the union of the two laminae
      (b) Transverse processes project laterally at either side from the junction of the lamina and the pedicle
      (c) Articular processes arise near the junction of the pedicle and the lamina—superior processes project upward; inferior processes project downward
   (2) Surfaces of the processes are smooth
      (a) Inferior articular processes of the vertebra fit into the superior articular processes below
      (b) Form true joints, but the contacts established serve to restrict movement
5. Distinguishing features
   a. Cervical region—triangular shape
      (1) All have foramina in the transverse process (upper six transmit the vertebral artery)
      (2) Spinous processes are short
         (a) C3 to C5 are bifurcated
         (b) C7 is long—prominence felt at the back of the neck
      (3) Have small bodies (except for C1 vertebra)
      (4) C1 vertebra (atlas)
         (a) No body
         (b) Anterior and posterior arch and two lateral masses
         (c) Superior articular processes articulate with the condyles of the occipital bone
      (5) C2 vertebra (axis)—process on the upper surface of the body (dens) forms a pivot about which the axis rotates
   b. Thoracic region

(1) Presence of facets for articulation with the ribs (distinguishing feature)
(2) Processes are larger and heavier than those of the cervical region
(3) Spinous process is directed downward at a sharp angle
(4) Circular vertebral foramen
   c. Lumbar region
      (1) Large and heavy bodies
      (2) Four transverse lines separate the bodies of the vertebrae on the pelvic surface
      (3) Triangular shape—fitted between the halves of the pelvis
      (4) Four pairs of dorsal sacral foramina communicate with four pairs of pelvic sacral foramina
   d. Sacral vertebrae
   e. Coccygeal vertebrae
      (1) Four to five modular pieces fused together
      (2) Triangular shape with the base above and the apex below
   f. Defects
      (1) Lordosis—exaggerated lumbar concavity
      (2) Scoliosis—lateral curvature of any region
      (3) Kyphosis—exaggerated convexity in the thoracic region
E. Bones of the thorax
   1. Sternum
      a. Forms the medial part of the anterior chest wall
      b. Manubrium (upper part)—clavicle and first rib articulate with the manubrium
      c. Body (middle blade)—second and tenth ribs articulate with the body via the costal cartilages
      d. Xiphoid (blunt cartilaginous tip)
   2. Ribs (12 pairs)
      a. Each rib articulates with both the body and the transverse process of its corresponding thoracic vertebra
      b. The second to ninth ribs articulate with the body of the vertebra above
      c. Ribs curve outward, forward, and then downward
      d. Anteriorly, each of the first seven ribs joins a costal cartilage that attaches to the sternum
      e. Next three ribs (eighth to tenth) join the cartilage of the rib above
      f. Eleventh and twelfth ribs do not attach to the sternum; are called "floating ribs"

Table 3-2 Appendicular skeleton

Upper extremity		Lower extremity

Shoulder
  Scapula
  Clavicle
	} Shoulder
	girdle
		Hip
		  Pelvic girdle
		Thigh
		  Femur

Arm
  Humerus
		Kneecap
		  Patella

Forearm
  Ulna, radius, carpals
  (wrist) (8 bones)
		Leg
		  Tibia, fibula, tarsals
		  (ankle) (7 bones)

Hand
  Metacarpals (5
  bones), phlanges
  (fingers) (14 bones)
		Foot
		  Metatarsals (5 bones),
		  phlanges (toes) (14
		  bones)

Appendicular Skeleton (Table 3-2)

A. Upper extremity
  1. Shoulder—clavicle and scapula
    a. Clavicle
      (1) Articulates with the manubrium at the sternal end
      (2) Articulates with the scapula at the lateral end
      (3) Slender S-shaped bone that extends horizontally across the upper part of the thorax
    b. Scapula
      (1) Triangular bone with the base upward and the apex downward
      (2) Lateral aspect contains the glenoid cavity that articulates with the head of the humerus
      (3) Spine extends across the upper part of the posterior surface; expands laterally and forms the acromion (forms point of shoulder)
      (4) Coracoid process projects anteriorly from the upper part of the neck of the scapula
  2. Arm (humerus)
    a. Consists of a shaft (diaphysis) and two ends (epiphyses)
    b. Proximal end has a head that articulates with the glenoid fossa of the scapula
    c. Greater and lesser tubercles lie below the head
      (1) Intertubercular groove is located between them; long tendon of the biceps attaches here
      (2) Surgical neck is located below the tubercles
    d. Radial groove runs obliquely on the posterior surface; radial nerve is located here
    e. Deltoid muscle attaches in a V-shaped area in the middle of the shaft, called the deltoid tuberosity
    f. Distal end has two projections, the medial and lateral epicondyles
      (1) Capitulum—articulates with the radius
      (2) Trochlea—articulates with the ulna
  3. Forearm
    a. Radius
      (1) Lateral bone of the forearm
      (2) Radial tuberosity is located below the head on the medial side
      (3) Distal end is broad for articulation with the wrist; has a styloid process on its lateral side
    b. Ulna
      (1) Medial side of the forearm
      (2) Conspicuous part of the elbow joint (olecranon)
      (3) Curved surface that articulates with the trochlea of the humerus is the trochlear notch
      (4) Lateral side is concave (radial notch); articulates with the head of the radius
      (5) Distal end contains the styloid process
  4. Hand
    a. Carpal bones (8)
      (1) Arranged in two rows of four
      (2) Scaphoid, lunate, triquetral, and pisiform (proximal row); trapezium, trapezoid, capitate, and hamate (distal row)
    b. Metacarpal bones (5)
      (1) Framework of the hand
      (2) Numbered 1 to 5 beginning on the lateral side
    c. Phalanges (14)
      (1) Fingers
      (2) Three phalanges in each finger; two phalanges in the thumb
B. Lower extremity
  1. Hip
    a. Constitutes the pelvic girdle
    b. United with the vertebral column
    c. Union of three parts that is marked by a cup-shaped cavity (acetabulum)
    d. Ilium

(1) Prominence of the hip
(2) Superior border is the crest
(3) Anterosuperior spine—projection at the anterior tip of the crest
(4) Corresponding projections on the posterior part are the posterosuperior and posteroinferior iliac spines
(5) Greater sciatic notch—located beneath the posterior part
(6) Most is a smooth concavity (iliac fossa)
(7) Posteriorly it is rough and articulates with the sacrum in the formation of the sacroiliac joint

e. Pubic bone
(1) Anterior part of the innominate bone
(2) Symphysis pubic—joining of the two pubic bones at the midline
(3) Body and two rami
(a) Body forms one fifth of the acetabulum
(b) Superior ramis extends from the body to the median plane; superior border forms the pubic crest
(c) Inferior ramus extends downward and meets with the ischium
(d) Pubic arch is formed by the inferior rami of both pubic bones

f. Ischium
(1) Forms the lower and back part of the innominate bone
(2) Body
(a) Forms two fifths of the acetabulum
(b) Ischial tuberosity—supports the body in a sitting position
(3) Ramus—passes upward to join the inferior ramus of the pubis; known as the obturator foramen

2. Pelvis
a. Formed by the right and left hip bones, sacrum, and coccyx
b. Greater pelvis
(1) Bounded by the ilia and lower lumbar vertebrae
(2) Gives support to the abdominal viscera
c. Lesser pelvis
(1) Brim of the pelvis corresponds to the sacral promontory
(2) Inferior outlet is bounded by the tip of the coccyx, ischial tuberosities, and inferior rami of the pubic bones
d. Female pelvis
(1) Shows adaptations related to functions as a birth canal
(2) Wide outlet
(3) Angle of the pubic arch is obtuse
e. Male pelvis
(1) Shows adaptations that contribute to power and speed
(2) Heart-shaped outlet
(3) Angle of the pubic arch is acute

3. Thigh
a. Femur—longest and strongest bone of the body
b. Proximal end has a rounded head that articulates with the acetabulum
c. Constricted portion—the neck
d. Greater and lesser trochanters
e. Slightly arched shaft; is concave posteriorly
(1) Linea aspera—strengthened by this prominent ridge
(2) Site of attachment for several muscles
f. Distal end has two condyles separated on the posterior side by the intercondyloid notch

4. Kneecap
a. Patella—sesamoid bone
b. Embedded in the tendon of the quadraceps muscle
c. Articulates with the femur

5. Leg
a. Tibia—medial bone
(1) Proximal end has two condyles that articulate with the femur
(2) Triangular shaft
(a) Anterior—shin
(b) Posterior—soleal line
(c) Distal—medial malleolus that articulates with the latus to form the ankle joint
b. Fibula—lateral bone
(1) Articulates with the lateral condyle of the tibia but does not enter the knee joint
(2) Distal end projects as the lateral malleolus

6. Ankle, foot, and toes
a. Adapted for supporting weight but similar in structure to the hand
b. Talus
(1) Occupies the uppermost and central position in the tarsus
(2) Distributes the body weight from the tibia above to the other tarsal bones
c. Calcaneus (heel)—located beneath the talus

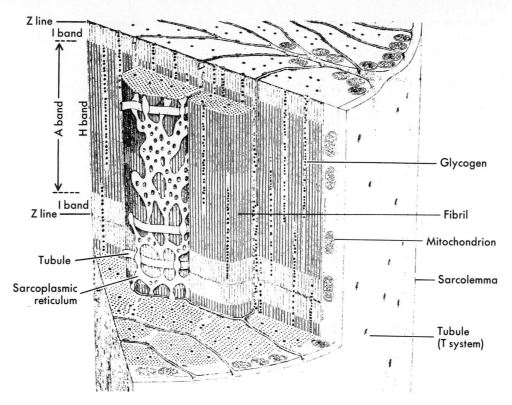

Z line
I band
A band
H band
I band
Z line
Tubule
Sarcoplasmic reticulum

Glycogen

Fibril

Mitochondrion

Sarcolemma

Tubule
(T system)

Fig. 3-10 Organization of myofibrils. (From Hoyle, G.: How is muscle turned on and off? Sci. Am. **222**:84, 1970. Copyright © 1970 by Scientific American, Inc. All rights reserved.)

d. Navicular—located in front of the talus on the medial side; articulates with three cuneiform bones distally

e. Cuboid—lies along the lateral border of the navicular bone

f. Metatarsals
   (1) First, second, and third metatarsals lie in front of the three cuneiform bones
   (2) Fourth and fifth metatarsals lie in front of the cuboid bone

g. Phalanges
   (1) Distal to the metatarsals
   (2) Two in the great toe; three in each of the other four toes

h. Longitudinal arches in the foot (2)
   (1) Lateral—formed by the calcaneus, talus, cuboid, and fourth and fifth metatarsal bones
   (2) Medial—formed by the calcaneus, talus, navicular, cuneiform, and first, second, and third metatarsal bones

i. Transverse arches—formed by the tarsal and metatarsal bones

Skeletal Muscular Tissue

A. Organization (Fig. 3-10; see also Fig. 2-14)
   1. Muscles as a whole are composed of various numbers of the fascicles
      a. Muscle fascicles are formed from grouping the skeletal muscle fibers (long, multinucleated cells and surrounded by endomysium) together and surrounding the muscle fibers with perimysium
      b. Muscle is formed by groups of the muscle fascicles bound together and surrounded with epimysium
      c. Epimysium and perimysium fuse together; form the junction between the muscle and the tendon
      d. Tendons fuse together with the periosteum of the bone; allow the muscles to produce traction of the bone
   2. Subcellular system of the muscle fibers consists of the tubules and fibrils
      a. Skeletal muscle fibers are composed of many longitudinally arranged myofibrils

(1) Sacroplasmic reticulum is analogous to the endoplasmic reticulum of other cells; contains Ca^{+2}

(2) T tubules communicate with the extracellular fluid of the fiber

(3) These systems provide a pathway for exchange of chemical material, which is important in muscle contraction

b. Myofibrils are formed by myofilaments
(1) Thin—actin
(2) Thick—myosin

c. Functional unit of the muscle is designated the sarcomere
(1) Relationship of the myofilaments forms several unique patterns
(a) Z line → Z line forms the sarcomere; distance between two Z lines contains the sarcomere unit; consists of only actin and is in the middle of the I band
(b) M line consists of only myosin; is in the middle of the A band
(c) I band contains actin that is lined up; shortens during contraction
(d) A band consists of actin and myosin that interdigitate; is bisected by the M line
(e) H zone appears in the A band when the muscle is relaxed

B. Muscular contraction
1. Myoneural junction
a. Unmyelinated end of a motor nerve almost touches a skeletal muscle fiber with its terminal buttons (end feet)
(1) Terminal buttons contain the transmitter substance acetylcholine
(2) Space between the nerve and muscle is the synaptic cleft
b. Nerve impulse that reaches the myoneural junction causes acetylcholine to be released into the synaptic cleft, causing increased permeability in the muscle and creating an action potential
c. Effect of acetylcholine is catabolized by the enzyme acetylcholinesterase to form choline and acetate
d. Action potential is sent to the deeper myofibrils via the T tubules
2. Muscle contraction
a. Calcium is released from the cisterns of the sacroplasmic reticulum; combines with the protein myosin to activate it

b. Cross-linkages are developed by projections from the myosin filament touching the actin filament
c. ATP, located on the myosin, is split so that energy can be released
d. Contraction mechanism is known as the ratchet theory, since the myosin filaments pull the actin filaments, thereby shortening the sarcomere

3. Energy for contraction
a. Muscles contain creatine phosphate that can be broken down by enzymatic activity to creatine, phosphate, and energy
b. Muscles also use glucose to form energy and pyruvic acid
c. Oxygen debt occurs in muscles when oxygen is not provided in sufficient amounts; pyruvic acid is changed to lactic acid if there is not enough oxygen

4. Muscle relaxation
a. Ca^{+2} is pumped into the sacroplasmic reticulum
b. Myosin projections are released from the actin filaments

Forms

A. Arrangement of muscle fibers may vary
1. Fusiform fibers consist of two tendons with a belly between the fibers parallel to the long axis
2. Pennate oblique fibers attach to a central tendon
a. Unipennate—approach central tendon from one side
b. Bipennate—approach central tendon from both sides
c. Circumpennate—cylindric muscle mass

B. Muscle power is proportional to the cross-sectional area; is measured at right angles to the long axis of the muscle fascicles

C. Attachments
1. Origin—attachment to a relatively immovable structure
2. Insertion—attachment to a relatively movable structure
3. Bones serve as levers and their joints as fulcrums; contraction of a muscle pulls the insertion end toward the origin of a muscle
4. Muscles generally act in groups
a. Agonists (prime movers)—give power for flexion
b. Synergists—assist the agonists and reduce unnecessary movement
c. Antagonists—are at rest while the agonists are contracting

D. Types of contraction
1. Isometric—muscle length is unchanged, but tension is developed
2. Isotonic—muscle length is shortened, and work is done

Physiologic Activities

A. Conditions of contraction
1. Electrical, chemical, or mechanical stimulant must be applied to a muscle for contraction to occur
2. If a stimulus is strong enough to cause a muscle fiber to contract, the entire muscle fiber (not just part of it) will contract (all-or-none law); strength of the stimulus will not change the response
3. Summation—muscles need to contract with varying amounts of force; therefore the number of muscle fibers that are stimulated and contract are in direct proportion to the force of the contraction
   a. Wave summations occur when a muscle fiber(s) contracts in rapid succession
   b. Strength of contraction will increase as the rate of stimulation increases

c. Tetanization—muscle twitches eventually fuse into a single contraction; has a shortened refractory period
4. Treppe—a muscle contracts more forcefully after it has been stimulated a few times (staircase phenomenon)
5. Fibrillation—muscle fibers contract randomly, producing an ineffective fluttering action

Description (Origin, Insertion, Function, and Innervation)

A. Muscles of facial expression (Table 3-3)
B. Muscles of mastication (Table 3-4)
C. Muscles that move the head (Table 3-5)
D. Muscles that move the shoulder (Table 3-6)
E. Muscles that move the chest wall (Table 3-7)
F. Muscles that move the upper arm (Table 3-8)
G. Muscles that move the lower arm (Table 3-9)
H. Muscles that move the hand (Table 3-10)
I. Muscles that move the trunk (Table 3-11)
J. Muscles that move the pelvic floor (Table 3-12)
K. Muscles that move the abdominal wall (Table 3-13)
L. Muscles that move the thigh (Table 3-14)
M. Muscles that move the lower leg (Table 3-15)
N. Muscles that move the foot (Table 3-16)

Text continued on p. 81.

Table 3-3 Muscles of facial expression

Muscle	Origin	Insertion	Function	Innervation
Epicranius (occipito-frontalis)	Occipital bone	Tissues of eyebrows	Raises eyebrows, wrinkles forehead horizontally	Cranial nerve VII
Corrugator supercilii	Frontal bone (super-ciliary ridge)	Skin of eyebrow	Wrinkles forehead vertically	Cranial nerve VII
Orbicularis oculi	Encircles eyelid		Closes eye	Cranial nerve VII
Procerus	Bridge of nose	Skin over epicranius	Narrows eye opening	Cranial nerve VII
Inferior labial depressor	Mandible	Skin of lower lip	Draws lower lip downward	Cranial nerve VII
Mentalis	Incisive fossa of mandible	Skin of chin	Raises and protrudes lower lip	Cranial nerve VII
Nasalis	Maxilla	Ala of nose	Compresses nasal aperture	Cranial nerve VII
Zygomaticus major	Zygomatic bone	Angle of mouth	Laughing (elevates angle of mouth)	Cranial nerve VII
Zygomaticus minor	Zygomatic bone	Upper lip	Elevates upper lip	Cranial nerve VII
Orbicularis oris	Encircles mouth		Draws lips together	Cranial nerve VII
Platysma	Fascia of upper part of deltoid and pectoralis major	Mandible (lower border) Skin around corners of mouth	Draws corners of mouth down—pouting	Cranial nerve VII
Buccinator	Maxillae	Skin of sides of mouth	Permits smiling Blowing, as in playing a trumpet	Cranial nerve VII

From Anthony, C.P., and Thibodeau, G.A.: Textbook of anatomy and physiology, ed. 11, St. Louis, 1983, The C.V. Mosby Co.

Table 3-4 Muscles of mastication

Muscle	Origin	Insertion	Function	Innervation
Masseter	Zygomatic arch	Mandible (external surface)	Closes jaw	Cranial nerve V
Temporal	Temporal bone	Mandible	Closes jaw	Cranial nerve V
Pterygoids (internal and external)	Undersurface of skull	Mandible (mesial surface)	Grate teeth	Cranial nerve V

From Anthony, C.P., and Thibodeau, G.A.: Textbook of anatomy and physiology, ed. 11, St. Louis, 1983, The C.V. Mosby Co.

Table 3-5 Muscles that move the head

Muscle	Origin	Insertion	Function	Innervation
Sternocleido-mastoid	Sternum Clavicle	Temporal bone (mastoid process)	Flexes head (prayer muscle) One muscle alone, rotates head toward opposite side; spasm of this muscle alone or associated with trapezius called torticollis or wryneck	Accessory nerve
Semispinalis capitis	Vertebrae (transverse processes of upper six thoracic, articular processes of lower four cervical)	Occipital bone (between superior and inferior nuchal lines)	Extends head; bends it laterally	First five cervical nerves
Splenius capitis	Ligamentum nuchae Vertebrae (spinous processes of upper three or four thoracic)	Temporal bone (mastoid process) Occipital bone	Extends head Bends and rotates head toward same side as contracting muscle	Second, third, and fourth cervical nerves
Longissimus capitis	Vertebrae (transverse processes of upper six thoracic, articular processes of lower four cervical)	Temporal bone (mastoid process)	Extends head Bends and rotates head toward contracting side	

From Anthony, C.P., and Thibodeau, G.A.: Textbook of anatomy and physiology, ed. 11, St. Louis, 1983, The C.V. Mosby Co.

Table 3-6 Muscles that move the shoulder

Muscle	Origin	Insertion	Function	Innervation
Trapezius	Occipital bone (protuberance)	Clavicle	Raises or lowers shoulders and shrugs them	Spinal accessory, second, third, and fourth cervical nerves
	Vertebrae (cervical and thoracic)	Scapula (spine and acromion)	Extends head when occiput acts as insertion	
Pectoralis minor	Ribs (second to fifth)	Scapula (coracoid)	Pulls shoulder down and forward	Medial and lateral anterior thoracic nerves
Serratus anterior	Ribs (upper eight or nine)	Scapula (anterior surface, vertebral border)	Pulls shoulder forward; abducts rotates it upward	Long thoracic nerve

From Anthony, C.P., and Thibodeau, G.A.: Textbook of anatomy and physiology, ed. 11, St. Louis, 1983, The C.V. Mosby Co.

Table 3-7   Muscles that move the chest wall

Muscle	Origin	Insertion	Function	Innervation
External intercostals	Rib (lower border; forward fibers)	Rib (upper border of rib below origin)	Elevate ribs	Intercostal nerves
Internal intercostals	Rib (inner surface, lower border; backward fibers)	Rib (upper border of rib below origin)	Probably depress ribs	Intercostal nerves
Diaphragm	Lower circumference of thorax (of rib cage)	Central tendon of diaphragm	Enlarges thorax, causing inspiration	Phrenic nerves

From Anthony C.P., and Thibodeau, G.A.: Textbook of anatomy and physiology, ed. 11, St. Louis, 1983, The C.V. Mosby Co.

Table 3-8   Muscles that move the upper arm

Muscle	Origin	Insertion	Function	Innervation
Pectoralis major	Clavicle (medial half) Sternum Costal cartilages of true ribs	Humerus (greater tubercle)	Flexes upper arm Adducts upper arm anteriorly; draws it across chest	Medial and lateral anterior thoracic nerves
Latissimus dorsi	Vertebrae (spines of lower thoracic, lumbar, and sacral) Ilium (crest) Lumbodorsal fascia	Humerus (intertubercular groove)	Extends upper arm Adducts upper arm posteriorly	Thoracodorsal nerve
Deltoid	Clavicle Scapula (spine and acromion)	Humerus (lateral side about halfway down — deltoid tubercle)	Abducts upper arm Assists in flexion and extension of upper arm	Axillary nerve
Coracobrachialis	Scapula (coracoid process)	Humerus (middle third, medial surface)	Adduction; assists in flexion and medial rotation of arm	Musculocutaneous nerve
Supraspinatus	Scapula (supraspinous fossa)	Humerus (greater tubercle)	Assists in abducting arm	Suprascapular nerve
Teres major	Scapula (lower part, axillary border)	Humerus (upper part, anterior surface)	Assists in extension, adduction, and medial rotation of arm	Lower subscapular nerve
Teres minor	Scapula (axillary border)	Humerus (greater tubercle)	Rotates arm outward	Axillary nerve
Infraspinatus	Scapula (infraspinatus border)	Humerus (greater tubercle)	Rotates arm outward	Suprascapular nerve

From Anthony, C.P., Thibodeau, G.A.: Textbook of anatomy and physiology, ed. 11, St. Louis, 1983, The C.V. Mosby Co.

Table 3-9 Muscles that move the lower arm

Muscle	Origin	Insertion	Function	Innervation
Biceps brachii	Scapula (supraglenoid tuberosity) Scapula (coracoid)	Radius (tubercle at proximal end)	Flexes supinated forearm Supinates forearm and hand	Musculocutaneous nerve
Brachialis	Humerus (distal half, anterior surface)	Ulna (front of coronoid process)	Flexes pronated forearm	Musculocutaneous nerve
Brachioradialis	Humerus (above lateral epicondyle)	Radius (styloid process)	Flexes semipronated or semisupinated forearm; supinates forearm and hand	Radial nerve
Triceps brachii	Scapula (infraglenoid tuberosity) Humerus (posterior surface— lateral head above radial groove; medial head, below)	Ulna (olecranon process)	Extends lower arm	Radial nerve
Pronator teres	Humerus (medial epicondyle) Ulna (coronoid process)	Radius (middle third of lateral surface)	Pronates and flexes forearm	Median nerve
Pronator quadratus	Ulna (distal fourth, anterior surface)	Radius (distal fourth, anterior surface)	Pronates forearm	Median nerve
Supinator	Humerus (lateral epicondyle) Ulna (proximal fifth)	Radius (proximal third)	Supinates forearm	Radial nerve

From Anthony, C.P., and Thibodeau, G.A.: Textbook of anatomy and physiology, ed. 11, St. Louis, 1983, The C.V. Mosby Co.

Table 3-10 Muscles that move the hand

Muscle	Origin	Insertion	Function	Innervation
Flexor carpi radialis	Humerus (medial epicondyle)	Second metacarpal (base of)	Flexes hand Flexes forearm	Median nerve
Palmaris longus	Humerus (medial epicondyle)	Fascia of palm	Flexes hand	Median nerve
Flexor carpi ulnaris	Humerus (medial epicondyle) Ulna (proximal two thirds)	Pisiform bone Third, fourth, and fifth metacarpals	Flexes hand Adducts hand	Ulnar nerve
Extensor carpi radialis longus	Humerus (ridge above lateral epicondyle)	Second metacarpal (base of)	Extends hand Abducts hand (moves toward thumb side when hand supinated)	Radial nerve
Extensor carpi radialis brevis	Humerus (lateral epicondyle)	Second, third metacarpals (bases of)	Extends hand	Radial nerve
Extensor carpi ulnaris	Humerus (lateral epicondyle) Ulna (proximal three fourths)	Fifth metacarpal (base of)	Extends hand Adducts hand (move toward little finger side when hand supinated)	Radial nerve

From Anthony, C.P., and Thibodeau, G.A.: Textbook of anatomy and physiology, ed. 11, St. Louis, 1983, The C.V. Mosby Co.

Table 3-11 Muscles that move the trunk

Muscle	Origin	Insertion	Function	Innervation
Sacrospinalis (erector spinae)			Extend spine; maintain erect posture of trunk Acting singly, abduct and rotate trunk	Posterior rami of first cervical to fifth lumbar spinal nerves
Lateral portion: Iliocostalis lumborum	Iliac crest, sacrum (posterior surface), and lumbar vertebrae (spinous processes)	Ribs, lower six		
Iliocostalis dorsi	Ribs, lower six	Ribs, upper six		
Iliocostalis cervicis	Ribs, upper six	Vertebrae, fourth to sixth cervical		
Medial portion: Longissimus dorsi	Same as iliocostalis lumborum	Vertebrae, thoracic ribs		
Longissimus cervicis	Vertebrae, upper six thoracic	Vertebrae, second to sixth cervical		
Longissimus capitis	Vertebrae, upper six thoracic and last four cervical	Temporal bone, mastoid process		
Quadratus lumborum (forms part of posterior abdominal wall)	Ilium (posterior part of crest) Vertebrae (lower three lumbar)	Ribs (twelfth) Vertebrae (transverse processes of first four lumbar)	Both muscles together extend spine One muscle alone abducts trunk toward side of contracting muscle	First three or four lumbar nerves
Iliopsoas	See muscles that move thigh		Flexes trunk	

From Anthony, C.P., and Thibodeau, G.A.: Textbook of anatomy and physiology, ed. 11, St. Louis, 1983, The C.V. Mosby Co.

Table 3-12 Muscles of the pelvic floor

Muscle	Origin	Insertion	Function	Innervation
Levator ani	Pubis (posterior surface) Ischium (spine)	Coccyx	Together form floor of pelvic cavity; support pelvic organs; if these muscles are badly torn at childbirth or become too relaxed, uterus or bladder may prolapse, that is, drop out	Pudendal nerve
Coccygeus (posterior continuation of levator ani)	Ischium (spine)	Coccyx Sacrum	Same as levator ani	Pudendal nerve

From Anthony, C.P., and Thibodeau, G.A.: Textbook of anatomy and physiology, ed. 11, St. Louis, 1983, The C.V. Mosby Co.

Table 3-13 Muscles that move the abdominal wall

Muscle	Origin	Insertion	Function	Innervation
External oblique	Ribs (lower eight)	Ossa coxae (iliac and pubis by way of inguinal ligament) Linea alba by way of an aponeurosis	Compresses abdomen Important postural function of all abdominal muscles is to pull front of pelvis upward, thereby flattening lumbar curve of spine; when these muscles lose their tone, common figure faults of protruding abdomen and lordosis develop	Lower seven intercostal nerves and iliohypogastric nerves
Internal oblique	Ossa coxae (iliac crest and inguinal ligament) Lumbodorsal fascia	Ribs (lower three) Pubic bone Linea alba	Same as external oblique	Last three intercostal nerves; iliohypogastric and ilioinguinal nerves
Tranversalis	Ribs (lower six) Ossa coxae (iliac crest, inguinal ligament) Lumbodorsal fascia	Pubic bone Linea alba	Same as external oblique	Last five intercostal nerves; iliohypogastric and ilioinguinal nerves
Rectus abdominis	Ossa coxae (pubic bone and symphysis pubis)	Ribs (costal cartilage of fifth, sixth, and seventh ribs) Sternum (xiphoid process)	Same as external oblique; because abdominal muscles compress abdominal cavity, they aid in straining, defecation, forced expiration, childbirth, etc.; abdominal muscles are antagonists of diaphragm, relaxing as it contracts and vice versa Flexes trunk	Last six intercostal

From Anthony, C.P., and Thibodeau, G.A.: Textbook of anatomy and physiology, ed. 11, St. Louis, 1983, The C.V. Mosby Co.

Table 3-14 Muscles that move the thigh

Muscle	Origin	Insertion	Function	Innervation
Iliopsoas (iliacus and psoas major)	Ilium (illiac fossa) Vertebrae (bodies of twelfth thoracic to fifth lumbar)	Femur (small trochanter)	Flexes thigh Flexes trunk (when femur acts as origin)	Femoral and second to fourth lumbar nerves
Rectus femoris	Ilium (anterior, inferior spine)	Tibia (by way of patellar tendon)	Flexes thigh Extends lower leg	Femoral nerve
Gluteal group				
Maximus	Ilium (crest and posterior surface) Sacrum and coccyx (posterior surface) Sacrotuberous ligament	Femur (gluteal tuberosity) Iliotibial tract	Extends thigh — rotates outward	Inferior gluteal nerve
Medius	Ilium (lateral surface)	Femur (greater trochanter)	Abducts thigh — rotates outward; stabilizes pelvis on femur	Superior gluteal nerve
Minimus	Ilium (lateral surface)	Femur (greater trochanter)	Abducts thigh; stabilizes pelvis on femur Rotates thigh medially	Superior gluteal nerve
Tensor fasciae latae	Ilium (anterior part of crest)	Tibia (by way of Iliotibial tract)	Abducts thigh Tightens iliotibial tract	Superior gluteal nerve
Piriformis	Vertebrae (front of sacrum)	Femur (medial aspect of greater trochanter)	Rotates thigh outward Abducts thigh Extends thigh	First or second sacral nerves
Adductor group				
Brevis	Pubic bone	Femur (linea aspera)	Adducts thigh	Obturator nerve
Longus	Pubic bone	Femur (linea aspera)	Adducts thigh	Obturator nerve
Magnus	Pubic bone	Femur (linea aspera)	Adducts thigh	Obturator nerve
Gracilis	Pubic bone (just below symphysis)	Tibia (medial surface behind sartorius)	Adducts thigh and flexes and adducts leg	Obturator nerve

From Anthony, C.P., and Thibodeau, G.A.: Textbook of anatomy and physiology, ed. 11, St. Louis, 1983, The C.V. Mosby Co.

Table 3-15 Muscles that move the lower leg

Muscle	Origin	Insertion	Function	Innervation
Quadriceps femoris group				
Rectus femoris	Ilium (anterior, inferior spine)	Tibia (by way of patellar tendon)	Flexes thigh Extends leg	Femoral nerve
Vastus lateralis	Femur (linea aspera)	Tibia (by way of patellar tendon)	Extends leg	Femoral nerve
Vastus medialis	Femur	Tibia (by way of patellar tendon)	Extends leg	Femoral nerve
Vastus intermedius	Femur (anterior surface)	Tibia (by way of patellar tendon)	Extends leg	Femoral nerve
Sartorius	Os innominatum (anterior, superior iliac spines)	Tibia (medial surface of upper end of shaft)	Adducts and flexes leg Permits crossing of legs tailor fashion	Femoral nerve
Hamstring group				
Biceps femoris	Ischium (tuberosity)	Fibula (head of)	Flexes leg	Hamstring nerve (branch of sciatic nerve)
	Femur (linea aspera)	Tibia (lateral condyle)	Extends thigh	Hamstring nerve
Semitendinosus	Ischium (tuberosity)	Tibia (proximal end, medial surface)	Extends thigh	Hamstring nerve
Semimembranosus	Ischium (tuberosity)	Tibia (medial condyle)	Extends thigh	Hamstring nerve

From Anthony, C.P., and Thibodeau, G.A.: Textbook of anatomy and physiology, ed. 11, St. Louis, 1983, The C.V. Mosby Co.

Table 3-16 Muscles that move the foot

Muscle	Origin	Insertion	Function	Innervation
Tibialis anterior	Tibia (lateral condyle of upper body)	Tarsal (first cuneiform) Metatarsal (bone of first)	Flexes foot Inverts foot	Common and deep peroneal nerves
Gastrocnemius	Femur (condyles)	Tarsal (calcaneus by way of Achilles tendon)	Extends foot Flexes lower leg	Tibial nerve (branch of sciatic nerve)
Soleus	Tibia (underneath gastrocnemius) Fibula	Tarsal (calaneus by way of Achilles tendon)	Extends foot (plantar flexion)	Tibial nerve
Peroneus longus	Tibia (lateral condyle) Fibula (head and shaft)	First cuneiform Base of first metatarsal	Extends foot (plantar flexion) Everts foot	Common peroneal nerve
Peroneus brevis	Fibula (lower two thirds of lateral surface of shaft)	Fifth metatarsal (tubercle, dorsal surface)	Everts foot Flexes foot	Superficial peroneal nerve
Tibialis posterior	Tibia (posterior surface) Fibula (posterior surface)	Navicular bone Cuboid bone All three cuneiforms Second and fourth metatarsals	Extends foot (plantar flexion) Inverts foot	Tibial nerve
Peroneus tertius	Fibula (distal third)	Fourth and fifth metatarsals (bases of)	Flexes foot Everts foot	Deep peroneal nerve

From Anthony, C.P., and Thibodeau, G.A.: Textbook of anatomy and physiology, ed. 11, St. Louis, 1983, The C.V. Mosby Co.

NERVOUS SYSTEM

A. Adapts to environmental influences by stimulating skeletal, cardiac, and smooth muscle; adaptation by the muscle system is almost immediate
1. Responds to various stimuli (chemical, electrical, mechanical, and thermal)
2. Stimulus must be at least at the threshold or liminal level; that is the weakest stimulus that will cause a response (Fig. 3-11)
   a. Subthreshold stimulus is below the threshold level and will not produce an effect
   b. Maximal stimulus causes the maximum response; if a higher stimulus is given, the same response will be produced
   c. Submaximal threshold is less than a maximal stimulus but greater than a threshold stimulus
3. Basic requirements for a stimulus to be effective
   a. It must be sufficient strength
   b. It must be applied for a minimal duration of time
   c. It must produce a rapid rate of change in the environment
B. Organized into various systems
1. Central nervous system (CNS) consists of the brain and spinal cord
2. Peripheral nervous system (PNS) contains the nerves to and from the body wall, which connect to the CNS; also known as the somatic division, since it is under voluntary control
3. Autonomic nervous system (ANS) is not under conscious control (involuntary); provides stimulus for the viscera and smooth and cardiac muscle
   a. Sympathetic division (thoracolumbar) involves motor (afferent) nerves from the ANS
   b. Parasympathetic division (craniosacral) involves motor (efferent) nerves from the ANS
4. Nerve cell is called a neuron
   a. Structure
      (1) Cell body or soma contains a nucleus (which has a distinct nucleal pattern); is not capable of reproducing nerve cells
      (2) Neurofibrils are threadlike fibers in the interior of the nerve cells; contain typical cytoplasm structures plus Nissl granules (clusters of ribonucleic acid [RNA])
      (3) Dendrite carries impulse toward the cell body under normal conditions

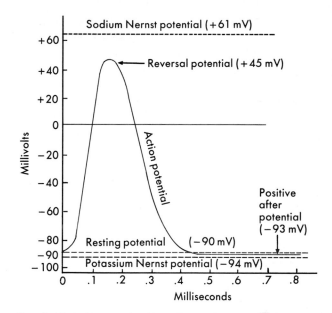

Fig. 3-11 Action potential. (From Guyton, A.C.: Textbook of medical physiology, ed. 6, Philadelphia, 1981, W.B. Saunders Co.)

      (4) Axon carries impulse away from the cell body and makes contact with the next cell at the button that contains chemicals in vesicles; release of chemicals starts impulse in the next neuron
      (5) Myelin sheath is a fatty substance around some cell axons; provides insulation
         (a) Myelin is laid down by Schwann cells in layers
         (b) Neuron must have a neurilemma to regenerate
         (c) Nodes of Ranvier are between myelin segments and are unmyelinated
   b. Neurons can carry impulses in different directions
      (1) Afferent neurons carry the sensory information to the CNS
      (2) Efferent neurons carry the motor information away from the CNS
      (3) Central or internuncial neurons are found entirely within the CNS; relay information within the system
   c. Neurons have various numbers of processes
      (1) Unipolar—one process off of the cell body
      (2) Bipolar—two distinct processes arising from opposite poles of the cell body

(3) Multipolar—contain several processes, usually an axon and three or more dendrites

C. Nerve impulse results from a change in the membrane potential (Fig. 3-12)
1. Membrane potential results from the concentration difference of two ions on the inside and outside of the nerve
2. Inside the axon membrane

$$[K^+] = 141 \text{ mEq/L}$$
$$[Na^+] = 10 \text{ mEq/L}$$ at rest

3. Outside the axon membrane

$$[K^+] = 4 \text{ mEq/L}$$
$$[Na^+] = 137 \text{ mEq/L}$$ at rest

4. Balance is mostly maintained by the sodium pump; potassium pump is not very important in this phenomenon, since the membrane is extremely permeable to potassium
5. A void of positive electrons is created on the inside; leads to a state of electronegativity that gives a reading of −65 mV to −85 mV on the voltmeter
   a. Creates the depolarization wave or nerve impulse (+35 mV)
   b. Law of forward conduction—impulse can leave in only one direction
6. Vesicles in the buttons are ruptured; various chemicals are released to carry the impulse to the next neuron
   a. Acetylcholine is released at all preganglionic fibers of the ANS, at all postganglionic fibers of the parasympathetic division, at some of the sympathetic fibers of the parasympathetic division, and at all of the motor neurons at the myoneural junction (cholinergic fibers)
   b. Acetylcholine is destroyed by acetylcholinesterase so nerve stimulation will be for a definite amount of time
   c. Norepinephrine is released by the adrenergic fibers (most of the sympathetic postganglionic nerve fibers)
   d. Norepinephrine is destroyed by monoamine oxidase
7. Immediately after the depolarization wave the nerve is repolarized because the membrane becomes impermeable to sodium ions, but potassium can diffuse back in the membrane; this high potassium concentration causes the positive electrons to migrate outward, creating electronegativity inside the membrane
8. Refractory period—nerve will not react to another stimulus

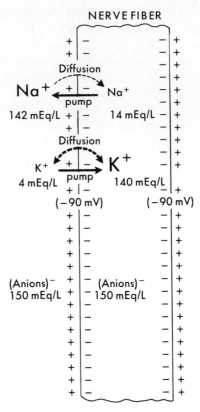

Fig. 3-12 Membrane potential. (From Guyton, A.C.: Textbook of medical physiology, ed. 6, Philadelphia, 1981, W.B. Saunders Co.)

   a. Absolute refractory period—will not react to any stimulus no matter how strong the stimulus; will extend through the depolarization stage
   b. Relative refractory phase—can produce a response if the stimulus is stronger than the original; starts at repolarization and prevents nerve impulses from piling up
9. Once an impulse begins, it remains constant throughout the nerve if it is healthy
   a. Greatest velocity will be over a coarse, myelinated nerve
   b. Least velocity will be over a fine, nonmyelinated nerve
   c. All-or-none principle in effect
   d. Graded response; the stronger the stimulus, the more impulses per second
10. Nerve impulses can be clocked by pressure, chemicals, or cold
   a. Sensory nerves are usually blocked before motor nerves
   b. Strychnine reduces resistance at the synapse; leads to convulsions
   c. Curare causes increased resistance at the synapse; produces paralysis

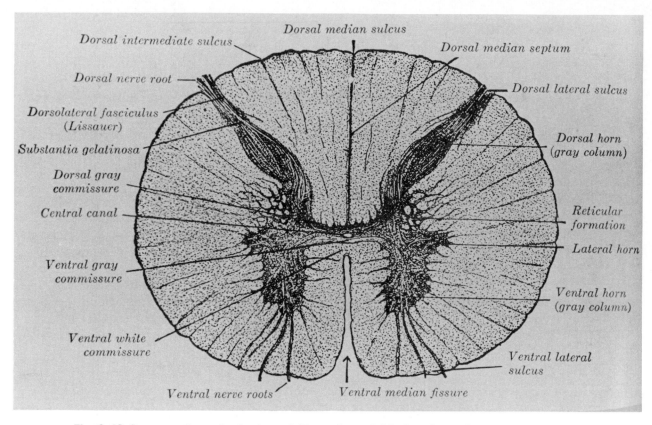

Dorsal median sulcus

Dorsal intermediate sulcus

Dorsal median septum

Dorsal nerve root

Dorsal lateral sulcus

Dorsolateral fasciculus (Lissauer)

Dorsal horn (gray column)

Substantia gelatinosa

Dorsal gray commissure

Reticular formation

Central canal

Lateral horn

Ventral gray commissure

Ventral horn (gray column)

Ventral white commissure

Ventral lateral sulcus

Ventral nerve roots

Ventral median fissure

Fig. 3-13 Cross section of spinal cord. (From Goss, C.M.: Gray's anatomy, American ed. 29, Philadelphia, 1973, Lea & Febiger.)

11. Nerves cannot store glycogen; need a constant supply of glycogen; can also function without oxygen for short periods

D. Spinal cord is approximately 45.8 cm long; occupies the upper two thirds of the vertebral canal
  1. Conus medullaris—pointed up where the spinal cord terminates between the L1 and L2 vertebrae
  2. Filum terminale—thin threadlike fiber from the coccyx to the spinal cord; acts as an anchor; has no nervous function
  3. Cauda equina—bundle of spinal nerve roots located below the L1 vertebra
  4. Has a unique structure in cross section (Fig. 3-13)

E. There are 31 pairs of spinal nerves; each has a dorsal (afferent) root and a ventral (efferent) root
  1. Spinal nerves come out of the spinal cord to form plexuses along the spinal cord except in the thoracic region
    a. Cervical plexus—first four cervical nerves innervate the muscles and skin of the upper chest; phrenic nerve originates here and innervates the diaphragm

    b. Brachial plexus—base of the neck; fifth to eighth cervical nerves and first thoracic nerve provide nerves to the shoulders and arms
      (1) Radial—lateral side of the arm
      (2) Medial—middle portion of the arm
      (3) Ulnar—medial side of the arm
    c. T2 to T12 compose the intercostal nerves; do not form a plexus
    d. Lumbrosacral plexus—includes L1 to S4
      (1) Lumbar portion—first four lumbar nerves contribute to the femoral nerve
      (2) Sacral portion—sacral nerves, last lumbar nerve, and coccygeal nerve supply the pelvis and legs; contribute to the sciatic nerve (largest nerve in the body)

F. Spinal cord acts as a relay and reflex center
  1. Reflex—unconscious response
  2. Reflex arc—structures over which the reflex impulses pass (Fig. 3-14)
  3. Conditioned reflex—becomes unconscious after repeated reinforcement (e.g., walking)
  4. Simple reflex—involves only one set of muscles

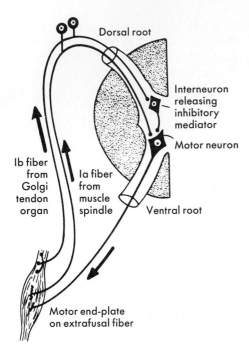

Fig. 3-14 Pathways responsible for stretch reflex. (From Ganong, W.F.: Review of medical physiology, ed. 11; copyright 1983 by Lange Medical Publications, Los Altos, Calif.)

5. Coordinated reflex—several reflexes performed in an orderly manner
6. Convulsive reflex—several reflexes performed in a random order
7. First-level spinal reflex—impulse enters the spinal cord and passes out of the same nerve
   a. Involves three neurons
      (1) Impulse picked up by the receptor and passed over to the afferent neuron (afferent neuron enters the spinal cord via the dorsal root)
      (2) In the posterior horn of the gray matter the afferent neuron synapses with the central or association neuron
      (3) Central neuron passes to the anterior horn and synapses with the efferent neuron
      (4) Efferent neuron leaves the spinal cord via the ventral root; passes to a muscle or gland and produces action
8. Second-level spinal reflex—impulse goes up or down the spinal cord; may involve the cerebellum or medulla
9. Third-level reflex—involves the cerebrum; most complex reflex arc

G. Fiber tracts are bundles of white fibers with the same origin (cell body location) and termination (axon button location) (Fig. 3-15)

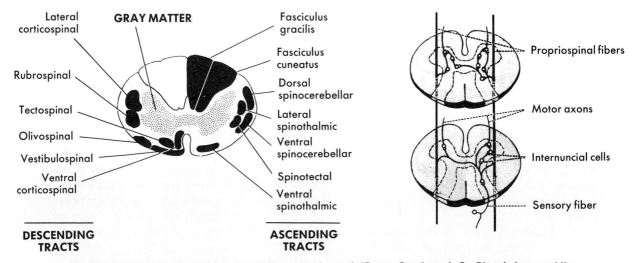

Fig. 3-15 Motor and sensory tracts in spinal cord. (From Guyton, A.C.: Physiology of the human body, ed. 5, Philadelphia, 1979, W.B. Saunders Co.)

1. All ascending fibers are afferent
   a. First-order neuron—associated with receptors; cell body located in the dorsal root ganglion
   b. Second-order neuron—passes up the spinal cord
   c. Third-order neuron—located in the brain; terminates in the outside layer of the cortex
2. All descending fibers are efferent
   a. Upper motor neurons—extend down the brain from the spinal cord and end in the ventral gray matter
   b. Lower motor neurons—cell body located in the ventral gray matter and goes out to muscles or glands
3. Ascending tracts
   a. Fasciculus gracilis—fibers from pressure and touch receptors; provides proprioception; involves first-order neurons
   b. Fasciculus cuneatus—first-order neurons pick up impulses from the skin; nerves travel up either side of the spinal cord to the medulla; make a synapse with a second-order neuron; this neuron crosses to the opposite side to the thalamus, synapses with a third-order neuron, and finally reaches the cerebral cortex
   c. Spinothalamic tract—second-order neurons cross over to the opposite side and can pass up the spinal cord
      (1) Ventral (nerves associated with touch)—synapses with the third-order neuron and ends in the cortex
      (2) Lateral (nerves associated with pain and temperature)—involves the second-order neurons that end in the thalamus
4. Descending tracts
   a. Lateral corticospinal—originates in the motor cortex; crosses over in the medulla and continues down the spinal cord on the opposite side (main mortor tract)
   b. Ventral corticospinal—crosses over (decussates) in the spinal cord; provides voluntary responses
   c. Rubrospinal—originates in the midbrain; decussates immediately and comes down on the opposite side of the brain (coordinates muscles to maintain balance)
H. Brain consists of four regions (Fig. 3-16)
   1. Cerebrum—seat of conscious activities; largest portion of brain; located most superiorly
      a. Cerebral cortex—thin, outside layer; gray color; consists of several layers of cells; convoluted surface
      b. Longitudinal fissure—divides into two hemispheres
      c. Corpus callosum—heavy band of white fibers; forms the floor of the longitudinal fissure
      d. Central fissure—posterior to the midline
      e. Frontal lobe—anterior to the central fissure
      f. Parietal lobe—posterior to the central fissure
      g. Temporal lobe—below the lateral fissure
      h. Occipital lobe—posterior part of the brain
      i. Broca's area—controls the muscular part of speech
      j. Somasthetic area—interprets body sensations
      k. Visual area—fibers from the medial part of the retina cross to opposite sides in the brain; fibers from the lateral portion do not cross
      l. Auditory area—superior central portion of the temporal lobe
      m. Prefrontal area—personality characteristics
      n. Asphasia—results from damage to the cerebral cortex
   2. Cerebellum—coordinates balance and equilibrium
      a. Cortex—consists of gray matter
      b. Vermis—bridgelike connection between the two hemispheres
      c. Arbor vitae—white matter in the cerebellum; similar to leaf veins
      d. Ataxia—results from damage to the cortex of the cerebellum
   3. Medulla oblongata—bulb of the spinal cord located inside the foramen magnum
      a. White on the outside; gray on the inside
      b. Controls three vital functions: cardiac, respiratory, and vasomotor
      c. Also controls mastication, salivation, swallowing, emesis, lacrimation, blinking, coughing, and sneezing
      d. Pons—ropelike mass of white fibers; connects the halves of the cerebellum
   4. Mesencephalon—short part of the brainstem above the pons—mostly white matter
      a. Tectum—four large ropelike masses
      b. Cerebral aquaduct—connects the third and fourth ventricles of the brain
      c. Corpora quadrigemina

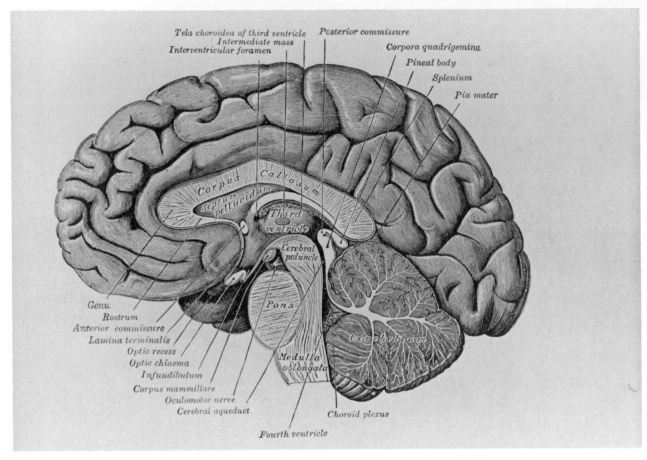

Fig. 3-16 Brain. (From Goss, C.M.: Gray's anatomy, American ed. 29, Philadelphia, 1973, Lea & Febiger.)

(1) Colliculus superior—inferior pair; synapse cranial nerves II and III

(2) Colliculus inferior—inferior pair; relay point of cranial nerve VIII

d. Cerebral peduncles—make up the ventral columns of white fibers

e. Reticular formation—acts as a clearing station for information; is associated with muscular movement; damage to this area results in coma

I. Meninges are the membranous coverings of the brain and spinal cord

1. Dura mater—double layers around the brain; single layer around the spinal cord including the cauda equina

2. Arachnoid—membrane just inside the dura mater; relatively thin; is attached via the arachnoid of cranial nerve VIII

3. Pia mater—soft covering that fits against the brain and spinal cord; contains an enormous amount of blood

   a. Leptomeninges—soft, delicate membrane; consists of the arachnoid and pia mater

   b. Subarachnoid space—threadlike structure where cerebrospinal fluid circulates; located between the pia mater and arachnoid

J. Cranial nerves are part of the PNS and originate at the base of the brain (Fig. 3-17); there are 12 pairs of cranial nerves, which can be referred to by name or by Roman numerals; can provide motor impulses, sensory impulses, or mixed impulses

1. Olfactory nerve (cranial nerve I)—provides the sensation of smell by innervating the olfactory epithelium of the nasal cavity

   a. Does not provide motor function

   b. Originates in the olfactory bulb of the brain; passes through the cribriform plate of the ethmoid bone

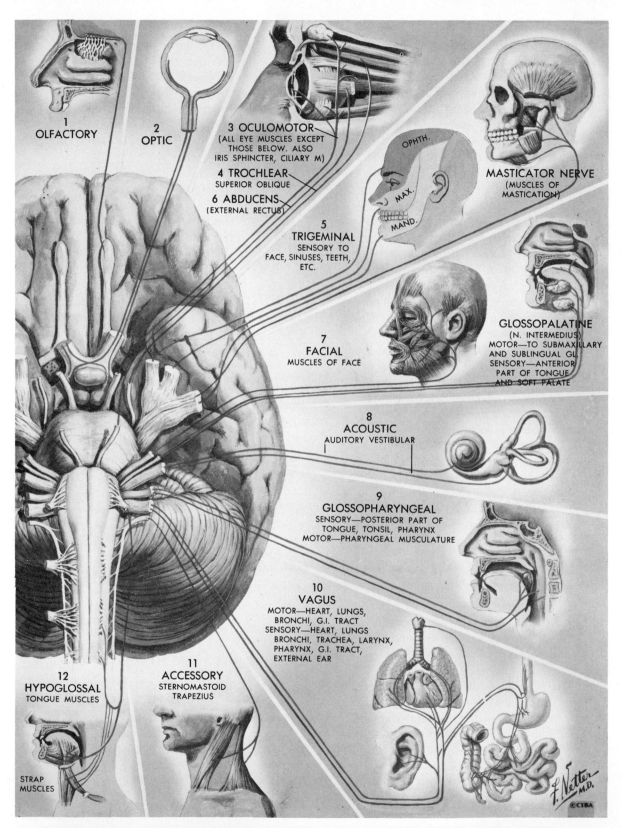

Fig. 3-17 Cranial nerves. (© Copyright 1972, CIBA Pharmaceutical Company, Division of CIBA-GEIGY Corporation. Reprinted with permission from The CIBA collection of medical illustrations, illustrated by Frank H. Netter, M.D. All rights reserved.)

2. Optic nerve (cranial nerve II)—innervates the retina of the eye with sensory neurons; provides the sensation of vision
   a. Does not provide motor function
   b. Originates from the base of the brain; forms two optic tracts that converge at the optic chiasma; passes through the optic canal (foramen)
3. Oculomotor nerve (cranial nerve III)—provides motor fiber for the ocular muscles and parasympathetic fibers for the ciliary gangion
   a. Primarily a motor nerve but contains some proprioceptive fibers from the brain
   b. Originates near the pons and enters the superior orbital fissure; has two divisions: superior and inferior
4. Trochlear nerve (cranial nerve IV)—smallest cranial nerve; supplies the superior oblique muscle of the eyeball
   a. Does not provide sensory function
   b. Originates near the optic tract; passes through the superior orbital fissure
5. Trigeminal nerve (cranial nerve V)—provides motor and sensory neurons
   a. Originates from two roots from the pons: a large sensory root and a small motor root
   b. Fibers are mixed in the trigeminal ganglion; produce three branches
      (1) Ophthalmic branch (cranial nerve V_1)—provides sensory fibers only; produces three nerves; passes through the superior orbital fissure
         (a) Lacrimal nerve
         (b) Nasociliary nerve
         (c) Frontal nerve
      (3) Maxillary branch (cranial nerve V_2)—provides sensory fibers only; produces several nerves; passes through the foramen rotundum to the pterygopalatine fossa (Table 3-17)
      (3) Mandibular branch (cranial nerve V_3)—provides motor and sensory fibers; produces several nerves; passes through the foramen ovale to the infratemporal fossa (Table 3-18)
6. Abducens nerve (cranial nerve VI)—provides motor fibers to the rectus lateralis muscle of the eyeball; passes through the superior orbital fissure
   a. Does not provide sensory fibers
   b. Originates at the inferior border of the pons

7. Facial nerve (cranial nerve VII)—has two roots of unequal size; provides motor and sensory fibers
   a. Originates at the base of the pons; emerges from the stylomastoid foramen
   b. Innervates the muscles of facial expression: the buccinator, platysma, stapedius, stylohyoid, and the posterior belly of the digastric muscles
   c. Provides fibers to the submandibular and sublingual salivary gland
   d. Provides the taste sensation in the anterior two thirds of the tongue (gives all sensations except bitter)
   e. Branches from the geniculate ganglion; greater petrosal nerve provides sensory fibers to the soft palate
   f. Branches from the pterygopalatine plexus; innervates the lacrimal glands and the mucous membrane of the nose and palate
   g. Branch of the facial nerve within the facial canal is the chorda tympani—unites with the lingual nerve (cranial nerve V_3) to provide taste to the anterior two thirds of the tongue
   h. Branches from the submandibular ganglion; innervates the submandibular and sublingual glands
   i. Branches of the facial nerve in the face and neck
      (1) Posterior auricular nerve supplies the occipital muscle
      (2) Digastric branch supplies the posterior belly of the digastric muscle
      (3) Stylohyoid branch supplies the stylohyoid muscle
      (4) Temporal branch supplies the frontalis, orbicularis oculi, and corrugator muscles
      (5) Zygomatic branches innervate the orbicularis oculi
      (6) Buccal branches supply the procerus, zygomaticus, levator labii superioris, buccinator, and orbicularis oris muscles
      (7) Mandibular branch supplies the muscles of the lower lip and chin
8. Acoustic nerve (cranial nerve VIII)—originates in the middle peduncle by the pons; passes through the internal auditory meatus
   a. Provides sensory nerve fibers only
   b. Vestibular nerve division innervates the semicircular canals of the ear; controls equilibrium
   c. Cochlear nerve innervates the cochlea; provides the sensation of sound

Table 3-17   Maxillary branch (V$_2$) of the trigeminal nerve

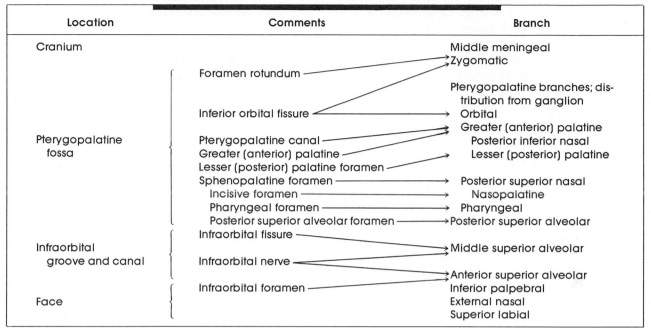

Location	Comments	Branch
Cranium		Middle meningeal
		Zygomatic
	Foramen rotundum	
		Pterygopalatine branches; distribution from ganglion
Pterygopalatine fossa	Inferior orbital fissure	Orbital
		Greater (anterior) palatine
	Pterygopalatine canal	Posterior inferior nasal
	Greater (anterior) palatine	Lesser (posterior) palatine
	Lesser (posterior) palatine foramen	
	Sphenopalatine foramen	Posterior superior nasal
	Incisive foramen	Nasopalatine
	Pharyngeal foramen	Pharyngeal
	Posterior superior alveolar foramen	Posterior superior alveolar
Infraorbital groove and canal	Infraorbital fissure	Middle superior alveolar
	Infraorbital nerve	Anterior superior alveolar
Face	Infraorbital foramen	Inferior palpebral
		External nasal
		Superior labial

Table 3-18   Mandibular branch (V$_3$) of the trigeminal nerve

Location	Comments	Branch
Main trunk	Foramen ovale	Nervus spinosus (ramus meninges)
	Foramen spinosum	Medial pterygoid (M)
		Tensor veli palatini
	Auditory tube	Tensor tympani (M)
Anterior division		Masseteric (M)
	Mandibular notch	Deep temporal (M)
		Lateral pterygoid (M)
		Long buccal (buccinator)
Posterior division		Auriculotemporal
		Otic ganglion — 6 branches
		Lingual nerve
		Chorda tympani (cranial nerve VII)
		Submandibular ganglion
		Hypoglossal (cranial nerve XII)
	Mandibular foramen	Inferior alveolar
	Mandibular canal	Mylohyoid (M)
		Dental branches
	Mental foramen	Mental and incisive (4)

M, Muscle.

9. Glossopharyngeal nerve (cranial nerve IX)—originates in the superior aspect of the medulla oblongata; passes through the jugular foramen
   a. Mixed nerve that provides taste to the posterior one third of the tongue, motor function to the muscles of the throat, and secretory fibers to the parotid salivary gland
   b. Tympanic nerve supplies the parotid gland and the mucous membrane covering of the middle ear; its continuation through the tensor tympani is known as the lesser petrosal nerve
   c. Carotid sinus nerve provides sensory fibers for the carotid sinus; main function is to monitor blood pressure
   d. Pharyngeal branches supply the muscular pharynx
   e. Tonsillar branch supplies the palatine tonsils
   f. Lingual branches innervate the circumvallate papillae
10. Vagus nerve (cranial nerve X)—has the widest distribution of any nerve in the body; is the dominant nerve to the heart; originates in the medulla oblongata; leaves the cranial cavity through the jugular foramen
    a. Provides sensory fibers to the larynx, lungs, arch of the aorta, and stomach; provides motor fibers to the heart, stomach, small intestine, larynx, esophagus, and gastric glands
    b. Right vagus nerve crosses the subclavian artery; forms the posterior pulmonary plexus by following the dorsal aspect of the lung; continues on to form the posterior vagus nerve
    c. Left vagus nerve passes between the left carotid and subclavian arteries; also forms a posterior pulmonary plexus on the dorsal surface of the lung; joins the right vagus nerve above the diaphragm to form the anterior vagus nerve
    d. Superior laryngeal nerve contributes motor and sensory fibers to the larynx
    e. Recurrent nerves—the right one loops under the subclavian artery and innervates the muscles of the larynx; the left one loops under the arch of the aorta and innervates all muscles of the larynx except one

f. Inferior cardiac branches innervate the cardiac muscle and great vessels
g. Esophageal branches innervate the esophagus
h. Branches continue through the abdominal cavity; form gastric, hepatic, and celiac branches
11. Accessory nerve (cranial nerve XI)—provides motor fibers to the muscles of the upper trunk region; consists of a cranial and spinal part
    a. Provides motor fibers to the muscles of the shoulder
    b. Cranial portion originates in the medulla oblongata and exits the cranial cavity through the jugular foramen; its fibers are distributed to the soft palate, pharynx, larynx, and esophagus
    c. Spinal part originates from the first five cervical segments of the spinal cord; pass up through the foramen magnum to join the cranial portion of cranial nerve XI; gives motor innervation to the sternocleidomastoid and trapezius muscles
12. Hypoglossal nerve (cranial nerve XII)—originates from the medulla oblongata and runs through the hypoglossal canal
    a. Provides motor fibers for the tongue muscles
    b. Forms the ansa cervicalis near the cricoid cartilage
K. ANS is the coordinator of internal actions; used to regulate (not initiate) the rate of internal action
   1. Sympathetic division (thoracolumbar) is located on either side of the spine
      a. Actions involve a great expenditure of energy
      b. Cell bodies of the preganglionic neurons are found in the gray matter of the spinal columns; are cholinergic in nature
      c. Cell bodies of the postganglionic neurons are found in the ganglia near the spinal cord; release norepinephrine as neurotransmitter substance fibers
   2. Parasympathetic division (craniosacral) is formed by nerves from the brain and sacrum
      a. This system is active except under stress
      b. Cell bodies of the preganglionic neurons are found in various nuclei of the brain and sacral segments of the spinal cord; use acetylcholine at the neurotransmitter junctions

Table 3-19 Autonomic nervous system

Visceral effector	Effect of sympathetic stimulation (neurotransmitter, norepinephrine unless otherwise stated)	Effect of parasympathetic stimulation (neurotransmitter, acetylcholine)
Heart	Increased rate and strength of heartbeat (beta receptors)	Decreased rate and strength of heartbeat
SMOOTH MUSCLE OF BLOOD VESSELS		
Skin blood vessels	Constriction (alpha receptors)	No parasympathetic fibers
Skeletal muscle blood vessels	Dilation (beta receptors)	No parasympathetic fibers
Coronary blood vessels	Dilation (beta receptors)	No parasympathetic fibers
Abdominal blood vessels	Constriction (alpha receptors)	No parasympathetic fibers
Blood vessels of external genitals	Ejaculation (contraction of smooth muscle in male ducts, e.g, epididymis and vas deferens)	Dilation of blood vessels causing erection in male
SMOOTH MUSCLE OF HOLLOW ORGANS AND SPHINCTERS		
Bronchi	Dilation (beta receptors)	Constriction
Digestive tract, except sphincters	Decreased peristalsis (beta receptors)	Increased peristalsis
Sphincters of digestive tract	Contraction (alpha receptors)	Relaxation
Urinary bladder	Relaxation (beta receptors)	Contraction
Urinary sphincters	Contraction (alpha receptors)	Relaxation
Eye		
Iris	Contraction of radial muscle; dilated pupil	Contraction of circular muscle; constricted pupil
Ciliary	Relaxation; accommodates for far vision	Contraction; accommodates for near vision
Hairs (pilomotor muscles)	Contraction produces goose pimples, or piloerection (alpha receptors)	No parasympathetic fibers
GLANDS		
Sweat	Increased sweat (neurotransmitter, acetylcholine)	No parasympathetic fibers
Digestive (salivary, gastric, etc.)	Decreased secretion of saliva; not known for others	Increased secretion of saliva
Pancreas, including islets	Decreased secretion	Increased secretion of pancreatic juice and insulin
Liver	Increased glycogenolysis (beta receptors); increases blood sugar level	No parasympathetic fibers
Adrenal medulla	Increased epinephrine secretion	No parasympathetic fibers

From Anthony, C.P., and Thibodeau, G.A.: Textbook of anatomy and physiology, ed. 11, St. Louis, 1983, The C.V. Mosby Co.

    c. Cell bodies of the postganglionic neurons are usually located near the organs that they innervate; release acetylcholine

3. Fight-or-flight mechanism prepares the body to deal with stresses; sympathetic and parasympathetic systems tend to produce opposite effects (Table 3-19)

SPECIAL SENSES

A. Eyeball is located in the orbital fossa for protection; is surrounded by fat
1. Eyelids—keep the eyes moist and clear; blinking reflex is controlled by the medulla
2. Eyelashes—shade the eyeball and protect it
3. Conjunctiva—thin mucous membrane that covers the front of the eye and lines the eyelid

4. Lacrimal glands—located bilaterally on the outer border of the orbital cavity; secrete about 1 ml of fluid per day; contain lysozyme to destroy bacteria
5. Nasolacrimal duct—carries fluid away from the gland
6. Contains intrinsic and extrinsic muscles of the eye
7. Parts of the eyeball
   a. Iris—colored part of the eye that is a circular diaphragm; regulates the amount of light that enters the eye
   b. Pupil—where light enters the eye; black in color
   c. Lens—biconvex disk without blood
   d. Sclera—white covering on the anterior aspect of the eye
   e. Vitreous body—colloid inside of the eyeball; maintains the shape
   f. Optic disk—located on the posterior surface of the eyeball; contains no rods or cones, only optic nerves
   g. Retina—contains cones in its center (fovea) and rods on the outer periphery
8. Physical process of forming an image on the retina is much like that used by a camera to produce a picture
   a. Light rays are bent as they enter the eye
   b. Lens adjust to the amount of light
   c. Light rays are converged on the fovea
   d. Rays cause changes in the chemistry of the rods and cones
   e. Optic nerve sends impulses to the occipital lobes of the brain
B. Ear controls the sense of hearing
   1. External ear consists of an ear flap
   2. Middle ear is separated by the tympanic membrane (eardrum); contains the malleus, incus, stapes, ossicles, and eustachian tube (to equalize pressure)
   3. Inner ear contains a vestibule, cochlea, and the semicircular canals
      a. Cranial nerve VIII innervates this structure
      b. Small hairs detect various frequencies and pitches; impulses are sent to the temporal lobes of the brain
      c. Semicircular canals maintain equilibrium
C. Tongue provides the sensation of taste
   1. Cranial nerve VII provides sensory fibers to the anterior two thirds of the tongue's tastebuds, fungiform, and foliate; sensations of sweet, sour, and salt are detected

2. Cranial nerve IX provides sensations of taste to the posterior one third of the tongue's circumvallate papillae; taste sensation of bitter is noted here
3. Food must be in solution in the mouth before the tastebuds can transfer the information to the brain
4. Most taste sensations are made up of various combinations of the four basic tastes
5. Olfactory system also provides sensory input to taste detection (cranial nerve I)
D. Olfactory sense is provided through the cranial nerve I
   1. Stimulates hairs (upper nasal cavity)
   2. Sensitive to slight odors
E. Sensation of touch is modulated by various nerve endings
   1. Meissner's corpuscles control the sensation of touch
   2. Pacinian corpuscles control the sensation of pressure
   3. Ruffini's corpuscles control the sensation of heat
   4. Krause's end bulbs control the sensation of cold
   5. Naked nerve fibers produce pain when stimulated

BLOOD

Blood is a connective tissue that originated from embryonic mesoderm
A. Serves the following body functions: nutrition, respiration, fluid balance, acid-base balance, excretion, protection, temperature regulation, and as an endocrine adjunct
   1. Whole blood has a specific gravity of 1.055 and a viscosity three to five times greater than that of water; makes up 9% of the total body; an adult has approximately 5 L of blood; pH remains fairly constant
   2. If whole blood is centrifuged in a test tube, various components can be separated out
      a. Plasma—clear straw color; at top (55%)
      b. White blood cells (WBCs)—white line in the center (less than 1%)
      c. Red blood cells (RBCs)—red color (45%)
   3. Hematocrit measures the volume of RBCs in blood by percent
      a. Women—less than 45%
      b. Men—greater than or equal to 45%
B. Consists of plasma and three cellular elements
   1. Erythrocytes (RBCs) transfer oxygen to the body and remove carbon dioxide
   2. Leukocytes (WBCs) are involved in the body's immune and protective function

3. Thrombocytes (platelets) are involved in blood coagulation
4. Plasma composes the fluid portion of the blood: 90% water plus 10% proteins and solids
   a. Serum albumin—important in maintaining osmotic pressure
   b. Globulins—important in maintaining osmotic pressure
   c. Fibrinogen—important for coagulation of blood; converted to fibrin to form the blood clot
   d. Nonprotein nitrogenous material (NPN)—amino acids and urea
   e. Nonnitrogenous materials—carbohydrates and fats
   f. Others—inorganic salts and bicarbonate buffers
C. Three types of cells (RBCs, WBCs, and platelets) in blood are unique in both their structure and functions
   1. Erythrocytes are biconcave disks that do not contain a nucleus; the advantages of a disk shape are that it allows for greater surface area for absorption and diffusion and allows for greater flexibility
      a. Cells stack up like coins (rouleaux formation) when they are out of circulation)
      b. Hematocrit is measured by a hemocytometer; is reported in millimeters cubed
         (1) Women—4.7 mm^3
         (2) Men—5.4 mm^3
      c. Elevation in the hematocrit is known as polycythemia; polycythemia vera is a serious pathologic condition pathologic condition that is often caused by a malignant tumor in the bone marrow and leads to sluggish blood, which damages the heart and other vessels
      d. Hemoglobin (Hb) is a functional part of the RBC and is a protein-pigment compound, a combination of acetic acid and glycine forms protoporphyrine; protoporphyrine plus one atom of iron produce the heme molecule; four heme molecules plus one globin form hemoglobin; each iron atom combines loosely with one molecule of oxygen to form oxyhemoglobin (HbO$_2$); this compound is very quick at combining and breaking down
         (1) Blood will appear bright scarlet if the tissue has less oxygen than the blood

         (2) Oxyhemoglobin breaks up and gives up the oxygen; becomes reduced hemoglobin (HHb), which looks blue through the tissue
         (3) Fetal hemoglobin (HbF) will pick up oxygen faster than adult hemoglobin (HbA)
      e. Formation of blood, erythropoiesis, occurs in the red bone marrow of the adult in the ribs, sternum, vertebrae, and angle of the mandible
      f. Effete RBCs are removed from circulation by the liver and spleen
   2. WBCs (leukocytes) average 7500/mm^3 in number
      a. An increase in WBCs is known as leukocytosis; a decrease is called leukopenia
      b. All WBCs have nuclei that aid in their identification
      c. Granulocytes are the most numerous
         (1) Neutrophils—most common with a polynuclear pattern; has an ameboid movement
         (2) Eosinophils—double-lobed nucleus with red granules; functions in detoxification
         (3) Basophils—S-shaped nucleus with blue granules; produces heparin
      d. Agranulocytes
         (1) Lymphocytes—large nucleus with a small amount of cytoplasm; involved in the immune system
         (2) Monocyte—C-shaped nucleus; function is to destroy necrotic tissue
   3. Thrombocytes (platelets) function in coagulation
      a. Fragments of megakaryocyte
      b. Average of 150,000 in the blood circulation
D. Blood clotting occurs when the platelets encounter rough, injured tissue (Fig. 3-18)
E. Erythrocytes carry antigens on their surfaces that make blood typing important; serum carries antibodies
   1. Type A blood carries the A agglutinogen; plasma carries the anti-B agglutinins
   2. Type B blood carries the B agglutinogen; plasma carries the anti-A agglutinins
   3. Type AB blood has the A and B agglutinogen; plasma does not carry any agglutinins
   4. Type O blood does not carry any agglutinogen; serum carries both the anti-A and anti-B agglutinins

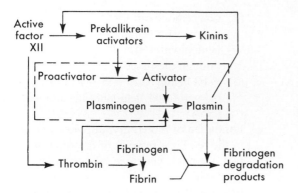

Fig. 3-18 Clotting scheme. (From Ganong, W.F.: Review of medical physiology, ed. 11; copyright 1983 by Lange Medical Publications, Los Altos, Calif.)

HEART

The heart is composed of cardiac muscle and serves to pump the blood through the circulatory system

A. Located behind the sternum; is the size of a human fist; the apex of the heart points down and to the left (Fig. 3-19)
1. Located in a space between the lungs in the thoracic cavity known as the *mediastinum*
2. Consists of four chambers: two atria and two ventricles
   a. Blood from the superior and inferior vena cava fills the right atria and passes into the right ventricle through the tricuspid valve (three flaps)
   b. From the right ventricle, the unoxygenated blood is sent to the lungs by passing through the semilunar valve and pulmonary artery
   c. Oxygenated blood is sent from the lungs to the left atria from the pulmonary veins; the left semilunar valve separates the left atria from the pulmonary veins
   d. From the left ventricle, the blood is sent to the aorta after passing through the mitral valve (two flaps) and the left ventricle
3. Heart wall consists of three layers
   a. Visceral pericardium or epicardium
   b. Myocardium—heaviest covering
   c. Endocardium—smooth continuous covering
   d. All valves and chambers are lined by endothelium
4. Valves of the heart are unique
   a. Antrioventricular (AV) valves—tough, fibrous tissue; open except when ventricles contract; hangs into the ventricle like a leaf; held in place by chordae tendinae at the edge of the valves
      (1) Tricuspid AV valve—three flaps form it

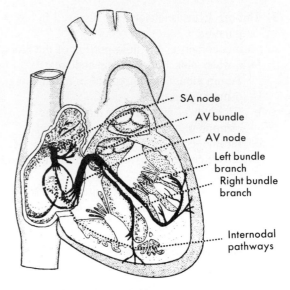

Fig. 3-19 Transmission of cardiac impulse. (From Guyton, A.C.: Physiology of the human body, ed. 5, Philadelphia, 1979, W.B. Saunders Co.)

      (2) Biscupid AV valve (mitral valve)—two parts form it
   b. Semilunar (SL) valves—pressure opens them, and reverse pressure closes them; remain closed until the ventricles contract
      (1) Pulmonary SL valve—located on the left
      (2) Aortic SL valve—located on the right
5. Heartbeat averages 70 to 72 beats per minute and cannot contract without nerve impulses; nerves regulate the rate of the beat
   a. Sinoatrial (SA) node—located in the wall of the right atrium near the superior vena cava; heartbeat begins here (Fig. 3-19)
      (1) From here, the action current spreads out and passes down to the fibrous layer and stops
      (2) Current goes through the AV node at the upper end of the interventricular septum
      (3) Modified cardiac muscle (bundle of His) divides into right and left branches
      (4) Along the AV bundle, fibers pass out into the cardiac muscle (Purkinje's fibers)
   b. Action current consists of the impulse starting at the SA node, spreads to the atria, passes to the AV node, is picked up and sent down through all the cardiac fibers from the Purkinje's fibers, and ends by spreading up over the ventricles; muscle contracts after the impulse spreads over the heart

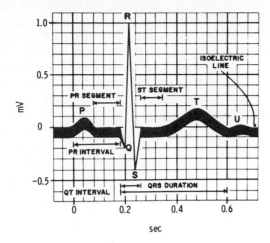

Fig. 3-20 QRS-T-P complex. (From Ganong, W.F.: Review of medical physiology, ed. 11; copyright 1983 by Lange Medical Publications, Los Altos, Calif.)

(1) Purkinje's fibers provide for uniform contraction

(2) If the AV node is blocked, ventricles will set up their own rhythm

5. Cardiac cycle consists of a relaxation-contraction cycle; lasts for approximately 0.8 seconds

a. SA node discharge begins the cycle

b. First isometric period—beginning of the atrial systole (contraction, very short in length); atria build up enough pressure to get the blood moving

c. Second isometric period—beginning of the atrial diastole (relaxation) and beginning of ventricular systole; AV valve is closed, and SL valve is open

d. At the beginning of ventricular systole the AV valve opens and the SL valve is closed

6. The heart sound is a ''lubb-dubb'' noise

a. First sound—AV valves close (louder, longer sound)

b. Second sound—SL valves close

c. Damage to the valves may yield stenosis (scarred), prolapse (limpness), or weakness (murmurs); dental hygienist may need to premedicate patients with antibiotics before starting any procedures that may produce a bacteremia; check with the guidelines established by the American Heart Association

7. Electrocardiogram is a record of the action current as it travels across the heart (Fig. 3-20)

a. P wave—depolarization of the atria

b. QRS complex—depolarization of the ventricles

c. T wave—repolarization of the ventricles

8. Starling's law—force of contraction is directly proportional to the initial tension of the muscle; allows for a more powerful contraction when blood piles up

a. Medulla—houses the cardiac control center

b. Right vagus nerve—most important nerve to the heart (goes to the SA node); left vagus nerve goes to the AV node

(1) Releases acetylcholine

(2) If the vagus nerve is injured, the heart rate increases

(3) Rapid vagus stimulation will stop the heart, but after a while vagal escape takes over and the heart begins to beat on its own

c. Sympathetic nervous system—first four thoracic spinal nerves (accessory nerves) contribute adrenergic fibers to the heart; affect the heart's irritability

(1) Stimulation leads to increased discharge from the SA node

(2) Produces more rapid, forceful contractions

9. Bainbridge's reflex—increase in the heart rate is initiated by an excess amount of blood returning to the right atrium; receptor cells in the right atrium are sensitive to pressure and stretch

a. Message is sent to the medulla via afferent fibers in the vagus nerve

b. This in turn causes efferent signals to be transmitted back through the vagus nerve

c. Final outcome will be to increase the heart rate and strength of the contractions

CIRCULATORY SYSTEM

The circulatory system involves the connection of the heart to the arteries, arterioles, capillaries, venules, and veins; the lymphatic system also interacts with this circulatory system

A. Arteries are thick-walled vessels that are elastic in nature; end in arterioles

1. Tunica adventitia is the outside layer; thicker in the large arteries; allows for stretch and recoil of the arteries

2. Tunica media contains the smooth muscle; circular pattern

3. Tunica intima is the innermost covering; continuous with the endocardium

4. Vasa vasorum are tiny capillaries that pass into the walls of the arteries and provide nourishment

B. Arteriole is the smallest branch of an artery; connected to venules by capillaries
C. Venules are connected to veins that carry blood toward the heart and carry unoxygenated blood (exception is the pulmonary vein)
D. Lymphatic system carries lymph; is involved in the maintenance of fluid pressure; contains lymph glands that filter out foreign particles
   1. Tissue fluid is located in the intracellular spaces and is derived from the blood; is constantly moving; similar to plasma without large proteins
   2. Lymph is tissue fluid that has been reabsorbed into the lymphatic vessels; these vessels begin blindly in the tissues; similar to capillaries except that they are much more permeable; lacteals are lymphatic capillaries in the intestines that are important for digestion
   3. Valves are necessary in the lymphatic system to keep fluid flowing in the right direction; most valves are located in the arms and legs where gravity is a problem
      a. If a person does not move around, lymph fluid will collect in the feet and hands
      b. Hydrostatic pressure forces fluid out
      c. Protein osmotic pressure tends to pick up fluid from the tissues
   4. Lymph nodes are spongy masses of tissue through which lymph filters; macrophages engulf foreign substances
   5. Lymphocytes are small WBCs that originate from stem cells
      a. T lymphocytes are involved in cell-mediated immunity
      b. B lymphocytes are involved in the humoral immune system
   6. Lymph nodes have more afferent vessels coming to the node than efferent vessels leaving the node
   7. An aggregate is a large number of lymph nodes in an area; usually named after a gland or organ
      a. Posterior auricular lymph nodes—located behind the ears
      b. Deep cervical lymph nodes—located around the sternocleidomastoid muscle
      c. Axillary lymph nodes—drain the chest and arm
      d. Inguinal lymph nodes—drain the legs
      e. Popliteal lymph nodes—located behind the knee
   8. Right lymphatic duct drains the upper right quadrant, right arm, and right side of the head and empties into the right subclavian vein
   9. Thoracic duct drains the rest of the body; begins at the cisterna chyli (bulblike enlargement at the L2 vertebra) and passes up the left side of the vertebral column through the aortic hiatus of the diaphragm into the left subclavian vein
   10. Lymphoidal tissue contains a spongelike network; found in various anatomic structures
      a. Spleen—contains the largest concentration of macrophages; the graveyard of RBCs
      b. Thymus—atrophies after puberty but is involved in the cell-mediated immune system
      c. Tonsils—located in the oral cavity
         (1) Palatine tonsils—located between the anterior and posterior pillars
         (2) Lingual tonsils—located on the posterior part of the tongue
         (3) Pharyngeal tonsils—located in the nasopharynx
         (4) Waldeyer's ring—formed by these structures; guards the opening to the digestive and respiratory systems
E. Veins have the same layers as arteries, except they are thinner
   1. Veins will collapse without blood
   2. Valves in the veins help to resist the forces of gravity
F. Capillaries connect small veins and small arteries; are lined by a thin layer of endothelium
   1. Metarterioles are the main pathways between the arterioles and venules; give rise to smaller capillary networks
   2. Networks have an average thickness of 1 μm
      a. Permeable to water but not to RBCs or large proteins
      b. Functional part of circulatory system; exchange center
   3. Capillaries can dilate or constrict, depending on the tissues' needs
   4. RBCs go through capillaries one cell at a time
   5. More active tissue has a greater number of capillaries
   6. Sinusoids are modified capillaries that are important in the liver, lymph nodes, and spleen
G. Arteriovenous shunt (anastomosis) is a large blood vessel that connects an arteriole and venule directly; thick walled; smooth muscle that surrounds it is controlled by a nerve
   1. Skin color is caused by blood in the capillaries and anastomoses; important for heat distribution
      a. Warm and red skin—capillaries constricted and anastomoses open

b. Warm and pale skin—capillaries constricted and anastomoses open

c. Cool and red skin—capillaries open and anastomoses closed

2. Only found in the hands, face, and toes where the body is exposed to weather

H. Arterial systemic circulation

1. Aorta arises from the left ventricle of the heart; first 5 cm is called the ascending aorta; two left and right coronary arteries branch off of it directly above the left semilunar valve and supply blood to the cardiac muscle

2. Aortic arch loops back over the top of the heart and left of the trachea; continues down in back of the heart; three arteries come off of the arch

a. Brachiocephalic artery—only a few centimeters in length

(1) Right subclavian artery (first branch) supplies blood to the right shoulder

(2) Right common carotid artery supplies blood to the right side of the head

b. Left common carotid artery supplies blood to the left side of the head

c. Left subclavian artery supplies branches to the upper chest and scapula

3. Descending aorta consists of the thoracic and abdominal sections of the aorta

a. Thoracic aorta starts after the left subclavian artery branches off the aortic arch and extends to the T4 vertebra; passes down and in front of the vertebral column and through the diaphragm

b. After it passes through the diaphragm, it is called the abdominal aorta; extends to the L4 vertebra; bifurcates into the left and right common iliac arteries

4. Carotid arteries supply the head; right carotid artery originates from the brachiocephalic artery; left carotid artery originates from the aortic arch (Fig. 3-21)

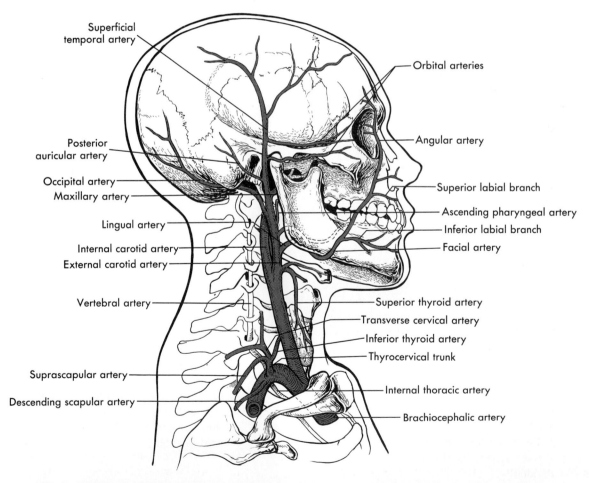

Fig. 3-21 Blood supply to head. (From McClintic, J.R.: Human anatomy, St. Louis, 1983, The C.V. Mosby Co.)

a. External carotid artery
   (1) Lingual artery—located from the branch to the tongue
   (2) Facial artery—comes out at an angle; serves the face
   (3) Occipital artery—located behind the scalp
   (4) Superficial temporal artery—main branch of the external carotid artery; moves into the scalp and toward the eye
   (5) External maxillary artery—branches off just below the ear; serves the face and part of the jaw; located in the mandibular canal and exits through the mental foramen
b. Internal carotid artery—supplies most of the blood for the brain and eye
   (1) Cervical part comes up the neck without branching; goes through the carotid foramen in the temporal bone
   (2) Ophthalmic artery supplies the eyeball, eye muscles, and lacrimal glands; middle cerebral artery provides blood for the temporal and lateral parietal lobes
   (3) Anterior cerebral artery passes forward through the longitudinal fissure where it joins other arteries to form the circle of Willis (Fig. 3-22)

5. Subclavian arteries provide blood to the shoulder and arms; left one comes from the aortic arch, right one from the brachiocephalic artery
   a. Pass over the first rib and under the clavicle
   b. Become the axillary artery as it passes through the shoulder region
   c. First branch off the subclavian artery is the vertebral artery, which passes up the neck through the transverse foramen of the cervical vertebrae and enters the skull through the foramen magnum; the two paired arteries join on the ventral side of the medulla and become the basilar artery (this artery joins branches from the internal carotid artery to form the circle of Willis) (Fig. 3-22)
   d. Axillary artery becomes the brachial artery at the humerus; moves along the medial surface across the elbow region and then divides

   (1) Radial artery moves along the radius and crosses it at the distal end (one can feel a pulse here); moves across the metacarpals and deep into the palm; forms a loop that connects with the ulnar artery
   (2) Ulnar artery travels down the medial surface of the forearm; becomes the superficial palmar artery that joins with the radial artery
   (3) Digital arteries supply the fingers and branch off from the palmar loop
6. Thoracic aorta gives off several branches
   a. Nine pairs of intercostal arteries serve the last nine ribs (subclavian artery serves the first three ribs)
   b. Two bronchial arteries supply the lungs
   c. One esophageal artery comes off the front part of the thoracic aorta and spreads into a network
   d. One or two superior phrenic arteries serve the upper surface of the diaphragm
7. Abdominal aorta gives rise to the visceral and parietal arteries
   a. Celiac artery—visceral artery that is 1.5 cm long and then divides
      (1) Left gastric artery—smallest branch to the stomach
      (2) Hepatic artery—supplies most of the blood to the liver; divides at the liver
         (a) Cystic artery—serves the gallbladder
         (b) Gastroduodenal artery—divides into the gastroepiploic artery (serves the stomach and pancreas) and the pancreaticoduodenal artery (serves the pancreas and duodenum)
      (3) Splenic artery—largest branch to the spleen
   b. Superior mesenteric artery—supplies all of the small intestine (except the duodenum) and superior ascending and transverse portions of the large intestine; comes off the front of the aorta below the celiac artery
   c. Inferior mesenteric artery—supplies blood for part of the transverse colon and all of the descending and sigmoid colon, rectum, and bladder

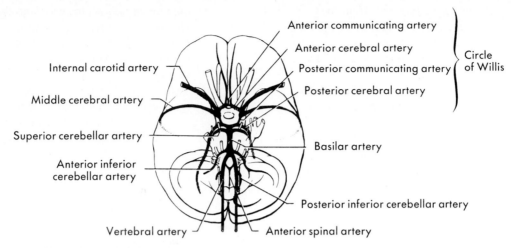

Fig. 3-22 Circle of Willis. (From Guyton, A.C.: Physiology of the human body, ed. 5, Philadelphia, 1979, W.B. Saunders Co.)

d. Renal artery—supplies the kidneys; located below the superior mesenteric artery
   (1) Right renal artery slightly longer and lower, since the aorta is slightly left of the midline
   (2) Enters the kidney at the hilus
e. Suprarenal artery—branches off the aorta above the renal artery (may be branches of the renal arteries)
f. Spermatic arteries—located below the renal arteries; pass through the inguinal canal
g. Ovarian arteries do not leave the abdominal cavity
h. Parietal artery branches off the thoracic aorta
   (1) Inferior phrenic artery—supplies the undersurface of the diaphragm
   (2) Lumbar arteries (four pairs)—opposite L1 to L4 vertebrae
   (3) Spinal arteries—serve the vertebral canal
i. Aorta terminates at the L4 vertebra
8. Aorta then divides and becomes the common iliac artery and then bifurcates again
   a. Internal iliac artery supplies the pelvic wall and viscera
   b. External iliac artery goes onto the leg
9. External iliac artery then passes over the pelvic brim and under the inguinal ligament; becomes the femoral artery
10. Just above the knee it becomes the popliteal artery and goes behind the knee to bifurcate
   a. Anterior tibial artery
   b. Posterior tibial artery

11. Anterior and posterior tibial arteries spread out at the ankle; become the dorsal artery of the foot
I. Venous systemic circulation
   1. Consists of one set of superficial veins and one set of deep veins
   2. Veins have a higher blood capacity than the arteries but have lower blood pressure and velocity than do the arteries
   3. Three sets of veins that connect to the heart
      a. Vena cava—serves the body; returns unoxygenated blood
      b. Coronary sinus—serves the heart; returns unoxygenated blood
      c. Pulmonary veins—serves the lung (two per lung); returns oxygenated blood to the left atria
   4. Superior vena cava begins at the level of the first rib; formed by two veins
      a. Left and right brachiocephalic veins (returns blood from the head, shoulders, and arms)
      b. Each brachiocephalic vein is a union of the internal jugular vein with the subclavian vein
   5. Jugular veins drain blood from the head
      a. External jugular vein drains the face and the scalp; is the union of three main veins (unite just below the ear and empties into the subclavian vein)
         (1) Superficial temporal vein
         (2) Posterior auricular vein
         (3) Posterior facial vein

b. Internal jugular vein returns from the internal carotid vein; originates in the skull
   (1) Begins as cerebral veins (drains cortex)
   (2) Superior sagittal sinus (center of falx cerebri)
   (3) Confluence of sinuses (just inside the external occipital protuberance)
   (4) Straight sinus (short vessel from the inferior sagittal sinus)—confluence of sinuses and passes laterally
   (5) Left and right transverse sinuses flow around the occipital bone to the temporal bone; become the sigmoid sinus, which eventually passes out the jugular foramen to become the internal jugular vein
6. Vertebral veins arise outside of the skull at the level of the atlas and pass through the transverse foramen to the subclavian artery
7. Arms and shoulders are drained by the deep veins that run alongside the arteries
   a. Palmar vein drains into the radial and ulnar veins, which drain into the brachial vein, which drains into the axillary vein, which drains into the subclavian vein
   b. Superficial veins—cephalic vein along the lateral forearm and arm drains into the axillary vein; basilic vein along the medial surface of the forearm drains into the brachial vein, which drains into the axillary vein
8. Inferior vena cava is formed by two common iliac veins at the L5 vertebra in front of the vertebral column; goes through the diaphragm via the caval opening
   a. Azygous vein branches off the inferior vena cava at the level of the renal veins; goes through the aortic hiatus of the diaphragm just above the heart and empties into the superior vena cava; picks up veins from the esophagus and bronchi
      (1) Esophageal vein
      (2) Bronchial vein
      (3) Intercostal vein
   b. Parietal veins—four pairs of lumbar veins, one sacral vein, and two inferior phrenic veins that empty into the inferior vena cava
   c. Renal veins (visceral) return blood from the kidneys; right renal vein is shorter than the left renal vein
   d. Ovarian or spermatic veins—located just below the renal veins
      (1) Paired veins
      (2) One set appears only in females, the other only in males
   e. Suprarenal veins—located from the adrenal glands to the inferior vena cava
   f. Hepatic vein returns blood from the liver to the inferior vena cava; part of the hepatic portal system
   g. Veins of the lower extremities
      (1) Deep veins have same names as the arteries; plantar vein drains into the anterior and posterior tibial veins, which drain into the popliteal veins, which drain into the femoral veins, which drain into the external iliac vein, which drains into the common iliac vein
      (2) Superficial veins
         (a) Great saphenous vein drains the dorsalis pedis area of the foot
         (b) Small saphenous vein drains the lateral side of the foot
         (c) Popliteal vein drains the lateral side of the leg
      (3) Connections exist between the deep and superficial veins along their paths

BLOOD PRESSURE

A. Pressure created by the force of the blood against the vessel walls in a closed system
   1. Highest in the arteries and lowest in the capillaries
   2. Pressure created in the veins is between the valves of the arteries and capillaries
B. Velocity of the blood flow is inversely related to the total cross-sectional area of the blood vessels
C. Five factors essential for maintaining the blood pressure
   1. An increase in cardiac output, especially ventricular systole, will lead to an increase in blood pressure
   2. The greater the peripheral resistance inside the blood vessels, the higher the blood pressure
   3. An increase in the volume of blood will cause an increase in blood pressure
   4. A decrease in the elasticity of the arterial walls will lead to an increase in blood pressure
   5. An increase in the viscosity of blood will cause an increase in blood pressure
D. Methods for measuring the pressure inside the vessel wall
   1. Direct method (uses a cannula)
      a. Cannula is inserted into a blood vessel
      b. When the pressure rises, a thin membrane inside of the cannula bulges outward; electric sensor detects the movement

c. Information regarding the rate and frequency of the movements produced on the membrane are recorded on a moving sheet of paper
2. Indirect method (involves the auscultatory method)
   a. Cuff with an inflatable bladder is placed around the upper arm
   b. Cuff is attached to either a mercury or aneroid monometer so the pressures can be measured
   c. Cuff is inflated until sounds can no longer be heard through a stethoscope that has been placed over the brachial artery
   d. Air is gradually released until the pressure in the cuff is great enough to close the artery during part of the arterial pressure cycle; Korotkoff sounds are heard
   e. Systolic pressure is noted when the Korotkoff sounds are first noted
   f. Diastolic pressure is noted when the Korotkoff sounds become muffled
   g. Blood pressure is reported with the systolic reading over the diastolic reading in millimeters of mercury (average 120 mm Hg/80 mm Hg)
   h. Pulse pressure is the difference between the systolic pressure and the diastolic pressure
3. Factors affecting the blood pressure
   a. Age (newborn 40 mm Hg/20 mm Hg)
      (1) Onset of puberty leads to a sharp increase in blood pressure
      (2) Continued increase in blood pressure as age increases; increase is greater in systolic reading
   b. Exercise can increase the blood pressure; rest can decrease the blood pressure
   c. Weight gain can cause an increase in the blood pressure, since the extra fat around the blood vessels will not allow them to expand; will also be more capillaries to serve the adipose tissue, leading to an increased amount of resistance created
   d. Disturbing emotions can cause a drop in blood pressure, leading to a decreased blood and oxygen supply to the brain and producing syncope (fainting)
   e. Pathologic changes can lead to hypertension
      (1) Primary or essential hypertension is seen with an increase in age usually resulting from a loss of elasticity in the arteries or atherosclerosis
      (2) Secondary or renal hypertension is more serious; usually associated with damaged kidneys

      (3) Essential hypertension has an unknown cause; exhibits a very strong hereditary tendency
      (4) As the blood passes through the various vessels, blood pressure changes
         (a) Average systolic pressure in the arteries—100 to 120 mm Hg
         (b) Average systolic pressure in the arterioles—30 to 70 mm Hg
         (c) Average systolic pressure in the capillaries—17 to 30 mm Hg
         (d) Average systolic pressure in the veins—0 to 17 mm Hg
E. Factors affecting pressure in the veins
   1. Force produced during ventricular contraction
   2. Vacuum created through the dilation of the ventricles
   3. Gravity and massaging action created by the contraction of the muscles
   4. Respiratory pump created during inhalation that causes a drop in pressure in the lungs and allows the blood to flow into the lungs
   5. Pressure almost at zero in the veins connected to the heart (therefore the blood flows through the veins toward the heart)
F. Blood pressure is controlled by the vasomotor center in the medulla; consists of two parts
   1. Vasoconstrictor system has a dominant role unless another stimulus overcomes it
   2. Vasodilator system is less dominant; even when it is in control, some vessels in the body remain constricted
G. Carotid sinus reflex also controls the blood pressure
   1. Carotid sinus is located where the internal and external carotid arteries branch
   2. Carotid sinus is composed of nerve endings that are sensitive to pressure; impulses are sent to the vasomotor system via the glossopharyngeal nerve (cranial nerve IX)
   3. Pressure on the sinus will result in vasodilation and a slowing of the heart rate
H. Marey's law states that there is an inverse relationship between the heart rate and the blood pressure
I. Chemical and hormonal regulators of blood pressure
   1. If body tissues are not receiving enough oxygen, the capillaries will automatically dilate
   2. Levels of carbon dioxide control both the rate of respiration and blood pressure
   3. Carbon dioxide acts to dilate the vessels and leads to a decrease in blood pressure

4. Angiotensin II is a very active enzyme that works on the arterioles to cause a rise in the blood pressure
   a. Stimulates the sympathetic nervous system
   b. Causes aldosterone to be released, which causes the kidneys to retain salt and water, thus causing an increase in blood pressure
   c. If the kidney becomes ischemic, this will lead to an increased production of renin that will intensify the effects of angiotensin II and aldosterone
5. Oxytocin, antidiuretic hormone, and epinephrine also raise the blood pressure

RESPIRATORY SYSTEM

The respiratory system performs two functions for the body: supplies oxygen to the tissues and removes carbon dioxide from the tissues
A. Respiration is the sum of the processes concerned with gaseous reception, distribution, and elimination; involves gaseous oxygen, carbon dioxide, and nitrogen
   1. External respiration—exchange of gases between the air sacs of the lungs and the bloodstream
   2. Internal respiration—exchange of gases between the bloodstream and tissue cells of the body
   3. Cellular respiration—use of oxygen within the cell

B. Respiratory quotient (RQ) is the ratio of the volume of carbon dioxide liberated to the volume of oxygen used
   1. RQ in the use of carbohydrates is 1
   2. RQ in the use of fats is 0.7
   3. RQ in the use of proteins is approximately 0.8
C. Respiratory tract begins at the nostril opening and extends to the alveoli of the lungs (Fig. 3-23)
   1. Air is drawn in through the nose, where it is warmed, humidified, and cleansed
   2. Nasal cavity is lined with olfactory epithelium in the sphenoethmoidal recess and by respiratory epithelium in the lower part
   3. Superior, middle, and inferior turbinates are located on the lateral surface of the nasal cavity
   4. Frontal, ethmoidal, maxillary, and sphenoidal paranasal sinuses empty into the nasal cavity
   5. Pharynx is the second part of the respiratory tract; starts at the base of the skull and extends to the esophagus; divided into three parts
      a. Nasopharynx—located behind the nasal cavity
         (1) Eustachian tube connects the middle ear with the pharynx; open only during swallowing; functions to equalize the pressure
         (2) Pharyngeal tonsils (adenoids)—located on the upper back wall of the nasopharynx; is a mass of lymphoid tissue

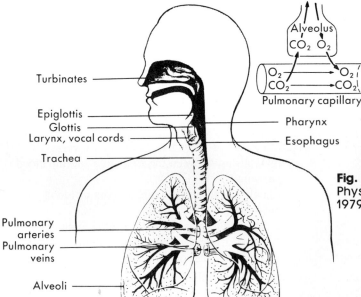

Fig. 3-23 Respiratory system. (From Guyton, A.C.: Physiology of the human body, ed. 5, Philadelphia, 1979, W.B. Saunders Co.)

b. Oropharynx extends from the soft palate to the base of the tongue; separated from the oral cavity by the palatine arches

c. Laryngopharynx extends from the hyoid bone to the larynx

6. Larynx is located at the base of the tongue; made up of nine cartilages: three single cartilages and three pairs of cartilage that are held together by membranes and ligaments

   a. Thyroid cartilage—largest cartilage; one on each side—fuse at the anterior surface to form one continuous cartilage; thyroid gland rests on the lower part of the cartilage

   b. Cricoid cartilage forms a signet-ring shape; attached by membranes to the upper part of the trachea

   c. Arytenoid cartilages—small, paired cartilages that are shaped like pyramids and located on the back of the larynx; serve as points of attachment for the vocal cords

   d. Other cartilages are the corniculate and cuneiform cartilages

   e. Epiglottis—large leaf-shaped cartilage that attaches to the thyroid cartilage and extends toward the base of the tongue; during swallowing the larynx comes up and the epiglottis folds over it to protect it

7. Vocal cords are folds of mucous membranes with elastic connective tissue at the edges

   a. Connective tissue tightens via the arytenoid cartilage; air passes through the glottis; vibrations for sounds are made from the true vocal cords

   b. False vocal cords protect against the entrance of food and water into the trachea

8. Trachea is approximately 12 cm long; located in front of the esophagus; composed of several C-shaped rings that prevent its collapse; lined with ciliated epithelium that beats upward

9. At the level of the T4 vertebra the trachea divides into left and right branches known as the primary bronchi

   a. Left primary bronchi is longer than the right; forms a sharp angle

   b. Right primary bronchi has a larger diameter than the left; comes off almost forming a straight line

10. Secondary bronchi branch off of the primary bronchi

    a. Three secondary bronchi for the right lung (one per lobe)

    b. Two secondary bronchi for the left lung (one per lobe)

11. Tertiary bronchi branch off the secondary bronchi; 10 tertiary bronchi per lung, since there are ten segments per lung

12. Bronchioles are smaller branches of the tertiary bronchi; surrounded by smooth muscle

    a. Terminal bronchioles—1 mm in diameter; do not contain cartilage for support; not involved in gaseous exchange

    b. Respiratory bronchioles—branch off of the terminal bronchioles; first site of diffusion of oxygen into the blood

13. Alveolar ducts branch off the respiratory bronchioles; alveolar sacs attach to the alveolar ducts

14. Surfactant is produced by pneumocytes

    a. Lipoprotein that is formed along the alveolar wall

    b. Acts to decrease surface tension and allows the lungs to expand

D. Two cone-shaped lungs in the thoracic cavity; base rests on the diaphragm, and the apex is located at the level of the clavicle

   1. Right lung has three lobes: superior, middle, and inferior; is larger than the left lung

   2. Left lung is smaller than the right lung, since two thirds of the heart is located on the left side and it contains only two lobes

   3. Ten bronchopulmonary segments per lung

      a. Each one has a branch from the tertiary bronchi

      b. Used as points of reference for surgery

   4. Cardiac notch is a depression on the medial surface of the lungs

   5. Point of attachment to a lung is designated as the hilus

      a. Blood vessels, bronchiole tree, and nerves enter at the hilus

      b. Hilus is located in the cardiac notch

   6. Pleura is the serous membrane surrounding the visceral and parietal layers of each lung

      a. Space between the two layers is the pleural cavity

      b. Lungs are not located in the pleural cavity

E. Mechanics of respiration involve changing the pressure in the lungs to cause inspiration or expiration (Fig. 3-24)

   1. Inspiration occurs when the air pressure in the lungs is decreased; causes the volume of the lungs to increase

      a. External intercostal muscles cause the ribs to elevate; increase the size of the chest cavity

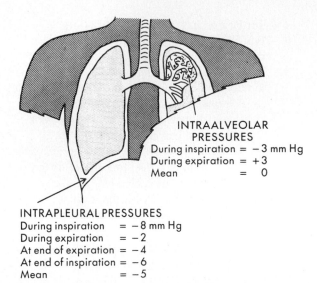

INTRAALVEOLAR
PRESSURES
During inspiration = −3 mm Hg
During expiration = +3
Mean   = 0

INTRAPLEURAL PRESSURES
During inspiration   = −8 mm Hg
During expiration   = −2
At end of expiration = −4
At end of inspiration = −6
Mean   = −5

Fig. 3-24 Alveolar and intraalveolar pressures in lung. (From Guyton, A.C.: Physiology of the human body, ed. 5, Philadelphia, 1979, W.B. Saunders Co.)

    b. Dome-shaped diaphragm (between the thoracic and abdominal cavity) pulls downward when contracted; will also increase the size of the chest cavity

2. Expiration is basically a passive movement; ribs fall down, and the diaphragm is pushed up by the abdominal viscera
    a. Abdominal muscles force the abdominal contents upward
    b. Internal intercostal muscles pull the ribs downward

3. During inspiration the enlargement of the thoracic cavity decreases the pressure in the alveoli to −3 mm Hg; therefore pulls air inside the lung; during expiration the opposite effects occur—the pressure in the alveoli increases to +3 mm Hg, pushing the air outside of the lung

4. Intrapleural pressure is always negative
    a. During inspiration the pressure is equal to −8 mm Hg
    b. During expiration the pressure is equal to −2 mm Hg

5. Differences in the alveolar and intrapleural pressures cause the lungs to pull away from the thoracic cage and cause a negative pressure

6. Malfunctions that can occur in the respiratory system
    a. Pneumothorax—when the chest wall is punctured, air enters the pleural cavity, causing the lung(s) to collapse

    b. Dyspnea—difficult or labored breathing
    c. Apnea—cessation of breathing
    d. Hypernea—increased respiration
    e. Orthopnea—person can breathe better in one position than another
    f. Cheyne-Stokes respiration—abnormal periodic respiration that consists of a long period of apnea followed by a short burst of hypernea followed by apnea

F. Normal lungs always contain air during breathing; amount of air can be measured with a spirometer
1. Tidal volume—air that passes in and out of the lungs
    a. Approximately 500 ml of air
    b. Normal rate of respiration is about 12 times per minute
2. Inspiratory capacity—amount of air that a person can take into the lungs beyond the amount brought in by the first breath; about 3000 ml
3. Expiratory reserve volume—amount of air that one can exhale after normal expiration; about 1100 ml
4. Residual volume—air that is left in the lungs after the most forceful expiration; about 1200 ml
5. Vital capacity—greatest amount of air that one can exchange in a forced respiration; approximately 4500 ml
6. Hering-Breuer reflex prevents overinflation of the lungs
    a. Pressure receptors located in the lungs are stimulated with inhalation and expansion
    b. Stimuli are sent over the afferent vagus nerve to the respiratory control centers
    c. When stimuli reach the critical level, inspiration ceases and expiration ceases (unless one holds his breath)
7. Carbon dioxide concentration in the blood is the most important stimulus; respiratory control center
    a. Direct—blood passes through the respiratory center
    b. Indirect—chemoreceptors in the aortic arch and carotid sinuses are stimulated by an increase in the carbon dioxide content, causing a nerve reflex to stimulate the respiratory center
    c. Four percent carbon dioxide in inhaled air leads to doubled respiratory rate; 20% carbon dioxide in inhaled air leads to loss of consciousness; 40% carbon dioxide in inhaled air leads to death

Table 3-20 Gaseous composition
of air involved in respiration

	Inspired (%)	Alveolar (%)	Expired (%)
Oxygen	20.84	13.6	16.3
Carbon dioxide	0.15	5.3	4
Nitrogen	79	75	79.7

Modified from Guyton, A.C., Physiology of the human body, ed. 5, Philadelphia, 1979, W.B. Saunders Co.

8. Cyanosis occurs when there is an excess amount of reduced hemoglobin (HHb) in the capillary circulation; causes the skin to turn blue
9. Anoxia occurs when an inadequate amount of oxygen is being received by the tissues
   a. Anoxic anoxia—decreased pressure in the lungs
   b. Anemic anoxia—blood has decreased oxygen-carrying power
   c. Stagnant anoxia—poor circulation
   d. Histiocytic anoxia—tissue cells are poisoned, making them incapable of picking up oxygen
G. Air that we breathe consists of several different gases and some water (Table 3-20)
   1. Each gas exerts pressure against the walls surrounding it (known as the partial pressure of a gaseous mixture); the greater the partial pressure of a gas, the greater the rate of diffusion of the gas through the pulmonary membrane
   2. Alveolar air constantly loses oxygen to the blood; blood allows diffusion of carbon dioxide into the alveolar air space
   3. Pulmonary membrane is thin; composed of surfactant and epithelial cells; allows for rapid diffusion of gases
   4. Gases pass through the membrane; follow the law of diffusion
   5. Oxygen is picked up in the blood (from the lungs) and forms oxyhemoglobin (HbO$_2$); blood leaving the lungs is saturated with oxygen and carries oxygen (20 ml oxygen/100 ml blood) to the tissues with decreased oxygen pressure; oxygen splits away from the hemoglobin and creates reduced hemoglobin; blood returning to the lungs has 15 ml oxygen/100 ml blood (Fig. 3-25)
   6. Oxygen is loaded and unloaded with the use of hemoglobin

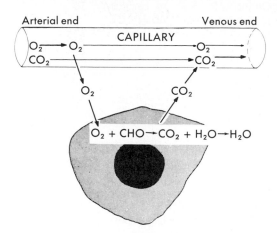

Fig. 3-25 Diffusion of oxygen from capillary to tissues. (From Guyton, A.C.: Physiology of the human body, ed. 5, Philadelphia, 1979, W.B. Saunders Co.)

   a. Loading tension (t_L)—oxygen tension in lungs will produce 97% saturation of blood; same as normal pressure in the lungs: 97 mm Hg
   b. Unloading tensions (t_U)—blood has given up 50% oxygen—oxygen pressure in tissues is approximately equal to 30 mm Hg; venous blood unloads faster than arterial blood (part of hemoglobin molecule)
7. When iron is in the ferric state, it is unable to carry and release oxygen normally (methemoglobin)
8. Carbon dioxide is carried away from the tissues to the lungs to be expired; most carbon dioxide is carried in the form of the bicarbonate ion (HCO$_3^-$); chloride shift uses carbonic anhydrase (c-a) to form carbonic acid

$$(CO_2 + H_2) \underset{}{\overset{c\text{-}a}{\rightleftarrows}} (H_2CO_3)$$

9. Small amounts of carbon dioxide are dissolved in the blood or carried away in carbaminohemoglobin

DIGESTIVE SYSTEM

A. Digestive or alimentary tract consists of a tube 6 m long from the mouth to the anus; selectively absorbs nutrients and water for the body (Fig. 3-26)
B. Mouth—location where food processing and digestion commences
   1. Secondary teeth (32 in the adult) tear and grind the food
   2. Tongue—fibromuscular organ that contains the taste buds; transmits the sensation of taste to the brain; rolls the food into a bolus for swallowing

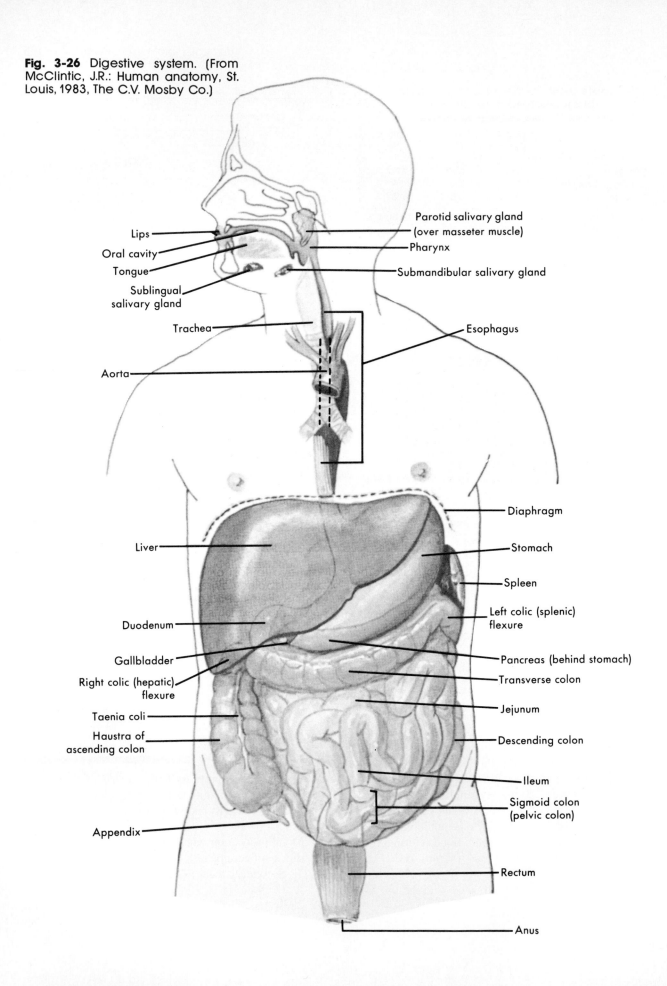

Fig. 3-26 Digestive system. (From McClintic, J.R.: Human anatomy, St. Louis, 1983, The C.V. Mosby Co.)

Lips

Oral cavity

Tongue

Sublingual salivary gland

Trachea

Aorta

Parotid salivary gland (over masseter muscle)

Pharynx

Submandibular salivary gland

Esophagus

Diaphragm

Liver

Stomach

Spleen

Left colic (splenic) flexure

Duodenum

Gallbladder

Right colic (hepatic) flexure

Taenia coli

Haustra of ascending colon

Appendix

Pancreas (behind stomach)

Transverse colon

Jejunum

Descending colon

Ileum

Sigmoid colon (pelvic colon)

Rectum

Anus

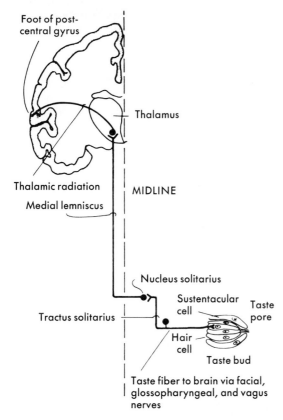

Foot of post-
central gyrus

Thalamus

Thalamic radiation

Medial lemniscus

MIDLINE

Nucleus solitarius

Sustentacular
cell

Taste
pore

Tractus solitarius

Hair
cell

Taste bud

Taste fiber to brain via facial,
glossopharyngeal, and vagus
nerves

Fig. 3-27 Taste pathways. (From Ganong, W.F.: Review of medical physiology, ed. 11; copyright 1983 by Lange Medical Publications, Los Altos, Calif.)

3. For the food to be rolled into a bolus, saliva must be added; saliva contains glycoproteins that enable the bolus to slip down the esophagus with greater ease; produced by three major paired glands and many minor glands (Fig. 3-27)
   a. Parotid glands are located in the preauricular region; saliva contains ptyalin that initiates digestion of starches; saliva travels down Stensen's duct, which opens opposite the second maxillary molar (serous secretion)
   b. Sublingual glands lie under the tongue and rest against the mandible in the sublingual fossa; saliva travels down Bartholin's duct and enters the oral cavity through Rivinus' ducts on the sublingual fold
   c. Submandibular glands lie on the medial surface of the mandible; saliva travels down the tortuous Wharton's duct and is released into the mouth at the sublingual caruncles (seromucous secretion)

4. Bolus of food is conducted from the mouth and pharynx to the esophagus, a muscular tube located posterior to the trachea and connected to the stomach
   a. During swallowing the soft palate is pushed back against the posterior pharyngeal wall, closing the passage to the nasopharynx
   b. Larynx is elevated; superior opening is protected by the epiglottis
C. Stomach is a dilated portion of the alimentary canal lying in the upper abdomen just under the diaphragm
  1. Several functions
   a. Stores food
   b. Digests—secretes pepsin, rennin, and gastric lipase
   c. Produces hydrochloric acid (parietal cells)
  2. Shaped like a J; internal surface is wrinkled (rugae)
   a. Cardiac portion—esophagus enters
   b. Body—main part
   c. Fundus—bulge at the upper end, left of the esophageal area
   d. Pyloric portion—narrows and connects with the small intestine
D. Small intestine—thin-walled muscular tube
  1. Three portions
   a. Duodenum—bile and pancreatic secretions are added to the small intestine; horseshoe-shaped
   b. Jejunum—greatest amount of absorption occurs here; 1.5 m long
   c. Ileum—connect with the large intestine; 2.4 m long
  2. Secretes several enzymes and substances
   a. Brunner's glands—located only in duodenum; secretes alkaline mucus
   b. Sucrase—acts on sucrose; end product is one molecule of glucose and one of fructose
   c. Maltase—acts on maltose; produces two molecules of glucose
   d. Lactase—acts on lactose; produces one molecule of glucose and one molecule of galactose
   e. Aminopeptidase—acts on the amino end of the protein chain; produces one amino acid and simpler proteins
   f. Dipeptidase—acts on dipeptides to produce two amino acids
   g. Enterokinase (coenzyme)—acts on trypsinogen to produce trypsin
   h. Secretin—hormone carried to the pancreas; stimulates the pancreas to produce watery pancreatic juice

      i. Enterogastrone—hormone carried to the stomach; produced when fatty foods are in the intestine; reduces gastric mobility

E. Large intestine—approximately 1.5 m long; divided into several divisions

  1. Cecum—blind pouch in the lower right quadrant; appendix attaches to the cecum; ileocecal sphincter separates the ileum from the cecum

  2. Colon

    a. Ascending—from the cecum to the hepatic flexure

    b. Transverse—from the hepatic flexure to the splenic flexure

    c. Descending—to the level of the pelvic bone, on the left side of the body

    d. Sigmoid—S-shaped curve

  3. Rectum—from the sigmoid colon down to the pelvic diaphragm

  4. Anus—3 cm in length (internal and external sphincters)

F. Pancreas—endocrine and exocrine gland

  1. Exocrine—acinar cells produce pancreatic juice that is collected by the pancreatic duct (Wirsung's duct) and carried away; joins the common bile duct to form Vater's ampulla, which penetrates the walls of the duodenum

  2. Endocrine—releases insulin that controls the blood glucose levels

G. Liver—largest and most active gland in the body

  1. Two main lobes and several lobules; lobules produce bile that is carried away and stored in the gallbladder

  2. Other functions

    a. Acts as a storehouse for glycogen

    b. Produces fibrinogen for blood clotting

    c. Synthesizes prothrombin with the aid of vitamin K

    d. Synthesizes some amino acids from simpler compounds

    e. Produces erythrocytes in the embryo and fetus

    f. Detoxifies nitrogenous waste

    g. Deaminates 50% to 60% of the absorbed amino acids

    h. Stores some cyanocobalamin (vitamin B_{12})

    i. Removes old erythrocytes and foreign substances by the action of the phagocytic Kupffer cells

    j. Stores iron, copper, and vitamins A and D

    k. Synthesizes and destroys uric acid

    l. Acts as a center for fat and carbohydrate metabolism

H. Digestion starts in the mouth; absorption of molecules occurs in the small intestine

  1. Functions of saliva in the oral cavity

    a. Lubricating—reduces friction

    b. Solvent—important for stimulation of taste buds

    c. Moistening—important for speech

    d. Cleansing—decreases bacterial population

    e. Buffering—helps to protect teeth from acid insults

    f. Minor digestion of starches

  2. Elevating the tongue causes the tongue to push the bolus of food toward the pharynx

  3. Wavelike contraction (peristalsis) keeps the bolus moving down the rest of the digestive system

  4. Food that is converted to a semifluid mass in the stomach is known as chyme

  5. Three phases of gastric digestion

    a. Cephalic—taste, smell, and sight of food stimulate the cerebral cortex; cause the salivary glands to produce saliva

    b. Gastric—food reaches the stomach, causing a copious flow of juices to form chyme

    c. Intestinal—chyme is in small intestines; causes enterogastrone to be released, which will inhibit gastric movement and secretion

  6. Davenport's theory of hydrochloric acid secretions in the stomach

    a. Parietal cells contain more carbonic anhydrase than the blood, which will form

$$H_2CO_3 \rightarrow H^+ + HCO_3$$

    b. Carbonate ion moves out into the blood and causes the chloride ions to shift back out of the blood into the interstitial spaces

    c. Chloride ion attaches to the free hydrogen ion to form hydrochloric acid (HCl)

  7. Mucus is also secreted in the stomach to protect against self-digestion

  8. Hydrochloric acid acts on pepsinogen to produce pepsin; converts milk protein and collagen to proteases and peptones

  9. Pancreas produces several enzymes that act on the chyme in the small intestine

    a. Lipase—acts on emulsified fats to form fatty acids and glycerol

    b. Amylase—acts on carbohydrates to form disaccharides

    c. Carboxypeptidase—works on the −COOH end of the protein chain to produce one amino acid and simpler proteins

d. Trypsinogen—inactive enzyme until the coenzyme enterokinase activates it to trypsin; splits large protein chains

e. Chymotrypsinogen—inactive enzyme until the coenzyme enterokinase activates it to chymotrypsin; acts on amino acids

10. After the enzymes have broken up the molecules (catabolism), they are selectively absorbed through the small intestine

    a. Amino acids are used to build new tissue or repair tissue; those not used are deamidized in the liver; ammonia formed is converted to urea and eliminated by the kidneys; nonnitrogenous portion may be oxidized to supply energy or synthesized to glucose (1 g of protein equals 4 calories); passes into the body via the blood capillaries in the villi

    b. Fats are oxidized to carbon dioxide and water with the released energy; fat not used can be stored in the liver or body and passed into the body via the lacteals of the lymphatic system (1 g of fat equals 9 calories)

    c. Carbohydrates may be oxidized in the tissue cells to supply energy or may be stored in the liver or muscles as glycogen; passes into the body via the blood capillaries in the villi

      (1) Glycogenesis—synthesis of glucose to glycogen

      (2) Glycogenolysis—hydrolysis of glycogen to glucose

      (3) One gram of carbohydrates equals 4 calories

11. Large intestine holds the fecal material that is not absorbed; reabsorbs water to maintain the internal environment

I. Kidneys

1. Important because they also excrete waste products from metabolism and maintain the water and acid-base balance in the body

2. Paired bean-shaped organs on either side of the vertebral column

    a. Renal artery and vein and the ureter (which attaches to the bladder) attach to the center of the kidney at the hilus

    b. Outer part of the kidney is designated the cortex and the inner part the medulla

      (1) Medulla consists of several pyramids

      (2) Apices of the pyramids project into the calyces

    c. Nephron is the functional unit of the kidney (Fig. 3-28)

    d. Renal circulation is renal arteries to interlobar artery to arcuate artery to glomerulus to efferent arterioles to secondary capillary network to interlobular vein to arcuate vein to interlobar vein to renal vein

3. Kidney connected to the bladder by the ureters

    a. Are approximately 27 cm long

    b. Urine flows down the ureters via peristalsis

4. Bladder lies behind the symphysis pubis; serves as a reservoir for the urine

    a. Smooth muscle (detrusor muscle) readjusts constantly to the amount of urine entering

    b. Three orifices form a trigone

5. Urethra connects the bladder to the exterior

    a. Female urethra is approximately 4 cm long

    b. Male urethra is approximately 20 cm long

6. Urine is a liquid with unique properties

    a. Colored by bile segments

    b. pH varies from 4.5 to 9

    c. Specific gravity varies from 1.015 to 1.025

    d. Amount excreted daily is approximately 1400 ml

    e. Consists of 95% water and solids

      (1) Urea, uric acid, creatinine, and urea

      (2) Sodium chloride and various phosphates and sulfates

7. Blood is filtered first in the glomeruli

    a. Ultrafiltrate of water and nonprotein solutes pass through the glomerular membranes into Bowman's capsule and then into the proximal tubules

    b. Filtration rate is determined by the filtration pressure, which is equal to the blood pressure in the glomerulus minus the sum of the protein osmotic pressure plus the intercapsular pressure

      (1) Approximately 75 liters of blood flow through the kidney per hour

      (2) Most of the filtrate is reabsorbed before reaching the collecting tubules

    c. Ultrafiltrate is modified as it passes through the tubules via reabsorption and secretion

      (1) Proximal convoluted tubule—all glucose and some sodium, chloride, potassium, bicarbonate, and hydrogen ions are reabsorbed in the blood

      (2) Loop of Henle—more precise adjustment of the sodium concentration is made

      (3) Distal collecting tubule—final adjustment is made in the levels of the sodium ions, acids, bases, and water

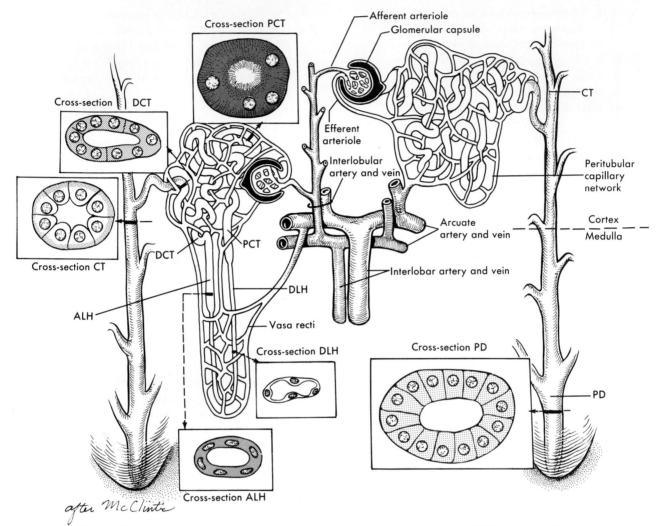

Fig. 3-28 Nephron. (From McClintic, J.R.: Human anatomy, St. Louis, 1983, The C.V. Mosby Co.)

d. Waste products are not reabsorbed
e. Adjustments of the sodium/potassium and calcium/phosphorus ratios are done in the distal convoluted tubules under the influence of aldosterone and the parathyroid gland
f. Hydrogen ions are exchanged in the distal convoluted tubules so that the pH levels are controlled
g. Water levels are also regulated in the distal convoluted tubules, depending on the amount of the antidiuretic hormone in the body

ENDOCRINE SYSTEM

The endocrine system consists of several glands that secrete hormones
A. Functions (Fig. 3-29)
   1. Composed of a number of glands that play a major role in supplementing the effect of the nervous system, in regulating the rate of various physiologic processes, and in maintaining the constancy of the internal environment of the body
   2. Glands
      a. Do not secrete their products into ducts; instead are secreted into the system
      b. Product of an endocrine gland is called a hormone

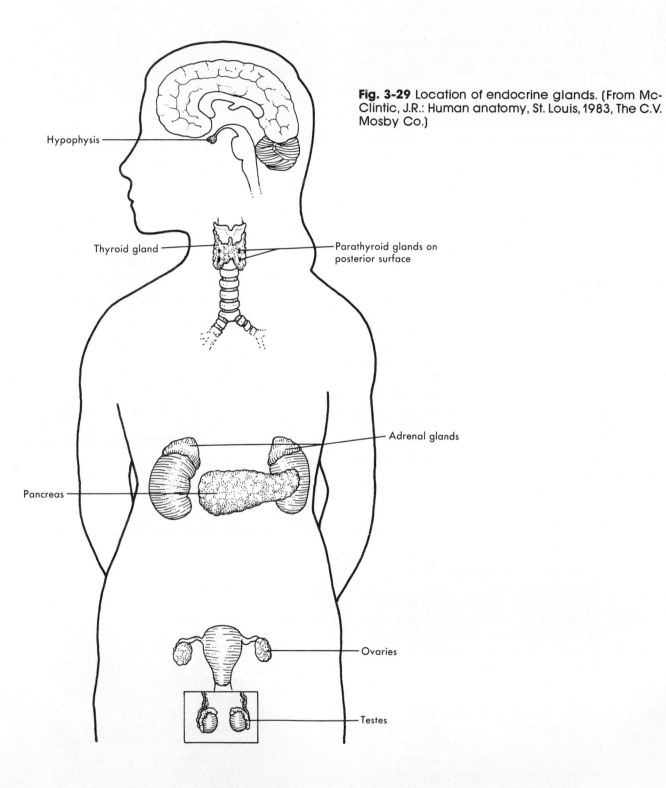

Fig. 3-29 Location of endocrine glands. (From Mc-Clintic, J.R.: Human anatomy, St. Louis, 1983, The C.V. Mosby Co.)

Hypophysis

Thyroid gland

Parathyroid glands on posterior surface

Adrenal glands

Pancreas

Ovaries

Testes

(1) Ectodermally derived endocrines secrete amine hormones

(2) Mesodermally derived endocrines secrete steroid hormones

(3) Endodermally derived endocrines secrete protein hormones

3. Hormones secreted by the endocrine system

   a. Main regulators of metabolism, reproduction, and maintenance of fluid and electrolyte balance and acid-base balance

   b. Produce slow and long-lasting responses in target cells

B. Control of endocrine secretion

  1. Blood levels of specific inorganic substances

  2. Total osmolarity of blood

  3. Blood levels of organic substances

  4. Positive and negative feedback

  5. Chemicals produced by nerve cells

  6. Nervous stimulation

C. Pituitary gland (Table 3-21)

  1. Located in the sella turcica of the sphenoid bone

  2. Composed of a portion derived from the roof of the oral cavity (adenohypophysis) and a portion from the hypothalmus (neurohypophysis)

  3. Arterial blood supply is derived mainly from the superior and inferior hypophyseal arteries

  4. Hypophyseal portal veins arise from the capillaries of the median eminence of the hypothalamus

  5. Veins empty into the sinusoid in the pars distalis

  6. Hypophysis receives its nerve supply from the sympathetic plexus around the carotid artery

  7. Adenohypophysis

   a. Contains three types of cells (pars distalis)

    (1) Acidophils—stain red-orange from an orange G or purplish red from an azocarmine stain

    (2) Basophils—stain blue from a periodic acid-Schiff's stain

    (3) Chromophobes—stain little if at all

   b. Growth hormone (somatotropin)

    (1) Produced by acidophils

    (2) Stimulates growth of both bone and soft tissues

    (3) Causes cells to shift from using carbohydrate to using fat for energy

    (4) Excess production of growth hormone

     (a) Pituitary gigantism—before epiphysial closure; large size but proportionally balanced

Table 3-21 Divisions of the hypophysis

Major divisions	Subdivisions
Adenohypophysis	Pars distalis
	Pars tuberalis
	Pars intermedia
Neurohypophysis	Infundibulum
	Neural lobe

     (b) Acromegaly—full-grown adult; characterized by enlarged hands, feet, and jaws

    (5) Deficient secretion of growth hormone

     (a) Pituitary dwarfism—develops during skeletal development; diminuitive size but proportionally balanced

     (b) Simmond's disease—develops during adult years; presents with premature aging and cachexia

   c. Prolactin (lactogenic hormone)

    (1) Produced by acidophils

    (2) Stimulates milk production by the mammary glands

     (a) Secreted during pregnancy—breast development

     (b) Secreted after delivery of child—lactation

    (3) Stimulates progesterone secretion by corpus luteum

   d. Adrenocorticotropic hormone (ACTH)

    (1) Secreted by basophils; also possibly secreted by chromophobes

    (2) Controls the synthetic and secretory activity of the two inner zones of the adrenal cortex

    (3) Atrophy of the adrenal cortex results in Addison's disease; can result in death because of a loss of sodium in the extracellular fluid

    (4) Hypertrophy of the adrenal cortex results in Cushing's syndrome; characterized by moon face, hirsutism, and possible hypertension

   e. Thyroid-stimulating hormone (TSH)

    (1) Secreted by basophils

    (2) Affects thyroid gland activity (accumulation of material, synthesis, and secretion)

    (3) Hypersecretion results in Grave's disease

    (4) Hyposecretion results in cretinism (young) or myxedema (adult)

    f. Luteinizing hormone (LH)
      (1) Secreted by basophils
      (2) Also classified as a gonadotropin
      (3) Female
        (a) Forms corpus luteum in the ovary
        (b) Causes corpus luteum to secrete progesterone
        (c) Necessary for ovulation and implantation of the zygote
      (4) Male
        (a) Interstitial cell—stimulating hormone
        (b) Stimulates the production of testosterone by the interstitial cells of the seminiferous tubules
    g. Follicle-stimulating hormone (FSH)
      (1) Female—controls maturation of primary follicles to vesicular follicles
      (2) Male—controls spermatogenesis
    h. Pars intermedia has no proven function in mammals
    i. Pars tuberalis has no proven function in mammals
  8. Neurohypophysis
    a. Contains pituicytes
      (1) Axons, with their cell bodies in the hypothalamus, terminate on or near the pituicytes
      (2) Hypothalamus produces the hormones and passes them over a nerve tract to be stored or released from the neurohypophysis
    b. Antidiuretic hormone (ADH)
      (1) Acts on the kidney to decrease urine formation
      (2) Acts on smooth muscle of arteries and arterioles; increases blood pressure
      (3) Hyposecretion of ADH results in diabetes insipidus
        (a) Polyuria
        (b) Polydipsia
        (c) Polyphagia
      (4) Release is controlled by osmosensitive cells in the hypothalamus
    c. Oxytocin
      (1) Secreted during parturition; affects the uterus
      (2) Aids milk ejection of the mammary glands
D. Thyroid gland
  1. Consists of two lobes that are interconnected by an isthmus; located on the ventral surface of the trachea; superior border is the thyroid cartilage; inferior border is the sixth tracheal ring

  2. Receives approximately 120 ml of blood per minute, which is supplied by the superior thyroid arteries (from the external carotid arteries) and by the inferior thyroid arteries (from the subclavian arteries); capillary system of the gland drains into the superior and middle thyroid veins to the internal jugular veins to the inferior thyroid veins to the left brachiocephalic vein
  3. Receives sympathetic fibers from the inferior and superior ganglia and parasympathetic fibers from branches of the vagus nerve
  4. Thyroxine (T_4) and triiodothyronine (T_3), which are iodinated amino acids, secreted by the follicles of the gland
    a. T_3 is more potent than T_4, but the thyroid contains more T_4 (under normal conditions)
    b. T_3 and T_4 must attach to a plasma protein in the circulating blood
    c. If T_3 and T_4 are to be stored, thin thyroglobulin is formed in the follicular colloid
    d. Effects of T_4
      (1) Accelerates catabolic reactions of glycolysis
      (2) Necessary for proper development of the brain
      (3) Controls metabolism by affecting glycogen levels; can control urine production
      (4) Influences cardiac metabolism
  5. Secretes calcitonin in response to high plasma concentrations of calcium and phosphate; can cause increased absorption of minerals by the kidneys; can increase mineralization of bones
  6. Effects of thyroid hormones on oral structures
    a. Injection of T_4 in newborn rats causes marked acceleration in the rate of eruption of the incisor teeth; can also affect eruption of the molars[1]
    b. Large doses of thyroid hormone given to guinea pigs affected the odontoblasts; dentin formation was adversely affected[1]
    c. Children with cretinism may exhibit a small dental arch; exfoliation patterns of the teeth are delayed
E. Parathyroid gland
  1. Variable number of parathyroid glands in the human; most people have two pairs, but the range varies from one to three pairs
  2. Small in size (approximately 5 mm); usually located on the posterior side of the thyroid gland

3. Composed of two types of cells
   a. Chief cells—produce parathyroid hormone (PTH)
   b. Oxyphil cells—reserve cells capable of producing PTH
4. Parathyroid hormone
   a. Controls serum calcium, magnesium, and phosphate levels
   b. Decreased calcium concentration in the blood stimulates secretion
   c. Affects the gut, bone, and kidneys
      (1) Gut—causes increased absorption of calcium, magnesium, and phosphate
      (2) Bone—stimulates osteoclasts; causes calcium and phosphate to be released into the blood
      (3) Kidney—causes increased calcium and phosphate reabsorption and increased phosphate excretion
   d. Disorders caused by unregulated PTH levels
      (1) Hyperparathyroidism (von Recklinghausen's disease)
         (a) Extremely high blood calcium levels, leading to muscular weakness
         (b) Cysts in the bones may develop (osteitis fibrosa cystica)
      (2) Hypoparathyroidism (tetany)—extremely low blood calcium levels, leading to muscular rigidity and convulsion
   e. Effects of PTH on oral structures
      (1) Hypoparathyroidism during tooth development produces defects in the matrix, mineralization in the enamel and dentin, and delays in eruption
      (2) Hyperparathyroidism, seen radiographically, shows loss of the lamina dura; alveolar bone can become osteoporotic with no change in density of the teeth
F. Pancreas gland
   1. Single gland that extends horizontally across the posterior abdominal wall on the left side
   2. Consists of three parts
      a. Head—duodenal portion
      b. Body—between the head and tail
      c. Tail—splenic portion
   3. Has an exocrine and endocrine function
      a. Exocrine—trypsin and trypsinogen (digestive functions)
      b. Endocrine—α-cells, glucagon (controls blood glucose; β-cells (controls insulin levels)

4. Insulin
   a. Complex protein hormone that is secreted in response to a rise in the blood glucose level
   b. Effects
      (1) Causes glycogenesis in the liver (conversion of glucose to glycogen)
      (2) Stimulates cells to take up glucose
      (3) Increase in blood glucose levels (caused by a lack of insulin) can lead to infection and bacteremias when bacteria are introduced into the blood system
5. Glucagon—secreted by α-cells in response to a fall in the blood glucose level; causes glycogenolysis (conversion of glycogen to glucose) in the liver
6. Diabetes mellitus can be caused by an insulin deficiency
   a. Signs and symptoms
      (1) Hyperglycemia—high blood glucose level
      (2) Glucosuria—kidney tubules cannot reabsorb all of the glucose, and the excess appears in the urine
      (3) Ketoacidosis—body uses fats as the main source of energy; ketone levels increase; acidosis can result from overtaxed buffering systems
      (4) Polyuria—excess water is lost with glucose in urine
      (5) Polydipsia—loss of water triggers thirst
      (6) Polyphagia—glucose loss triggers a desire to eat
   b. If the β-cells are destroyed, the patient must receive insulin and control diet
   c. If some β-cells survive, oral sulfonylurea compounds may be prescribed to stimulate the β-cells
7. Hypoglycemia can develop from low blood glucose levels; can result from insulin shock, islet tumors, and starvation
   a. Mainly affects the brain
   b. Can also lower the body temperature, disturb respiration, and depress the reflexes
G. Adrenal glands
   1. These paired glands are located on the top of each kidney; adrenal cortex develops from the embryologic mesoderm; adrenal medulla develops from the neural ectoderm
   2. Adrenal cortex secretes several hormones that can be classified as steroids
      a. Cells located in the zona glomerulosa secrete mineralocorticoids (aldosterone and corticosterone) that regulate electrolytes in the extracellular fluids

(1) Sodium is reabsorbed into the blood from the glomerular filtrate

(2) Potassium (a positive ion) is lost in the urine because of the electronegativity created by the reabsorption of sodium in the kidney tubules

(3) Chloride (a negative ion) is reabsorbed from the glomerular filtrate because of the electronegativity created by the reabsorption of sodium in the kidney tubules

b. Secretion of aldosterone is regulated in response to changes in the extracellular fluid; decreased sodium concentration produces a weak effect on the cortex to increase secretion, causes the kidneys to secrete renin that stimulates the release of angiotensin in the cortex, and causes the pituitary gland to release ACTH

c. Addison's disease is caused by the hyposecretion of aldosterone and cortisol

(1) Causes brown pigmentation of the skin

(2) Causes hypotension

d. Cells located in the zona fasiculata secrete glucocorticoids (cortisol) that affect the body's metabolic system

(1) Glucocorticoid secretion causes an increased concentration of the blood glucose

(2) Cortisol causes a decrease in the quantity of protein in most tissues and an increase in protein in the liver

(3) Cortisol can stabilize lysozymes and therefore inhibit cell death

(4) Cushing's syndrome can manifest from an increase in glucocorticoids

(a) Moon face

(b) Buffalo hump on shoulders

(c) Fat abdomen

e. Cells located in the zona reticularis secrete androgens and produce masculine features; excess production in women can lead to masculine features

REPRODUCTIVE SYSTEM

Male

A. Testes

1. Two ovoid bodies that lie in the scrotum

2. Suspended in the inguinal region by the spermatic cord

3. Sperm is formed and stored in the seminiferous tubules of the testes

4. Testosterone is produced in the testes

5. Epididymis is adjacent to the testes in the scrotum

a. Acts as a storage reservoir for sperm along with the seminiferous tubules

b. Sperm may live for as long as a month in both the epididymis and tubules

6. If the testes have failed to descend in an infant, the condition is referred to as cryptorchism

B. Vas deferens

1. Conducts sperm from the epididymis to the urethra

2. Acts as a storage site for sperm

C. Urethra

1. Passageway for semen from the vas deferens through the penis

2. Passageway for urine from the bladder through the penis

3. Ends at the urinary meatus, which is the opening in the glans penis through which urine and semen are excreted

D. Seminal vesicles

1. Membranous pouches located posterior to the bladder

2. Produces a secretion that contains fructose, amino acids, and mucus

3. Secretes mucoid material into the upper end of the vas deferens

E. Prostate gland

1. Located inferior to the bladder

2. Secretes an alkaline fluid to activate the sperm

3. Secretes its milky fluid into the vas deferens

F. Bulbourethral glands (Cowper's glands)

1. Located inferior to the prostate gland

2. Secretes a mucous secretion into the urethra that precedes ejaculation; aids in lubrication

G. Penis

1. Organ of copulation that is divided into a shaft and glans penis

a. Glans penis is the most sensitive portion of the penis

b. Foreskin covers the glans penis (removed by circumcision)

2. Erective tissue (corpus cavernosum) surrounds the penile urethra; causes erection when engorged with blood

H. Sperm

1. Spermatozoa formed in the testes

2. Contains head, neck, body, and tail

a. Head contains the genetic material of the male

b. Tail provides motility through flagella movement

c. Sperms moves through the female genital tract to seek the ovum at a velocity of approximately 1 to 4 mm per minute

3. Spermatogenesis
   a. After a spermatogonium has been divided by mitosis for the last time, it increases in size and forms a primary spermatocyte
   b. Primary spermatocyte is divided by meiosis to form secondary spermatocyte with haploid number of chromosomes (23)
   c. Division of the secondary spermatocytes results in spermatids being formed
   d. Spermatids are transformed into motile cells called spermatozoa

I. Physiology of ejaculation
   1. Erection is the stiffening of a flaccid penis
   2. Rhythmic peristalsis in the genital ducts during orgasm causes semen to be propelled through the epididymis, vas deferens, seminal ducts, and urethra
   3. Semen is a thick, whitish fluid of high viscosity
      a. Between 2.5 and 5 ml are secreted at ejaculation
      b. Each milliliter contains 10 to 150 million sperm
      c. Sperm usually move at about 3 mm/min

J. Hormonal influences
   1. Hormones are essential to the mechanism of reproduction and to the development and maintenance of secondary sex characteristics
   2. Anterior pituitary gland secretes FSH and LH, which cause growth and function of the testes at puberty
   3. Secondary sex characteristics in the male that appear during adolescence
      a. Deepening of voice; widening of musculature of chest and shoulders
      b. Growth of facial and body hair

Female

A. Pelvis
   1. Contains the reproductive organs, bladder, and rectum
   2. Shaped like a funnel with a wide mouth
   3. Divided into true and false pelvis by the inlet or brim; sacral promontory and ileopectineal lines are dividing points between the true and false pelvis
   4. Forms part of the birth canal
   5. Perineum, vagina, muscles, and ligaments form the soft structures of the pelvis
      a. Retain pelvic organs in place
      b. During labor direct presenting part of the infant forward

B. Ovaries
   1. Flat, oval-shaped bodies about 2.5 cm long
   2. Supported in the pelvis by the broad ligament and suspensory ligament
   3. Three types of follicles located in the ovaries
      a. Primordial follicles—contain a primary oocyte
         (1) Present at birth
         (2) Follicles finish first maturation under the influence of FSH
      b. Growing follicles—contain a mature ovum and spaces that contain fluid
      c. Mature follicles—seen bulging from the surface of the ovary

C. Fallopian tubes (oviducts)
   1. Lie in the folds of the broad ligaments
   2. Fimbriae (fingerlike projections) located at the ovarian ends; isthmus portion is connected to the uterus
   3. Important events occurring in the fallopian tube—fertilization of the ovum by a spermatozoa, segmentation, and formation of the blastocyst

D. Uterus
   1. Hollow organ with thick muscular walls
   2. Located behind the bladder and in front of the rectum
   3. Pear-shaped; divided into three parts
      a. Fundus—rounded upper part
      b. Body—narrows from the fundus
      c. Cervix—tapering projection
   4. Muscular layers
      a. Endometrium—one layer of ciliated columnar cells except for lower one third of the cervical canal where it changes to stratified squamous epithelium; contains glands and a good blood supply
      b. Myometrium—contains smooth muscle and large blood vessels
      c. Exometrium—contains the pelvic peritoneum
   5. Serves as the womb for a developing fetus

E. External genitalia
   1. Vagina—female organ of copulation
      a. Muscular, membranous orifice; 7.6 to 12.7 cm long
      b. Connects the uterus to the external surface (vaginal orifice)
      c. Serves as the birth canal for the delivery of a baby
   2. Mons pubis—rounded eminence in front of the pubic symphysis
   3. Labia majora—two longitudinal folds; protects the inner vulva
   4. Labia minora—two inner folds; smaller; protects the clitoris
   5. Clitoris
      a. Homologue of the penis in the male
      b. Can increase in size with sexual stimulation

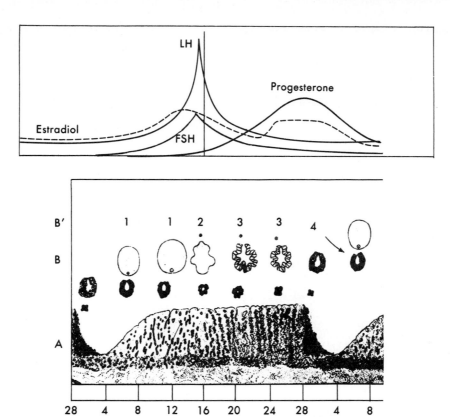

Fig. 3-30 Relationship of pituitary gonadotropins and ovarian hormones to follicular development and uterine changes. (From McClintic, J.R.: Human anatomy, St. Louis, 1983, The C.V. Mosby Co.)

F. Perineum contains the structures found between the pubic symphysis and the coccyx

G. Mammary glands
 1. Composed of compound alveolar glands
 2. Secrete milk to the nipples under the influence of the lactogenic hormone from the pituitary gland
 3. Pigmented circular region (areolar surrounds the nipple)
 4. Active glandular growth occurs during pregnancy to prepare the mammary glands to produce milk (lactation)

H. Hormonal cycle (Fig. 3-30)
 1. Begins at puberty and ends at menopause
 2. FSH is secreted by the anterior pituitary gland; activates the primary graafian follicle
 3. Maturing follicle produces estrogen; causes the endometrium to become engorged with blood and prepares it to receive the fertilized ovum
 4. Both hormones (FSH and estrogen) allow the ova to mature
 5. Mature ovum is released into the fallopian tube by a ruptured graafian follicle; LH assists ovulation; follicle forms the corpus luteum and secretes progesterone

 6. Increased progestogen levels reduce FSH and increase LH; cause the corpus luteum to secrete progesterone
  a. Stimulates uterus to store glycogen and increases the uterine blood supply
  b. Corpus luteum begins to involute as a result of lowered FSH levels
 7. Menstrual cycle lasts 21 to 35 days
  a. Menstruation begins if the ovum is not fertilized
  b. If fertilization occurs, the placenta will secrete chorionic gonadotropin that will maintain the corpus luteum; estrogens and progesterone will also continue to be secreted and will maintain the rich vascular supply in the endometrium for the developing embryo

I. Secondary sex characteristics that develop in response to estrogen and progesterone secretion during puberty
 1. Widening of hips
 2. Breast and genital enlargement
 3. Growth of axillary and pubic hair

REFERENCE

1. Jenkins, G.N.: The physiology and biochemistry of the mouth, ed. 4, Oxford, 1978, Blackwell Scientific Publications Ltd.

SUGGESTED READINGS

Anthony, C.P., and Thibodeau, G.A.: Textbook of anatomy and physiology, ed. 11, St. Louis, 1983, The C.V. Mosby Co.

The Ciba collection of medical illustrations, vol. I, The nervous system, Summit, N.J., 1972, Ciba Pharmaceutical Products, Inc.

Ganong, W.F.: Review of medical physiology, ed. 11, Los Altos, Calif., 1983, Lange Medical Publications.

Goss, C.M., editor: Gray's anatomy, American ed. 29, Philadelphia, 1973, Lea & Febiger.

Guyton, A.C.: Physiology of the human body, ed. 5, Philadelphia, 1979, W.B. Saunders Co.

Guyton, A.C.: Textbook of medical physiology, ed. 6, Philadelphia, 1981, W.B. Saunders Co.

Hoyle, G.: How is muscle turned on and off? Sci. Am. **22:**84, April 1970.

Junqueira, L.C., and Carneiro, J.: Basic histology, ed. 4, Los Altos, Calif., 1983, Lange Medical Publications.

McClintic, J.R.: Human anatomy, St. Louis, 1983, The C.V. Mosby Co.

Squier, C.A., Johnson, N.W., and Hopps, R.A.: Human oral mucosa: development, structure and function, Oxford, 1976, Blackwell Scientific Publications.

Review Questions

1 Which of the following adjectives describes the relationship of the hand to the head when a human is in anatomic position?
1. Ventral
2. Dorsal
3. Caudal
4. Cephalic
5. Posterior

2 Which one of the following planes divides the body into right and left halves?
1. Sagittal plane
2. Median plane
3. Coronal plane
4. Transverse plane
5. Horizontal plane

3 Which of the following body cavities contains the lungs?
1. Pleural cavity
2. Pericardial cavity
3. Vertebral cavity
4. Cranial cavity
5. Abdominopelvic cavity

4 Which of the following statements *best* describes the cell membrane?
1. It is permeable to all substances
2. It has a $3:2$ ratio of lipids to proteins
3. It has 8 Å pores in its surface that allow large lipids to pass through
4. It does not exclude substances from entering
5. It is a bipolar membrane

Situation: Mr. Barker is undergoing radiation therapy to the head and neck for squamous cell carcinoma of the pharyngeal tonsils. Questions 5 to 8 refer to this situation.

5 If radiation affects those cells that are rapidly dividing (i.e., going though mitosis) and the carcinoma cells are in metaphase, what activities in the cell would one expect to see?
1. Nuclear envelope disappearing
2. Spindle fibers developing
3. Genetic material replicating
4. Centrioles replicating
5. Chromatids lining up at the center

6 The pharyngeal, palatine, and lingual tonsils form a certain arrangement known as
1. Circle of Willis
2. Waldeyer's ring
3. Peyer's patches
4. Inguinal nodes
5. Meissner's corpuscles

7 Where are the pharyngeal tonsils located?
1. In the groin area
2. At the base of the tongue
3. Between the anterior and posterior pillars of the oral cavity
4. In the neck
5. In the posterior wall of the upper pharynx

8 During a postradiation therapy appointment the dental hygienist notices that a milky white fluid can be expressed from Stensen's duct orifice on palpation. This would indicate an infection in which gland or structure?
1. Submandibular gland
2. Lacrimal gland
3. Sublingual gland
4. Parotid gland
5. Pharyngeal tonsils

---

9 Which of the following factors will increase the rate of diffusion?
1. Decreasing the concentration differences
2. Increasing the distance
3. Decreasing the temperature
4. Decreasing the square root of the molecular substance
5. Decreasing the cross-sectional area of the chamber

10 An erythrocyte that is placed in a hypotonic solution will exhibit which of the following characteristics?
1. No change
2. Adsorption
3. Lysis
4. Crenation
5. Diapedesis

11 The lateral ptyergoid muscle is which type of muscle?
1. Voluntary, striated
2. Involuntary, striated
3. Involuntary, smooth
4. Voluntary, smooth
5. None of the above

12 What are the origin and insertion of the lateral ptygergoid muscles?
1. Origin, zygomatic process; insertion, coronoid process
2. Origin, greater wing of the sphenoid; insertion, condyloid process of the mandible
3. Origin, pterygoid fossa; insertion, posterior body of the ramus
4. Origin, temporal fossa; insertion, coronoid process
5. Origin, hyoid bone; insertion, tongue

13 The lateral pterygoid muscles are part of which of the following groups of muscles?
1. Cranial muscles
2. Facial expression muscles
3. Mastication muscles
4. Extrinsic muscles of the tongue
5. Muscles of the larynx

14 Which of the following nerves innervates the lateral pterygoid muscle?
1. Cranial nerve I
2. Cranial nerve V
3. Cranial nerve VII
4. Cranial nerve XII
5. Cervical spinal nerves I to III

15 From which foramen in the skull does the cranial nerve that innervates the lateral pterygoid exit?
1. Foramen rotundum
2. Foramen ovale
3. Foramen magnum
4. Foramen spinosum
5. Foramen lacerum

16 The lateral pterygoid muscle is involved in the movement of the temporomandibular joint. What type of articulation exists in this joint?
1. Syndesmosis
2. Gomphosis
3. Synchondrosis
4. Cartilaginous joint
5. Synovial joint

Situation: During the update of the medical history, Mr. Bates tells the dental hygienist that he is taking chlorothiazide (Diuril), 500 mg two times a day, and potassium chloride (Klorvess), a potassium supplement. Mr. Bates also reports that he has recovered from a fractured femur in the last 6 months. Questions 17 to 20 refer to this situation.

17 Potassium chloride (Klorvess) is taken with chlorothiazide (Diuril) to prevent hypokalemia (decreased blood potassium levels). What is the normal potassium concentration in the extracellular fluid?
1. 142 mEq/L
2. 5 mEq/L
3. 103 mEq/L
4. 10 mEq/L
5. Less than 1 mEq/L

18 During the intraoral examination the dental hygienist notices that Mr. Bates is experiencing xerostomia. What gland is responsible for contributing to xerostomia?
1. Lacrimal gland
2. Adrenal gland
3. Pituitary gland
4. Sebaceous gland
5. Salivary gland

19 Chlorothiazide (Diuril) inhibits the tubular reabsorption of sodium and other electrolytes, thus causing diuresis. Where does this process occur?
1. In the pituitary gland
2. In the pancreas
3. In the colon
4. In the kidney
5. In the bladder

20 On further questioning, the dental hygienist learns that a pin was used to set the femur near the greater trochanter. What is a trochanter?
1. A sharp prominence
2. A large rounded projection
3. A ridge
4. A sinus
5. A large prominence

Situation: Ms. Evers reports to the dental hygienist that she had a traumatic injury to the temporal bone and that her hearing and equilibrium have been affected. Questions 21 to 23 refer to this situation.

21 The traumatic injury suffered by Ms. Evers most likely involved which portion of the temporal bone?
1. Zygomatic process
2. Petrous portion
3. Mastoid portion
4. Glenoid fossa
5. Styloid process   /MANDIBULAR

22 Where is the glenoid fossa located?
1. On the face
2. Behind the ear
3. On the floor of the cranium
4. Above the ear
5. Anterior and medial to the external auditory meatus

23 Equilibrium is detected by which of the following structures in the ear?
1. Stapes
2. Tympanic membrane
3. Eustachian tube
4. Incus
5. Semicircular canals

24 What is the name of the fossa located on the posterior surface at the distal end of the humerus?
1. Olecranon fossa
2. Mandibular fossa
3. Infraspinous fossa
4. Subscapular fossa
5. Coronoid fossa

25 What is the name given to the small fingernail-like bone forming part of the medial wall of the orbital cavity?
1. Vomer
2. Calvaria
3. Xiphoid
4. Lacrimal
5. Sphenoid

26 Which vertebra has a process on its body that forms a pivot with an adjacent vertebra?
1. C1
2. C2
3. T2
4. L1
5. Coccygeal

27 Which bones form the fingers?
1. Clavicles
2. Radii
3. Carpals
4. Metacarpals
5. Phlanges

28 The following definition describes which of the following bones?
"It is the longest and strongest bone of the body, and its proximal end has a rounded head that articulates with the acetabulum."
1. Femur
2. Patella
3. Tibia
4. Fibula
5. Calcaneous

29 What is the name given to the functional unit of the muscle?
1. Epimysium
2. Endomysium
3. Perimysium
4. Sarcomere
5. Myoneural junction

30 Which one of the following muscles raises the eyebrow?
1. Epicranius
2. Corrugator supercilia
3. Orbicularis oculi
4. Procerus
5. Mentalis

31 Which one of the following muscles closes the eye?
1. Epicranius
2. Corrugator supercilia
3. Orbicularis oculi
4. Procerus
5. Mentalis

32 What are the origin and insertion locations of the platysma muscle?
1. Origin, maxillae; insertion, skin of the sides of the mouth
2. Origin, zygomatic bone; insertion, upper lip
3. Origin, fascia of the deltoid; insertion, lower border of the mandible
4. Origin, maxilla; insertion, ala of the nose
5. Origin, zygomatic bone; insertion, angle of the mouth

33 Relating to nerve impulses, studies of the membrane potential and action potential show that
1. In the nerve cell the nerve impulse always occurs immediately after passage of the action current
2. Inactivation of the membrane, as repolarization begins, is only permeable to the Na^+ ions and not to the K^+ ions
3. The sodium pump is activated as soon as the membrane becomes activated by a threshold stimulus
4. Depolarization is accompanied by a reversal potential of +110 to +120 mV
5. None of the above

34 Which of the following types of neurons carry sensory information?
1. Afferent
2. Efferent
3. Internuncial
4. Multipolar
5. Schwann cells

35 Where is norepinephrine released?
1. In the preganglionic fibers of the autonomic nervous system
2. In the postganglionic fibers of the parasympathetic nervous system
3. In the preganglionic fibers of the sympathetic nervous system
4. In the postganglionic fibers of the sympathetic nervous system
5. None of the above

36 The phrenic nerve innervates the diaphragm. In what portion of the spinal cord is the origin of this nerve?
1. C1 to C4
2. C3 to C5
3. C5 to C8, T1
4. T2 to T12
5. L1 to S4

37 Which of the following descending spinal tracts coordinates the muscles to maintain balance?
1. Fasciculus gracilis
2. Fasciculus cuneatus
3. Spinothalamic
4. Lateral corticospinal
5. Rubrospinal

38 What is the name given for damage to the cortex of the cerebral cortex?
1. Diplopia
2. Aphasia
3. Ataxia
4. Cyanosis
5. Paroxysm

39 The ciliary ganglion is located just behind the eyeball. It receives preganglionic fibers by way of
1. Cranial nerve I
2. Cranial nerve III
3. Cranial nerve V
4. Cranial nerve VII
5. Cranial nerve XII

40 All preganglionic fibers of the parasympathetic division arise from which of the following?
1. Brain and lumbar region of the spinal cord
2. Lumbar and thoracic regions of the spinal cord
3. Thoracic and sacral regions of the spinal cord
4. Brain and thoracic region of the spinal cord
5. Brain and sacral region of the spinal cord

41 Where is the image formed on the eyeball?
1. Retina
2. Iris
3. Pupil
4. Lens
5. Sclera

42 von Willebrand's disease involves deficiencies in clotting factors. Which mineral is necessary to convert prothrombin to thrombin?
1. Copper
2. Calcium
3. Sodium
4. Chloride
5. Potassium

43 The heart contains four sets of valves that act to direct and regulate the flow of blood through the heart. Which fibrous cords extend from the papillary muscles to the edges of the atrioventricular valves?
1. Chordae tendineae
2. Popliteus muscle
3. Pericardium
4. Myocardium
5. Endocardium

44 The QRS complex on the electrocardiogram represents which of the following phenomenon of the action current as it travels across the heart?
1. Depolarization of the atria
2. Depolarization of the ventricles
3. Repolarization of the atria
4. Repolarization of the ventricles
5. None of the above because it is represented on the phonogram

45 What is the name of the structure that guards the opening to the digestive system and is composed of tonsillar tissue?
1. Circle of Willis
2. Cisterna chyli
3. Chordae tendineae
4. Vitreous body
5. Waldeyer's ring

46 The first of three arteries that arise from the aortic arch is the
1. Left subclavian artery
2. Left common carotid artery
3. Right subclavian artery
4. Right common carotid artery
5. Brachiocephalic artery

47 Which of the following arteries does *not* originate from the external carotid artery?
1. Ophthalmic artery
2. Lingual artery
3. Facial artery
4. Occipital artery
5. Superficial temporal artery

48 The vertebral arteries pass upward through the transverse foramina and enter the skull through the foramen magnum. Inside the skull the two vertebral arteries join to form one artery, the
1. Brachiocephalic artery
2. Superficial temporal artery
3. External carotid artery
4. Basilar artery
5. Internal carotid artery

49 What vein arises from the inferior vena cava, passes upward through the aortic hiatus of the diaphragm, and then terminates by emptying into the superior vena cava just above the heart?
1. Brachiocephalic vein
2. Common iliac vein
3. Radial vein
4. Azygos vein
5. Portal vein

50 The larynx is the so-called voice box and is made up of nine cartilages, the largest of which is the
1. Thyroid cartilage
2. Cricoid cartilage
3. Arytenoid cartilage
4. Corniculate cartilage
5. Cuneiform cartilage

51 The mechanics of respiration involve several sets of muscles; however, normally about 80% of the movement of air is accounted for by the movement of the
1. Abdominal muscles
2. Internal intercostal muscles
3. External intercostal muscles
4. Pleura
5. Diaphragm

52 Normal, quiet respiration is referred to as eupnea. Difficult or labored breathing and a very slow rate of respiration are referred to as
1. Dyspnea and bradypnea
2. Apnea and pneumothorax
3. Hypernea and anoxia
4. Orthopnea and tachypnea
5. Cheyne-Stokes respiration and cyanosis

53 Which of the following factors allow for rapid diffusion of gases through the pulmonary membrane
(a) It is thin
(b) It contains epithelial cells
(c) It contains cilia
(d) It contains surfactant
1. a and c
2. b and d
3. a, c, and d
4. a, b, and d
5. All of the above

54 When oxygen is split away from the hemoglobin molecule, it will form
1. Oxyhemoglobin
2. Methemoglobin
3. Reduced hemoglobin
4. Carbaminohemoglobin
5. Carbonic anhydrase

55 The sublingual salivary gland is located in which of the following regions with saliva released through which duct(s)?
1. Preauricular; Rivinus' ducts
2. Preauricular; sublingual caruncles
3. Preauricular; Stensen's duct
4. Sublingual fossa; Stensen's duct
5. Sublingual fossa; Rivinus' ducts

56 What is the name for the bulge at the upper end of the stomach?
1. Cardiac portion
2. Body
3. Fundus
4. Pyloric portion
5. Rugae

57 Which of the following accurately describes the renal circulation?
1. Arcuate artery → interlobar artery → renal artery → glomerulus → efferent arterioles → secondary capillary network → interlobular vein → renal vein → interlobar vein → arcuate vein
2. Renal artery → interlobular artery → arcuate artery → glomerulus → efferent arterioles → secondary capillary network → interlobular vein → arcuate vein → interlobar vein → renal vein
3. Renal artery → glomerulus → arcuate vein → interlobular vein → renal vein
4. Interlobar artery → arcuate artery → renal artery → glomerulus → efferent arterioles → secondary capillary network → interlobular vein → arcuate vein → interlobar vein → renal vein
5. Renal vein → interlobar vein → arcuate vein → interlobar vein → secondary capillary network → efferent arterioles → glomerulus → arcuate artery → interlobar artery → renal artery

58 Which of the following properties is(are) true concerning urine?
(a) Urine is colored by blood pigments
(b) pH varies from 1 to 4
(c) Specific gravity varies from 1.015 to 1.025
(d) Amount excreted daily is approximately 1400 ml
1. a only
2. b and d
3. c and d
4. a, b, and c
5. All of the above

Situation: A woman has a recall oral prophylaxis examination. During the assessment of the patient the dental hygienist notes that the patient has an enlarged mandible, hands, and feet. The patient cannot hear in either ear and reports that the dentures seem too small. Questions 59 and 60 relate to this assessment.

59 This patient most likely is suffering from an imbalance of which pituitary hormone?
1. Somatotropin
2. Prolactin
3. Adrenocorticotropic hormone
4. Thyroid-stimulating hormone
5. Luteinizing hormone

60 From what pathologic state is this patient suffering?
1. Pituitary dwarfism
2. Grave's disease
3. Myxedema
4. Acromegaly
5. Cushing's disease

---

61 Which of the following hormones is produced by a maturing follicle in the ovary?
1. Estrogen
2. Testosterone
3. Follicle-stimulating hormone
4. Luteinizing hormone
5. Thyroid-stimulating hormone

62 Which structure acts as a storage reservoir for sperm in the male?
1. Urethra
2. Testes
3. Epididymis
4. Vas deferens
5. Prostate

Answers and Rationales

1. (3) When a human is in anatomic position (standing with the arms at the sides), the hand is caudal in relation to the head.
   (1) Ventral refers to the anterior surface.
   (2) Dorsal refers to the posterior surface.
   (4) Cephalic refers to the upper extremity (toward the head).
   (5) Posterior refers to the back.
2. (2) A median plane is a sagittal plane that divides the body into right and left halves.
   (1) A sagittal plane divides the body or any of its parts into right and left sides.
   (3) A coronal plane divides the body into anterior and posterior portions.
   (4) A transverse plane is a crosswise plane.
   (5) A horizontal plane is synonymous with a transverse plane.
3. (1) The pleural cavity contains the lungs.
   (2) The heart is in the pericardial cavity.
   (3) The vertebrae and spinal column are in the vertebral cavity.
   (4) The cranial cavity is formed by the bones of the skull and contains the brain.
   (5) The abdominopelvic cavity contains the small and large intestines, stomach, spleen, pancreas, gallbladder, bladder, and reproductive organs.
4. (5) The cell membrane consists of a central core of lipids between two layers of protein.
   (1) The permeability of the cell membrane may be varied.
   (2) The cell membrane has a 3:2 ratio of proteins to lipids.
   (3) The cell membrane has 8 Å pores that allow diffusion of small lipid-insoluble substances.
   (4) The cell membrane is semipermeable.
5. (5) During radiation therapy for squamous cell carcinoma, the chromatids in the cell line up during metaphase.
   (1) The nuclear envelope disappears during prophase.
   (2) Spinal fibers develop during prophase.
   (3) Replication of the genetic material occurs during interphase.
   (4) The centrioles are replicated during telophase.
6. (2) Waldeyer's ring is a ring of tonsillar tissue that forms around the openings of the respiratory and digestive tracts.
   (1) The circle of Willis is formed in the blood supply to the brain.
   (3) Peyer's patches are lymphoid aggregates in the ileum.
   (4) Inguinal lymph nodes are concentrated in the groin.
   (5) Meissner's corpuscles provide the sensation of touch.

For each question the correct answer and rationale are listed first. The other choices are presented in order with the reasons why they are not correct.

7. (5) The pharyngeal tonsils are located in the nasopharynx.
   (1) The inguinal nodes are located in the groin area.
   (2) The lingual tonsils are located at the base of the tongue.
   (3) The palatine tonsils are located between the anterior and posterior pillars of the oral cavity.
   (4) The cervical lymph nodes are located in the neck.
8. (4) The parotid gland empties into Stensen's duct.
   (1) The submandibular gland empties into Wharton's duct.
   (2) The lacrimal gland produces tears for the eye.
   (3) The sublingual gland empties into Bartholin's duct.
   (5) The pharyngeal tonsils do not have ducts.
9. (4) Decreasing the square root of the molecular substance will increase the rate of diffusion.
   (1) Decreasing the concentration differences will decrease the rate of diffusion.
   (2) Increasing the distance will decrease the rate of diffusion.
   (3) Decreasing the temperature will decrease the rate of diffusion.
   (5) Decreasing the cross-sectional area of the chamber will decrease the rate of diffusion.
10. (3) An erythrocyte placed in a solution of sodium chloride less than 0.9% concentration will lyse.
    (1) No change would occur if it were in an isotonic solution.
    (2) Adsorption refers to the sticking together of a gas, liquid, or substance.
    (4) Crenation would occur if it were in a hypertonic solution.
    (5) Diapedesis is a phenomenon demonstrated by white blood cells when they move through tissue spaces.
11. (1) The lateral pterygoids are classified as skeletal muscles, which are voluntary, striated muscles.
    (2) Involuntary, striated muscle describes cardiac muscle.
    (3) Involuntary, smooth muscle describes visceral muscle.
    (4) Voluntary, smooth muscle tissue does not fall into this classification.
    (5) Answer 1 is correct.
12. (2) The greater wing of the sphenoid is the origin and the condyloid process of the mandible is the insertion of the lateral pterygoid muscle.
    (1) The zygomatic process is the origin and the coronoid process is the insertion of the masseter muscle.
    (3) The pterygoid fossa is the origin and the posterior body of the ramus is the insertion of the medial pterygoid muscle.
    (4) The temporal fossa is the origin and the coronoid process is the insertion of the temporalis muscle.
    (5) The hyoid bone is the origin and the tongue is the insertion of the hyoglossus muscle.
13. (3) The lateral pterygoid muscles are part of the group of muscles of mastication that also includes the temporalis, medial pterygoid, and masseter muscles.
    (1) The lateral pterygoid muscles are not muscles of the scalp.

(2) The lateral pterygoid muscles are not used for facial expressions.
(4) The lateral pterygoid muscles are not part of the fibromuscular tongue.
(5) The lateral pterygoid muscles are not part of the larynx.
14. (2) The trigeminal nerve of cranial nerve V innervates the muscles of mastication, which include the lateral pterygoid muscles.
    (1) The olfactory nerve of cranial nerve I provides sensory innervation only.
    (3) The facial nerve of cranial nerve VII innervates the muscles of facial expression.
    (4) The hypoglossal nerve of cranial nerve XII innervates the muscles of the tongue.
    (5) Cervical spinal nerves I and III innervate the infrahyoid group of muscles.
15. (2) Cranial nerve V_3 exits through the foramen ovale.
    (1) Cranial nerve V_2 exits through the foramen rotundum.
    (3) The spinal column exits through the foramen magnum.
    (4) An artery to the meninges is transmitted to the foramen spinosum.
    (5) The internal carotid artery passes through the foramen lacerum.
16. (5) The temporomandibular joint is a synovial joint, which has bones that may be separated by disks and are attached by ligaments.
    (1) Syndesmosis is a fibrous joint, which is two bones united by interosseous ligaments.
    (2) Gomphosis is a fibrous joint, which is the insertion of a cone-shaped process into a socket.
    (3) Synchondrosis is a cartilaginous joint, which is when the ends of the bones are approximated by hyaline cartilage.
    (4) A cartilaginous joint contains no joint cavity, and contiguous bones are united by cartilage.
17. (2) A concentration of 5 mEq/L is the normal concentration of potassium in the extracellular fluid.
    (1) A concentration of 142 mEq/L is the $[Na^+]$ in the extracellular fluid.
    (3) A concentration of 103 mEq/L is the $[Cl^-]$ in the extracellular fluid.
    (4) A concentration of 10 mEq/L is the $[Na^+]$ in the intracellular fluid.
    (5) A concentration of less than 1 mEq/L is the $[Ca^{+2}]$ in the intracellular fluid.
18. (5) Xerostomia is dryness of the oral cavity and is produced by the salivary glands.
    (1) Lacrimal glands produce tears; a lack of secretion would cause xerophthalmia.
    (2) The adrenal gland is an endocrine gland that secretes mineralocorticoids, gluccocorticoids, androgens, and epinephrine.
    (3) The pituitary gland is an endocrine gland that secretes gonadotropins, thyroid-stimulating hormone, adrenocorticotropic hormone, and growth hormone.
    (4) Sebaceous glands secrete oily sebum and are usually located in the skin.

19. (4) The process of tubular reabsorption occurs in convoluted tubules of the kidney.
    (1) The pituitary gland controls hydration levels by secreting an antidiuretic hormone.
    (2) The pancreas secretes enzymes and insulin used for metabolism.
    (3) The colon absorbs water but does not contain tubules.
    (5) The bladder stores urine.

20. (5) A trochanter is one of the two bony prominences on the proximal end of the femur.
    (1) A sharp prominence on a bone is called a spine.
    (2) A large, rounded projection on a bone is called a tuberosity.
    (3) A ridge is a projection on the surface of a bone, such as the femur, that gives attachment to a muscle.
    (4) A sinus is a cavity within a bone.

21. (2) The petrous portion of the temporal bone contains the organs of hearing and equilibrium.
    (1) The zygomatic process forms part of the zygomatic arch on the face.
    (3) The mastoid portion is located behind the ear.
    (4) The glenoid fossa is located at the place where the mandible articulates with the skeleton.
    (5) The styloid process is located anterior to the mastoid process.

22. (5) The glenoid fossa is the site of articulation of the condyle to form the temporomandibular joint.
    (1) The face contains the facial bones and zygomatic arch.
    (2) The mastoid portion of the temporal bone is located behind the ear.
    (3) The petrous portion of the temporal bone is located on the floor of the cranium.
    (4) The squamous portion of the temporal bone is located above the ear.

23. (5) The semicircular canals detect movements caused by changes in fluid pressures within the canals.
    (1) The stapes are auditory ossicles.
    (2) The tympanic membrane is involved in transmitting sound waves.
    (3) The eustachian tube opens to the nasopharynx to equalize pressure.
    (4) The incus is an auditory ossicle.

24. (1) The olecranon fossa is the posterior deep depression located above the articular surfaces.
    (2) The mandibular fossa is located on the temporal bone just anterior to the external acoustic meatus.
    (3) The infraspinous fossa is a large, shallow depression on the dorsal surface of the scapula.
    (4) The subscapula fossa is located on the anterior surface of the scapula.
    (5) The coronoid fossa is the anterior depression above the articular surfaces of the humerus.

25. (4) The lacrimal bones form part of the medial surface of the orbital cavity.
    (1) The vomer is a plowshare-shaped bone forming the lower part of the nasal septum.
    (2) Calvarium is the name given to the domelike superior portion of the skull.

(3) The xiphoid is part of the sternum.
(5) The sphenoid is the butterfly-shaped bone of the skull.

26. (2) The C2 vertebra has a process on the upper surface of the body (dens), which forms a pivot about which the C1 vertebra rotates.
    (1) The atlas (C1 vertebra) articulates with the condyles of the occipital bone.
    (3) The thoracic vertebrae have articulations for the ribs.
    (4) The lumbar vertebrae have heavy bodies that support the weight of the total body.
    (5) The coccygeal vertebrae are fused together.

27. (5) There are 14 phalanges per hand, and they form the fingers.
    (1) The clavicles form part of the shoulder girdles.
    (2) The radii form part of the forearm.
    (3) The carpals form the wrist.
    (4) The metacarpals form the palm of the hand.

28. (1) The femur forms the thigh and is the longest and strongest bone of the body.
    (2) The patella is a sesamoid bone and forms the kneecap.
    (3) The tibia is the medial bone of the leg and approximates with the femur.
    (4) The fibula is the lateral bone of the leg and articulates with the tibia.
    (5) The calcaneous is located beneath the talus and forms the heel.

29. (4) The functional unit of a muscle is the sarcomere and is located between two Z lines of a myofibril.
    (1) The epimysium is the most external connective tissue layer on the muscle.
    (2) The endomysium ties individual fibers together.
    (3) The perimysium is a covering that forms muscle fascicles.
    (5) The myoneural junction consists of the end of a nerve fiber and is located in close approximation to a bundle of muscles.

30. (1) The epicranius is the muscle of facial expression that raises the eyebrow.
    (2) The corrugator supercilia muscle wrinkles the forehead vertically.
    (3) The orbicularis oculi muscle encircles the eyelid and closes the eye.
    (4) The procerus muscle narrows the eye opening.
    (5) The mentalis muscle protrudes the lower lip.

31. (3) The orbicularis oculi muscle encircles the eyelid and closes the eye.
    (1) The epicranius muscle raises the eyebrow.
    (2) The corrugator supercili muscle wrinkles the forehead vertically.
    (4) The procerus muscle narrows the eye opening.
    (5) The mentalis muscle protrudes the lower lip.

32. (3) The fascia of the deltoid is the origin and the lower border of the mandible is the insertion of the platysma muscle.
    (1) The maxilla is the origin and the skin of the sides of the mouth is the insertion of the buccinator muscle.
    (2) The zygomatic bone is the origin and the upper lip is the insertion of the zygomaticus minor muscle.

(4) The maxilla is the origin and the ala of the nose is the insertion of the nasalis muscle.

(5) The zygomatic bone is the origin and the angle of the mouth is the insertion of the zygomaticus major muscle.

33. (2) Inactivation of the neuron membrane, as repolarization begins, is only permeable to the Na⁺ ions and not to the K⁺ ions, which explains repolarization.

(1) The action current must be of sufficient strength for the nerve impulse to occur.

(3) The sodium pump is turned off as soon as the membrane becomes activated by a threshold stimulus.

(4) Depolarization is accompanied by a reversal potential of +35 mV to +40 mV.

(5) Statement 2 is correct.

34. (1) Afferent neurons carry the sensory information to the central nervous system.

(2) Efferent neurons carry the motor information away from the central nervous system.

(3) Internuncial neurons are found within the spinal column and relay information.

(4) Multipolar neurons are neurons that have several processes.

(5) Schwann cells lay myelin around the axons of the nerves.

35. (4) The sympathetic postganglionic fibers (also classified as adrenergic fibers) release norepinephrine.

(1) The preganglionic fibers of the autonomic nervous system are cholinergic fibers and use acetylocholine.

(2) The postganglionic fibers of the parasympathetic nervous system are cholinergic fibers and use acetylcholine.

(3) The preganglionic fibers of the sympathetic nervous system are cholinergic fibers and use acetylcholine.

(5) Statement 4 is correct.

36. (2) The phrenic nerve originates from C3 to C5.

(1) C1 to C4 form the cervical plexus.

(3) C5 to C8 and T1 form the brachial plexus.

(4) T2 to T12 form the intercostal nerves.

(5) All four lumbar nerves and sacral nerves form the lumbrosacral plexus.

37. (5) The rubrospinal tract originates in the midbrain, decussates immediately, and comes down on the opposite side of the brain.

(1) Fasciculus gracilis is an ascending fiber tract.

(2) Fasciculus cuneatus is an ascending fiber tract.

(3) The spinothalmic tract is an ascending fiber tract.

(4) The lateral corticospinal tract is a descending tract and is the main motor tract.

38. (2) Aphasia indicates damage to the cerebral cortex.

(1) Diplopia indicates double vision.

(3) Ataxia indicates damage to the cortex of the cerebellum.

(4) Cyanosis indicates that the tissues are not receiving adequate oxygen.

(5) Paroxysm describes a sudden attack of symptoms.

39. (2) The oculomotor nerve (cranial nerve III) controls almost all of the eye muscles of the iris sphincter and the lacrimal gland.

(1) The olfactory nerve (cranial nerve I) controls the sensation of smell.

(3) The trigeminal nerve (cranial nerve V) provides sensations to the face, sinuses, and teeth.

(4) The facial nerve (cranial nerve VII) innervates the muscles of the face.

(5) The hypoglossal nerve (cranial nerve XII) innervates the muscles of the tongue.

40. (5) The parasympathetic (craniosacral) division is formed by nerves from the brain and sacrum and is active except when under stress.

(1) The brain contributes nerves to the parasympathetic division; the lumbar region contributes nerves to the sympathetic division.

(2) The sympathetic division (thoracolumbar region) is located on either side of the spine.

(3) The thoracic region contributes nerves to the sympathetic division; the sacral region contributes nerves to the parasympathetic division.

(4) The brain contributes nerves to the parasympathetic division; the thoracic region contributes nerves to the sympathetic division.

41. (1) The physical process of forming an image on the retina is much like that used by a camera to produce a picture.

(2) The iris is the colored part of the eye.

(3) Light enters the eye at the pupil.

(4) The lens is a biconvex disk that bends light rays.

(5) The white covering on the anterior aspect of the eye is the sclera.

42. (2) Calcium is necessary to convert prothrombin to thrombin.

(1) Copper aids in the synthesis of hemoglobin in the bone marrow.

(3) Sodium is important in kidney function.

(4) Chloride is important in kidney function.

(5) Potassium is not important in the conversion of prothrombin to thrombin.

43. (1) The atrioventricular valve hangs into the ventricle like a leaf and is held in place by the chordae tendineae.

(2) The popliteus muscle is one of the deep muscles of the back of the leg.

(3) The pericardium makes up part of the heart wall.

(4) The myocardium is the heaviest covering of the heart wall.

(5) The endocardium is the smooth continuous covering of the heart wall.

44. (2) Depolarization of the ventricles is represented by the QRS complex on the electrocardiogram.

(1) Depolarization of the atria is represented by the P wave.

(3) Repolarization of the atria will not show up without the use of special equipment.

(4) Repolarization of the ventricles is represented by the T wave.

(5) The QRS complex is detected on the electrocardiogram.

45. (5) Waldeyer's ring is formed by the palatine, lingual, and pharyngeal tonsils.

    (1) The circle of Willis is formed by blood vessels in the brain.

    (2) The cisterna chyli is a bulblike enlargement at the L2 vertebra and is part of the thoracic duct.

    (3) Chordae tendineae are fibrous chords that extend from the papillary muscles to the edges of the atrioventricular valves in the heart.

    (4) The vitrous body is a transparent jellylike substance that fills the interior of the eyeball behind the lens.

46. (5) The brachiocephalic artery is only a few centimeters in length and is the first branch off the aortic arch.

    (1) The left subclavian artery is the third branch and supplies blood to the scapula and upper chest.

    (2) The left common carotid artery supplies blood to the left side of the head and is the second branch off of the aortic arch.

    (3) The right subclavian artery is the first branch off of the branchiocephalic artery.

    (4) The right common carotid artery is a branch off of the branchiocephalic artery.

47. (1) The ophthalmic artery originates from the internal carotid artery.

    (2) The lingual artery branches from the external carotid and serves the tongue.

    (3) The facial artery branches from the external carotid and serves the face.

    (4) The occipital artery is the main branch of the external carotid.

    (5) The superficial temporal artery branches from the external carotid and serves the face and part of the jaw.

48. (4) The basilar artery joins branches from the internal carotid artery to form the circle of Willis.

    (1) The branchiocephalic artery branches off of the aortic arch.

    (2) The superficial temporal artery branches off of the external carotid artery.

    (3) The external carotid artery branches off of the carotid artery.

    (5) The internal carotid artery branches off of the carotid artery.

49. (4) The azygos vein also picks up veins from the esophagus and bronchi.

    (1) The brachiocephalic veins unite to form the superior vena cava.

    (2) The common iliac veins unite to form the inferior vena cava.

    (3) The radial vein is a deep vein located on the lateral side of the arm.

    (5) The portal vein is the main vein of the hepatic-portal system.

50. (1) There are two thyroid cartilages, one on each side, that fuse at the anterior surface to form one continuous cartilage.

    (2) The cricoid cartilage is signet-ring shaped and is attached by membranes to the upper part of the trachea.

    (3) The arytenoid cartilages are shaped like pyramids and are located on the back of the larynx.

    (4) The corniculate cartilages are two tiny cones, one placed on the apex of each arytenoid cartilage.

    (5) The cuneiform cartilages are two tiny rods placed in the mucous membrane fold and joins the arytenoids to the epiglottis.

51. (5) The dome-shaped diaphragm pulls downward when contracted and will increase the size of the chest cavity.

    (1) The abdominal muscles force the abdominal contents upward during expiration.

    (2) The internal intercostal muscles pull the ribs downward during expiration.

    (3) The external intercostal muscles cause the ribs to elevate during inspiration.

    (4) The pleura is the serous membrane surrounding the visceral and parietal layers of each lung.

52. (1) Dyspnea occurs during difficult breathing; bradypnea is a slow rate of respiration.

    (2) Apnea is the cessation of breathing; pneumothorax is created when the chest wall is punctured.

    (3) Hypernea is the increase in respiration; anoxia occurs when an inadequate amount of oxygen is being received by the tissues.

    (4) Orthopnea occurs when a person can breathe better in one position than another; tachypnea is an increased rate of respiration.

    (5) Cheyne-Stokes respiration consists of abnormal periodic respiration; cyanosis occurs when there is an excess amount of reduced hemoglobin in the capillary circulation.

53. (4) The pulmonary membrane is thin and is composed of surfactant and epithelial cells.

    (1) The pulmonary membrane does not contain cilia.

    (2) True, but its thin design also contributes to the rapid diffusion of gases.

    (3) The pulmonary membrane does not contain cilia but does contain epithelial cells.

    (5) The pulmonary membrane does not contain cilia.

54. (3) Reduced hemoglobin (HHb) is created when the oxygen is split away from the hemoglobin.

    (1) Oxyhemoglobin (Hbo$_2$) is formed when the hemoglobin molecule picks up oxygen in the blood (from the lungs).

    (2) When iron is in the ferric state, it is unable to release oxygen normally.

    (4) Small amounts of carbon dioxide are dissolved in the blood or carried away in carbaminoglobin.

    (5) The chloride shift uses carbonic anhydrase to form carbonic acid.

55. (5) The sublingual glands lie under the tongue, and saliva enters the oral cavity through Rivinus' ducts on the sublingual fold.
    (1) The parotid gland is in the preauricular region, but the saliva from the sublingual gland enters through Rivinus' ducts.
    (2) The parotid gland is in the preauricular region, but saliva from the submandibular glands enters the oral cavity through the sublingual caruncles.
    (3) These two terms describe the parotid gland.
    (4) The sublingual gland is located in the sublingual fossa, but the parotid gland excretes saliva through Stensen's duct.

56. (3) The fundus is located to the left of the esophageal area.
    (1) The cardiac portion of the stomach is where the esophagus enters the stomach.
    (2) The body is the main part of the stomach.
    (4) The pyloric portion of the stomach is where it narrows and connects with the small intestine.
    (5) The rugae are the "wrinkles" on the internal surface of the stomach that increase its surface area.

57. (2) This order of arteries and veins most accurately reflects the blood flow through the xephron.
    (1) The renal artery comes before the interlobar artery, and blood flows through the arcuate vein before it reaches the interlobar vein.
    (3) The interlobular vein comes before the arcuate vein. Also this list of blood vessels is not as complete as answer 2.
    (4) Blood reaches the interlobular artery after it has passed through the renal artery and then the arcuate artery.
    (5) This list suggests that blood flows from the veins and then to the arteries. The reverse list would be correct.

58. (3) The specific gravity of urine ranges from 1.015 to 1.025, and approximately 1400 ml are excreted per day.
    (1) The urine is colored by bile pigments.
    (2) The pH varies from 4.5 to 9, and approximately 1400 ml are excreted per day.
    (4) That is the correct range for the specific gravity, but the urine is colored by bile pigments and the pH varies from 4.5 to 9.

    (5) Answers c and d are correct, but the urine is *not* colored by blood pigments and its pH varies from 4.5 to 9.

59. (1) Somatotropin stimulates growth of both bone and soft tissues.
    (2) Prolactin stimulates milk production by the mammary glands.
    (3) Adenocorticotropic hormone controls the synthetic and secretory activity of the inner two zones of the adrenal cortex.
    (4) Thyroid-stimulating hormone affects thyroid activity.
    (5) Luteinizing hormone is a gonadotropin that is necessary for the implantation of the zygote in the female.

60. (4) Acromegaly is caused by the release of somatotropin after the epiphyses of the bones have closed.
    (1) Pituitary dwarfism is caused by the hyposecretion of somatotropin before the epiphyses of the bones have closed.
    (2) Grave's disease is caused by hypersecretion of thyroid-stimulating hormone.
    (3) Myxedema is caused by hyposecretion of thyroid-stimulating hormone in adults.
    (5) Cushing's syndrome manifests with a moon face, hirsutism, and possible hypertension.

61. (1) Estrogen stimulates the endometrium to become engorged with blood.
    (2) Testosterone is produced in the testes of the male.
    (3) Follicle-stimulating hormone is released by the anterior pituitary, which in turn activates the primary graafian follicle.
    (4) Luteinizing hormone causes the corpus luteum to secrete progesterone.
    (5) Thyroid-stimulating hormone has the thyroid gland as its target organ.

62. (3) Sperm may remain alive for as long as a month in both the epididymis and the tubules.
    (1) The urethra is the passageway for semen from the vas deferens through the penis.
    (2) The testes produce sperm and testosterone.
    (4) The vas deferens conducts sperm from the epididymis.
    (5) The prostate secretes an alkaline fluid that activates sperm.

CHAPTER 4

Dental Anatomy and Root Morphology

DONALD E. ISSELHARD

Dental anatomy is one of the fundamental dental sciences on which the clinical practice of the dental hygienist is based. With a thorough knowledge of the clinical structures of the oral cavity, dental anatomy, and root morphology, the dental hygienist is able to assess patient oral health status, distinguish normal from abnormal, and use essential terminology and charting systems for effective communication with other dental professionals. Moreover, knowledge of root morphology is essential for the development of proficiency in scaling and root planning—skills critical to the dental hygienist's role in oral health promotion, disease control, and periodontal health maintenance. This chapter addresses basic dental anatomy including structures of the oral cavity, dental nomenclature, anatomy and root morphology of the primary and permanent dentitions, and eruption sequences.

ORAL CAVITY – BASIC STRUCTURES

A. Vestibule—space between the lips and cheeks on one side and by the teeth and gingiva on the other side
 1. Labial frenum—thin fold of tissue that extends from the midline of the lip to the mucosa covering the jaw; found within the vestibule (maxillary and mandibular)
 2. Buccal frenum—thin folds of tissue that attach the cheek to the mucosa of the jaws; found within the vestibule (maxillary and mandibular) in the area of the premolars
B. Lips—junction between the face and oral cavity
 1. Lined by moist mucous membrane on the inside of the oral cavity and by skin on the outside
  a. Labia (lips) form the anterior border of the vestibule
   (1) Labium superius—upper lip
   (2) Labium inferius—lower lip
  b. Philtrum—midline vertical indentation of the skin below the nasal septum
  c. Commissure—junction of the upper and lower lips at the corners of the mouth

 2. May be reddish brown because of melanin pigmentation in dark-skinned individuals
 3. Vermilion zone—reddish tissue that lies in an area of transition where the lip joins the face
 4. Mucobuccal or mucolabial fold—composed of alveolar mucosa; extends from the lips or cheeks to attached gingiva; as alveolar mucosa it is soft, thin, and loosely attached to the underlying bone; transition between the vestibule and oral cavity proper; joins these two at the mucogingival junction; darker red in color than gingiva because it is nonkeratinized
C. Cheeks—covered by shiny mucous membrane on the inside and skin on the outside; form the lateral border of the vestibule
 1. Fordyce's granules or spots—small yellowish elevations that are isolated sebaceous glands inside the lips and cheeks; these glands are embedded in the mucous membrane as a result of the fusion of the upper and lower parts of the cheek during embryonic development
 2. Stensen's duct—opening of the parotid salivary gland; appears bilaterally as a small elevation of tissue on the inside of the cheek opposite the maxillary first molar
D. Oral cavity proper—area from the teeth or alveolar ridges to the hard and soft palate, where it ends posteriorly at the palatine tonsils; in the mandibular area the tongue occupies the middle section
E. Gingiva—stratified squamous epithelium that surrounds the teeth and is firmly attached to the alveolar bone; extends from the mucogingival junction (fold) across the alveolar ridges and also covers the hard palate; varies in color from coral pink to brown or is spotted with brown according to the skin coloring of the individual
 1. Free or marginal gingiva—unattached gingival tissue that surrounds the teeth and joins the attached gingiva at the gingival groove; forms the wall of the gingival crevice

2. Attached gingiva—gingival tissue that is firmly attached to the underlying bone and joins the alveolar mucosa at the mucogingival junction
3. Interdental papilla—gingival tissue found between teeth in the interproximal area
4. Alveolar mucosa—nonkeratinized oral mucosa that covers the alveolar process

F. Alveolar arches—bony processes or ridges in the maxilla and mandible that hold the teeth; provide anchorage for roots of teeth within their alveolar processes
1. Maxillary tuberosity—bony protuberance behind the last maxillary molar
2. Retromolar area—triangular bony prominence behind the last mandibular molar
3. Exostoses—bony growths on the facial cortical plate or hard palate of the maxilla and sometimes on the facial or lingual cortical plate of bone on the mandible (e.g., palatine tori [torus palatinus] and mandibular tori)

G. Roof of the mouth—divided into the hard and soft palates
1. Hard palate—anterior portion of the roof of the mouth from the lingual aspect of the maxillary incisors to the third-molar area; covered by firmly attached gingiva that is grayish red because of keratinization
   a. Incisive papilla—bulge of tissue at the midline immediately lingual to the central incisors; carries the nasopalatine nerve, which innervates the soft tissue lingual to the maxillary anterior teeth
   b. Palatine rugae—series of irregular tissue ridges radiating in a web-shaped pattern behind the maxillary anterior incisors; usually at least four rows
   c. Palatine raphe—narrow, slightly elevated ridge that runs from the incisive papilla posteriorly to the end of the hard palate; joins the right and left maxillae
2. Soft palate—extends from the hard palate laterally to the hamular process of the medial pterygoid plate and posteriorly to the uvula; usually redder in appearance than the hard palate; pharynx is behind the soft palate
   a. Uvula—small fleshy tissue projecting downward from the midline of the posterior border of the soft palate
   b. Anterior palatine pillar—fold of tissue that can be seen at the back of the mouth extending from the soft palate to the base of the tongue

   c. Posterior palatine pillar—fold of tissue that extends from the soft palate downward toward the pharynx
   d. Palatine tonsil—lymphoid tissue located bilaterally between the anterior and posterior palatine pillars
   e. Oropharyngeal isthmus—opening into the pharynx
   f. Pterygomandibular raphe—outside of the soft palate; separates the soft palate from the cheek; extends from the buccinator muscle to the superior constrictor of the pharynx; can be seen extending from the retromolar area

H. Floor of the mouth—area of the oral cavity that lies beneath the tongue; covered by smooth, shiny lining mucosa; large blood vessels are visible
1. Lingual frenum—also called frenulum; attaches the ventral side of the tongue to the floor of the mouth
2. Sublingual caruncle—papilla located on the right and left sublingual folds; contains a pair of openings from ducts (Wharton's duct) of the submandibular gland and the major sublingual duct of the sublingual gland
3. Sublingual folds or plica sublingualis—begin from the sublingual caruncle and run posteriorly in a V-shaped direction along the floor of the mouth; house the openings of ducts from the underlying salivary glands

I. Tongue—located within the curve of the mandible; broad, flat muscular organ of speech and taste; grayish red; rough because of the presence of numerous papillae on the dorsal surface
1. Papillae
   a. Circumvallate or vallate papillae—V-shaped row of 8 to 12 large mushroom-shaped, raised papillae located on the posterodorsal surface of the tongue in front of the sulcus terminalis; surrounded by a trough containing von Ebner's glands; taste buds are present in large numbers
   b. Fungiform papillae—large red raised projections primarily at the sides and apex of the dorsal surface of the tongue; bear taste buds
   c. Filiform papillae—threadlike projections covering the anterior two thirds of the dorsal surface of the tongue
   d. Foliate papillae—projections, inconsistent in size and number, found near the posterior border of the tongue; bear taste buds and excretory ducts from von Ebner's glands

2. Lingual tonsils—mass of lymphoid tissue immediately behind the circumvallate papillae on the most posterior aspect of the dorsum of the tongue
3. Foramen cecum—pit on the posterior midline of the dorsum of the tongue; marks the point where the stalk of the thyroglossal duct originated

BASIC NOMENCLATURE

Classification of Dentitions

A. Diphyodont—having two different dentitions in a lifetime—primary dentition and permanent dentition—such as that found in humans
   1. Succedaneous—replace primary teeth
   2. Nonsuccedaneous—permanent molars
B. Dentitions
   1. Primary or deciduous dentition—set of 20 teeth (10 maxillary and 10 mandibular) that erupt during ages 6 months to 2 years
   2. Mixed dentition—both primary and permanent teeth present at the same time; occurs during ages 6 to 12 years
   3. Permanent dentition—set of 32 teeth (16 maxillary and 16 mandibular) that erupt during ages 6 to 21 years

Classification of Teeth and Dental Formula

A. Primary or deciduous teeth

Incisors	I	$\frac{2}{2}$
Canines	C	$\frac{1}{1}$
Molars	M	$\frac{2}{2}$

B. Permanent teeth

Incisors	I	$\frac{2}{2}$
Canines	C	$\frac{1}{1}$
Premolars	P	$\frac{2}{2}$
Molars	M	$\frac{3}{3}$

Numbering Systems

A. Palmer notation—dental charting method used in graphically representing the teeth; mouth is divided into four quadrants ┼; each quadrant has its own bracket (e.g., ⌋, ∟, ⌐, Γ)
   1. Permanent dentition uses the numbers *1* to *8*
   2. Primary or deciduous dentition uses the letters *a* to *e*
   3. Examples— ⌋ is the permanent maxillary right central incisor; *l̲a̲* is the primary mandibular left central incisor

B. Universal numbering system—dental charting method used in graphically representing the teeth; uses Arabic numerals
   1. Each permanent tooth is assigned a number from 1 to 32
   2. Each primary tooth is assigned a letter from A to T
   3. System begins from the most posterior molar on the maxillary right, extends across the maxillary arch to the most posterior mandibular left molar, and goes back across the mandibular arch
   4. Examples—*16* is the permanent maxillary left third molar; *S* is the primary mandibular right first molar
C. FDI system (Federation Dentaire Internationale)—dental charting method used in graphically representing the teeth
   1. Permanent teeth are numbered from 1 to 8 in each quadrant as in the Palmer system; in addition, each quadrant has its own number—*1* is assigned to the maxillary right quadrant, *2* to the maxillary left quadrant, *3* to the mandibular left quadrant, and *4* to the mandibular right quadrant (e.g., *18* is the maxillary right central incisor)
   2. Primary dentition has the number *5* assigned to the maxillary right quadrant, *6* to the maxillary left, *7* to the mandibular left, and *8* to the mandibular right (e.g., *83* would be the primary mandibular right canine; *64* the primary mandibular left first molar; *48* the permanent mandibular right third molar; *17* the permanent maxillary right second molar)

DENTAL NOMENCLATURE – BASIC TERMINOLOGY

A. Parts of a tooth
   1. Crown
   2. Root
   3. Pulp
   4. Pulp cavity
B. Tissue making up a tooth
   1. Dentin—hard tissue surrounding the pulp and underlying the enamel and cementum; makes up the bulk of a tooth
   2. Enamel—hard, calcified tissue covering the anatomic crown of a tooth
   3. Cementum—bonelike connective tissue covering the anatomic root of a tooth
   4. Pulpal tissue—innermost tissue containing blood vessels, lymphatics, and nerves

C. Pulp cavity
  1. Pulp canal—portion of the pulp cavity in the root of the tooth
  2. Pulp chamber—central portion of the pulp cavity
  3. Pulp horns—extensions of the pulp chamber toward the cusps of lobes of teeth
D. Tooth surfaces
  1. Mesial—surface of the tooth that faces toward the midline
  2. Distal—surface of the tooth that faces away from the midline
  3. Lingual—surface of the tooth that faces toward the tongue
  4. Facial—surface of the tooth that faces toward the lips or cheeks
    a. Labial—facial surfaces of anterior teeth
    b. Buccal—facial surfaces of posterior teeth
  5. Incisal—biting edges of anterior teeth
  6. Occlusal—chewing surfaces of posterior teeth
E. Line angles—imaginary line formed by the junction of two crown surfaces
  1. Line angles for anterior teeth
    a. Distolabial
    b. Mesiolabial
    c. Distolingual
    d. Mesiolingual
    e. Linguoincisal
    f. Labioincisal
  2. Line angles for posterior teeth
    a. Distobuccal
    b. Mesiobuccal
    c. Distolingual
    d. Mesiolingual
    e. Distoocclusal
    f. Mesioocclusal
    g. Buccoocclusal
    h. Linguoocclusal
F. Point angles—point at which three surfaces of a tooth meet
  1. Point angles for anterior teeth
    a. Mesiolabioincisal
    b. Distolabioincisal
    c. Mesiolinguoincisal
    d. Distolinguoincisal
  2. Point angles for posterior teeth
    a. Mesiobuccoocclusal
    b. Distobuccoocclusal
    c. Mesiolinguoocclusal
    d. Distolinguoocclusal
G. Crown elevations
  1. Cusps—large, elevated points or peaks on the occlusal surfaces of molar and premolar teeth and on the incisal edges of canine teeth

  2. Cingulum—large rounded eminence on the cervical third of the lingual surface of the crown of an anterior tooth
  3. Tubercles—small rounded projections
  4. Ridges—elevated portions of a tooth that run in a line
    a. Marginal ridges—on incisor teeth the rounded borders of enamel that form the mesial and distal shoulders of the lingual surface; on posterior teeth the rounded borders of enamel that form the mesial and distal boundaries of the occlusal surface
    b. Triangular ridge—ridge from the cusp tip toward the central groove of the occlusal surface
    c. Transverse ridge—union of two triangular ridges: a buccal and a lingual cusp; ridge crosses the occlusal surface in a buccolingual direction
    d. Oblique ridge—special type of transverse ridge that crosses in an oblique direction from the distobuccal to mesiolingual cusps on maxillary molars
    e. Labial ridge—ridge that crosses the center of the labial surface of a canine tooth in a cervicoincisal direction
    f. Buccal ridge—ridge that crosses the center of the buccal surface of a premolar tooth in a cervicoocclusal direction
    g. Cervical ridge—ridge that crosses the cervical third of a crown in a mesiodistal direction
  5. Mamelons—small rounded projections of enamel on the incisal edges of newly erupted anterior teeth
H. Crown depressions
  1. Fossa—depression on the lingual surface of an anterior tooth and on the occlusal surface of a posterior tooth
  2. Sulcus—long, narrow depression on the occlusal surface of a posterior tooth; a groove is at the bottom of a sulcus
  3. Groove—narrow linear depression on the surface of a tooth, named according to location
    a. Developmental grooves—grooves that divide cusps or lobes from each other
    b. Supplemental grooves—irregular grooves that branch from a developmental groove; usually found on occlusal surfaces
  4. Pit—small depression where two or more developmental grooves join; deepest part of a fossa
I. Lobe—one of the primary anatomic divisions of a crown, usually separated by developmental grooves

J. Cervical line—demarcation where the enamel and cementum meet; also known as the cementoenamel junction (CEJ)

K. Dentinoenamel junction (DEJ)—where the enamel and dentin meet inside the tooth

L. Periodontium—supporting structures of the teeth
  1. Periodontal ligament
  2. Alveolar process
  3. Gingiva
  4. Cementum
  5. Dentogingival junction

M. Interproximal terminology
  1. Proximal area—surface area between two adjacent teeth in the same arch
  2. Proximal contact area—area of the proximal surface that actually contacts or touches the adjacent tooth
  3. Interproximal spaces—V-shaped spaces between the teeth formed by the proximal surfaces and their contact areas; these spaces are normally filled with gingival tissue called papillary gingiva or interdental papilla
  4. Embrasures (also called spillways and interdental spillways)—spaces between the teeth that widen from the contact areas facially and lingually
    a. Crowns of most teeth converge lingually, except for the maxillary first molar and the mandibular second premolar; other teeth are narrower mesiodistally on the lingual surfaces; therefore their lingual embrasures are wider than their facial embrasures
    b. Functions of embrasures
      (1) Shunt food away from the contact areas during mastication
      (2) Reduce the forces of occlusal trauma
      (3) Provide self-cleansing areas around the interproximal spaces
      (4) Allow stimulation to the gingiva by the frictional massage of food

N. Contact areas
  1. Facial view
    a. Contact areas of the anterior teeth are located closer to the incisal surfaces of the teeth
    b. Posterior teeth have their contact areas closer to the middle third of the teeth
    c. The more posterior the tooth, the more cervical the location of its contact area; the one exception is the distal contact area of the maxillary canine, which is located more cervical than that of the first or second premolar

  2. Occlusal view
    a. Contact areas of anterior teeth are located in the middle third between the labial and lingual surfaces
    b. Posterior teeth have contact areas slightly buccal to the center of the teeth
    c. Buccolingually, the lingual embrasures are wider than the facial embrasures; this is because, from their contact points outward, the teeth are narrower on the lingual than on the facial side

O. Heights of contour
  1. Height of contour is the area of greatest bulge on the facial and lingual surfaces of a tooth
  2. In anterior teeth the height of contour on both the labial and lingual surfaces is located in the cervical (gingival) third
  3. In posterior teeth on the buccal surface the height of contour is located in the cervical third
  4. In posterior teeth on the lingual surface the height of contour is located in the middle or occlusal third

P. Curvature of the cementoenamel junction (cervical line)
  1. Crowns of anterior teeth show greater curvature to the cervical line than do those of posterior teeth
  2. Amount of curvature of the mesial surface is greater than on the distal surface

Q. Roots—general characteristics
  1. Root of a tooth is widest at the cervical line and tapers toward the apex
  2. Length, shape, and number of roots are determined by the form and function of the tooth
  3. Roots and classification of teeth
    a. Incisors—usually have single, slender roots
    b. Canines
      (1) Usually have single, very long roots
      (2) Mandibular canines may, on rare occasion, be bifurcated
      (3) Have the longest roots of any teeth
    c. Premolars
      (1) Mandibular premolars have a single root
      (2) Maxillary premolars have a tendency to bifurcate
      (3) Maxillary first premolars usually have two roots: one buccal and one palatal
      (4) Mandibular second premolars occasionally have two roots but more often have a single root
    d. Molars
      (1) Multirooted
      (2) Maxillary molars are trifurcated with one lingual and two buccal roots

(3) Mandibular molars usually are bifurcated with one mesial and one distal root

(4) Third molars often have their roots fused except for the apices

(5) The more posterior the tooth, the shorter the root, the larger the crown/root ratio, and the closer the roots

ERUPTION

A. Primary or deciduous dentition
1. There are 20 primary teeth; 5 in each quadrant: 2 incisors (1 central and 1 lateral), 1 canine, and 2 molars (1 first and 1 second)
2. Primary dentition erupts into full occlusion by 3 years of age
3. By age 5 years the teeth should no longer be in proximal contact with each other because of the rapid growth of both arches
4. Primary dentition is important to ensure normal jaws and teeth and maintain space for the permanent teeth
5. As a general rule, individual mandibular teeth usually precede eruption of maxillary teeth
6. Period of primary dentition begins between ages 6 and 8 months with the eruption of the first primary tooth; this period ends with the eruption of the first permanent tooth
7. Sequence of tooth eruption—primary dentition (great individual variation)[1]

	Maxillary	Mandibular
Central incisor	7½ months	6 months
Lateral incisor	9 months	7 months
Canine	18 months	16 months
First molar	14 months	12 months
Second molar	24 months	20 months

8. Process of exfoliation (shedding of the primary teeth) is made possible because the roots of the primary teeth are resorbed by the pressure generated by the erupting permanent successors; pressure exerted by the eruption of the permanent teeth triggers osteoclastic cells to resorb not only the bone, but also the roots of the primary teeth
9. General characteristics
   a. Primary teeth are smaller than permanent teeth
   b. Primary teeth are whiter in color than permanent teeth
   c. Anterior teeth
      (1) Prominent cervical ridge on the facial surface of the crown
      (2) Root is long and narrow in proportion to the crown

(3) Labial surface is usually free of depressions

(4) Crown is narrow at the cervix

   d. Posterior teeth
      (1) Prominent cervical ridge
      (2) Coronal surface is usually free of depressions
      (3) Root furcation is near the cervical line
      (4) Roots are divergent

B. Mixed dentition
1. From 6 to 12 years of age, the primary teeth are gradually exfoliated and replaced by the permanent teeth
2. Both primary and permanent teeth are present; therefore a period of mixed dentition exists
3. As the jaws grow, spaces occur between the primary teeth; these spaces are called primate spaces
   a. Primate spaces play an important role in helping the permanent teeth come into proper occlusion
   b. If no primate spaces exist, crowding of the permanent teeth will more likely occur, since the anterior permanent teeth are larger than the primary teeth they are replacing

C. Permanent dentition
1. Period of mixed dentition ends after the last primary tooth is exfoliated
2. Permanent incisors, canines, and premolars all succeed primary teeth and therefore are called succedaneous teeth; permanent molars have no predecessors in the primary dentition
3. If a primary tooth was not formed, no succedaneous replacement will form; succedaneous teeth are formed from their primary predecessor's tooth buds
4. Anterior permanent teeth are positioned lingual to the primary anterior teeth; as eruption occurs, anterior permanent teeth move labially
5. Posterior permanent premolars are positioned between the bifurcations of the primary molars; posterior permanent molars erupt straight into the area occupied by the primary molars
6. Sequence of tooth eruption–permanent dentition (great individual variation)

Mandibular first molar	6-7 years
Maxillary first molar	6-7 years
Mandibular central incisor	6-7 years
Mandibular lateral incisor	7-8 years
Maxillary central incisor	7-8 years
Maxillary lateral incisor	8-9 years
Mandibular canine	9-10 years
First premolar	9-10 years
Second premolar	11-12 years
Maxillary canine	11-12 years
Second molar	11-13 years
Third molar	17-21 years

D. Essential differences between primary and permanent teeth
   1. Primary anterior teeth are smaller than their permanent successors in both crown and root portions
   2. Primary molars are wider mesiodistally than the permanent premolars that replace them
   3. Roots of primary teeth are narrower and longer in comparison with the crown length than the roots of permanent teeth; posterior primary teeth flare their roots in order to accommodate the permanent premolars
   4. Anatomic crowns of primary teeth are relatively short compared with their anatomic roots
   5. All of the primary teeth appear very bulbous buccolingually
   6. Crowns of primary teeth are more constricted at the cervix, since the root trunk is narrow and short
   7. Primary teeth are usually lighter in color than permanent teeth
   8. Buccal and lingual surfaces of primary molars taper occlusally above the cervical curvatures much more than do the permanent molar surfaces; this results in a much narrower occlusal table buccolingually
   9. There are faciocervical ridges of enamel on the primary anterior and molar teeth
   10. In primary teeth the pulp chambers are relatively large in comparison with the crowns that envelop them
   11. In primary teeth the pulp horns extend rather high occlusally, placing them much closer to the enamel than occurs in permanent teeth
   12. Dentin thickness between the pulp chambers and the enamel is much less in primary than in permanent teeth
   13. Enamel in primary teeth is relatively thin and has a consistent depth

PERMANENT DENTITION

Incisors

General Characteristics

A. There are eight permanent incisors: four maxillary (upper) and four mandibular (lower)
B. Maxillary group consists of two central and two lateral incisors, as does the mandibular group
C. Incisal two thirds appear flattened on labial and lingual sides
D. Incisors have a biting edge called an incisal edge; they have no cusps

Maxillary Central Incisors

A. Crown
   1. Greater crown/root ratio (crown larger; root about the same as or smaller than that of the lateral incisor)
   2. Maxillary central incisor is the widest mesiodistally of any of the anterior teeth; crown is wider mesiodistally than faciolingually
   3. Mesioincisal angle is relatively sharp (90-degree angle), with the contact area in the incisal third
   4. Lingual fossa is broad and smooth with a well-developed cingulum
   5. Distoincisal angle is more rounded than the mesioincisal angle, with the contact area at the junction of the incisal and middle thirds
   6. Incisal margin may have mamelons
   7. Facial surface may show two developmental lines running vertically and separating the three facial lobes
   8. Imbrication lines—faint cervically curved lines on the facial surface, running mesiodistally along the cervical third of the crown, are usually present
B. Root
   1. Single conical root, relatively straight and tapering to a rounded apex
   2. Triangular in cross section; broader on the facial side
   3. Length is 1½ times the crown length
   4. Two anomalies that sometimes occur are a short root or an unusually long crown
   5. No grooves or depressions appear along the root

Maxillary Lateral Incisors

A. Crown
   1. Lesser crown/root ratio (crown smaller; root about the same as that of the central incisor)
   2. Mesioincisal angle is more rounded than that of the central incisor, with the contact area at the junction of the middle and incisal thirds
   3. Small cingulum, often with a lingual pit
   4. Distoincisal angle is more rounded than the mesioincisal angle, with the contact area in the middle third
   5. Lateral incisor is smaller in all dimensions than the central incisor except for the root length, which may be as long
   6. As with all mandibular and maxillary incisors, three mamelons may be present
   7. Lateral incisor is relatively longer incisocervically and narrower mesiodistally than the central incisor; in all other ways the lateral

incisor appears to resemble the central incisor; is just a smaller, more rounded, anatomically more pronounced version of the central incisor

8. Lateral incisor is more likely to have lingual pits, lingual tubercles, a more pronounced cingulum, and a more prominent incisal edge; is likely to be more convex labially and lingually

B. Root
1. Maxillary lateral incisor, like the central incisor, has a single conical root; in comparison, the lateral incisor's root appears narrower and longer
2. Apex of the root is sharper; apical third may be deflected toward the distal aspect
3. No grooves or depressions are present

C. Anomalies
1. Peg-shaped lateral incisor, a common anomaly, is a very small cone-shaped tooth with no development on the mesial or distal portions of the crown
2. Corkscrew type of lateral incisor, with the enamel twisted around the crown, a developmental anomaly, is sometimes associated with prenatal infections
3. Maxillary lateral incisors are the most congenitally missing of the anterior teeth; are also the most varied in appearance, anomalies, size, and shape of all anterior teeth

Mandibular Central Incisors

A. Crown
1. Smaller than that of the maxillary central or lateral incisor; mandibular central incisor is the smallest permanent tooth
2. Wider faciolingually than mesiodistally; occludes only with one opposing tooth (the maxillary central incisor) because it is so much smaller mesiodistally than the maxillary central incisor
3. Compared with the maxillary incisor, the structures of the mandibular incisor are less prominent (e.g., the cingulum is smaller, the lingual margins are poorly formed, and no lingual pits or grooves are present)
4. Incisal edge wears on the labial surface
5. Both the mesioincisal angle and the distoincisal angle are relatively sharp and almost identical, making this tooth the most symmetric tooth in the mouth
6. Both the mesial and distal contact areas are in the incisal third
7. Mandibular central incisor is one of two teeth in the mouth that occlude with only one opposing tooth (the other is the maxillary third molar)

B. Root
1. Single, straight, symmetrically shaped root
2. Apex does not usually point in any specific direction; rather, is more likely to be straight up and down
3. Oval in cross section
4. May appear longer compared with the crown

Mandibular Lateral Incisors

A. Crown
1. Mandibular lateral incisor appears to have the same form as the mandibular central incisor except that the lateral incisor is bigger in all dimensions than the central incisor
2. Distoincisal line angle is more rounded than the mesioincisal line angle
3. Contact area on the distal surface is at the junction of the incisal and middle thirds, whereas the contact area on the mesial surface is in the incisal third
4. Incisal edge curves toward the lingual in its distal portion
5. Cingulum is displaced slightly toward the distal surface
6. Compared with the maxillary incisor, the structure of the mandibular incisor is less prominent (e.g., the cingulum is smaller, the lingual margins are poorly formed, and no lingual pit or grooves are present)

B. Root
1. Usually straight root
2. Slightly wider, thicker, and longer than that of the mandibular central incisor
3. Apex may point toward the labial or distal aspect
4. Proximal grooves are commonly found on the root surface, giving the appearance of a double root
5. May appear longer compared with the crown

Canines
General Characteristics

A. The four maxillary and mandibular permanent canines, one on each side of the jaw, are the longest teeth in the mouth
B. Their position at the corners of the mouth have earned them the title of "cornerstones of the mouth"
C. Canines have the longest roots of any teeth; these roots are embedded in thick bony anchorage
D. Extra-heavy labial bony eminence protects the canine from lateral displacement; this projection of bone is called the canine eminence

E. Like the incisors, the canines are formed from four lobes: three labial and one lingual; they have much more developed lingual and middle facial lobes; middle lobe extension results in formation of a single cusp

F. Lingual lobe is much thicker than in the incisors; canines are therefore much wider labiolingually than incisors and have a much more developed cingulum

Maxillary Canines

A. Crown
   1. Longest tooth in the mouth
   2. Cingulum shows greater development than in the incisors, with two lingual fossae, an extremely developed lingual cusp ridge, and an occasional lingual pit
   3. Mesial contact area is at the junction of the incisal and middle thirds
   4. Distal contact area is at the middle third
   5. Distal surface is more convex than the mesial surface, and there is a concavity from the distal contact area to the cervical line
   6. Distal marginal ridge is more highly developed than the mesial marginal ridge

B. Root
   1. Longest root of any of the teeth or at least as long as that of the mandibular canine
   2. Triangular in cross section
   3. There is a developmental groove (longitudinal groove) on the mesial and distal aspects of the root

Mandibular Canines

A. Crown (in comparison with that of the maxillary canine)
   1. Mandibular canine is narrower, less developed, and somewhat smaller; its cingulum is less developed, and the marginal ridges are less prominent
   2. Mandibular canine crown is narrower mesiodistally
   3. Mandibular canine crown length is as long as that of the maxillary canine and is sometimes even longer
   4. Labiolingual measurement of the crown and root is usually less than that of the maxillary canine
   5. Lingual surface of the mandibular canine is smoother, the cingulum is less developed, and the marginal ridges are less prominent than those of the maxillary canine; lingual surface resembles that of the mandibular anterior incisor
   6. Cusp of the mandibular canine is less well developed

B. Root
   1. Longest mandibular root; second in length only to that of maxillary canine; may be as long as that of a maxillary canine
   2. Wide labiolingually and narrow mesiodistally
   3. Some specimens show a bifurcated root in the apical third
   4. Mandibular canine is the anterior tooth most likely to have a bifurcated root; when the root is bifurcated, one branch is labial and the other lingual
   5. Single-rooted form is much more common; if deep longitudinal grooves are present on the proximal surfaces of the root, there tend to be two root canals even if they join together at the apex

Premolars

General Characteristics

A. Permanent premolars succeed the primary molars

B. Term *premolar* implies that these teeth are immediately before the molars

C. Premolars are a transition in shape and function between the anterior teeth and the molars

D. Premolars have at least one buccal and one lingual cusp

E. Mandibular second premolar may have two lingual cusps

F. Maxillary premolars
   1. Maxillary first premolars have two cusps: one buccal and one lingual
   2. Maxillary premolars may have either a single or a bifurcated root
   3. Most maxillary first premolars have two roots and two pulp canals; even when only one root is present, two pulp canals can usually be found; it is not uncommon for maxillary second premolars to also have two roots; however, there is usually only one
   4. Mesial and distal contact areas are more nearly equal in their height
   5. All maxillary posterior premolars have their cusp tips centered over their roots

G. Mandibular premolars
   1. Mandibular first premolars have many of the characteristics of the mandibular canines
   2. Mandibular premolars have a short buccal cusp, which is the only part that occludes with the maxillary teeth
   3. Lingual cusps of the mandibular premolars are small and afunctional compared with the larger lingual cusps of the maxillary premolars
   4. Lingual cusps of the mandibular premolars are not centered over their roots; rather, they are lingual to their roots

Maxillary First Premolars

A. Crown
1. From the facial view, the maxillary premolar has the appearance of the maxillary canine, but it is shorter as well as narrower mesiodistally
2. Buccal cusp is longer than the lingual cusp
3. Mesial marginal groove extends from the mesial marginal ridge of the mesial surface of the crown; it crosses the mesial marginal ridge and runs from the occlusal to the middle third of the crown
4. Mesial developmental depression is located cervically to the mesial contact area
5. All maxillary first premolars have their cusp tips centered over their roots

B. Root
1. Root may be either single or bifurcated
2. Bifurcated root form is far more common, but even in the single root form, two root canals are usually present
3. Bifurcated root form consists of one buccal (facial) and one palatal (lingual) root
4. On the single-rooted form grooves are usually present on the mesial and distal aspects of the root; these grooves run lengthwise and give the appearance of trying to divide the root into two

Maxillary Second Premolars

A. Crown
1. As with the first premolar, both the lingual and buccal cusps are centered over their roots
2. Buccal cusp of the second premolar is more nearly equal the size of the lingual cusp; buccal cusp is less pointed than that on the first premolar
3. No depression is present on the mesial or distal crown surfaces
4. Mesial marginal groove is present that is similar to the distal marginal groove, but usually it does not cross the ridge
5. From the occlusal view, the second premolar is more bilaterally symmetric than the first premolar
6. From the occlusal view, there is a transverse ridge formed by the buccal triangular ridge and the lingual triangular ridge
7. Central groove is short, with frequent and numerous supplemental grooves
8. Central groove ends in the mesial and distal triangular fossae
9. Second premolar is less angular and more rounded in appearance than the first premolar; also varied more than the first premolar in size, shape, groove pattern, etc.

B. Root
1. Usually single root with a longitudinal groove on the mesial surface and a deeper longitudinal groove on the distal surface; groove gives the appearance of trying to divide the root into two: buccally and lingually
2. Usually there is only one root canal, but often a divided canal occurs in at least a portion of the root
3. Bifurcated root similar to that of the first premolar is common; this form has two root canals
4. Root tapers to the apex, which may be bent distally

Mandibular First Premolars

A. Crown
1. Like the maxillary premolar, this premolar has two cusps: one buccal and one lingual
2. This tooth develops from four lobes; three lobes form the buccal cusp, and one lobe forms the small lingual cusp
3. Occlusal surface slopes toward the lingual side in a cervical direction
4. Mesial and distal contact areas are located in the middle third
5. Distal marginal ridge is more developed than the mesial marginal ridge
6. A mesial and a distal pit lie on each side of the lingual triangular ridge of the buccal cusp; significance of these pits is their susceptibility to caries
7. These are the only premolars (maxillary or mandibular) that may have a transverse ridge that does not cross an occlusal developmental groove
8. Triangular ridge of the buccal cusp slopes toward the center of the occlusal surface; triangular ridge of the lingual cusp is nearly horizontal
9. Frequently a depression or groove crosses the mesial marginal ridge on the lingual third of the tooth; this is the most striking characteristic of this tooth; because of the extreme lingual location, this groove is called the mesiolingual developmental groove; no such groove exists on the distal marginal ridge
10. Great variation exists in the occlusal morphology of the mandibular first premolar

B. Root
1. Single root occupied by a single root canal
2. Mesial and distal root surfaces are usually slightly convex; if a longitudinal groove is present, it may be deep or shallow

3. In cross section the root is convex buccally and narrow lingually
4. From the facial aspect the tip of the root is often bent distally

Mandibular Second Premolars

A. Crown
1. Mandibular second premolar is always larger than the mandibular first premolar; buccal cusp is shorter and rounded; root is longer
2. Lingual cusps of the second premolar are much more developed; both marginal ridges are higher
3. Two common forms of this tooth: three-cusp type and two-cusp type, with one pulp horn in each cusp
4. This is the only premolar that may be formed from five lobes; three lobes form the large buccal cusp, and one lobe forms each of the two small lingual cusps (three-cusp variety only)
5. Three-cusp type is the most common; has Y-shaped groove pattern
6. Two-cusp type can have either a U- or H-shaped groove pattern; usually two fossae—mesial and distal—are present, each with its own pit
7. Three-cusp form has a mesiolingual cusp and a distolingual cusp; mesiolingual cusp is usually the wider and longer of the two cusps, which are divided by a lingual groove

B. Root
1. Single root of the second premolar is larger and longer than that of the first premolar; is sometimes bifurcated, but this is rare
2. Root of the mandibular second premolar is similar to that of the first premolar; is longer and wider buccolingually
3. Has no tendency to bifurcate, as the mandibular first premolar sometimes does
4. Most likely premolar to consistently have only one root

Molars

General Characteristics

A. The 12 permanent molars are the largest and strongest teeth in the mouth by virtue of their crown bulk size and their root anchorage in bone
B. Molars are referred to as accessional or nonsuccedaneous teeth because they do not replace any primary teeth
C. Maxillary molars
  1. Maxillary first molars are normally the largest teeth in the maxillary arch
  2. Occlusal surface normally exhibits three to five cusps, at least two of which are buccal cusps
  3. Maxillary molars are usually trifurcated
  4. First molar is the largest of the three maxillary molars; second and third molars are progressively smaller
  5. Maxillary molars are usually wider buccolingually than mesiodistally or are about the same in dimension
  6. Maxillary molars have a distal oblique groove
D. Mandibular molars
  1. Permanent mandibular molars are the largest mandibular teeth; as with the maxillary molars, the second and third molars are progressively smaller than the first molar
  2. Crowns of mandibular molars are shorter cervicoocclusally than those of the teeth anterior to them
  3. Crowns are wider mesiodistally than buccolingually
  4. Mandibular molars are bifurcated and have two roots: one buccal and one lingual
  5. Mandibular molars have four major cusps and sometimes a minor fifth one

Maxillary First Molars

A. Crown
1. Lingual groove extends from the center of the lingual surface occlusally, between the two lingual cusps, where it curves sharply to the distal side and becomes the distal oblique groove
2. Mesiolingual cusp is the largest of the four functional cusps; the two buccal cusps are next in size and are nearly equal to each other; distolingual cusp is the smaller of the functional cusps
3. Maxillary first molar usually has an afunctional fifth cusp called the cusp or tubercle of Carabelli; this cusp is found on the lingual surface of the mesiolingual cusp
4. Oblique ridge is a transverse ridge peculiar to maxillary molars
5. From the occlusal view, the crown is roughly a parallelogram with two acute angles (mesiobuccal and distolingual) and two obtuse angles (distobuccal and mesiolingual)
6. Broad, shallow depression can sometimes be observed in the center of the cervical third of the mesial surface
7. Buccal groove separates the buccal cusps and sometimes terminates in a buccal pit
B. Root
1. Three roots—mesiobuccal, distobuccal, and lingual—connected to a single root trunk

2. Lingual root is the largest and longest; mesiobuccal root is the next largest; distobuccal root is the smallest, shortest, and weakest
3. Mesiobuccal root may house two root canals itself; each of the other two roots has one root canal
4. The two small root canals in one small root make root canal therapy particularly difficult
5. Longitudinal depressions can be found on the mesial surface of the mesiobuccal root and on the lingual surface of the lingual root; distobuccal root is convex without longitudinal depression
6. Mesiobuccal and distobuccal roots are widely separated and are often curved distally

Maxillary Second Molars

A. Crown
   1. Shorter occlusocervically and narrower mesiodistally than in the first molar; third molar continues to be smaller in all crown proportions, including buccolingually
   2. Shows supplemental grooves and pits
   3. Oblique ridge is less prominent than in the first molar
   4. Cusp of Carabelli usually disappears on the second molar
   5. Distolingual cusp is less developed on the second molar; mesiobuccal cusp is larger and longer than the distobuccal cusp
   6. Buccal groove, shorter than the buccal groove of the first molar, separates the buccal cusps; buccal pit is less frequently observed
B. Root
   1. Roots are shorter and closer together than those of the first molar; greater distal inclination of the buccal roots can be observed
   2. Each of the three roots usually has only one root canal

Maxillary Third Molars

A. Crown
   1. Maxillary third molar varies more than any other maxillary tooth in size, shape, and anatomic form; varies so much that it may be congenitally missing
   2. Third molar shows more supplemental and accidental grooves than do the other maxillary molars; overall appearance of the occlusal surface is wrinkled
   3. Oblique ridge is even less prominent or even missing entirely, since the distolingual cusp is markedly diminished or completely absent

4. Occlusal outline becomes more heart shaped with the demise of the distolingual cusp
B. Root
   1. Jaw does not have room to accommodate all of the teeth; therefore maxillary third molars usually exhibit poor root development
   2. Three roots: mesiobuccal, distobuccal, and lingual; have a tendency to be fused and extremely short
   3. Roots have a tendency to curve at their apex
   4. Furcation may be only a short distance cervically from the apices of the roots

Mandibular First Molars

A. Crown
   1. Mandibular first molar is usually the first permanent tooth to erupt
   2. This is the only mandibular molar to consistently have five cusps: mesiobuccal, distobuccal, mesiolingual, distolingual, and distal; the two buccal and two lingual cusps are major cusps; distal cusp is a minor cusp
   3. The two lingual cusps are almost the same size
   4. Tooth is wider on the buccal than on the lingual surface because of the presence of the distal cusp, which is located more on the buccal surface than on the lingual surface
   5. Buccal surface has two grooves: one distobuccal and one mesiobuccal; lingual surface has a lingual groove that separates the mesiolingual and distolingual cusps
   6. Mesiobuccal groove frequently terminates in a deep pit on the buccal surface
   7. On the occlusal surface there are three fossae: a central fossa, a mesial triangular fossa, and a distal triangular fossa; deep pits may be found at the base of each fossa
   8. Several principal grooves are found on the occlusal surface: a central groove, a mesial buccal groove, a distal buccal groove, and a lingual groove; there are numerous supplemental grooves
   9. On the occlusal surface a transverse ridge is formed by the triangular ridges of the mesiobuccal cusp and the mesiolingual cusp; a transverse ridge is also formed by the triangular ridges of the distobuccal cusp and the distolingual cusp
B. Root
   1. Two roots: one distal and one mesial; mesial root is broad buccolingually; distal root is less broad and more pointed at the apex

2. Mesial root has two root canals (one buccal and one lingual); distal root has only one
3. These two roots are widely separated
4. Mesial root is the longer and larger of the two
5. Furcation area is near the cervical line because of a short root trunk
6. Deep depression can be observed from the cervical line to the apex on the mesial surface of the mesial root; distal surface may be convex or have a shallow longitudinal depression
7. Buccolingual depression occurs on the root trunk above the bifurcation; ridge of cementum often crosses the space in the root bifurcation
8. From the buccal view, the roots curve distally

Mandibular Second Molars

A. Crown
1. Mandibular second molar resembles the mandibular first molar buccally and lingually except that the fifth cusp is usually absent
2. All four cusps of the mandibular second molar are nearly equal in size; however, from the buccal view, the tips of the mesiolingual and distolingual cusps can be seen behind the mesiobuccal and distobuccal cusps
3. Second molar is more rectangular than the first molar
4. Lingual surface has a lingual groove that separates the mesiolingual and distolingual cusps; buccal surface has a buccal groove that separates the mesiobuccal and distobuccal cusps
B. Root
1. The two roots are shorter, closer together, and more distally inclined than in the first molar
2. Each of the two roots usually has one root canal
3. Furcation area is near the cervical line because of a short root trunk
4. Buccolingual depression occurs on the root trunk above the bifurcation
5. Longitudinal depression can be observed on the broad mesial root surface

Mandibular Third Molars

A. Crown
1. Like the maxillary third molar, the mandibular third molar is irregular and unpredictable
2. Crown is usually shorter in all dimensions than in the first and second molars
B. Root
1. Roots are usually shorter, inclined distally, and very close together to the point of being fused

PRIMARY DENTITION
Incisors
Maxillary Central Incisors
A. Crown
1. Mesiodistal diameter is greater than its cervicoincisal length (the opposite is true of the permanent central incisor)
2. No mamelons or grooves are visible; incisal edge is nearly straight
3. Cervical ridges of enamel give the appearance of a bulging cervical ridge; these cervical ridges are on the labial and lingual surfaces
B. Root
1. Is overhung by the cervical ridges, giving the tooth the appearance of tapering drastically at the area of the cervical line
2. About twice the length of the crown; tapers evenly toward the apex
3. Mesial concavity is present on the root; distal surface is generally convex

Maxillary Lateral Incisors
A. Crown
1. Smaller in all dimensions, except that the cervicoincisal length is greater than its mesiodistal width; in all other ways is similar in appearance to the central incisor
2. Like the central incisor, no developmental grooves are present on the labial surface, but the lingual fossa is deeper, and the marginal ridges are more pronounced
B. Root
1. Longer, more tapered, and less blunt at the apex than the root of the central incisor
2. Appears much longer in proportion to the crown as compared with the central incisor

Mandibular Central Incisors
A. Crown
1. Mamelons or grooves are visible
2. Appears wide in comparison with its permanent successor
3. Mesial and distal sides taper evenly from the contact areas
4. From the lingual aspect the marginal ridges are less pronounced than those of the primary maxillary incisors
B. Root
1. Long and slender; tapers to a pointed apex
2. No developmental depressions can be observed on either the mesial or the distal root surface
3. May be two to three times the height of the crown; very narrow and conical

Mandiblar Lateral Incisors

A. Crown
   1. Wider and longer with a more developed cingulum than that of the central incisors
   2. Labiolingually, central and lateral incisors are about equal in measurement
   3. Incisal ridge tends to slope distally; distal margin is more rounded and bulges more than the mesial margin
B. Root—has a distal longitudinal groove and a mesial depression running lengthwise

Canines

Maxillary Canines

A. Crown
   1. Bulkier than the primary incisor crown in every aspect
   2. More constricted at the cervix in relation to its mesiodistal width and more convex on its mesial and distal surfaces
   3. Facial lobes are well developed; sharp cusp is evident
B. Root—about twice as long as the crown; more slender than that of its permanent successor

Mandibular Canines

A. Crown
   1. Compared with that of the maxillary canine, the labial face is much flatter, with shallow developmental grooves
   2. Distal cusp ridge is longer than that on the maxillary canine
   3. Crown is much narrower labiolingually than that on the maxillary canine
   4. Lingual features are less prominent than those of the maxillary canine
B. Root
   1. Long, narrow root almost twice the length of the crown
   2. Shorter and more tapered than that of the maxillary canine

Molars

Maxillary First Molars

A. Crown
   1. Unlike that of any other primary or permanent tooth; wider buccolingually than mesiolingually
   2. Only two major cusps: one mesiobuccal and one mesiolingual
   3. Distolingual cusp is small and rounded, if present at all
   4. One type of primary maxillary first molar has only three cusps: one lingual and two buccal
   5. No cusp of Carabelli is present
   6. Prominent cervical ridge is present on the facial surface
   7. Crown converges toward the cervical line from its contact areas; this convergence is rather abrupt and ends where the crown joins a rather short root trunk
B. Root
   1. Three roots; lingual root is the largest
   2. Roots flare greatly in order to accommodate the permanent premolar
   3. Root trunk is extremely short; roots themselves are long, slender, and widely divergent

Maxillary Second Molars

A. Crown
   1. Primary maxillary second molar resembles the permanent maxillary first molar, although it is much smaller
   2. From the buccal view, two well-developed buccal cusps, with a buccal groove between them, are visible
   3. As on a primary first molar, the crown is narrow at its cervix as compared with its mesiodistal measurement at the contact area
   4. Primary second molar is much larger than the primary first molar in both crown and root formation
   5. The two buccal cusps are about equal in size
   6. There are four major cusps and a fifth supplemental cusp. the cusp of Carabelli
B. Root
   1. Root trunk is not as short as in the first molar but is much shorter than in the permanent tooth
   2. Three roots flared widely apart; lingual root is the longest; distobuccal root is the shortest

Mandibular First Molars

A. Crown
   1. Like the maxillary first molar, this tooth is unlike any other primary or permanent tooth
   2. Crown is wider mesiodistally than buccolingually, like that of the permanent mandibular molars
   3. Two rather distinct buccal cusps; mesial cusp is much larger than the distal cusp
   4. Two lingual cusps; mesial cusp is again much larger than the distal cusp; the two larger mesial cusps give this tooth a rhomboid occlusal outline

5. Most characteristic feature of this tooth is an extremely bulbous curvature on its buccal surface at the cervical third; this extreme buccocervical convexity can easily be seen on the mesial view and causes the occlusal table to appear rather narrow from cusp tip to cusp tip

B. Root
   1. Two roots flared wide apart: one mesial and one distal; mesial root is very flat and broad with a centrally located developmental depression
   2. Mesial root has two canals: one buccal canal and one lingual canal
   3. Apex is very blunt to the point of being flat
   4. Distal root is thinner and shorter and tapers more apically than the mesial root; has one root canal

Mandibular Second Molars

A. Crown
   1. Primary mandibular second molar resembles the permanent mandibular first molar except that it is smaller and has the typical primary molar constriction at the cervix of the crown
   2. Roots are longer in proportion; crown is shorter than that of the permanent molar
   3. Like the permanent first molar, this tooth has three buccal cusps, all of which are nearly equal in size; there are two lingual cusps—mesiolingual and distolingual—which are not as wide as the three buccal cusps; tooth converges lingually

B. Root
   1. Roots are about twice as long as the crown
   2. Roots are long and slender, flare widely almost immediately below the cervical line
   3. Mesial root is broad, flat, and blunted at the apex; houses two canals—unlike the roots of the maxillary primary molars, which have only one canal per root
   4. Mesial root is longer and bigger than the distal root

REFERENCE

1. Sicher, H., and Bhaskar, S.N.: Orban's oral histology and embryology, ed. 7., St. Louis, 1972, The C.V. Mosby Co.

SUGGESTED READINGS

Brand, R., and Isselhard, D.E.: Anatomy of orofacial structures, ed. 3, St. Louis, 1986, The C.V. Mosby Co.

Permar, D.: An outline for dental anatomy, Philadelphia, 1975, Lea & Febiger.

Review Questions

1 The period of deciduous dentition begins
   1. At age 6 years
   2. When the first deciduous tooth erupts
   3. Before the first teeth ever erupt
   4. At birth
   5. At conception

2 The period of mixed dentition exists
   1. When the third molars erupt
   2. Before the eruption of the permanent incisors
   3. Before the age of 6 years
   4. After the age of 12 years
   5. None of the above

3 The line that demarcates the junction of the enamel and the cementum is called
   1. The cervical line
   2. The cementoenamel junction
   3. The CEJ
   4. All of the above
   5. None of the above

4 The junction of three surfaces is called a
   1. Line angle
   2. Marginal ridge
   3. Point angle
   4. Triangular ridge
   5. Transverse ridge

5 Facially, the mandibular second premolar most closely resembles the
   1. Canine
   2. Maxillary second premolar
   3. Mandibular first premolar
   4. Maxillary first premolar
   5. None of these

6 A small depression in the enamel of a tooth occurring at the end of a developmental groove or at the junction of two or more developmental grooves is known as a
   1. Fissure
   2. Sulcus
   3. Pit
   4. Fossa
   5. Tubercle

7 Which of the following is an example of a line angle?
   1. Mesiolabioincisal
   2. Buccolingual
   3. Mesiodistal
   4. Labioincisal
   5. Incisoocclusal

8 The roots of teeth are generally
   1. Tapered the most at the cervical third
   2. Widest at the apex
   3. Widest at the cervical third
   4. Narrowest at the cervical third
   5. None of the above

9 Which teeth in the dental arch show the greatest difference between the position of the mesial and distal contact areas?
1. Maxillary premolars
2. Maxillary canines
3. Third molars
4. Mandibular incisors
5. Mandibular molars

10 The greatest height of contour of the lingual surface of a molar or premolar is located in the
1. Cervical third
2. Middle third
3. Occlusal third
4. Gingival third
5. Cervical and gingival thirds

11 The follicles of developing succedaneous teeth are in what relationship to the deciduous teeth they replace?
1. The anterior teeth are beneath the root, and the posterior teeth are in the furcation
2. The anterior teeth are in a lingual relationship, and the posterior teeth are in the furcation
3. Both the anterior and the posterior teeth are lingual to their predecessors' roots
4. Both the anterior and the posterior teeth are buccal to the deciduous roots
5. None of the above

12 Root resorption of deciduous teeth begins
1. Immediately after eruption
2. Shortly after root completion
3. A year after root completion
4. A year before exfoliation
5. At least 1 or 2 years before exfoliation

13 A lingual pit is more likely to be present on a
1. Maxillary central
2. Maxillary lateral
3. Mandibular central
4. Maxillary canine
5. Mandibular canine

14 A 7-year-old enters the office with only six permanent teeth. Which of the following is most likely true?
1. Four of the permanent teeth are incisors
2. The child has delayed eruption
3. Two permanent teeth have been extracted
4. Four of the permanent teeth are first molars
5. Three of the permanent teeth are maxillary, and three are mandibular

15 The last permanent incisors to erupt are most likely the
1. Maxillary centrals
2. Mandibular laterals
3. Maxillary laterals
4. Mandibular canines
5. Mandibular third molars

16 The longest teeth in the mouth are most likely the
1. Maxillary canines
2. Mandibular canines
3. Maxillary first molars
4. Central incisors
5. Maxillary first premolars

17 The canine eminence is
1. An osseous structure surrounding the canine root on the labial aspect
2. The labial ridge on the crown of the canine
3. The lingual ridge on the crown of the canine
4. Associated with the mandibular canine only
5. A deep depression in the bone distal to the canine

18 Which are succedaneous teeth?
1. Deciduous incisors
2. Permanent canine and incisors
3. Permanent premolars
4. Permanent molars
5. Permanent canines, incisors, and premolars

19 The facial surfaces of maxillary molars build up calculus faster than most teeth because
1. Stensen's duct opens just opposite the molars
2. Wharton's duct opens just opposite the molars
3. The sublingual gland opens into this area
4. No salivary gland is present in this area
5. The submaxillary gland opens into this area

20 Before scaling a maxillary canine, what anatomic facts concerning the tooth should one review?
1. A proximal groove is present on the mesial surface
2. A proximal groove is present on the distal surface
3. Proximal groove are present on both the mesial and the distal surfaces
4. A mesial developmental depression is present on the crown
5. Mesial and distal proximal grooves and a mesial developmental depression are present

21 Which of the following is least likely to have a bifurcated root?
1. Maxillary first premolar
2. Maxillary second premolar
3. Deciduous mandibular molar
4. Mandibular canine
5. Maxillary canine

22 An unerupted canine shows a dark radiolucent area at the end of a half-formed maxillary canine root. The patient is 9 years old. Which of the following statements is most probably true?
1. The patient must be given antibiotics
2. The patient does not necessarily have an abscess but should be followed up with a radiograph once a month to be sure
3. This is normal for an unerupted tooth
4. This is normal for an incompletely formed root
5. The possibility of an abscess indicates a monthly follow-up and antibiotic therapy as a preventive measure

23 The cusp of Carabelli of a maxillary first molar may be
1. The largest cusp
2. The fourth largest cusp
3. Located on the distolingual cusp
4. Located on the mesiobuccal cusp
5. Absent

Answers and Rationales

1. (2) The period of deciduous dentition begins with the eruption of the first deciduous central incisors at about 6 months after birth.
   (1) The period of deciduous dentition ends and the period of mixed dentition begins with the eruption of the first permanent molars at about age 6 years
   (3) Sometimes teeth are present at birth, but these are not deciduous teeth and are therefore not apart of the period of deciduous dentition.
   (4) The period of deciduous dentition does not begin at birth, but with the eruption of the first deciduous tooth.
   (5) The period of deciduous dentition does not begin at conception, but with the eruption of the first deciduous tooth.

2. (2) The mixed dentition begins with the eruption of the permanent teeth. The first of these to erupt at age 6 years are the first molars, followed by the incisors.
   (1) The third molars do not erupt until late in the period of permanent dentition.
   (3) Generally, mixed dentition begins at age 6 years.
   (4) Mixed dentition ends with the exfoliation of the last deciduous teeth, sometime between the ages of 12 and 13 years.
   (5) The correct answer is 2.

3. (4) *Cervical line, cementoenamel junction,* and *CEJ* are synonymous terms.
   (1) The cervical line is the line between the root and the crown.
   (2) The cementoenamel junction is where the cementum joins the enamel.
   (3) *CEJ* is an abbreviation for *cementoenamel junction.*
   (5) The correct answer is 4.

4. (3) By definition, a point angle is the junction of three surfaces.
   (1) A line angle is the junction of two surfaces.
   (2) A marginal ridge is an elevation of enamel forming the proximal margins of the tooth on the occlusal or lingual surface.
   (4) A triangular ridge extends from the cusp point to the central groove or the occlusal surface.
   (5) A transverse ridge is formed by the union of two triangular ridges.

5. (3) From the facial view, the mandibular first and second premolars are very similar. It is from the lingual view that they differ.
   (1) The lower premolars do have a resemblance to the lower canines from the facial view, but they resemble each other more.

6. (3) A pit is a small depression at the end of a developmental groove.
   (1) A fissure is a long, deep depression usually found on the occlusal or buccal surface.
   (2) A sulcus is a long, valley depression between the ridges and the cusps.
   (4) A fossa is a wide, shallow depression on the tooth surface.
   (5) A tubercle is a small elevation of enamel on a surface of the crown of a tooth.

7. (4) A line angle is the junction of two surfaces. The only two surfaces listed that could form a line angle are the labial and incisal surfaces.
   (1) The mesiolabioincisal is a point angle.
   (2) The buccal and lingual surfaces are direct opposites and could never meet on the same tooth.
   (3) The mesial and distal surfaces are direct opposites and could never meet to form a line angle.
   (5) The incisal and occlusal surfaces cannot meet on the same tooth to form a line angle.

8. (3) The widest part of a root is always at the cervical third where the root joins the crown.
   (1) The root is thicker at the cervical third.
   (2) The narrowest area is always at the apex, or tip, of the root.
   (4) The root is narrowest at the apex.
   (5) The correct answer is 3.

9. (2) Of the choices listed, only the maxillary canines show a difference in the locations of the distal and mesial contact areas. The other choices all have their contact areas at about the same level.
   (1) The maxillary premolars have their contacts near the same level.
   (3) The mesial and distal contact areas of the third molars are at the same level.
   (4) The mandibular central incisor is the most symmetric of the teeth, and it is often impossible to tell the right from the left for that reason.
   (5) The contact points on the mandibular molars are at about the same level.

10. (2) The height of contour refers to the widest part of the tooth. The widest or greatest height of contour of the lingual surface in all posterior teeth is in the middle third.
    (1) The cervical third has the greatest height of contour for molars and premolars on the facial surface.
    (3) The occlusal third tapers in toward the buccal third.
    (4) The gingival third is also the greatest height contour for molars and premolars on the facial surface.
    (5) The cervical third and gingival third are the same height.

For each question the correct answer and rationale are listed first. The other choices are presented in order with the reasons why they are not correct.

(2) The maxillary second premolars resemble the canines more than the lower premolars.
(4) The maxillary first premolars resemble the canines more than the mandibular premolars.
(5) The correct answer is 3.

11. (2) The anterior teeth are in a lingual relationship, and the posterior teeth are in the furcation. As the permanent anterior teeth erupt, the tongue pushes them labially.
   (1) The anterior teeth are lingual to the roots of their deciduous predecessors.
   (3) The posterior teeth are in the furcation of their predecessors' roots.
   (4) Neither the anterior nor the posterior teeth are buccal to the deciduous roots.
   (5) The correct answer is 2.

12. (5) The tooth root begins to resorb 1 or 2 years before exfoliation.
   (1) The root does not begin to resorb until at least 3 years after eruption.
   (2) The root does not begin to resorb until almost 2 years after root completion.
   (3) The first teeth to be resorbed are the mandibular central incisors. Resorption of their roots begins 2½ years before they are exfoliated.
   (4) Most deciduous teeth begin resorption of their roots 1½ years or more before they are exfoliated.

13. (2) A lingual pit is more likely to be present on a maxillary lateral.
   (1) A maxillary central occasionally has a lingual pit.
   (3) A mandibular central rarely has a lingual pit.
   (4) A maxillary canine has a lingual pit more often than a maxillary central, but less often than a maxillary lateral.
   (5) A mandibular canine rarely has a lingual pit.

14. (4) Four of the permanent teeth are first molars, since the permanent first molars erupt before the central incisors.
   (1) Only two of the permanent teeth would be incisors. The permanent centrals start to erupt at about age 7.
   (2) The child's eruption pattern appears to be normal.
   (3) There is no evidence that any teeth have been extracted.
   (5) Teeth usually erupt in pairs—two lower centrals, then two upper centrals, etc.

15. (3) The maxillary laterals are the last permanent incisors to erupt.
   (1) The maxillary centrals are sometimes the first permanent incisors to erupt, but the mandibular centrals are more commonly first.
   (2) The mandibular laterals are sometimes the last incisors to erupt, but normally the mandibular teeth erupt before the maxillary teeth.
   (4) Canines are not incisors.
   (5) Third molars are not incisors.

16. (1) The maxillary canines are usually the longest teeth in the mouth.
   (2) The roots or crowns of the mandibular canines could be as long as the roots or crowns of the maxillary canines, but usually the mandibular canines are shorter than the maxillary canines in total length.

(3) First molars are longer than other molars but are not as long as canines.
   (4) Central incisors are not as long as canines.
   (5) Premolars are not as long as canines.

17. (1) The canine eminence is an osseous bony structure covering the labial aspect of the canine root.
   (2) The canine eminence is concerned with bone structure, not tooth structure.
   (3) The canine eminence is concerned with bone structure, not tooth structure.
   (4) The canine eminence is usually associated with the maxillary canine.
   (5) The eminence is a convexity, not a depression.

18. (5) Succedaneous teeth are permanent teeth that succeed, or replace, deciduous teeth.
   (1) Deciduous teeth are not succedaneous.
   (2) Permanent canines and incisors are succedaneous teeth but so are permanent premolars.
   (3) Permanent premolars are succedaneous teeth, but so are permanent canines and incisors.
   (4) Permanent molars are not succedaneous teeth, since they do not replace primary teeth.

19. (1) Stensen's duct is the opening of the parotid duct just opposite the maxillary first molars.
   (2) Wharton's duct is the opening for the submandibular gland.
   (3) The sublingual gland opens under the tongue.
   (4) The parotid gland is present in this area.
   (5) The submaxillary gland and the sublingual gland are the same.

20. (3) The mesial and distal developmental grooves seem to divide the canine root into two parts. If this groove is deep, scaling becomes much more difficult.
   (1) The mesial groove extends from the cervical line halfway to the apex.
   (2) The distal groove may be even deeper than the mesial groove.
   (4) The crown may have a flat or sometimes concave area above the contact area, but it should not be a problem during scaling.
   (5) Only the mesial and distal grooves could provide difficulty during scaling.

21. (5) The maxillary canine is the least likely of those listed to have a bifurcated root.
   (1) The maxillary first premolar is more frequently bifurcated than not.
   (2) The maxillary second premolar is very commonly bifurcated.
   (3) The deciduous mandibular molar is almost always bifurcated.
   (4) While the mandibular canine is normally a single-rooted tooth, it is the most commonly bifurcated anterior tooth and is not considered a rarity.

22. (4) All incompletely formed roots will exhibit a radiolucent area, since the roots in the area are not calcified.
    (1) Antibiotics are totally inappropriate.
    (2) Radiographic follow-up is totally unnecessary.
    (3) This is normal for an unerupted tooth whose root has not finished calcification.
    (5) Since the radiolucent area is not an abscess, antibiotics are unnecessary.

23. (5) The cusp of Carabelli is not always present on maxillary molars.
    (1) When present, this fifth cusp, as it is sometimes called, is the smallest of the five cusps.
    (2) The cusp of Carabelli is so small that it is more appropriately referred to as a tubercle and not a cusp.
    (3) It is located on the lingual aspect of the mesiolingual cusp.
    (4) It is located on the lingual aspect of the mesiolingual cusp.

CHAPTER 5

Oral Radiology

NANCY B. WEBB

K. CY WHALEY

One aspect of the practice of dental hygiene essential for total patient care is the delivery of comprehensive oral radiologic services to aid in the prevention and treatment of oral disease.

Knowledge and skill in applying that knowledge are critical for the safe use of radiation in the dental care setting. Therefore special emphasis is given to radiation physics, production, biology, protection, and ethics; radiographic imaging techniques and receptor systems; radiographic film processing and quality assurance procedures; and radiographic anatomy and principles of interpretation.

GENERAL CONSIDERATIONS
Radiation Physics

A. Emission or propagation of energy in the form of wave or particles[5]
B. Types of radiation
   1. Particulate radiations
      a. Particles that have both mass and energy
      b. Some particles may have a positive, negative, or neutral charge
      c. Cannot reach speed of light
      d. Examples—neutrons, protons, electrons, α-particles, and β-particles
   2. Electromagnetic radiations
      a. Definitions
         (1) Wavelength—distance from one crest of a wave to the next; wavelength of the electromagnetic radiations ranges from 10^6 to 10^{-16} m
         (2) Frequency—number of crests passing a particular point per unit of time and measured in Hertz (Hz); 1 Hz is equal to 1 cycle/sec; frequency of the electromagnetic radiations ranges from 10^2 to 10^{24} Hz
         (3) Photon and quantum—term used to designate a single unit or bundle of energy

         (4) Energy—ability to work; energy of the electromagnetic radiations is measured in electron volts (eV); ranges from 10^{-12} to 10^{10} eV (1 keV is equal to 1000 eV)
      b. Characteristics
         (1) Bundles of energy that have neither mass nor charge
         (2) Electric and magnetic fields are associated with the travel of the electromagnetic energy through space
         (3) Electromagnetic energies exist over a wide range of magnitudes; are termed the electromagnetic spectrum
         (4) Interaction of electromagnetic radiation with matter may be described in terms of wave and particle behavior
         (5) Electromagnetic spectrum is measured according to frequency, energy, and wavelength
      c. Examples—radiowaves, microwaves, infrared, visible light, ultraviolet light, x-rays, gamma rays, and cosmic rays
   3. Ionizing radiations
      a. Definitions
         (1) Ion—charged particle; either positive or negative
         (2) Ion pair—positive ion and negative ion
         (3) Ionization—process by which radiant energy removes an orbital electron from an atom to yield an ion pair
         (4) Ionizing radiations—those particulate and electromagnetic radiations with sufficient energy to cause ionization of atoms; radiation must have energy greater than the electron-binding energy
      b. Biologic significance—damage of biologic systems results from the ionization process
      c. Examples—α-particles, β-particles, x-rays, and gamma rays

C. Sources of radiation
1. Natural background radiation is the greatest contributor to population exposure from radiation
a. Naturally occurring radionuclides in the soil (a radionuclide is an unstable atom that decays by emitting particles and energy from the nucleus to become electrically stable; deposited within the human body through the inhalation of air, food, and water)
b. Cosmic radiations from outer space
2. Healing arts
a. Radiopharmaceutical agents
b. X-radiation
3. Production and use of nuclear energy
a. Atmospheric weapons tests
b. Nuclear power reactors
4. Research facilities
a. High-voltage x-ray machines
b. Particle accelerators
c. Diffraction units
d. Electron microscopes
5. Consumer and industrial products may contain radioactive materials or use ionizing radiation
a. Building materials
b. Luminous dial watches
6. Miscellaneous sources
a. Transportation of radioactive materials
b. Cosmic radiations received by airline passengers[2]

Discovery of X-Radiation

A. Crookes tube
1. Developed by Sir William Crookes
2. Also known as a cathode ray tube
3. Evacuated glass tube with two electrodes (cathode and anode) through which an electrical current is passed
B. Wilhelm Conrad Roentgen
1. Accidentally discovered x-rays on November 8, 1895
2. Was investigating properties of the cathode ray using a Crookes tube and discovered the following properties of cathode rays
a. Electrically negative particles
b. Travel only a few centimeters in air
c. Can cause a fluorescent screen to glow
3. Roentgen enclosed the Crookes tube with black paper; noticed glowing of fluorescent material on a workbench several feet away; termed the unknown ray X

X-Ray Machines

A. Types
1. Intraoral units are designed to provide sufficient x-ray output for standard intraoral radiographs: bitewing, periapical, and occlusal
a. X-ray beam is restricted to provide exposure of small anatomic sites
b. Kilovolt peak (kVp) and milliamperage (mA) settings may be constant or variable, depending on the manufacturer
2. Extraoral units are designed to provide greater x-ray output as required by the extraoral procedures; x-ray beam is larger to accommodate larger anatomic areas under study
B. Components of the x-ray unit
1. Generator—device that supplies electrical power to the x-ray tube
a. Transformer[3]
(1) Device that changes the potential difference of the incoming electrical energy to any desired level
(2) Consists of two wire coils wound around opposite sides of an iron ring
(3) Current flows through the primary coil; creates a magnetic field in the iron ring
(4) Magnetic field then induces a current in the second coil
(5) Voltage in the two circuits is proportional to the number of turns in the two coils
(6) An increase in the voltage must be accompanied by a corresponding decrease in the current
b. Types of transformers
(1) Step-up transformer has more turns in the secondary coil than in the primary coil, which increases the voltage; used to supply voltage to the high-voltage (kilovolt peak) tube circuit
(2) Step-down transformer has fewer turns in the second coil than in the primary coil, which decreases the voltage; used to supply voltage to the filament (milliamperage) circuit
(3) Auto-transformer is a special type of transformer because the primary and secondary windings are incorporated into a single winding
(a) Has a number of connections called electrical taps located along the length of the coil

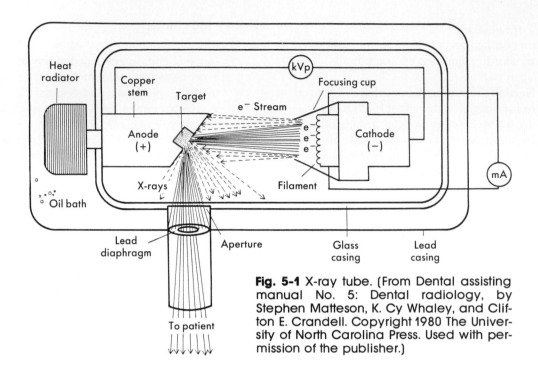

Fig. 5-1 X-ray tube. (From Dental assisting manual No. 5: Dental radiology, by Stephen Matteson, K. Cy Whaley, and Clifton E. Crandell. Copyright 1980 The University of North Carolina Press. Used with permission of the publisher.)

    (b) Designed to supply voltage of varying magnitude to several different circuits of the x-ray machine (i.e., filament circuit and high-voltage tube circuit)

2. X-ray tube (Fig. 5-1)
  a. Protective housing
    (1) Lead-lined metal casing for the x-ray tube designed to prevent excessive radiation exposure and electrical shock
    (2) Limits the amount of leakage radiation escaping from the unit
    (3) Provides mechanical support for the x-ray tube and protection from rough handling
  b. Cooling system
    (1) Oil is sealed in the protective housing and surrounds the x-ray tube
    (2) Serves as both a thermal cushion and electrical insulator
  c. Glass envelope
    (1) Usually made of Pyrex glass to withstand high heat produced
    (2) Surrounds the electrodes of the x-ray tube to provide a vacuum
    (3) Window is a thin segment of the glass that allows maximum emission of x-rays and minimum absorption by the glass (also called the aperture)

  d. Cathode
    (1) Electrically negative portion of the x-ray tube
    (2) Composed of the filament and focusing cup
    (3) Filament is a coil of tungsten wire; filament is embedded in the focusing cup, which is negatively charged
    (4) Electrical current is passed through the coil
    (5) Atoms of wire absorb thermal energy, and some of the outer shell electrons acquire enough energy to move a small distance away; process is termed thermionic emission
    (6) *Therm* means heat; *ionic* relates to the atoms ionized in the filament and *emission,* since electrons are emitted from the filament
    (7) Heating (amount of current flowing) of the filament is controlled by the step-down transformer, which is regulated by the milliamperage control
    (8) Since like charges repel, the electron beam is directed to a small area of the anode
    (9) Electrons "boiled off" by thermionic emission are referred to as the electron cloud

e. Anode
    (1) Electrically positive portion of the x-ray tube
    (2) Composed of the target and copper stem
    (3) Portion of the target bombarded by the electrons is termed the focal spot
    (4) Tungsten is used as the target material because of the high atomic number that yields higher efficiency in x-ray production plus higher-energy x-ray photons; conducts heat well; has a high melting point (3380° C)
    (5) Target is embedded into the copper stem, which functions to conduct heat away
    (6) Anode receives the electrons from the cathode; conducts them back to the high-voltage section
f. Filtration
    (1) Process of selectively removing x-rays from the beam
    (2) Total filtration is the result of inherent and added filtration
    (3) Inherent filtration is the filtering of the beam by the glass envelope
    (4) Added filtration occurs by placing metal disks (usually aluminum) within the path of the x-ray beam
    (5) Low-energy, nonpenetrating x-rays are removed from the beam
g. Diaphragm—lead disk with a circular or rectangular opening attached to the x-ray tube head to restrict the size of the x-ray beam

3. Console
  a. Description—exposure factors (milliamperage, kilovolt peak, and exposure time) are set and electrical circuits are activated using the controls located on the x-ray machine console
  b. Function
    (1) May control up to three x-ray tube heads
    (2) Usually, settings of 10 or 15 mA are available; kilovolt peak settings range from 50 to 90 kVp
    (3) Depending on the machine type, the automatic timer is adjusted in impulses or seconds
    (4) Exposure switch is depressed to initiate the emission of x-radiation

    (5) Emission of x-radiation from the machine is noted by an audible "chirping" sound and the glowing of the exposure indicator light
    (6) Console should be located adjacent to the x-ray cubicle so that continuous observation of the patient is possible; however, the operator should be protected from any radiation exposure

Production of X-Radiation

A. X-ray machine preparation
  1. Initial process for x-radiation production is achieved by the activation of the on-off switch located on the unit console; this process completes the filament circuit, and the filament is heated
  2. Appropriate milliamperage, kilovolt peak, and exposure time are set using controls located on the unit console
    a. Milliamperage control, which is connected to the milliamperage-filament circuit (step-down transformer), allows for the warming of the cathode filament and determines the number of electrons available for x-ray production; the higher the milliamperage, the hotter the filament becomes, resulting in a greater number of available electrons
    b. Kilovolt peak control, which is connected to the high-voltage circuit (step-up transformer), establishes the high voltage needed for x-ray production (65,000 to 90,000 volts); this also provides that the anode is positively charged and the cathode is negatively charged for the attraction and high-speed acceleration of electrons from the cathode to the anode; the higher the kilovolt peak setting, the greater the speed of acceleration of electrons from the cathode to the anode
    c. Exposure timer establishes the time during which electrons are available for bombardment of the target material
B. Electronics of x-ray production
  1. X-rays are produced by the interactions that occur when high-speed electrons strike a target material
  2. Phenomenon of x-ray production occurs only when the exposure switch on the console is depressed, thereby completing the high-voltage circuit

a. Heated filament provides electrons for x-ray production by thermionic emission

b. Thermionic emission occurs when electrons absorb sufficient thermal energy (from the milliamperage circuit), which allows for the electrons' short movement away from the filament; commonly referred to as a "boiling off" of electrons; electron cloud surrounding the filament is formed

c. Closure of the high-voltage circuit creates an electrical potential difference, whereby electrons are attracted from the negative cathode to the positive anode

d. The one-directional flow of electrons (from the negative cathode to the positive anode) is influenced by the focusing cup of the cathode; electrons are repelled away from the negatively charged focusing cup, since like charges repel; this mechanism controls the size and shape of the electron stream

C. Electron-target interactions

1. Electron stream is directed at a small portion of the target, referred to as the focal spot

2. Actual production of x-radiation occurs by the interaction of the accelerating electrons and the target atoms

   a. Accelerating electrons have variable kinetic energy because the electrical power source for the x-ray unit is an alternating current

   b. Example—at 70 kVp the current begins at 0, rises to the peak (potential) of 70, then is followed by a return to 0; only a small number of electrons leaving the cathode will possess the peak energy; most electrons will be leaving the cathode when the current is rising from or returning to 0

   c. A variety of x-ray photon energies will be emitted from the unit as a result of the alternating current

3. Two types of interactions for x-ray production

   a. Bremsstrahlung radiation (Fig. 5-2)

      (1) Also known as general radiation or braking radiation

      (2) Accelerating electron passes near the nucleus of the target atom and is slowed down by the attraction of the nucleus

      (3) Slowing-down process results in a transference of the electron's kinetic energy into x-ray energy plus a change in the traveling direction of the electron

      (4) Energy of the photon produced is dependent on the amount of kinetic energy transferred

      (5) Electron may give up its energy in stages, yielding photons of various energy levels

      (6) The closer the accelerating electron passes by the nucleus, the greater the nuclear attraction, thereby yielding greater energy transference and higher photon energy

   b. Characteristic radiation (Fig. 5-3 and Table 5-1)

      (1) Also known as discrete radiation

      (2) Radiation is characteristic of the target material

      (3) Steps for characteristic radiation production involve ionization of the target atom by removing an orbital electron and restabilization of the atom by shifting orbital electrons

      (4) During restabilization of the ionized atom the hole created by the ejected orbital electron is filled by an outer-shell electron; movement of the outer-shell electron results in the transference of electron-binding energy into x-ray energy

      (5) Energy of the resulting characteristic x-ray photon is a result of the difference in the binding energies of the orbital electrons involved

      (6) Example—transference of a P-shell electron to a K-shell vacancy yields a photon energy of 69.5 keV for a tungsten atom)

D. Emanation of the x-ray beam from the tube

1. X-rays are isotropically emitted from a point source (focal spot); however, only a small portion is allowed to exit the machine and be used for image production

2. X-ray beam emitted is described as polychromatic, meaning a range in the photon energies

3. Long-wavelength, low-energy x-ray photons have less penetrating ability and are commonly referred to as soft rays; short-wavelength, high-energy x-ray photons have greater penetrating ability and are commonly referred to as hard rays

4. Characteristics of the x-ray beam emitted from the tube are altered for various reasons

   a. Soft, nonpenetrating, nonradiographic, image-producing x-rays are removed by filtration

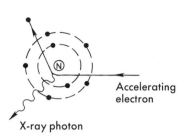

Fig. 5-2 Bremmstrahlung interaction. (Redrawn from Christensen, E.E., Curry T.S. III, and Dowdy, J.E.: An introduction to the physics of diagnostic radiology, ed. 2, Philadelphia, 1978, Lea & Febiger.)

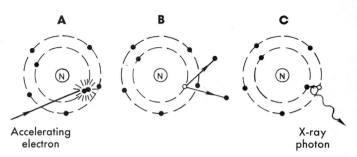

Fig. 5-3 Characteristic interaction. **A,** Collision of accelerating electron and orbital electron. **B,** Vacancy of inner shell. **C,** Shifting of outer-shell electron to inner vacancy with generation of x-ray photon. (Redrawn from Christensen, E.E., Curry, T.S. III, and Dowdy, J.E.: An introduction to the physics of diagnostic radiology, ed. 2, Philadelphia, 1978, Lea & Febiger.)

Table 5-1 Characteristic x-rays of tungsten and their effective energies (keV)

Characteristic x ray	Electron transition from					Effective energy
	L shell	*M* shell	*N* shell	*O* shell	*P* shell	
K	57.1	66.7	68.9	69.4	69.5	69
L		9.3	11.5	12.0	12.1	12
M			2.2	2.7	2.8	2
N				0.52	0.6	0.6
O					0.08	0.08

From Bushong, S.C.: Radiologic science for technologists: physics, biology, and protection, ed. 3, St. Louis, 1984, The C.V. Mosby Co.

  b. Mean photon energy of the x-ray beam increases following filtration (removal of low-energy photons), yielding a ''harder beam''
  c. Field size of the x-ray beam is restricted (collimated) to match the image receptor size
  d. Preceding factors provide a reduction in patient radiation exposure
E. Characteristics of x-rays
  1. Are a portion of the electromagnetic spectrum
  2. Pure energy without mass nor charge
  3. Travel at the speed of light (186,000 miles/sec)
  4. Affect photographic emulsion
  5. Cause fluorescence of certain chemicals
  6. Can adversely affect biologic tissues

Interactions of X-Rays with Matter

A. Considerations[4]
  1. When x-ray photons interact with matter, they may either be absorbed or scattered
    a. If an incident (initial) photon is absorbed, it ceases to exist
    b. If an incident photon is scattered, its direction of travel is altered; does not aid in formation of the radiographic image and only increases film density; scattered radiation causes film fog (or noise) that destroys image quality
  2. Attenuation (removal) of x-ray photons from the beam as they travel through matter (tissue) is determined by the intensity (energy) of the radiation and the density, atomic number, and electrons per gram of the matter
    a. As the energy of the radiation increases, the number of photons passing through the matter increases

    b. As the density, atomic number, or electrons per gram of the material increase, the number of photons passing through the matter decreases

3. Definitions[5]
    a. Primary radiation—photons coming directly from the target of the x-ray tube
    b. Secondary radiation—radiation resulting from the interaction of primary radiation and matter
    c. Scattered radiation—one form of secondary radiation in which the direction of travel was altered

B. Types of interactions
1. No interaction
    a. Refers to the passing of x-ray photons through a material without any alteration of the photon or the material
    b. Photons proceed to expose the silver halide crystals of the film emulsion
2. Thompson scattering
    a. Also termed unmodified or coherent scattering
    b. Refers to the interaction of an incident photon passing near an outer-shell electron and being scattered without losing energy
    c. Incident photon causes the electron to vibrate
    d. Incident photon ceases to exist, and a new photon of identical energy is released from the vibrating electron
    e. Direction of travel of the Thompson scattered photon is different from that of the incident photon
    f. In the diagnostic energy range Thompson scattering accounts for 5% of the total interactions
3. Photoelectric effect
    a. Results from an incident photon colliding with a tightly bound inner-shell electron
    b. Incident photon ceases to exist; electron is ejected as a recoil electron (or photoelectron)
    c. Ionization of the atom occurs; ejected electron leaves a vacancy in the shell that must be filled
    d. Low-energy characteristic radiation is produced by the shifting of an outer-shell electron to the inner vacancy
    e. In the diagnostic energy range the photoelectric effect accounts for 75% of the interactions

4. Compton effect
    a. Results from an incident photon colliding with a loosely bound outer-shell electron
    b. Incident photon gives up part of its energy in the ejection of the orbiting electron
    c. Ionization of the atom occurs
    d. Direction of travel of the incident photon is changed; its energy is reduced
    e. Energy of the Compton scattered x-ray is equal to the difference between the energy of the incident photon and the energy imparted to the ejected electron
    f. Scattered photon and ejected electron may have sufficient energy to undergo many more ionizing interactions before losing their entire energy
    g. Compton scattered x-radiations may exit the patient's tissues and cause film fog
    h. In the diagnostic energy range Compton scattering accounts for 20% of the interactions

C. Image formation and differential attenuation
1. Radiographic image formation is dependent on differential attenuation of x-ray photons from the primary beam by the patient's tissues
2. If all photons exited the patient (no absorption), the film would be totally exposed; if all photons were attenuated (absorbed), the film would be unexposed
3. X-ray photons in the primary beam are in a uniform distribution
4. As a result of the Thompson, Compton, and photoelectric interactions, x-ray photons are removed from the beam
5. Distribution of transmitted photons represents the patient's tissues
6. Variances in attenuating ability of the tissues produce radiographic contrast
7. As previously stated, attenuation is dependent on the intensity (energy) of the radiation plus the density, atomic number, and electrons per gram of the tissue
8. Example—when the kilovolt peak setting is increased, more x-rays are produced and the mean energy of the beam is increased; x-ray photons with higher energy have greater penetrating ability; at a 50 kVp setting many photons are unable to pass through the structures, and a high-contrast radiographic image is obtained; at a 90 kVp setting many photons are able to pass through the structures, and a low-contrast radiographic image is obtained (NOTE: As the kilovolt peak is increased, the exposure time must be decreased to prevent overexposure to provide a film of acceptable density)

9. Generally as the density, atomic number, and electrons per gram of tissue increases, the number of attenuated photons increases; gold, amalgam, enamel, dentin, cementum, and bone attenuate photons to a great extent and are radiopaque structures; bone marrow spaces, sinuses, pulps, and periodontal ligament spaces do not attenuate photons and are radiolucent structures

Interactions of Ionizing Radiation on Cells, Tissues, and Organs

A. Definitions
  1. Whole-body exposure (total body)—each gram of tissue in the entire body absorbs equal amounts of radiation
  2. Specific-area exposure (localized)—each gram of tissue of the body in the specific area irradiated absorbs equal amounts of radiation; (e.g., facial exposure from four bitewing radiographs)
  3. Direct effect—transfer of energy by the ionization mechanism from an x-ray photon to a biologically critical molecule such as deoxyribonucleic aid (DNA)
  4. Indirect effect—transfer of energy by the ionization mechanism from an x-ray photon to a noncritical molecule, which in turn delivers the energy to the biologically critical molecule
  5. Generic effect—mutations of future generations; results from exposure of the reproductive cells yielding alterations in the genetic code
  6. Somatic effect—refers to injury observed in the person being irradiated
  7. Latent period—time between the exposure and the development of the biologic effect
  8. Acute effects (short-term or early)—effects that may occur minutes, hours, or weeks after the exposure; usually result from high doses of whole-body exposure
  9. Chronic effects (long-term or late)—effects observed years after the original exposure
B. Units of radiation measurement
  1. Roentgen (R) is a unit of radiation exposure or intensity
    a. One roentgen is that amount of x-radiation or gamma radiation that will produce 2.08 $\times 10^9$ ion pairs in 1 cc of air
    b. International System of Units (SI unit) for exposure is defined as electrical charge per unit mass of air

$$1 \text{ R} = 2.58 \times 10^{-4} \text{ coulomb (C)/kg}$$

2. Rad (rad) is the unit of an absorbed dose; 1 rad is equal to 100 ergs of energy from any type of radiation per gram of absorbing material; SI unit for absorbed dose is the gray (Gy); 1 Gy is equal to 100 rad; 1 Gy is equal to 1 joule (J)/kg
3. Rem (rem) is the unit of dose equivalent and refers to the occupational dose received by radiation workers
  a. Some radiations are more damaging than x-rays; rem facilitates comparisons among the biologic effects of various radiations
  b. Rem is the product of the absorbed dose in rad times the quality factors (QF), indicating the relative biologic effectiveness
  c. SI unit for dose equivalent is the seivert (Sv); 1 seivert is equal to 100 rad
4. Curie (Ci) is the unit of radioactivity; refers to the quantity of radioactive material and *not* the radiation emitted by radioactive decay; 1 Ci is equal to that quantity of material in which 3.7 $\times 10^{10}$ atoms disintegrate per second; SI unit for radioactivity is the becquerel (Bq); 1 Ci is equal to 3.7 $\times 10^{10}$ Bq
C. Radiation dose-response relationships
  1. Applications
    a. Design of radiation therapeutic treatment routines for patients with malignant disease
    b. To provide information on low-dose irradiation effects
  2. Characteristics of dose-response relationships
    a. Linear—response is directly proportional to the dose
    b. Nonlinear—response is not directly proportional to the dose
    c. Nonthreshold—any dose, regardless of its size, is expected to produce a response
    d. Threshold—from zero to a particular point, no response would be expected; above the threshold point any dose will produce a response
D. Biologic responses to irradiation
  1. Considerations
    a. Radiation exposure is harmful to all living tissues and should be used cautiously
    b. Although the interaction between x-rays and tissues occurs at the atomic level, it is theorized that observable human radiation injury results from molecular derangement of macromolecules and water
    c. Injury to cells, tissues, and organs occurs at the time of exposure but may require hours, days, or generations for manifestation
    d. Radiation injury is induced immediately following the interaction of x-rays and tissues; caused by ionization

e. Ionization
  (1) Refers to the excitation of orbital electrons in an atom and to the deposition of energy in the tissues
  (2) Occurs when the atoms of a molecule are separated into charged atomic particles (e.g., table salt; NaCl yields $Na^+ + Cl^-$ when mixed in H_2O)
  (3) May cause a breakage in the molecule or relocation of the atom in the molecule
  (4) Altered molecules may function improperly or cease to function altogether

2. Radiation effects on cells
  a. Two types of cells in the human body
    (1) Genetic cells are the oogonium of the female and the spermatogonium of the male
    (2) Somatic cells comprise all other cells
  b. Nucleus of proliferating somatic and genetic cells is considered to be the most sensitive area of the cell to the ionizing effects
    (1) Exposure to the nucleus results in cell inhibition
    (2) Most sensitive sites within the cell's nucleus are the DNA and chromosomes
    (3) Chromosome aberrations in somatic cells are observed during the metaphase stage of mitosis (cell division); changes in genetic material can occur during meiosis or reduction division
      (a) Chromosomes control the growth, development, and maintenance of the cell
      (b) Sufficient radiation damage to the DNA may yield visible or invisible chromosome aberrations that may lead to cell death or malfunction
      (c) Tissue or organ destruction occurs when several cells are damaged and not sufficiently repaired by the body's repair mechanism
      (d) DNA damage can result in an uncontrolled, rapid proliferation of cells, the principal characteristic of radiation-induced malignant disease
      (e) Genetic cell or germ cell injury may be observed only in future generations (ranging from increased susceptibility to disease to birth defects to cancer)

c. Cells found to be the most sensitive to radiation exposure are young, rapidly dividing, nondifferentiated cells such as those of the developing fetus
d. Cell responses to irradiation
  (1) Cell death refers to the immediate or delayed death of a cell following excessive exposure to a lethal dose
  (2) Swelling of the cell results from interference of fluid exchange through the cell wall
  (3) Alterations in specific cell function, such as the production of a protein or enzyme of changed chemical composition, can also occur following excessive exposure
  (4) Cell aberration results from damage occurring during mitosis or meiosis

3. Radiolysis of water
  a. Yields radicals that combine to form hydrogen peroxide
  b. Hydrogen peroxide is a toxic agent to living tissues; is an indirect damaging effect of ionizing radiation

4. Biologic effects on tissues and organs
  a. Bergonié-Tribondeau law of radiosensitivity
    (1) The more mature a cell is, the more resistant it is to radiation
    (2) The younger tissues and organs are, the greater the radiosensitivity is
    (3) The higher the metabolic activity is, the higher the radiosensitivity is
    (4) The greater the proliferation rate for cells and the growth rate for tissues, the greater the radiosensitivity
    (5) The more differentiated (or specialized in function) a cell is, the more radioresistant it is
  b. Degree of tissue sensitivity in rank order
    (1) Reproductive (most sensitive)
    (2) Lymphatic
    (3) Circulatory
    (4) Endocrine
    (5) Respiratory
    (6) Digestive
    (7) Nervous
  c. Determinants of the radiosensitivity of an organ[3]
    (1) Function of the organ to the body
    (2) Rate at which cells mature and are turned over in the organ
    (3) Inherent radiosensitivity of the cell type
  d. Organ tissues considered critical because of their sensitivity are skin, thyroid, eye, and hemopoietic and genetic tissue

e. The most radiosensitive area of tissues and organs is the endothelial cell layer, which lines the capillary walls

f. Repeated exposure to the capillary network leads to functional impairment observed as a decline in performance and reduction in defense against infection

g. Continued low-dose exposure negatively affects the repair mechanism; overloading of the repair system by time or amount of exposure can result in somatic or genetic damage

5. Repair and accumulation of radiation effects

a. Most injury resulting from low-dose radiation exposure is repaired within the cells, tissues, and organs (depending on the relative biologic damaging ability of the radiation)

b. Repeated exposure may lead to some unrepaired effects that accumulate in the exposed tissues

c. Accumulated radiation effect accelerates and increases the probability of inducing cancer and the normal aging process; high doses result in a more rapid expression of the effects

Image Receptors

A. Definition

1. Serve as a mechanism for transferring information contained in an attenuated remnant x-ray beam into a visible image

2. For dental radiology, an image receptor is either a piece of x-ray film or the combination of film and an intensifying screen

B. Types

1. Classified as either direct or indirect imaging systems

2. Direct imaging refers to the exposure of the x-ray film by the interaction of the photographic emulsion and remnant x-ray beam

3. Indirect imaging refers to the exposure of the x-ray film primarily by the light emitted from an intensifying screen and, to a lesser extent, by the remnant x-ray beam

C. Radiographic film

1. X-ray film used with direct and indirect imaging systems is similar in composition

2. Quality control procedures are followed during the manufacture of film for standardization

3. Film composition

a. Base material must possess dimensional stability to withstand processing procedures; cellulose acetate is used

b. Adhesive is applied evenly to the base; used to provide for uniform attachment of the emulsion to the base

c. Emulsion consists of the gelatin and silver halide crystals; records the information within the x-ray beam

d. Protective coating is applied to protect the emulsion from scratching

4. Film classifications

a. Intraoral and extraoral film refers to the designated use of the film

(1) Intraoral means the film is placed within the oral cavity (e.g., bitewing or periapical)

(2) Extraoral refers to film placed outside of the mouth for exposure of large areas (e.g., panoramic or cephalometric)

b. Screen film is characteristically a much slower film with a thinner emulsion layer and is used with an intensifying screen (e.g., panoramic film); nonscreen film refers to film exposed by x-rays alone and has a thicker emulsion to increase its sensitivity to radiation

c. Speed refers to the film's responsiveness to x-radiation and is directly related to image visibility

(1) Fast film has larger silver halide crystals and decreased image resolution

(2) Slow film has smaller silver halide crystals and increased image resolution

(3) Traditionally, speed ranges have been designated from A to F, with A being the slowest

(4) Radiation hygiene factors prevent A- to C-speed films from being commercially available for patient use; D- and E-speed films are available for use

d. Size—variable sizes are available for both screen and nonscreen film

(1) Nonscreen film

(a) No. 0—22 × 35 mm

(b) No. 1—24 × 40 mm

(c) No. 2—32 × 41 mm

(d) No. 3—27 × 54 mm

(e) No. 4—57 × 76 mm

(2) Screen film

(a) 4 × 5 in

(b) 5 × 12 in

(c) 8 × 10 in

e. Use
  (1) Nonscreen films are used for periapical, bitewing, and occlusal radiographic projections
  (2) Screen films are used for extraoral projections such as the panoramic and cephalometric projections
f. Intraoral nonscreen film is available in single or double film packets; double film packets provide a duplicate radiograph for patient records
5. Packet construction of intraoral films
  a. Light-tight, leak-proof wrapping protects the film from light and the patient's saliva
  b. Black protective paper is used for additional protection of the film from light and saliva
  c. Lead foil is inserted between the black paper and the outer wrapping for packet stability and protection of tissues from excessive radiation exposures
  d. Double or single films are enclosed
6. Intensifying screens
  a. Housed inside a light-tight cassette
  b. Used as a component of the indirect imaging systems to reduce patient exposure to x-radiation for study of large anatomic areas
  c. Screen construction
    (1) Base material may be composed of high-grade cardboard, polyester, or metal; must be sturdy and moisture resistant; should not interfere with phosphorescence of the phosphor layer
    (2) Reflective layer, coated onto the base material, may be either magnesium oxide or titanium dioxide; redirects light toward the film to increase the efficiency of the film
    (3) Phosphor layer
      (a) Composed of phosphorescent crystals (e.g., calcium tungstate or rare earth crystals); crystals convert the energy of the remnant x-ray beam into visible light; visible light is used to expose the film
      (b) Phosphorescent crystals
        [1] Have a higher atomic number to increase the probability of their interaction with the x-ray photons
        [2] Should emit a large amount of light per interaction
        [3] Should emit light of proper wavelength to match sensitivity of the film to light
        [4] Should stop emitting light once the x-ray exposure has been terminated
    (4) Protective coating is applied to the phosphor layer to prevent abrasion of the phosphor and must be transparent to light
  d. Calcium tungstate phosphor
    (1) Emits blue light
    (2) Traditionally used in the phosphor layer of the intensifying screen
  e. Rare earth phosphors
    (1) Primarily emit green light
    (2) Represent recent research in indirect imaging systems
    (3) Use gadolinium oxysulfide or lanthanum oxysulfide
    (4) Respond more efficiently to x-radiation; result in a significant decrease in patient exposure
7. Extraoral film identification methods
  a. Lead letter (R or L) is attached to the tube-side surface of the cassette but positioned away from the structures of interest; can be used to record the date and patient's name
  b. Radiopaque tape is also available for recording the patient's name and date
  c. Light flasher units are used to record the patient's name, date, and so on, into the image before processing
D. Film care storage methods
  1. Must be stored away from heat, moisture, chemical vapors, and radiation
  2. Should be stored by emulsion date so that the oldest films are used first
E. Latent image formation
  1. Film considerations
    a. Crystals within the emulsion are composed of positive silver ions and negative bromide and iodide ions
    b. Crystals contain imperfections
      (1) Free interstitial silver ions
      (2) Iodine atoms within bromine sites yield physical distortion of crystals
      (3) Crystals are chemically sensitized by sulfur compounds bound to the surface
    c. Irregularities of crystals are termed latent image sites; trap recoil electrons to begin image-formation process
  2. Silver halide crystals are irradiated

3. X-ray photons are absorbed by bromide ions; bromide ions are converted to bromine atoms; process produces high-speed recoil electrons and scattered photons
4. High-speed recoil electrons travel through crystal with the ability to dislodge other electrons
5. High-speed recoil electrons are trapped by latent image sites (crystal imperfections); impart a negative charge to the site
6. Free interstitial silver ions are attracted to the negatively charged latent image site
7. Atom of metallic silver is produced by the combination of the trapped electron and silver ion
8. When photons interact with bromide ions, the process occurs
9. Accumulation of silver atoms at the latent image sites (crystal imperfection sites) comprises the latent (invisible) image
10. Crystals with metal silver deposits are subject to chemical reduction by the developer solution during film processing
11. Individual crystals are completely reduced to metallic silver or not at all during film-processing procedures
12. Crystals not exposed to radiation are removed from the emulsion by the fixer solution
13. Visible image is a result of the variations in the number of exposed and reduced crystals

DARKROOM TECHNIQUES — RADIOGRAPHIC FILM PROCESSING

A. Chemical solutions
   1. Developer
      a. Reducing agent (hydroquinone or elon)—functions to reduce the latent image–containing silver bromide crystals to black metallic silver
      b. Alkalizer (sodium carbonate)—provides the required alkaline medium for the reducer to work; softens and swells the gelatin of the emulsion to allow reducers to reach the silver bromide crystals
      c. Preservative (sodium sulfite)—slows the oxidation of the solution to prolong its life span
      d. Restrainer (potassium bromide)—slows down the action of the chemicals
   2. Fixer
      a. Clearing or fixing agent (sodium or ammonium thiosulfate)—removes the unexposed or undeveloped crystals from the emulsion

   b. Acidifier (acetic acid)—provides the required acidity so the fixing solutions can work; stops the action of the developer
   c. Preservative (sodium sulfite)—slows the oxidation of the solution to prolong its life span
   d. Hardener (potassium aluminum)—shrinks and hardens the emulsion
   e. Vehicle (distilled water)—used to mix the chemicals

B. Processing methods
   1. Basic procedure of film processing
      a. Developing—reduces latent image–containing silver bromide crystals to black metallic silver
      b. Rinsing—washes away excess developer solution to avoid contamination and neutralization of the fixer
      c. Fixing—removes the unexposed or undeveloped crystals from the emulsion
      d. Washing—removes the fixer solution to avoid staining the film
      e. Drying—removes water from the emulsion; prepares the film for viewing
   2. Time-temperature method
      a. Recommended scientific method for film processing
      b. Optimum amount of reduction of silver bromide crystals occurs
      c. Developer activity is dependent on the temperature of the solution
      d. Less activity occurs at lower temperatures; greater activity occurs at higher temperatures
      e. Optimum results are obtained at 20° C (68° F) (Table 5-2)
   3. Sight method*
      a. Not a recommended method of film processing
      b. Films are removed periodically from the developer solution, examined under a safelight to determine the presence of visible images, then placed in a fixer solution
      c. Disadvantages
         (1) Lack of quality control
         (2) Nonstandardized procedures
         (3) Radiographic density of variable range

---

*We do not recommend this method and have described it only for completeness of the topic area, since the practice of sight development does occur.

Table 5-2 Time-temperature processing

Temperature of developer (°F)	Time in developer (min)
60	8
65	5½
68	4½ optimum
70	4
75	3
80	2¼

From Dental assisting manual No. 5: Dental radiology, by Stephen Matteson, K. Cy Whaley, and Clifton E. Crandell. Copyright 1980 The University of North Carolina Press. Used with permission of the publisher.

4. Manual method
   a. Films are placed on racks and hand dipped in solutions
   b. Normally associated with the time-temperature method
5. Automatic method
   a. Films are carried from solution to solution and through the dryer by a roller assembly
   b. Completed in 5 to 7 minutes
   c. Advantages over manual processing method
      (1) Standardized procedure
      (2) Solutions of proper strength provided
      (3) Temperature solutions controlled
      (4) Processing time regulated
      (5) Increased number of films can be processed
      (6) Reduction in processing time
6. Rapid processing method
   a. Sometimes referred to as ''hot processing''
   b. Accomplished by use of high-temperature solutions or concentrated solutions at room temperature
   c. Completed in 1 minute or less
   d. Film quality is less than that obtained with standard methods
   e. Recommended in endodontic or emergency procedures
7. Wet reading
   a. Immediate evaluation of radiographic technique and dental disease
   b. Often used in manual processing
   c. Minimum fixing time of 3 minutes required before viewing films
   d. For archival quality films, normal time-temperature processing procedures must be resumed as soon as possible
C. Darkroom design and requirements[5]
   1. Location and size
      a. Located near rooms where x-ray units are placed
      b. Minimum of 16 square feet for one person to work
      c. Size-determining factors
         (1) Number of radiographs to be processed
         (2) Number of personnel using the darkroom
         (3) Processing method(s) used (i.e., manual, automatic, or both)
         (4) Space for duplicating, drying, and storage
      d. Light-tight room
      e. Door with an inside lock to prevent accidental white light exposure of films
   2. Lighting
      a. Illuminating safelight
         (1) Any illumination that will not expose x-ray film
         (2) Determining factors include x-ray film sensitivity to light, film position, and intensity of light
         (3) Usually 10- 15-watt bulb with filter (e.g., Wratten 6B) placed 3 to 4 feet away from working surface
         (4) Panoramic and other extraoral films are more sensitive to light than intraoral films; therefore the safelight must accommodate the film sensitivity
      b. Overhead white light
         (1) Provides adequate illumination for the room
         (2) Switch is positioned in the room to avoid accidental white light exposure of films during processing
      c. Viewing safelight—mounted on the wall behind the processing tanks for wet readings (after films have been in the fixer solution for 3 minutes)
      d. X-ray viewbox—for wet readings
      e. Outside warning light
         (1) To prevent accidental entry of personnel during film-processing procedures
         (2) Should be wired to the safelight so that both are on at the same time
   3. Plumbing
      a. Hot and cold water supply for time-temperature processing
      b. Adequate drainage
      c. Thermostatically controlled intake valve to maintain constant temperatures of solutions
      d. Constant water flow for automatic processors must be considered
      e. Noncorrosive pipes to withstand chemicals
      f. Large sink with gooseneck faucet needed to accommodate cleaning procedures

4. Darkroom contents
   a. Processing tanks
   b. Processing solutions
   c. Timer
   d. Thermometer
   e. Film hangers
   f. Dryer
   g. Stirring paddles for solutions
   h. Cleaning supplies
5. Record keeping
   a. Inventory of chemicals
   b. Dates of solution changes
   c. Film identification records
      (1) Patient's name
      (2) Number of films
      (3) Rack numbers
      (4) Date of film exposure and processing
6. Silver retrieval sources
   a. Old; no longer used or needed for radiographs
   b. Exhausted fixer solution (units may be purchased for the precipitation of silver)
   c. Lead foil may be sold for scrap
D. Film-processing errors
   1. Fogged films
      a. Causes
         (1) Unsafe darkroom illumination
         (2) Safelight too close to the working surface
         (3) Overactive chemicals (freshly made)
         (4) Exposure to scattered radiation
      b. Corrective action
         (1) Check safelight filter for cracks
         (2) Check appropriate filter for film sensitivity
         (3) Check wattage of the light bulb in the safelight
         (4) Check distance of the safelight from the working surface
   2. Underdeveloped films
      a. Causes
         (1) Temperature of developer solution too cool
         (2) Insufficient developing time
         (3) Developer solution exhausted
      b. Corrective action
         (1) Check developer temperature with a thermometer
         (2) Check developing time with an accurate timing device
         (3) Replace old developer solution

3. Overdeveloped films
   a. Causes
      (1) Temperature of developer solution too high
      (2) Excessive developing time used
      (3) Overactive solutions (no restrainer chemical)
   b. Corrective action
      (1) Check developer temperature with a thermometer
      (2) Check developing time with an accurate timing device
      (3) Check chemistry of solutions and mixing procedures
4. Developer cut off
   a. Caused by film that is partially immersed in the developer solution
   b. Corrective actions
      (1) Check height of the developer solution in the tank
      (2) Add replenishment to the developer solution if necessary
      (3) Do not attach films to the top clip of the developing rack
5. Clear films
   a. Causes
      (1) Film placed in the fixer solution first, which removed all silver bromide crystals
      (2) Excessive washing to cause removal of emulsion
   b. Corrective actions
      (1) Label solution tanks
      (2) Post appropriate processing procedures in the darkroom
      (3) Remove films from wash after appropriate time
6. Stained films
   a. Developer stains
      (1) Dark overdeveloped areas caused by contamination of the film with developer solution before the normal processing cycle
      (2) Corrected by keeping the darkroom work area clean, preventing dripping or splashing of the developer solution on the work counter, and washing hands if handling solutions
   b. Fixer stains
      (1) Clear or light spots on the film that result from contamination of the film by fixer solutions before the normal processing cycle; corrected by keeping the work area clean to avoid dripping and splashing of the fixer solution on the counter

(2) Brown or yellow stains result from insufficient fixing time or insufficient washing time for removal of fixer chemicals from the film emulsion; corrected by employing appropriate film-processing procedures

c. Fluoride artifacts
   (1) Dark areas on the film caused by contamination of the film with fluoride
   (2) Corrected by washing hands to remove fluoride before unwrapping film

d. Saliva stains
   (1) Dark areas on the film
   (2) Corrected by wiping saliva from the film after removal from the oral cavity and preventing the black protective paper from sticking to the emulsion

e. Green film
   (1) Film emulsion not in contact with processing chemicals
   (2) Corrected by separating double film packets

7. Reticulation of emulsion
   a. Caused by transferring the film from one solution to another with extreme changes in temperature
   b. Corrected by monitoring solution temperatures

8. Torn or scratched films
   a. Caused by the emulsion that is in contact with rough objects or the sides of the tanks while wet
   b. Corrected by monitoring placement of the film in the processing tanks

9. Lost films
   a. Causes
      (1) Film not securely attached to the rack (manual processing)
      (2) Film did not proceed through the roller assembly properly (automatic processing)
   b. Corrective actions
      (1) Repair the manual rack, and securely fasten the film
      (2) Repair the roller assembly if defective, and review the method of film insertion

10. Air bubbles
    a. Caused by air bubbles caught on the film emulsion when placed in the developer solution
    b. Corrected by agitating the film rack for 5 seconds to release air bubbles

11. Static electricity
    a. Caused by removing the film from the packet or cassette during winter, which yields dark streaks on the film
    b. Corrected by carefully removing the film from the packet

12. Light leaks
    a. Cause
       (1) Film packet covering is torn
       (2) Accidental opening of the packet under the white light
       (3) Failure to cover the film-processing tanks during the procedure
       (4) Failure to allow the film to be fully accepted by the rollers for automatic processing before turning on the white light
       (5) Cuffs of the daylight loader of the automatic processor not tight enough around the arms; light enters during the unwrapping of the film
    b. Corrective action
       (1) Follow proper procedures
       (2) Examine the daylight loader cuffs for secure fit

E. Film duplication
   1. Purpose
      a. To provide copies of radiographs to dental insurance companies
      b. To forward the patient's treatment records to the new dentist
      c. To use in dental malpractice cases
   2. Equipment
      a. Radiographic duplicating film
         (1) Base—blue-tinted polyester base
         (2) Solarized emulsion
            (a) Emulsion composed of gelatin and silver bromide crystals
            (b) Refers to the phenomenon in which more light exposure of the film yields a decrease in film density and less light exposure of the film yields an increase in film density
            (c) Often the term *direct positive* is used
         (3) Antihalation coating
            (a) Layer of gelatin containing a dye
            (b) Process of halation occurs when the light passing through the film and into the air is reflected back toward the emulsion, causing unsharp edges
            (c) Dye absorbs the reflected light to prevent image unsharpness
            (d) Dye is washed away during film processing

b. Film-duplicating printer
   (1) Box-type device with a glass top, adjustable timer, and ultraviolet light source
   (2) Printing area of variable size; dependent on dealer and model type
3. Procedure
   a. Original radiographs are positioned on the glass top
   b. Right and left sides are identified
   c. Under safelight conditions, remove the duplicating film from the box; place the solarized emulsion side down over the film
   d. Appropriate exposure time is selected; ultraviolet light passes through the original radiographs to expose the duplicating film
   e. Duplicating film is processed by either manual or automatic processing such as that used for normal dental radiographs
4. Duplication errors
   a. Light duplicate film results from overexposure of the duplicating film
   b. Dark duplicate film results from underexposure of the duplicating film
   c. Poor definition of the film results from loss of intimate contact between the original and copy film

ORAL RADIOGRAPHIC TECHNIQUES
Description of the Radiographic Image

A. Definitions
   1. Radiolucent—black to dark gray areas on the radiograph resulting from more exposure of the film by radiation passing through the less dense anatomic structures
   2. Radiopaque—white to light gray areas on the radiograph resulting from less exposure of the film by radiation being absorbed by the dense anatomic structures
   3. Radiographic density—overall blackening of a radiograph; density is read with a densitometer
   4. Radiographic contrast—differences in densities of adjacent areas of the radiograph
      a. Long-scale contrast (also called low contrast)—scale with many shades of gray resulting from the small differences in densities; obtained with a high kilovolt peak technique
      b. Short-scale contrast (also called high contrast)—scale with few shades of gray resulting from a large difference in densities; obtained with a low kilovolt peak technique
   5. Detail (definition)—degree of clarity on a radiograph
   6. Resolution—ability to record separate images of small objects that are placed close together
   7. Sharpness—ability of the x-ray film to define an edge
   8. Fog—overall gray appearance yielding a lower film contrast; results from exposure of the film by scattered radiation or exposure by unsafe illumination of the darkroom
B. Factors affecting visualized radiographic image
   1. Exposure time
      a. Directly proportional to film density
      b. Increased exposure time provides more x-ray photons to interact with the emulsion
   2. Milliamperage
      a. Directly proportional to film density
      b. Increased milliamperage yields more heat in the filament; produces more electrons by thermionic emission, which yields more x-ray photons
      c. With more x-rays produced, more x-rays interact with the film emulsion
   3. Kilovolt potential
      a. Directly proportional to film density; a higher kilovolt peak technique yields a more penetrating x-ray beam, and a greater number of x-ray photons are produced; therefore more of the film emulsion is exposed
      b. Inversely proportional to film contrast; decreased kilovolt peak yields film with high contrast, since the beam has less penetrating ability; increased kilovolt peak yields film with low contrast, since the beam has more penetrating ability
   4. Collimation
      a. Inversely proportional to film density; increased collimation of the x-ray beam decreases density because there is a reduction in the number of scattered photons that cause film fog
      b. Directly proportional to film contrast; with less scattered photons causing fog, the contrast is higher (short scale)
   5. Filtration—inversely proportional to film density; the greater the filtration of the x-ray beam, the fewer photons available to penetrate the patient and interact with the film

6. Target-to-film distance
   a. Inversely proportional to film density
   b. Based on the phenomenon of the inverse square law

$$\frac{I_1}{I_2} = \frac{d_2{}^2}{d_1{}^2}$$

   where I_1 is the intensity at the first distance (d_1) from the source, and I_2 is the intensity at the second distance (d_2) from the source
      (1) States that the intensity of the x-ray beam is inversely proportional to the square of the distance
      (2) Rapid decrease in intensity results from the spreading out of the x-ray photons over a larger area as they move farther from the source
      (3) Example—if the intensity of an x-ray beam is 400 milliroentgens (mR) at 36 inches, then at 72 inches (double the distance) the intensity is only one fourth as great and is 100 mR
   c. To maintain film density when switching from a short target-to-film distance to a long target-to-film distance, the milliamperage or exposure time must be increased
7. Patient-object thickness—inversely proportional to film density; as thickness increases, more of the beam is attenuated, yielding a decrease in film density
8. Patient-object density—inversely proportional to film density; more of the beam is attenuated by the patient, yielding a decrease in film density

Radiographic Techniques

A. Shadow-casting principles
   1. Smallest focal spot (x-ray source) as possible
      a. Yields more parallel x-ray photons
      b. Reduces penumbra
      c. Enhances image sharpness
   2. Longest focal spot (x-ray source–to–object [tooth] distance) as possible
      a. Results in use of more parallel x-ray photons
      b. Decreases image magnification
      c. Enhances image sharpness
   3. Shortest object (tooth)–to-film distance as possible
      a. Decreases image magnification
      b. Enhances image sharpness
   4. Object (tooth) and film should be in a parallel relationship; reduces image distortion (e.g., elongation and foreshortening)
      5. X-ray beam should be perpendicular to the tooth and film; reduces image distortion
B. Intraoral procedures
   1. Paralleling technique
      a. Theory
         (1) Introduced by McCormack
         (2) Yields radiographs with a minimum of image distortion
         (3) Minimizes the superimposition of adjacent oral structures
         (4) Commonly referred to as the long-cone technique or right-angle technique
         (5) Applies shadow-casting principles Nos. 1, 2, 4, and 5
      b. Application (Fig. 5-4)
         (1) Film packet is placed parallel with the long axis of the tooth and perpendicular to the horizontal axis of the tooth
         (2) X-ray beam is directed perpendicular to the long axis of the tooth and image receptor (film)
         (3) X-ray beam is directed through the interproximal spaces
         (4) X-ray beam centered over the anatomic structures and image receptor
   2. Bisecting-the-angle technique
      a. Theory
         (1) Introduced by Cieszynski
         (2) Applies the rule of isometry (correct length of the tooth image obtained if the x-ray beam is perpendicular to the bisector of the angle formed by the plane of the film and the long axis of the tooth)

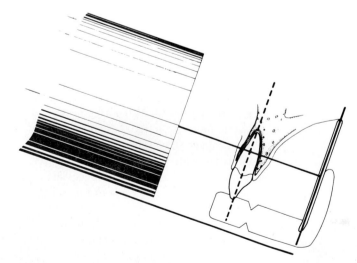

Fig. 5-4 Paralleling technique. (From Whaley, K.C.: Intraoral radiography: the paralleling technique, Chapel Hill, 1977, University of North Carolina.)

(3) Commonly referred to as the short-cone technique

(4) Does not use shadow-casting principles Nos. 4 and 5 as listed under *A* (p. 164)

b. Application (Fig. 5-5)

(1) Film packet is placed against the teeth

(2) X-ray beam is directed perpendicular to the imaginary bisector of the angle formed by the plane of the film and the long axis of the tooth

(3) X-ray beam is directed through the interproximal spaces

(4) X-ray beam is centered over the anatomic structures and image receptor

3. Intraoral radiographic techniques

a. Periapical projection demonstrates the entire tooth and surrounding structures (Fig. 5-6); indications are

(1) Periodontal involvement

(2) Suspected impaction

(3) Congenitally missing teeth

(4) Defective restorative work

(5) Localized sensitivity

(6) Suspected pathologic condition (e.g., caries and periapical involvement)

(7) Injury or trauma to the oral cavity

(8) Endodontic therapy

(9) No previous radiographs

(10) On request by the dentist

b. Bitewing projection demonstrates anatomic crowns of the maxillary and mandibular teeth plus height of the alveolar bone (Fig. 5-7); indications are

(1) Carious lesions

(2) Localized periodontal involvement

(3) No previous radiographs

(4) On request by the dentist

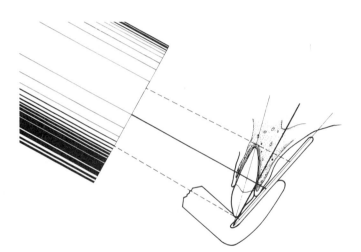

Fig. 5-5 Bisecting-the-angle technique. (From Whaley, K.C.: Intraoral radiography: the paralleling technique, Chapel Hill, 1977, University of North Carolina.)

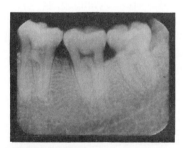

Fig. 5-6 Periapical radiograph.

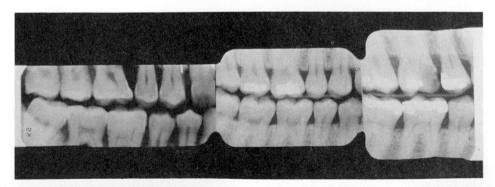

Fig. 5-7 Bitewing radiographs. *Left to right:* Long horizontal bitewing, standard horizontal bitewing, and vertical bitewing.

c. Occlusal projection demonstrates the large anatomic region or entire arch (Fig. 5-8); indications are
   (1) Localization of objects
   (2) Trauma
   (3) Supernumerary teeth
   (4) Image margins of the large pathologic lesions
d. Complete radiographic survey is a combination of periapical and bitewing projections that image entire dentition with the number of projections variable (Fig. 5-9)

4. Intraoral film holding devices are used to stabilize the film position, reduce the film movement during exposure, and eliminate the need for the patient to hold the film

C. Intraoral technique errors (Fig. 5-10)
   1. Typical packet placement errors involve improper positioning of the film behind the teeth of interest and failure to achieve shadow-casting principles
   2. Vertical angulation
      a. Typical vertical angulation errors with the paralleling technique are visualized as missing apical or coronal structures
      b. Typical vertical angulation errors with the bisecting-the-angle technique are visualized as foreshortened or elongated structures
   3. Horizontal overlap
      a. Visualized as the radiopaque density resulting from the superimposition of adjacent interproximal tooth surfaces
      b. Commonly occurs by directing the beam from an excessive mesial or distal horizontal position
   4. Centering
      a. Visualized as a clear area on the film
      b. Results from improper coverage of the image receptor by the x-ray beam

D. Extraoral procedures are considered supplemental projections and are used when evaluating a variety of maxillofacial conditions
   1. Lateral oblique mandible projection is used for visualizing the mandible from the canine region posteriorly to the mandibular body and ramus (Fig. 5-11)
      a. Technique
         (1) Occlusal plane is perpendicular to the plane of the film
         (2) X-ray beam is centered over the area of interest
         (3) Cone is directed 25 degrees to the negative

b. Indications—to evaluate radiolucencies and radiopacities seen on other projections, third molars, and trauma-related conditions and to determine the extent of pathologic lesions

2. Temporomandibular joint (TMJ)—transcranial projection is traditionally the most preferred method of imaging the TMJ area; provides visualization of the neck and condylar head of the mandible and the TMJ space without superimposition of adjacent structures (Fig. 5-12)
   a. Technique
      (1) Midsagittal plane and film are parallel
      (2) X-ray beam is directed transcranially 25 to 30 degrees to the positive
      (3) X-ray beam exits at the joint space of interest, which is against the film
   b. Indication—TMJ dysfunction

3. Waters' projection is a supplemental extraoral projection used primarily for visualization of the maxillary sinuses with minimal superimposition of other anatomic structures (Fig. 5-13)
   a. Technique
      (1) Patient is in an anteroposterior position facing the film cassette
      (2) Chin is extended, establishing a perpendicular mentomeatal line (line formed by the external auditory meatus and the mental region of the chin)
      (3) X-ray beam is directed perpendicular to the film and parallel to the mentomeatal line
      (4) Structures shown include the maxilla, maxillary sinuses, zygomatic arches, and orbital rims
   b. Indications include trauma and visualization of "cloudy" radiopaque sinuses

4. Cephalometric projection is used primarily during orthodontic treatment to measure changes in the cranial bones and by oral surgeons involved in maxillofacial reconstruction (Fig. 5-14)
   a. Technique
      (1) Cephalostat with earpost is used to allow for reproduction of patient position at subsequent examinations
      (2) Patient is instructed to look straight ahead in a natural position
      (3) Midsagittal plane-to-film distance of 11.5 cm is used
      (4) Target-to-film distance of 1.5 m is used
      (5) Placement of a wedge filter in the path of the x-ray beam provides a soft tissue outline *Text continued on p. 172.*

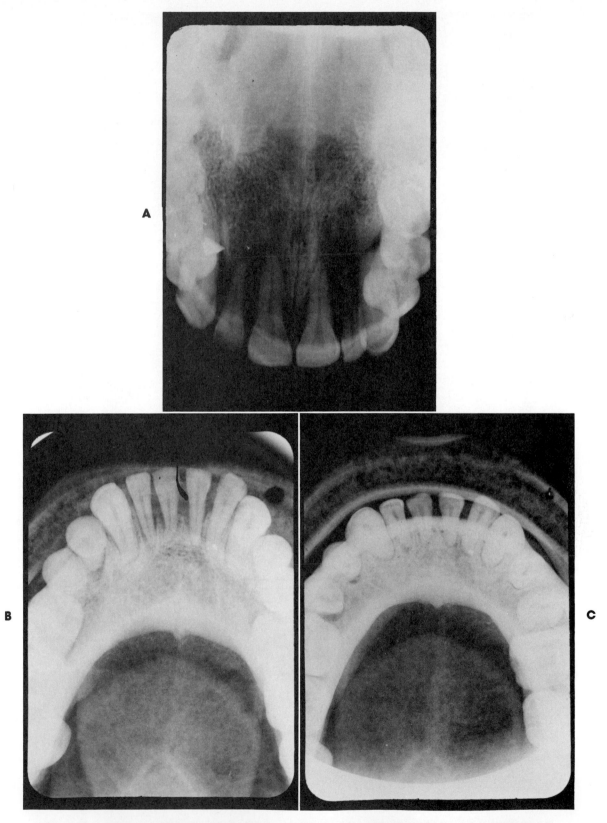

Fig. 5-8 Occlusal radiographs. **A,** Topographic occlusal radiograph of maxillary arch. **B,** Topographic occlusal radiography of mandibular arch. **C,** Cross-sectional occlusal radiograph of mandibular arch.

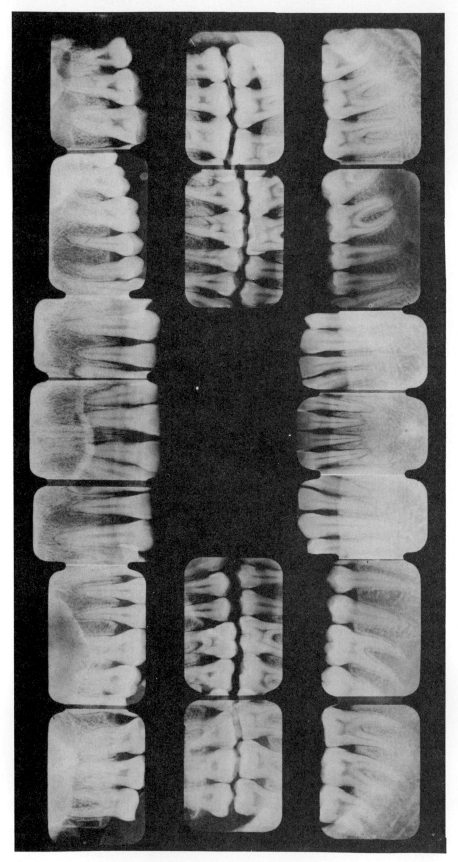

Fig. 5-9 Full-mouth radiographic survey. (From Dental assisting manual No. 5: Dental radiology, by Stephen Matteson, K. Cy Whaley, and Clifton E. Crandell. Copyright 1980 The University of North Carolina Press. Used with permission of the publisher.)

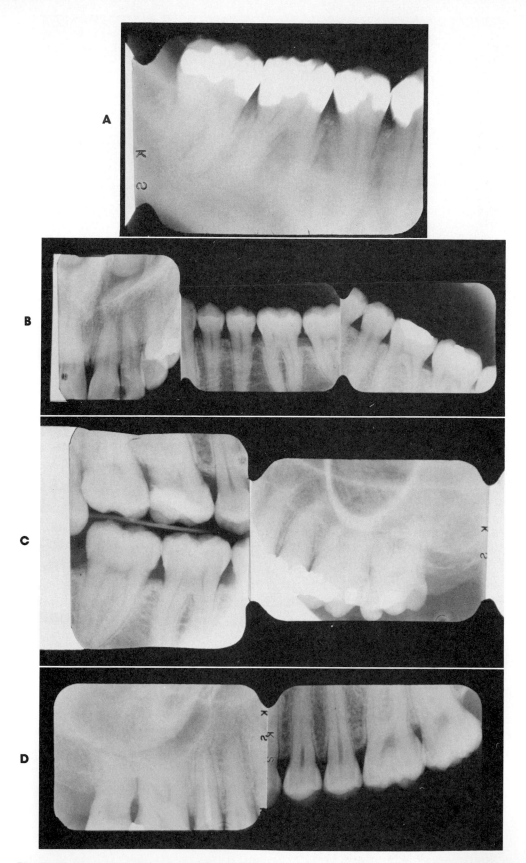

Fig. 5-10 Intraoral technique errors. **A,** Motion. **B,** Packet placement. *Left to right:* Packet off center, packet too high, and packet tilted. **C,** Cone cut. **D,** Vertical angulation (with paralleling technique). Excessive vertical angulation projects crowns off image receptor *(left);* insufficient vertical angulation projects apices off image receptor *(right).*

Continued.

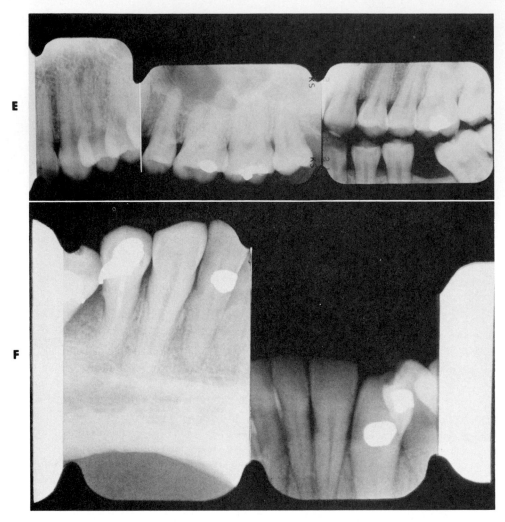

Fig. 5-10, cont'd E, Horizontal overlap. **F,** Combination of errors. Object and film not parallel and excessive vertical angulation *(left);* Packet positioned too high and insufficient vertical angulation *(right).*

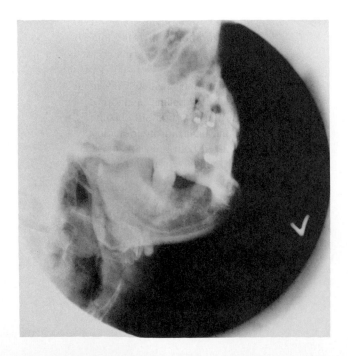

Fig. 5-11 Lateral oblique mandible.

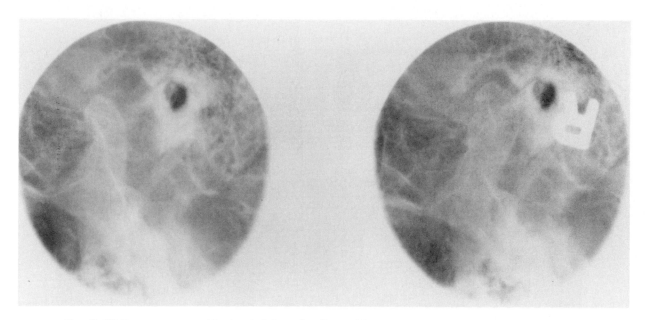

Fig. 5-12 Temporomandibular joint projection of transcranial projection. Open *(left)*; closed *(right)*.

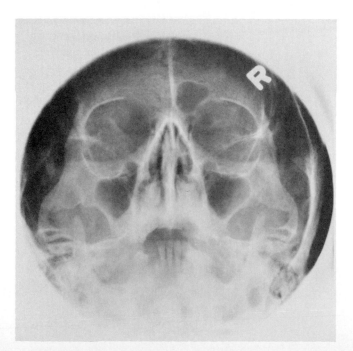

Fig. 5-13 Waters' projection.

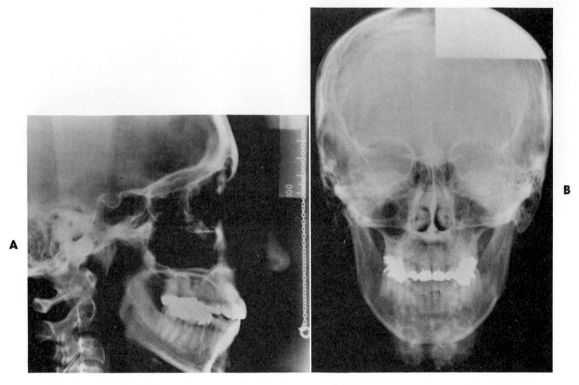

Fig. 5-14 A, Lateral cephalometric projection. **B,** Posteroanterior cephalometric projection.

b. Indications
(1) Orthodontic patients
(2) Maxillofacial reconstructive patients
(3) Evaluation of pedodontic patients
5. Panoramic radiography (Fig. 5-15)
a. Single radiograph, usually 5 by 12 inches, which records both the maxillary and mandibular arches; all of the mandible (from condyle to condyle) and all of the maxillae (up to the middle third of the orbit) are imaged on a single film
b. Types
(1) Split image provides two lateral projections of the jaws; clear vertical strip of unexposed film is in the center of the radiograph; anterior structures, from approximately canine to canine, are imaged twice
(2) Continuous image provides an uninterrupted view of the jaws without anterior redundancies
c. Image production
(1) Based on the principle of tomography

(2) Tomography is the radiographic technique that permits visualization of structures in a chosen plane or layer within an object while intentionally blurring out the images above and below the selected plane
(3) Tomographic process is accomplished by moving the film and x-ray source parallel to each other and in opposite directions while the patient remains stationary
(4) Layer or plane of interest is termed the focal trough (the plane of acceptable focus)
(5) Curved, horseshoe focal trough is needed to image the jaw; chin rest represents the focal trough
(6) Curved focal trough is obtained by connecting the x-ray tube and the film carriage assembly and then circling them around the object such that the x-ray beam rotates around a pivot point
(7) Depending on the machine design, the pivot points may be stationary or moving

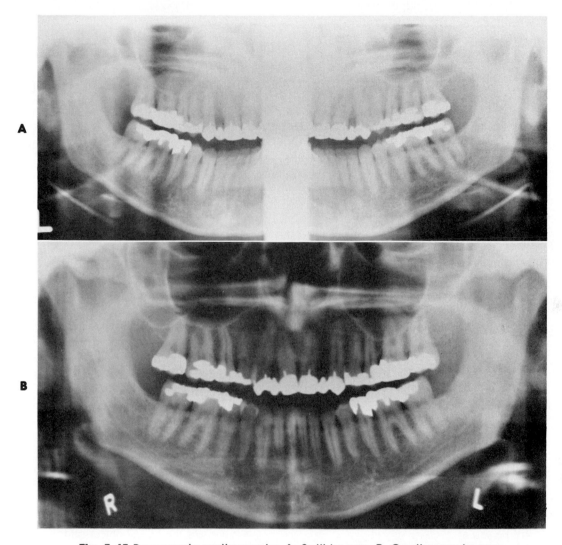

Fig. 5-15 Panoramic radiographs. **A,** Split image. **B,** Continuous image.

d. Technique
  (1) Always refer to the manufacturer's directions for specific operating procedures
  (2) Film cassette is loaded into the unit
  (3) Patient is positioned in the unit so that the midsagittal plane is perpendicular to the floor and the occlusal plane is parallel with the floor
  (4) Dental arches are separated by the patient closing on a cotton roll or similar device (e.g., bite rod)
  (5) Patient's head is stabilized
  (6) Width of the patient's head (in centimeters) is used to determine the kilovoltage setting
  (7) Exposure is made, and film is processed by either the automatic or the manual method
e. Indications
  (1) As a survey film
  (2) Trauma to facial structures
  (3) Evaluation of growth and development
  (4) Evaluation of extensive pathoses
6. Panoramic technique errors
a. Patient movement during the exposure cycle yields a blurred image that is not diagnostically useful
b. Patient-positioning errors
  (1) When the patient's chin is positioned in front of the focal trough (closer to the film assembly), those structures will be blurred and diminished in size

(2) When the patient's chin is positioned behind the focal trough (farther from the film assembly), those structures will be blurred and magnified in size

(3) When the patient's chin is tilted upward, the resulting radiograph will appear to "frown"; in addition, the dense bony palatal structures will absorb much of the radiant beam, causing the maxillary anterior teeth to be obscured or faintly imaged

(4) When the patient's chin is tilted downward, the resulting radiograph will appear to "smile"

(5) When the patient's midline is not centered and is turned too far to the right, more teeth will be imaged on the right and the teeth of the left will be magnified

(6) When the patient's midline is not centered and is turned too far to the left, more teeth will be imaged on the left and the teeth on the right will be magnified

(7) If the tube head–film carriage assembly is positioned too low, the superior structures will not be imaged and the chin rest will be imaged excessively

(8) If the tube head–film carriage assembly is positioned too high, the superior structures will be imaged excessively and the inferior border of the mandible will be absent

c. Operator errors
   (1) Exposure errors
      (a) Double exposure of the film
      (b) Insufficient kilovolt peak producing less dense (light) radiographs
      (c) Failure to depress the exposure switch through the entire cycle
   (2) Processing errors—refer to the section on film processing
   (3) Lead apron and thyroid collar artifacts are radiopaque densities; if the protective device is positioned within the path of the x-ray beam, then the beam is absorbed and anatomic structures are obliterated
   (4) Metallic object artifacts are seen as radiopaque densities and result from failure to remove objects such as earrings, bobby pins, glasses, and partial dentures; often ghost images are present

d. Equipment errors—failure of the equipment to function properly may yield no image, a partial image, or an extremely blurred image

E. Radiographic localization methods
   1. Purpose—periapical and bitewing projections image the teeth and bone in the superoinferior and anteroposterior dimensions; relative buccolingual position of structures is often required for diagnosis and treatment planning in a variety of clinical situations
   2. Indications
      a. Impacted teeth
      b. Supernumerary teeth
      c. Foreign objects
      d. Fractures or trauma
      e. Pathologic lesions
      f. Endodontic therapy
      g. Sialoliths
   3. Methods
      a. Definitive evaluation
         (1) Based on shadow-casting principle No. 3 (the shortest object to the film distance improves image sharpness)
         (2) Radiographic film is positioned lingually; therefore more lingually positioned objects have better radiographic sharpness
         (3) Additional radiographs are not necessary, which decrease the patient's radiation exposure
      b. Clark's technique (Fig. 5-16)
         (1) Also referred to as te tube shift method or the buccal object rule
         (2) Requires a second periapical radiograph with an alteration of 20 degrees in either the vertical or horizontal angulation
         (3) Key phrase is "same on lingual, opposite on buccal," the SLOB rule[9]
         (4) In comparison of the initial and second radiograph, the buccal object will appear to have moved in the opposite direction as the tube shift
         (5) In comparison of the initial and second radiograph, the lingual object will appear to have moved in the same direction as the tube shift
      c. Miller's technique (Fig. 5-17)
         (1) Also referred to as the right-angle method
         (2) Requires a second radiograph taken at a right angle to the initial radiograph
         (3) Intraorally, the cross-sectional occlusal radiograph provides the buccolingual dimension

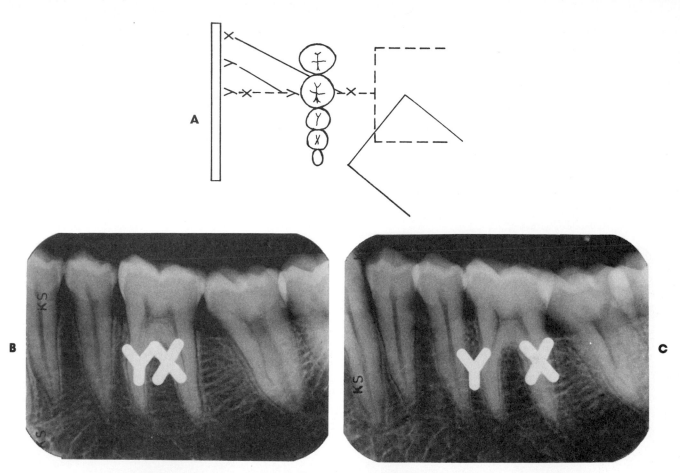

Fig. 5-16 Localization using Clark's technique. NOTE: Dotted-line cone represents standard angulation to yield overlap of first molar and objects; solid-line cone represents mesial cone shift to yield visual separation of first molar and objects. **B,** Radiograph taken with standard angulation yielding superimposition of first molar and lead letters X and Y. **C,** Radiograph taken with mesial cone shift yielding separation of first molar and lead letters X and Y. X is facially positioned and appears to move opposite tube shift. Y is lingually positioned and appears to move with tube shift.

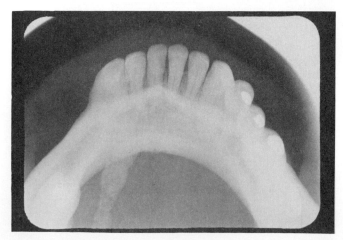

Fig. 5-17 Cross-sectional occlusal radiograph illustrating lingually positioned radiopacity.

d. Panoramic
   (1) Requires use of a split-image panoramic radiograph in which the anterior regions are imaged twice (e.g., S.S. White Panorex)
   (2) Anterior structures are imaged with two different horizontal angulations as a result of the split-image radiograph
   (3) Relative movement of the object is compared with the adjacent structures from one side of the film to the other
   (4) Key phrase is "same on lingual; opposite on buccal," the SLOB rule[9]
   (5) Buccal object will appear to have moved in the opposite direction of the clinician's viewing movement
   (6) Lingual object will appear to have moved in the same direction as the clinician's viewing movement (Fig. 5-18)

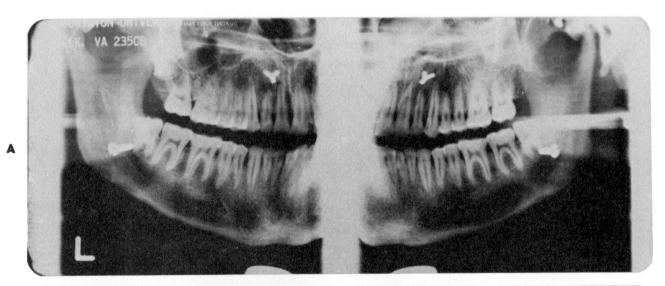

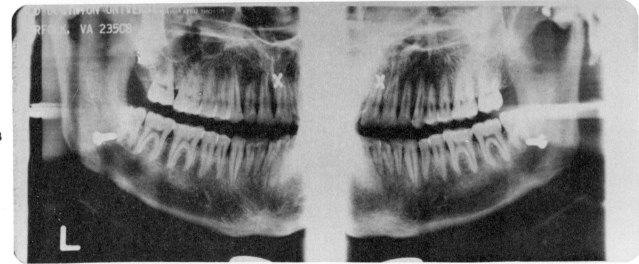

Fig. 5-18 Localization with split-image panoramic radiograph and SLOB rule. **A,** Lead letter *Y* is located lingually and appears to move in same direction as viewer's movement. **B,** Lead letter *X* is located facially and appears to move in opposite direction of viewer's movement.

Film Mounting

A. Purpose—provides a systematic approach for viewing and evaluating radiographs with placement of the radiograph in a holding device according to anatomic considerations

B. Mount construction—made of either cardboard or plasticlike material; available with windows for placement of radiographs in various number and size combinations

C. Mounting procedures
   1. Intraoral radiographs
      a. Labial mounting
         (1) Raised portion of embossed dot is toward the viewer
         (2) Patient's left side is the viewer's right side
         (3) Orientation is that the viewer is facing the patient
      b. Lingual mounting
         (1) Raised portion of embossed dot is away from the viewer
         (2) Patient's left side is the viewer's left side
         (3) Orientation is that the viewer is on the patient's tongue
   2. Extraoral radiographs
      a. During film exposure the side(s) under examination should be identified with a lead letter (*R* or *L*) placed on the film cassette
      b. Radiographs may be placed on an illuminating viewbox with orientation so that the viewer is facing the patient or that the viewer is on the patient's tongue

Radiographic Anatomy

A. General considerations
   1. Radiographic examination is an essential component to the total assessment of the patient's dental health
   2. When viewing dental radiographs, one must be able to distinguish between normal and abnormal appearances of radiographic anatomic conditions
   3. Occasionally, normal or a variation of a normal anatomic condition may be confused for dental disease; therefore the clinical examination is mandatory
   4. Radiographic evidence of dental disease is observed as an abnormal radiolucency or radiopacity in the radiographic image
   5. Most often evidence of caries, periodontal disease, and periapical inflammations are observed in dental radiographs; developmental disturbances, traumatic injuries, and neoplastic lesions are also observed
   6. Dental hygienist must be able to identify normal tooth and bony structure anatomic conditions to distinguish between signs of disease and variations of normal

B. Tooth anatomy
   1. Radiographic appearance is distinguished by the variations in radiographic densities
   2. Dense tooth structure (i.e., enamel) appears radiopaque; less dense tooth structure (i.e., pulp chamber) appears radiolucent
   3. Radiographic appearance of the tooth and supporting structures is seen in Fig. 5-19

C. Radiographic anatomy of the maxilla (Fig. 5-20)
   1. Nasopalatine foramen—oval radiolucency between the maxillary central incisors; provides passage for the nasopalatine nerve and artery; when superimposed over the apex of an incisor, it is often confused with periapical disease
   2. Median palatine suture—radiolucent line extending vertically between the maxillary incisors; may be confused as a fracture line, nutrient canal, or fistula tract
   3. Nasal fossae—two radiolucent densities observed superior to the central incisors outlining the nasal walls
   4. Nasal septum—radiopaque density representing the bony division of the nasal cavities
   5. Anterior nasal spine—increased radiopacity adjacent and superior to the incisive foramen

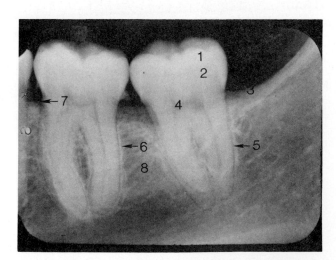

Fig. 5-19 Tooth anatomy. *1*, Enamel; *2*, dentin; *3*, cementum; *4*, pulp; *5*, periodontal membrane; *6*, lamina dura; *7*, alveolar crest; *8*, trabeculae.

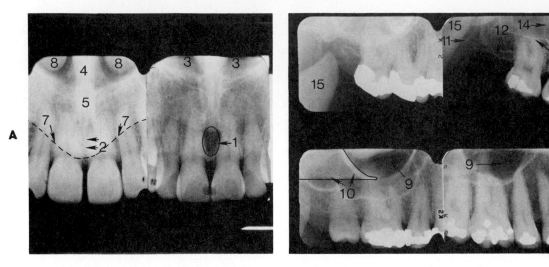

Fig. 5-20 Maxillary anatomy. **A,** *1,* Nasopalatine foramen; *2,* median palatine suture; *3,* nasal fossa; *4,* nasal septum; *5,* anterior nasal spine; *7,* soft tissue outline of nose *(dotted line); 8,* turbinates. **B,** *9,* Maxillary sinus; *10,* zygomatic process; *11,* hamular process; *12,* maxillary tuberosity; *13,* floor of sinus; *14,* sinus septum; *15,* coronoid process.

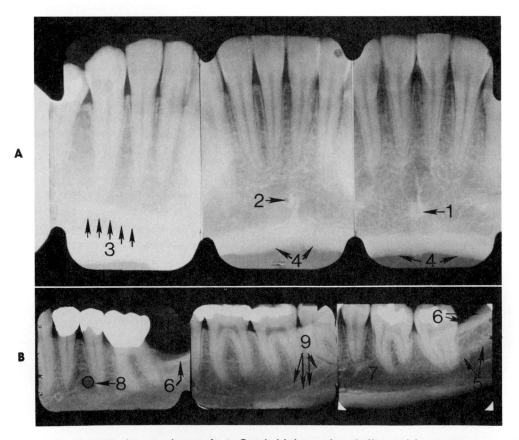

Fig. 5-21 Mandibular anatomy. **A,** *1,* Genial tubercules; *2,* lingual foramen; *3,* mental ridge; *4,* inferior border of mandible. **B,** *5,* Internal oblique ridge; *6,* external oblique ridge; *7,* submandibular fossa; *8,* mental foramen; *9,* mandibular canal.

6. Typical Y formation—Y-shaped radiopacity created by the radiopaque lines that outline the nasal floor and anterior portion of the maxillary sinus
7. Maxillary sinus—bilateral radiolucency originating at the canine region and extending posteriorly; outlined by a radiopaque wall; represents the maxillary sinus air space
8. Nutrient canals—thin radiolucent lines often confused as fracture lines; generally seen in the maxillary sinus area
9. Zygomatic process (arch)—radiopaque structure observed superior to the maxillary posterior teeth that joins the maxilla, frontal, and temporal bones
10. Maxillary tuberosity—most distal region of the maxilla and appears as a raised alveolar bony ridge
11. Hamular process—radiopaque spine located on the medial pterygoid plate
12. Lateral pterygoid plate—radiopaque extension of the sphenoid bone
13. Maxillary torus—radiopaque density superior to the apices seen in some patients

D. Radiographic anatomy of the mandible (Fig. 5-21)
1. Genial tubercles—radiopaque spines (often seen as a circle) located inferior to the mandibular central incisors; serve as the attachment of the geniohyoid and genioglossus muscles
2. Lingual foramen—small radiolucency in the center of the genial tubercles for the passage of nerves and vessels
3. Nutrient canals—narrow radiolucent lines observed in the mandibular anterior regions
4. Mental ridge—radiopaque density (lines) corresponding to the raised bone level along the anterior aspect of the mandible
5. Inferior border of the mandible—radiopaque density representing the dense cortical bone
6. Internal oblique ridge (mylohyoid line)—radiopaque line representing a ridge of bone on the lingual surface of the mandible, which serves as the attachment of the mylohyoid muscles
7. External oblique ridge—radiopaque ridge created by the raised bony surface on the facial side of the mandible for the attachment of the buccinator muscle; superior to the internal oblique ridge
8. Submandibular fossa—radiolucent area in the posterior body of the mandible that represents the lingual depression for the submandibular salivary gland

9. Mental foramen—circular radiolucency on the facial aspect of the mandible near the apex of the second premolar for the exit of the mental nerve; often mistaken for a periapical pathologic condition of the premolars
10. Mandibular canal—radiolucent horizontal canal in the mandible through which the interior alveolar nerve and artery pass; extends anteriorly from the mandibular foramen on the lingual aspect of the ramus through the body and terminates at the mental foramen
11. Mandibular torus—radiopacity below the apices and seen on some patients

E. Radiographic appearance of tooth development—radiography of the developing dentition normally includes most of the 20 primary or deciduous teeth and, depending on the age of the child, evidence of the development of the 32 permanent teeth (Fig. 5-22)
F. Panoramic anatomy (Fig. 5-23) and artifacts (Fig. 5-24)
G. Restorations (Fig. 5-25)
1. Metallic (gold, amalgam)
2. Nonmetallic (composite, gutta-percha, etc.)

Radiographic Interpretation

A. Systematic approach
1. Mounting of radiographs
2. Placement of radiographs on the illuminating viewbox (labial mounting recommended)
3. Masking out of extraneous light around films and dimming of room light
4. Evaluation of technical quality of films
   a. Should be free of technical errors and artifacts
   b. Should adequately image anatomic regions of interest
5. Dentition evaluation
   a. Begin assessment at tooth No. 1 and proceed to tooth No. 32 (if present, continue with *A* through *T*)
   b. Order of evaluation
      (1) Presence or absence of tooth
      (2) Size of teeth
      (3) Shape of teeth
      (4) Eruption and location of teeth
      (5) Presence of restorative materials
      (6) Signs of pathoses (abnormal radiolucencies and radiopacities)

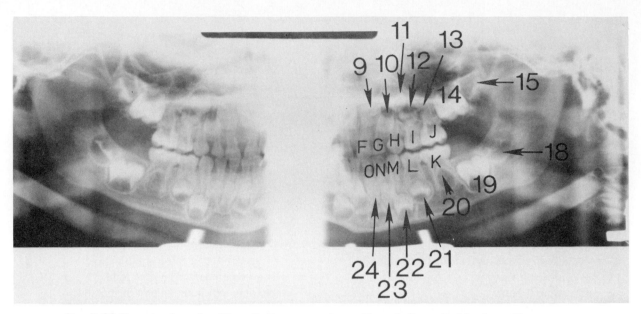

Fig. 5-22 Developing dentition. *9,* Permanent maxillary left central incisor; *10,* permanent maxillary left lateral incisor; *11,* permanent maxillary left canine; *12,* permanent maxillary left first premolar; *13,* permanent maxillary left second premolar; *14,* permanent maxillary left first molar; *15,* permanent maxillary left second molar; *18,* permanent mandibular left second molar; *19,* permanent mandibular left first molar; *20,* permanent mandibular left second premolar; *21,* permanent mandibular left first premolar; *22,* permanent mandibular left canine; *23,* permanent mandibular left lateral incisor; *24,* permanent mandibular left central incisor; *F,* primary maxillary left central incisor; *G,* primary maxillary left lateral incisor; *H,* primary maxillary left canine; *I,* primary maxillary left first molar; *J,* primary maxillary left second molar; *K,* primary mandibular left second molar; *L,* primary mandibular left canine; *N,* primary mandibular left lateral incisor; *O,* primary mandibular left central incisor. (Courtesy Dr. Henry Fields, Department of Pedodontics, University of North Carolina School of Dentistry, Chapel Hill, N.C.)

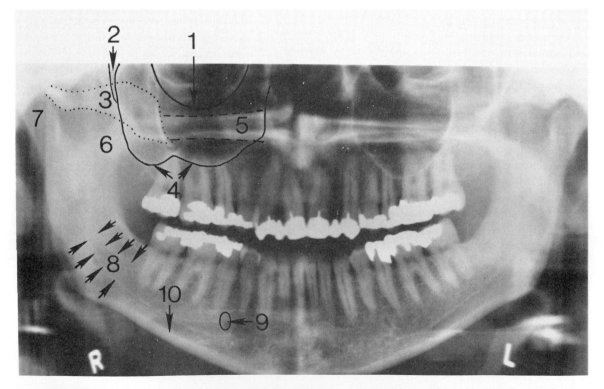

Fig. 5-23 Panoramic anatomy. *1,* Orbital floor; *2,* pterygoid maxillary fissure; *3,* zygomatic arch; *4,* walls of maxillary sinus; *5,* palate; *6,* coronoid process; *7,* mandibular condyle; *8,* mandibular canal, *9,* mental foramen; *10,* inferior border of mandible.

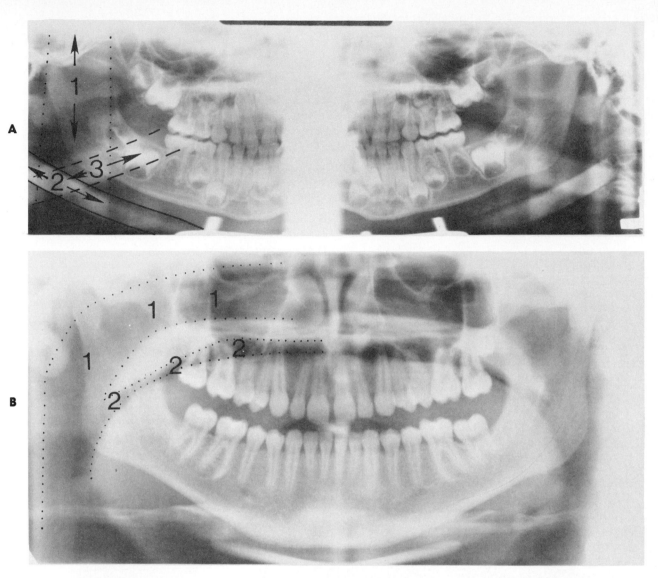

Fig. 5-24 Panoramic artifacts. **A,** *1,* Pancentric head positioner; *2,* chin rest of right side; *3,* shadow of chin rest of left side. **B,** *1,* Nasopharyngeal airspace; *2,* palatal glossal air space. (Courtesy Dr. Henry Fields, Department of Pedodontics, University of North Carolina School of Dentistry, Chapel Hill, N.C.)

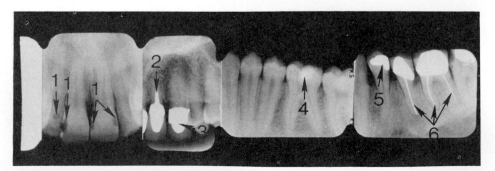

Fig. 5-25 Restorative materials. *1,* Radiolucent esthetic restorations; *2,* post and core with porcelain fused to metal crown; *3,* porcelain fused to metal crown; *4,* temporary restoration; *5,* metallic restoration (amalgam); *6,* root canal filling material.

6. Supporting structure evaluation
   a. Periodontal membrane (ligament) space
   b. Lamina dura
   c. Bone trabecular pattern
   d. Cortical plates
   e. Alveolar bone height
   f. Sinuses (when present)
   g. Orbits (when present)
   h. Sign of pathoses (abnormal radiolucencies and radiopacities)
B. Developmental disturbances (Fig. 5-26)
C. Inflammatory responses (Fig. 5-27)
D. Traumatic injuries (Fig. 5-28)
E. Neoplastic conditions (Fig. 5-29)
F. Caries and bone loss (Fig. 5-30)

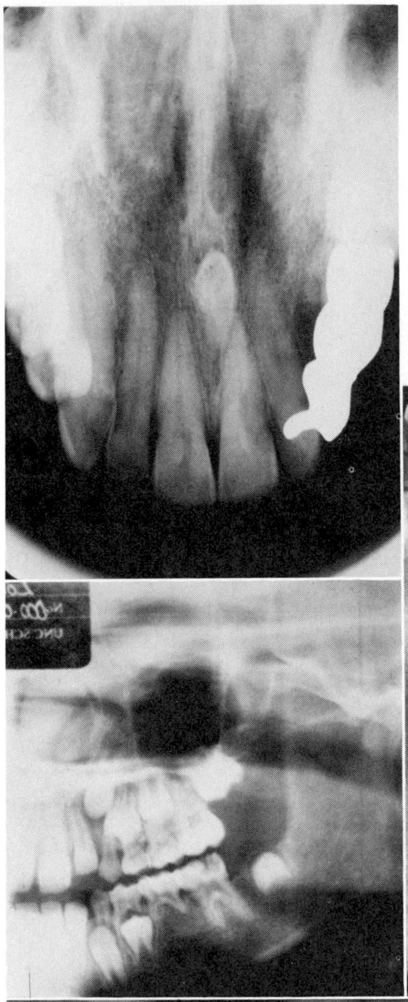

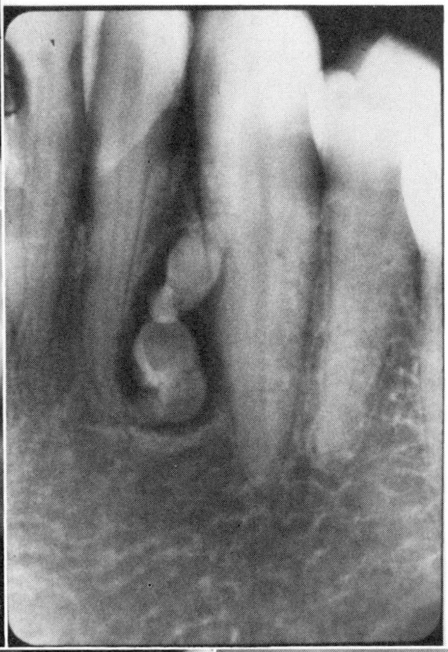

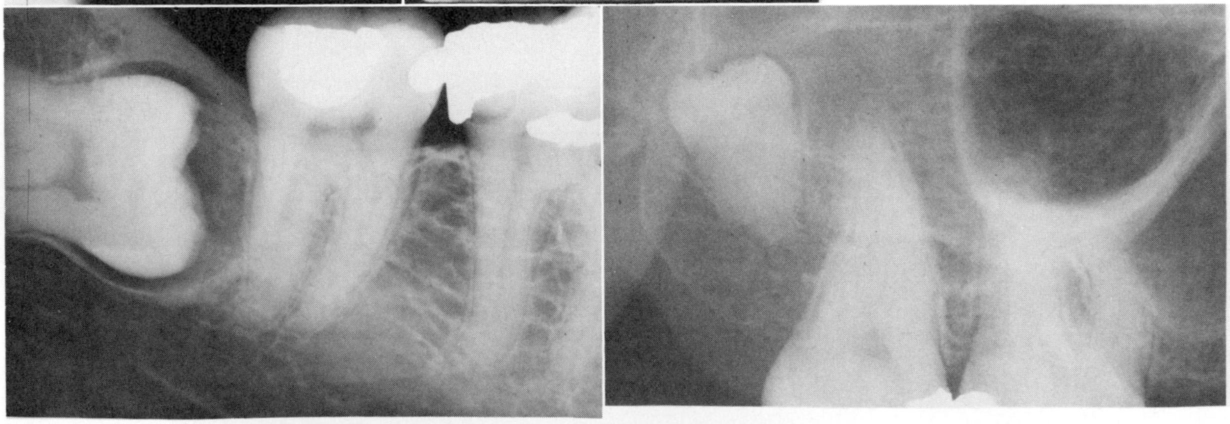

Fig. 5-26 Developmental disturbances. **A,** Supranumerary tooth (mesiodens). **B,** Tooth No. 20 is congenitally missing, and deciduous tooth K is retained. **C,** Compound odontoma. **D,** Dentigerous cyst. **E,** Impacted third molar.

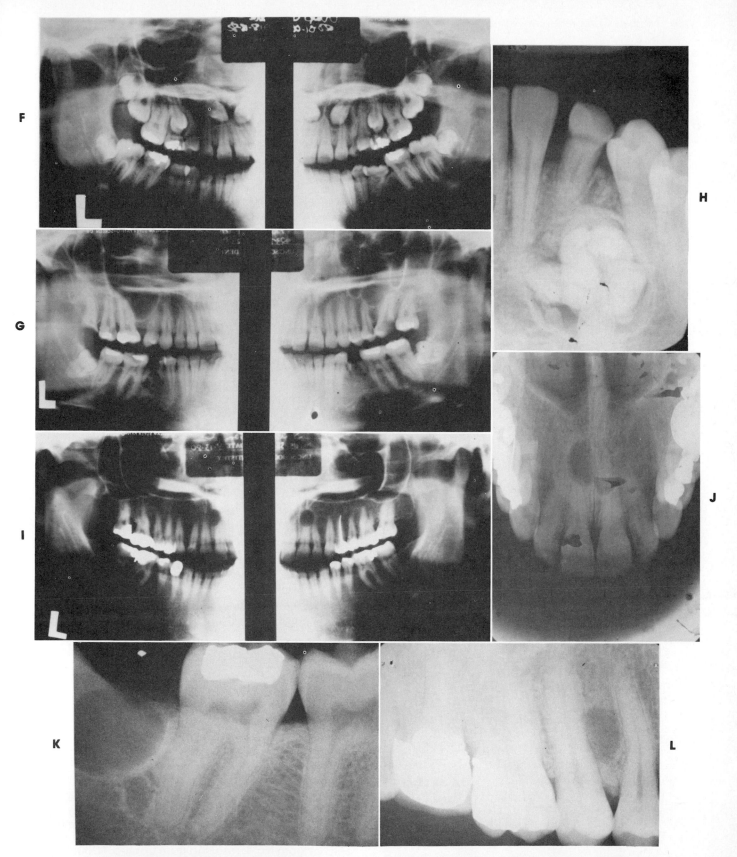

Fig. 5-26, cont'd F, Missing tooth No. 20 *(left); multiple impactions (right).* **G,** Congenitally missing teeth Nos. 20 and 29 *(left);* right and left maxillary sinus pneumatization *(right).* **H,** Compound odontoma. **I,** Panoramic view of incisive canal cyst. **J,** Occlusal view of incisive canal cyst. **K,** Primordial cyst. **L,** Lateral periodontal cyst. (Courtesy Dr. Donald Tyndall and Dr. Stephen Matteson, Department of Oral Diagnosis, University of North Carolina School of Dentistry, Chapel Hill, N.C.)

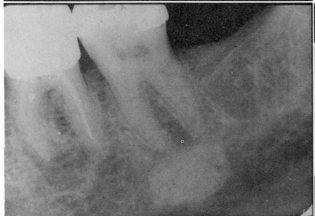

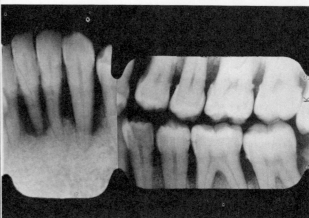

Fig. 5-27 Inflammatory responses. **A,** Periapical radiolucencies. **B,** Condensing osteitis apical to tooth No. 18. **C,** Extensive bone loss resulting from periodontal disease.

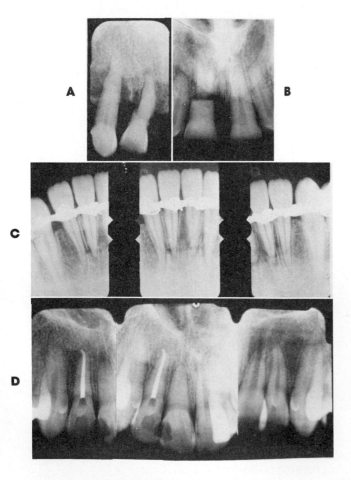

Fig. 5-28 Traumatic responses. **A,** Root fracture. **B,** Root fracture of tooth No. 8. **C,** Alveolar fracture. **D,** Pulp of tooth No. 8 is obliterated resulting from trauma; apical root resorption and widening of pulp of tooth No. 9 resulting from trauma. (Courtesy Dr. Donald Tyndall and Dr. Stephen Matteson, Department of Oral Diagnosis, University of North Carolina School of Dentistry, Chapel Hill, N.C.)

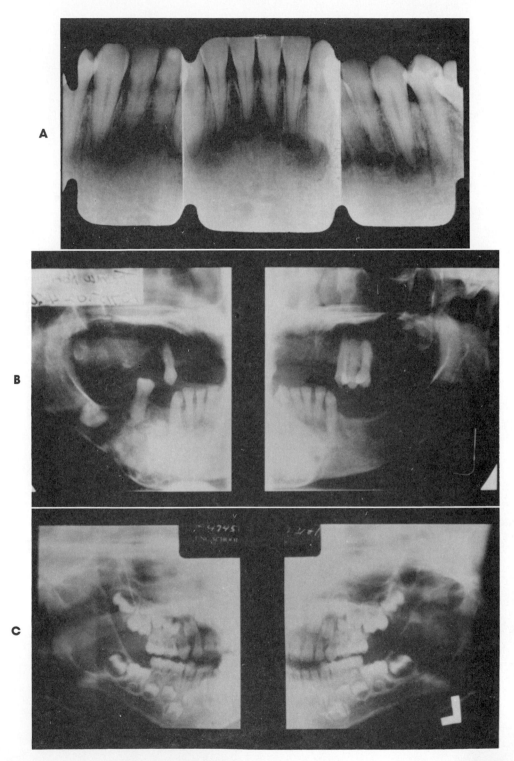

Fig. 5-29 Radiographic appearances of neoplastic and systemic diseases. **A,** Cementoma, stage I. **B,** Multiple cementoma, stage III. **C,** Cherubism.   *Continued.*

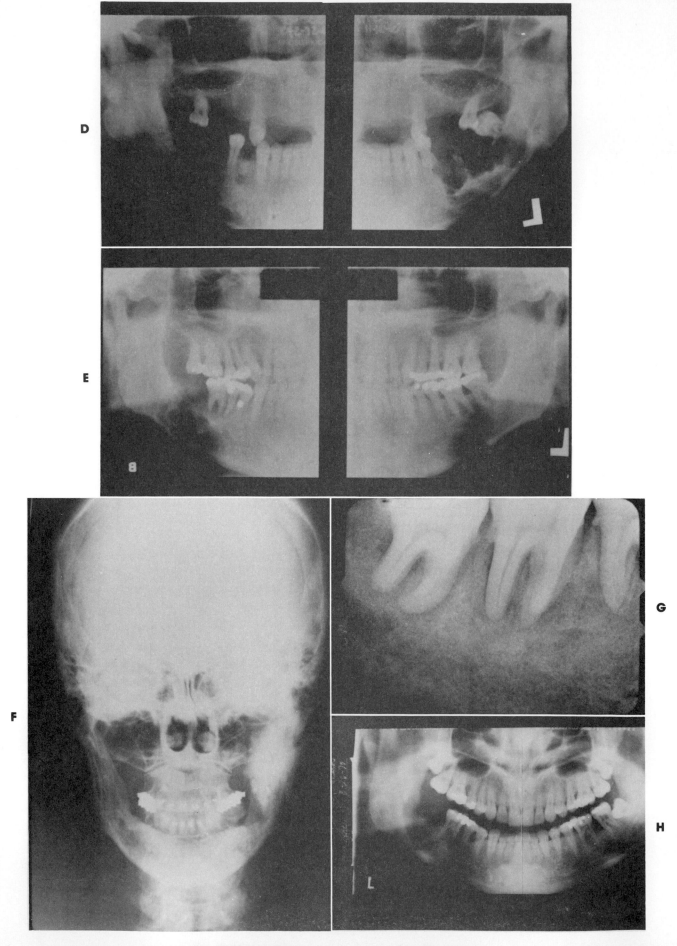

Fig. 5-29, cont'd For legend see opposite page.

Fig. 5-29, cont'd D, Ameloblastoma. **E,** Chondrosarcoma. **F,** Osteogenic sarcoma. **G,** Hyperparathyroidism. **H,** Histiocytosis X of left mandible. (Courtesy Dr. John R. Jacoway, Section of Oral Pathology, University of North Carolina School of Dentistry, Chapel Hill, N.C.)

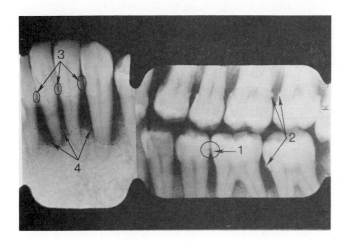

Fig. 5-30 Caries and bone loss. *1,* Interproximal caries; *2,* calculus deposits; *3,* heavy calculus deposits; *4,* height of alveolar bone following resorption.

Xeroradiography

A. Process
   1. A photoconductive selenium plate is inserted into a light-tight cassette and is used as the image receptor
   2. Selenium plate is sensitized by the deposition of a uniform positive charge on its surface
   3. Cassette is placed in a plastic bag for protection against saliva
   4. Cassette is positioned intraorally with the charged surface facing the tube
   5. Exposure is made; photo receptor surface is discharged in proportion to the attenuated x-ray beam
   6. Latent image is a pattern of positive charges
   7. Cassette is placed into an automatic xeroradiographic processing unit whereby the latent image is made visible by a liquid toner
   8. Liquid toner is dried; clear adhesive tape is used to lift the toner off the selenium plate
   9. Process is completed by the lamination of the tape to a translucent backing; image is then dispensed from the unit
   10. Following the automatic cleaning of the residual toner and sterilization with ultraviolet light, the selenium plate and cassette are ready for reuse

B. Comparison of xeroradiographic imaging with conventional dental film
   1. Xeroradiography uses a positively charged selenium plate; conventional methods use film with silver halide emulsion as the image receptor system
   2. Xeroradiographic selenium plate is reusable; dental film is not
   3. Xeroradiography requires between one third and one half the radiation exposure time of conventional dental films
   4. Xeroradiography images are dry and ready for viewing approximately 25 seconds after insertion of the cassette into the automatic xeroradiographic processing unit; automatic processing of dental film requires 5 to 7 minutes for a dry, ready-to-read film; manual processing procedures require 1 hour or longer for a dry, ready-to-read film
   5. Xeroradiography does not require a darkroom or plumbing
   6. Xeroradiographs are processed immediately after exposure
   7. Xeroradiographs may be viewed as a photograph or on a viewbox; dental films must be viewed on a viewbox
   8. Xeroradiographs have the unique property of edge enhancement; "edge enhancement is the ability to amplify the contrast at the interface between two structures even when there is only minimal subject contrast"[3]; this allows for the visualization of very small objects with small differences in the density

9. Xeroradiographs provide better resolution of the teeth (particularly at the dentoenamel junction), periodontal ligament, pulp canals, trabecular bone, and minute calculus deposits
10. Xeroradiographs have a greater exposure latitude that reduces retakes because of incorrect exposure time and, most important, a wider range of tissue densities are imaged at once

Quality Assurance

A. Definition—"refers to the routine and special procedures developed to ensure that the final product is of consistently high quality"[3]
B. Components of a quality assurance program
   1. Operator/technician competence
      a. Self-evaluation of radiographs for technique analysis
      b. Peer review of radiographs for technique analysis
      c. Continuing education courses
   2. Equipment inspections by state and local radiation regulatory agencies
      a. Timer accuracy; milliamperage accuracy
      b. Collimation and alignment of the x-ray beam
      c. Leakage radiation
      d. Mechanical support of unit
   3. Quality assurance procedures for film processing
      a. Periodic evaluation of the darkroom
         (1) Check for light leaks
         (2) Check safelight illumination for cracks in the filter, bulb wattage, and safety (penny test)
         (3) Penny test for safelight evaluation involves the placement of a coin on an unwrapped, unexposed film under a safelight for 2 to 3 minutes; if the coin outline is present on the processed film, corrective action is necessary
      b. Periodic cleaning, maintenance, and daily monitoring of the processing equipment
         (1) Weekly cleaning of the automatic roller assembly and manual racks is appropriate to prevent debris buildup and artifacts on films
         (2) Records of unit cleaning should be kept
         (3) Scheduled maintenance and preventive maintenance are necessary for optimum equipment operation
         (4) Solution temperatures should be monitored daily
         (5) Solutions should be replenished daily
         (6) Sensitometric analysis for fog, speed, and contrast should be determined and recorded

ETHICAL CONSIDERATIONS REGARDING THE USE OF IONIZING RADIATION

A. Regulatory agencies
   1. International Commission on Radiological Protection (ICRP)
   2. National Council on Radiation Protection and Measurements (NCRP)
   3. Nuclear Regulatory Commission (NRC)
   4. Bureau of Radiological Health (BRH) of the Food and Drug Administration
   5. State and local agencies
   6. American Dental Association
   7. American Academy of Dental Radiology
B. Authorization for radiographic procedures
   1. "Radiographic examination(s) must be ordered only after a review of the medical, oral and dental histories and following a clinical examination. Such examination(s) must be based on the needs of the patient for diagnostic, treatment planning and preventive services. Radiographic examination(s) must not be secured for administrative purposes"[1]
   2. Only a licensed physician or dentist may prescribe radiographic services
C. Radiation protection
   1. Cardinal principles of radiation protection[3]
      a. "Keep the *time* of exposure to radiation short"
      b. "Maintain a large *distance* between the source of radiation and the exposed person"
      c. "Insert *shielding* material between the source and the exposed person"
   2. ALARA concept—those individuals working with radiation should attempt to keep all radiation exposure *as low as* reasonably *a*chievable
   3. Maximum permissible dose (MPD) (Table 5-3)
      a. "The maximum dose of radiation that in light of present knowledge would *not* be expected to produce significant radiation effects"[3]
      b. Specified for the occupational exposure received by the radiation worker (e.g., dental personnel working with radiation)
      c. Assumes a linear, nonthreshold dose-response relationship

Table 5-3 Maximum permissible dose

Group	MPD
Radiation workers	
Combined whole-body occupational exposure	
Prospective annual limit	5 rem in any given year
Retrospective annual limit	10 to 15 rem in any given year
Long-term accumulation to age N years	5 ($N - 18$) rem
Skin	15 rem in any given year
Hands	75 rem in any given year (25 rem per quarter)
Forearms	30 rem in any given year (10 rem per quarter)
Other organs, tissues, and organs systems	15 rem in any given year (5 rem per quarter)
Pregnant women (with respect to fetus)	0.5 rem in gestation period
Public or occasionally exposed individuals	0.5 rem in any given year
Students	0.1 rem in any given year
General population	
Genetic	0.17 rem average per year
Somatic	0.17 rem average per year

From Bushong, S.C.: Radiologic science for technologists; physics, biology, and protection, ed. 3, St. Louis, 1984, The C.V. Mosby Co.

    d. Annual MPD for occupationally exposed workers is 5 rem or 5000 mrem (or 50 mSv)

    e. Cumulative MPD for occupationally exposed persons (whole-body exposure)

      (1) Formula is

$$MPD = 5\ (N - 18)\ \text{rem}$$

        where N equals age in years

      (2) Persons younger than age 18 should not be employed as radiation workers

      (3) Older workers, not previously exposed, may exceed the 5 rem/yr limit if the cumulative limit is not exceeded

    f. Nonoccupational exposure (whole body) is 10% of that for the radiation worker (500 mrem/yr or 5 mSv/yr)

  4. Reduction of unnecessary patient dose

    a. Eliminate unnecessary examinations

    b. Eliminate repeat examinations

    c. Use proper radiographic technique factors

    d. Use as fast an image receptor system as possible

    e. Position patient and film properly

    f. Shielding specific areas (gonads and thyroid)

  5. Reduction of occupational exposure

    a. Protective shielding and apparel

    b. Distance from source

    c. Never hold patient or film

    d. Personnel monitoring devices and reports

D. Personnel monitoring devices

  1. Film badge

    a. Description—small piece of film sandwiched between the metal filters inside a plastic holder

    b. Film density is proportional to the exposure received

    c. Not accurate below 20 mR (read as minimal "M"), but higher exposures are accurately reported

    d. Filters are usually made of copper and aluminum

    e. Advantages

      (1) Inexpensive

      (2) Easy to handle

      (3) Easy to process

      (4) Reasonably accurate

    f. Disadvantages

      (1) Cannot be worn for periods longer than 1 month

      (2) Film subject to fogging

      (3) Limited sensitivity

  2. Thermoluminescent dosimeters (TLD)

    a. Lithium fluoride crystals absorb x-ray energy

    b. Ionizing radiation excites (raises the energy) the outer-shell electrons of the crystal

    c. When the lithium fluoride crystals are heated, the excited electrons fall back to the normal orbital state and emit light

    d. Light emitted is proportional to the radiation exposure

    e. Advantages

      (1) More sensitive and accurate than film monitors

      (2) Not affected by humidity

      (3) Can be worn for 3 months

    f. Disadvantage—more costly than film monitors

E. Documentation of patient's radiographic exposure
   1. In addition to the record of dental treatment rendered, the dental chart should provide appropriate space for a separate listing of radiographic services
   2. All radiographic exposures, both acceptable and nonacceptable, should be entered sequentially and cumulatively
   3. Essential information for radiographic services
      a. Date of radiographic examination
      b. Number of radiographs
      c. Type of radiographs
      d. Number and type of retake radiographs
      e. Exposure factors used
         (1) Kilovoltage
         (2) Milliamperage
         (3) Exposure time
         (4) Target-to-film distance
         (5) Image receptor system and relative speed[1]
F. Documentation of patient's refusal of radiographic services
   1. Patient must be informed of the possible diagnostic information and possible risks from the radiographic procedure
   2. Patient should be informed of all protection procedures employed (i.e., equipment standards, quality assurance, standard darkroom procedures, protective shielding, and operator competency)
   3. For legal purposes patient should sign refusal-for-radiographic-services form to release dental personnel of any responsibility
   4. Refusal form must be kept in patient's dental record

REFERENCES

1. American Dental Association, Commission on Dental Accreditation: Guidelines for evaluating radiograph curriculum and instruction, Chicago, 1981, The Association.
2. Assembly of Life Sciences, National Research Council, Division of Medical Sciences, Committee on the Biological Effects of Ionizing Radiations: The effects on populations on exposure to low levels of ionizing radiation: 1980, Washington, D.C., 1980, National Academy Press.
3. Bushong, S.C.: Radiologic science for technologists: physics, biology, and protection, ed. 3, St. Louis, 1984, The C.V. Mosby Co.
4. Christensen, E.E., Curry, T.S. III, and Dowdey, J.E.: An introduction to the physics of diagnostic radiology, ed. 2, Philadelphia, 1978, Lea & Febiger.
5. Frommer, H.H.: Radiology for dental auxiliaries, ed. 3, St. Louis, 1983, The C.V. Mosby Co.
6. Gratt, B.M., Sickles, E.A., and Armitage, G.C.: Use of dental xeroradiographs in periodontics: comparison with conventional radiographs, J. Periodontol. **51:**1, Jan. 1980.
7. Gratt, B.M., et al.: Xeroradiography of dental structures. IV. Image properties of a dedicated intraoral system, Oral Surg. **50:**572, 1980.
8. Jeromin, L.S., et al.: Xeroradiography for intraoral dental radiology, Oral Surg. **49:**178, 1980.
9. Langlais, R.P., Langland, O.E., and Morris, C.R.: Radiographic localization techniques, Dent. Radiogr. Photogr. **52**(4):67, 1979.
10. McNulty, B.: Xeroradiography adds new dimension to intraoral imaging, Rep. No. 1850, Quintessence Int. **11:**1, Feb. 1980.
11. Xerox Medical Systems, Xerox 110, Dental x-ray imaging system, Pasadena, Calif.

Review Questions

1 Which of the following is *not* a characteristic of electro-magnetic radiations?
1. They have magnetic fields
2. They are particles with mass and energy
3. They have electrical fields
4. Energies cover a wide range
5. They may cause biologic damage

2 Which of the following is *not* an example of ionizing radiations?
1. Radiowaves
2. α-Particles
3. X-rays
4. Gamma rays
5. β-Particles

3 The interaction of an incident photon passing near an outer-shell electron and being scattered without losing energy is termed
1. Characteristic effect
2. Photoelectric effect
3. Compton scatter
4. Thompson scatter
5. Bremsstrahlung scatter

4 Bremsstrahlung radiation refers to
1. The acceleration of photons through the nucleus of a target
2. A slowing process of accelerated electrons and transference of kinetic energy to x-ray photons
3. The speeding process that occurs during the transference of an electron's kinetic energy into x-ray energy
4. The monochromatic energy released by the incident photon as it interacts with a tungsten target
5. A shifting of the outer-shell electrons to inner vacancies in the target atom

5 The term *rad* refers to
1. Energy absorbed per gram of material
2. Ionization of air by x-radiation
3. Ionization of air by gamma radiation
4. Occupational exposure
5. Amount of radioactive element

6 Radiation dose received by dental personnel is measured in
1. Coulombs per kilogram
2. Rem
3. Rad
4. Gray
5. Roentgen

7 A step-up transformer
(a) Has fewer turns in the secondary coil
(b) Has more turns in the secondary coil
(c) Supplies voltage to the kilovolt peak circuit
(d) Supplies voltage to the milliamperage circuit
(e) Supplies voltage to the filament
1. a only
2. a and c
3. a and d
4. b and c
5. b and e

8 The electrically negative portion of the x-ray tube is the
1. Anode
2. Cathode
3. Copper stem
4. Target
5. Metal casing

9 The milliamperage controls the
1. Heating of the target
2. Heating of the filament
3. Energy of electrons during movement from the anode to the cathode
4. Energy of electrons during movement from the cathode to the anode
5. The quality of the x-ray beam spectrum

10 With all other technique factors constant, an increase in exposure time from 30 to 48 impulses would
1. Increase film density
2. Decrease film density
3. Increase photon energy
4. Decrease photon energy
5. Increase photon wavelength

11 Duplicate radiographs with low density result from
1. Underexposure of the duplicating film
2. Overexposure of the duplicating film
3. Overdevelopment of the duplicating film
4. The antihalation coating of the duplicating film
5. Loss of intimate contact of the duplicating film with the original

12 A radiograph with long-scale contrast would
(a) Have small differences in densities
(b) Have large differences in densities
(c) Be obtained with low kilovolt peak techniques
(d) Be obtained with high kilovolt peak techniques
(e) Have few shades of gray
(f) Have many shades of gray
1. b, c, and e
2. a, d, and f
3. b, c, and e
4. b, c, and f
5. b, d, and e

13 If the intensity of an x-ray beam is 100 mR at 16 inches, then at 8 inches the intensity would be
1. 25 mR
2. 50 mR
3. 75 mR
4. 200 mR
5. 400 mR

14 Which technique provides the relative buccolingual position of a salivary stone in the submandibular gland?
1. Bitewing radiograph
2. Periapical radiograph
3. Panoramic radiograph
4. Mandibular cross-sectional occlusal radiograph
5. Maxillary topographic occlusal radiograph

15 Evaluation of the periapical pathologic condition is accomplished best with which radiographic projection?
1. Bitewing radiograph
2. Periapical radiograph
3. Lateral cephalometric radiograph
4. Cross-sectional occlusal radiograph
5. Waters' view radiograph

16 Which of the following is an advantage of panoramic images?
1. Increased detail over intraoral films
2. Decreased overlap in premolar regions
3. The entire dentition is seen on a single film
4. They use direct imaging
5. They reduce exosure of the thyroid gland

17 With a direct imaging receptor system, the x-ray film is
1. Exposed by intensifying screens
2. Exposed by heat
3. Exposed by the x-ray photons only
4. Exposed by the light photons only
5. Exposed by both the light and the x-ray photons

18 The speed of a direct imaging system is primarily determined by the
1. Size of the silver halide crystal
2. Size of the calcium tungstate crystals
3. Size of the gadolinium oxysulfide crystals
4. Concentration of the calcium tungstate crystals
5. Concentration of the gadolinium oxysulfide crystals

19 The exposure time used for a xeroradiograph is
1. One half the time used for Kodak D-speed film
2. Equal to the time used for Kodak D-speed film
3. One and one-half times greater than the time used for Kodak D-speed film
4. Two times greater than the time used for Kodak D-speed film
5. Four times greater than the time used for Kodak D-speed film

20 The latent image refers to the
1. Observed changes within the emulsion after exposure
2. Calcium tungstate fluorescence
3. Activation of the reflective layer
4. Accumulation of silver atoms at the crystal imperfection sites
5. Visible image observed after film processing

21 Which of the following is *not* a component of an intensifying screen?
1. Base material
2. Lead foil
3. Phosphor layer
4. Protective coating
5. Reflective layer

22 Which of the following is true regarding the lingual mounting of intraoral radiographs?
1. The embossed dot faces upward
2. The patient's left side is the viewer's right side
3. Orientation is that the viewer is facing the patient
4. A lead letter *L* is placed on the film packet before exposure
5. The patient's right side is the viewer's right side

23 Which of the following statements is *false* regarding the authorization of dental radiographic procedures?
1. Radiographic examinations must not be secured for administrative purposes
2. Dental hygienists may prescribe dental radiographic services
3. Radiographic services should be ordered only after complete clinical examination and review of the patient's history
4. Licensed physicians may prescribe dental radiographic services
5. Licensed dentists may prescribe dental radiographic services

Question 24 refers to Fig. 5-31.

24 The bilateral horizontal radiopaque lines overlapping the apices of the canines are termed the
1. Nutrient canals
2. Mental ridges
3. Inferior border of the mandible
4. Genial tubercles
5. Mandibular canal

Question 25 refers to Fig. 5-32.

25 The curved radiopaque density obstructing visualization of the molar apices is the
1. Coronoid process
2. Maxillary sinus
3. Hamular process
4. Maxillary tuberosity
5. Zygomatic process

Questions 26 to 28 refer to Fig. 5-33.

26 The small circular radiolucency identified by *A* is the
1. Mental foramen
2. Genial tubercles
3. Nutrient canals
4. Trabecular space
5. Lingual foramen

27 The radiopaque structure identified by *B* is the
1. Mental ridge
2. Inferior border of the mandible
3. Submandibular fossa
4. External oblique ridge
5. Internal oblique ridge

28 The small circular radiopaque density identified by the black lines is the
1. Genial tubercles
2. Incisive canal
3. Mental foramen
4. Torus
5. Nutrient canal

Questions 29 to 32 refer to Fig. 5-34.

29 The radiopaque structure identified by *A* is the
1. Mandibular condyle
2. Hamular process
3. Maxillary tuberosity
4. Coronoid process of the mandible
5. Zygomatic process

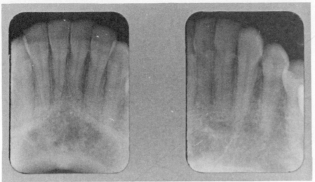

Fig. 5-31

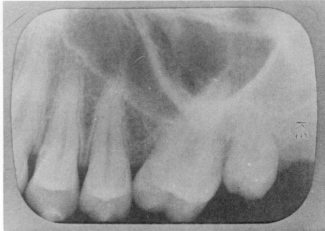

Fig. 5-32

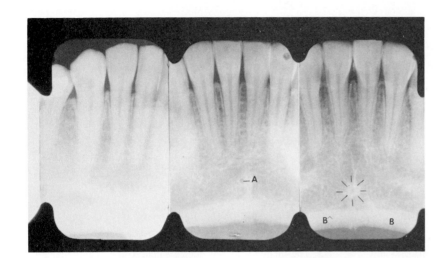

Fig. 5-33

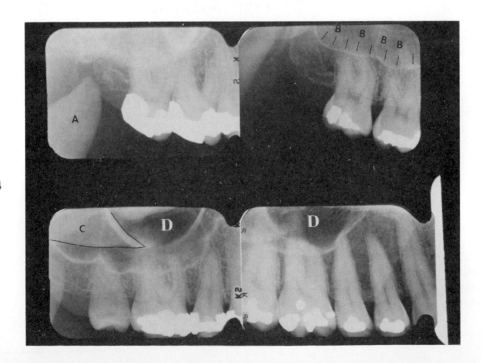

Fig. 5-34

30 The thin radiopaque line identified by the black lines and *B* is the
1. Palate
2. Median nasal septum
3. Lamina dura
4. Floor of the maxillary sinus
5. Nutrient canal

31 The radiopacity identified by the black lines and *C* is the
1. Inferior border of the maxillary sinus
2. Zygomatic process
3. Coronoid process of the mandible
4. Palate
5. Maxillary tuberosity

32 The large radiolucent structure identified by *D* is the
1. Nasal fossa
2. Maxillary sinus
3. Palatine torus
4. Condensing osteitis
5. Periapical abscess

Questions 33 to 36 refer to Fig. 5-35.

33 The radiolucency enclosed within the circle identified by *A* is the
1. Lingual foramen
2. Mandibular canal
3. Periapical abscess
4. Mental foramen
5. Submandibular fossa

34 The dense radiopaque area identified by *B* is
1. Cone cut
2. Gutta-percha
3. A gold crown
4. An esthetic restoration
5. A pontic

35 The horizontal radiolucent line running posterior to anterior identified by *C* is
1. The mental canal
2. The submandibular foss
3. The mandibular canal
4. A fracture line
5. The internal oblique ridge

36 The radiopaque density identified by the vertical lines and *D* is the
1. Internal oblique ridge
2. Mylohyoid line
3. External oblique ridge
4. Nutrient canal
5. Mandibular canal

Questions 37 to 41 refer to Fig. 5-36.

37 The vertical radiopaque line outlining the root identified by *A* is the
1. Periodontal membrane
2. Lamina dura
3. Fracture line
4. Hypercementosis
5. Nutrient canal

38 The radiopaque density extending from the distal of tooth No. 19 and identified by *B* is
1. Hypercementosis
2. An enamel pearl
3. Calculus
4. Incipient caries
5. A bone spicule

39 The radiolucent line outlining the root and identified by *C* is the
1. Nutrient canal
2. Fracture line
3. Lamina dura
4. Periodontal membrane
5. Pulp canal

40 The radiopaque region identified by *D* is
1. Enamel
2. Dentin
3. Pulp
4. Dental plaque
5. An esthetic restoration

41 The radiolucent region identified by *E* is
1. Pulp
2. Furcation involvement
3. Dentin
4. Cervical burnout
5. Periodontal membrane

Questions 42 to 44 refer to Fig. 5-37.

42 The radiopaque structure identified by *A* is the
1. Zygomatic arch
2. Auditory canal
3. Mandibular condyle
4. Maxillary tuberosity
5. Coronoid process

43 The bilateral radiolucencies apical to the mandibular premolars and identified by *B* is the
1. Incisive foramen
2. Lingual foramen
3. Submandibular fossa
4. Trabeculae
5. Mental foramen

44 The bilateral radiolucent area outlined by the dotted line is
1. The maxillary sinus
2. The Palate
3. The palatoglossal airspace
4. A pancentric head positioner artifact
5. The nasal fossa

Question 45 refers to Fig. 5-38.

45 The radiopaque structure identified by the arrow is most likely
1. A periapical abscess
2. Condensing osteitis
3. A supernumerary molar
4. A retained root tip
5. An impacted third molar

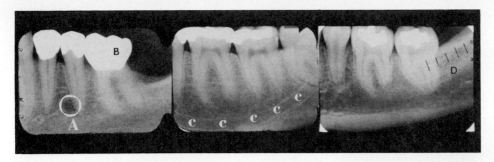

Fig. 5-35

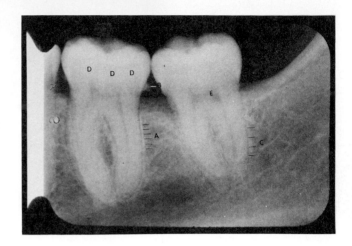

Fig. 5-36

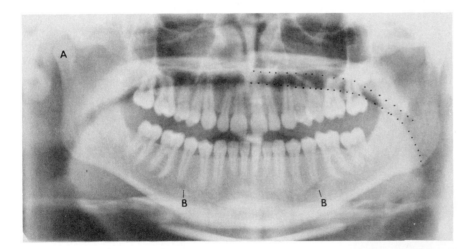

Fig. 5-37

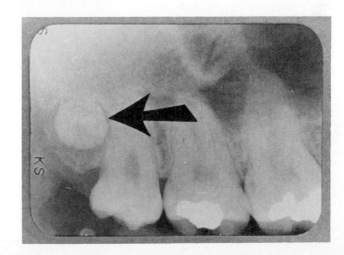

Fig. 5-38

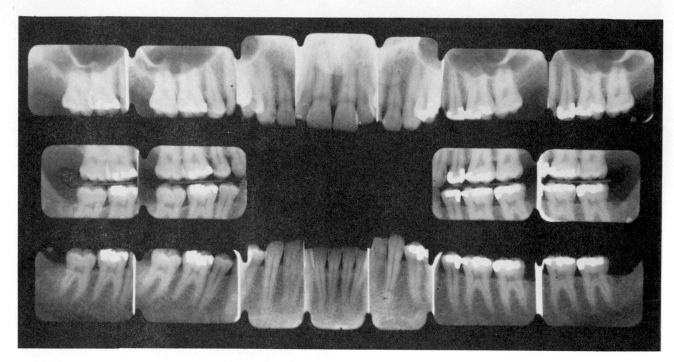

Fig. 5-39

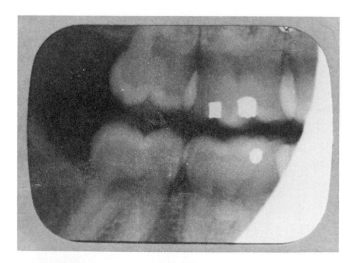

Fig. 5-40

Question 46 refers to Fig. 5-39.

46 Dental caries may be seen on
    (a) Tooth No. 2
    (b) Tooth No. 4
    (c) Tooth No. 8
    (d) Tooth No. 11
    (e) Tooth No. 22
    (f) Tooth No. 23
    (g) Tooth No. 30
    1. a, c, and d
    2. b and d
    3. b, e, and f
    4. e, f, and g
    5. g only

Question 47 refers to Fig. 5-40.

47 The radiographic technique errors present on the molar bitewing radiograph are
    (a) Cone cut
    (b) Horizontal overlap
    (c) Tilting of the film packet
    (d) Underexposure
    (e) Foreshortening
    1. a only
    2. a and b
    3. b and d
    4. c and e
    5. c, d, and e

48 The most radiosensitive site to ionizing effects within the cell is (are)
1. The cell wall
2. DNA and chromosomes
3. Cell proteins
4. Enzymes
5. Ribosomes

49 The cumulative maximum permissible dose (MPD) for a dental hygienist age 30, is
1. 0.5 rem
2. 5 rem
3. 10 rem
4. 60 rem
5. 132 rem

50 Which of the following is an advantage of a thermoluminescent dosimeter (TLD) over a film badge?
1. A TLD is less expensive than a film badge
2. A TLD is sensitive to humidity
3. A TLD is less accurate than a film badge
4. A TLD is subject to fogging
5. A TLD can be worn for 3 months

51 Time-temperature film-processing procedures provide a mechanism for patient protection by
1. Ensuring optimum clearing of the latent image–containing crystals
2. Ensuring optimum reduction of the latent image–containing crystals
3. Providing auxiliary opportunity for sight development
4. Allowing overexposure and underdevelopment of films
5. Allowing underexposure and overdevelopment of films

52 The reduction of the latent image–containing silver halide crystals is achieved by which chemical?
1. Potassium alum
2. Hydroquinone
3. Sodium sulfite
4. Ammonium thiosulfate
5. Potassium bromide

53 The clearing agent in the fixer solution is
1. Acetic acid
2. Potassium alum
3. Distilled water
4. Sodium sulfite
5. Ammonium thiosulfate

54 A minimal fixing time of _____ is required before viewing films for a wet reading
1. 2 minutes
2. 3 minutes
3. 4 minutes
4. 5 minutes
5. 6 minutes

55 The recommended distance between the darkroom safelight and the working surface is
1. 2 feet
2. 4 feet
3. 5 feet
4. 6 feet
5. 7 feet

Answers and Rationales

1. (2) Particulate radiations have mass and energy; electromagnetic radiations do not.
   (1) Magnetic fields are characteristics of electromagnetic radiations.
   (3) Electromagnetic radiations have electric fields.
   (4) Energies cover a wide range in electromagnetic radiations.
   (5) Electromagnetic radiations may cause biologic damage.

2. (1) Radiowaves have insufficient energy to cause the ionization process.
   (2) α-Particles have sufficient energy to cause ionization.
   (3) X-rays have sufficient energy to cause ionization.
   (4) Gamma rays have sufficient energy to cause ionization.
   (5) β-Particles have sufficient energy to cause ionization.

3. (4) Thompson scatter is a change in direction without loss of energy by the x-ray photon.
   (1) Characteristic effect does not exist.
   (2) Photoelectric effect is interaction of a photon with an inner-shell electron.
   (3) Compton scatter is interaction of a photon and an outer-shell electron.
   (5) Bremsstrahlung scatter is not a form of scatter radiation.

4. (2) Bremsstrahlung radiation results when an accelerated electron passes near the nucleus of the target atom, slowed by nuclear attraction, and kinetic energy is transferred to x-ray photon energy.
   (1) Electrons, rather than photons, pass thorugh the nucleus of the target.
   (3) Kinetic energy occurs by the slowing down process, not the speedingup process.
   (4) Polychromatic energy is generated by bremsstrahlung interaction.
   (5) Characteristic radiation is produced by the shifting of electrons in the target atom.

5. (1) The rad refers to radiation absorbed dose.
   (2) Ionization of air by radiation refers to the roentgen unit of measure.
   (3) Ionization of air by radiation refers to the roentgen unit of measure.
   (4) The rem unit of measurement refers to occupational exposure.
   (5) Curie is the unit of radioactivity.

For each question the correct answer and rationale are listed first. The other choices are presented in order with the reasons why they are not correct.

6. (2) Occupational dose is measured in rem.
   (1) Coulombs per kilogram is the standard international (SI) unit for radiation intensity.
   (3) Rad is the unit for absorbed dose.
   (4) Gray is the SI unit for absorbed dose.
   (5) Roentgen is the unit for radiation intensity.
7. (4) The step-up transformer has more turns in the secondary coil and supplies voltage to the kilovolt peak circuit.
   (1) The step-down transformer has fewer turns in the secondary coil.
   (2) The step-down transformer has fewer turns in the secondary coil; selection c is a correct statement.
   (3) The milliamperage circuit receives voltage from the step-down transformer.
   (5) The filament receives voltage from the step-down transformer.
8. (2) The cathode is the electrically negative portion of the x-ray tube.
   (1) The anode is the electrically positive portion of the x-ray tube.
   (3) The copper stem is a portion of the anode.
   (4) The target is located in the anode portion of the x-ray tube.
   (5) The metal casing houses the x-ray tube.
9. (2) The heating of the filament is determined by the milliamperage selector.
   (1) The target is not heated as a part of x-ray production.
   (3) The movement of electrons during x-ray production is from the cathode to the anode.
   (4) The kilovolt peak determines the energy of electron movement across the x-ray tube.
   (5) The kilovolt peak determines the quality of the x-ray beam spectrum.
10. (1) With increased exposure time, more crystals in film emulsion are exposed.
    (2) Decreased density results from decreased exposure time.
    (3) Increased photon energy results from an increased kilovolt peak.
    (4) Decreased photon energy results from a decreased kilovolt peak.
    (5) Increased photon wavelength results from a decreased kilovolt peak.
11. (2) Duplicating film is a direct positive film, so overexposure will yield a light duplicate film.
    (1) Underexposure yields a dark duplicate.
    (3) Overdevelopment yields a dark duplicate.
    (4) Antihalation coating prevents image unsharpness.
    (5) Loss of contact causes image unsharpness.
12. (2) Long-scale contrast radiographic images have small differences in densities (a), are obtained with high kilovolt peak techniques (d), and have many shades of gray (f).
    (1) Selection a refers to long-scale contrast radiographic images, and selections c and e refer to short-scale contrast radiographic images.
    (3) These selections refer to short-scale contrast radiographic images.

(4) Selections b and c refer to short-scale contrast radiographic images. Selection f refers to long-scale contrast radiographic images.
(5) Selections b and e refer to short-scale contrast radiographic images. Selection d refers to long-scale contrast radiographic images.
13. (5) According to the inverse square law, if the distance is reduced by half, then the intensity would be four times as great, in this case 400 mR.
    (1) Twenty-five milliroentgens is an incorrect solution of the inverse square law.
    (2) Fifty milliroentgens is an incorrect solution of the inverse square law.
    (3) Seventy-five milliroentgens is an incorrect solution of the inverse square law.
    (4) Two hundred milliroentgens is an incorrect solution of the inverse square law.
14. (4) The mandibular cross-sectional occlusal radiograph is exposed with the central ray perpendicular to the mandibular occlusal plane.
    (1) A bitewing radiograph provides an anteroposterior and superoinferior position.
    (2) The periapical radiograph provides an anteroposterior and superoinferior position.
    (3) The panoramic radiograph provides an anteroposterior and superoinferior position.
    (5) A maxillary topographic occlusal radiograph does not image the submandibular gland.
15. (2) A periapical intraoral radiograph provides better detail of the periapical region.
    (1) A bitewing radiograph shows alveolar crest and interproximal surfaces.
    (3) A lateral cephalometric radiograph is used for orthodontic diagnosis.
    (4) A cross-sectional occlusal radiograph distorts periapical regions.
    (5) Waters' view radiograph is used in the diagnosis of the maxillary sinus.
16. (3) A panoramic film may be used as a scout film because the entire dentition is observed on a single film.
    (1) A panoramic film has decreased detail.
    (2) A panoramic view has increased overlap in premolar regions.
    (4) Panoramic films use an indirect imaging system.
    (5) Because of machine geometry, the thyroid gland may receive primary and secondary exposure during panoramic exposures.
17. (3) With a direct imaging system, the film is exposed by the x-ray photons only.
    (1) Intensifying screens refer to the indirect imaging system.
    (2) Heat is not used to expose film.
    (4) Light photons are not singularly used to expose dental film.
    (5) Light and x-ray photons refer to the indirect imaging system.
18. (1) The larger the size of the silver halide crystal, the faster the speed of the direct imaging system.

(2) The size of the calcium tungstate crystals refers to an indirect imaging system speed; as the size and concentration of the crystals increase, the indirect imaging system increases.

(3) The size of gadolinium oxysulfide crystals refers to the indirect imaging system speed.

(4) The concentration of calcium tungstate crystals refers to the indirect imaging system speed.

(5) The concentration of gadolinium oxysulfide crystals refers to the indirect imaging system speed.

19. (1) Xeroradiography requires one third to one half of the exposure time of conventional dental film (Kodak D-speed film).

(2) Equal exposure time is excessive exposure time for xeroradiographs.

(3) One and one-half times greater exposure is excessive for xeroradiographs.

(4) Two times greater exposure is excessive for xeroradiographs.

(5) Four times greater exposure is excessive for xeroradiographs.

20. (4) Silver halide crystals contain imperfections that trap recoil electrons that impart a negative charge to the site. The negative site then attracts free interstitial silver ions that form the latent image.

(1) The latent image within the crystals cannot be seen after film exposure but only after processing.

(2) Calcium tungstate fluorescence does not refer to latent image.

(3) Activation of the reflective layer does not refer to latent image.

(5) The latent image is invisible.

21. (2) Lead foil is used in intraoral film packet construction to absorb remnant beam for patient protection.

(1) Base material is a component of the intensifying screen.

(3) The phosphor layer is a component of the intensifying screen.

(4) A protective coating is a component of the intensifying screen.

(5) The reflective layer is a component of the intensifying screen.

22. (5) With lingual mounting, orientation is that the viewer is on the patient's tongue.

(1) The dot facing upward refers to labial mounting.

(2) When the patient's left side is the viewer's right side, this refers to labial mounting.

(3) The viewer facing the patient refers to labial mounting.

(4) Lead letters *R* and *L* refer to right and left and are placed on extraoral cassettes for orientation purposes.

23. (2) Dental hygienists may *not* prescribe dental radiographic services.

(1) Radiographic examinations must be ordered only after a review of the medical, oral, and dental histories and following a clinical examination. A licensed physician or dentist may prescribe dental radiographic services.

(3) Radiographs are ordered only after complete clinical examinations and a review of the patient's history is made.

(4) Licensed physicians may prescribe dental radiographic services.

(5) Licensed dentists may prescribe dental radiographic services.

24. (2) Mental ridges may appear as opaque lines and represent increased thickness of cortical bone on the facial aspect of the mandible.

(1) Nutrient canals are radiolucent.

(3) The inferior border of the mandible is the most inferior radiopaque structure.

(4) Genial tubercles are seen as circular radiopaque structures inferior to the central incisors.

(5) The mandibular canal is radiolucent and inferior to the posterior teeth.

25. (5) The zygomatic process often appears superimposed over the molar apices and most often when the bisecting-the-angle technique is used.

(1) The coronoid process is part of the mandibular anatomy.

(2) The maxillary sinus is radiolucent.

(3) The hamular process is posterior and extends inferior to the maxillary tuberosity.

(4) The maxillary tuberosity is posterior to the third molar.

26. (5) The lingual foramen is a small circular radiolucency located inferior to the mandibular central incisors.

(1) The mental foramen is located in the mandibular premolar region.

(2) The genial tubercles are radiopaque.

(3) The nutrient canals are vertical radiolucent lines.

(4) The trabecular space has a honeycomb appearance.

27. (2) The inferior border of the mandible is a very dense and wide radiopaque band representing cortical bone.

(1) The mental ridge is seen as a less dense radiopaque line just inferior to the mandibular incisors and canines.

(3) The submandibular fossa is radiolucent.

(4) The external oblique ridge is located in the posterior region.

(5) The internal oblique ridge is located in the posterior region.

28. (1) Genial tubercles are radiopaque structures inferior to the mandibular central incisors and surround the lingual foramen.

(2) The incisive canal is located on the maxillae.

(3) The mental foramen is radiolucent.

(4) A torus is a large radiopacity.

(5) A nutrient canal is radiolucent.

29. (4) The coronoid process of the mandible may be seen on maxillary molar projections.

(1) The mandibular condyle is located within the glenoid fossa and is not seen on periapical radiographs.

(2) The hamular process is a small radiopaque projection.

(3) The maxillary tuberosity is distal to the most posterior molar.

(5) The zygomatic process is seen superior to the maxillary molars.

30. (4) The floor of the maxillary sinus is seen as a thin radiopaque line.
    (1) The palate is seen as a dense radiopaque band.
    (2) The median nasal septum is a vertical radiopaque band superior to the maxillary central incisors.
    (3) The lamina dura outlines the teeth.
    (5) A nutrient canal is radiolucent.
31. (2) The zygomatic process is superimposed on the sinus with use of the bisecting-the-angle technique and appears as a radiopaque density.
    (1) The inferior border of the sinus is a thin radiopaque line.
    (3) The coronoid process of the mandible is usually inferior to zygomatic process and is in the lower distal corner of film.
    (4) The palate is an opacity in the superior aspect of film.
    (5) The tuberosity is an opacity distal to the last molar.
32. (2) The maxillary sinus is located superior to the molars.
    (1) The nasal fossa is superior to the maxillary central incisors.
    (3) A palatine torus is radiopaque.
    (4) Condensing osteitis is radiopaque.
    (5) The tooth is nonpathologic; therefore the radiolucent area is not an abscess.
33. (4) The mental foramen is located in the mandibular premolar region.
    (1) The lingual foramen is located apical to the mandibular central incisors.
    (2) The mandibular canal is a horizontal radiolucent line.
    (3) The tooth is asymptomatic.
    (5) The submandibular fossa is a large radiolucent area apical to the mandibular molars.
34. (3) Gold crowns are radiopaque.
    (1) Cone cut is seen as a radiopacity with a curved border.
    (2) Gutta-percha fills the root canals.
    (4) Most esthetic restorations are radiolucent.
    (5) A pontic replaces a missing tooth.
35. (3) The mandibular canal is located apical to premolars and molars.
    (1) The mental canal is located at the terminal end of the mandibular canal at the mental foramen.
    (2) The submandibular fossa is a large diffuse radiolucency.
    (4) A fracture line is a narrow radiolucency.
    (5) The internal oblique ridge is radiopaque.
36. (3) The external oblique ridge is a dense line that extends forward from the ramus of the mandible and crosses coronal portions of the molar.
    (1) The internal oblique ridge is often apical to the mandibular molars.
    (2) The mylohyoid line is often apical to the mandibular molars.
    (4) A nutrient canal is radiolucent.
    (5) The mandibular canal is radiolucent.

37. (2) Lamina dura is dense bone lining the socket and is seen as a radiopaque line.
    (1) The periodontal membrane is radiolucent.
    (3) A fracture line is radiolucent.
    (4) Hypercementosis is a localized circular radiopacity.
    (5) A nutrient canal is radiolucent.
38. (3) Calculus appears as a radiopaque projection.
    (1) Hypercementosis is a circular radiopacity associated with a root.
    (2) An enamel pearl is a radiopaque structure near the cementoenamel junction.
    (4) Incipent caries is radiolucent.
    (5) Bone spicules would not be attached to a coronal structure.
39. (4) The periodontal membrane is the thin radiolucency outlining the root.
    (1) A nutrient canal would not be seen between the tooth and lamina dura.
    (2) No evidence of trauma is visualized.
    (3) The lamina dura is radiopaque.
    (5) The pulp canal is within the center of the root.
40. (2) Dentin is a radiopaque density enclosed by more opaque appearance of enamel.
    (1) Enamel is the most opaque of natural tooth structures.
    (3) Pulp is radiolucent.
    (4) Dental plaque is not seen radiographically.
    (5) Esthetic restorations are radiolucent.
41. (1) Pulp is the most radiolucent area within the tooth.
    (2) Furcation involvement is not evident.
    (3) Dentin is radiopaque.
    (4) Cervical burnout shows a radiolucent area at the cementoenamel junction.
    (5) The periodontal membrane is the radiolucency outlining the tooth.
42. (3) The mandibular condyle is a radiopaque projection of the superoposterior portion of the mandible.
    (1) The zygomatic arch is superior to the condyle.
    (2) The auditory canal is radiolucent.
    (4) The maxillary tuberosity is an opaque area distal to the last molar.
    (5) The coronoid process is a radiopaque projection of the superoposterior portion of the mandible and is anterior to the condyle.
43. (5) The mental foramen is the radiolucent area near the mandibular premolar apical region.
    (1) The incisive foramen is a radiolucent area on the maxilla.
    (2) The lingual foramen is a radiolucency inferior to the mandibular incisors.
    (3) The submandibular fossa is a large, ill-defined radiolucency inferior to the mandibular molars.
    (4) Trabeculae have a honey-combed appearance and appear throughout the alveolar bone.

44. (3) The palatoglossal air space is a radiolucent area corresponding to the space between the tongue and palate.
    (1) The maxillary sinus is a contained circular radiolucency.
    (2) The palate is radiopaque.
    (4) A pancentric head positioner artifact is radiopaque.
    (5) Nasal fossae are small radiolucencies apical to the maxillary incisors.
45. (3) All permanent molars are erupted, and the opaque density is a supernumerary molar.
    (1) A periapical abscess appears radiolucent.
    (2) Condensing osteitis does not have tooth structure appearance.
    (4) A retained root tip would appear smaller and less opaque.
    (5) The third molar is erupted.
46. (2) Dental caries are seen on the distal surfaces of teeth Nos. 4 and 11.
    (1) No radiographic lesions are observed on teeth Nos. 2 and 8.
    (3) No radiographic lesions are observed on teeth Nos. 22 and 23.
    (4) No radiographic lesions are observed on teeth Nos. 22, 23, and 30.
    (5) No radiographic lesion is observed on tooth No. 30.
47. (2) Cone cutting results from inadequate coverage of the image receptor by the beam of radiation, whereas horizontal overlap results from incorrect mesiodistal angulation of the beam of radiation.
    (1) Overlap, as well as cone cut, is exhibited.
    (3) Underexposure yields film with decreased density.
    (4) Tilting of the film packet results in an uneven distribution of the maxillary and mandibular structures, whereas foreshortening is a result of excessive vertical angulation.
    (5) The film does not exhibit tilting of the film packet, underexposure, or foreshortening of images.
48. (2) The DNA and chromosomes are the most biologically radiosensitive sites within the cell.
    (1) The cell wall is sensitive but less than DNA and the chromosomes.
    (3) Cell proteins are sensitive but less than DNA and the chromosomes.
    (4) Enzymes are sensitive but less than DNA and the chromosomes.
    (5) Ribosomes are sensitive but less than DNA and the chromosomes.
49. (4) The formula for the cumulative MPD for an occupationally exposed worker is 5 (N − 18) rem where N equals age in years. For a dental hygienist age 30, 5 (30 − 18) rem = 60 rem.
    (1) The yearly MPD for occasionally exposed individuals is 0.5 rem.
    (2) The yearly MPD for occupationally exposed individuals is 5 rem.
    (3) An incorrect solution to the formula is 10 rem.
    (5) An incorrect solution to the formula is 132 rem.
50. (5) A thermoluminescent dosimeter (TLD) can be worn for 3 months, whereas a film badge is accurate for only 1 month.
    (1) A film badge is less expensive than a TLD.
    (2) A film badge is sensitive to humidity.
    (3) A film badge is less accurate than a TLD.
    (4) A film badge is subject to fogging.
51. (2) Time-temperature processing indicates the time required to correctly develop film in relation to solution temperature. This eliminates retake procedures because of a processing error.
    (1) Clearing is a function of the fixer, and nonlatent image-containing crystals should be cleared (removed).
    (3) Sight development is not a recommended procedure.
    (4) Overexposure of film increases patient dose.
    (5) Correct technique factors (milliamperage, kilovolt peak, and time) should be used to provide properly exposed film.
52. (2) Hydroquinone, elon, and the developer chemicals reduce the latent image–containing crystals into metallic silver.
    (1) Potassium alum is a component of the fixer solution.
    (3) Sodium sulfite is the preservative agent in the developer and fixer solutions.
    (4) Ammonium thiosulfate is a component of the fixer solution.
    (5) Potassium bromide is the restrainer agent in the developer solution.
53. (5) Ammonium thiosulfate serves to remove the unexposed and unreduced silver halide crystals.
    (1) Acetic acid stops the activity of the developer.
    (2) Potassium alum shrinks and hardens the emulsion.
    (3) Distilled water serves as the solvent for the fixer solution.
    (4) Sodium sulfite is the preservative agent.
54. (2) Three minutes is the minimal fixing time required before a wet reading.
    (1) Two minutes is insufficient time.
    (3) It is not essential to wait 4 minutes before viewing wet films.
    (4) It is not essential to wait 5 minutes before viewing wet films.
    (5) It is not essential to wait 6 minutes before viewing films for a wet reading.
55. (2) The recommended distance between the safelight and the working surface is 4 feet based on the inverse square law.
    (1) Two feet would increase film fog.
    (3) Five feet would reduce the amount of light available to perform film-processing procedures.
    (4) Six feet would reduce the amount of light available to perform film-processing procedures.
    (5) Seven feet would reduce the amount of light available to perform film-processing procedures.

CHAPTER 6

Oral Pathology

OLGA A. C. IBSEN

One important skill of the dental hygienist is to be able to identify pathologic conditions and bring these findings to the attention of the dentist for definitive diagnosis, treatment, or referral. A knowledge of pathology also is critical for protecting oneself from disease transmission, for use as background preparation in managing emergency situations, and for planning and implementing dental hygiene treatment plans congruent with the health conditions of the patient.

To assume this responsibility, the dental hygienist must be able to differentiate between normal and abnormal findings and relate significant health history information to clinical, histologic, and radiographic findings. Although the dental hygienist is not responsible for the dental diagnosis, skill in the use of the diagnostic method is essential.

In this chapter the review of pathologic conditions and anomalies is outlined according to etiology, age and sex considerations, location, clinical features, radiographic appearance, laboratory tests/findings, histologic characteristics, and treatment/prognosis.

BENIGN LESIONS OF SOFT TISSUE ORIGIN

General Characteristics

A. Etiology—unknown
B. Age and sex vary with the type of lesion
C. Clinical features
   1. Sharp line of demarcation outlines the lesion
   2. Lesion has a sessile or pedunculate base
   3. Lesion is easily palpable
D. Histologic characteristics depend on the lesion (e.g., a lipoma is composed of fat cells)
E. Lesion grows slowly, which contributes to an evaluation of a benign state
F. Lesion is removed surgically and usually does not recur

Fibroma

A. Etiology—unknown
B. Age and sex affected—all ages affected (30 to 50 years most common age); males and females equally affected

C. Location
   1. Buccal mucosa, gingiva, floor of the mouth, palate, tongue, lips
   2. When on the gingiva and palate, the lesion lacks mobility and ease of palpation
D. Clinical features
   1. Smooth surface; round, ovoid, or elliptic shape
   2. Well-defined pale pink projection
   3. Size varies from the common size of a few millimeters to several centimeters
   4. Consistency varies from firm and resilient to soft, spongy, and easily palpable
E. Histologic characteristics
   1. Bundles of interlacing collagenous fibers are interspersed with fibroblasts, fibrocytes, and small blood vessels
   2. Outer portion of the lesion is covered by a layer of stratified squamous epithelium
F. Treatment/prognosis
   1. Conservative surgical excision
   2. Seldom recurs

Irritative Fibroma

A. Etiology—mild irritant causes a pyogenic granuloma, which scars down to an irritative fibroma
B. Age and sex affected—50% between 20 and 50 years; males and females equally affected
C. Location—anywhere on the soft tissues: buccal mucosa, fauces, tongue, gingiva, or floor of the mouth
D. Clinical features
   1. Pink to red color
   2. Round or semicircular shape
   3. Up to 2 cm in size
   4. Sessile or pedunculate base
E. Histologic characteristics
   1. Chronic hyperkeratosis; dense collagen and scar tissue covered with normal epithelium
   2. Contains fewer fibroblasts than a fibroma; inflammatory cells
F. Treatment—complete excision

Papilloma

A. Etiology—unknown; long duration; slow development
B. Age and sex affected—50% between 20 to 50 years; males and females equally affected
C. Location—usually on the lips, labial or buccal mucosa, tongue, or palate
D. Clinical features
  1. Cauliflower-like or wartlike surface
  2. Grayish or white color
  3. Well-delineated growth with a pedunculate base; fingerlike projections
E. Histologic characteristics
  1. Composed primarily of long, fingerlike projections of squamous epithelium
  2. ''Acanthosis'' of epithelium—increase in thickness of cells covered by a keratin layer
F. Treatment/prognosis
  1. Excision
  2. Does not recur

Wart (Verruca Vulgaris)

A. Etiology—virus
B. Age and sex affected—all ages; males and females equally affected
C. Location—skin (hands), buccal mucosa, lips, tongue
D. Clinical features
  1. Differs from a papilloma in that warts grow faster, are more often a multiple lesion, are smaller, and develop in a shorter time
  2. Heals alone, since it is of viral origin
  3. Self-inoculated (finger to mouth)
E. Histologic characteristics
  1. Contains large clear squamous cells with large dark intranuclear inclusions
  2. Church-spiral effect
  3. Papillary acanthosis
F. Treatment—excision if necessary; lateral lipping of the epithelium undermines it, and the wart falls off

Hemangioma

A. Etiology—congenital origin; proliferation of blood cells
B. Age and sex affected—present at birth or by the end of the first year; more common in females (2:1)
C. Location—buccal mucosa, labial mucosa, tongue, vermilion of the lip
D. Clinical features
  1. Flat or raised, well-circumscribed lesion of mucosa
  2. Deep red or bluish red color

  3. Pressure produces a pallor to the lesion; when released, the lesion again appears bluish red
  4. Two types
    a. Venus or capillary—small to moderate size; soft
    b. Cavernous—located on the tongue and buccal mucosa; 2 or more cm in diameter; exhibits an impressive protrusion of tissue; deep purple; soft or semifirm
E. Histologic characteristics
  1. Venus or capillary—many small capillaries lined by a single layer of endothelial cells supported by a connective tissue stroma of varying density; endothelial cell proliferation
  2. Cavernous—large dilated blood sinuses with thin walls, each having an endothelial lining; sinusoidal spaces filled with blood and lymphatic vessels
F. Treatment/prognosis
  1. Treatment depends on the size and/or location
    a. Nonintervention in cases where remission has occurred
    b. Surgical removal
    c. Radiation in infants or young children
    d. Sclerosing agents (sodium morrhuate or psylliate) injected into the lesion
    e. Electrocauterization
    f. Carbon dioxide snow (cryotherapy)
    g. Compression
  2. Prognosis excellent; does not become malignant; does not recur

Lipoma

A. Etiology—unknown; rare
B. Age and sex affected—all ages; males and females equally affected
C. Location—tongue, buccal mucosa, mucobuccal folds, gingiva
D. Clinical features
  1. Single or lobulated, well-defined, painless
  2. Sessile or pedunculate base
  3. Soft to palpation
  4. Yellowish color
E. Histologic characteristics
  1. Circumscribed mass of mature fat cells with collagen strands and a few blood vessels
  2. Thin epithelium
  3. If fibrous connective tissue forms a more significant part of the lesion, it is called a fibrolipoma
F. Treatment/prognosis
  1. Surgical excision
  2. Recurrence is rare

INFLAMMATORY TUMORS (GRANULOMAS)

General Characteristics

A. Growth or enlargement of tissue composed mainly of inflammatory cells
B. Account for the major portion of all mouth tumors
C. Benign tumors

Pyogenic Granuloma

A. Etiology—chronic irritants (calculus, poor restorative margins)
B. Age and sex affected—more common in 15- to 45-year age range; more common in females (3:1), perhaps related to increased estrogen levels
C. Location—anterior maxillary labial gingiva; buccal mucosa
D. Clinical features
   1. Protrusive mass growing outward with a pedunculate, sessile, or lobulate base
   2. Red, rather than pink, surface; appearing like a pregnancy tumor
   3. Soft and spongy; freely movable; bleeds easily
   4. Sixty-five percent are ulcerated
   5. Can scar down to an irritative fibroma—fibrogranuloma
E. Histologic characteristics
   1. Epithelium, if present, is thin
   2. Rich in capillaries with proliferation of endothelial cells, which form blood vessels
   3. Contains polymorphonuclear leukocytes, acute and chronic inflammatory cells, plasma cells, and lymphocytes
   4. Has histologic characteristics similar to those of a pregnancy tumor
F. Treatment/prognosis
   1. Removal of the irritant
   2. Excision of the lesion
   3. If cells infiltrate the underlying tissue, 5% to 10% will recur

Pseudopapillomatosis (Inflammatory Papillary Hyperplasia or Palatal Inflammatory Hyperplasia)

A. Etiology—chronic irritation to the palate caused by the suction chamber of a denture; excessive pressure of an ill-fitting denture; poor denture hygiene
B. Age and sex affected—denture wearers usually over 40 years of age; males and females equally affected
C. Location—usually on the palate
D. Clinical features
   1. Closely clustered projections (papillary processes) 1 to 4 mm in diameter
   2. Round, smooth glistening red surface
   3. Varying degrees of inflammation present
E. Histologic characteristics
   1. Small vertical projections, each composed of parakeratotic or orthokeratotic stratified squamous epithelium and a central core of connective tissue
   2. Epithelial proliferation
   3. Infiltrated with inflammatory cells
F. Treatment/prognosis
   1. Surgical excision via curettage
   2. Electrosurgery preceding new denture construction
   3. Denture removed at night to rest tissues
   4. Prognosis good

Epulis Fissuratum (Epulis Granulomatosa or Redundant Tissue)

A. Etiology—irritation caused by a denture flange producing a proliferation of tissue
B. Age and sex affected—40- to 50-year age range; slightly more common in females
C. Location—mucobuccal folds; alveolar ridge in anterior regions along the denture flange line
D. Clinical features
   1. Exophytic or elongated protrusion of tissue under or around the denture flange—linear irritative fibroma
   2. Pink to reddish color
   3. Firm to palpation
E. Histologic characteristics
   1. Excessive bulk of dense fibrous connective tissue covered by stratified squamous epithelium
   2. Connective tissue composed of coarse bundles of collagen fibers with a few fibroblasts or blood vessels (unless inflammation is present)
F. Treatment/prognosis
   1. Removal of the irritant
   2. Correction of the denture flange
   3. Surgical excision of the lesion
   4. Prognosis excellent if the cause is corrected

Peripheral Giant Cell Granuloma

A. Etiology—local irritant or trauma
B. Age and sex affected—either very young, 20- to 35-year age group, or elderly (edentulous); more common in females (2:1)
C. Location
   1. Gingiva or alveolar process, anterior to the molars
   2. Fifty-five percent occur in the mandible, 45% in the maxilla
   3. In edentulous patients, it occurs on the crest of the ridge

D. Clinical features
  1. Outwardly growing lesion 0.5 to 1.5 cm in diameter
  2. Red or pink color
  3. Pedunculate or sessile base
  4. Arises from a deeper area in the tissue than does a pyogenic granuloma or fibroma
E. Radiographic appearance—radiolucent "cuffing" or erosion of bone
F. Histologic characteristics
  1. Composed of a delicate reticular and fibrillar connective tissue stroma containing a large number of ovoid or spindle-shaped young connective tissue cells
  2. Multinucleated giant cells
  3. Proliferation of collagen and blood vessels
  4. Can infiltrate bone, but does not metastasize
  5. Appears to originate from the periodontal ligament or mucoperiostium
G. Treatment/prognosis
  1. Surgical removal of the entire base to eliminate recurrence
  2. Five to ten percent recur

Central Giant Cell Reparative Granuloma

A. Etiology—trauma caused by a fall or blow
B. Age and sex affected—children and young adults; more common in females (2:1)
C. Location
  1. Sixty-six percent occur in the mandible, 33% in the maxilla
  2. Anterior segment of the arch crossing the midline
D. Clinical features
  1. Appears as a swelling or bulge resulting from expansion of cortical plates
  2. No symptoms, so may be discovered accidentally
E. Radiographic appearance
  1. Large or small radiolucent area with diffuse margins that are sometimes smooth, with faint trabeculae
  2. Displacement of teeth
  3. Root resorption
F. Histologic characteristics
  1. Loose fibrillar connective tissue with many fibroblasts
  2. Rich vascularity
  3. Foreign-body multinucleated giant cells
G. Treatment/prognosis
  1. Surgical excision or curettage; no radiation therapy
  2. Invariably fills with new bone and heals

Pulpal Granuloma

A. Etiology—large carious lesion
B. Age and sex affected—children and young adults; males and females equally affected
C. Location
  1. Usually in primary molars or permanent first molars
  2. Can occur in any tooth with a large carious lesion
D. Clinical features
  1. Red to pink outgrowth of tissue protruding from the crown of a large open carious lesion
  2. Lesion is not painful
E. Histologic characteristics
  1. Originates from pulpal tissue
  2. Contains acute and chronic inflammatory cells, plasma cells, and lymphocytes
F. Treatment/prognosis
  1. Extraction of the tooth involved or root canal therapy plus full restorative coverage depending on the extent of the lesion
  2. Prognosis good; no complications

Internal Resorption

A. Etiology—not clear; theories include
  1. Trauma
  2. Irritative factors
  3. Chronic pulpal inflammation
B. Age and sex affected—any age; males and females equally affected
C. Location—usually found in permanent dentition within the tooth
D. Clinical features
  1. Dentin immediately surrounding the pulp in the area of resorption is destroyed
  2. Crown appears pink ("pink tooth") because of the vascularity of the lesion within
E. Radiographic appearance—well-defined radiolucent lesion in close proximity to the pulp canal
F. Histologic characteristics—highly vascularized chronic inflammatory tissue
G. Treatment—endodontic therapy if perforation of the root has not occurred; otherwise, extraction of the tooth

Periapical Granuloma

A. Etiology—caries or deep restorations
B. Age and sex affected—any age; males and females equally affected
C. Location—apex of the tooth
D. Clinical features
  1. Nonvital tooth
  2. Fistula or parulis may be present if the condition has been chronic

E. Radiographic appearance—well-defined circular radiolucent lesion at the apex of the tooth involved

F. Histologic characteristics—contains proliferating endothelial cells and young fibroblasts

G. Treatment—endodontic therapy or extraction of the tooth

BENIGN INTRAOSSEOUS NEOPLASMS

General Characteristics

A. Etiology—generally unknown

B. Onset—gradual with slow development or enlargement

C. Early stages—asymptomatic

D. With expansion of the lesion, malocclusion may occur; bone tenderness on palpation; cortical bone may become thin

Osteoma

A. Etiology—generally unknown, but may be caused by irritation or inflammation

B. Age and sex affected—more common in young adults, but can be found at any age; males and females equally affected

C. Location—endosteal or periosteal; rarely found in the maxilla or mandible

D. Clinical features—patient may be unaware of the lesion, since it grows slowly; considerable growth must occur before cortical plates expand

E. Radiographic appearance—well-circumscribed radiopaque mass that is indistinguishable from scar bone; panoramic or lateral plate radiograph may be needed to view the lesion in its entirety

F. Histologic characteristics—extremely dense, compact bone or coarse, cancellous bone

G. Treatment/prognosis
   1. If it interferes with normal physiologic speech or eating, the lesion should be removed surgically
   2. Does not recur after surgical removal

Chondroma

A. Etiology—unknown

B. Age and sex affected—any age; males and females equally affected

C. Location
   1. Maxilla—anterior area
   2. Mandible—posterior to the canines
   3. May involve the body of the mandible or the coronoid or condylar process

D. Clinical features
   1. Painless
   2. Slow, progressive swelling of the jaw may loosen or malposition teeth
   3. Tendency toward malignancy

E. Radiographic appearance—irregular radiolucent or mottled area in bone; may displace surrounding teeth or cause root resorption

F. Histologic characteristics
   1. Mass of hyaline cartilage with areas of calcification or necrosis
   2. Cartilage cells are small and have one nucleus
   3. Large biopsy sample must be made, since the lesion is similar to a malignant chondrosarcoma

G. Treatment/prognosis
   1. Nonconservative surgical removal; tumor resistant to radiation therapy
   2. Periodic evaluation necessary to detect recurrence or possible malignant transformation

Myxoma

A. Etiology—unknown; originates from mesenchymal tissue of the tooth germ

B. Age and sex affected—any age; males and females equally affected

C. Location—maxilla or mandible only (because of its origin)

D. Clinical features—deep-situated lesion

E. Radiographic appearance
   1. Numerous small radiolucencies occurring in groups, giving a "honeycomb" appearance
   2. May be large and multilocular
   3. May show displaced teeth, mandibular canal, and antrum (may also invade the antrum)
   4. Peripheral borders are irregular, diffuse, and not well defined

F. Histologic characteristics
   1. Loose-textured tissue containing delicate reticulin fibers and mucoid material
   2. Contains stellate, spindle-shaped cells
   3. Tumor is not encapsulated and may invade surrounding tissues
   4. Does not metastasize

G. Treatment/prognosis
   1. Surgical removal
   2. Recurrence is common

Exostosis

Torus Palatinus

A. Etiology—unknown; possibly a hereditary factor

B. Age and sex affected—any age, but peak incidence is before 30 years; more common in females (2:1)

C. Location—midline of the hard palate

D. Clinical features
   1. Bony hard protuberance in the midline in a variety of shapes—nodular, lobular, smooth
   2. Occurs in 20% to 25% of the U.S. population
   3. Ulcerated if traumatized by coarse foods or a toothbrush

E. Radiographic appearance—dense radiopaque area
F. Histologic characteristics—dense, compact bone
G. Treatment—surgical removal if it interferes with a prosthodontic appliance

Torus Mandibularis

A. Etiology—unknown; possibly a hereditary factor
B. Age and sex affected—any age, but first observed in patients under 30 years of age; more common in females (2:1)
C. Location—lingual surface of the mandible above the mylohyoid line in the area of the bicuspids or premolars
D. Clinical features
   1. Bony hard protuberance varying in size and shape
   2. Slow growing—usually unnoticed
   3. Bilateral incidence more common (80%)
E. Radiographic appearance—dense radiopaque area
F. Histologic characteristics—dense, compact bone
G. Treatment—surgical excision if it interferes with a prosthodontic appliance

Odontoma

A. Etiology—unknown; theories include
   1. Infection
   2. Local trauma
   3. Inherited trait
   4. Mutant gene
   5. Interference postnatally with genetic control of tooth development
B. Age and sex affected—any age; males and females equally affected
C. Location—maxilla or mandible, usually between the roots of teeth
D. Clinical features
   1. Usually small; asymptomatic
   2. Cyst involvement may occur
E. Radiographic appearance—irregular mass of calcified material (''toothlike structures'') surrounded by a narrow radiolucent band with a smooth outer periphery; ranges from radiolucency to radiopacity
F. Histologic characteristics—tumor in which epithelial and mesenchymal cells show differentiation, resulting in abnormal enamel and dentin formation
G. Treatment/prognosis
   1. Surgical removal
   2. Prognosis good; rare recurrence

GINGIVAL FIBROMATOSIS
General Characteristics

A. Enlargement of gingival tissue sometimes covering the teeth
B. Contains a proliferation of dense fibrous connective tissue
C. Classification includes
   1. Irritative fibromatosis—localized areas associated with extraneous irritants
   2. Hereditary fibromatosis—generalized enlargement of gingival tissue

Irritative Fibromatosis

A. Etiology—irritant such as mouth breathing, orthodontic appliances, heavy plaque, calculus, debris, overhanging fillings, or ill-fitting prosthodontic appliances
B. Age and sex affected—any age; males and females equally affected
C. Location—localized areas on interproximal papillae; in mouth breathers, on upper and lower anterior labial gingivae
D. Clinical features—solitary round, smooth-surfaced, pink enlargement of papillae, well attached to surrounding structures
E. Histologic characteristics—proliferation of dense fibrous connective tissue with an increase in the number of fibroblasts
F. Treatment/prognosis
   1. Removal of the irritant
   2. Improved oral hygiene
   3. Gingivectomy in severe cases
   4. Prognosis excellent

Hereditary Fibromatosis

A. Etiology
   1. Hereditary; believed to have genetic or developmental involvement or be related to hormonal imbalances
   2. Contributing factors include poor oral hygiene, food impaction, calculus, and malocclusion
B. Age and sex affected—within the first 5 years of age; at the eruption of permanent teeth; slightly more common in females
C. Location—excessive enlargement of interproximal gingival tissues throughout the mouth
D. Clinical features
   1. Two varieties
      a. Symmetric type—diffuse smooth-surfaced, pink, firm tissue in interproximal papillae
      b. Nodular type—multiple protruding pink, stippled firm masses; labial and buccal areas most affected; teeth may be displaced; occurs after eruption of permanent teeth

2. Primary teeth especially are affected; often mistaken for "unerupted teeth," since teeth may be completely covered by tissue overgrowth
E. Histologic characteristics—bundles of fibrous connective tissue with fibroblasts and fibrocytes (depending on the formative stage)
F. Treatment/prognosis
   1. Excision
   2. Rigid home care
   3. Recurrence is common

ULCERATIVE DISEASES
General Characteristics

A. Ulcer—formed by destruction of epithelium and some underlying tissue
B. Factors aiding in the diagnosis of ulcers occurring in the oral cavity
   1. Number and size
   2. Location
   3. Depth
   4. Borders
   5. Personal, medical, and drug histories
C. Etiology—not always known
D. Can be classified as acute or chronic conditions
   1. Acute ulcerative conditions include traumatic ulcers, acute necrotizing ulcerative gingivitis (ANUG), recurrent ulcerative stomatitis (RUS), allergic reactions, and viral ulcerations
   2. Chronic ulcerative conditions include those caused by or associated with systemic diseases such as leukemia, colitis, malnutrition, tuberculosis, syphilis, sickle cell anemia, and drug toxicity

Traumatic Ulcer

A. Etiology—various types of trauma
   1. Physical—biting the mucosa, denture irritation, toothbrush injury, sharp tooth, fractured filling
   2. Chemical—mouth rinse, phenol, topical medication used to treat a "toothache"
   3. Thermal—hot foods ("pizza burn")
   4. Electrical
B. Age and sex affected—any age; males and females equally affected
C. Location—lateral border of the tongue, buccal mucosa, lips, palate (especially tori)
D. Clinical features
   1. Small, single, oval or round shape
   2. Flat or slightly depressed
   3. Covered by necrotic membrane and surrounded by an inflammatory halo

4. Painful for 2 to 5 days
5. Heals within 10 days
E. Histologic characteristics
   1. Loss of continuity of surface epithelium
   2. Fibrinous exudate covering exposed connective tissue
   3. Infiltration of polymorphonuclear leukocytes in connective tissue
   4. Fibroblastic activity can be prominent
F. Treatment/prognosis
   1. Removal of the irritant
   2. Orabase with benzocaine to relieve symptoms (or Kenalog in Orabase)
   3. Denture adhesive to protect the area
   4. Anesthetic-type mouth rinse to relieve discomfort
   5. Antibacterial mouth rinse to reduce or eliminate secondary infection
   6. Hydrogen peroxide rinses
   7. Tetracycline suspension (120 ml/1 tsp/4 hr)
   8. Tincture of Benzoin compound
   9. Prognosis good

Acute Necrotizing Ulcerative Gingivitis (ANUG)

A. Etiology
   1. Anerobic bacteria, fusiform bacilli
   2. *Borrelia vincentii,* a spirochete
   3. Contributory factors
      a. Systemic—fatigue, poor hygiene, stress, malnutrition
      b. Local—poor restorations, gingivitis, poor oral hygiene, heavy smoking
B. Age and sex affected—any age, usually 17 to 35 years; males and females equally affected
C. Location—free gingival margin, crest of gingiva, interdental papillae
D. Clinical features
   1. Acute gingivitis with extensive necrosis
   2. Craters form with punched-out interdental papillae
   3. Mouth odor, pain, bleeding, bad taste
   4. Headaches, low-grade fever
   5. Regional lymphadenopathy
E. Histologic characteristics
   1. Ulcerated stratified squamous epithelium
   2. Thick fibrinous exudate containing polymorphonuclear leukocytes
   3. Lack of keratinization
   4. Connective tissue infiltrated by dense numbers of polymorphonuclear leukocytes

F. Treatment/prognosis
   1. Hydrogen peroxide rinses (three to four times a day for 2 weeks)
   2. Penicillin (500 mg four times a day for 5 to 7 days) is the drug of choice when systemic complications occur
   3. Thorough scaling, curettage, and root planing (may require a topical or local anesthetic)
   4. Home care to improve oral hygiene (toothbrushing, flossing, rubber tip stimulation)
   5. Can recur if the patient lacks good home care or is predisposed to contributory factors

Recurrent Ulcerative Stomatitis (RUS, Recurrent Aphthous Stomatitis)

A. Etiology
   1. Theories
      a. *Streptococcus sanguis* (L-form)
      b. Autoimmune response of oral epithelium
      c. Nutritional deficiencies
      d. Inherited predisposition
   2. Contributory factors
      a. Hormonal imbalance
      b. Endocrine conditions—premenstrual (incidence increases), pregnancy (eruptions occur after delivery)
      c. Psychologic—anxiety, depression, acute emotional problems
      d. Allergic—asthma, hay fever, food, drug
B. Age and sex affected—first episode occurs in the 20s; more common in females
C. Location—buccal and labial mucosa, soft palate, pharynx, tongue
D. Clinical features
   1. Oval or round shape with a red halo having a distinct border
   2. Range from 1 to 100 in number (3 to 10 most common)
   3. Size—0.5 to 1 cm
   4. Pain, tenderness, discomfort
   5. Interference with function—speech, eating
   6. Contributory factors include low-grade fever and localized lymphadenopathy
E. Laboratory tests/findings—blood tests and cultures for exclusions
F. Histologic characteristics—superficial erosion of soft tissue covered by a membrane
G. Treatment/prognosis—self-limiting, healing in 10 to 12 days; recurrence is common

Recurrent Scarifying Ulcerative Stomatitis (RSUS, Periadenitis Mucosa Necrotica Recurrens, Mikulicz' Aphthae, Sutton's Disease, Major Aphthous Ulcer)

A. Etiology
   1. Autoimmune response of oral epithelium
   2. L-form *Streptococcus sanguis*
B. Age and sex affected—usually adults; more common in females
C. Location—oral cavity, buccal mucosa, tongue, soft palate, lips, posterior fauces
D. Clinical features
   1. Multiple large ulcers, 1 to 10 in number, 2 cm in diameter
   2. Craterlike formations with irregular shapes
   3. Lesions last 5 to 6 weeks, producing scars at healing that are firm and grayish or pale pink
   4. Very painful
   5. Occur at frequent intervals
E. Histologic characteristics
   1. Fibrinopurulent membrane covering the ulcerated area
   2. Necrotic epithelium
   3. Intense inflammatory cell infiltration in connective tissue
   4. Neutrophils and lymphocytes present
   5. Granulation tissue at the base of the lesion
   6. Microscopic picture is nonspecific; conclusive diagnosis cannot be made without thorough clinical and historical data
F. Treatment/prognosis
   1. Tetracycline mouthwash (250 mg) taken in doses of 5 ml four times a day for 5 to 7 days
   2. Topical application of corticosteroids
   3. Orabase
   4. Recurrence is common; patient seldom without an ulcer; remission periods of 2 to 3 months; long-term problem

Chronic Benign Mucosal Pemphigoid (Benign Mucous Membrane Pemphigoid, Ocular Pemphigus)

A. Etiology—unknown
B. Age and sex affected—40 to 55 years; more common in females (2:1)
C. Location
   1. Mucous membranes—nose, larynx, vulva, mouth, eye tissues, vagina, anus (ocular most severe)
   2. Only 30% are skin lesions
D. Clinical features
   1. Bullous lesion appears; thick walled; takes 24 to 48 hours to rupture

2. After rupture, the surface is eroded, raw
3. Lesions heal by scar formation
4. Gingiva exhibits persistent erythema long after the lesion heals

E. Histologic characteristics
   1. Vesicles and bullae are subepithelial
   2. No evidence of acantholysis—degeneration of cohesive elements of cells (bridges)

F. Treatment/prognosis
   1. Mild forms—no treatment
   2. With bullous eruptions or conjunctival involvement, use systemic corticosteroids
   3. Long duration of lesions, extending many years; few remissions

Herpes

See Chapter 7, section on herpes

Primary Herpes

A. Etiology
   1. Virus—herpes simplex
   2. Transmission—droplet infection; direct contact and highly contagious

B. Age and sex affected—2 to 11 years (85%), not younger than 6 months; males and females equally affected

C. Location—lips, gingiva, tongue, pharynx, floor of the mouth, buccal mucosa

D. Clinical features
   1. Systemic symptoms
      a. Abrupt onset of fever
      b. Headache, irritability
      c. Pain on swallowing—pharyngitis
      d. Regional lymphadenopathy
   2. Oral symptoms
      a. Hypertrophic gingivitis
      b. Painful ulcers 1 to 3 mm in size; filled with yellowish fluid
      c. Shallow craters covered by white or yellow plaque; bright red margins—"halo"
      d. Third to seventh day most acute

E. Laboratory tests/findings
   1. Rabbit eye test—virus injected into a rabbit eye; keratoconjunctivitis results; results take several days
   2. Embryonated egg—"pock" formation occurs; results take several days; expensive
   3. Cytologic smear—ulcer scraped and stained; multinucleated cells observed; not dependable
   4. Serologic—first sample taken before fourth day; second sample taken within 7 to 21 days to see if antibodies are present

F. Histologic characteristics
   1. Vesicle is an intraepithelial blister filled with fluid
   2. Degenerating cells show "ballooning" or intranuclear inclusions (Lipschütz' bodies)
   3. Displacement of chromatin
   4. When the vesicle ruptures, the surface of the tissue is covered by exudate composed of fibrin, polymorphonuclear leukocytes, and degenerated cells

G. Treatment/prognosis
   1. Symptomatic therapy—bed rest, fluids, mouthwash; antibiotics on the third day to prevent secondary infections (especially in patients with rheumatic fever)
   2. Self-limiting, healing in 7 to 14 days (21 at most)

Herpes Labialis (Cold Sore)

A. Etiology
   1. Residual form of primary herpesvirus
   2. Contributory factors
      a. Exposure to sunlight
      b. Trauma
      c. Menstruation, pregnancy
      d. Upper respiratory tract infection
      e. Emotional stress, anxiety, fatigue
      f. Allergic reactions
      g. Systemic diseases, gastrointestinal upset

B. Age and sex affected—adults; males and females equally affected

C. Location
   1. Lips—most common
   2. Intraorally—hard palate, attached gingiva, alveolar ridge

D. Clinical features
   1. Burning sensation, feeling of tightness, swelling, and soreness where the vesicle eventually appears
   2. Small lesion or several in clusters
   3. Gray to white vesicles rupture, leaving a red "halo"
   4. Lip vesicles covered with a brownish crust when dried
   5. Pain and discomfort varies

E. Histologic characteristics
   1. Ballooning degeneration; chromatin margination
   2. Lipschütz' bodies; multinucleated giant cells
   3. Isolation of herpes simplex virus

F. Treatment/prognosis
   1. Topical remedies—camphor, calamine lotions, *Lactobacillus* tablets
   2. Vitamin supplements
   3. Self-limiting, healing in 7 to 10 days

Herpes Zoster (Shingles)

A. Etiology
  1. Varicella virus, which causes chickenpox; injury to the dorsal nerve root
  2. Contributory factors
     a. Systemic disease
     b. Drug toxicity
     c. Malnutrition
     d. Trauma to cranial nerve V (oral)
     e. Extreme fatigue
B. Age and sex affected—adults, usually over 50 years; males and females equally affected
C. Location—skin or mucosa supplied by the affected nerve
D. Clinical features
  1. Clusters of vesicles along the pathway of the nerve
  2. Inflammation with severe pain, itching, and burning preceding vesicle eruption
  3. Unilateral distribution
E. Treatment/prognosis
  1. Propoxyphene (Darvon), meperidine (Demerol), or morphine to control pain
  2. Topical anesthetics; Orabase
  3. Antiseptic mouthwashes
  4. Radiation—three treatments of 150 rad to involved dorsal root ganglia to reduce pain
  5. Prognosis good if cranial nerve V involvement (healing in 2 to 3 weeks); involvement of other nerve ganglia may be long lasting

Herpangina (Aphthous Pharyngitis)

A. Etiology—coxsackievirus A
B. Age and sex affected—children 6 months to 8 years; males and females equally affected
C. Location—posterior hard or soft palate, tongue, fauces (pillars), uvula, tonsils
D. Clinical features
  1. Systemic symptoms
     a. Comparatively mild and short duration
     b. Sore throat
     c. Fever—101° to 105° F—peaks in 2 days
     d. Headache
     e. Vomiting
     f. No lymphadenopathy—differs from primary herpes
  2. Oral symptoms
     a. Eight to 12 small ulcers with a gray base and inflamed periphery
     b. Numerous small vesicles precede the ulcers—often overlooked
     c. Slightly painful and sometimes difficult to swallow
     d. Sudden onset
     e. Erythematous pharynx

E. Laboratory tests/findings—throat scrapings and stool specimens to isolate coxsackievirus
F. Treatment/prognosis
  1. Aspirin for fever
  2. Bed rest
  3. Self-limiting with few complications

Infectious Mononucleosis (Glandular Fever)

A. Etiology
  1. Unknown; possibly Epstein-Barr (EB) virus
  2. Transmission—intimate oral exchange of saliva—"kissing disease"
B. Age and sex affected—children and young adults; males and females equally affected
C. Clinical features
  1. Systemic symptoms
     a. Fever, chills
     b. Sore throat, cough
     c. Headache
     d. Nausea, vomiting
     e. Lymphadenopathy—cervical lymph nodes
  2. Oral symptoms
     a. Acute gingivitis and stomatitis
     b. Inflamed attached gingiva
     c. Ulcerations similar to those of herpes or herpangina
     d. Purpura spots beneath the epithelium (thrombocytopenia means a decrease in the number of platelets)
     e. Edema of the soft palate and uvula
D. Laboratory tests/findings
  1. Blood count may indicate anemia, thrombocytopenia, or lymphocytosis, but lymphocytosis is very characteristic
  2. Increased heterophil antibody titer—1:56 normal; 1:4096 positive for mononucleosis (Paul-Bunnell test)
  3. Sharp increase in the number of white blood cells
E. Treatment/prognosis
  1. Antibiotics
  2. Bed rest
  3. Nutritional diet
  4. Course runs 2 to 4 weeks

SKIN DISEASES
General Characteristics

A. Characterized by various forms and sizes of ulcerative eruptions
B. Lesions may appear first or during the course of the disease
C. Reaction simulates an allergic-type reaction

Erythema Multiforme

A. Etiology
  1. Unknown
  2. Possibly allergy, toxicity, viral or bacterial infection, drug intake
  3. May be preceded by herpes simplex infection
B. Age and sex affected—young adults 20 to 40 years; more common in black males
C. Location
  1. Extremities—hands, feet, arms, legs
  2. Skin—macular, papular, or bullous eruptions ("target" or "bull's-eye" lesions)
  3. Mouth—lips, buccal mucosa, tongue
D. Clinical features
  1. Systemic symptoms
    a. Abrupt onset
    b. Fatigue, malaise, fever
    c. Previous occurrences
    d. Has been associated with terminal cancer, nephritis, and typhoid fever
    e. May be a toxic reaction to an iodide, bromide, salicylate, or antibiotic
  2. Oral symptoms
    a. Painful lesions
    b. Macules, papules, or vesicles ulcerate and bleed easily
    c. Have a raw tissue base with a grayish necrotic slough
    d. Irregular shape; surrounded by a band of inflammation; encrustations
    e. Edema of the lips
E. Laboratory tests/findings—biopsy for differential diagnosis
F. Histologic characteristics
  1. Zone of severe liquefaction degeneration in upper layers of epithelium
  2. Intraepithelial vesicle formation and thinning
  3. Absence of a basement membrane
  4. Dilation of capillaries and lymphatic vessels in the surface layer of connective tissue
  5. Varying degree of inflammatory cell infiltration
G. Treatment/prognosis
  1. Removal of the cause if known
  2. Topical or systemic applications of corticosteroids
  3. Antibacterial, mild mouthwashes (e.g., hydrogen peroxide)
  4. Liquid diet—Metracal, Nutriment, Instant Breakfast
  5. Antibiotics if secondary infection is present
  6. Antihistamines if an allergic response
  7. Lesions remain 2 to 4 weeks; can recur

Stevens-Johnson Syndrome

Severe bullous form of erythema multiforme
A. Etiology—unknown; possibly viral
B. Age and sex affected—children and young adults under 25 years; more common in males; history of previous similar illness
C. Location—oral cavity, skin, eyes, genitalia
D. Clinical features
  1. Oral symptoms—bullae rupture, leaving thick white or yellow exudate; eating becomes impossible
  2. Skin lesions—severe, numerous; cover wide areas of the body (face, chest, abdomen)
  3. Eye involvement—severe conjunctivitis, photophobia, corneal ulceration
E. Treatment/prognosis
  1. Antibiotics and corticosteroids to control severity
  2. 1- to 4-week duration
  3. Prognosis good; some fatalities because of pneumonia

Behçet's Syndrome (Behçet's Triad, Behçet's Triple Complex)

Variant of erythema multiforme
A. Etiology—unknown; theories include
  1. Viral, hormonal, or metabolic origin
  2. Toxic mechanism
  3. Pleuropneumonia-like organisms (PPLOs)
  4. Mycoplasma (bacteria having no cell walls)
B. Age and sex affected—10 to 40 years; more common in males (6:1)
C. Location—triad location
  1. Oral cavity—97%
  2. Eyes
  3. Genitalia
D. Clinical features
  1. Oral lesions
    a. Painful ulcerations
    b. Large ulcers surrounded by a red border; covered with gray or yellow exudate
    c. Similar to those of recurrent ulcerative stomatitis and erythema multiforme
  2. Eye lesions
    a. Begin with photophobia and irritation
    b. Purulent conjunctivitis and uveitis
    c. Healing may be followed by scarification and consequent blindness
    d. Hypopyon (pus in the anterior chamber of the eye between the iris and cornea) in severe cases

3. Genital lesions
   a. In females—painful ulcerations in the vulval folds, labia majora, and vaginal canal
   b. In males—painful ulcerations on the scrotum and penis
4. Systemic symptoms
   a. Occasionally fever, pallor
   b. Complications can involve the central nervous, cardiac, and pulmonary systems
E. Laboratory tests/findings
   1. Excessive gamma globulin in the blood
   2. Leukocytosis with eosinophilia
   3. Elevated sedimentation rate
F. Histologic characteristics
   1. Endothelial proliferation in lesions
   2. Other characteristics similar to those of recurrent ulcerative stomatitis in oral tissues
G. Treatment/prognosis
   1. Similar treatment as for erythema multiforme
   2. Lesions last 2 to 4 weeks
   3. Disease is long lasting with remission periods
   4. Complications may result in fatalities

Pemphigus Vulgaris

A. Etiology—unknown; theories include viral or streptococcal origin
B. Age and sex affected—adults over 30 years (usually between 40 and 50 years); more common in white females
C. Location—oral cavity, eyes, skin
D. Clinical features
   1. Oral lesions appear first
   2. Blisters, vesicles, or bullae collapse as soon as they are formed
      a. Vary in shape and size (from several millimeters to centimeters)
      b. Ragged peripheral borders; flat or shallow; base intensely red and raw; may extend into the lips with crusting
   3. Filmy necrotic slough of tissue can be detached from underlying tissue
   4. Neighboring soft tissue appears normal
   5. Nikolsky's sign present—epithelial tissue separates under light pressure
   6. Pain may be severe with the patient unable to eat
   7. Salivation is profuse; mouth odor
E. Laboratory tests/findings
   1. Blood chemistry shows a decrease in the serum sodium level
   2. Biopsy—most conclusive

F. Histologic characteristics
   1. Vesicle or bulla entirely intraepithelial above the basal layer, producing a distinctive "split"
   2. Prevesicular edema weakens the junction
   3. Intercellular bridges between epithelial cells disappear with loss of cohesiveness
   4. Clumps of epithelial cells lie free within the vesicular space
   5. Tzanck cells present—swelling of nuclei
   6. Increase in RNA in the cytoplasm
   7. Scarcity of inflammatory cell infiltration
G. Treatment/prognosis
   1. Corticosteroids and antibiotics to control secondary infections
   2. When lesions are present, prednisolone, 100 to 175 mg/day reduced to 10 mg/day after the lesions disappear
   3. Germicidal or tetracycline suspension mouth rinses
   4. Prognosis poor in severe cases; patients with mild cases recover within a few days or weeks

WHITE LESIONS
General Characteristics

A. May be keratotic or hyperkeratotic
B. Vary from simple lesions to diffuse coverage; smooth to rough surfaces; elevated to flat
C. Firmly attached to mucous membranes
D. Color—white, grayish white, yellowish white
E. Painless

Stomatitis Nicotina (Nicotine Stomatitis)

A. Etiology—heavy smoking; "pipe smoker's palate"
B. Age and sex affected—adults 30 to 50 years; more common in males
C. Location—posterior hard and soft palates
D. Clinical features
   1. Begins with redness and inflammation of the minor salivary duct orifice; 4 to 5 mm in size
   2. Diffuse grayish white, thickened coating with a red center in each tiny nodule (indicates an inflamed, dilated, or partially occluded duct orifice)
   3. Fissures or cracks around the nodules create an overall wrinkled appearance
E. Histologic characteristics
   1. Hyperkeratosis
   2. Thickening of epithelium adjacent to the orifice
F. Treatment/prognosis
   1. Stop smoking—condition is reversible
   2. Prognosis good if the patient permanently ceases smoking

Linea Alba

A. Etiology—pattern of occlusion may be contributory
B. Age and sex affected—any age; males and females equally affected
C. Location—buccal mucosa along the occlusal plane; usually bilateral
D. Clinical features
   1. Pink to grayish velvety swelling or clustering of tissue along the line of occlusion
   2. Localized, single line in thickness
E. Histologic characteristics—localized intracellular edema (leukoedema)
F. Treatment/prognosis—no treatment required; nonpathogenic

Leukoedema

A. Etiology—unknown; possibly a hereditary factor or defect in maturation of squamous epithelium
B. Age and sex affected—average age, 45 years; males and females equally affected; blacks more affected (80% of incidence)
C. Location—buccal and labial mucosa; bilateral; extending to the inside of the lips
D. Clinical features
   1. Soft, spongy, velvety, filmy opalescence of buccal mucosa
   2. Later becomes grayish white with a coarsely wrinkled surface
E. Histologic characteristics
   1. Intracellular edema of prickle cells (spinous layer)
   2. Increased thickness of epithelium with a superficial parakeratotic layer several cells thick
   3. Broad rete pegs that appear irregularly elongated
   4. Does not produce keratin
F. Treatment/prognosis—no treatment required; nonpathogenic

Chronic Discoid Lupus Erythematosus

A. Etiology—unknown; theories include
   1. Genetic origin
   2. Form of tuberculosis
   3. Associated with foci of infection
   4. Toxic agents
B. Age and sex affected—30 to 40 years; more common in females (3:1)
C. Location
   1. Oral mucosa—buccal
   2. Skin—face, chest, back, bridge of the nose, extremities

D. Clinical features
   1. Slow onset
   2. Oral lesions usually precede skin lesions
      a. Vary in size; may have butterfly configuration
      b. Superficial, painful ulcerations with crusting or bleeding; no actual scale as on skin lesions
      c. Margins not sharply demarcated but show a narrow zone of keratinization
   3. Skin lesions—rough and circular with red or purple macules; scales form; butterfly configuration on the bridge of the nose
   4. Scarred appearance shows the duration of the disease
   5. Fissuring of the tongue
E. Laboratory tests/findings—blood tests are definitive; reveal
   1. Lupus erythematosus cell inclusion phenomenon
   2. Anemia; leukopenia; thrombocytopenia
   3. Elevated sedimentation rate and serum gamma globulin level
   4. Positive Coombs test
F. Histologic characteristics
   1. Hyperkeratosis or hyperparakeratosis alternating with areas of epithelial atrophy
   2. Acanthosis
   3. Pseudoepitheliomatous hyperplasia
   4. Necrosis of the basal cell layer; thickening of the basement membrane
   5. Diffuse infiltration of lymphocytes in the corium
G. Treatment/prognosis
   1. Corticosteroid therapy
   2. Periods of remission

Familial White Folded Dysplasia (Spongy Nevus)

A. Etiology—hereditary; autosomal dominant trait
B. Age and sex affected—progressive from childhood to adulthood; males and females equally affected
C. Location—buccal mucosa, palate, gingiva, tongue, lips (inner surface)
D. Clinical features
   1. Mucosa thickened
   2. Lesions diffuse and generalized
   3. Grayish white; soft, spongy, velvety
   4. Early years—tissues smooth and flat
   5. Adolescence—tissues become increasingly folded or corrugated; appear opalescent-white when the lesion peaks

E. Histologic characteristics
   1. Epithelium thickened with both hyperkeratosis and acanthosis
   2. Basal cell layer intact
   3. Cells of the spinous layer toward the surface exhibit intracellular edema with pyknotic nuclei
   4. Lack of differentiation of epithelial cells beyond the parabasal level
F. Treatment/prognosis
   1. No treatment required
   2. Prognosis excellent; no clinical complications

Lichen Planus

A. Etiology—emotional stress, nervousness
B. Age and sex affected—adults; more common in females
C. Location—skin, buccal mucosa, tongue
D. Clinical features
   1. Size—small (several millimeters to centimeters)
   2. Varied patterns/forms
      a. Reticular pattern
         (1) Narrow, slightly elevated lines forming a mesh, net, or lacelike pattern
         (2) Mucous membrane between the lace pattern appears normal in color and texture
         (3) Whitish, grayish
      b. Papular pattern
         (1) Small, pinhead, raised, glistening papules; scattered or clustered
         (2) Coalescence
         (3) Radiating striae appear at the periphery
      c. Plaque pattern
         (1) Solid grayish or whitish raised patch
         (2) Varies in size and shape
         (3) Often simulates hyperkeratosis or leukoplakia
      d. Erosive or ulcerative form
         (1) Located on the buccal mucosa
         (2) Begins as an erosive, flat, or depressed lesion
         (3) Intensely red, blotching pattern
         (4) Preceded by bullous lesions or ulcerations
      e. Atrophic form
         (1) Smooth, red, poorly defined areas
         (2) Peripheral striae evident
   3. Gingival involvement
      a. Rare; similar to desquamative gingivitis
      b. Barely detectable, disrupted, patterned, diffuse or patchy papules
      c. Denuded and painful

E. Histologic characteristics
   1. Hyperparakeratosis or hyperorthokeratosis
   2. Thickened spinous layer (acanthosis) and granular layer
   3. Intracellular edema of cells in the spinous layer
   4. Necrosis or degeneration of the basal cell layer with a thin band of eosinophilic coagulum in its place
   5. Infiltration of lymphocytes into connective tissue
F. Treatment/prognosis
   1. Bicotin T—three or four times a day
   2. Vitamin B complex therapy
   3. Corticosteroids to decrease ulcerations and inflammation
   4. Niacinamide—200 mg/day
   5. Lesions are self-limiting, healing spontaneously over months or years; not considered a premalignant lesion

Keratoses

Includes hyperkeratosis and leukoplakia
A. Etiology
   1. Local factors (80% of incidence)—constant, low-grade irritation (e.g., from cheek biting, a denture clasp/flange, a sharp filling, or a fractured cusp)
   2. Systemic factors
      a. Vitamin A deficiency
      b. Hyperestrogen medication over a prolonged period
      c. Tertiary syphilis causing keratosis of the tongue
      d. Alcoholism, malabsorptive syndromes
      e. Cirrhosis of the liver
      f. Ulcerative colitis
   3. Combination of local and systemic factors
B. Age and sex affected—over 40 years; more common in males
C. Location—anywhere in the oral cavity
D. Clinical features
   1. Hyperkeratosis
      a. Flat, smooth, soft lesion with a diffuse boundary
      b. Three layers of epithelium affected: granular, prickle, and basal
      c. Fissures or ulcerations rare
   2. Leukoplakia
      a. White elevated patch with a rough surface and discrete border
      b. Fissures and erosion present
      c. Three to five percent of cases are true leukoplakia; rest are hyperkeratosis

E. Laboratory tests/findings—biopsy most conclusive; repeated if indicated
F. Histologic characteristics
   1. Hyperkeratosis
      a. Abnormal layer of keratin/parakeratosis where not normally found; thickness of keratin in areas where normally found (e.g., attached gingiva)
      b. Normal underlying epithelial cells
   2. Leukoplakia
      a. Dyskeratosis in underlying squamous epithelium; disorientation and intermingling of cell layers (dysplasia)
        (1) Increased, abnormal mitosis of the basal layer
        (2) Individual cell keratinization; epithelial pearls in the spinous layer
        (3) Alterations in the nuclear/cytoplasmic ratio
        (4) Loss of polarity; disorientation of cells; hyperchromatism
        (5) Large, prominent nuclei, almost equal in size to the cell
      b. Abnormal cell size, shape, and stain
      c. Outside layer is keratin
      d. Considered a premalignant lesion
      e. Histologic diagnosis is definitive
G. Treatment/prognosis
   1. Hyperkeratosis
      a. Removal of the irritant
      b. Surgical excision if small; if large, high doses of vitamin A for 6 weeks
      c. Slowly induced with a prolonged duration
   2. Leukoplakia
      a. Surgical excision or stripping
      b. Electrocoagulation
      c. Vitamin B therapy
      d. Radiation therapy discouraged
      e. More rapid development with a shorter duration than that of hyperkeratosis

MALIGNANT NEOPLASMS OF THE MOUTH

Mouth Cancer

A. Etiology—unknown; possibly viral
B. Age and sex affected—45 to 55 years and over; more common in males (4:1)
C. Location—98% begin in soft tissues
   1. Maxilla or mandible—2%
   2. Lips—25% to 35%; mostly the lower lip
   3. Tongue—25%; lateral borders at the junction of the middle and third sections; dorsum or posterior area; early metastases
   4. Floor of the mouth—20%
   5. Buccal mucosa, other areas—25%

D. Clinical features
   1. Hard, firm lesion in soft tissue; feels anchored to underlying tissue
   2. Stages
      a. Stage I—early; asymptomatic
      b. Stage II—intermediate; bone tenderness, pain, unexplained toothache, numbness or tingling, sudden looseness of teeth
      c. Stage III—advanced; pain and ulcerations from loss of blood; lesion moves around teeth under palpation
E. Radiographic appearance
   1. Diffuse radiolucency with irregular borders after 40% to 60% of the bone has been destroyed; penetration into the cortex
   2. Resorption of tooth roots; expansion between teeth
F. Laboratory tests/findings
   1. Exfoliative cytology—not always accurate
   2. Biopsy
      a. Incisional—removal of a piece of tissue
      b. Excisional—removal of the entire mass
G. Histologic characteristics
   1. Proliferation of abnormal cells; nucleus denser and larger
   2. Invasive to underlying tissues; metastasizes to lymph nodes, etc.
   3. Types—fugating, infiltrating, papillary (growth in lateral direction)
H. Treatment/prognosis
   1. Surgical excision, radiation, and/or chemotherapy
   2. Treatment and prognosis depend on the site and size of the tumor, the presence or absence of metastasis, the histologic grade, and the age and health of the patient

Mixed Tumor (Pleomorphic Adenoma)

A. Etiology—unknown
B. Age and sex affected—any age; males and females equally affected
C. Location
   1. Ninety-five percent occur around the mouth
   2. Parotid gland
   3. Hard or soft palate
D. Clinical features
   1. Parotid gland involvement
      a. Tumor arises from secreting cells of parotid gland
      b. Parotid gland is most frequent site of mixed tumors
      c. Single nodular mass with sharp borders; firm and hard to palpation
      d. Slow growing over months or years

2. Palatal involvement
   a. Located on either side of the midline
   b. Fleshy growth similar to a fibroma
   c. Ulceration; cystic variety
   d. Intraosseous (moves bone and teeth)
E. Histologic characteristics
   1. Benign, but some are locally invasive (salivary glands)
   2. Epithelial origin
F. Treatment/prognosis
   1. Surgical excision
   2. Recurrence rate—35%

CYSTIC DISEASES
General Characteristics

A. True cyst is
   1. Abnormal sac or space found in hard or soft tissue
   2. Lined by epithelium and enclosed within a capsule of connective tissue
   3. Space often filled with fluid or fragments of tissues
B. Cysts are classified according to
   1. Size
   2. Location
   3. Etiology
   4. Histologic components

Radicular Cyst (Root-End Cyst, Apical Periodontal Cyst)

A. Etiology
   1. Caries
   2. Trauma
   3. Deep restoration causing pulpitis and periapical inflammation
B. Age and sex affected—any age; males and females equally affected
C. Location—apex of the tooth
D. Clinical features
   1. Nonvital tooth
   2. Small and asymptomatic
E. Radiographic appearance—round or ovoid, well-defined radiolucent area 1 to 2 cm in size
F. Histologic characteristics—stratified aquamous epithelium
G. Treatment
   1. Extraction of the tooth
   2. Surgical procedure for removal of the cyst sac

Residual Cyst

A. Etiology
   1. Radicular cyst not removed after extraction of a tooth
   2. Open socket with debris acting as a stimulus

B. Age and sex affected—any age; males and females equally affected
C. Location
   1. Apices of teeth
   2. Near the alveolar ridge in edentulous mouths
D. Clinical features—small and asymptomatic
E. Radiographic appearance—well-defined radiolucent area
F. Histologic characteristics—stratified squamous epithelium lining a space or lumen
G. Treatment—removal of the cyst

Lateral Periodontal Cyst

A. Etiology—theories include
   1. Resulted from a dentigerous cyst
   2. Epithelial remnants of the periodontal ligament
   3. Remnants of dental lamina
   4. Trauma
B. Age and sex affected—adults; males and females equally affected
C. Location—between roots of teeth Nos. 21 and 22; 27 and 28
D. Clinical features
   1. Teeth are vital
   2. Asymptomatic, no bulge
E. Radiographic appearance—small (1 cm), well-defined ovoid or elliptic radiolucent area found between teeth
F. Histologic characteristics—cystic sac composed of stratified squamous epithelial lining and a connective tissue wall
G. Treatment—surgical removal without extraction of the surrounding teeth

Developmental Cysts

A. Etiology—entrapped epithelial cells between embryonic processes of bones at fissures
B. Age and sex affected—adults; males and females equally affected
C. Location—names are based on location
   1. Median mandibular cyst
   2. Globulomaxillary cyst
   3. Nasoalveolar cyst
   4. Median alveolar cyst
   5. Median palatal cyst
   6. Cyst of incisive papilla
   7. Nasopalatine or incisive canal cyst
D. Clinical features
   1. Vary in size from no evidence of a lesion to a bulge or expansion of bone
   2. All teeth vital

E. Radiographic appearance—well-defined radiolucent area
   1. Globulomaxillary cyst located between a maxillary lateral incisor and canine often is pear shaped
   2. Incisal canal cyst is heart shaped
F. Histologic characteristics
   1. Median mandibular cyst in the midline of the mandible is the only fissural cyst with all stratified squamous epithelium
   2. Fissural cysts of the maxilla have glandular tissue or mucous glands involved
G. Treatment/prognosis
   1. Enucleation of the cystic sac
   2. Prognosis excellent

Primordial Cyst

A. Etiology—neoplastic; arises from epithelium of the enamel organ or from primordial epithelium
B. Age and sex affected—under 25 years; males and females equally affected
C. Location—mandibular third molar space or posterior to an erupted mandibular third molar
D. Clinical features
   1. Tooth never present in the space occupied by the cyst
   2. Size varies from small to quite large
E. Radiographic appearance—radiolucent, well-defined oval lesion; can be multilocular
F. Histologic characteristics
   1. Four to eight cells of stratified squamous epithelium
   2. No rete pegs
   3. Parallel bundles of collagen fibers
G. Treatment/prognosis
   1. Surgical removal of bone in the area by curettage
   2. Can develop into an ameloblastoma

Dentigerous Cyst (Follicular Cyst)

A. Etiology—from reduced enamel epithelium after the crown of the tooth is completely formed (unerupted or impacted tooth); accumulation of fluid between the crown and reduced enamel epithelium
B. Age and sex affected—25 years; males and females equally affected
C. Location
   1. Mandibular third molar area—often extending to and destroying the ramus
   2. Maxillary canine region

D. Clinical features
   1. Always associated with the crown of an imbedded or unerupted tooth
   2. Aggressive lesion causing expansion of bone and extreme displacement of teeth
   3. Painful
E. Radiographic appearance—smooth, unilocular radiolucency, larger than 4 mm, extending from the crown to the reduced enamel epithelium
F. Histologic characteristics—stratified squamous epithelium lining the lumen; surrounded by a thin connective tissue wall
G. Treatment—enucleatium of the cystic sac

Peripheral or Soft Tissue Cysts

Ranula

A. Etiology
   1. Blockage or obstruction (by a salivary stone) of an accessory salivary gland duct
   2. Trauma
B. Age and sex affected—any age; males and females equally affected
C. Location—floor of the mouth, under the tongue, past the midline
D. Clinical features
   1. Translucent, bluish, round, smooth-surfaced bulge 1 to 3 cm in diameter
   2. Semifirm
   3. Increases in size between meals; decreases immediately after a meal
E. Radiographic appearance—radiopaque calculi in the duct area
F. Histologic characteristics—epithelium lining is present
G. Treatment/prognosis
   1. Surgical excision
   2. Can recur

Mucocele

A. Etiology
   1. Obstruction of a minor salivary gland duct
   2. Trauma to the salivary duct by lip biting or pinching
B. Age and sex affected—under 30 years; males and females equally affected
C. Location—most common on the lower lip; can occur on the palate, buccal mucosa, or tongue
D. Clinical features
   1. Blisterlike raised, circumscribed vesicle; pinhead to 1 cm in size
   2. Translucent and bluish
   3. Firm, movable to palpation
   4. Straw-colored fluid can be aspirated

E. Histologic characteristics
1. Cavity rarely lined by a thin layer of epithelium; therefore not a true cyst
2. Wall composed of fibrous connective tissue lining and fibroblasts
3. Numerous polymorphonuclear leukocytes present
4. Lumen filled with many leukocytes and mononuclear phagocytes
F. Treatment/prognosis
1. Excision of the lesion and associated gland
2. Recurrence is possible

Soft Tissue Developmental Cysts

Thyroglossal Duct Cyst

A. Etiology—developmental, between the embryonic thyroglossal tract; caused by a draining infection or trauma to lymphoid tissues
B. Age and sex affected—usually young persons, but can occur at any age; more common in females
C. Location—midline of the tongue to the neck
D. Clinical features
1. Firm, cystic mass; round or oval shape; few millimeters to several centimeters in size
2. As swelling develops slowly, a fistula may form
3. Swallowing becomes difficult (dysphagia)
E. Histologic characteristics
1. Lining of stratified squamous epithelium or other types of epithelial tissue
2. Connective tissue wall may contain lymphoid or thyroid tissue and mucous glands
F. Treatment—complete surgical excision after a thyroid scan

Branchial Cleft Cyst (Lateral Cervical Cyst)

A. Etiology—theories include
1. Epithelial remnants of embryonic branchial arches
2. Epithelium entrapped in lymph nodes in the branchial arch region
3. Not related to the branchial arches
B. Age and sex affected—children and young adults; males and females equally affected
C. Location
1. Lateral aspect of the second branchial arch; lateral aspect of the upper neck
2. Usually close to the anterior border of the sternocleidomastoid muscle
3. Area from the clavicle to the parotid gland
D. Clinical features
1. Slow growing; asymptomatic
2. Circumscribed, movable mass

E. Histologic characteristics
1. Lined by stratified squamous epithelium; lymphoid tissue in the wall
2. May contain pseudostratified columnar epithelium
F. Treatment—surgical removal

Epidermoid Cyst

A. Etiology
1. From epithelial cells entrapped in closure lines of soft tissue during fetal development
2. Trauma
B. Age and sex affected—young persons; males and females equally affected
C. Location
1. Floor of the mouth above the geniohyoid muscle
2. Mucobuccal folds
3. Geniohyoid muscle
D. Clinical features—round, well-defined, semifirm palpable mass
E. Histologic characteristics—stratified squamous epithelium lining with a fibrous tissue wall
F. Treatment—remove surgically

Dermoid Cyst

A. Etiology—from epithelial cells entrapped in closure lines of soft tissue during fetal life
B. Age and sex affected—young adults (depends on the stage); males and females equally affected
C. Location—floor of the mouth; submaxillary or sublingual area
D. Clinical features
1. Semifirm to hard (dependent on contents)
2. Two or more centimeters in diameter
3. Fistula may form for drainage
E. Histologic characteristics
1. Stratified squamous epithelial lining with a fibrous connective tissue wall
2. May contain sebaceous glands, hair follicles, and sweat glands
F. Treatment—surgical removal

Bone Cysts

Aneurysmal Bone Cyst

A. Etiology—theories include
1. Arterial venus shunt—caused by a benign fibroosseous lesion in the area, altering blood vessels; this theory is most widely believed and accepted
2. Trauma—trauma ruptures a blood vessel with blood accumulating outside of the wall; resorbs bone

B. Age and sex affected—under 20 years; males and females equally affected
C. Location
1. Over 50% occur in the long bones or vertebral column
2. When occurrence is in the jaws, the mandible is the more frequent site (2:1)
D. Clinical features
1. May be asymptomatic or a slight to moderate well-defined bulge
2. Tenderness, pain on motion; may limit movement
E. Radiographic appearance—hazy, gray radiolucent area; appears cystic, with a "soap bubble" effect
F. Histologic characteristics
1. Walls of fibrous connective tissue
2. Many cavernous or sinusoidal spaces filled with blood
3. Young fibroblasts in the connective tissue stroma
4. Multinucleated giant cells—similar to those of a giant cell granuloma
G. Treatment
1. Surgical exploration—on entering, if excessive bleeding is encountered, surgical enucleation and thorough curettage
2. Radical surgery
3. Low-radiation therapy—least preferred because of the possibility of a radiation sarcoma developing

Traumatic Bone Cyst (Hemorrhagic Cyst, Idiopathic Bone)

A. Etiology—theories include
1. Intramedullary hemorrhage following trauma; altered bone prevents fibroblasts and/or endothelial cells from entering the hemorrhage; clot does not form; blood never organizes, leaving a void within the bone
2. Necrotizing infection
3. Degeneration of a benign tumor
4. Bone did not develop in the area
B. Age and sex affected—around 18 years (75% in the second decade); males and females equally affected
C. Location—most frequent in the mandible
D. Clinical features—asymptomatic (discovered through radiographic examination)
E. Radiographic appearance—radiolucent area 1 to 7 cm in diameter; round, oval, elliptic, multilocular; projections extend between roots of teeth; lamina dura appears intact

F. Histologic characteristics
1. Thin connective tissue membrane lining the cavity; no epithelial lining
2. Center is a void
G. Treatment/prognosis
1. Surgical intervention to establish bleeding
2. Lesion heals within a year

Lingual Mandibular Bone Concavity (Stafne's Bone Cyst)

A. Etiology—developmental; salivary gland extends laterally into the mandible
B. Age and sex affected—young persons; slightly more common in males
C. Location—angle of the mandible below the inferior alveolar canal; anterior mandible
D. Clinical features—asymptomatic; occasionally bilateral
E. Radiographic, appearance—well-defined ovoid radiolucency 1 to 3 cm in diameter
F. Histologic characteristics—lymphoid, fat, submaxillary salivary gland tissues; striated muscle
G. Treatment/prognosis
1. Surgical intervention to determine contents; once diagnosed, leave alone
2. Prognosis excellent; no complications

BLOOD DYSCRASIAS
General Characteristics

A. Disease with most numerous types of dyscrasias
B. Important to know normal blood levels and chemistries in order to make differential diagnosis
C. Anemias (most common type of blood dyscrasia) are categorized according to etiology
1. Blood loss
2. Excessive destruction of red blood cells because of a congenital or hemolytic condition
3. Decrease in production of red blood cells
4. Associated with congenital diseases

Sickle Cell Anemia

A. Etiology—hereditary; hemolytic
B. Age and sex affected—before 30 years; more common in females; predominantly affects black race (1 in 600)
C. Clinical features—systemic symptoms
1. Weakness, easily fatigued; pallor of tissues
2. Shortness of breath; nausea, vomiting
3. Pain in joints
D. Radiographic appearance
1. Perpendicular trabeculations radiating outward, giving a "hair-on-end" appearance to the skull
2. Decrease of trabeculae in the jaws with large marrow spaces
3. Lamina dura not affected

E. Laboratory tests/findings
  1. Red blood cell count reduced to 1,000,000/ mm^3 (normal—4 to 6,000,000/mm^3)
  2. Decrease in the hemoglobin level (normal— males, 13.5 to 18 g/dl; females, 12 to 16 g/dl
F. Histologic characteristics
  1. Crescent-shaped erythrocytes caused by hemoglobin S or binucleation
  2. Atypical chromatin distribution
G. Treatment/prognosis
  1. Transfusions of whole blood
  2. Prognosis unpredictable; many fatalities

Erythroblastosis Fetalis (Rh Anemia)

A. Etiology
  1. Congenital
  2. Antibody of the mother's Rh factor reacts against the fetal Rh factor, causing destruction of fetal blood
B. Age and sex affected—newborn (firstborn usually is not affected; chances increase with each birth); Rh factor more common in females
C. Clinical features
  1. Systemic symptoms
    a. Infants stillborn
    b. Those that live have anemia and jaundice
  2. Oral symptoms
    a. Primary teeth have a green, brown, or blue hue in enamel because of blood pigments; bilirubin
    b. Enamel hypoplasia
D. Laboratory tests/findings
  1. Red blood cell count—1,000,000/mm^3 to normal
  2. Large number of nuclcated red blood cells in circulating blood
  3. Icterus (jaundice) index may reach 100 units (normal—4 to 6 units)
  4. Positive direct Coombs test
E. Treatment/prognosis
  1. No treatment necessary for teeth, since deciduous
  2. If undetected, infants may be stillborn

Pernicious Anemia (Primary Anemia, Addison's Anemia, Biermer's Anemia)

A. Etiology—failure to secrete intrinsic factor (substance found in normal gastric juices; responsible for absorption of extrinsic factor—vitamin B$_{12}$
B. Age and sex affected—rarely before 30 years (increases with advancing age; in the United States, more common in males; in Scandinavia, more common in females

C. Clinical features
  1. Systemic symptoms
    a. General weakness, dizziness, pallor
    b. Numbness or tingling of extremities
    c. Nausea, vomiting, diarrhea; abdominal pain
    d. Loss of appetite and weight
  2. Oral symptoms
    a. Sore, painful, "beefy-red" tongue (glossitis)
      (1) Shallow ulcers
      (2) Atrophy of papillae ("bald tongue," Hunter's glossitis, Moeller's glossitis)
    b. Distorted taste
    c. Pallor of the oral mucosa
D. Laboratory tests/findings
  1. Red blood cell count—1,000,000/mm^3
  2. Irregularly shaped red blood cells
  3. Decrease in leukocytes
  4. Achlorhydria—lack of gastric hydrochloric acid secretion
E. Histologic characteristics
  1. Buccal scrapings show enlarged, irregularly shaped nuclei
  2. Variation in size of erythrocytes
F. Treatment/prognosis
  1. Vitamin B$_{12}$ (5 μg/day)
  2. Increased dietary intake of folic acid (leafy green vegetables, organ meats, wheat cereals)
  3. Five to ten percent of patients develop gastric carcinoma

Plummer-Vinson Syndrome (Iron Deficiency Anemia)

A. Etiology—iron deficiency caused by
  1. Chronic blood loss (e.g., profuse menstruation)
  2. Inadequate dietary intake
  3. Faulty iron absorption
  4. Increased iron requirements (e.g., infancy, pregnancy)
B. Age and sex affected—40 to 50 years; more common in females (5% to 30% female incidence in United States; 50% female incidence in other countries)
C. Clinical features
  1. Systemic symptoms
    a. Lemon-tinted skin; pallor
    b. Difficulty in swallowing (dysphagia)
    c. Brittle fingernails
    d. Enlarged spleen (splenomegaly) (20% to 30% of cases)
    e. Absence of free hydrochloric acid in the stomach

2. Oral symptoms
   a. Cheilosis
   b. Smooth, red, painful tongue with atrophy of filiform and fungiform papillae
D. Histologic characteristics
   1. Altered exfoliated squamous epithelial cells of the tongue and soft tissues
   2. Deficiency of keratinized cells
   3. Abnormal cell maturation; enlarged nuclei
E. Treatment
   1. Iron, vitamin B complex therapy
   2. High-protein diet

Aplastic Anemia
Primary Aplastic Anemia
A. Etiology—unknown
B. Age and sex affected—young adults; males and females equally affected
C. Clinical features—oral symptoms
   1. Spontaneous bleeding
   2. Petechiae
   3. Purpuric spots
   4. Gingival infection
   5. Pallor of oral tissues
D. Laboratory tests/findings
   1. Reduction in the number of all blood cells (pancytopenia)
   2. Reduction in the number of red blood cells (anemia)
   3. Reduction in the number of white blood cells (leukopenia)
   4. Reduction in the number of platelets (thrombocytopenia)
   5. Bone marrow changes
E. Treatment/prognosis
   1. Blood transfusions
   2. Antibiotics
   3. Rapid destruction; usually fatal

Secondary Aplastic Anemia
A. Etiology
   1. Exposure to a drug or chemical substance
   2. Exposure to radiant energy—x-rays, radium, or radioactive isotopes
B. Age and sex affected—any age; males and females equally affected
C. Clinical features—same as in primary aplastic anemia
D. Treatment/prognosis
   1. Remove cause
   2. Support therapy
   3. Prognosis good

Thalassemia (Cooley's Anemia, Erythroblastic Anemia)
A. Etiology—hereditary and racial
   1. Defect in the component controlling the rate of synthesis of adult hemoglobin
   2. Transmitted by autosomal recessive trait
   3. Racial predilection—Mediterranean countries
B. Age and sex affected—within the first 2 years (homozygous); later in childhood, mild form (heterozygous); males and females equally affected
C. Clinical features
   1. Systemic symptoms
      a. Yellow pallor of the skin
      b. Enlarged spleen (splenomegaly); enlarged liver (hepatomegaly)
      c. Mongoloid facial features
         (1) Sunken nose bridge
         (2) Protruding zygoma
         (3) Slanting eyes
   2. Oral symptoms
      a. Malocclusion; protrusion of the maxillary anterior teeth
      b. Pallor of the mucosa
D. Radiographic appearance
   1. Peculiar trabecular pattern of the maxilla and mandible—"salt-and-pepper" effect
   2. Mild osteoporosis of the jaws
   3. Thinning of lamina dura
E. Laboratory tests/findings
   1. Elevated white blood cell count—10,000 to 25,000/mm^3
   2. Elevated serum bilirubin level
   3. Decreased hemoglobin level
F. Histologic characteristics—bone marrow shows cellular hyperplasia
G. Treatment/prognosis
   1. Splectomy and periodic blood transfusions provide temporary remissions
   2. Prognosis poor

Polycythemia
General Characteristics
A. Abnormal increase in the number of red blood cells
B. Increased hemoglobin level
C. Three forms
   1. Relative polycythemia—temporary increase in the number of red blood cells caused by shock, a severe burn, or excessive loss of body fluids
   2. Primary polycythemia
   3. Secondary polycythemia

Primary Polycythemia (Polycythemia Vera, Erythremia)

A. Etiology—unknown; possibly familial

B. Age and sex affected—over 40 years; more common in males

C. Clinical features
1. Systemic symptoms
   a. Headache, dizziness, weakness
   b. Enlarged, painful spleen
   c. Gastric complaints; peptic ulcers
   d. Tips of fingers cyanotic
   e. Nose bleeds easily (epistaxis)
2. Oral symptoms
   a. Oral mucosa deep red to purple because of the decreased hemoglobin level
   b. Gingivae swollen and spongy; bleed easily
   c. Submucosal petechiae

D. Laboratory tests/findings
1. Red blood cell count elevated to 10,000,000 to 12,000,000/mm^3
2. Increase in
   a. Hemoglobin content
   b. Blood viscosity
   c. Platelet and white blood cell count
   d. Hematocrit value

E. Treatment/prognosis
1. Nonspecific treatment; phenylhydrazine to destroy or interfere with production of red blood cells
2. Radioactive isotope phosphorus
3. Therapy provides only temporary remissions

Secondary Polycythemia (Erythrocytosis)

A. Etiology
1. Bone marrow anoxia (lack of oxygen) caused by
   a. Pulmonary dysfunction
   b. Heart disease
   c. High altitudes
   d. Carbon monoxide poisoning
2. Production of stimulatory factors such as drugs or chemicals

B. Other characteristics and features similar to those of primary polycythemia

Agranulocytosis

A. Etiology
1. Primary form—unknown
2. Secondary form—drug ingestion or allergic reaction

B. Age and sex affected—any age; more common in adults; more common in females

C. Clinical features
1. Systemic symptoms
   a. Sudden onset
   b. High fever, chills, sore throat
   c. Malaise, weakness
   d. Skin is jaundiced
2. Oral symptoms
   a. Infection in the oral cavity
   b. Regional lymphadenitis
   c. Ulcerations of the tonsils, pharynx, palate, and gingiva
   d. Hemorrhage occurs, especially from the gingiva
   e. Excessive salivation

D. Laboratory tests/findings—severe decrease or absence of granulocytes or polymorphonuclear cells; bone marrow has few or no granulocytes

E. Histologic characteristics
1. Necrosis of the gingiva, sulcus, free gingiva, periodontal ligament, alveolar bone
2. Rapid destruction of supporting structures of teeth

F. Treatment
1. All dental surgical procedures should be avoided
2. Removal of the causative drug or agent
3. Antibiotics
4. Transfusions

Cyclic Neutropenia

A. Etiology—unknown, possibly hormonal or allergic factors

B. Age and sex affected—infants and young children; males and females equally affected

C. Clinical features
1. Systemic symptoms
   a. General weakness
   b. Fever, sore throat, headache
   c. Regional lymphadenopathy
2. Oral symptoms
   a. Severe gingivitis, stomatitis, periodontitis
   b. Ulcerations
   c. Mild to severe loss of alveolar bone

D. Laboratory tests/findings
1. Periodic depression of granulocytes
2. Neutrophils may completely disappear in the acute stage

E. Treatment/prognosis
1. Nonspecific
2. Splenectomy sometimes beneficial
3. Remission periods

Leukemia

General Characteristics
A. Malignant neoplasm involving blood-forming cells
B. Excessive proliferation of white blood cells in the immature state
C. Etiology—unknown; theories include
   1. Infections
   2. Virus
   3. Chronic exposure to chemicals or radiation
   4. Patients with Down syndrome (mongoloidism) have a high incidence
   5. Chromosome abnormalities present

Acute Leukemia
A. Age and sex affected—children and young adults; males and females equally affected
B. Clinical features
   1. Systemic symptoms
      a. Sudden onset
      b. Weakness, fever, headache, infection
      c. Swelling of lymph nodes—often the first sign
      d. Hemorrhages on the skin and mucous membranes—caused by a decrease in the number of platelets
      e. Enlargement of organs—spleen, liver, kidney
      f. Bone and joint pain
   2. Oral symptoms
      a. Purpuric spots
      b. Severe gingival enlargement; red, soft, spongy; spontaneous bleeding
      c. Sometimes similar to Vincent's infection—ulcerations, blunted papillae, necrosis, odor
      d. Pallor of tissues
      e. Toothache caused by invasion and necrosis of the pulp
      f. Mobility of teeth caused by a breakdown of the periodontal membrane and supporting structures
C. Laboratory tests/findings
   1. Both anemia and thrombocytopenia present
   2. Prolonged bleeding and coagulation times
   3. White blood cell count elevated to 100,000/mm^3
D. Treatment/prognosis
   1. Transfusions
   2. Antibiotics
   3. Corticosteroids and antimetabolites provide periods of remission
   4. Fatal in 2 to 3 months

Chronic Leukemia
A. Age and sex affected—middle age or older; males and females equally affected
B. Clinical features
   1. Systemic symptoms
      a. Very slow onset—disease may be present for weeks or months before symptoms lead to diagnosis
      b. Pallor
      c. Lymph node enlargement in the chronic lymphatic type; not in the myeloid type
      d. Xerostomia (dry mouth)
      e. Petechiae on the skin with nodules of leukemic cells
      f. Destructive bone lesions—result in fracture
   2. Oral symptoms
      a. Gingival tissues may be normal for some time, then become tender and enlarged
      b. Pallor of the gingiva and lips
      c. Purpuric spots
      d. Enlarged lymph nodes
C. Laboratory tests/findings
   1. Anemia and thrombocytopenia sometimes present
   2. White blood cell count—500,000/mm^3 (95% of the total number of blood cells)
   3. Shift to the left in maturity of the cells
   4. Differential count elevated in the cell type involved
D. Treatment/prognosis
   1. Radiation therapy to the marrow, spleen, and lymph nodes
   2. Chemotherapy
   3. Remissions occur
   4. Untreated, fatal in 2 to 3 years; if treated, fatal in 5 to 7 years

Purpura

General Characteristics
A. Purplish discoloration of the skin and mucous membranes resulting from spontaneous escape of blood into tissues
B. Caused by
   1. Defect or deficiency in blood platelets (thrombocytopenic purpura)
   2. Unexplained increase in capillary fragility (vascular or nonthrombocytopenic purpura)

Thrombocytopenic Purpura (Werlhof's Disease)
A. Etiology
   1. Primary—unknown; autoimmune mechanism in which the patient is immunized against his or her own platelets

2. Secondary—caused by a variety of conditions, including
   a. Drug toxicity
   b. Allergic reactions
   c. Infectious diseases
   d. Malignant neoplasms
B. Age and sex affected—primary in childhood; secondary at any age; males and females equally affected
C. Clinical features
   1. Systemic symptoms
      a. Spontaneous hemorrhagic lesions on the skin; vary in size (petechiae, ecchymoses, hematomas)
      b. Patient bruises easily
      c. Bleeding via the urinary tract
      d. Bleeding from the nose (epistaxis)
      e. Spleen not palpable
   2. Oral symptoms
      a. Profuse gingival hemorrhage
      b. Clustered petechiae 1 mm or less in size
D. Laboratory tests/findings
   1. Severe reduction in the platelet count—below 60,000/mm^3 (normal—150,000 to 400,000/mm^3)
   2. Bleeding time prolonged to 1 or more hours
   3. Positive capillary fragility test
E. Treatment
   1. Corticosteroids
   2. Transfusions
   3. Bed rest
   4. For secondary form—eliminate cause; splenectomy

Vascular Purpura (Nonthrombocytopenic Purpura)

A. Etiology—results from a variety of conditions that produce capillary fragility: infectious diseases, drug history, etc.
B. Clinical features—platelet count normal; other symptoms similar to those of thrombocytopenic purpura

Hemophilia

A. Etiology
   1. Hereditary; sex linked, occurring only in males
   2. Defect carried by the X chromosome
   3. Transmitted through unaffected daughters to grandsons; sons are normal and not carriers
B. Age and sex affected—present at birth, but symptoms may not appear until later; males only (except with type C)

C. Clinical features
   1. Systemic symptoms
      a. Clotting deficiency produces persistent bleeding
      b. Massive hematomas
      c. Three forms—differ in blood-clotting factor
         (1) Type A—most common; antihemophilic globulin (AHG) factor
         (2) Type B—plasma thromboplastin component (PTC) factor
         (3) Type C—plasma thromboplastin antecedent (PTA); less severe bleeding; not sex linked
   2. Oral symptoms
      a. Gingival hemorrhage
      b. Prolonged hemorrhage following tooth eruption, exfoliation, or extraction
D. Laboratory tests/findings
   1. Prolonged coagulation and venous clotting times
   2. Normal bleeding time and blood cell count
E. Treatment
   1. Hospitalization for transfusions of whole blood
   2. Topical coagulants

FIBROUS DISEASES (DYSPLASIA) ▬▬▬

General Characteristics

A. Rare diseases affecting bones
B. Produce swelling of bones with deformities in some forms of disease
C. Varient forms—all of unknown etiology

Monostotic Fibrous Dysplasia

A. Etiology—unknown; theories include
   1. Local infection
   2. Trauma
B. Age and sex affected—children and young adults; slightly higher incidence in females
C. Location
   1. Ribs—most common site
   2. Mandible, maxilla
   3. Can affect any bone
D. Clinical features
   1. Painless swelling; enlargement of the jaw involving the buccal plate
   2. Can cause malposition, tipping, or displacement of the dentition
   3. In the maxilla lesions are not clearly outlined, since they extend into the sinus or the floor of the orbit

E. Histologic characteristics
   1. Proliferating fibroblasts in the stroma of woven collagen fibers
   2. Irregularly shaped trabeculae; some are C shape
F. Treatment/prognosis
   1. Surgical removal of the deformed area
   2. Radiation therapy contraindicated, since malignant transformations reported
   3. Rarely fatal

Polyostotic Fibrous Dysplasia

A. Etiology—unknown
B. Age and sex affected—childhood; more common in females (3:1)
C. Location
   1. Long bones; often unilateral
   2. Bones of the face and skull
   3. Clavicles
   4. Pelvic bones
D. Clinical features
   1. Systemic symptoms
      a. Painless to slight pain; may be unnoticed
      b. Bowing of long bones
      c. Irregular, pigmented spots on the skin
      d. Females may reach premature puberty at age 2 or 3 years
      e. Dysfunction of the endocrine system—pituitary, thyroid, and parathyroid glands
   2. Oral symptoms
      a. Expansion and deformity of the jaws
      b. Disturbed eruption pattern caused by endocrine dysfunction
E. Radiographic appearance—irregular bone trabeculae; expansion of cortical bone; sometimes a multilocular cystic appearance with several radiolucencies
F. Laboratory tests/findings
   1. Serum alkaline phosphatase level sometimes elevated
   2. Moderately elevated basal metabolic rate
G. Histologic characteristics
   1. Fibrillar connective tissue
   2. Many trabeculae
   3. Irregularly shaped, coarse-woven fibers
   4. Osteocytes
H. Treatment/prognosis
   1. Surgical removal of the deformity
   2. No treatment for minor involvement
   3. Known fatal cases

Albright's Syndrome

Variant of polyostotic fibrous dysplasia
A. Etiology—unknown
B. Age and sex affected—young persons; males and females equally affected
C. Location—same as for polyostotic fibrous dysplasia
D. Clinical features and other characteristics—same as for polyostotic fibrous dysplasia

Cherubism (Familial Fibrous Disease of the Jaws)

A. Etiology—hereditary; autosomal dominant gene
B. Age and sex affected—onset at birth or early childhood; more common in males
C. Location—only in the maxilla and mandible (more common in the mandible)
D. Clinical features
   1. Bilateral enlargement of the jaws; usually posterior area involving the ramus; firm and hard to palpation
   2. Taut facial skin; downward pull of the eyelids; ''cherubic'' appearance
   3. Regional lymphadenopathy
   4. Has been mistaken for an ameloblastoma or multilocular cyst
   5. Primary dentition may be prematurely shed at age 3 years
   6. Permanent dentition often defective; absence of teeth (anodontia); lack of eruption of the teeth present
E. Radiographic appearance—bilateral thinning of cortical plates; numerous unerupted, displaced teeth in cystlike spaces
F. Laboratory tests/findings—all blood levels normal
G. Histologic characteristics
   1. Fibrous tissue proliferation
   2. Numerous large multinucleated giant cells in a loose, delicate, fibrous connective tissue stroma
   3. Fibroblasts; small blood vessels
   4. Epithelial remnants from developing teeth scattered throughout
H. Treatment/prognosis
   1. Self-limiting; remission at 8 to 10 years of age
   2. No surgical intervention
   3. Prognosis good; rare malignant transformation

Cementoma (Cementoblastoma, Periapical Cemental Dysplasia, Periapical Fibrous Dysplasia, Fibrocementoma)

A. Etiology—unknown; theories include
   1. Chronic trauma
   2. Infection of a tooth
   3. Past history of syphilis
   4. Endocrine or hormonal imbalance

B. Age and sex affected—mid-30s; more common in females (15:1) and blacks (8:1)
C. Location
1. Mandible; rare in the maxilla
2. Anterior incisor region
3. Apex of teeth; in or near the periodontal ligament
D. Clinical features
1. Benign, slow-growing multiple lesions
2. Asymptomatic; teeth in the affected area vital
E. Radiographic appearance—depends on the stage of development
1. Osteolytic—radiolucent lesion
2. Cementoblastic—lucent with some opacities
3. Mature—cementum and/or bone densely opaque with a thin rim of lucency
F. Laboratory tests/findings—normal blood levels
G. Histologic characteristics
1. Increase in connective tissue cells of the periodontal ligament
2. Normal bone replaced with a fibrous mass; varying amounts of calcified material within
H. Treatment/prognosis
1. Self-limiting; no treatment necessary
2. Prognosis good; no complications

Paget's Disease (Osteitis Deformans, Osteitis Hyperplastica)

A. Etiology—unknown; theories include
1. Hereditary
2. Vascular involvement; arteriosclerosis
3. History of syphilis; inflammatory response
4. Endocrine imbalance
B. Age and sex affected—over 50 years; more common in males (3:1)
C. Location—bones, including the maxilla and mandible
D. Clinical features
1. Systemic symptoms
a. Symptoms develop slowly
b. Enlargement of bones—spine, femur, tibia, skull (change in hat size)
c. Affected bones are warm to the touch as a result of increased vascularity
d. Severe headache, deafness, dizziness; bone neuralgia
2. Oral symptoms
a. Enlarged maxilla; spread of the dentition
b. No change in enamel or dentin
E. Radiographic appearance
1. Irregular radiolucent and radiopaque areas, giving a cotton wool appearance
2. Root resorption; hypercementosis; lamina dura may be completely absent

F. Laboratory tests/findings
1. Serum calcium and phosphorus levels are normal
2. Serum alkaline phosphatase level is elevated; serum acid phosphatase level is normal
G. Histologic characteristics—characterized by both bone resorption and bone deposition
1. Areas of resorption—osteoclast activity
2. Areas of deposition—osteoblast activity
3. Areas of both resorption and deposition— osteoclasts and osteoblasts present; give mosaic appearance
H. Treatment/prognosis
1. No treatment
2. Fifteen percent develop into sarcomas; prognosis poor

METABOLIC BONE DISEASES
General Characteristics

A. Associated with metabolic disturbances, deficiencies, or excesses
B. Disease can be caused by an internal cellular change or dietary or nutritional intake

Hyperparathyroidism

A. Etiology
1. Primary hyperparathyroidism—parathyroid gland produces an excessive quantity of parathyroid hormone
2. Secondary hyperparathyroidism—accompanies other systemic diseases such as renal disturbances, rickets, or extensive bone tumors
B. Age and sex affected—middle age; more common in females (3:1)
C. Clinical features
1. Systemic symptoms
a. Rare disease with bone pain, joint stiffness, and resorption of bone with spontaneous fractures
b. Urinary tract stones caused by increased calcium in urine
c. Weakness, fatigue, constipation
2. Oral symptoms
a. Resembles a giant cell tumor or cyst
b. Diffuse bone loss causing malocclusion and shifting of teeth
D. Radiographic appearance
1. Cystlike radiolucencies found posteriorly in the jaws; "ground glass" appearance
2. Lamina dura lost or sketchy

E. Laboratory tests/findings
1. Loss of calcium replaced by fibrous tissue
2. Serum calcium level elevated above normal
F. Histologic characteristics
1. Osteoclastic resorption of trabeculae of spongiosa bone
2. Fibrosis of marrow spaces
3. Fibroblasts replace resorbed bone
G. Treatment—surgical excision of the parathyroid gland

Osteoporosis

A. Etiology
1. Calcium deficiencies over a long period of time
2. Factors producing deficiency
   a. Congenital
   b. Vitamin C deficiency; general malnutrition
   c. Senility
B. Age and sex affected—elderly; most common in postmenopausal females
C. Clinical features—systemic symptoms
1. Lower back pain
2. Pathologic fractures
3. Loss of stature; deformities
D. Radiographic appearance—localized or diffuse radiolucencies
E. Laboratory tests/findings—serum calcium, phosphorus, and alkaline phosphatase levels are normal
F. Histologic characteristics—resorption of bone, which increases with age
G. Treatment—estrogen therapy; calcium supplements

Osteomalacia

A. Etiology
1. Deficiency or impaired absorption of Vitamin D (produces osteomalacia in adults; rickets in children)
2. Urinary loss of calcium and phosphorus in renal function
3. Fanconi syndrome—group of diseases related to renal tubular function
B. Age affected—adults
C. Clinical features
1. Loss of calcification of bone; soft bone
   a. Generalized weakness
   b. Bone pain and tenderness; fractures
   c. Affects gait
2. Polyuria—urine output greatly increased
3. Polydipsia—severe thirst
4. No oral symptoms

D. Radiographic appearance
1. Generalized demineralization of bone; "milkman's syndrome"
2. Lamina dura of teeth may be absent
3. Radiopaque renal calculi in the kidney
E. Laboratory tests/findings
1. Low serum calcium and phosphorus levels
2. Serum alkaline phosphorus level elevated
F. Treatment
1. Increased dosage of vitamin D; if malabsorption, water-soluble, synthetic vitamin D can be given
2. Calcium supplements

Rickets

A. Etiology
1. Deficiency of vitamin D, phosphorus, and calcium
2. Form of osteomalacia; failure of calcification of cartilage and bone
B. Age affected—young children
C. Clinical features
1. Systemic symptoms
   a. Pliable bones; bowlegs, knock-knees
   b. Muscle pain
   c. Enlarged skull, spinal curvature
   d. Enlarged liver and spleen
2. Oral symptoms
   a. Retardation of tooth eruption
   b. Malposition of teeth
   c. Retardation of growth of the mandible; Class II malocclusion
D. Treatment—increased dietary intake of vitamin D, calcium, and phosphorus; supplements

Histiocytosis X (Reticuloses)
General Characteristics
A. Etiology—unknown
B. Cells accumulate in granulomatous masses
C. Includes a group of three diseases characterized by proliferation of histiocytes or reticulocytes of the reticuloendothelial system

Letterer-Siwe Disease (Acute or Subacute)
A. Age affected—first 2 years of life
B. Clinical features
1. Skin rash on the trunk, scalp, and extremities
2. Persistent low-grade fever; malaise, irritability
3. Splenomegaly, hepatomegaly
4. Anemia
5. Oral lesions—not common
C. Prognosis—invariably fatal

Hand-Schüller-Christian Disease (Chronic Disseminated)

A. Age affected—early life; more common in males
B. Clinical features
  1. Systemic symptoms—classic triad
    a. Skull and jaws affected (see radiographic appearance)
    b. Diabetes insipidus—result of pituitary dysfunction
    c. Exophthalmos—bulging eyes caused by massive infiltration of reticulocytes
  2. Oral symptoms
    a. Sore mouth without lesions
    b. Halitosis, unpleasant taste
    c. Loose, sore teeth
    d. Failure to heal after extractions
C. Radiographic appearance—radiolucencies in the skull and jaws
D. Treatment/prognosis
  1. Curettage
  2. Radiation therapy
  3. Cytotoxic drugs
  4. Prognosis poor; many fatalities

Eosinophilic Granuloma (Localized)

A. Age and sex affected—older children and young adults; more common in males (2:1)
B. Clinical features
  1. Most benign variety of histiocytosis X
  2. May be asymptomatic; local pain, swelling, tenderness
  3. Sore mouth, fetid breath, loosening of teeth, swollen gingiva
C. Radiographic appearance—irregular radiolucencies, single or multiple; well-defined, resembling a cyst
D. Treatment/prognosis
  1. Curettage
  2. Radiation therapy
  3. Prognosis good

ABNORMALITIES OF TEETH

Loss of Tooth Structure

Attrition

A. Etiology—wearing away of tooth surfaces by active, physiologic forces
  1. Mastication
  2. Bruxism
  3. Occlusion—heavy biting forces
  4. Diet—coarse foods; tobacco chewing
B. Clinical features
  1. Polished facets
  2. Flat incisal edge
  3. Discolored surface
  4. Exposed dentin

Abrasion

A. Etiology—wearing away of tooth structure through abnormal mechanical processes
  1. Toothbrushing
  2. Dentifrices
B. Clinical features
  1. V-shaped wedge at the cervical margin; common in the cuspid and premolar areas
  2. Recession of gingiva creates sensitivity
  3. Pipe smoking abrades where the pipe rests
  4. Notching associated with carpenters and tailors who hold tacks, nails, and pins between their teeth

Erosion

A. Etiology—loss resulting from chemical action
  1. Acid or low-pH fluid intake
  2. Acidic foods habitually used over long periods of time
B. Clinical features
  1. Usually found on labial or buccal surfaces
  2. "Wear" depressions or etchings on cervical or occlusal surfaces
  3. Hypersensitivity of teeth affected

Dental Caries

A. Etiology
  1. Primarily *Streptococcus mutans*
  2. *Lactobacillus acidophilus*—produce acid that reacts with sugars
B. Age and sex affected—highest incidence before 25 years; males and females equally affected
C. Clinical features
  1. Any crown surface affected—most common
    a. Occlusal pits and fissures
    b. Interproximal surfaces
  2. Explorer sticks in a pit, groove, or accessible surface, indicating a lesion has formed
  3. Mesial and distal lesions not observable clinically until large; create a grayish shadow in the area of the marginal ridge
D. Radiographic appearance—radiolucent areas in enamel; extend into dentin and then pulp as the lesion progresses.
E. Laboratory tests/findings—caries activity test (Snyder)
F. Treatment—restorative dentistry: composite, amalgam, or gold

Developmental Defects Affecting Enamel and Dentin

Amelogenesis Imperfecta (Hereditary Enamel Dysplasia, Hereditary Brown Enamel, Hereditary Brown Opalescent Teeth)

A. Etiology—malfunction of the tooth germ
B. Produces two types
  1. Enamel hypoplasia—defect in formation of the matrix
    a. Etiology—hereditary; environmental such as nutritional deficiency, congenital syphilis, high fever, birth injuries
    b. Enamel of primary and permanent teeth appear pitted; vertical grooving; deficiency in thickness (aplasia); yellow to dark brown; open contacts; occlusal wear
    c. Radiographic appearance—enamel absent or very thin layer over tips of cusps and interproximal areas
    d. Histologic characteristics—thin, defective enamel; few enamel prisms; no lamellae
    e. Treatment—restorations; crowns; bonding
  2. Enamel hypocalcification—defect in mineralization of the formed matrix
    a. Etiology—autosomal trait
    b. Enamel yellow to dark brown; chalky and breaks down easily
    c. Radiographic appearance—tooth shape normal; enamel and dentin have same radiodensity, which makes it difficult to differentiate
    d. Histologic characteristics—broadening of interprismatic substance; distinct enamel prisms; enamel low in mineral content
    e. Treatment—restorations; crowns; bonding

Dentinogenesis Imperfecta (Hereditary Opalescent Dentin)

A. Etiology
  1. Hereditary
  2. Disturbance of dentin formation
    a. Affects mesodermal component
    b. Enamel remains normal
B. Clinical features
  1. Teeth appear "opalescent," a translucent hue
  2. Gray to bluish brown color
  3. Distinct constriction at the cementoenamel junction
C. Radiographic appearance
  1. Partial or total obliteration of pulp chambers and root canals

  2. Roots are short, blunted, and sometimes fractured
  3. Cementum, periodontal membrane, and alveolar bone appear normal
D. Histologic characteristics
  1. Mesoderm disturbance
  2. Dentin composed of irregular tubules; uncalcified matrix
  3. Tubules large in width; few in number
  4. Odontoblasts degenerate easily within the matrix
  5. Decrease in inorganic content
E. Treatment—cast metal crowns; caution needed with partial appliances because of root fractures

Developmental Defects Affecting Tooth Shape

Dilaceration

Sharp bend or curve in the root of a formed tooth
A. Etiology—trauma during tooth development
  1. Calcified area displaced
  2. Amount of tooth formed at the time of trauma will affect the angle or curve in the root; usually affects the apical third of the root
B. Radiographic appearance—bend in the root
C. Treatment—none

Fusion

Union of two normally separated tooth germs
A. Etiology—physical force or abnormal pressure; hereditary tendency
B. Clinical features
  1. If the defect occurs early in development, one large tooth
  2. If the defect occurs later, fusion of roots only
  3. Dentin always confluent
  4. Can occur in both deciduous and permanent dentitions
  5. Can occur between two normal teeth or one normal tooth and one supernumerary tooth
C. Radiographic appearance—can have separate or fused root canals
D. Treatment—usually none; hemisection for a crown or bridge if necessary

Gemination

Division of a single tooth germ by invagination; results in incomplete formation of two teeth
A. Etiology—possibly trauma; hereditary tendency
B. Can affect deciduous dentition
C. Usually have two completely or incompletely separate crowns with one root; one root canal

Concrescence

Fusion that occurs after root formation completed; roots united by cementum
A. Etiology—traumatic injury; crowding of teeth with resorption of interdental bone
B. Radiographic appearance—establishes diagnosis, since teeth are joined at the root surfaces and cannot be observed clinically

Dens in Dente

Tooth within a tooth
A. Etiology—increased localized external pressure; growth retardation
B. Location—maxillary lateral incisor in the area of the lingual pit
C. Frequently bilateral
D. Radiographic appearance—small tooth within the pulp chamber
E. Treatment—none unless the pulp becomes inflamed or necrotic

Natal Teeth

Teeth present at birth
A. Etiology—develop from
  1. Part of dental lamina before the deciduous bud or
  2. Bud of accessory dental lamina
  3. May represent a dental lamina cyst
B. Location—usually found in the mandibular anterior incisor area
C. Histologic characteristics—hornified epithelial structures without roots (therefore not true teeth)
D. Treatment/prognosis
  1. Removal (after determining they are not prematurely erupted deciduous teeth)
  2. Prognosis excellent; no complications

Developmental Defects Affecting the Number of Teeth

Anodontia

Missing teeth
A. Etiology—no tooth germ developed
B. Two forms
  1. Total anodontia
    a. Rare condition—all teeth missing
    b. May involve both deciduous and permanent dentitions
    c. Usually associated with hereditary ectodermal dysplasia
  2. Partial anodontia
    a. Rather common
    b. Teeth usually affected include third molars and maxillary lateral incisors
    c. Familial/hereditary tendency

Supernumerary Teeth

More than the normal number of teeth
A. Etiology—additional tooth buds arise from dental lamina; hereditary
B. Classification
  1. Mesiodent (mesiodens)—most common; cone-shaped crown; short root; located between the maxillary centrals
  2. Maxillary fourth molar—distal to the third molar; occasionally find a mandibular fourth molar
  3. Maxillary paramolar—usually a small molar; located buccally or lingually in the area of the maxillary molars
C. Treatment—none; observe for cystic transition; remove when interfere with normal dentition

Developmental Defects Affecting Tooth Size

Macrodontia

Abnormally large tooth; rare; possibly a result of fusion

Microdontia

Abnormally small tooth; maxillary lateral incisor and third molar most commonly affected

ABNORMALITIES OF ORAL SOFT TISSUES

Abnormalities Affecting Mucous Membranes or Skin

Amalgam Tattoo
A. Etiology—dust or particle of an amalgam restoration embedded in the mucosa or gingiva
B. Clinical features—blue to purplish area near an amalgam restoration
C. Radiographic appearance—radiopaque
D. Treatment—none unless inflammation results

Melanin

Dark pigmentation of the gingiva or mucosa
A. Etiology—hereditary; dark-complexioned races most commonly affected
B. Treatment—none, since tissue is healthy

Angular Stomatitis
A. Etiology
  1. Idiopathic
  2. Nutritional deficiency
  3. Denture irritation
  4. Infections

B. Clinical features—inflammation and cracking at the corners of the lips; extend into facial skin

C. Histologic characteristics—inflammatory cells

D. Treatment—dependent on the etiology: improve the diet; correct the vertical dimension of the denture

Fordyce's Granules

A. Etiology—developmental; aberrant sebaceous glands

B. Clinical features
   1. Affects the vermilion of the lips and buccal mucosa
   2. Yellow, slightly raised spots a few millimeters in size

C. Histologic characteristics—glandular tissue; not pathologic

D. Treatment—none

Abnormalities Affecting the Tongue

Geographic Tongue (Benign Migratory Glossitis)

A. Etiology—unknown; theories include
   1. Nutritional deficiency
   2. Hereditary
   3. Psychogenic origin

B. Age and sex affected—any age, but more common in children and young adults; males and females equally affected

C. Clinical features
   1. Fungiform papillae appear as red, mushroomlike projections
   2. Condition assumes variations in shape, giving a maplike appearance
   3. Discomfort

D. Histologic characteristics—characteristic inflammatory cells; keratotic cells around the borders of the lesion

E. Treatment—none

Black Hairy Tongue

A. Etiology—irritation to filiform papillae caused by
   1. Smoking
   2. Alcohol
   3. Hydrogen peroxide
   4. Antacid liquids

B. Clinical features—brownish to black appearance on the dorsum or middle third of the tongue

C. Histologic characteristics—elongation of filiform papillae; characteristic inflammatory cells

D. Treatment/prognosis
   1. Brushing or scraping of the tongue
   2. Prognosis good; totally reversible

SUGGESTED READINGS

Bhaskar, S.N.: Synopsis of oral pathology, ed. 6, St. Louis, 1981, The C.V. Mosby Co.

Eversole, L.R.: Clinical outline of oral pathology, ed. 2, Philadelphia, 1984, Lea & Febiger.

Kerr, D.A., Ash, M.M., Jr., and Millard, H.D.: Oral diagnosis, St. Louis, 1983, The C.V. Mosby Co.

Lynch, M.A., Brightman, V.J., and Greenberg, M.S., editors: Burket's oral medicine, ed. 8, Philadelphia, 1984, J.B. Lippincott Co.

Rose, L.F., and Kaye, D.: Internal medicine for dentistry, St. Louis, 1983, The C.V. Mosby Co.

Scopp, I.W.: Oral medicine: a clinical approach with basic science correlation, ed. 2, St. Louis, 1973, The C.V. Mosby Co.

Shafer, W.G., Hine, M.K., and Levy, B.M.: A textbook of oral pathology, ed. 4, Philadelphia, 1983, W.B. Saunders Co.

Smith, R.M., Turner, J.E., and Robbins, M.L.: Atlas of oral pathology, St. Louis, 1981, The C.V. Mosby Co.

Wood, N.K., and Goaz, P.W.: Differential diagnosis of oral lesions, ed. 2, St. Louis, 1980, The C.V. Mosby Co.

Zegarelli, E.V., Kutscher, A.H., and Hyman, G.A.: Diagnosis of diseases of the mouth and jaws, ed. 2, Philadelphia, 1978, Lea & Febiger.

Review Questions

1 In which of the following would you *not* be able to use the radiographic diagnostic method?
1. Caries
2. To determine supernumerary teeth
3. Odontoma
4. Fibroma
5. Cementoma

2 Which one of the diagnostic methods listed is most reliable and ensures the highest degree of accuracy?
1. Surgical
2. Differential
3. Therapeutic
4. Clinical
5. Historical

3 Which of the following does *not* define the term *pathogenesis?*
1. How the lesion begins
2. Behavior of the lesion
3. Clinical picture of the lesion
4. Development of the lesion
5. Evolution of the lesion

4 A pyogenic granuloma is known to *scar down* to a (an)
1. Pregnancy tumor
2. Fibrogranuloma
3. Lipoma
4. Osteoma
5. Odontoma

5 The patient is a 28-year-old woman. A gingival lesion between the maxillary central and lateral incisors is bright red, soft, and spongy; it bleeds easily; and it is caused by an irritant. The histology report shows proliferation of inflammatory cells and thin epithelium. It is likely that the lesion is
1. A fibroma
2. A pyogenic granuloma
3. Redundant tissue
4. A papilloma
5. Pseudopapillomatosis

6 Which one of the following cysts has the potential of developing into an ameloblastoma?
1. Lateral periodontal cyst
2. Primordial cyst
3. Stafne's bone cyst
4. Residual cyst
5. Traumatic bone cyst

7 Clinical examination reveals a possible leukoplakia. The first course of action should be
1. To perform a biopsy
2. To perform surgical stripping
3. To give the patient vitamin A therapy
4. To have the patient return in 1 month to check the growth
5. To perform a blood test

8 Which one of the following tests is *not* used for pemphigus?
1. Pels-Macht
2. Tzanck test
3. Rabbit eye
4. Nikolsky's sign
5. Immunofluorescent test

9 The palatal condition of an elderly patient *primarily* caused by chronic irritation from the suction chamber of a denture would be
1. A fibroma
2. A papilloma
3. Pseudopapillomatosis
4. A median palatal cyst
5. Primary aplastic anemia

10 A lesion found on the buccal mucosa of a 30-year-old white woman is pink, well-defined, and soft to palpation. It has been slow growing and histologically consists of collagenous fibers, fibroblasts, and fibrocytes, but no fat cells or bone. It has a pendunculate base. The lesion is likely a
1. Fibrosarcoma
2. Fibroma
3. Fibrolipoma
4. Fibroosteoma
5. Papilloma

11 A radiolucent lesion in the posterior part of the mandible, anterior to the angle, has radiographic features of a cyst. After surgical intervention, the histology report shows submaxillary salivary gland tissue. One may conclude the lesion is
1. A residual cyst
2. A traumatic bone cyst
3. Stoffer's bone cyst
4. A lingual mandibular bone concavity
5. An ameloblastoma

12 A cyst commonly found in the floor of the mouth changes size between meals. Clinically, it has a bluish hue. It may be caused by
1. A decayed tooth
2. Blockage of a major salivary duct
3. Failure of developmental fusion of the branchial arches
4. Medications that cause xerostomia
5. Chemotherapy

13 Pleuropneumonia-like organisms (PPLOs), mycoplasmas, severe systemic complications, and a triad of symptom locations (oral, eye, and genital) in a male patient are specifically indicative of
1. Erythema multiforme
2. Stevens-Johnson syndrome
3. Beçhet's syndrome
4. Recurrent ulcerative stomatitis (RUS)
5. Acquired immune deficiency syndrome (AIDS)

14 For which one of the following is the etiology definitely known?
1. Papilloma
2. Torus
3. Granuloma
4. Lipoma
5. Polyostotic fibrous dysplasia

15 In the histology report for a granuloma the following cells are found in abundance
1. Mesenchymal cells
2. Squamous epithelial cells
3. Osteoblasts
4. Fibroblasts
5. Osteoclasts

16 There are two types of hereditary gingival fibromatosis. The one that is significant *after* the eruption of permanent teeth is
1. Nodular
2. Symmetric
3. Chemical
4. Epithelial
5. Skeletal

17 An intraoral examination shows a clinical picture of punched-out papillae. The patient complains of pain and a bad taste. The history indicates that the patient's diet is poor and that he has been under stress. The course of action would be to
1. Do a culture and laboratory study
2. Apply a therapeutic diagnosis and debride the mouth, do a light curettage, recommend hydrogen peroxide mouth rinse, and reappoint
3. Immediately refer the patient to a periodontist
4. Do a complete prophylaxis, which would include extensive root planing and curettage
5. Send patient for a complete blood cell count

18 The histology reports for leukoplakia should show *all* of the following *except*
1. Dyskeratosis
2. Acanthosis
3. Large nuclei
4. Some necrosis
5. Osteoclasts

19 Which one of the following is *most* important to the pathologist when a chondroma is in question?
1. A complete personal history of the patient
2. Complete removal of the tumor in question
3. Submission of a large-enough sample of tissue for histologic study, since a chondroma resembles a malignant chondrosarcoma
4. Radiographs of all large bones
5. Employment of radiation and chemotherapy

20 The clinical picture of this lesion is a well-defined yellowish blisterlike eruption. It is a rare, benign neoplasm. The histology report shows a predominance of fat cells. One may conclude the lesion is a (an)
1. Papilloma
2. Osteoma
3. Lipoma
4. Fibroma
5. Myxoma

21 A tooth involved with a cyst is discovered to be *not* vital on pulp testing. The cyst is probably
1. A residual cyst
2. A lateral periodontal cyst
3. A radicular cyst
4. A dentigerous cyst
5. Stafne's bone cyst

22 Which one of the following is very characteristic of pemphigus vulgaris?
1. Nikolsky's sign
2. Black females
3. Drug reaction etiology
4. White males
5. Positive rabbit eye test

23 The clinical picture reveals a palpable benign tumor in the anterior midline of the palate. The tumor arises from deeper tissue and seems to originate from the periodontal ligament. The radiograph shows the lesion infiltrating bone but no metastasis. The patient is a 35-year-old woman. A possible diagnosis is a (an)
1. Peripheral giant cell granuloma
2. Lipoma
3. Torus palatinus
4. Irritative fibroma
5. Pregnancy tumor

24 The clinical picture of this lesion shows a severe drug reaction, with the lips especially affected. There are also skin "bull's-eye" lesions, which had an abrupt onset. The diagnosis would most likely be
1. Lichen planus
2. Herpes
3. Erythema multiforme
4. Mononucleosis
5. Acquired immune deficiency syndrome (AIDS)

25 Which one of the following cysts is the result of extracting a tooth without the cystic sac?
1. Radicular cyst
2. Residual cyst
3. Periodontal cyst
4. Primordial cyst
5. Traumatic bone cyst

26 The dental hygienist observes a clinical picture of gingival fibromatosis resulting from a chemical reaction from phenytoin (Dilantin) therapy. Which one of the following statements is correct?
1. The patient should stop taking the drug
2. There is an overgrowth of connective tissue
3. There is an overgrowth of epithelium
4. A gingivectomy would "cure" the condition
5. The condition is related to hereditary fibromatosis

27 Which one of the following diagnostic methods should be applied to establish the diagnosis of stomatitis nicotina?
1. Surgical
2. Radiographic
3. Laboratory
4. Clinical and historical
5. Therapeutic

28 Clinically, this white cauliflower-like lesion is similar to a wart. The histology report shows long fingerlike projections of epithelium. The etiology is unknown. One could suspect
1. Verruca vulgaris
2. Papilloma
3. Hyperkeratotic fibroma
4. Linea alba
5. Melanoma

29 The location specifically important in diagnosing a lateral periodontal cyst is

1. $\underline{4, 3 \mid 3, 4}$
2. $\underline{1 \mid 1}$
3. $\overline{4, 3 \mid 3, 4}$
4. $\overline{8 \mid 8}$
5. $\underline{8 \mid 8}$

30 A platelet count of 150,000 to 400,000/mm³ of blood could *not* be indicative of

1. Thrombocytopenia
2. Anemia
3. Leukemia
4. Nonthrombocytopenia
5. Mononucleosis

31 Which one of the following is *not* a true characteristic of acute necrotizing ulcerative gingivitis (ANUG)?

1. Punched-out papillae and craters
2. Hyperkeratinization
3. Odor
4. Pain and bleeding
5. Necrotic slough of epithelium

32 The most accepted theory in the etiology of Beçhet's syndrome is

1. Viral origin
2. Metabolic origin
3. Pleuropneumonia-like organisms (PPLOs)
4. Hormonal origin
5. Sexual transmission

33 Which of the following makes Beçhet's syndrome different from recurrent ulcerative stomatitis (RUS)?

1. Skin and eye lesions
2. A triad of locations of lesions (oral, eye, and genital)
3. Exudate from lesions
4. Mesenchymal proliferations
5. Osteoclastic activity

34 Herpangina is caused by

1. Chickenpox virus
2. Coxsackievirus
3. Epstein-Barr (EB) virus
4. Varicella
5. Pleuropneumonia-like organisms (PPLOs)

35 In treatment of fibrous dysplasia, which one of the following would *not* be advised?

1. Radiation
2. Surgery
3. Chemotherapy
4. Bone marrow depressants
5. Transplants

36 Precocious puberty is *most* characteristic of which of the following?

1. Jaffe's syndrome
2. Monostotic fibrous dysplasia
3. Polyostotic fibrous dysplasia
4. Albright's syndrome
5. Paget's disease

37 The most conclusive diagnostic approach to a malignant lesion is

1. Complete excision
2. Radiation therapy
3. Biopsy
4. Chemotherapy
5. Stripping

38 The radiographic appearance of a malignant lesion in bone will

1. Show destruction at the earliest stages
2. Show destruction when 10% to 20% of the bone is destroyed
3. Show destruction when 40% to 60% of the bone is destroyed
4. Never be fully determined
5. Go from radiopaque to radiolucent

39 Achlorhydria, inability to absorb vitamin B_{12}, and lack of folic acid are characteristic of

1. Thrombocytopenia
2. Hypervitaminosis
3. Pernicious anemia
4. Hyperkeratosis
5. Herpes

40 Bone marrow anoxia occurs in

1. Secondary polycythemia
2. Pernicious anemia
3. Thalassemia
4. Aplastic anemia
5. Thrombocytopenia

41 Which one of the following is referred to as "Mediterranean anemia"?

1. Acute anemia
2. Thalassemia
3. Aplastic anemia
4. Thrombocytopenia
5. Acquired immune deficiency syndrome (AIDS)

42 In leukopenia, which cell type is *predominantly* involved?

1. Erythrocytes
2. Granulocytes
3. Eosinophils
4. Monocytes
5. Osteocytes

43 Which of the following cysts is involved with nonvital teeth?

1. Nasoalveolar cyst
2. Lateral periodontal cyst
3. Radicular cyst
4. Cyst of the incisive papilla
5. Stafne's bone cyst

44 Which cyst could develop into an ameloblastoma?

1. Residual cyst
2. Primordial cyst
3. Median mandibular cyst
4. Lateral periodontal cyst
5. Radicular cyst

45 A tooth was extracted with a cyst left behind. The cyst would be a
1. Residual cyst
2. Primordial cyst
3. Radicular cyst
4. Dentigerous cyst
5. Lateral periodontal cyst

46 A radicular cyst is *most* often caused by
1. Deep fillings
2. Trauma
3. Primary occlusal traumatism
4. Caries
5. Food impaction

47 Epulis fissuratum is caused by
1. A denture flange
2. The suction chamber of a denture
3. An allergic reaction to acrylic material
4. Denture cleaners
5. Poor oral hygiene

48 Sickle cell anemia is of hereditary origin and is common to what race?
1. White
2. Indian
3. Mediterranean
4. Black
5. Oriental

49 A patient with achlorhydria has
1. A low blood glucose level
2. A lack of hydrochloric acid
3. Too much hydrochloric acid
4. Dry mouth
5. Multiple skin lesions

50 A patient with leukopenia has a (an)
1. Decrease in the number of white blood cells
2. Increase in the number of white blood cells
3. Decrease in the number of red blood cells
4. Decrease in the number of platelets
5. Increase in the number of platelets

Answers and Rationales

1. (4) A fibroma is composed of soft tissue and does not appear radiographically.
   (1) Caries appear radiolucent.
   (2) Supernumerary teeth appear radiopaque.
   (3) An odontoma appears radiopaque.
   (5) An early cementoma appears radiolucent and then radiopaque.

2. (2) Differential diagnosis is the most complete and combines all of the other diagnostic methods.
   (1) Surgical diagnostic methods contribute only a part of the information.
   (3) Therapeutic methods contribute only a minute evaluative approach.
   (4) Clinical methods show the visible picture only.
   (5) Historical methods may show only the age, sex, and race, which may often be noncontributory.

3. (3) The clinical picture itself has nothing to do with the pathogenesis or growth of the lesion in question.
   (1) How the lesion begins is of vital importance; was the onset gradual or acute?
   (2) How the lesion behaves in terms of growth, expansion, etc., is of extreme importance.
   (4) The development of the lesion also describes its progression.
   (5) The evolution of the lesion is really the same as its development.

4. (2) A fibrogranuloma is often referred to as the healing stage of a pyogenic granuloma and contains fibrous cells and granulation tissue.
   (1) *Pregnancy tumor* is another name for a pyogenic granuloma.
   (3) A lipoma is composed primarily of fat cells.
   (4) An osteoma is composed of dense, compact bone.
   (5) An odontoma is composed of tooth structures.

5. (2) *Pyogenic granuloma* is another name for a pregnancy tumor, and all of the diagnostic factors presented contribute to this diagnosis.
   (1) A fibroma is composed of fibroblasts and fibrocytes, has no sex predilection, and is usually observed in patients between the ages of 30 and 50 years.
   (3) Redundant tissue is associated with a denture flange.
   (4) A papilloma is white in color and rare; there is no sex predilection.
   (5) Pseudopapillomatosis is associated with the suction chamber of a denture.

For each question the correct answer and rationale are listed first. The other choices are presented in order with the reasons why they are not correct.

6. (2) Primordial cysts are neoplastic in nature, and the location in the posterior part of the mandible is also contributory.
   (1) Lateral periodontal cysts are found in the mandibular premolar area.
   (3) Stafne's bone cysts are found in the posterior part of the mandible, are composed of salivary gland tissues, and are completely benign in nature.
   (4) A residual cyst is a "remnant" of a radicular cyst that is usually caused by caries.
   (5) Traumatic bone cysts are related to trauma. Surgical intervention stimulates healing within a year.

7. (1) Biopsy findings are the most contributory diagnostic factor for a possible leukoplakia.
   (2) Surgical stripping is performed for hyperkeratosis.
   (3) Vitamin A therapy also assists in hyperkeratosis.
   (4) If leukoplakia is suspected, 1 month is far too long for the patient to wait and return.
   (5) A blood test will be noncontributory.

8. (3) The rabbit eye test is used for primary herpes.
   (1) The Pels-Macht test is used to determine pemphigus.
   (2) The Tzanck test is used to determine pemphigus.
   (4) Nikolsky's sign is used to determine pemphigus.
   (5) The immunofluorescent test is used to determine pemphigus.

9. (3) Pseudopapillomatosis is caused by chronic irritation of the palate from the poor suction of a denture.
   (1) A fibroma has little or nothing to do with a denture, unless irritation from a partial denture clasp irritates the buccal mucosa, where fibromas are often found.
   (2) A papilloma is rare, white, and not related to a denture or to the age of the patient.
   (4) A median palatal cyst is developmental and has nothing to do with dentures.
   (5) Primary aplastic anemia is found in young adults and has nothing to do with dentures.

10. (2) A fibroma primarily consists of fibroblasts and fibrocytes.
    (1) A fibrosarcoma has bone cells.
    (3) A fibrolipoma has fat cells.
    (4) A fibroosteoma has bone cells.
    (5) A papilloma has acanthosis of the epithelium.

11. (4) A lingual mandibular bone concavity is also called Stafne's bone cyst and is composed of salivary gland tissue.
    (1) A residual cyst is "left over" from a radicular cyst, which is found anywhere in the dentition and caused by caries.
    (2) A traumatic bone cyst has no salivary gland tissue. When opened, it is a void. After surgical intervention, the bone fills in within a year.
    (3) Stoffer's bone cyst is a distractor for the alternate term applied to a lingual mandibular bone concavity: *Stafne's bone cyst.*
    (5) An ameloblastoma is found in the same location but does not have salivary gland tissue. It is a very aggressive and pathologic lesion that invades surrounding tissues.

12. (2) Blockage of a major salivary duct usually causes the formation of a ranula, which has the clinical characteristics described.
    (1) A decayed tooth would not produce a blue cystic lesion in the floor of the mouth.
    (3) A ranula is not a developmental cyst; it is usually caused by trauma.
    (4) Dry mouth has nothing to do with cystic formation when related to medications. Medications do not cause cysts.
    (5) Chemotherapy may cause dry mouth, but dry mouth does not cause blue cystic lesions.

13. (3) Beçhet's syndrome is specifically characterized by the triad of oral, eye, and genital symptoms.
    (1) Erythema multiforme does not have genital and eye lesions.
    (2) Stevens-Johnson syndrome is a severe form of erythema multiforme.
    (4) RUS has oral lesions, but not eye or genital lesions.
    (5) AIDS has nothing to do with the triad of symptoms and characteristics described.

14. (3) A granuloma is caused by an irritant.
    (1) Papilloma—the etiology is unknown.
    (2) Torus—the etiology is unknown.
    (4) Lipoma—the etiology is unknown.
    (5) Polyostotic fibrous dysplasia—the etiology is unknown.

15. (4) Fibroblasts and endothelial cells are found in abundance in a granuloma.
    (1) Mesenchyme is an embryonic form of connective tissue.
    (2) Epithelial cells are very few in number in a granuloma.
    (3) Osteoblasts are found in areas of bone formation.
    (5) Osteoclasts are found in areas where bone is being resorbed.

16. (1) Nodular hereditary gingival fibromatosis is significant only after the eruption of permanent teeth.
    (2) Symmetric is also a type of gingival fibromatosis but has no relation to the dentitions.
    (3) Chemical type is related to phenytoin (Dilantin) and is not hereditary.
    (4) Epithelial type is a distractor because in fibromatosis, only the connective tissue proliferates.
    (5) Skeletal type relates to muscles and is not hereditary; the etiology is unknown.

17. (2) Basically one would suspect acute necrotizing ulcerative gingivitis (ANUG) and treat the patient with a therapeutic approach.
    (1) A culture and any laboratory study would be a waste of time, since the culture would show anerobic bacteria, confirming ANUG.
    (3) A periodontist would use the same therapeutic approach, considering the clinical and contributory signs.
    (4) Considering the patient's condition, a complete prophylaxis would be impossible and would demonstrate poor judgment in the case.
    (5) A complete blood cell count would be noncontributory in treating the patient.

18. (5) Osteoclasts would not be visible in a case of suspected leukoplakia, since they are involved in bone formation; in leukoplakia, soft tissue is involved.
    (1) Dyskeratosis is a histologic sign of leukoplakia.
    (2) Acanthosis is a histologic sign of leukoplakia.
    (3) Large nuclei are histologic signs of leukoplakia.
    (4) Some necrosis is a sign of leukoplakia.

19. (3) Since the lesion is so similar to a malignancy, the histology report is of vital importance.
    (1) A personal history is noncontributory, since there is no age or sex predilection in a chondroma.
    (2) Complete removal of something that one is not sure of should never be performed without a thorough diagnostic evaluation.
    (4) Radiographs of all large bones is unnecessary and exposes the patient to radiation; noncontributory information would result.
    (5) The tumor is resistant to radiation therapy.

20. (3) A lipoma is composed of fat cells.
    (1) A papilloma is composed of epithelial cells.
    (2) An osteoma is composed of dense, compact bone.
    (4) A fibroma is composed of fibrous cells.
    (5) A myxoma is composed of loose-textured tissues of delicate reticulin fibers.

21. (3) A radicular cyst is most often caused by caries, and the tooth involved would most likely be nonvital.
    (1) A residual cyst is not associated with a tooth present in the mouth. It results when a radicular cyst is left behind after extraction of the offending tooth.
    (2) Lateral periodontal cysts are always associated with vital teeth.
    (4) A dentigerous cyst is observed in the area of unerupted third molars or is associated with unerupted supernumerary teeth.
    (5) Stafne's bone cyst is not associated with a tooth. It is observed in the mandible and is composed of salivary gland tissues.

22. (1) Nikolsky's sign, in which an air syringe can "blow" the epithelium away from the connective tissue, is one of the most characteristic signs of pemphigus vulgaris.
    (2) There is no sex or racial predilection in pemphigus vulgaris.
    (3) The etiology of pemphigus vulgaris is unknown or may be viral.
    (4) There is no sex or racial predilection in pemphigus vulgaris.
    (5) The rabbit eye test is performed for herpes.

23. (1) All of the characteristics described indicate the presence of a peripheral giant cell granuloma.
    (2) A lipoma is composed of fat cells and is rare and yellowish in color.
    (3) A torus palatinus is a bony hard nonpalpable lesion, is often hereditary, and does not "infiltrate."
    (4) An irritative fibroma is really an inflammatory lesion and the "scar-down" results of a pyogenic granuloma. It is composed only of soft tissues.
    (5) A pregnancy tumor is the same as a pyogenic granuloma and is an inflammatory tumor.

24. (3) Erythema multiforme is caused by a severe drug reaction with an acute onset that seemingly is almost an allergic type of reaction. The bull's-eye description of the lesion is very characteristic.
    (1) Lichen planus is not associated with a drug reaction.
    (2) Herpes is viral in origin.
    (4) Mononucleosis has an etiology that is unknown or possibly related to the Epstein-Barr (EB) virus.
    (5) AIDS is not associated with a drug etiology.

25. (2) The residual cyst is the "leftover" of a radicular cyst when the offending tooth has been extracted with the cyst left behind. It is usually observed on the alveolar ridge.
    (1) The radicular cyst is caused by caries and is found at the apex of the tooth involved.
    (3) A periodontal cyst is found between teeth, and the associated teeth are vital.
    (4) A primordial cyst is neoplastic in nature and is found where a tooth was never formed.
    (5) A traumatic bone cyst is related to trauma; it is often asymptomatic but shows radiographically as a well-defined radiolucent lesion. With surgical intervention the area fills in with new bone.

26. (2) An overgrowth of connective tissue is present in gingival fibromatosis.
    (1) The patient should never stop medication, but the physician may elect to substitute an equally effective drug.
    (3) There is never an overgrowth of epithelium.
    (4) A gingivectomy would temporarily enhance esthetics; however, since the drug is causing the condition, it would return as long as the patient uses the medication.
    (5) The condition is caused by the drug and has nothing to do with other types of fibromatosis.

27. (4) Stomatitis nicotina is an easily detectable pathologic condition when observed clinically, with its hyperkeratosis of the palate and marked inflammation of the salivary duct orifice. These clinical signs, coupled with the history of a patient who smokes a pipe (heat in the pipe causes the hyperkeratosis), make the diagnosis certain.
    (1) Surgical intervention would not be necessary if the irritant, the pipe, were removed and the tissues responded.
    (2) Radiographic diagnosis would be noncontributory, since the soft tissues of the palate are affected.
    (3) A laboratory test would be noncontributory.
    (5) A therapeutic diagnosis would be secondary to first determining the clinical and historical pictures. Vitamin A therapy may assist the reduction of hyperkeratosis.

28. (2) *Papilloma* is always defined as a cauliflower-like lesion similar to a wart. Its etiology is unknown, but warts are caused by a virus.
    (1) *Verruca vulgaris* is another name for a wart.
    (3) A fibroma may occasionally have some hyperkeratosis, but not as a rule. Its etiology is unknown, and it is not a white lesion.

(4) Linea alba is a "white line" that runs along the occlusal plane of the buccal mucosa. It is not considered a lesion per se.

(5) A melanoma is a black malignant lesion. It is one of the most aggressive lesions and is often fatal.

29. (1) The mandibular cuspid and premolar areas are the primary locations for a lateral periodontal cyst.

(2) An incisal canal cyst might be observed between the maxillary central incisors.

(3) A globulomaxillary cyst, which is developmental in nature, might be found in the area of the maxillary cuspid.

(4) A dentigerous cyst, Stafne's bone cyst, or an ameloblastoma, could be found in the mandibular third molar area.

(5) The maxillary third molar area is not a prime location for any cyst.

30. (1) There is a marked decrease in the platelet count in thrombocytopenia—a count of $60,000/mm^3$. The numbers given are normal values for platelets.

(2) The number of red blood cells is severely decreased in anemia.

(3) There is an increase in the number of white blood cells in leukemia.

(4) In nonthrombocytopenic purpura, the platelet count is normal. The bleeding tendency is a result of the fragility of the capillary walls.

(5) There is an increase in the total white blood cell count in mononucleosis. Cells called Downey cells are found in abundance. Mononucleosis can be mistaken for leukemia, but the Paul-Bunnell heterophil test will be positive in mononucleosis.

31. (2) Hyperkeratinization is never found in ANUG, because there is such destruction of the epithelium.

(1) Punched-out papillae and craters are characteristics of ANUG.

(3) Odor is a characteristic of ANUG.

(4) Pain and bleeding are characteristics of ANUG.

(5) Necrosis of epithelium is a characteristic of ANUG.

32. (3) PPLOs are the most widely accepted theory concerning the etiology of Beçhet's syndrome.

(1) A viral etiology is also suspected.

(2) Metabolic etiologic factors may also play a role.

(4) There is a hormonal association, since the disease occurs more often in males (6:1).

(5) Sexual transmission has no relation to the etiology, although the genitalia are affected with lesions.

33. (2) The triad of locations of lesions involving oral, eye, and genital areas is specifically characteristic.

(1) Skin and eye lesions without genital involvement do not provide the triad of locations.

(3) There can be exudate from all types of lesions in RUS or Beçhet's syndrome.

(4) Histologically, the epithelial tissues are involved; however, in Beçhet's syndrome, there is also endothelial proliferation that is not observed in RUS.

(5) There is no bone activity in either disease; all are soft tissue involvements.

34. (2) The coxsackievirus A is the cause of herpangina.

(1) The chickenpox virus causes herpes zoster.

(3) The EB virus is associated with infectious mononucleosis.

(4) *Varicella virus* is another name for the chickenpox virus, which causes herpes zoster.

(5) PPLOs are the organisms associated with Beçhet's syndrome.

35. (1) Radiation therapy has triggered malignant transformation in cases of fibrous dysplasia.

(2) Surgery is often the mode of treatment.

(3) Chemotherapy has not been reported.

(4) Bone marrow depressants are not administered; however, bone recontouring via surgery is usually performed for esthetics.

(5) Any type of transplant or resection is seldom indicated.

36. (4) Albright's syndrome is a variant of polyostotic fibrous dysplasia, with precocious puberty in girls being the strongest diagnostic factor.

(1) Jaffe's syndrome is a *severe* form of polyostotic fibrous dysplasia.

(2) Monostotic fibrous dysplasia does not exhibit precocious puberty.

(3) "Regular" polyostotic fibrous dysplasia does not exhibit precocious puberty.

(5) Paget's disease does not exhibit precocious puberty, since the disease occurs more commonly in men over 50 years of age.

37. (3) If a determination has been made that a lesion may be malignant, the next step toward a conclusive diagnosis is to perform a biopsy. If the biopsy findings are negative but the clinician still believes that the lesion could be malignant because of its other characteristics, a second biopsy should be performed.

(1) Complete excision of an undiagnosed lesion should not be performed.

(2) Radiation therapy is not indicated, especially with an unconfirmed diagnosis.

(4) Chemotherapy is not a diagnostic method.

(5) Stripping is usually done in cases of hyperkeratosis.

38. (3) At least 40% to 60% of the bone involved must be destroyed before it can be seen radiographically.

(1) During the earliest stages nothing is observed radiographically.

(2) A 10% to 20% bone loss is still too little to identify a malignant lesion.

(4) Bone destruction can be observed radiographically in the 40% to 60% bone loss stage.

(5) There will not be a change from dense radiopacity to radiolucency. The lesion will become more and more radiolucent.

39. (3) Lack of hydrochloric acid, vitamin B_{12}, and folic acid are all related to pernicious anemia. The secretion of intrinsic factor (hydrochloric acid) does not occur, therefore preventing B_{12} from being absorbed.

(1) Thrombocytopenia produces a decrease in the number of platelets.

(2) Hypervitaminosis indicates an excess of a particular vitamin.

(4) Hyperkeratosis indicates thickening of, and the formation of a protective layer of cells over, the epithelium.

(5) Herpes is caused by a virus and has nothing to do with vitamins or gastric secretion.

40. (1) Bone marrow anoxia, caused by a particular irritant, occurs in secondary polycythemia.

(2) The etiology of pernicious anemia is related to the lack of hydrochloric acid in the stomach and B_{12} absorption.

(3) In thalassemia, the bone marrow shows cellular hyperplasia.

(4) There is marrow disfunction in aplastic anemia.

(5) There is a decrease of the number of platelets in thrombocytopenia.

41. (2) Thalassemia is often referred to as "Mediterranean anemia" because of the racial predilection.

(1) Acute anemia usually results from an automobile accident.

(3) Aplastic anemia has no location predilection, and the etiology is unknown.

(4) Thrombocytopenia shows a decrease in the number of platelets.

(5) *AIDS* does not refer to any form of anemia.

42. (2) Granulocytes are found in abundance in leukopenia, although there is a reduction in the number of *all* white blood cells.

(1) Erythrocytes form red blood cells.

(3) Eosinophils are few in number in the normal blood, but with a decrease in the total number of white blood cells, their number also is decreased.

(4) Large mononuclear leukocytes in the blood having a great deal of protoplasm are not involved in leukopenia.

(5) Osteocytes are bone-forming cells and have nothing to do with the blood.

43. (3) A radicular cyst is caused by caries; the tooth involved is usually nonvital.

(1) A nasoalveolar cyst is developmental.

(2) A lateral periodontal cyst is found between teeth that are vital.

(4) A cyst of the incisive papilla is developmental.

(5) Stafne's bone cyst involves salivary gland tissues; the dentition is not affected.

44. (2) A primordial cyst is neoplastic in nature and therefore has the potential of developing into an ameloblastoma.

(1) A residual cyst is a remnant of a radicular cyst that was not removed.

(3) A median mandibular cyst is developmental.

(4) A lateral periodontal cyst is not aggressive and is usually found in the mandibular cuspid and premolar areas.

(5) A radicular cyst is associated with a tooth and caused by caries.

45. (1) A residual cyst is the cystic sac left behind after a radicular cyst was incompletely removed. Usually the offending tooth is extracted with the cyst left on the alveolar ridge.

(2) A primordial cyst is a neoplastic cyst found *in place* of a tooth.

(3) A radicular cyst is found at the apex of a tooth and is generally caused by caries.

(4) A dentigerous cyst is a neoplastic cyst usually found around the crown of an unerupted tooth. The mandibular third molar or a supernumerary tooth is the most common location.

(5) A lateral periodontal cyst is found between teeth, with the teeth involved all being vital.

46. (4) Caries is the most common etiologic factor in a radicular cyst.

(1) A deep filling may trigger pulpitis, which stimulates periapical pathology.

(2) Trauma does not usually cause a radicular cyst.

(3) Primary occlusal traumatism is a secondary etiologic factor in a radicular cyst.

(5) Food impaction does not cause a cyst.

47. (1) A denture flange irritating the ridge area causes epulis fissuratum, or redundant tissue.

(2) Poor suction in the palatal chamber causes pseudopapillomatosis.

(3) An allergic reaction to the acrylic, would occur all over the mucosa, not in a specific area.

(4) Denture cleaners help maintain good denture hygiene and prevent tissue response.

(5) Poor oral or denture hygiene can contribute to any oral condition or denture response but is not the primary etiologic factor in epulis fissuratum.

48. (4) One in 600 blacks have sickle cell anemia.

(1) Sickle cell anemia is rarely found in whites.

(2) Sickle cell anemia has not been reported in the Indian race.

(3) Sickle cell anemia is not a Mediterranean disease, as is thalassemia.

(5) Sickle cell anemia has not been reported in the Oriental race.

49. (2) Achlorhydria is a lack of production of intrinsic factor (hydrochloric acid) in the stomach.

(1) A low blood glucose level has nothing to do with the problem.

(3) A lack of production, not an increase in production, of hydrochloric acid occurs in achlorhydria.

(4) Hydrochloric acid production is not related to xerostomia.

(5) Skin lesions are not related to a lack of intrinsic factor.

50. (1) Leukopenia is an abnormality in the blood showing a marked decrease in the number of white blood cells, particularly the granulocytes.

(2) There is no increase in the number of white blood cells.

(3) The number of red blood cells is not changed.

(4) The number of platelets is not changed.

(5) The number of platelets is not changed.

CHAPTER 7

Microbiology and Prevention
of Disease Transmission

JAN SHANER GREENLEE

The practice of dental hygiene involves the risk of contracting diseases such as hepatitis, tuberculosis, respiratory tract infections, and herpes. Self-protection and reducing the possibilities for transmitting disease to patients are responsibilities of the dental hygienist. To recognize disease entities and understand the rationale for aseptic procedures, a basic knowledge of microbiology is required.

The microbiology review covers microbial classification, structure, functions, relationships, and methods of observation. Major diseases caused by microbes are organized by systems. Microbiology of the oral cavity describes the normal oral flora, the microbial structure of plaque, and microbial aspects of oral diseases. Clinical application in dental hygiene practice details sources of contamination and aseptic preparation of the dental unit, instruments, and radiographic equipment. Protective measures for patients, including maximum precautions for the high-risk patient, and dental health professionals are outlined.

General Microbiology

MICROORGANISMS
General Considerations
A. Present in most environments
B. Exhibit characteristics common to all biologic systems: reproduction, metabolism, growth, irritability, adaptability, mutation, and organization
C. Classification of medically important microorganisms
  1. Kingdom Procaryotae
    a. Division I—photobacteria
    b. Division II—nonphotosynthetic bacteria (scotobacteria)
      (1) Class I
        (a) Bacteria
        (b) Includes most bacteria that are human pathogens
      (2) Class II
        (a) Obligatory intracellular parasites of living eucaryotic cells
        (b) Rickettsiae, chlamydiae
      (3) Class III
        (a) Scotobacteria that do not possess cell walls
        (b) Includes the genus *Mycoplasma*
  2. Kingdom Mycetidae
    a. Fungi
    b. Classified by types of spores produced
  3. Viruses
    a. Classification is still evolving but based on
      (1) Type and properties of nucleic acid
      (2) Morphology of nucleoproteins
      (3) Presence and properties of envelopes
    b. Obligatory intracellular parasites
    c. Do not have a true cellular form
    d. Replicate only inside living cells
  4. Protozoa
    a. Members of Kingdom Protista
    b. Unicellular animals
    c. Eucaryotes
    d. Most that cause human disease are parasites of the alimentary tract or hemolymphatic system
  5. Helminths
    a. Members of Kingdom Animalia
    b. Multicellular organisms
    c. Generally parasites of the human alimentary tract or hemolymphatic system
D. Nomenclature—the binomial system
  1. Two-word designation
    a. Genus and species
    b. First word capitalized and both words italicized (e.g., *Escherichia coli*)
  2. Devised by Carolus Linnaeus

Methods of Observation

A. Most commonly used units of measurement
1. Micrometer (μm $= 10^{-6}$ m)
2. Nanometer (nm $= 10^{-9}$ m)
3. Angstrom unit (Å $= 10^{-10}$ m)
4. Millimeter (mm $= 10^{-3}$ m)
5. Centimeter (cm $= 10^{-2}$ m)

B. Light microscopes illuminate objects by visible light
1. Bright-field microscopy
   a. Simple microscopes
   b. Compound microscopes consist of at least two lens systems
      (1) Objective
         (a) Magnifies the specimen and is close to it
         (b) Low power, high power, and oil immersion
      (2) Ocular
         (a) Eyepiece
         (b) Magnifies the image produced by the objective lens
2. Dark-field microscopy
   a. Specimens seen as bright objects against a dark background
   b. Used for examination of unstained microorganisms, hanging-drop preparations, and colloidal solutions
   c. Advantage—allows a view of living bacteria undisturbed in size or shape by fixing and staining techniques
3. Fluorescence microscopy
   a. Used to visualize objects that fluoresce or emit light when exposed to light of a different wavelength
   b. Ultraviolet light, fluorescent chemicals, and special filter systems required
   c. Commonly used in the medical field to track antigen-antibody reactions
4. Phase microscopy
   a. Useful in examining transparent, living cells, including their internal structure, in a fluid medium
   b. Variations in density between the microbes and surrounding medium are capitalized on to increase the contrast between the two
5. Specimen preparation
   a. Viewing living organisms
      (1) Methods
         (a) Hanging drop
         (b) Temporary wet mount
      (2) Advantages
         (a) Maintain shape of organisms
         (b) Useful to determine size, shape, motility, and reactions to chemicals or immune sera

   b. Staining
      (1) Procedure
         (a) Thin films of microorganisms are spread on a glass slide and allowed to dry (smear)
         (b) Films are fixed, either by a chemical fixative or by passing through a flame; this coagulates the protein and kills the cell
         (c) Dyes or stains are applied to the smear to allow for greater visualization; allows some differentiation of species
         (d) Fixation process tends to reduce the size of cells; dye addition tends to increase the size of cells
      (2) Types of dyes
         (a) Acidic or negative is used to stain cytoplasmic materials
         (b) Basic or positive is used to stain nuclear components
      (3) Simple staining procedures
         (a) Uses a single dye (e.g., carbolfuchsin, crystal violet, methylene blue, or safranin)
         (b) Used to show shapes, sizes, arrangements of bacterial cells, and presence of spores
      (4) Differential staining procedures
         (a) More than one dye preparation used
         (b) Most common methods
            [1] Gram stain differentiates microorganisms based on color as gram positive (purple or blue) or gram negative (red); certain characteristics of microorganisms appear correlated to their staining reactions: cell wall thickness, chemical composition, and sensitivity to penicillin; useful in diagnosis of infectious diseases
            [2] Acid-fast stain is used to differentiate mycobacteria (e.g., *Mycobacterium leprae* and *Mycobacterium tuberculosis*) from other bacteria; organisms resist decolorization with an acidic solution of alcohol after being stained with a basic dye

[3] Spore stain is used to identify spore-producing bacteria such as those belonging to the genera *Bacillus* and *Clostridium*

(c) Used for preliminary bacterial grouping

C. Electron microscopy
1. Electrons used as a source of illumination
2. Higher magnification and better resolving power available than with a light microscope
3. Types
   a. Transmission electron microscope
   b. High-voltage electron microscope
   c. Scanning electron microscope

Procaryotic (Bacterial) Cell Structure and Function (Table 7-1)

A. Bacterial morphology
1. Cocci (singular, coccus)
   a. Spherical shape
   b. Occur in pairs (diplococci), chains (streptococci), four-in-a-square arrangement (tetrad), eight cells in a cubic arrangement (sarcinae), and irregular clusters (staphylococci)
2. Bacilli (singular, bacillus)
   a. Cylindric or rodlike
   b. Occur in pairs (diplobacilli), chains (streptobacilli), and small, rounded rods (coccobacilli)
3. Spirilla (singular, spirillum)
   a. Spiral
   b. Vary in number and fullness of turns
   c. Vibrios are portions of a spiral
B. Bacterial surface structures
1. Appendages
   a. Flagella
      (1) Responsible for motility; motility must be distinguished from brownian movement, which is caused by bacteria being hit by molecules in their surrounding medium; flagella enable bacteria to move toward more favorable environments (e.g., toward nutrients [chemotaxis])
      (2) Composed of protein called flagellin
      (3) Thinner than those of eucaryotic cells
   b. Pili
      (1) Enable bacteria to adhere to surfaces (e.g., *Neisseria gonorrhoeae*)
      (2) Attach to other bacteria before deoxyribonucleic acid (DNA) transfer
      (3) Serve as receptor sites for bacterial viruses

c. Axial filaments
   (1) Aid in motility
   (2) Spirochetes move by this method
2. Surface adherents
   a. Capsules
      (1) Organized masses of polysaccharides and/or polypeptides
      (2) Encapsulation protects pathogenic organisms from drugs, phagocytosis, and bactericidal factors
      (3) Some bacteria needing capsules to maintain virulence include *Streptococcus pneumoniae* and *Streptococcus mutans*
   b. Slimes are unorganized masses of material similar to capsular material
3. Cell wall
   a. Functions
      (1) Determines and maintains the shape of the microorganism
      (2) Provides support for flagella
      (3) Prevents rupture of the cell resulting from osmotic pressure differences on either side of the cell wall
   b. Composed of the macromolecule peptidoglycan
   c. Comparison of gram-negative and gram-positive cell walls
      (1) Gram-negative cell walls are more complex
      (2) Gram-negative cell walls have a thinner peptidoglycan structure
      (3) Gram-negative cell walls are more easily broken by mechanical forces; susceptible to lysis by antibody, complement, and streptomycin
      (4) Gram-positive cell walls are susceptible to action of lysozyme and penicillin
4. Cell envelope
   a. Includes all external structures and appendages, including the capsule, pili, flagella, cell wall, and cytoplasmic membrane
   b. Properties confer staining characteristics
C. Interior cell structures
1. Plasma membrane
   a. Functions
      (1) Osmotic barrier passively regulating movement of materials in and out of the cell
      (2) Active transport
      (3) Aids in energy production capability of the cell
   b. Lies adjacent to and beneath the cell wall

Table 7-1 Procaryotic organelles and their functions

Structure	Properties, functions, activities	Major chemical components
Akinete	1. Limited protection? 2. Resting cell (spore) 3. Nitrogen fixation?	General components of a blue-green procaryotic cell
Axial filament	Movement in spiral types of organisms	Protein
Capsule	Protection against phagocytosis and certain drugs	Polysaccharides, polypeptides
Carboxysome	Utilization of carbon dioxide	Protein
Cell membrane	1. Selective barrier between the cell's interior and exterior 2. Biosynthesis 3. Chromosome separation	Protein, fatty acids, no sterols
Cell wall	1. Encloses procaryotic cell 2. Provides shape and mechanical protection 3. Contains bacterial virus receptor sites	Amino sugar (N-acetylglucosamine and N-acetylmuramic acid), protein, lipopolysaccharides
Chlorobium vesicle	Photosynthesis	Protein, lipid, photosynthetic pigment
Cyst	1. Limited protection? 2. Resting stage	General components of procaryotic cell
Endospore	1. Protection against physical heat, pH changes and drying 2. Cellular differentiation 3. Reproduction, for some blue-green bacteria*	General components of procaryotic cell plus calcium and dipicolinic acid DPA
Flagellum	Movement	Protein
Gas vesicle	1. Regulates buoyancy 2. Light shielding	Protein, common gases
Genome (nuclear region, or nucleoplasm)	Contains all of the genetic information of the procaryote	Deoxyribonucleic acid
Heterocyst	Nitrogen fixation	Protein, lipid
Mesosome	1. Nucleoplasm division 2. Sporulation 3. Biosynthesis 4. Cell wall formation	Protein, lipid
Metachromatic granules	Storage of reserve nutrients	Nucleic acids, lipid, protein, phosphate
Plasmid	Carries genetic factors associated with drug resistance and certain metabolic enzymes	Extrachromosomal DNA
Pilus	1. Attachment 2. Transfer of genetic material 3. Receptor sites for viruses	Protein
Ribosome	Protein synthesis	Protein, ribosomal RNA
Spine	Unknown	Protein
Thylakoid	Photosynthesis	Protein, lipid, photosynthetic pigment

Reprinted with permission of Macmillan Publishing Company from Microbiology, third edition, by George A. Wistreich and Max D. Lechtman. Copyright © 1980 Glencoe Publishing Company (a Division of Macmillan, Inc.).
*Endospores of blue-green bacteria differ both in chemical composition and function from those of other procaryotes.

2. Mesosomes
    a. Occur primarily in gram-positive species
    b. Associated with cell wall formation, division of nuclear material, cellular respiration, and spore formation

3. Genetic material or genome
    a. Procaryotes lack the distinct nucleus of eucaryotes

Table 7-2 Eucaryotic organelles and their functions

Organelle	Associated functions and activities
Cell membrane	1. Transport of substances into and out of cells 2. In some cells, engulfment of foreign material (phago-cytosis) 3. Pinocytosis
Cell wall	1. Found only in plants, im-parts shape and strength to the cell 2. Protection against certain osmotic imbalances
Chloroplast	Photosynthesis
Cilium	Motion, or movement of sub-stances past the ciliated cell
Endoplasmic reticulum	Protein synthesis
Flagellum	Propulsion
Golgi apparatus	1. Transfer of proteins and other cellular components to a secretory cell's ex-terior 2. Storage and packing struc-ture for cellular products
Microbody, or peroxisome	Enzymatic activities
Microtubule	1. Cell transport of materials 2. Development and mainte-nance of cell shape 3. Cell division 4. Ciliary and flagellar move-ment
Mitochondrion	Synthesis of the energy-rich compound adenosine tri-phosphate (ATP)
Nucleolus	Major site for the formation of ribosomal components
Nucleus	1. Control of cellular physio-logical process 2. Transfer of hereditary fac-tors to subsequent gen-erations
Ribosome	Protein synthesis
Vacuoles	1. Locations of water 2. Storage site for certain amino acids, carbohy-drates, and proteins 3. Dumping ground for cellu-lar wastes

Reprinted with permission of Macmillan Publishing Company from Microbiology, third edition, by George A. Wistreich and Max D. Lechtman. Copyright © 1980 Glencoe Publishing Company (a Division of Macmillan, Inc.).

b. Single chromosome is composed of a single molecule of DNA, existing as a closed loop not enclosed by a nuclear membrane; located in the nucleoplasm of the cell

c. Additional genetic material is found in plasmids that are extrachromosomal DNA molecules; they carry information that determines drug resistance or sensitivity

4. Ribosomes
   a. Function in synthesis of protein
   b. Composed of ribosomal protein and ribosomal ribonucleic acid (RNA)

5. Photosynthetic apparatus

6. Inclusions
   a. Accumulations of reserve storage materials
   b. Include polysaccharide granules: starch and glycogen

D. Endospores
   1. Dormant structures formed within gram-positive bacterial cells
   2. Formed during a process called sporulation: disintegration of parent cell releases endospore; then called exospore or free spore
   3. Can remain in a spore state for years; exhibit unusual resistance to heat, drying, chemical disinfection, and radiation
   4. Spores can transform back into a vegetative cell through a process called germination
   5. Ability of bacteria to produce endospores is restricted mainly to the genera *Bacillus* and *Clostridium*

Eucaryotic Cell Structure and Function (Table 7-2)

A. More complex than a procaryotic cell; typical of fungi, protozoa, and certain algae; has a distinct nucleus bounded by a nuclear membrane, a nucleolus, and membrane-bound organelles

B. Animal cells
   1. Cell membrane
      a. Surrounds the cell and interconnects with the cell's internal membrane systems
      b. Functions
         (1) Regulates the passage of substances in and out of the cell through active and passive transport
         (2) Involved with phagocytosis, tumor formation, drug sensitivity, and immune response

2. Nucleus
   a. Controls the cell's physiologic and reproductive processes
   b. Composition
      (1) Nuclear membrane
      (2) Nucleoplasm
      (3) Nucleoli (involved in RNA synthesis)
      (4) Chromosomes (composed of DNA)
      (5) Nucleoprotein (chromatin)
3. Internal structures
   a. Mitochondria are involved with adenosine triphosphate (ATP) or energy production
   b. Endoplasmic reticulum (ER)
      (1) Network of membranes involved with chemical reactions, storage, and transportation
      (2) Rough ER has ribosomes attached
   c. Golgi apparatus
   d. Lysosomes contain digestive enzymes
   e. Microtubules
C. Plant cells
   1. Have some of the same organelles as animal cells, including cell membrane, nucleus, nucleolus, mitochondria, and endoplasmic reticulum
   2. Cell wall is simpler in structure; major component is the polysaccharide cellulose
   3. Plastids
      a. Chromoplasts impart color to flowers, fruits, and leaves
      b. Chloroplasts are necessary for photosynthesis
      c. Leukoplastids are colorless and store starch
   4. Vacuoles

Microbial Growth and Cultivation

A. Definitions
   1. Culture media—nutrient preparations used to cultivate microorganisms
   2. In vitro techniques—procedures using nonliving materials in a culture vessel
   3. In vivo techniques—procedures using living cells or entire animals or plants
   4. Colony—resulting accumulation of bacteria on a medium
B. Conditions affecting growth
   1. Nutrition available
      a. Heterotrophic organisms
         (1) Require organic compounds as sources of carbon and energy
         (2) Most commonly cultured on a medium of glucose
      b. Autotrophic organisms
         (1) Use inorganic compounds such as carbon dioxide

(2) Thrive in soils and bodies of water
   c. Hypotrophic organisms
      (1) Obligate intracellular parasites; grow only within a living host cell
      (2) Include the viruses and rickettsiae
2. Gaseous requirements
   a. Aerobes require oxygen
   b. Microaerophilic organisms need low concentrations of oxygen
   c. Anaerobes do not need oxygen
   d. Obligate (strict) anaerobes cannot tolerate any free oxygen
   e. Facultative anaerobes will grow in the presence or absence of oxygen
3. Thermal conditions (Fig. 7-1)
   a. Most bacteria grow over a range of temperatures
      (1) Psychrophiles—0° to 20° C (32° to 68° F)
      (2) Mesophiles—20° to 45° C (68° to 113° F)
      (3) Thermophiles—45° to 90° C or above (113° to 194° F or above)
   b. Minimal, maximal, and optimal requirements are the organisms' cardinal temperatures

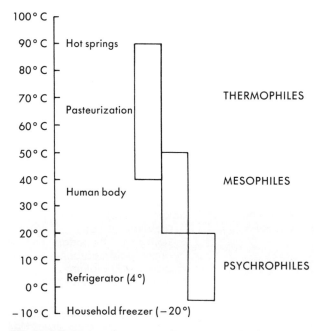

Fig. 7-1 Temperature growth range of microorganisms. Organisms in each category cannot grow over entire range for group. (Adapted from Microbiology, 2nd edition, by Eugene W. Nester et al. Copyright © 1973, 1978 by Holt, Rinehart & Winston. Reprinted by permission of Holt, Rinehart & Winston, CBS College Publishing.)

4. Acidity or alkalinity (pH)
   a. Most bacteria grow best near a neutral pH, between 6 and 7.5
   b. Acidic or alkaline solutions can be disinfecting agents
5. Minerals needed include sulfur and phosphorus
6. Nitrogen is derived from proteins and their products
7. Osmotic pressure
   a. Bacterial cell is 80% water
   b. Needs constant contact with a water supply
8. Certain vitamins and growth factors

C. Types of media
1. Synthetic media have a known amount of chemical compounds
2. Rich complex media have a poorly defined amount of nutrient material
3. Differential media
   a. Contain combinations of nutrients and pH indicators to produce visual differentiation of several microorganisms
   b. Example—blood agar is an enriched medium that allows streptococci to leave different signs on the medium; green discoloration around colonies means α-hemolytic streptococcus, clear zones mean β-hemolysis, and no effect means γ-hemolysis
4. Selective media
   a. Allow interference with or prevention of certain microorganisms' growth while permitting others to grow
   b. Dyes and antibiotics make the media selective
5. Selective and differential media
   a. Combine properties of the preceding two types of media
   b. Examples—mannitol salt agar and MacConkey agar
6. Media for anaerobic microorganisms have reducing agents to create anaerobic conditions

D. Pure culture techniques
1. Used to isolate and identify a bacterial species
2. Methods
   a. Pour-plate technique
      (1) Cool the melted agar-containing medium
      (2) Inoculate the medium
         (a) Use the loop or needle to transfer the organism
         (b) Pass the loop through the flame and heat to redness
         (c) Flame edges of tubes from which cultures are taken before and after removal of the organism
      (3) Pour the inoculated medium into a sterile Petri dish
      (4) Allow the medium to solidify
      (5) Incubate at the desired temperature
   b. Streak-plate technique
      (1) Spread a loopful of material containing organisms over the surface of the solidified agar
      (2) Streaking methods are shown in Figs. 7-2 and 7-3

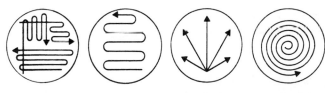

Fig. 7-2 Representative streaking patterns. (Reprinted with permission of Macmillan Publishing Company from Microbiology, third edition, by George A. Wistreich and Max D. Lechtman. Copyright © 1980 Glencoe Publishing Company [a Division of Macmillan, Inc.].)

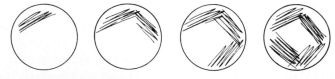

Fig. 7-3 Clock-plate method of streaking. (Reprinted with permission of Macmillan Publishing Company from Microbiology, third edition, by George A. Wistreich and Max D. Lechtman. Copyright © 1980 Glencoe Publishing Company [a Division of Macmillan, Inc.].)

E. Bacterial growth
   1. Most bacteria reproduce by binary fission (i.e., two new cells are produced by one parent cell)
   2. Growth on the culture medium
      a. Typical growth curve results
      b. Phases
         (1) Lag phase—no increase in cell number, but the cell size increases
         (2) Logarithmic phase—cell number increases in geometric progression; generation time is the average time for the cell to divide
         (3) Stationary phase—total number of viable cells is constant
         (4) Death phase—number of viable cells decreases
   3. Measurement of growth
      a. Made by observing an increase in mass or numbers
      b. Cell mass can be measured by dry weight, chemical analysis, and turbidity
      c. Cell numbers can be measured by viable counts; estimates are expressed as colony-forming units (CFU) (for bacteria) or plaque-forming units (PFU) (for viruses)

Microbial Metabolism and Cell Regulation

A. Metabolism
   1. Definition—set of chemical reactions by which cells maintain life
   2. Phases
      a. Anabolism
         (1) Constructive, building-up period; energy-consuming phase
         (2) Macromolecules such as nucleic acids, lipids, and polysaccharides are synthesized
      b. Catabolism
         (1) Breaking-down phase
         (2) Complex compounds are broken down, releasing energy in the form of ATP molecules
   3. Energy storage and transfer
      a. Conserved as chemical energy in ATP
      b. May be transported by electrons (electron transport system)
      c. Energy produced through oxidation-reduction reactions
         (1) Aerobic oxidation (respiration)
         (2) Anaerobic oxidation (fermentation)
   4. Metabolic pathways
      a. Series of steps to complete biochemical process

      b. Glycolytic pathway
         (1) Most important way carbohydrates are metabolized
         (2) Converts glucose to pyruvic acid
         (3) Anaerobic fermentation process
      c. Tricarboxylic acid (Krebs) cycle
         (1) Follows the glycolytic pathway
         (2) Responsible for complete oxidation of glucose
         (3) Important to aerobic bacteria
   5. Protein synthesis
      a. DNA directs formation of proteins aided by various types of RNA
      b. Transcription
         (1) Messenger RNA (mRNA) is formed
         (2) Carries genetic code from DNA
      c. Translation
         (1) Information on mRNA is decoded into series of amino acids at the ribosomes
         (2) Forms protein molecules
   6. Metabolic control
      a. Largely by enzymatic control
      b. Types of enzymes
         (1) Constitutive—always present in the cell
         (2) Inducible—produced only when the product to be degraded (inducer) is in the environment
      c. Types of regulation
         (1) Catabolite repression
            (a) Related to levels of cyclic adenosine monophosphate (cAMP)
            (b) Reduces unnecessary synthesis of enzymes
         (2) Allosteric enzymes
            (a) Direct regulation of action of enzymes by enzymes
            (b) Result in an immediate slowdown of end products of reactions
            (c) Are those subject to such immediate control
         (3) Feedback inhibition—accumulation of end products inhibits enzyme activity
         (4) Operons—clusters of genes that can regulate metabolic processes

Microbial Genetics

A. Bacteria are haploid; they contain a single set of unpaired chromosomes
B. Genetic recombination
   1. Definition—exchange of genetic material between members of different bacterial genera and species

2. Methods
   a. Transformation results in genetic change caused by soluble extracts of DNA
   b. Conjugation is the transfer of genetic material between two living bacteria that are in physical contact
   c. Sexduction (F-duction) involves transfer of genetic material by an extrachromosomal genetic particle, or F particle, to a cell lacking this particle
   d. Transduction occurs when a bacterial virus (bacteriophage) transfers genetic material
   e. Lysogenic or viral conversions refer to genetic changes that can occur in bacteria as a result of viral infection, including toxin production or antigenic changes
   f. Plasmids (small extrachromosomal DNA) can replicate independently
C. Mutations
   1. Result in changes in DNA strand sequence
   2. Can be caused by agents such as ultraviolet light, radiation, nitrous acid, and mustard gas

Microbial Relationships

A. Syntrophism
   1. Organisms are not intimately associated with each other but benefit from each other
   2. Examples—yogurt production and organisms feeding in soil where decaying plant material is found
B. Competition
   1. Interaction between organisms resulting from a demand for nutrients and energy that exceeds immediate supply
   2. Example—molds such as *Penicillum* compete by secreting substances toxic to other organisms
C. Predation controls the population by predators feeding on another species, the prey
D. Symbiosis
   1. Two different forms of life coexist in an intimate ecologic relationship
   2. Forms
      a. Mutualism
         (1) Both members benefit
         (2) Examples—termites and lichens
      b. Commensalism
         (1) Only one organism benefits, and the other neither benefits nor is harmed
         (2) Examples—higher organisms and their intestinal microorganisms; normal oral bacteria
      (3) Under certain circumstances, commensals can become pathogenic and are then called opportunists
   c. Parasitism
      (1) One organism benefits at the expense of the other
      (2) Example—disease-producing microorganisms

Bacteria

Bacteria are described in Table 7-3

Fungi

A. Description
   1. Eucaryotic
   2. Nonphotosynthetic
   3. Larger than bacteria
   4. Grow well in dark, moist environments
   5. Heterotrophic saprophytes use preexisting organic products, either living or dead
   6. Few species are pathogenic to humans
B. Forms
   1. Molds
      a. Do not have true roots, stems, or leaves
      b. Structural unit is the hypha; hyphae result in a cobweblike growth called mycelium
      c. Reproduce by spores
   2. Yeasts
      a. Oval or spherical
      b. Produce moist, shiny colonies
      c. Reproduce asexually by producing new buds or daughter cells
   3. Dimorphism
      a. Some fungi exhibit two forms
      b. May appear as yeasts or molds
C. Classification
   1. Ascomycetes or sac fungi
      a. Live in aquatic or moist land environments
      b. Include yeasts that leaven bread and ferment beer and wine
   2. Basidiomycetes include bracket fungi of trees, mushrooms, rusts, and smuts
   3. Deuteromycetes
      a. Several are medically important, including the genus *Penicillium,* source of the antibiotic
      b. Pathogenic members cause two types of human infections, (e.g., those involving superficial structures such as the skin, nails, and hair [ringworm and thrush] and those affecting deeper tissues)
   4. Oomycetes cause destructive plant diseases such as potato blight

Table 7-3 Description of bacteria*

Category	General description	Representative genera
Phototrophic bacteria	Gram-negative, spherical or rod-shaped bacteria; multiplication is by binary fission and/or budding; they are photosynthetic without producing oxygen; pigments are purple, purple-violet, red, orange-brown, brown, or green	*Chromatium, Rhodomicrobium*
Gliding bacteria	Gram-negative rods typically embedded in a tough slime coat; they are capable of a slow gliding movement; reproduction is by binary fission; gliding bacteria sometimes form colorful fruiting bodies	*Beggiatoa, Cytophaga, Leucothrix*
Sheathed bacteria	Gram-negative rods that occur in chains within a thin sheath; they sometimes have a holdfast cell for attachment to surfaces	*Crenothrix, Leptothrix, Sphaerotilus*
Budding and/or appendaged bacteria	Bacteria with rod-, oval-, egg-, or bean-shaped filamentous growth; multiplication is by budding or binary fission; these bacteria sometimes have a holdfast cell	*Caulobacter, Hyphomicrobium*
Spirochetes	Slender, flexible, coiled cells; they may occur in chains and exhibit transverse fission	*Borrelia, Cristispira, Leptospira,† Treponema†*
Spiral and curved bacteria	Rigid, helically curved rods with less than one complete turn to many turns	*Bdellovibrio,† Campylocabacter,† Microcyclus, Spirillum†*
Gram-negative aerobic rods and cocci	Rods that are usually motile, with polar flagella; bluntly rod-shaped to oval cells, some of which are motile by polar or peritrichous flagella and some of which are cyst formers; and rods and cocci that require high concentrations of sodium chloride for growth	*Acetobacter, Alcaligenes,† Agrobacterium, Azotobacter, Bordetella,† Brucella,† Francisella,† Halobacterium, Pseudomonas†*
Gram-negative facultatively anaerobic rods	Straight and curved rods; some are nonmotile; others are motile by polar or peritrichate flagella; all members are nonsporeformers; some have special growth requirements	*Citrobacter,† Edwardsiella, Enterobacter,† Escherichia,† Haemophilus,† Klebsiella,† Pasteurella,† Salmonella,† Serratia,† Shigella,† Streptobacillus,† Vibrio,† Yersinia†*
Gram-negative anaerobic rods	Strict (obligate) anaerobic, non-spore-forming organisms; some members are motile; pleomorphism (variation in shape) occurs	*Bacteroides,† Desulfovibrio, Fusobacterium, Leptotrichia*
Gram-negative cocci and coccal bacilli	Cocci, characteristically occuring in pairs; adjacent sides of the cells may be flattened; organisms are not flagellated	*Acinetobacter,† Branhamella,† Moraxella,† Neisseria†*
Gram-negative anaerobic cocci	Cocci of variable size and characteristically in pairs; they are not flagellated	*Veillonella†*
Gram-negative chemolithotrophic bacteria	Pleomorphic rods; these organisms use inorganic materials for energy	*Nitrobacter, Nitrococcus, Thiobacillus*
Methane-producing bacteria	Rods or cocci; some members are Gram-positive, others are Gram-negative; all are anaerobic and produce methane	*Methanobacterium, Methanococcus, Methanosarcina*
Gram-positive cocci	Various arrangements of cocci that are aerobic, facultative, or anaerobic	*Aerococcus,† Micrococcus, Peptococcus, Sarcina, Staphylococcus,† Streptococcus†*
Endospore-forming rods and cocci	Members are aerobic, facultatively anaerobic, or anaerobic; most members are Gram-positive	*Bacillus, Clostridium,† Sporosarcina*

*Based on the divisions and descriptions in Buchanan, R.E., and Gibbons, N.E., editors: Bergey's manual of determinative bacteriology, ed. 8, Baltimore, 1974, Williams & Wilkins.
†Medically important species are contained in this genera.

Table 7-3   Description of bacteria — cont'd

Category	General description	Representative genera
Gram-positive asporogenous (non-spore-forming) rod-shaped bacteria	Members may be aerobic, facultatively anaerobic, or anaerobic	*Erysipelothrix,*† *Lactobacillus, Listeria*†
Actinomycetes and related organisms	Rods or pleomorphic rods, with filamentous and branching filaments; included are aerobic, facultatively anaerobic, and anaerobic rods; these organisms are usually Gram-positive, and some are acid-alcohol-fast (acid-fast)	*Actinomyces,*† *Arachnia, Arthrobacter, Bifidobacterium,*† *Corynebacterium,*† *Mycobacterium*†, *Nocardia,*† *Propionibacterium, Streptomyces*
Rickettsia	The majority of cells are Gram-negative coccoid or pleomorphic rods; most are obligate intracellular parasites transmitted by arthropods	*Chlamydia,*† *Cowdria, Coxiella,*† *Ehrlichia, Neorickettsia, Rickettsia,*† *Rickettsiella, Rochalimaea,*† *Symbiotes*
Mycoplasma	Highly pleomorphic, Gram-negative organisms that contain no cell wall; they reproduce by fission, by production of many small bodies, or by budding; members may be aerobic, facultatively (adaptable) anaerobic, or anaerobic	*Acholeplasma, Mycoplasma,*† *Spiroplasma, Thermoplasma*

5. Zygomycetes include the common bread mold, *Rhizopus nigricans*
6. Myxomycetes or slime molds are parasitic and injure plants such as cauliflower, radish, and turnip

Protozoa

A. Description
   1. Unicellular
   2. Eucaryotic
   3. Motile
   4. Require organic food
   5. Many can form cysts
      a. Protective resting stage
      b. Can serve as a site for division or spreading of pathogenic protozoans (e.g., *Entamoeba histolytica,* which causes amoebic dysentery)
B. Classification
   1. Ciliata
      a. Most highly developed forms of unicellular organisms
      b. Includes *Paramecium*
   2. Sarcodina includes *Amoebae*
   3. Mastigophora includes agent of African sleeping sickness
   4. Sporozoa includes agents of malaria and toxoplasmosis

Algae

A. Description
   1. Photosynthetic, aquatic organisms
   2. Eucaryotic cells
   3. Part of plankton population
   4. Important part of food chains
   5. Cause of environmental problems (e.g., algal blooms and algal toxins)
B. Classification
   1. Green algae
   2. Golden brown algae and diatoms
   3. Euglenoids
   4. Brown algae
   5. Dinoflagellates
   6. Red algae
   7. Lichens—symbiotic relationship between certain blue-green bacteria or green algae and fungi

Viruses

A. Properties of a mature virus particle or virion
   1. Has a single type of nucleic acid, RNA or DNA, that contains genetic material, or a genome
   2. Absence of cellular structures
   3. Nucleic acid is surrounded by a protein outer coat, the capsid; nucleic acid and capsid compose the nucleocapsid

Table 7-4 Major animal virus groups and their properties

Virus group*	Type of nucleic acid	Enveloped	General properties
Adenovirus	DNA	No	Found in several animal species, including humans, associated with respiratory infections and with tumors in laboratory animals
Herpetovirus	DNA	Yes	Important causative agents of human disease such as chickenpox, infectious mononucleosis, and infections of the skin and mucous membranes
Papovavirus	DNA	No	Causes warts; used in the study of tumor development
Parvovirus	DNA	No	Satellite viruses that are incapable of replication except in presence of a helper virus
Poxvirus	DNA	No	Found in several animal species, including humans; examples of infections include smallpox and molluscum contagiosum; all viruses affect the skin
Arenavirus	RNA	Yes	Particles contain cellular ribosomes; viruses cause natural inapparent infections of rodents
Bunyavirus	RNA	Yes	Viruses are spread by a variety of arthropods (arboviruses)
Coronavirus	RNA	No	Includes several agents of the common cold
Orthromyxovirus	RNA	Yes	Includes the influenza virus
Paramyxovirus	RNA	Yes	Many produce human childhood diseases such as measles and mumps and localized respiratory infections
Picornavirus	RNA	No	Includes several agents of diseases such as poliomyelitis, rashes, meningitis, and mild upper respiratory infections
Reovirus	RNA	No	All are spread by arthropods; many have yet to be associated with specific diseases
Retrovirus	RNA	No	Group includes tumor- and cancer-causing agents
Rhabdovirus	RNA	Yes	Group includes large bullet-shaped viruses such as the agents for rabies and vesicular stomatitis
Togavirus	RNA	Yes	Arthropod-spread diseases, including yellow fever and several nervous system diseases

Reprinted with permission of Macmillan Publishing Company from Microbiology, third edition, by George A. Wistreich and Max D. Lechtman. Copyright © 1980 Glencoe Publishing Company (a Division of Macmillan, Inc.).
*Several new viruses, as well as some unclassified viruses, may require the formation of new groups.

4. Viral nucleic acid controls new virus production or replication
5. Obligate intracellular parasites
6. Lack components for energy production and protein synthesis
B. Classification
  1. Bacteriophages (bacterial viruses)
    a. Contain either RNA or DNA
    b. Virulent or lytic viruses infect and destroy host cells
    c. Temperate viruses can cause lysis or integrate their DNA into the host cell
      (1) If they integrate, they are referred to as a prophage, and a stable association is established between the host and virus
      (2) Bacterial cell containing a prophage is called lysogenic; during the prophage phase cellular changes can occur
  2. Animal viruses (Table 7-4)
    a. Effects range from mild skin rashes to tumor formation

    b. Destructive effects to cells are termed cytopathic
  3. Plant viruses (most contain RNA)
  4. Viroids
    a. Smallest infectious agents known
    b. Found mainly in plants
C. Viral interference
  1. Definition—cells infected by one virus resist challenge by a second virus
  2. Mechanisms
    a. First virus alters the surface of the host cell so the second virus cannot attach
    b. First virus stimulates production of interferons by the host cell
      (1) Glycoproteins
      (2) Released from macrophages and lymphocytes
      (3) Induce state of resistance to viruses
D. Viral replication
  1. Uses biosynthetic mechanisms of the host cell

Table 7-5 Conditions or factors involved in bacterial opportunistic infections

Predisposing condition and/or factor	Bacteria	Infection or disease state
Abdominal and other forms of surgery	*Bacteroides fragilis*	Blood poisoning (septicemia)
	Streptococcus spp.	Blood poisoning and lung disease
Alcoholism	*Haemophilus* spp.	Infection of brain coverings (meningitis)
	Klebsiella pneumoniae	Lung disease (pneumonia)
	Mycobacterium tuberculosis	Tuberculosis
Antimicrobial therapy	*Escherichia coli, Proteus vulgaris, Serratia marcescens*	Urinary tract infection
	Staphylococcus aureus	Blood poisoning (septicemia)
Breaks in skin, wounds, burns, etc.	*Acinetobacter calcoaceticus, Bacteroides, Clostridium* spp.	Blood poisoning
	Pseudomonas spp., *Staphylococcus aureus, Streptococcus* spp.	Blood poisoning, lung infection
Diabetes mellitus	Anaerobes	Foot ulcers
	Haemophilus spp.	Infection of brain coverings
	Nocardia spp., *Streptococcus pneumoniae*	Lung infection
Immunosuppression	*Corynebacterium* spp.	Lung infection
	Escherichia coli	Urinary tract infection
	Staphylococcus aureus	Blood poisoning
Malnutrition	*Mycobacterium tuberculosis*	Tuberculosis
Malignancies (various types of cancer)	*Aeromonas hydrophilia, Clostridium perfringens* and other clostridia, *Citrobacter* spp., *Escherichia coli,* and *Pseudomonas* spp.	Blood poisoning and lung infections
Sickle cell disease	*Haemophilus* and *Yersinia* spp.	Blood poisoning
Transplants	*Arizona* spp.	Blood poisoning
	Mycobacterium spp.	Lung infection
	Mycobacterium tuberculosis	Tuberculosis

2. Phases
   a. Attachment to the host cell
   b. Penetration
   c. Intracellular replication
   d. Release
E. Slow virus diseases
   1. Caused by viruses or viruslike agents
   2. Characteristics
      a. Incubation periods of months or years
      b. Prolonged course; may extend over a lifetime
   3. Examples
      a. Subacute sclerosing panencephalitis (SSPE)
      b. Progressive multifocal leukoencephalopathy (PML)
F. Role of virus in cancer
   1. Oncogenous viruses can induce various types of cancer (RNA- or DNA-type viruses)
   2. Process unclear
   3. No direct, conclusive evidence yet that human cancers are caused by viruses

MICROBIAL VIRULENCE AND DISEASE TRANSFER

A. Definitions
   1. Pathogenicity—ability to cause disease
   2. Pathogen—disease-producing virus or other microorganism
   3. Opportunist—organism that has the potential to produce infection but not to directly invade the host tissue; situations contributing to opportunism include alcoholism, genetic defects, antibiotic use, and immunosuppressive therapy (Table 7-5)
   4. Virulence—measure of the degree of pathogenicity; properties that determine an organism's pathogenicity include invasiveness, ability to multiply in the host, and toxin production
   5. Infection—invasion of the tissue by a pathogenic microorganism and multiplication of the organism
      a. Localized—organism remains in a particular area

b. Generalized or systemic—microorganism invades the bloodstream and lymphatic system
c. Mixed—involves more than one organism
d. Acute—runs a rapid course; terminates abruptly
e. Chronic—slow onset; infection of long duration
f. Primary—original infection
g. Secondary—one that follows a primary infection and is often caused by an opportunist
h. Toxemia—presence of toxin in the blood
i. Subclinical—no symptoms recognized
j. Focal—localized in one area and spreads elsewhere
k. Bacteremia—presence of bacteria in the bloodstream
6. Infectious disease—interference with the normal functioning of the host; proof by Koch's postulates
a. Microorganism present in every case of disease
b. Microorganism grows in pure culture from the diseased host
c. Same disease reproduced when pure culture is inoculated into the healthy host
d. Microorganism recovered from the inoculated host

B. Toxin production
1. Exotoxins
a. Soluble substances secreted by bacteria
b. Clinically significant exotoxins are associated with botulism, tetanus, diphtheria, gas gangrene, scarlet fever, and staphylococcal food poisoning
2. Endotoxins
a. Lipopolysaccharides—components of bacterial cell walls
b. Most commonly from gram-negative bacteria
c. Pathologic affects
(1) Fever
(2) Interference with hemostatic mechanisms of blood
(3) Shock
(4) Activation of the complement system

C. Transmission of disease
1. Reservoir of infection—all potential sources of the disease agent
a. Active cases of infectious disease
b. Carriers are persons harboring infectious agents
(1) Asymptomatic carrier—harbors agent without showing ill effects (e.g., chronic carrier of hepatitis B)

(2) Incubatory carrier—has beginning state of disease but is still without symptoms
(3) Convalescent carrier—recovering but still able to transmit disease
c. Animals and birds
d. Environmental sources include water, food, soil, and dust
e. Endogenous infection is one in which the causative organism is derived from the host's own microflora
2. Portals of exit are sources of infectious body fluids
a. Gastrointestinal tract
b. Genitourinary system
c. Oral region
d. Respiratory tract
e. Blood and blood derivatives
f. Skin lesions
3. Routes of transmission
a. Direct contact through contact with lesions (e.g., hand contact)
b. Indirect contact
(1) Contaminated food or water
(2) Inanimate objects called fomites (e.g., equipment and patient records)
(3) Air- and dust-borne organisms
(a) Talking, sneezing, and coughing
(b) Redistribution of room dust
(c) Aerosol production in the dental operatory
(4) Accidental inoculation by a contaminated needle or instrument
(5) Arthropods including ticks, lice, fleas, mosquitoes, and cockroaches

Disease Barriers

A. Normal or indigenous flora
1. Includes beneficial microorganisms and pathogens
2. When ecologic balance is disturbed, infection can occur (e.g., antibiotic therapy may result in *Candida albicans* infection)
B. Nonspecific resistance
1. Mechanical and chemical barriers (Table 7-6)
a. Intact skin
b. Intact mucous membranes
c. Nasal hairs
d. Coughing and sneezing reflexes
e. Tears and eyelashes
f. Secretions and microorganisms of the gastrointestinal system

Table 7-6 Host defense mechanisms against microbial invasion

Normal host defense	Altering agent or disease	Possible mechanism
Physical barriers, e.g., skin and mucous membrane	Burns, trauma, surgery, infection or inflammatory disease	Provides new portals of entry for micro-organisms Altered physiologic defense, e.g., depressed cough reflex, deficient ciliary action in respiratory tract, defective clearing mechanism in lung, predispose to pulmonary infection
	Foreign body, prostheses	Acts as nidus for infection, provide new entry portals or cause obstruction with stasis and infection
	Diagnostic procedures	Provides new portals of entry for micro-organisms
	Urinary tract and intravenous catheters	Provides new portals of entry or acts as nidus of infection
	Antimetabolites or radiation	Injures rapidly growing cells (e.g., in gastrointestinal tract) to produce ulceration, bleeding and subsequent portals of entry
	Local ischemia	Alters permeability of skin or mucous membrane to produce new portals of entry, e.g., in diabetes
Normal flora	Burns, trauma	Alters normal skin flora by changing skin ecology and physicochemical properties
	Hospitalization	Host becomes colonized with new or resistant organisms
	Antibiotics	Alters normal microbial flora of skin, mucous membranes, respiratory and gastrointestinal tracts
	Heroin	Mechanism unclear; appears to alter nasal flora
Inflammatory response	Diabetes mellitus	Defects in chemotaxis and phagocytosis aggravated by marked acidosis
	Cirrhosis	Depressed chemotaxis due to serum inhibitor
	Alcohol	Defects in leukocyte mobilization, lung macrophage antibacterial activity
	Sickle cell disease	Deficiency of opsonizing antibody and probable abnormality of the alternate pathway of complement, relative asplenia
	Intrinsic leukocyte abnormalities (e.g., lazy leukocyte syndrome)	Chemotactic leukocyte defect
	Chronic granulomatous disease, myeloperoxidase deficiency	Defects in intracellular killing
	Corticosteroids, radiation and antimetabolites	Various defects in leukocyte mobilization, complement
	Hematopoietic (e.g., leukemia)	Quantitative or qualitative deficiency of polymorphonuclear cells
Immunologic system Humoral system	Multiple myeloma and chronic lymphatic leukemia	Decrease in normal immunoglobins, delayed and defective antibody response to antigenic stimuli or production of various amounts of abnormal immunoglobulins
	Extremes of age	During first 3 mo-6 mo, infant dependent on maternal antibody, possible decrease in delayed immune response in elderly
	Nephrotic syndrome, protein losing enteropathy	Excessive loss of immunoglobulins
	Ataxia telangiectasia, chronic obstructive pulmonary disease, Wiskott-Aldrich syndrome, dysproteinemia, systemic lupus erythematosis	Defective synthesis or excessive catabolism of different classes of protein and abnormalities of complement system
Cell-mediated system	Hodgkin's Disease Uremia Sarcoidosis Systemic lupus erythematosis Corticosteroids and antimetabolites Combined deficiency states	Depression of delayed hypersensitivity

From McGhee, J.R., Michalek, S.M., and Cassell, G.H., editors: Dental microbiology, New York, 1982, Harper & Row, Publishers, Inc.

2. Blood and lymphatics
   a. Leukocytes—proportionate number changes in response to infection
      (1) Granulocytes (basophils, eosinophils, neutrophils, or polymorphonuclear leukocytes)
      (2) Agranulocytes (lymphocytes and monocytes)
   b. Lymphatic system transports white blood cells and removes foreign cells and tissue debris
      (1) Consists of lymphatic vessels, lymph fluid, nodes, and lymphocytes
      (2) Reticuloendothelial system (RES)— macrophages that digest foreign and host substances
3. Phagocytosis
   a. Digestion of the invading matter
   b. Accomplished by granulocytes, monocytes, and macrophages

4. Inflammation
   a. Produced by disease agents or irritants such as chemicals, heat, or mechanical injury
   b. Cardinal signs include heat, pain, redness, swelling, and loss of function
   c. Pus formation possible
5. Antimicrobial substances
   a. Chemicals available in animal fluid and tissue
   b. Complement, histone, lysozyme, and interferon
C. Immunity (Fig. 7-4)
   1. Development of a degree of resistance to infectious agents; accomplished by the production of specific antibodies or immunoglobulins to the introduction of foreign agents or antigens
   2. Immune responses
      a. Humoral immunity—β-lymphocytes involved with specific antibody synthesis

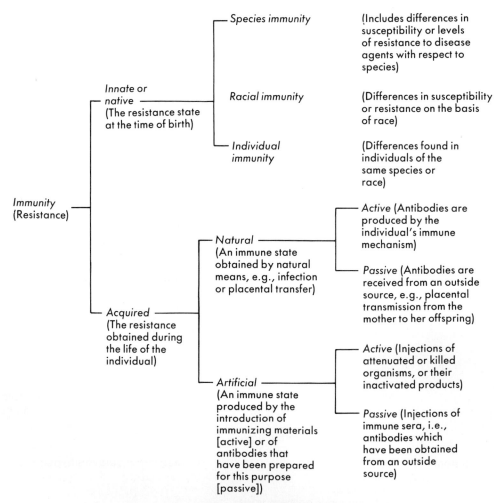

Fig. 7-4 States of immunity. (Reprinted with permission of Macmillan Publishing Company from Microbiology, third edition, by George A. Wistreich and Max D. Lechtman. Copyright © 1980 Glencoe Publishing Company [a Division of Macmillan, Inc.].)

b. Cell-mediated immunity
  (1) Involves T lymphocytes interacting directly with foreign substances, especially those on cell surfaces
  (2) Includes situations such as the tuberculin response, rejection of foreign tissue, and activation of macrophages

Immunodeficiency

A. Inability of the immune system to perform normally; properly functioning system recognizes and destroys that which is foreign, or non-self
B. Results in increased susceptibility to infection
C. Types
  1. Primary—congenital
  2. Secondary—acquired
D. Hypersensitivity or allergy is an exaggerated response to specific substances; inciting agent is the allergen
  1. Type I (classic, immediate)
    a. Includes asthma, anaphylactic shock, hay fever, and hives
    b. Rapid release of histamines and serotonin
  2. Type II (cytotoxic)
    a. Results in cell destruction
    b. Mother-infant Rh incompatability, blood transfusion reactions
  3. Type III (immune-complex mediated)
    a. Soluble antigens and immunoglobulins combine
    b. Serum sickness, Arthus reaction
  4. Type IV (cell mediated, delayed)
    a. Depends on T-lymphocyte reactions
    b. Includes contact dermatitis from chemicals (e.g., formaldehyde), metals (e.g., mercury), poison ivy, and graft rejection
E. Autoimmune diseases (autoallergic)
  1. Self-antigens stimulate the production of antibodies or sensitized lymphocytes
  2. May be part of type IV hyrpersensitivity
  3. Includes systemic lupus erythematosus and rheumatoid arthritis
F. Acquired immune deficiency syndrome (AIDS)
  1. Definition—disease at least moderately predictive of a defect in cell-mediated immunity occurring in a person with no known cause of diminished resistance to that disease; cellular immunity is profoundly suppressed, allowing development of opportunistic infections and cancers[41,51]
  2. Irreversible acquired defect[21]
  3. Etiology unknown[21,51]; evidence strong for viral, transmissible agent[21,37]
    a. Human T-cell leukemia virus (HTLV) III virus; a retrovirus
    b. Defect in the β-cells and T cells of the immune system leads to
      (1) Propagation of neoplastic cells
      (2) Establishment of opportunistic infections
  4. High fatality rate; 50%, possibly higher[21,41]
  5. Suggested route of transmission is through the blood or body fluids[41]; similar to hepatitis B virus
  6. Symptoms are nonspecific, highly variable
    a. General malaise
    b. Fever
    c. Swollen lymph nodes
    d. Weight loss
    e. Opportunistic infections
      (1) Kaposi's sarcoma—skin lesions; may be oral; multiple small reddish blue, purple, or hyperpigmented brown papules, plaques, or modules (Fig. 7-5)
      (2) Cytomegalovirus (CMV)—frequently involves the eye, causing retinal lesions
      (3) Hepatitis B
      (4) *Pneumocystis carinii*
      (5) Oral and esophageal infection from *C. albicans*
      (6) Herpes simplex viruses I and II[41]
  7. Incidence/prevalence
    a. Since the disease was identified in 1981, 4000 cases have been reported in the United States
    b. Incidence is doubling every 6 months
    c. Mortality is over 60%
    d. High-risk groups
      (1) Male homosexuals
      (2) Intravenous drug users
      (3) Haitian immigrants
      (4) Frequent recipients of blood or blood products (e.g., hemophiliac patients)
      (5) Female prostitutes
      (6) Infants of parents with AIDS
      (7) Female sexual partners of male patients with AIDS[41]
    e. Dental personnel may be at risk if transmission proves to be similar to that of hepatitis B virus
  8. Treatment
    a. No known cure
    b. Just now developing a vaccine for prevention and a blood test for detection of the virus

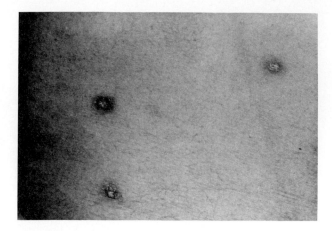

Fig. 7-5 Kaposi's spots. (Courtesy Dr. Charles Barr, Beth Israel Medical Center, New York.)

9. Oral manifestations
   a. Herpetic lesions
   b. Oral candidiasis
   c. Kaposi's spots (Fig. 7-5)
G. Immunosuppression
   1. Used as an adjunct to renal transplantation and other organ grafts; also used for the treatment of immunologically mediated disease
   2. Examples of drugs used include corticosteroids, azathioprine, and cyclophosphamide; common complication is infection

Infections of the Skin, Nails, and Hair

A. Bacterial infections
   1. Tetanus
      a. Agent is *Clostridium tetani;* spores germinate in the wound and produce tetanus-causing toxin
      b. Incubation period is 7 to 10 days
      c. Symptoms
         (1) Trismus (stiff jaw); eventually locked jaw
         (2) Spasms of facial muscles
         (3) Dysphagia
         (4) Difficulty in breathing
      d. Antitoxin given following injury
   2. Leprosy
      a. Agent is *Mycobacterium leprae*
      b. Transmitted by prolonged direct contact or inhalation of organisms
      c. Incubation period is 1 to 5 years or longer
      d. Symptoms
         (1) Skin lesions
         (2) Oral lesions are tumorlike masses of tissue involving the oral lining, tongue, lips, or palate

3. *Pseudomonas aeruginosa* infections
   a. Low pathogenicity for humans, except in debilitated patients; may develop from changes in normal flora or immune mechanisms (e.g., from the use of antibiotics or drugs suppressing antibody production)
   b. Water and soil parasite; multiplies in standing water (overnight) in dental unit waterlines as chlorine dissipates from the water
   c. Resultant infections
      (1) Skin infections
      (2) Bacteremia
      (3) Endocarditis
      (4) Pneumonia
      (5) Meningitis
      (6) Pyelonephritis
4. Staphylococcal infections
   a. Main agent is *Staphylococcus aureus*
   b. Causes acute suppurative inflammation (pus) such as furuncles (boils) and carbuncles
   c. Impetigo is transmitted through direct contact
   d. Most *S. aureus* strains are resistant to penicillin
5. Streptococcal infections
   a. Known for secondary invasion; capable of infecting all areas of the body
   b. Scarlet fever
      (1) Acute inflammation of the upper respiratory tract
      (2) Generalized rash caused by erythrogenic exotoxin
      (3) Oral mucosa is red; "strawberry tongue"
      (4) Caused by the β-hemolytic group A streptococci
   c. Consequences from group A streptococcal infections include rheumatic fever and hemorrhagic glomerulonephritis
B. Fungal infections
   1. Various forms of ringworm or tinea
      a. Agents are dermatophytes
      b. Symptoms
         (1) Inflammatory response, especially at the border of lesions
         (2) Dermatophytes' antigens can cause an allergic response
   2. Candidiasis
      a. Agent is *C. albicans*
         (1) Opportunistic pathogen
         (2) Normal inhabitant of the skin and mucosal surfaces

b. Predisposing factors
   (1) Diabetes mellitus
   (2) Pregnancy
   (3) Obesity
   (4) Vitamin deficiency
   (5) Use of broad-spectrum antibiotics
   (6) Immunologic defects
c. Oral candidiasis or thrush
   (1) Lesions are soft, grayish white; strip off, leaving raw bleeding surfaces
   (2) Occurs mostly in infants and in elderly persons
   (3) Lesions common on the buccal mucosa, tongue, and soft palate
   (4) Complaints of thirst and metallic taste
d. Angular cheilitis or perlèche
   (1) Infection in corners of the mouth
   (2) Can also be caused by *S. aureus*
e. Denture stomatitis or denture sore mouth
   (1) Chronic atrophic candidiasis
   (2) Palatal mucosa inflamed under the full denture

C. Viral infections
1. Herpesvirus hominis (herpes simplex)
   a. Types
      (1) Type I—generally above the waist; commonly found in and around the mouth
      (2) Type II—herpes genitalis
   b. Primary infection with type I
      (1) Usually in children
      (2) Frequently asymptomatic
      (3) Clinical manifestations
         (a) Most commonly acute gingivostomatitis—fever, malaise, lymphadenopathy, and anorexia; red, edematous gingiva and adjacent mucosa; lesions are vesicles with yellowish contents that rupture and ulcerate; bright margin of erythema; sharply defined; pain may be severe; duration of about 7 days; self-limiting
         (b) Herpetic whitlow—infection of fingers (cuticle is common site); can be caused by herpes simplex type I or II; abrupt onset; local irritation, tenderness, edema, erythema, and vesicles; difficult to differentiate from bacterial pyoderma caused by staphylococci
         (c) Ocular herpes
   c. Recurrent secondary infections by type I
      (1) Virus now latent but permanently established in nerve ganglia (carrier)
      (2) Host resistance is reduced (e.g., by stress, sun, or colds)
      (3) Herpes labialis is the most common clinical manifestation of recurrent infection
         (a) Cold sores, fever blisters
         (b) Vesicles on an erythematous base
         (c) Prodromal burning and hyperesthesia
         (d) Swollen lymph nodes
      (4) Intraoral lesions
         (a) Usually found on the bound-down mucosa or hard palate; gingival lesions common
         (b) Small, discrete lesions; vesicles of clear fluid; ulcerate with a red base
      (5) May also involve the eye
         (a) Conjunctiva and cornea
         (b) Repeated attacks may result in blindness
   d. Transmission
      (1) Direct contact, including kissing, touching hands, and sexual relations
         (a) Through oral and ocular secretions
         (b) Present in saliva even in apparent good health[43]
      (2) Indirect contact (e.g., fomites)
2. Varicella-zoster virus
   a. Chickenpox (varicella)
      (1) Probably transmitted by inhalation of droplets
      (2) Incubation period of 2 weeks
      (3) Oral lesions may occur throughout the mouth and appear like small canker sores or aphthae; vesicles rupture quickly
   b. Shingles (herpes zoster)
      (1) Chickenpox and shingles represent different forms of infection with the same agent
      (2) Reinvasion or recurrence of varicella-zoster virus; infection of a person with partial immunity from previous infection
      (3) Virus resides in ganglia; usually affects sensory nerves (thoracic area is the most often involved; ophthalmic division of the trigeminal nerve is the next most involved)
      (4) Mostly found in adults
      (5) Symptoms
         (a) Pain
         (b) Rash and vesicles along the nerve trunk
3. Warts (papilloma virus)

4. Measles
   a. Usually contracted by the spread of respiratory secretions
   b. Bacterial secondary infections occur, such as middle ear infections or pneumonia
   c. Symptoms
      (1) Koplik's spots
         (a) Small bluish white spots with a red surrounding zone; cannot be wiped off
         (b) Occur on the buccal mucosa opposite the molars
      (2) Followed by a diffuse skin rash and fever
5. German measles (rubella)
   a. Mild disease, except in pregnant women it may cause fetal defects
   b. Symptoms
      (1) Fever and rash lasting 2 to 3 days
      (2) Swollen sublingual and cervical lymph glands
6. Smallpox (variola)
   a. Transmitted through the respiratory tract and skin of active cases
   b. Symptoms
      (1) Generalized skin rash; develops into vesicles
      (2) Red areas on mucous membranes of the mouth then ulcerate; tongue can be involved

Infections of the Respiratory Tract

Upper Respiratory System Infections
A. Bacterial infections
   1. Diphtheria
      a. Agent is *Corynebacterium diphtheriae*
      b. Damage caused by the systemic distribution of toxin
      c. Pseudomembrane forms on tonsils
   2. Otitis media
      a. Agents are *S. aureus, Haemophilus influenzae,* and *Streptococcus pneumoniae*
      b. Infection of the middle ear
   3. Sinusitis—agents usually are *S. pneumoniae* and *H. influenzae*
   4. Streptococcal sore throat ("strep" throat)
      a. Agent is *Streptococcus pyogenes*
      b. Transmitted by the respiratory route and contaminated food, water, and milk
      c. Symptoms
         (1) Severe inflammation of the throat and tonsils
         (2) Gray or yellowish white throat

B. Viral infections
   1. Common cold
      a. Majority caused by agents such as rhinovirus, coronavirus, and respiratory synctial virus
      b. High viral counts found in respiratory secretions, saliva, and on hands; washing hands removes rhinovirus
   2. Croup
      a. Agents are adenovirus, orthomyxovirus, paramyxoviruses, and respiratory synechial virus
      b. May be severe and life threatening

Lower Respiratory System Infections
A. Bacterial infections
   1. Bacterial pneumonia
      a. Inflammation of the lungs
      b. Caused by several species
      c. Legionnaire's disease
         (1) Agent is *Legionnella pneumophila*
         (2) Influenza-like illness with pneumonia
         (3) Complications include renal failure, gastrointestinal hemorrhage, and respiratory failure
      d. Pneumococcal pneumonia
         (1) Most common agent is *S. pneumoniae*
         (2) Spread by droplets from nasal or pharyngeal secretions
         (3) Person may contract the disease or become an asymptomatic carrier
         (4) Predisposing factors include viral infections of the upper respiratory tract, pulmonary edema, age, diabetes, and fatigue
         (5) Symptoms include sudden onset of high fever, chills, chest pain, dry cough, and rust-colored sputum
   2. Tuberculosis
      a. Agent is *Mycobacterium tuberculosis*
         (1) Killed by heat
         (2) Resistant to drying and chemical germicides
         (3) Generally attacks the lungs
      b. Transmitted by inhalation of droplets, ingestion, or direct inoculation; disseminated by coughing, sneezing, or contaminated dust
      c. Predisposing factors
         (1) Advanced age
         (2) Chronic alcoholism
         (3) Poor nutrition
         (4) Diabetes mellitus
         (5) Prolonged stress

d. Incubation period is generally 28 to 42 days; can be as long as 6 months

e. Symptoms vary but include
   (1) Fever
   (2) General discomfort
   (3) Weight loss
   (4) Tubercle formation (nodule in lung tissue)
   (5) Night sweats
   (6) Persistent cough
   (7) Oral lesions may appear as an ulcerated lesion on the tongue or mucosa (rare)

f. Diagnosis by a skin test and a radiograph

g. Indochinese refugees have a high incidence of tuberculosis

3. Whooping cough (pertussis)
   a. Agent is *Bordetella pertussis*
   b. Transmitted by inhalation of droplets
   c. Spasmodic coughing and gasping noise with inhalation

4. Psittacosis
   a. Agent is *Chlamydia psittaci*
   b. Transmission
      (1) Humans infected by inhaling dust contaminated with excreta of infected birds
      (2) Symptoms in humans include fever and pneumonitis; spread from the lungs to the spleen, brain, or other organs; mild, coldlike illness; may be asymptomatic
      (3) Many birds including parakeets, canaries, lovebirds, and cockatoos can suffer from this disease

B. Fungal infections
   1. Histoplasmosis
      a. Agent is *Histoplasma capsulatum*
      b. Transmitted by spores, especially in excreta of wild birds, poultry, and bats
      c. Symptoms
         (1) Asymptomatic or mild infection of the lung
         (2) Acute severe pulmonary infection
         (3) Chronic pulmonary disease
   2. Coccidioidomycosis
      a. Agent is *Coccidioides immitis*
      b. Transmitted by inhalation of dust or soil containing arthrospores
      c. Three forms include acute, chronic, and disseminated
      d. Symptoms
         (1) Skin lesions are common
         (2) Meningitis

3. Blastomycosis
   a. Agent is *Blastomyces dermatitidis*
   b. Endemic in dogs and humans
   c. Three forms include primary pulmonary, primary cutaneous, and disseminated
   d. Symptoms
      (1) Enlarged lymph nodes
      (2) Fever, cough, and general discomfort
      (3) Oral mucosa may have lesions in the disseminated form

C. Influenza virus infection
   1. Agents are orthomyxoviruses
   2. Secondary infection by *S. aureus, H. infleunzae, S. pyogenes,* and *S. pneumoniae;* may result in bronchitis and pneumonia
   3. Transmitted by inhalation of contaminated air
   4. Virus attaches to the respiratory epithelium
   5. Soft palate is usually inflamed

Infections of the Gastrointestinal Tract

A. Bacterial infections
   1. Cholera
      a. Agent is *Vibrio cholerae*
      b. Severe diarrhea
      c. Transmitted in unsanitary living conditions
   2. Salmonellosis
      a. Agent includes several species of *Salmonella*
      b. Active infection (food poisoning) produced by organisms
      c. Transmitted through contaminated food or water
      d. Sudden onset often associated with group meals (e.g., wedding receptions or banquets)
      e. Symptoms include abdominal pain, diarrhea, dizziness, fever, headache, nausea, and vomiting
   3. Shigellosis (bacillary dysentery)
      a. Agents are *Shigella dysenteriae* and *Shigella flexneri*
      b. Transmitted through contaminated food or water
      c. Complications include carrier state, perforation of the large intestine, and massive bleeding
   4. Diarrhea caused by *Escherichia coli*
      a. Member of the normal intestinal flora
      b. Cause of traveler's diarrhea when exposed to different strains of *E. coli*
      c. Cause of infant epidemic diarrhea
   5. Typhoid fever
      a. Agent is *Salmonella typhi*
      b. Transmitted through contaminated food or water

    c. Symptoms include fever, severe headache, abdominal pain, and abdominal rash

    d. Complications include carrier state, relapses, inflammation of the gallbladder, and intestinal bleeding

  6. Food poisoning

    a. Results from toxins produced by bacteria

    b. Botulism

      (1) Agent is *Clostridium botulinum*

        (a) Regularly contaminates human, plant, and animal food products

        (b) Produces a deadly toxin that acts on nerves

      (2) Incubation period is from 12 to 96 hours

      (3) Transmitted through improperly preserved foods and uncooked fish and meats; foods do not appear contaminated

      (4) Symptoms include difficulty in speaking, blurred vision, inability to swallow, heart failure, and respiratory paralysis

      (5) Infant botulism results from ingestion of spores occurring in dust and foods

    c. Staphylococcal food poisoning

      (1) Toxin produced by staphylococci (usually *S. aureus*) in unrefrigerated foods such as dairy products, custard, cream-filled products, fish, or processed meats

      (2) Incubation period is from 1 to 6 hours

      (3) Symptoms include abdominal cramps, chills, bluish coloration of the skin, diarrhea, nausea, and headache

      (4) Complications or death is rare

    d. Perfringens poisoning

      (1) Agent is *Clostridium perfringens*

      (2) Incubation period is 18 hours

      (3) Symptoms are similar to those of staphylococcal food poisoning

B. Viral infections

  1. Cytomegalovirus (CMV) inclusion disease

    a. Salivary gland viruses

    b. Infants can acquire CMV congenitally; results in developmental malformations in the fetus

    c. Symptoms include hepatitis, decreased number of blood platelets, increased size of the liver and spleen, and loss of sight

  2. Viral hepatitis (Table 7-7)

    a. Inflammation of the liver

    b. Often impossible to distinguish clinically among the types of viral hepatitis

    c. Occupational hazard for medical and dental personnel

    d. Hepatitis A (formerly infectious hepatitis)

      (1) Terminology

        (a) Hepatitis A virus (HAV)

        (b) Antibody to hepatitis A virus (anti-HAV)

      (2) Transmission

        (a) Oral-fecal route in unsanitary conditions; contaminated food and water

        (b) Rarely through the blood

      (3) Incubation period is from 15 to 40 days

        (a) Communicability diminishes after jaundice

        (b) Usually occurs in children and young adults

      (4) Symptoms

        (a) Preicteric (before jaundice appears) —similar to influenza; fever, headache, nausea, vomiting, fatigue, and abdominal pain

        (b) Icteric—jaundice (rare in children); other symptoms continue

        (c) Anicteric—without jaundice; two to three times more prevalent than icteric state; symptoms resemble those of influenza

      (5) Recovery and immunity

        (a) Anti-HAV is usually in the blood 2 weeks after onset

        (b) Most individuals recover completely in 4 to 6 weeks

        (c) Immunity develops following recovery

        (d) No carrier state develops

      (6) Passive immunization

        (a) Immune globulin for prevention in susceptible persons exposed to hepatitis A

        (b) Given within the first few days after exposure

    e. Hepatitis B (serum hepatitis)

      (1) Terminology

        (a) Hepatitis B virus (HBV)

        (b) Hepatitis B surface antigen (HB_sAg) (Australia antigen)—serologic indicator found in the blood during an acute, chronic, or carrier state of hepatitis B

        (c) Hepatitis B core antigen (HB_cAg)

Table 7-7 Comparison of viral hepatitis: types A, B, and NANB

	Type A	Type B	Type NANB
Etiologic agent	HAV	HBV	Not yet defined
Antigen-antibody systems	HAV; anti-HA	HB_sAg; anti-HB_s HB_cAg; anti-HB_c HB_eAg; anti-HB_e	Not yet defined
Principal transmission route	Predominantly fecal-oral	Predominantly parenteral	Predominantly parenteral via transfusions
Incubation period	2 to 5 weeks	2 to 6 months	Similar to type B
Age preference	Predominantly children and young adults	Any age but uncommon under age 15 years	Probably similar to type B
Seasonal incidence	Fall and winter	None	None
Severity	Usually mild	Occasionally severe	Occasionally severe
Complications	Rare	Yes	Yes
Immunity conferred following infection	Probably lifetime	Probably lifetime	Probably lifetime
Immune globulin (IG) prophylaxis	IG usually effective	IG has variable effectiveness; hepatitis B IG usuly effective	Unknown
Vaccine available	No	Yes	No
Carrier state	No	Yes, in 5% to 10% of patients	Probably, but not yet defined

From Little, J.W., and Falace, D.A.: Dental management of the medically compromised patient, ed. 2, St. Louis, 1984, The C.V. Mosby Co.

(d) Hepatitis B e antigen (HB_eAg) —considered an indicator of infectivity; may indicate development of chronic liver disease

(e) Antibody to HB_sAg (anti-HB_s or HB_sAb)—present after clinical or subclinical infection; represents immunity

(f) Antibody to HB_cAg (anti-HB_c or HB_cAb)—found during the active phase of acute hepatitis; "with anti-HB_s" means immunity

(g) Antibody to HB_eAg (anti-HB_e or HB_eAb)—indicates a low infectivity rate but not necessarily complete elimination of infectivity

(2) Transmission

(a) Infected blood or serum through parenteral inoculation (e.g., blood transfusions, contaminated dental or medical instruments, needles and syringes used by drug abusers, and accidental self-inoculation by health care professionals)

(b) Other body fluids, including saliva, semen, tears, urine, sweat, and nasopharyngeal secretions

(c) Oral or sexual contact or other close personal contact

(d) Coughing or sneezing and aerosols

(e) Salivary transmission by way of hands, instruments, and other equipment is important in the practice of dental hygiene

(3) Incubation

(a) Between 60 and 160 days

(b) Presence of HB_sAg indicates ability to be infective

(4) Symptoms

(a) Similar to hepatitis A

(b) Slower in onset; longer duration

(c) More severe, debilitating

(d) Person may have subclinical disease and remain undiagnosed

(e) May result in chronic liver disease; strong evidence for link between chronic hepatitis B infection and liver cancer[7]

(5) Recovery

(a) Development of anti-HB_s indicates immunity

(b) Between 5% and 10% of those infected develop a chronic carrier state; HB_sAg still present after 6 months; person can remain a carrier for as long as 25 years; carriers are usually asymptomatic and often undetected

(6) High-risk individuals
    (a) Persons with a history of hepatitis or jaundice
    (b) Patients receiving renal dialysis or hemodialysis
    (c) Patients with hemophilia or leukemia and other patients who have received many blood transfusions
    (d) Blood bank and hemodialysis technicians
    (e) Drug addicts who inject themselves
    (f) Dentists and health care workers with frequent blood contact
    (g) Family and close associates of patients and carriers of hepatitis or drug addicts[12]
    (h) Male homosexuals and prostitutes
    (i) Institutionalized persons, particularly those with Down syndrome, and prisoners
    (j) Persons exposed to hepatitis B in the past 6 months
    (k) Military personnel
    (l) Patients receiving long-term immunosuppressive therapy
    (m) Residents of areas with a high incidence of hepatitis, particularly Indochinese refugees
(7) Immunization
    (a) Active results from hepatitis B vaccine (Heptavax-B)
    (b) Passive results from hepatitis B immune globulin (HBIg); used for postexposure prophylaxis; preferably within 24 to 48 hours; partially effective[7]
f. Non-A hepatitis, non-B hepatitis
  (1) Transmitted through blood transfusions
  (2) Agent not yet identified
  (3) Symptoms similar to hepatitis A and B
  (4) Carrier state can develop

Infections of the Circulatory System

Diseases of the Heart

A. Rheumatic fever and rheumatic heart disease
  1. Rheumatic fever—hypersensitivity state developing after streptococcal infection; associated with β-hemolytic group A streptococci
  2. Heart valves become inflamed; subsequent abnormal growths of connective tissue; scarring of valves occurs, resulting in rheumatic heart disease

Table 7-8 Underlying heart disease in patients with infective endocarditis

Underlying heart disease	Percent
Rheumatic heart disease	45
Congenital heart disease	10
Arteriosclerosis, prosthetic heart valves, calcific murmurs of undetermined etiology	35
No apparent cardiac abnormalities	10

From McGhee, J.R., Michalek, S.M., and Cassell, G.H., editors: Dental microbiology, New York, 1982, Harper & Row, Publishers, Inc.

  3. Heart valve damage
    a. Stenosis—narrowing of the valve opening
    b. Valvular insufficiency—failure of the valve to close completely
  4. Antibiotic premedication is necessary before dental treatment
B. Infectious endocarditis (Table 7-8)
  1. Inflammatory condition of the heart; microbial colonization of the endothelial membrane that covers the inner surface of the heart and valves
  2. Predisposing factors
    a. Heart valves scarred by rheumatic fever
    b. Valves altered by congenital malformations
    c. Arteriosclerosis
    d. Patients who have had cardiac surgery (valve replacement)
    e. Narcotic abusers
    f. Patients with low resistance to infection
  3. Dental procedures that may allow bacteria to enter the bloodstream (bacteremia) and lodge in the heart valves
    a. Surgical procedures, extractions, periodontal surgery, and administration of a local anesthesic
    b. Endodontics
    c. Deep scaling, curettage
  3. Agents
    a. Oral streptococci account for more than 50% of the cases
      (1) Three species predominate: *S. mitis, S. sanguis,* and *S. mutans*
      (2) Production of extracellular glucans; aids adherence to the heart valves
    b. *Staphylococcus eidermidis* has become more common in endocarditis
  4. Symptoms
    (a) Prolonged fever
    (b) Changing heart murmur
    (c) Bacterial growths on valves
    (d) May result in death
  5. Antibiotic prophylaxis recommended for all dental procedures likely to cause bleeding

Other Microbial Diseases of the Circulatory System

A. Bacterial infections
1. Tularemia
   a. Agent is *Francisella tularensis*
   b. Transmitted by flies, ticks, contaminated water, and carcasses of infected animals
   c. Enlargement of lymph nodes
2. Rickettsial infections
   a. Obligate, intracellular parasites
   b. Transmitted by arthropods such as fleas, lice, mites, and ticks
   c. Rocky Mountain spotted fever (tick vector)
   d. Endemic typhus (flea borne, common in rats)
   e. Rickettsialpox (mouse mite vector)
   f. Symptoms
      (1) High fever
      (2) Inflammatory reaction at the site of the insect bite
      (3) Generalized rash
      (4) Variety of systemic manifestations; most involve the circulatory system
B. Protozoan infections—malaria
1. Spread by *Anopheles* mosquitoes
2. Symptoms include shaking, chills, fever, headache, and nausea
C. Infectious mononucleosis
1. Agent is Epstein-Barr (EB) virus
2. Acute leukemia-like infection
3. Involves the lymph nodes and spleen; increase in lymphocytes
4. Primarily found in young adults
5. Transmitted by kissing or sharing drinking glasses
6. Symptoms include mild jaundice, fever, enlarged and tender lymph nodes, sore throat, bleeding gingiva, and general weakness

Infections of the Reproductive and Urinary System

Urinary Tract Infections

A. Agents
1. Usually caused by normal intestinal flora and coliforms
2. *E. coli, P. aeruginosa, S. aureus, Streptococcus faecalis,* and *C. albicans*
3. In culture, presence of more than 100,000 bacteria per milliliter of urine is strongly indicative of infection
B. Predisposing conditions
1. Diabetes mellitus
2. Neurologic diseases (e.g., polio and spinal cord injury)

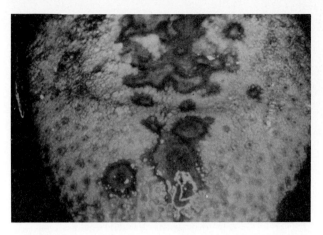

Fig. 7-6 Gonococcal glossitis. (Courtesy Beverly Entwistle, Department of Applied Dentistry, University of Colorado School of Dentistry, Denver, Colo.)

3. Lesions (e.g., kidney stones) interfering with urine flow
4. Eclampsia of pregnancy
C. Symptoms
1. Blood in urine
2. Accumulation of fluid in tissue
3. Pain
4. Kidney enlargement
5. Blood loss and resultant anemia

Reproductive System Infections

A. Puerperal (childbirth) sepsis
1. Infection in the genital tract in women following childbirth
2. Agents are anaerobic streptococci, clostridia, and *E. coli*
B. Venereal diseases
1. Gonorrhea
   a. Agent is *Neisseria gonorrhoeae,* a gram-negative aerobic bacteria
      (1) Highly infectious
      (2) Grow primarily in the genitourinary tract; possess pili that allow attachment to mucosal cells
      (3) Sometimes found in the pharynx; localized yellow or gray-white raised patches or generalized lesions with a gray membrane; membrane sloughs, leaving a bright area; seen on the gingiva, tongue, and soft palate; may have itching or burning.
      (4) Gonococcal glossitis (Fig. 7-6)
      (5) Destroyed by drying and temperature changes

b. Incidence/prevalence
   (1) Most frequently reported infectious disease in the United States
   (2) Increased 100% in 14 years
   (3) Incidence is 443/100,000 population
   (4) Cases reported more often in men (3:1), probably because of subtle and often undiagnosed symptoms in women
c. Transmission
   (1) Primarily direct sexual contact
   (2) Newborn's eyes may be infected on passing through the birth canal (ophthalmia neonatorum); use of silver nitrate or antibiotic after birth reduces incidence
   (3) Type of host epithelium influences invasiveness
       (a) Columnar and transitional epithelium highly susceptible
       (b) Stratified squamous epithelium highly resistant
d. Symptoms
   (1) Men experience painful, frequent urination and mucous and pus-containing discharge
   (2) Women frequently do not have symptoms; may have urethral or vaginal discharge, backache, or abdominal pain
   (3) Both men and women experience pharyngitis, glossitis, or stomatitis including some areas of ulceration (see Fig. 15-13)
e. Complications include sterility, endocarditis, meningitis, and the carrier state
f. Use of oral contraceptives increases the possibility of infection by creating more favorable growth conditions for *N. gonorrhoeae*

2. Syphilis
   a. Agent is *Treponema pallidum*
      (1) Spirochete, anaerobic
      (2) Outside the body, *T. pallidum* is vulnerable to physical and chemical agents; easily killed by heat, drying, and exposure to oxygen, soap, and water
   b. Incidence/prevalence
      (1) Third most frequently reported infectious disease in the United States
      (2) Between 1977 and 1980, 34% increase
   c. Transmission
      (1) Direct contact with lesions in primary and secondary stages; lesions may be oral, genital, or skin
      (2) *T. pallidum* can pass through abraded skin and intact mucous membranes
      (3) Organisms gain access to the circulatory system; affect all organs; rapidly spread to the lymphatic system and bloodstream
      (4) Congenital syphilis occurs when *T. pallidum* crosses the placenta
   d. Symptoms (Fig. 7-7)
      (1) Primary stage
          (a) Chancre—single granulomatous lesion; often asymptomatic; common on the lips; may involve the tongue and oral mucosa; highly contagious; occurs 2 to 3 weeks after exposure and lasts 3 to 5 weeks; red, small, elevated nodule; heals spontaneously; no scarring
          (b) After contact local disinfection ineffective because of the immediate rapid spread of organisms
      (2) Secondary stage
          (a) Appears 6 to 8 weeks after exposure; patient can be asymptomatic for 2 to 6 months and then have secondary lesions appear
          (b) Flulike symptoms
          (c) Skin rashes—maculopapular rash on the face, hands, and feet
          (d) Mucous patches on the lips, soft palate, and tongue—painless shallow ulcers; grayish white areas may be removed, leaving red areas of erosion; highly contagious
          (e) Swollen lymph nodes
      (3) Tertiary stage
          (a) Gumma—inflammatory granulomatous lesion with a central zone of necrosis; may be on the tongue, palate (perforation), or facial bones; soft, swollen areas or tumors; not contagious and usually asymptomatic
          (b) Often takes 5 to 20 years to develop
          (c) Involvement of the central nervous system and spinal cord leads to paresis, loss of fine muscle coordination, or personality changes
          (d) Involvement of the cardiovascular system—major cause of death
      (4) Congenital syphilis
          (a) Hutchinson's incisors—notched, bell-shaped (Fig. 7-8)

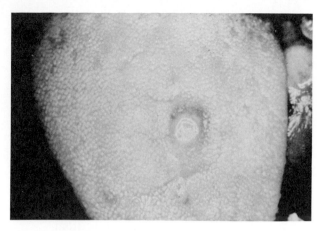

Fig. 7-7 Chancre lesion of primary syphilis. (Courtesy Beverly Entwistle, Department of applied Dentistry, University of Colorado School of Dentistry, Denver, Colo.)

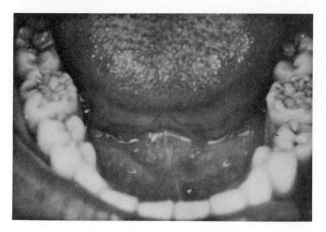

Fig. 7-9 "Mulberry molars" of congenital syphilis. (Courtesy Beverly Entwistle, Department of Applied Dentistry, University of Colorado School of Dentistry, Denver, Colo.)

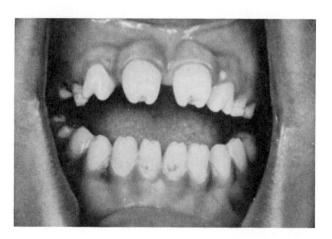

Fig. 7-8 Hutchinson's incisors of congenital syphilis. (Courtesy Beverly Entwistle, Department of Applied Dentistry, University of Colorado School of Dentistry, Denver, Colo.)

       (b) "Mulberry molars"—first molars are irregular with poorly developed cusps (Fig. 7-9)
       (c) Skin, mucous membrane lesions
       (d) High mortality
  3. *Herpesvirus hominis* (herpes simplex)
    a. Type II—herpes genitalis (genital herpes)
    b. Transmitted by sexual contact
    c. Lesions appear 2 to 7 days after exposure
    d. Lesions appear in or on the genitalia and skin
    e. Lesions may ulcerate early and be painful or crust over

    f. Fever, lymphadenopathy
    g. Initial lesions subside and heal in 3 to 5 weeks
    h. Recurrent lesions are less severe (itching, burning, and vesicle formation with healing in 10 to 14 days)
    i. Highly infectious
    j. Primary and recurrent infections
      (1) Most (90%) primary infections are subclinical
      (2) Recurrent infections in women often serve as a source of neonatal herpes
      (3) Cervical herpes may be related to the development of cervical carcinoma

Infections of the Central Nervous System

A. Typical symptoms
  1. Fever
  2. General weakness
  3. Headache
  4. Stiff neck
B. Bacterial infections
  1. Meningitis
    a. Inflammation of protective membranes around the brain and spinal cord
    b. Most common bacterial agents
      (1) *S. pneumoniae*
      (2) *H. influenzae*
  2. Meningococcal meningitis (cerebrospinal fever)
    a. Agent is *Neisseria meningitidis*
    b. Transmitted by inhalation of droplets
    c. Able to cause death for humans faster than any other infectious agent (within 2 hours)

C. Viral infections
  1. Aseptic (nonbacterial) meningitis
     a. Agents are coxsackieviruses, ECHO viruses, and poliomyelitis virus
     b. Primarily observed in children
  2. Poliomyelitis (infantile paralysis)
     a. Agent is poliomyelitis virus
     b. Transmitted via the mouth and intestines
     c. Effects
        (1) Acute inflammation of the meninges; invasion and destruction of the motor neurons
        (2) May range from a mild illness to paralysis
  3. Rabies (hydrophobia)
     a. Agent is rabies virus
     b. Transmitted via saliva from the bite of a rabid animal; usually involves wild mammals
     c. Incubation period is from 4 to 6 weeks or longer
     d. Symptoms include visual difficulties, painful throat spasms, convulsions, and respiratory paralysis
  4. Viral encephalitis
     a. Agents are arboviruses
        (1) Replicate in and spread by arthropods, usually mosquitoes or ticks
        (2) Cause extensive nervous tissue damage and encephalitis
     b. Incubation period is from 4 to 21 days
     c. Symptoms include fever, chills, nausea, fatigue, drowsiness, pain and stiffness of the neck, general disorientation, blindness, deafness, and paralysis
D. Protozan infection—Toxoplasmosis
  1. Agent is *Toxoplasma gondii*
  2. Sources
     a. Infected cat feces
     b. Contaminated raw meat
     c. Contaminated soil
     d. Rodents (cats may eat infected mice)
  3. Transmission
     a. Inhaling or ingesting cysts when handling cat litter or sandboxes frequented by the infected cat
     b. Eating raw meat
     c. Through the placenta (especially important for pregnant women not to eat raw or undercooked meat and not to handle litter boxes)

  4. Symptoms
     a. Resembles infectious mononucleosis in adults
     b. Newborns contracting in utero
        (1) Fever
        (2) Convulsions
        (3) Enlarged spleen
        (4) Central nervous defects causing blindness and mental retardation
E. Fungal infection—cryptococcosis
  1. Agent is *Cryptococcus neoformans*
  2. Transmission
     a. Pigeon droppings promote growth of fungus
     b. Human infection thought to be from inhalation of dehydrated yeasts
  3. Symptoms
     a. Meningitis most common; often associated with diabetes mellitus, immunodeficiency, or corticosteroid treatment
     b. Pulmonary disease
     c. Disseminated disease can affect the adrenal glands, skin, liver, and kidneys

Infections of the Eye

A. Bacterial diseases
  1. Streptococcal infections
     a. Main agent is *S. pneumoniae*
     b. Infections
        (1) Conjunctivitis
           (a) Irritation around the eyelid
           (b) Symptoms include tearing, swelling, redness, and discharge
           (c) Incubation period is from 24 to 27 hours
        (2) Corneal ulcer
        (3) Keratitis (inflammation of the cornea)
        (4) Postoperative infections
  2. Staphylococcal infections
     a. Most common causative agents of eye infections
     b. Main agent is *S. aureus*
     c. Infections
        (1) Conjunctivitis
        (2) Styes
        (3) Keratitis
        (4) Postoperative infections
  3. Pinkeye (acute mucopurulent conjunctivitis)
     a. Agent is *Haemophilus aegypticus*
     b. Incubation period is from 1 to 4 days
     c. Highly contagious
     d. Symptoms include abundant discharge, redness, extreme swelling of the eyelids; bleeding within the conjunctiva can occur

B. Viral diseases
1. Herpes corneae
   a. Agent is *Herpesvirus hominis* (herpes simplex virus type I)
   b. Unilateral ulcer on the conjunctiva or cornea
   c. May be a primary or recurrent lesion
      (1) Recurrent type is more common
      (2) Keratitis is associated with recurrent herpes
      (3) Herpetic conjunctivitis is commonly found in children
2. Conjunctivitis caused by Newcastle disease virus
3. Epidemic keratoconjunctivitis (EKC)
   a. Agent is adenovirus, types 7 and 8
   b. Transmission
      (1) Direct contact with respiratory or ocular secretions
      (2) Possibly swimming pools
      (3) Infection by dust and dirt in factories following injury

Helminths (Worms) as Human Parasites

A. Nematodes (roundworms)
1. Hookworm infection
   a. Adult worm lives in the human small intestine
   b. Transmitted through contaminated soil; infection acquired through the soles of the feet
   c. Generally found in the southern part of the United States and in Central and South America
   d. Symptoms include iron deficiency anemia, abdominal pain, and protein deficiency; mild infections are asymptomatic
2. Pinworm (seatworm, *Enterobius vermicularis* infection)
   a. Adult worm lives in the intestine
   b. More common in children
   c. Tickling or intense itching in the perianal area
   d. Transmission
      (1) Ingestion of larvae
      (2) Handling of fomites (infected bedding and clothes)
      (3) Contaminated hands
      (4) Inhalation of eggs
3. Trichinosis
   a. Adult worm lives in the intestine
   b. Transmitted by eating improperly cooked or inadequately processed pork

c. Symptoms include diarrhea, muscular pain, and nervous disorders; many light infections are asymptomatic

B. Platyhelminths (flatworms)
1. Tapeworms (cestodes)
   a. Adult worm lives in the intestine
   b. Transmitted by contaminated or inadequately cooked beef, pork, lamb, or fish
   c. Symptoms include nausea and abdominal discomfort; many cases are asymptomatic or have poorly defined symptoms
2. Flukes (trematodes)
   a. Adults can live in the liver, lungs, bladder, or large intestine, causing various diseases
   b. Transmitted by inadequately cooked or contaminated fish, vegetation, or crayfish; also by swimming or working in contaminated water

Microbiology of the Oral Cavity

NORMAL ORAL FLORA

A. Composition (Table 7-9)
1. Flora of mucous membranes
   a. Different types of surfaces affect the number and variety of organisms present
   b. Streptococci (gram-positive cocci)
      (1) *Streptococcus salivarius*
      (2) *Streptococcus mitis*
   c. Staphylococci (gram-positive cocci)
      (1) *S. aureus*
      (2) *S. epidermidis*
   d. Veillonellae (anaerobic gram-negative cocci)
   e. Neisseriae (gram-negative cocci)
2. Tongue
   a. Papillae allow for a large surface area for colonization
   b. *S. salivarius* (gram-positive cocci) composes one third of bacteria
   c. Veillonellae (gram-negative diphtheroids) compose one third of bacteria
   d. One third composed of *S. milleri* and *S. mitis* (gram-positive cocci) and *Propionibacterium, Bacteroides, Peptostreptococcus,* and *Peptococcus* (anaerobes)
3. Saliva
   a. Organisms derived mainly from the dorsum of the tongue and plaque
   b. Streptococci
   c. Veillonellae
   d. Neisseriae

Table 7-9 Description of the oral microbiota

Description	Gram stain	Generic name	Preferred oral site(s)*
Cocci	Positive	*Streptococcus*	
		S. faecalis	G
		S. mitis (mitior)	M, S, D, T, G
		S. mutans	D
		S. salivarius	T = S, M
		S. sanguis	D, M, S, T, G
		S. milleri	G, D, T
		Staphylococcus	
		S. epidermidis	
		S. aureus	T, G
		Peptostreptococcus species	
	Negative	*Neisseria*	S (low)
		N. flavescens	
		N. mucosa	
		N. sicca (pharyngis)	
		N. subflava	
Anaerobic cocci	Negative	*Veillonella*	T = G = S
		V. alcalescens	
		V. parvula	
Anaerobic bacilli	Negative	*Bacteroides*	
		B. melaninogenicus	G
		B. saccharolyticus	
		B. oralis	G, D, T
		B. (Eikenella) corrodens	
		B. (Capnocytophaga) ochraceus	
		Fusobacterium	G, D, T
		F. nucleatum	
		F. plauti	
		Leptotrichia	
		L. buccalis	
		Selenomonas	
		S. sputigena (Spirillum sputigena)	
Asporogenous rod-shaped bacteria	Positive	*Lactobacillus* species	G = S
Facultative anaerobic bacilli	Negative	*Haemophilus*	
		H. influenza	
		H. parainfluenza	
		Actinobacillus	
		A. actinomycetemcomitans	
Endospore-forming bacteria	Positive	*Clostridium* species	G
Actinomycetes and related organisms	Positive	*Corynebacterium* species	
		Propionibacteria	
		P. acnes	
		Actinomyces	G, D
		A. israelii	
		A. naeslundii	
		A. odontolyticus	
		A. viscosus	
		Arachnia propionica	
		Bacterionema	
		B. matruchotii	D, G
		Rothia (Nocardia)	
		R. dentocariosa	

From McCracken, A.W., and Cawson R. A.: Clinical and oral microbiology, Washington, D.C., 1983, Hemisphere Publishing Corp.
*The letters designate the site(s) where the organism is predominantly found. If more than one site, they are given in decreasing order of preference; *G*, gingival area; *D*, dental plaque; *T*, tongue; *M*, mucosa; *S*, saliva.

Table 7-9 Description of the oral microbiota—cont'd

Description	Gram stain	Generic name	Preferred oral site(s)
Spiral and curved bacteria	Negative	*Campylobacter* *C. sputorum*	G
The spirochetes		*Treponema* *T. vincentii (Borrelia vincentii)* *T. buccale (Borrelia buccale)* *T. denticola* *T. macrodentium* *T. mucosum* *T. orale* *T. scoliodontum*	G
The mycoplasmas		*Mycoplasma* *M. salivarium* *M. orale*	G
The yeasts		*Candida* *C. albicans*	
The protozoa		*Entamoeba* *E. gingivalis* *Trichomonas* *T. tenax*	
The viruses		*Herpes* *Herpesvirus hominis*	

e. *Haemophilus* organisms

f. Yeasts (90% are *C. albicans*)

g. Viruses

  (1) Not part of the normal flora but present temporarily in disease or asymptomatic infections

  (2) *Herpesvirus hominis* most frequently isolated virus

4. Tooth surfaces (plaque)

  a. Four main areas of dental plaque formation

    (1) Interproximal surfaces

      (a) Inaccessible to routine oral hygiene

      (b) Plaque bacteria can proliferate undisturbed

      (c) Common site for caries

    (2) Occlusal pits and fissures

      (a) Morphologic condition allows for proliferation

      (b) Common site for caries

    (3) Gingival sulcus is an area of stagnation and bacterial proliferation

    (4) Remaining coronal surfaces

      (a) Can be covered with plaque if oral hygiene is absent

      (b) Plaque formation limited by the cleansing action of saliva, soft tissue movement, and the action of food particles

B. Factors influencing microbial composition

  1. Nutrient requirements

    a. Most need carbohydrates

    b. Organic amino acids

    c. Nitrogen

    d. Carbon dioxide

    e. Minerals

  2. Nutrient sources

    a. Exogenous sources include the host's diet, especially dietary sugar needed for acid and polysaccharide production

    b. Endogenous sources

      (1) Saliva

      (2) Gingival exudate

      (3) Epithelial cells and leukocytes

      (4) Flora continues to exist even when humans and animals are fed by a stomach tube

      (5) Certain bacteria use metabolic by-products from other bacteria

  3. pH requirements

    a. Dietary sugars provide a selective force favoring predominance of certain organisms that tolerate an acidic medium

    b. Strains of *S. mutans,* related streptococci, and lactobacilli are both acidogenic (produce acid) and aciduric (tolerate low pH values)

4. Oxygen concentration—plaque is a predominantly anaerobic mass, even on exposed surfaces
5. Microbial interactions
   a. Presence of normal flora inhibits pathogenic colonization
   b. Interspecies antagonisms—acid-producing and hydrogen peroxide–producing–bacteria inhibit staphylococci and corynebacteria; acid producers include *S. mutans*, *S. salivarius*, *Streptococcus sanguis*, and lactobacilli; hydrogen peroxide producers include *S. mitis*, *S. sanguis*, and viridans streptococci
   c. Bacteria yield virulent phages that may inhibit other bacteria
   d. Microbial aggregation
      (1) Certain species undergo reactions between cell surfaces
      (2) Such reactions may contribute to the formation and accumulation of plaque
6. Saliva
   a. Flow rate bears some relationship to caries susceptibility
   b. Rate of secretion is correlated to the buffering capacity
   c. Components aid in bacterial attachment to teeth
   d. Immunologic and nonimmunologic components may adversely affect attachment to teeth or inhibit bacterial growth
      (1) High molecular weight glycoproteins inhibit adherence
      (2) Antibacterial components include lysozyme, lactoperoxidase, and lactoferrin
      (3) Secretory IgA inhibits microbial attachment
   e. Flow of saliva removes bacteria from oral surfaces

Development of Oral Microflora

A. Oral cavity usually sterile at birth
B. Number of organisms increases 6 to 10 hours after birth
C. At 12 months most children have
   1. Streptococcus
      a. *S. salivarius* is first oral streptococcus
      b. *S. mutans* and *S. sanguis* are not established until teeth erupt
      c. *S. mutans* disappears when full-month extractions occur; reappears with dentures
   2. Staphylococcus
   3. *Veillonella* organisms

   4. *Neisseria* organisms
   5. *Actinomyces* organisms
   6. Lactobacilli
   7. *Nocardia* organisms
   8. *Fusobacterium* organisms
D. Preschool-age child
   1. Resembles flora of adult
   2. *Bacteroides melaninogenicus* and spirochetes not common

BACTERIAL DENTAL PLAQUE

(See Chapter 11, section on bacterial dental plaque)
A. Definition
   1. Deposit formed by the colonization of teeth by members of the normal oral flora
   2. Complex of bacteria in the matrix mainly of bacterial polysaccharides
B. Stages of formation
   1. Cell-free pellicle
      a. High molecular weight salivary glycoproteins
      b. Quickly colonized by bacteria
   2. Bacterial colonization
      a. Streptococci show early dominance
      b. *S. sanguis* is usually one of the first colonizers, but lactobacilli, nocardiae, veillonellae, or neisseriae may be found in the beginning
      c. Filamentous bacteria appear in 7 to 14 days
      d. Complexity increases
      e. Respiration becomes increasingly anaerobic (increase in *Bacteroides* and *Fusobacterium* organisms)
C. Factors affecting adherence and retention
   1. Salivary glycoprotein
      a. Affinity for hydroxyapatite
      b. Causes bacteria to aggregate
   2. Specific bacterial attachment mechanisms
      a. Electrostatic forces
      b. Bacterial surface components bind to the pellicle
   3. Bacterial competition
      a. Relative numbers of a species may affect colonization patterns
      b. *S. sanguis* has a stronger affinity for enamel than *S. mutans;* fewer numbers of *S. mutans* are in saliva and available to compete for tooth sites
   4. Bacterial interactions—some evidence that *S. mutans* and *S. sanguis* are antagonistic; often one predominates
   5. Natural local cleansing activity and retentive areas
   6. Diet

D. Plaque polysaccharides
 1. Extracellular
    a. Glucans
       (1) Synthesized from sucrose
       (2) Properties
           (a) Insoluble
           (b) May mediate attachment of bacteria to dental tissues
           (c) May serve as nutrient reserves
           (d) May entrap bacterial enzymes or metabolic products
           (e) Ability of *S. mutans* to produce glucans appears essential for cariogenicity
       (3) Produced by *S. mutans, S. sanguis, S. salivarius, Lactobacillus casei, Lactobacillus acidophilus,* and *Neisseria* organisms
    b. Levans (fructans)
       (1) Soluble
       (2) Reserve nutrients
       (3) Produced by *Actinomyces viscosus, S. mutans, S. salivarius,* and *Rothia dentocariosa*
 2. Intracellular
    a. Glycogen-like
    b. Function seems to be a reserve source of carbohydrate
    c. Synthesized by *S. mutans* and many noncariogenic bacteria
E. Microbial composition of plaque
 1. Factors affecting composition
    a. Site sampled
    b. Oral hygiene
    c. Diet
    d. Maturity of plaque
    e. Host factors
       (1) Age
       (2) Salivary flow
       (3) Tooth and gingival crevice morphology
       (4) Disease status
 2. Bacterial composition of supragingival (supramarginal) plaque (Table 7-10)
    a. Thin layer; 1 to 20 cells thick
    b. Mostly gram-positive facultative anaerobic organisms
    c. Most prominent organisms are *S. sanguis* and *A. viscosus*
    d. Other species found include *Actinomyces naeslundii, Actinomyces israelli, Bacteroides oralis, R. dentocariosa, S. mitis, S. mutans* and *Veillonella, Neisseria,* and *Fusobacterium* organisms

Table 7-10 Predominant cultivable bacteria of dental plaque in periodontal health

Bacteria*	Stain and Morphology
Streptococcus sanguis	Gram + cocci
Actinomyces viscosus	Gram + rod or filament
Actinomyces naeslundii	Gram + rod or filament
Other *Streptococcus* sp.	Gram + cocci
Actinomyces israelii	Gram + filament
Veillonella parvula	Gram − cocci

From McGhee, J.R., Michalek, S.M., and Cassell, G.H., editors: Dental microbiology, New York, 1982, Harper & Row, Publishers, Inc.
*Listed in approximate rank order beginning with the most numerous.

 3. Bacterial composition of normal gingival crevice plaque
    a. Quantity and species relatively constant; proportions of species vary among people and even within the same mouth
    b. Streptococci
    c. *Actinomyces* organisms
    d. Some motile rods, filamentous forms (*Nocardia* and *Corynebacterium* organisms and *R. dentocariosa*)
 4. Bacterial composition in periodontally healthy elderly persons
    a. Characterized by a high level of resistance to disease
    b. Gram-positive bacteria, especially streptococci, which compose 50% of bacteria
    c. Gram-negative anaerobes and/or facultative rods (30%)
       (1) *Bacteroides* organisms
       (2) *Fusobacterium* organisms
       (3) *Bacteroides (Capnocytophaga) ochraceus*
 5. Calculus
    a. Microbes similar to those of the gingival crevice area
    b. Main role in periodontal disease is to serve as a collection site for more bacteria

DENTAL CARIES

A. Prerequisites for caries development
 1. Cariogenic bacteria
 2. Supply of substrate for acid production
 3. Susceptible host
B. Cariogenic bacteria
 1. Essential properties
    a. Acidogenic and aciduric; acid must be produced and low pH maintained for a long period
    b. Ability to attach to tooth surfaces

    c. Formation of protective matrix
    d. Proteolytic activity
  2. Streptococci
    a. *S. mutans*
      (1) Most strongly cariogenic bacteria in animals
      (2) Hard surfaces are a prerequisite for presence; organisms disappear if teeth are extracted; reappear with dentures
      (3) Can maintain acid production at a lower pH than other streptococci; rapidly produces low pH from sugar
      (4) Produces insoluble glucans
      (5) High-sucrose diet is generally associated with an increased *S. mutans* population
      (6) Usually found in early stages of plaque formation
      (7) Association of *S. mutans* with human caries is based on epidemiologic findings, but these findings are conflicting
    b. *S. sanguis*
      (1) Produces glucans
      (2) Some strains are cariogenic in animals
      (3) Colonizes teeth earlier and more widely than *S. mutans*
    c. *S. mitior*
      (1) Synthesizes intracellular polysaccharides
      (2) Cariogenic in animals
    d. *S. milleri*
      (1) Cariogenic in animals
      (2) Generally found near the gingival crevice
    e. *S. salivarius*
      (1) Usually has a strong affinity for oral soft tissues
      (2) Not thought to be cariogenic
  3. Lactobacilli
    a. Present in large numbers in saliva but in small numbers in plaque
    b. Increase in number in the mouth when the sugar content in the diet is high
      (1) Sites in the mouth where sugar is retained
      (2) Carious lesions act as retention sites
    c. Strongly acidogenic and aciduric
    d. Cariogenic in animals; found mainly in fissures
    e. Evidence for causative role in human caries does not appear to be strong
  4. Actinomycetes
    a. *A. viscosus* and *A. naeslundii* cause root-surface caries in animals
    b. Present in plaque

C. Acid production in plaque
  1. Decalcification of teeth occurs by acids produced through bacterial fermentation
  2. Cariogenic plaque, when exposed to sugar, shows a decrease in pH that is low enough to decalcify enamel within minutes; pH returns to resting levels after approximately 45 minutes; even though sugar is washed away by saliva, pH can remain at a low level for 20 minutes[31]
  3. Important features of the acid production process
    a. Rapidity with which sugars diffuse into plaque
    b. Speed at which pH is lowered
    c. Slow return of pH to resting levels
  4. More lactic acid present than any other acid
D. Bacterial substrates and diet
  1. Sucrose
    a. Main substrate for cariogenic bacteria
    b. Readily enters bacterial plaque
    c. Metabolized to form acids and glucans
    d. Essential for caries production in animals
    e. Epidemiologic evidence established its role in human caries
    f. High cariogenic effect when eaten at frequent intervals
    g. High cariogenic effect when retained on teeth for a long period
  2. Starches
    a. Low cariogenicity
    b. Larger molecules than sucrose; may be less available to bacteria
    c. Can increase the cariogenicity of sugar by enhancing the adhesiveness of sugar when the two are combined in foods, such as in cookies and cakes
E. Host factors
  1. Tooth surface
    a. Influence of the genetic contribution to resistant tooth structure is unclear
    b. Nutrition during tooth development can affect structure and, theoretically, resistance
    c. Addition of fluoride to the water supply reduces caries prevalence
  2. Saliva
    a. Functions affecting the carious process
      (1) Clearance of food
      (2) Buffer activity
      (3) Contributions to plaque
      (4) Bacterial aggregation
      (5) Antibacterial functions
    b. Rate of flow and buffering abilities
      (1) As flow rate increases, pH rises
      (2) High salivary flow rates and buffering are associated with low caries activity

INFLAMMATORY PERIODONTAL DISEASES

A. Types
1. Gingivitis (Table 7-11)
   a. Inflammation of gingiva is related to the accumulation of bacterial plaque
   b. Early gingivitis
      (1) Plaque is thicker and more complex than in health; 100 to 300 cells thick
      (2) *Actinomyces* organisms predominate
      (3) Mostly gram-positive organisms
   c. Chronic gingivitis
      (1) Gram-negative organisms increase
      (2) Presence of *Veillonella, Fusobacterium,* and *Bacteroides* organisms
2. Periodontitis
   a. Extension of inflammatory changes into deeper periodontal structures with resulting bone loss
   b. Pockets provide a favorable environment for bacteria
   c. Different bacterial populations associated with destructive periodontitis have been described[31,47] (Table 7-12)

Table 7-11 Predominant cultivable bacteria in experimental and naturally occurring gingivitis

Bacteria*	Stain and morphology
Actinomyces naeslundii	Gram + rod or filament
Veillonella parvula	Gram − cocci
Actinomyces viscosus	Gram + rod or filament
Streptococcus intermedius	Gram + cocci
Streptococcus sanguis	Gram + cocci
Actinomyces odontolyticus	Gram + rod or filament
Fusobacterium nucleatum	Gram − rod
Capnocytophaga gingivalis	Gram − rod
Bacteroides melaninogenicus ss. intermedius	Gram − rod
Streptococcus morbillorum	Gram + rod
Lactobacillus sp	Gram + rod
Hemophilus sp	Gram − rod
Treponema sp	Spiral

From McGhee, J.R., Michalek, S.M., and Cassell, G.H., editors: Dental microbiology, New York, 1982, Harper & Row, Publishers, Inc.
*Not ranked by frequency

Table 7-12 Predominant cultivable bacteria in periodontitis

Bacteria	Supra/Sub*	Stain and morphology
Fusobacterium nucleatum	+ + +/+ + +	Gram − rod
Eubacterium nodatum	±/+ + +	Gram + rod
Eubacterium timidum	+/+ + +	Gram + rod
Bacteroides melaninogenicus ss. intermedius	+ +/+ +	Gram − rod
Actinomyces naeslundii	+ +/+	Gram + rod
Streptococcus sanguis	+ +/+	Gram + rod
Peptostreptococcus micros	+/+ +	Gram + cocci
Actinomyces israelii	+/+	Gram + rod
Bacteroides melaninogenicus ss. melaninogenicus	+ +/+ +	Gram − rod
Capnocytophaga gingivalis	+ +/±	Gram − rod
Eubacterium brachy	−/+	Gram + rod
Proprionibacterium acnes	+/+	Gram + rod
Bacteroides gingivalis†	+/+	Gram − rod
Streptococcus intermedius	+/+	Gram + cocci
Selenomonas sputigena	±/+	Gram − rod
Lactobacillus species	±/+	Gram + rod
Treponema species	+/+ +	Spiral

From McGhee, J.R., Michalek, S.M., Cassell, G.H., editors: Dental microbiology, New York, 1982, Harper & Row, Publishers, Inc.
*Approximate relative frequency of occurrence and numerical prominence in supragingival flora/same estimate in subginigval flora in samples from subjects with periodontitis; + + +, most frequent, −, generally absent.
†Formerly *B. asaccharolyticus*

d. Controversy exists as to predominance and numbers of
   (1) *Bacteroides gingivalis* (formerly *B. asaccharolyticus*
   (2) *Eikenella corrodens*
   (3) *Eubacterium nodation, Eubacterium timidium,* and *Eubacterium brachy*
   (4) *Fusobacterium nucleatum*
   (5) Anaerobic vibrios
   (6) ''Gelatin-loving'' *Bacteroides* organisms

3. Juvenile periodontitis
   a. Controversial etiology
   b. Two groups of gram-negative anaerobic rods are prominent in cases
      (1) *Capnocytophaga*[30,31,36,45,50]
      (2) *Actinobacillus actinomycetem-comitans*
   c. Severe periodontal destruction starting early in life

4. Acute necrotizing ulcerative gingivitis (ANUG)
   a. Anaerobic infection of gingival margins causing ulceration and, if allowed to progress, destruction of gingivae and underlying bone
   b. Appears to be opportunistic infection based on the predisposing factors
   c. Proliferation of fusiforms and spirochetes
      (1) *Fusobacterium nucleatum*
      (2) Spirochetes difficult to cultivate; may be *Borrelia vincentii*

B. Plaque and periodontal disease
   1. Factors determining the severity of periodontal disease
      a. Level of oral hygiene
      b. Nature of bacterial flora of plaque
      c. Host resistance
   2. Evidence supports a microbial etiology of periodontal disease
      a. Difficulties in determining specific bacterial cause
      b. Increasing evidence that plaque associated with gingivitis and periodontitis of varying degrees of severity has different bacterial populations
      c. Current approaches
         (1) Establish the predominant cultivable flora of plaques associated with various degrees of disease
         (2) Assess the nature of the bacterial population in plaque at different oral sites
         (3) Quantify the kinds and relative numbers of bacteria present, especially of the more potentially pathogenic flora

3. Pathogenic mechanisms of plaque bacteria
   a. Attachment mechanisms
      (1) Attachment to the tooth surface may depend on gram-positive (e.g., *Streptococcus* and *Actinomyces*) organisms
      (2) *Bacteriodes gingivalis* and *F. nucleatum* adhere to oral epithelial cells
   b. Products of bacteria
      (1) Bacteria themselves do not invade tissue
      (2) Products may result in tissue destruction
         (a) Endotoxins
         (b) Enzymes (collagenase, lysozyme, and hyaluronidase)

4. Immunologic aspects of periodontal disease
   a. Bacteria of plaque are antigenic in varying degrees; present a challenge to the immune system
   b. Immune responses are just as likely to be protective as they are injurious to tissue
   c. A variety of mechanisms of tissue destruction have been suggested; no confirmation at this time of their participation in periodontal tissue destruction in humans
   d. Participation of the humoral immune system
      (1) Lymphocytes and plasma cells are the predominant cells in the gingiva in the vicinity of plaque
      (2) Antibody production is stimulated
      (3) Complement system is activated
         (a) Mediates inflammatory response and immunologic reactions
         (b) Evidence that complement is activated by plaque bacteria, either by endotoxin (lipopolysaccharide) or by bacterial antigen-antibody complexes
         (c) Involved with chemotaxis (directed migration of inflammatory cells)
   e. Participation of the cell-mediated immune system
      (1) Evidence of cell-mediated immunity in response to plaque bacteria has been reported in humans[31]
      (2) Conflicting reports when correlating the cell-mediated reactivity with the severity of periodontal disease
      (3) Clinically not possible to distinguish between cell-mediated immunity (resistance) and delayed hypersensitivity (damaging) reactions in humans; both reactions depend on the same cellular participants

PERIAPICAL INFECTIONS AND ORAL-FACIAL TISSUE INFECTIONS ▰▰▰

A. Infections
  1. Abscesses (periodontal and periapical)
  2. Postsurgical and extraction wound infections
  3. Endodontically involved infections
  4. Sinus tract infections
  5. Cellulitis
  6. Traumatic injuries
  7. Osteomyelitis
  8. Postextraction alveolar osteitis (dry socket)
  9. Pericoronitis
  10. Periodontally involved infections
B. Bacteria cultivated from such infections (Tables 7-13 and 7-14)
  1. Most common
    a. *Bacteroides* organisms
    b. *Fusobacterium* organisms
    c. *Peptostreptococcus*
    d. *S. mitis*
    e. *S. salivarius*
    f. *S. faecalis*

Table 7-13 Predominating bacteria detected in 120 pyogenic oral infections

Organism	Frequency of occurrence
Streptococcus species	50%
S. pyogenes	0%
Staphylococcus aureus	4%
Coliforms	14%
Bacteroides species	37%
Fusobacterium species	2%
Anaerobic gram-positive cocci	8%
Anaerobic gram-positive rods	6%

From McGhee, J.R., Michalek, S.M., and Cassell, G.H., editors: Dental microbiology, New York, 1982, Harper & Row, Publishers, Inc.

Table 7-14 Predominant organisms detected in 126 samples from acute oral-facial infections

Lesion category	Anaerobic organisms	Aerobic organisms
Abscess (46/126) 37%*	*Bacteroides melaninogenicus* (16/46) 16%† *B. melaninogenicus* ss. *melaninogenicus* (3/46) 7% *B. melaninogenicus* ss. *intermedius* (1/46) 2% *Bacteroides asaccharolyticus* (2/46) 4% *Bacteroides uniformis* (1/46) 2% *Bacteroides* sp. (19/46) 42% *Fusobacterium nucleatum* (2/46) 4% *Fusobacterium* sp. (1/46) 2% *Veillonella parvula* (3/46) 7% *Streptococcus intermedius* (2/46) 4% *Peptostreptococcus parvula* (1/46) 2% *Peptostreptococcus anaerobius* (1/46) 2% *Peptostreptococcus micros* (1/46) 2% *Peptostreptococcus* sp. (1/46) 2% *Propionibacterium acnes* (1/46) 2% Anaerobic gram positive rods (2/46) 4%	*Streptococcus mitis* (1/46) 2% *Streptococcus viridans* (26/46) 57% *Streptococcus fecalis* (1/46) 2% *Streptococcus group B* (1/46) 2% *Staphylococcus aureus* (1/46) 2% *Klebsiella pneumoniae* (3/46) 7%
Post-surgical and extraction wounds (32/126) 25%	*B. melaninogenicus* ss. *melaninogenicus* (3/32) 9% *B. melaninogenicus* ss. *intermedius* (1/32) 3% *Bactercoides asaccharolyticus* (1/32) 3% *Bacteroides* sp. (6/32) 19% *Veillonella parvula* (1/32) 3% *Streptococcus intermedius* (3/32) 9% *Actinomyces viscosus* (1/32) 3%	*Streptococcus mitis* (2/32) 6% *Streptococcus sanguis* (1/32) 3% *Streptococcus viridans* (10/32) 31% *Streptococcus, group B* (1/32) 3% *Staphylococcus aureus* (3/32) 9% *Eikenella corrodens* (3/32) 9% *Pseudomonas aeruginosa* (2/32) 6% *Enterobacter cloacae* (1/32) 3% *Enterobacter aerogenes* (2/32) 6% *Escherichia coli* (2/32) 6% *Klebsiella oxytoxa* (1/32) 3% *Klebsiella pneumoniae* (1/32) 3% *Klebsiella* sp. (1/32) 3%

From McGhee, J.R., Michalek, S.M., and Cassell, G.H., editors: Dental microbiology, New York, 1982, Harper & Row, Publishers, Inc.
*(Number of lesions out of total specimens) and percentage
†(Number of specimens from which isolated in each lesion category) and percentage

Table 7-14 Predominant organisms detected in 126 samples
from acute oral-facial infections — cont'd

Lesion category	Anaerobic organisms	Aerobic organisms
Endodontically involved infections (25/126) 20%	*Bacteroides melaninogenicus* (1/25) 4% *B. melaninogenicus ss. intermedius* (1/25) 4% *Bacteroides uniformis* (1/25) 4% *Bacteroides capillosus* (1/25) 4% *Bacteroides* sp. (4/25) 16% *Fusobacterium nucleatum* (1/25) 4% *Veillonella parvula* (1/25) 4% *Streptococcus intermedius* (1/25) 4% *Peptococcus saccharolyticus* (1/25) 4% *Actinomyces odontolyticus* (1/25) 4% *Actinomyces* sp. (1/25) 4% Anaerobic gram positive rods (2/25) 8%	*Streptococcus sanguis* (1/25) 4% *Streptococcus viridans* (12/25) 48% *Streptococcus fecalis* (2/25) 8% *Klebsiella pneumoniae* (1/25) 4%
Sinus tracts (16/126) 13%	*Bacteroides melaninogenicus* (2/16) 13% *Bacteroides asaccharolyticus* (1/16) 6% *Bacteroides capillosus* (1/16) 6% *Bacteroides* sp. (1/16) 6% *Capnocytophaga* sp. (1/16) 6% *Streptococcus intermedius* (1/16) 6% *Peptococcus saccharolyticus* (1/16) 6% *Peptostreptococcus anaerobius* (1/16) 6% *Actinomyces* sp. (2/16) 13% *Veillonella parvula* (1/16) 6%	*Streptococcus viridans* (6/16) 38% *Eikenella corrodens* (1/16) 6% *Pseudomonas aeruginosa* (1/16) 6% *Klebsiella pneumoniae* (2/16) 13%
Cellulitis (10/126) 8%	*Bacteroides melaninogenicus* (2/10) 20% *Bacteroides asaccharolyticus* (1/10) 10% *Bacteroides* sp. (3/10) 30% *Fusobacterium nucleatum* (1/10) 10% *Peptostreptococcus* sp. (1/10) 10% Anaerobic gram positive rods (1/10) 10%	*Streptococcus viridans* (8/10) 80%
Surface Lesion (6/126) 5%		*Candida albicans* (3/6) 50% normal flora only: (*Streptococcus* and *Neisseria* sp. (3/6) 50%
Traumatic injuries (6/126) 5%	*Bacteroides melaninogenicus* (2/6) 33% *Bacteroides* sp. (1/6) 17% *Capnocytophaga* sp. (1/6) 17% *Actinomyces* sp. (1/6) 17%	*Streptococcus mitis* (1/6) 17% *Streptococcus viridans* (1/6) 17% *Klebsiella oxytoca* (1/6) 17%
Osteomyelitis (5/126) 4%	*B. melaninogenicus ss. intermedius* (1/5) 20% *Bacteroides asaccharolyticus* (1/5) 20% *Bacteroides ureolyticus* (1/5) 20% *Bacteroides* sp. (1/5) 20% *Capnocytophaga* sp. (1/5) 20% *Peptococcus saccharolytics* (1/5) 20% *Actinomyces* sp. (1/5) 20%	*Streptococcus viridans* (2/5) 40%
Cyst related infections (3/126) 2%		*Streptococcus mitis* (1/3) 33% *Streptococcus viridans* (2/3) 67%
Periodontally involved infections (2/126) 2%	*Bacteroides* sp. (2/2) 100%	
Human bite (1/126) 0.8%		*Streptococcus mitis* (1/1) 100% *Streptococcus sanguis* (1/1) 100%

2. Least common
   a. *S. pyogenes*
   b. *S. aureus*
   c. When either of these do occur, the organisms can produce severe oral-facial infections

OPPORTUNISTIC INFECTIONS OF THE ORAL CAVITY

A. Definition—organisms that take advantage of a compromised situation in the host and subsequently invade and cause infection
B. Actinomycosis
   1. Agent is *A. israelii*
      a. Gram-positive bacteria
      b. Member of the normal oral and intestinal flora
   2. Noncontagious, progressive
   3. Usually occurs after trauma (e.g., tooth extraction or facial fracture)
   4. Symptoms
      a. Facial swelling, most commonly in soft tissues below the angle of the jaw
      b. Small, chronic, superficial mass
      c. Abscess with sinus and chronic discharge develops
C. Ludwig's angina
   1. Mixed infection
      a. *S. pyogenes, S. aureus,* and spirochetes
      b. Often caused by the normal oral flora gaining access through the infected tooth
   2. Symptoms
      a. Rapidly spreading, diffuse bilateral cellulitis of the floor of the mouth and neck
      b. Swelling may block air passages
      c. Fever and malaise
   3. Predisposing factors
      a. Infected mandibular molars
      b. Thin lingual cortical plate of the mandible
D. Pseudomonas species can enter wounds when the air-water syringe is used
E. Candidiasis
F. Staphylococci
   1. Normal flora of the skin, oral cavity, and anterior nares
   2. Important pathogens
      a. *S. aureus*
      b. *S. epidermidis*

3. Infections
   a. Localized
      (1) Cellulitis
      (2) Carbuncles
   b. Systemic
      (1) Endocarditis
      (2) Pneumonia
   c. Mandibular osteomyelitis
   d. Acute suppurative parotitis
E. Other oral diseases
   1. Mumps (acute epidemic parotitis)
      a. Agent is mumps virus
      b. Symptoms
         (1) Painful, swollen parotid or submaxillary glands
         (2) Fever and malaise
         (3) Papilla of Stensen's duct is red and swollen
      c. Prevention through vaccine
   2. Herpangina (vesicular pharyngitis)
      a. Agent is coxsackievirus A
      b. Primarily occurs in children
      c. Symptoms
         (1) Fever
         (2) Vomiting
         (3) Vesicles and later ulcers on the mucous membrane of the throat, palate, or tongue
      d. Recovery in 7 to 10 days; complications rare
   3. Recurrent apthous ulcers
      a. Etiology unknown; evidence suggests immunologic role
      b. Appearance
         (1) Canker sore, small ulcer
         (2) Covered by pseudomembrane
         (3) Surrounding erythematous halo
         (4) Occur on the nonkeratinized mucosa
      c. Heal within 1 week without scarring
   4. Hand, foot, and mouth disease
      a. Agent is coxsackievirus A
         (1) Highly infectious
         (2) Typically affects many children, particularly in schools
      b. Symptoms
         (1) Vesicular stomatitis and rash
         (2) Affects the buccal mucosa, tongue, gingiva, lips, hands, and feet
         (3) Pain

PREVENTION OF DISEASE TRANSMISSION IN DENTISTRY ▰▰▰▰▰

General Considerations

A. Sources of contamination in the dental operatory
1. Dust-borne organisms
2. Aerosols created by
   a. Breathing, speaking, coughing, and sneezing[52]
   b. Prophylaxis angles, cups, and brushes
   c. Handpieces
   d. Ultrasonic scalers
   e. Air-water syringe[27,32,33,35]—capillary action and splatter contaminate the ends and insides of tips[16]
3. Dental unit water
   a. Normally occurring aquatic bacteria (e.g., *P. aeruginosa*)
   b. Microorganisms from saliva[3]
   c. High concentrations of bacteria found in water from handpieces, air-water syringes, and ultrasonic scalers[1,24,44]
4. Suction devices
   a. Residues of infected material form
   b. Lead to permanent bacterial growth on the insides of tubes[26]

B. Transmission
1. Direct droplet transfer from the patient to the clinician or from the clinician to the patient
2. Direct contact by the hands and instruments used on the patient
3. Indirect transfer by way of the hands to equipment, instruments, and records
4. Organisms from the oral cavity enter the air of the operatory and are indirectly transferred[52]

C. Autogenous infection
1. Local or systemic posttreatment infections caused by introducing the microflora of patients into injured tissues[15]
2. May develop if the host's defense mechanisms are modified
3. Examples of possible infections
   a. Bacteremia
   b. Abscess at the site of injection
   c. Infections developing after oral surgery or treatment of fractures
4. Prevention
   a. Antibiotic premedication where indicated
   b. Lower the oral microbial count by rinsing with an antibacterial rinse (e.g., iodophore mouthwashes)
   c. Preparation of the injection site
      (1) Block saliva with cotton rolls
      (2) Apply a topical antiseptic (e.g., iodophore solutions with 1% iodine)[15,52]

D. Pathogens transmissible through the oral cavity (Table 7-15)

E. Definitions
1. Sterilization—any process, chemical or physical, that destroys or removes all forms of life, including bacterial spores and viruses[18,52,53]
2. Disinfection—any process, chemical or physical, that kills pathogenic organisms but not necessarily spores; disinfectants are agents applied to inanimate objects for the purpose of disinfection; antiseptics are applied to living tissues[18,52,53]
3. Sanitization—process of reducing microbial populations to levels judged to be safe by public health requirements; generally refers to a cleaning process of inanimate objects[18,52,53]
4. -cide—suffix used to indicate agents that kill[53]; germicide indicates chemical agents that kill most vegetative bacteria, especially pathogens, but not all spore forms; terms *viricide, fungicide,* and *sporicide* refer to products that kill viruses, fungi, and spores, respectively[15,18]
5. -static—suffix used to indicate agents that prevent growth but do not necessarily kill organisms[53]
6. Sepsis—condition in which pathogenic microorganisms are present[52]
7. Asepsis—condition in which living pathogenic microorganisms are absent[52]
8. Aseptic technique—describes procedures followed to avoid infection or microbial contamination[18,48,52]

Preparation of the Operatory and Unit

A. General cleaning procedures
1. Construction of the operatory
   a. Floors and walls easily cleaned
   b. Carpet free
   c. Sinks and soap dispensers with knee- or foot-operated controls[19]
   d. Hoses made of plastic, not cloth[12]
2. Disinfect walls at regular intervals[10]
3. Scrub floors daily with a phenol product (e.g., Lysol) or quaternary ammonium compound[18]
4. Scrub dust-collecting surfaces on or above the chair seat level daily
   a. Before the first patient
   b. Agent—phenol disinfectant or 70% alcohol
   c. Spray surfaces with the disinfectant and wipe with paper towels[12]
5. Do not eat, have eating utensils, or clean up eating utensils in treatment areas[10,52]

Table 7-15 Principal pathogenic organisms of oral transmission

Agent	Disease produced	Route or mode of transmission	Incubation period	Communicability	Estimated survival at 25° C (77° F)
Hepatitis A virus	"Infectious" hepatitis Chronic liver disease	Fecal-oral Blood during acute stage Food, water, shellfish	2-6 weeks	2-3 weeks before onset of jaundice through 8 days after	Months
Hepatitis B virus	"Serum" hepatitis Chronic liver disease	Blood Saliva Semen All other body fluids	2-6 months	Before, during, and after clinical signs Carrier state: indefinite	Months
Herpes simplex virus type I	Herpes labialis (fever blister, cold sores) Acute herpetic gingivostomatitis Keratoconjunctivitis Finger lesion (whitlow)	Saliva Direct contact Vesicles Indirect contact	14-16 days; up to 21 days	Carrier state in persons with latent virus One day before onset to 6 days after macules appear; until all lesions are crusted	Seconds or minutes
Mycobacterium tuberculosis	Tuberculosis	Droplet nuclei Sputum Saliva	Up to 6 months	Long, repeated exposure usually needed	Days to weeks
Influenza viruses	Influenza	Droplet nuclei Nasal discharge	24-72 hours	3 days from clinical onset	Hours
Herpes zoster	Shingles	Saliva Vesicles	2-3 weeks	4 days before lesions; until all lesions are crusted	Hours to days
β-Hemolytic streptococci (Streptococcus pyogenes)	Tonsillitis Strep throat Scarlet fever Impetigo Rheumatic fever	Droplet nuclei Direct contact Saliva, secretions	1-3 days	24 hours when treated 10-21 days when untreated Carrier state	
Staphylococcus aureus	Abscesses Postoperative infections Boils (furuncle) Impetigo Bacterial pneumonia	Saliva Exudates Skin contact Angular cheilitis	4-10 days; variable	As long as lesions drain and carrier state persists	Days
Treponema pallidum	Syphilis	Direct contact Transplacental	Primary: 10-90 days Secondary: 2 weeks-6 months Tertiary: years, decades	Variable and indefinite Highly infectious during the chancre stage Mucous patches of oral mucosa are highly infectious	Seconds

Continued.

Data from Wilkens, E.M.: Clinical practice of the dental hygienist, ed. 5, Philadelphia, 1983, Lea & Febiger; and Crawford, J.J.: Clinical asepsis in dentistry, ed. 2, Mesquite, Tex., 1978, R.A. Kolstad.

Table 7-15 Principal pathogenic organisms of oral transmission—cont'd

Agent	Disease produced	Route or mode of transmission	Incubation period	Communicability	Estimated survival at 25° C (77° F)
Neisseria gonorrhoeae	Gonorrhea	Direct contact Indirect contact Skin Saliva	2-5 days usually; may be 9 days or longer	During incubation period and continued for months or years	Seconds
Rubeola (RNA paramyxovirus)	Rubeola (measles)	Droplet nuclei Direct contact (saliva) Dust	9-14 days (10 days to fever, 14 days to rash)	4 days before to 5 days after rash appears	
Rubella (togavirus)	Rubella (German measles)	Droplet nuclei Direct contact (saliva) Dust	14-21 days	From early signs of illness to 7 days after rash Highly communicable	
Mumps virus (myxovirus)	Infectious or epidemic parotitis (Mumps)	Droplet nuclei Direct contact (saliva)	14-28 days	From 1-7 days before symptoms until 9 days after swelling has gone	Hours
Varicella virus	Chickenpox	Direct contact Indirect contact Droplet nuclei	14-16 days	5 days before appearance of rash until crusting of vesicles	
Poliovirus	Poliomyelitis	Direct contact Saliva Droplet nuclei	7-14 days	Most infectious 7-10 days before and after onset of symptoms	
Respiratory viruses (rhinovirus, coronavirus, respiratory synctial virus)	Common cold, croup, minor upper respiratory tract illness (fever, sore throat, swollen lymph nodes, cough)	Droplet nuclei (saliva, nasal secretions)	1-14 days	Usually requires close contact	Hours

6. Monitor waste disposal
   a. Do not allow saliva or blood-coated material to accumulate on the bracket tray
   b. Tape a small bag to the back of the dental unit; when full, seal and dispose
   c. Line trash cans with plastic or paper bags
   d. When the trash can is full, seal and send for incineration[29]

B. Surface disinfection
   1. Strategy
      a. Identify and list surfaces that will be touched during treatment; post the list in the operatory to increase effectiveness and efficiency[15]
      b. Devise methods to avoid contact with objects that must be handled
         (1) Use disposable covers (e.g., patient napkins, aluminum foil, and plastic wrap) secured with tape
         (2) Pick up small objects with gauze or paper towels; open drawers in the same manner
         (3) Have sterile pliers or forceps available on each tray to gather additional instruments or gauze during treatment[11,12,40]
         (4) Disinfect surfaces that will be directly touched[12,15,28]
   2. Typical list of surfaces to disinfect
      a. All hose ends
      b. Supports for handpiece, air-water syringe, and suction devices
      c. Chair
      d. Control switches (chair, light, and ultrasonic scalers)
      e. Cuspidor
         (1) Use paper towels saturated with a disinfectant
         (2) Disinfect outside first, then inside
         (3) Wash hands before disinfecting other items, or disinfect the cuspidor last
      f. Sink handles (if manually operated)
      g. Soap dispenser (if manually operated)
      h. Instrument tray (if cannot be sterilized)
      i. Lamp handle
      j. Blood pressure equipment
      k. Miscellaneous items such as the floss dispenser and cotton pellet dispenser[15,52]
   3. Chemical disinfectants for surface disinfection
      a. Must be effective in killing vegetative forms of pathogenic organisms, influenza and enteroviruses, and the tubercle bacillus within 30 minutes[6]

   b. Quaternary ammonium compounds, alcohols, and phenolic compounds are unacceptable for surface disinfection[6,12]
   c. Recommended chemicals
      (1) Approved effective agents described in section on instrument care
      (2) Iodophor solutions
         (a) Only one has been approved by the Environmental Protection Agency (EPA) for disinfection: Wescodyne (dilute as specified by the manufacturer)[15]
         (b) May use a solution of iodine surgical scrub (e.g., Vestal Iodine Scrub) and 70% isopropyl alcohol; 1:20 dilution (0.05% or 500 parts per million [ppm] of available iodine)[16]; stronger solution (1:1 dilution) recommended for a patient with a known communicable disease or carrier state[12,52]
         (c) Does not stain metal; may stain painted and pastel surfaces
         (d) Residual film of the iodine-effective antibacterial and antiviral agent[14,46,52]
         (e) Can remove an iodine film with alcohol after 3 minutes if the film is unacceptable or unattractive[52]
         (f) Dilutions kept in dark glass containers remain stable up to 1 month[16]
         (g) Effectiveness needs further evaluation[16]
      (3) Sodium hypochlorite
         (a) Bleach, 5%, diluted 1:100 with water (0.05% to 0.5% or 500 to 5000 ppm sodium hypochlorite)[16,18,46]
         (b) Corrosive to metal
         (c) May injure skin
         (d) Preferred for hospital disinfective use[16]
         (e) Hypochlorite, 0.5%, acceptable for surface clean up after a patient with suspected hepatitis; leave the solution on for 30 minutes, then remove with alcohol[15]
      (4) Glutaraldehyde, 2%, activated
         (a) Expensive
         (b) Can irritate skin

d. Do not store gauze in chemicals[52]
   (1) Effectiveness of the agent is reduced over a long period (e.g., all day)
   (2) Put dry sponges in a cup for each use
   (3) Store the disinfecting solution in a separate bottle (e.g., empty the mouthwash bottle and soap dispenser) and wet gauze before use
e. Characteristics of the ideal disinfectant for dentistry[16,18]
   (1) Sporicidal, tuberculocidal, and viricidal in the times stated for each
   (2) Effective in 3 minutes or less for surfaces
   (3) Nonirritating to the skin and eyes
   (4) Nonstaining
   (5) Reasonable cost
   (6) Stable shelf life when diluted for use
   (7) Retains most of its stability and activity in the presence of organic matter and in heavy use for the periods described
   (8) Good penetrating and cleaning ability
   (9) Not damaging to painted, plastic, or metal surfaces
   (10) If used for instrument disinfection, disinfection or sporicidal action should be readily verifiable
f. Tests of effectiveness of chemical disinfectants
   (1) Phenol coefficient test—compares activity of a product with the killing power of phenol
   (2) Use-dilution test—devised to establish appropriate dilutions of a germicide for actual conditions
4. Procedure for disinfecting surfaces
   a. Effectiveness is a result of two actions
      (1) Mechanical scrubbing—most important goal[15]
      (2) Chemical inactivation of microorganisms[15]
   b. Use several large gauze sponges (at least 4 by 4 inches) saturated with a disinfectant
   c. Scrub vigorously
   d. If spraying disinfectant, must follow up with scrubbing
   e. Moist contact time of 3 to 30 minutes
      (1) Three minutes in low-risk situations
      (2) Thirty minutes for heavily contaminated surfaces or after infectious or high-risk patients[17,52]
C. Aerosol reduction
   1. Use air and water separately instead of a combined spray[3,32,34]

2. Use a rubber cup instead of brushes for polishing[29]; use a toothbrush for occlusal surfaces
3. Use laminar air flow[15,39]
4. Use high-volume suction
   a. Keep suction equipment free of bacterial growth
   b. Pass 1 gallon of diluted household detergent through all suction systems at the end of each day[12]
D. Dental unit water
   1. Often contaminated with gram-negative bacteria (e.g., Enterobacteriaceae and Pseudomonadaceae families, which can be infectious in patients with altered resistance)
   2. If present, replace the water-retraction valve in the handpiece with an antiretraction valve; until 1981 most units were fitted with retraction valves to prevent water dripping; also can draw saliva and aerosols back up the waterline when the handpiece is stopped*
   3. Screen filters are less conducive to trapping debris; replace porous stone or ultrafine metal filters[3,9]
   4. Flush waterlines at the beginning of each day for several minutes to reduce bacterial counts (handpiece, air-water syringe, and ultrasonic scalers)[12,15,52]
   5. Between patients, flush waterlines for 1 minute[15]
   6. Sterile water should be used for surgery and irrigating pockets[52]
   7. Test the water spray for bacterial contamination
      a. Corrective action recommended if more than 10 colony-forming units/ml[3]
      b. Place 0.1 ml water on the blood-agar plate; incubate 48 hours at 37° C (98.6° F)[1]
E. Handpieces, prophylaxis angles, contraangles, and air-water syringes
   1. Sterilizing these pieces of equipment is recommended[12,13,15,52]
      a. Follow the manufacturer's instructions
      b. Most manufacturers now make such equipment so that it can be sterilized
      c. For effective routine sterilization, one or more is needed for each operatory[15,52]
      d. For angles and handpieces
         (1) Disassemble before sterilization
         (2) Clean with grease solvent
         (3) Sterilize
         (4) Lubricate
         (5) Reassemble[15]

---

*References 3, 12, 14, 15, 46, 52.

2. Nonautoclavable handpieces, angles, and air-water syringes
   a. Temporary, stopgap usage until equipment can be replaced with equipment that can be sterilized
   b. Scrub at a sink with hypochlorite or iodophore detergent[15,46,52]
   c. If equipment does not reach the sink, scrub twice with sponges soaked in a disinfectant (iodine surgical scrub or hypochlorite)
   d. If feasible, wrap sponges soaked in detergent around the equipment and leave in place 30 minutes (e.g., cover with a finger cot)[15,52]

Instrument Care

A. Instrument cleaning
   1. Handle contaminated instruments with heavy household rubber gloves[15,52]
   2. Use an area separate from the operatory to clean instruments; splatter occurs and increases the potential of environmental pathogens[4]
   3. Clean and dry before sterilization
      a. Organic debris acts as a barrier to the sterilant
      b. Water interferes with dry heat effects and ethylene oxide[12]
   4. If time lapses before cleaning, rinse in cold water; soak in warm water with blood solvent or detergent[52]
      a. Do not use ordinary soap, because it can form insoluble alkalis that protect bacteria from sterilization[38]
      b. Prevents adherence of organic debris
      c. Prevents rust and discoloration[52]
   5. Ultrasonic instrument cleaning
      a. Preferred method
      b. Advantages
         (1) Cleans more thoroughly
         (2) Less chance of injury
         (3) Less time consuming
         (4) Less splatter of aerosols
         (5) Penetrates grooves in instruments[15,52]
      c. Procedure
         (1) Follow the manufacturer's instructions on solutions to be used
         (2) Dismantle instruments
         (3) Do not overload; keep the unit covered
         (4) Time from 1 to 10 minutes, depending on the unit, solution, and material being cleaned; consult the manufacturer's instructions
         (5) Rinse instruments and dry (by towel or air)

(6) Change the solution daily
(7) Wipe the unit with 1% sodium hypochlorite[52]
(8) Perform terminal disinfection (i.e., soaking in recommended chemical disinfectant for 30 minutes; recommended by some authorities; remove instruments promptly and sterilize; discard solution preferably after each use[15])

   d. Action of ultrasonic cleaning
      (1) Ultrasonic vibrations initiate cavitation; minute bubbles are produced; bubbles expand and collapse, creating vacuum areas that are responsible for cleaning by dislodging, dispersing, or dissolving the material on instruments
      (2) Cleans by physical agitation and chemical dissolution[52]
   6. Manual scrubbing
      a. Scrub with a stiff brush; concentrate on grooved areas
      b. Use detergent, not soap
      c. Rinse and dry
      d. Sterilize brushes; do not mix with brushes used for hand cleansing
      e. Disadvantages
         (1) Splatter
         (2) Injury
         (3) Time consuming[52]

B. Instrument packaging
   1. Instrument arrangement for sterilization
      a. Wrap
         (1) Materials vary according to the type of sterilization method (Table 7-16)
         (2) All surgical and infrequently used items[15]
      b. Place on an open tray and sterilize
         (1) Transfer with sterile forceps or cotton pliers to storage areas or treatment areas after sterilization
         (2) Store away from aerosols, dust, and contaminated fingers
         (3) Disinfect storage drawers and shelves weekly[12,13,46]
         (4) If prepared trays are used, store behind glass and in drawers and cover with plastic wrap[28]
         (5) Trays with fitted covers—covers need to be ajar during sterilization[52]
   2. Packaging suggestions
      a. Cover sharp points of instruments (cotton roll, gauze, and x-ray envelopes)[4,15,52]
      b. Heat-seal or tape bags; do not staple[4]

Table 7-16 Suggestions for packaging materials to be used in sterilizers

Sterilizer	Packaging materials	Comments
Autoclave	Muslin, paper, steam-permeable plastic, nylon	Open trays may be used. No closed containers.
Dry heat	Paper, aluminum foil, metal or glass containers, certain nylon bags	Cloth may char. Heavy wraps and large tight containers extend sterilization time.
Ethylene oxide	Any plastic wrap, light paper, light cloth wrap	No closed glass or metal containers.
Formaldehyde alcohol vapor	Light weight paper bags, nylon, steam-permeable plastic, unwrapped instruments preferred	No closed containers. Avoid use of paper and autoclave tape with high content of sulfur. Sulfur causes sterilizing chamber to turn black and may damage internal components of unit.
All systems		Two layers of cloth packaging provides maximum protection against contamination incurred in storage. More than two layers slows sterilization and may prevent killing of pathogens.

Data from Crawford, J.J.: Clinical asepsis in dentistry, ed. 2, Mesquite, Tex., 1978, R.A. Kolsted; and Crawford, J.J.: status of instrument sterilizers and sterilization devices, Unpublished report to the American Dental Association, 1978.

Table 7-17 Suitable methods for sterilizing common dental instruments and items

Materials	Steam autoclave*	Dry heat oven	Chemical vapor	Ethylene oxide
General hand instruments				
Stainless steel	1	1	1	2
Carbon steel	3	1	1	2
Mirrors	2	1	1	2
Burs†				
Steel	2	1	1	2
Carbon steel	3	1	1	2
Tungsten-carbide	2	1	2	2
Stones				
Diamond	2	1	1	2
Polishing	1	2	1	2
Sharpening	2	1	2	2
Polishing wheels and disks				
Rubber	2	4	3	2
Garnet and cuttle	4	3	3	2
Rag	1	2	2	2
Rubber dam equipment				
Carbon or carbide steel clamps	3	1	1	2
Stainless steel clamps	1	1	1	2
Punches	3	1	1	2
Plastic frames	3	4	4	2
Metal frames	1	1	1	2
Pluggers and condensers	1	1	1	2
Glass slabs	1	2	1	2

Key to Methods
1 = Preferred method with minimum risk of damage.
2 = Materials should withstand treatment with minimum risk of damage.
3 = Treatment is usually not suitable and may damage materials; manufacturer should be consulted.
4 = Materials are likely to be damaged or process may be ineffective.

From American Dental Association Council on Dental Materials, Instruments, and Equipment (prepared by Crawford, J.J., Whitacre, R.J., and Middaugh, D.G.): Current status of sterilization instruments, devices, and methods for the dental office, J. Am. Dent. Assoc. 102:683, 1981. Copyright by the American Dental Association. Reprinted by permission.
*Chemical protection of certain nonstainless instruments may permit steam autoclaving. A rust-preventive dip (1% sodium nitrate) is recommended before sterilization.
†Steel burs may also be sterilized in a hot salt endodontic sterilizer for 15 to 20 seconds at 475° F (246° C), but the process may not be suitable for carbide burs.
‡Some common latch-type contraangles cannot withstand repeated heat sterilization; short, heat-sterilizable contraangle handpieces are now available.

Table 7-17 Suitable methods for sterilizing common dental instruments and items — cont'd

Materials	Steam autoclave*	Dry heat oven	Chemical vapor	Ethylene oxide
Dappen dishes	1	2	1	2
Handpieces‡				
High speed	3	3	3	2
Low speed straight	3	3	3	2
Prophy angles	2	2	2	2
Contraangles	4	4	4	2
X-ray equipment				
Plastic film holders, columating devices	3	4	4	2
Stainless steel surgical instruments	1	1	2	2
Ultrasonic scaling tips	2	4	4	2
Electrosurgical tips and handles	4	4	4	4
Needles				
Disposable (do not reuse)	4	4	4	4
Reusable	2	2	4	4
Impression trays				
Aluminum	1	2	1	2
metal, chromeplated	1	1	1	2
Custom acrylic resin	4	4	4	2
Plastic (discarding is preferred)	4	4	4	2
Fluoride gel trays				
Heat-resistant plastic	1	4	3	2
Nonheat-resistant plastic	4	4	4	2
Orthodontic pliers				
High quality stainless	1	1	1	2
Low quality stainless	4	1	1	2
With plastic parts	4	4	3	1
Endodontic instruments				
Reamers and files, broaches, stainless metal handles	1	1	1	1
Nonstainless, metal handles	4	1	1	1
Stainless with plastic handles	3	3	3	1

c. Label or date packages
  (1) Instruments in autoclave bags remain sterile approximately 2 weeks
  (2) For indefinite storage, use aluminum foil[28]
C. Sterilization methods (Table 7-17)
  1. All items used intraorally should be sterilized[3]
  2. Steam sterilization
    a. Action
      (1) Moist heat coagulates protein; pressure serves only to elevate temperature[52]
      (2) Steam must be able to penetrate
        (a) Air must be adequately removed to allow steam penetration and heat transfer
        (b) Steam travels vertically
        (c) Pack loosely; arrange load to allow free passage of steam
        (d) Place jars on sides[5,28,52]

b. Application to dental equipment
  (1) Recommended for
    (a) High-quality stainless steel instruments
    (b) Brushes
    (c) Many prophylaxis angles, contraangles, and handpieces
    (d) Glass slabs, Dappen dishes, and sharpening stones (dry these first)[12]
  (2) Not recommended for
    (a) Rubber goods—may deteriorate (discard prophylaxis cups, since they do not withstand autoclaving well)
    (b) Carbon steel—low-quality steel may rust; can use corrosion inhibitor (e.g., 1% sodium nitrite)
    (c) Some orthodontic pliers
    (d) Most plastics[5,15,52]

c. Operation
(1) Autoclave at 121° C (250° F) at 15 pounds pressure for 15 minutes
(2) Autoclave at 134° C (270° F) at 30 pounds pressure for 3 to 7 minutes
(3) For wrapped instruments, add 5 to 10 minutes
(4) Heavy loads may require twice the time[52]
(5) Timing begins when the temperature gauge reaches the recommended temperature[5]
d. Care of the autoclave
(1) Daily
(a) Maintain the level of distilled water
(b) Wash the interior with a mild detergent
(c) Clean the removable plug, screen, or strainer[52]
(2) Weekly
(a) Follow the manufacturer's instructions
(b) Flush the chamber with an appropriate cleaning solution[52]
3. Dry heat
a. Action
(1) Oxidation of cell parts
(2) Heat conducted from the exterior surface to the interior of the object; time required for heat penetration varies among materials[52]
b. Application to dental equipment
(1) Does not rust
(2) Recommended for
(a) Dry metal instruments including carbon steel instruments
(b) Closed, nonporous containers
(c) Oils and powders[13,52]
(d) Burs[4]
(e) Glass slabs, Dappen dishes, and sharpening stones[15]
(f) Orthodontic pliers[15]
(g) Metal impression trays—caution: solder melts above 170° C (338° F)[15]
(3) Not recommended for
(a) Liquids
(b) Rubber
(c) Plastics
(d) Cotton
(e) Paper[13]

c. Operation
(1) Sterilize at 160° to 171° C (320° to 340° F) for 1 to 2 hours[15]
(2) Timing variation occurs
(a) Start timing when materials are at the sterilization temperature; may take 15 to 60 minutes
(b) Sterilization then occurs in 30 minutes
(c) Total time in preheated oven is 45 to 90 minutes[15,52]
(d) Dependent on contents and wrapping[15,52]
(3) Verification of temperature
(a) Oven thermometer only indicates the oven temperature, not the instruments' temperature
(b) Load temperature should be checked with a thermocouple and pyrometer[15]
3. Unsaturated formaldehyde alcohol vapor pressure
a. Action
(1) Permeation of heated formaldehyde and alcohol vapor acts as a sterilant[52]
(2) Alcohols, formaldehyde, ketone, water, and acetone heated under pressure to produce gas[15]
b. Application to dental equipment
(1) Does not rust
(2) Instruments dry at the end of the cycle
(3) Recommended for any dry metal instruments
(4) Not recommended for
(a) Most plastics
(b) Rubber items
(c) Liquids
(d) Heavy loads of cloth goods[4,13]
c. Operation
(1) Sterilize at 127° to 132° C (260° to 270° F) with 20 to 40 pounds pressure (follow the manufacturer's directions) for 20 minutes[52]
(2) Start timing after the correct temperature is reached[15]
(3) Heavy wrapping and large loads greatly increase time[15]
(4) Need the manufacturer's chemical solution
(5) Heavy, tightly wrapped packages do not allow vapor penetration (e.g., muslin packs will not sterilize)[15,52]
(6) Adequate ventilation required[13]

4. Ethylene oxide
   a. Action
     (1) Ethylene oxide vapor destroys all organisms given enough time[15,52]
     (2) Has unusual powers of penetration of organic material[16]
   b. Application to dental equipment
     (1) Nearly all materials can withstand ethylene oxide sterilization[15,52]
     (2) Some plastics may degrade after repeated exposure[12,13]
   c. Operation
     (1) Sterilize at room temperature for 8 to 10 hours[3,12,13]
     (2) Sterilize at 50° C (120° F) for 2 to 3 hours; short-cycle units are expensive
     (3) Preferably overnight processing
     (4) Well-ventilated area required[52]
     (5) Aeration of materials after sterilization
       (a) Metal instruments can be used immediately
       (b) Aerate absorbent materials (plastics and rubber) for 1 to 2 days[15,16]

D. Verification of sterilization
   1. Needed because failure of sterilization can occur as a result of
     a. Overloading
     b. Improper packaging
     c. Improper timing[15]
     d. Improper unit operation
     e. Unit failure
     f. With autoclave, not cleaning the air-exit screen of the chamber[15]
   2. Methods
     a. Color-change tape
       (1) Not proof of sterilization
       (2) Distinguishes those instruments that have been in the sterilizer from those that have not[15]
       (3) Use on each pack or in each load
       (4) Date tape and resterilize when necessary
     b. Indicator strips
       (1) Indicate heat, steam, or gas reached inside of the load for prolonged time and probable sterilization
       (2) Sensitive to certain combinations of exposure; cannot be relied on for proof of sterility[4,12,13,42]
       (3) Provide a warning of gross sterilizer malfunction
       (4) Use with each load or pack

   c. Spore tests
     (1) Most reliable test of sterilization
     (2) Test the dental office sterilizer weekly[12,13,15]
     (3) Use to test a new machine or after repairs[52]
     (4) Steam and chemical vapor—use spores of *Bacillus stearothermophilus*[12]
     (5) Dry heat and ethylene oxide—use spores of *Bacillus subtilis*[4,12,13,46]

E. Disinfection procedures
   1. Use
     a. Stopgap measure until sterilization equipment is purchased
     b. Emergency situation (e.g., failure of sterilization equipment)[15, 52]
   2. Immersion in boiling water
     a. Begin timing for 30 minutes when vigorous boiling begins
     b. If instruments are added during cycle, begin timing again
     c. Add antirust tablets or 1% sodium nitrite[5,15,52]
   3. Chemical disinfection
     a. Limitations
       (1) No cold chemical agent can be considered a substitute for sterilization by steam, dry heat, chemical vapor, or ethylene oxide[52]
       (2) No liquid disinfectants are available that are harmless to metals and destroy spores in 10 to 30 minutes; liquid germicides presently available to act as sterilants at room temperature require exposures (6 to 10 hours) too long for practicality in the dental office[15]
       (3) No automatic control over timing of disinfection[12,15]
       (4) Verification not possible
       (5) Poor penetration of crevices of instruments and plastics
       (6) Difficult to judge expiration of the solution
       (7) Expense of the least corrosive agents
       (8) Cannot produce sterile packages[15]
       (9) Not timesaving when compared with steam autoclaving or vapor pressure[16]

(10) Solutions may be diluted or inactivated by water, other soaps, and chemicals
    b. Recommended disinfectants for instruments
        (1) Glutaraldehyde, 2%, activated
            (a) Kills most bacteria and viruses (possibly the hepatitis virus)* in 30 minutes
            (b) Sporicidal in 10 hours
            (c) Effectiveness limited to 2 weeks[18,52]
            (d) Rinse instruments thoroughly
            (e) May corrode carbon steel instruments if left over 24 hours[52]
            (f) Can irritate the skin and eyes
            (g) Expensive[18]
        (2) Sodium hypochlorite
            (a) Household bleach, 5%, diluted 1:100 with water[18,46,52]
            (b) Solutions of 500 to 5000 ppm have been recommended to control hepatitis B[8,9,18]
            (c) Soak for 30 minutes
            (d) Change the solution daily[18]
            (e) Corrodes metal instruments
            (f) Useful for plastics but may deteriorate eventually
            (g) Can harm the skin, eyes, and clothing; strong odor
            (h) Deteriorates on standing[52]
            (i) Low cost[18,52]
        (3) Iodophor solutions
            (a) Iodine is released slowly to provide antibacterial and antiviral action[18,52]
            (b) Iodophor solution is prepared in 1:20 dilution of iodine surgical scrub (1 part) with 70% isopropyl alcohol (20 parts)[6,12,46] (iodine scrubs, e.g., povidone-iodine [Vestal, Betadine])
            (c) Soak 30 minutes
            (d) Evidence supports effectiveness of Wescodyne diluted as manufacturer suggests (with water, not alcohol) against hepatitis B virus[15]; Wescodyne is the only iodophor registered with the EPA as a disinfectant
            (e) Corrodes metal instruments
            (f) Some people may be sensitive to iodine

            (g) Can remove residual iodine with alcohol[52]
            (h) Change the solution daily[18]
            (i) Low cost[18]
        (4) New chemicals on the market that claim sporicidal activity are the most likely to be effective against hepatitis B virus and tuberculosis
    c. Unacceptable agents for instrument disinfection
        (1) Quaternary ammonium compounds (e.g., benzalkonium chloride)
            (a) Lack tuberculocidal and broad viricidal activity[16]
            (b) Limitations in penetrating organic debris[16]
            (c) Unstable[15]
        (2) Phenolic compounds
            (a) Tuberculocidal
            (b) Not effective against hepatitis B virus or spores[18]
            (c) Cannot be relied on to penetrate organic debris[16]
        (3) Alcohols
            (a) Evaporate too quickly[16,52]
            (b) Tuberculocidal but will not inactivate hepatitis B virus or kill spores[18]
    d. Procedure
        (1) Handle and clean instruments as recommended before sterilization
        (2) Soak for a minimum of 30 minutes[18]
        (3) Do not add instruments without starting timing over[52]
        (4) Remove instruments with sterile forceps
        (5) Rinse and dry
F. Sterilization center design
    1. Linear progression
    2. Separation of sterile and nonsterile items
    3. Refer to Fig. 7-10
        a. Contaminated instruments are brought to area *A,* scrubbed in sink *1,* and placed in the ultrasonic cleaning unit
        b. Plastic instruments are placed in hypochlorite
        c. Metallic instruments that cannot be sterilized are placed in glutaraldehyde
        d. After appropriate soaking time, remove instruments with sterile forceps and rinse in sink *2*
        e. Other instruments are packaged in area *B* and sterilized
        f. Sterile instruments are returned to storage areas; if unwrapped, instruments are handled with sterile forceps[28]

*Research[9] has shown hepatitis B virus not to be as resistant to disinfectant chemicals as once thought. However, laboratory conditions are not equivalent to chemical practice conditions. Also, penetration of organic debris and crevices is more reliable by heat or gas sterilization. Chemical disinfection cannot be verified.

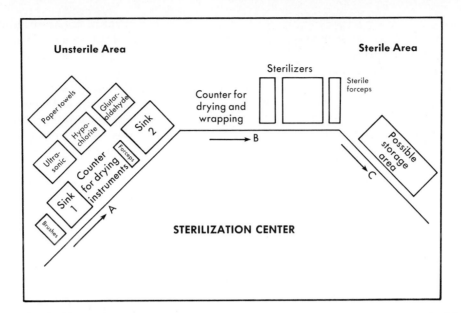

Fig. 7-10 Design of sterilization center. Sequential arrangement recommended by Dr. R. Kilstad during continuing education seminar in Williamsburg, Va., Jan. 31, 1981. (From Greenlee, J.S. Reprinted from Dental Hygiene, (R) The Journal of the American Dental Hygienists Association, volume 57, number 12, 1983.)

Radiographic Equipment

A. Surface disinfection
   1. Any part of the radiographic unit touched should be scrubbed; may include control knobs and the machine head and cone
   2. Alternative is to use disposable covers
B. Instruments
   1. Metal intraoral—autoclave or dry heat
   2. Plastic intraoral—ethylene oxide; if ethylene oxide is not available, disinfect in one of the recommended chemical disinfectants
   3. Use disposable radiographic holders
C. Plastic film packets
   1. Wipe twice with iodophore detergent diluted 1:1 with isopropyl alcohol on a gauze sponge and rinse
   2. For patients with hepatitis or other communicable diseases
      a. Rinse and soak film 30 minutes in iodophore detergent
      b. Wash hands with iodophore detergent
      c. Rinse, dry, and process the film
D. Paper film packets
   1. Cannot be soaked or wiped
   2. Can wrap with plastic before use
      a. After exposure, remove the film aseptically
      b. Discard the plastic covering
      c. Wash hands with iodophore detergent before processing the film[14,17]

Protection of Dental Personnel

A. Immunizations and testing
   1. Test every 6 to 12 months for HB_sAg and anti-HB_s[12,52]
      a. If found to be a carrier, one may practice as long as there is no epidemiologic evidence of transmission[11,17] or when released by a physician[52]
      b. If a carrier, one must routinely wear gloves[16,28]
   2. Annual tuberculin test[52]
   3. Immunization available for hepatitis B[52]
B. Clinical dress
   1. Design
      a. Wear neat, simple clothes
      b. If smocks are worn, wear closed to protect street clothes underneath[15,52]
      c. Wear short sleeves
      d. Use a cover (e.g., plastic apron) during procedures creating great amounts of aerosols and splatter (e.g., when using an ultrasonic scaling instrument)[52]
   2. Care of clothing
      a. Do not wear clinical clothing outside of the clinical setting, because this practice takes contamination home[15,52]
      b. Launder separately from other clothing, with bleach if possible[12,14,42]

C. Hair
  1. Keep away from treatment areas because it can become heavily contaminated[15]
  2. Cover, including facial hair, during surgical procedures[15]
  3. Wash daily
D. No jewelry worn on hands or wrists[15,52]
E. Facial protection (wash face frequently[12,14,46])
  1. Masks
    a. Recommended for all appointments; many diseases are transmitted when no clinical signs are apparent[52]
    b. Minimal guidelines for wearing masks
      (1) Patient's medical history shows a possible infection or carrier state
      (2) Current infection of dental personnel
      (3) Aerosol production (air-water syringe, handpieces, prophylaxis angles, and ultrasonic instruments)
      (4) All surgical procedures
      (5) Protection of facial hair from splatter[15,52]
    c. Use
      (1) Tie on before washing hands[52]
      (2) Change when damp—no longer effective[52]
    d. Type—glass fiber or synthetic fiber most effective[15,16,33]
  2. Glasses—indications
    a. For all procedures for dental personnel
      (1) To prevent injury
      (2) To prevent infection[14,15]
    b. For each patient
      (1) Patients may use their own glasses
      (2) Glasses provided by dental personnel should
        (a) Be lightweight
        (b) Be shatterproof
        (c) Afford wide coverage
        (d) Be easily disinfected
      (3) Disinfect glasses after each patient
        (a) Rinse abrasives off before cleaning
        (b) Rub with or soak in an acceptable disinfectant[52]
F. Gloves
  1. Routine use of gloves is recommended by many[12,15,16,52]
    a. Rationale
      (1) Impossible to detect all patients who carry infections such as hepatitis or tuberculosis or who are in the incubation stage of disease[15,52]
      (2) Common small breaks in skin and nails go unnoticed

      (3) Frequent handwashing necessary in dentistry; causes drying and irritation, increasing the chance for breaks in skin[15]
      (4) Transient disease agents are not completely and consistently removed by rapid handwashing between patients
      (5) Most hand cleansers have too narrow a spectrum to destroy all viral or bacterial agents
      (6) Cleansers with a broad spectrum of activity (e.g., iodine) are often too drying for most dental personnel[15]
      (7) Gloves can be washed cleaner than bare hands using two latherings and rinsings in 20 to 30 seconds[12,15,18]
    b. Minimal guidelines for wearing gloves
      (1) All surgical procedures
      (2) Any treatment that causes bleeding
      (3) Initial intraoral and extraoral examinations
      (4) Patient has a facial or oral lesion (e.g., herpes or syphilitic lesion)
      (5) Clinician has breaks or cuts on hands
      (6) Patient has a history suggestive of, or symptoms or signs of, systemic infection[12,16]
      (7) Clinician tests positive for HB_sAg[3,52]
  2. Procedure
    a. Wash hands before putting on gloves
      (1) Bacteria multiply under gloves
      (2) Potential for tears to occur in gloves
    b. If possible, use disposable gloves and change between patients[16,52]
    c. If gloves are worn for consecutive appointments, lather and rinse two or three times between patients[52]
    d. Wash gloves before removing
      (1) Reduces possible contamination to the clinician's hands
      (2) Clean reusable gloves before sterilization[52]
G. Handwashing
  1. Rationale
    a. Reduces bacterial flora to a minimum[15]
    b. Prevents organisms acquired from the patient from becoming resident flora[52]
    c. Cannot sterilize the skin
    d. Most important actions of handwashing are friction of rubbing and rinsing with water to remove microbes[15,52]
    e. Use of an antiseptic aids in destruction of bacteria[52]

2. Methods of handwashing
   a. Short scrub
      (1) Recommended before the first patient of the day[28,52]
      (2) Stroke-count or time method
      (3) Method
         (a) Wet hands, wrists, and forearms; apply antiseptic soap and lather; leave water running
         (b) Clean under nails with an orangewood stick from a sterile package; rinse from fingers to wrists; lather hands and arms again
         (c) Use a sterile brush to scrub all surfaces from fingers to forearms; scrub each surface five times
         (d) Rinse hands thoroughly from fingers to forearms
         (e) Dry with paper towels, one for each hand, from hands to forearms
         (f) Maintain cleanliness by touching only sterile or disinfected surfaces and instruments[52]
   b. Normal handwashing
      (1) Used between patients[25,28]
      (2) Method
         (a) Wet hands and wrists
         (b) Dispense approximately 1 ml of liquid cleanser
         (c) Lather, rubbing all surfaces vigorously
         (d) Rinse thoroughly from fingertips to hands
         (e) Repeat three times
         (f) Dry with paper towels[12,15,52]
   c. Surgical hand scrub
      (1) Used before surgery
      (2) Procedure usually posted over scrub sinks
3. Recommendations
   a. Do not use a brush on hands more than once a day because it can be irritating to the skin[28]
   b. Sterilize brushes after each use
   c. If the sink does not have foot- or knee-operated controls, use paper towels to turn off after handwashing
   d. If using cloth towels for drying, use a new one for each patient
   e. Keep nails short and clean and cuticles well groomed to prevent breaks[52]

4. Soaps
   a. Use liquid soap[16,28]
   b. Iodophore preparation recommended
      (1) Iodine, 1%—broadest-spectrum chemical added to hand cleansers
      (2) Irritating to some in prolonged, heavy use such as in the dental office[15,16]
   c. Other recommendations
      (1) Chlorhexidine (Hibiclens)
         (a) Effective bactericidal agent
         (b) Mild cleanser
         (c) Not tuberculocidal; limited viricidal action[15]
      (2) Other liquid preparations with bacteriostatic chemicals
         (a) Evaluate for individual preference according to cost, gentleness, and effectiveness
         (b) Choose cleansers that do not irritate hands to preserve the natural defense of the intact skin[15]

Patient Precautions

A. Medical history
   1. Review for past infections that can develop a carrier state
   2. Review for current disease or recent exposure to infectious diseases
   3. Possible actions
      a. Reschedule patient
      b. Refer for diagnostic tests
         (1) If the patient is suspected of being a carrier of hepatitis B, screen by radioimmunoassay for HB_sAg[52]
         (2) If the patient is suspected of having tuberculosis, refer to a physician for tuberculin testing and examination[46]
      c. Use protective measures for dental staff
   4. Limitations—in studies comparing serologic information with medical histories completed by patients, it was found that medical histories are not sufficient to identify a significant proportion of individuals who are carriers of HB_sAg[48,49]
B. Disinfection of prosthetic devices
   1. Disinfect before taking to the laboratory and before returning to the patient
   2. Procedure
      a. Place the prosthetic appliance in a plastic self-sealing bag containing hypochlorite (1:20 aqueous-dilution) or 1:5 mix of iodine surgical scrub in water; hypochlorite will damage chromium cobalt

b. Place in an ultrasonic cleaning unit
c. Time for cleaning varies from 3 to 30 minutes, depending on contamination
d. Rinse well after disinfecting[12,13,46]

Maximal Precautions

A. Indications
1. Patient positive for HB_sAg
2. Patient suspected of having or diagnosed as having AIDS[2,20,41]
B. Advance preparations
1. Have handpieces, prophylaxis angles, contraangles, and air-water syringes that can be sterilized
2. Treat the patient in an enclosed, confined treatment room; have all materials needed in the room to prevent the need for traffic
3. Use disposable materials when possible
4. Use unit hoses of smooth plastic for easy disinfection
5. Check valves in handpiece waterlines
6. Disinfect and drape all surfaces
   a. Cover the entire dental chair (e.g., with a plastic painter's drop cloth)
   b. Cover control switches with plastic
   c. Cover the bracket table, supports for handpieces, suction, and air-water syringe with plastic or aluminum foil
   d. Cover the air-water syringe handles, lamp handle, and radiographic head and controls
7. Schedule the patient at the end of the day to allow time for preparation and clean up
8. Have extra packs of sterilized scalers and curettes to prevent the need for sharpening equipment
9. Place radiographs on the viewbox and cover with transparent plastic
C. Dental personnel preparation
1. Wear a disposable paper gown or cloth gown that can be sterilized; cover hair
2. Wear safety glasses with a side shield that can be disinfected
3. Wear two pairs of surgical gloves
4. Wear two surgical tie-on masks
D. Patient preparation
1. Cover hair with a disposable cap
2. Use a disposable drape over clothing
3. Provide protective glasses

E. Treatment considerations
1. Touch only draped or covered areas
2. Avoid procedures that have a high risk of injury to hands
3. Avoid high-aerosolization procedures
4. Use a disposable radiographic film holder
5. Submerge the exposed plastic film in iodine scrub diluted with isopropyl alcohol (1:1) for 30 minutes; rinse and dry before processing
F. Posttreatment procedures
1. Place all instruments and reusable wraps directly in the sterilizer; after sterilization, clean and sterilize a second time
2. Place all disposable covers and materials in a bag for direct incineration or sterilize first
3. Soak prosthetic devices, appliances, and rubber-base impressions in iodine surgical scrub diluted 1:1 with isopropyl alcohol for 30 minutes; handle alginate impressions with gloves; pour stone models and sterilize with ethylene oxide
4. Disinfect any surfaces touched, but not draped, with iodine surgical scrub diluted 1:1 with isopropyl alcohol or 0.5% solution of hypochlorite; keep wet for 30 minutes; then rinse well with alcohol or water
5. Disinfect glasses in undiluted iodine surgical scrub
6. Wash face and hands with undiluted iodine scrub, lather, and rinse three times[2,12,46,52]
G. Accidental exposure to hepatitis B
1. Examples
   a. Accidental needle stick
   b. Accidental puncture or cut with instrument
2. Patient status—known to be HB_sAg positive
   a. Clinician (if not immune to hepatitis B) should receive hepatitis B immune globulin (HBIg) as soon as possible, preferably within 48 hours; clinician should receive second dose after 30 days[12,23]
   b. Clinician should have a blood test in six months to verify presence or absence of HB_sAg and anti-HB_s[28]
3. Patient status: unknown
   a. Request that the patient have a blood test for HB_sAg
   b. If results are negative, nothing more is necessary
   c. If positive for HB_sAg, follow steps outlined above[12,23,28]

REFERENCES ▪▪▪▪▪▪▪▪▪▪

1. Abel, L.C., et al.: Studies on dental aerobiology. IV. Bacterial contamination of water delivered by dental units, J. Dent. Res. **50**:1567, 1971.
2. Acquired immune deficiency syndrome (AIDS): Precautions for clinical and laboratory staffs, MMWR **31**:577, 1982.
3. American Dental Association Council on Dental Materials and Devices and Council on Dental Therapeutics: Infection control in the dental office, Can. Dent. Hyg. **13**(1):18, 1979.
4. American Dental Association Council on Dental Materials, Instruments, and Equipment (prepared by Crawford, J.J., Whitacre, R.J., and Middaugh, D.G.): Current status of sterilization instruments, devices, and methods for the dental office, J. Am. Dent. Assoc. **102**:683, 1981.
5. American Dental Association Council on Dental Therapeutics: Sterilization or disinfection of dental instruments. In Accepted dental therapeutics, ed. 37, Chicago, 1977, The Association.
6. American Dental Association Council on Dental Therapeutics: Quaternary ammonium compounds not acceptable for disinfection of instruments and environmental surfaces in dentistry, J. Am. Dent. Assoc. **97**:855, 1978.
7. Barker, L.F., and Dodd, R.Y.: Viral hepatitis. In Viral infections in oral medicine, New York, 1982, Elsevier Science Publishing Co., Inc.
8. Bond, W.W., et al.: Viral hepatitis B: aspects of environmental control, Health Sci. **14**:235, 1977.
9. Bond, W.W., et al.: Inactivation of hepatitis B virus by intermediate-to-high-level disinfectant chemicals, J. Clin. Microbiol. **18**:535, 1983.
10. Commission on Dental Practice: Recommendations for hygiene in dental practice, Int. Dent. J. **29**:72, 1979.
11. Crawford, J.J.: New light on the transmissibility of viral hepatitis in dental practice and its control, J. Am. Dent. Assoc. **91**:829, 1975.
12. Crawford, J.J.: Clinical asepsis in dentistry, ed. 2, Mesquite, Tex., 1978, R.A. Kolstad.
13. Crawford, J.J.: Status of instrument sterilizers and sterilization devices, Unpublished report to the American Dental Association, 1978.
14. Crawford, J.J.: Office sterilization and asepsis procedures in endodontics, Dent. Clin. North Am. **23**:717, 1979.
15. Crawford, J.J.: Sterilization, disinfection, and asepsis in dentistry. In McGhee, J.R., Michalek, S.M., and Cassell, G.H., editors: Dental microbiology, New York, 1982, Harper & Row, Publishers, Inc.
16. Crawford, J.J.: Sterilization, disinfection, and asepsis in dentistry. In Block, S.S., editor: Disinfection, sterilization, and preservation, ed. 3, Philadelphia, 1983, Lea & Febiger.
17. Crawford, J.J., and Fine, J.: Infection control in hospital dentistry. In Hooley, J.R., and Daun, L.G., editors: Hospital dental practice, St. Louis, 1980, The C.V. Mosby Co.
18. Crawford, J.J., and Jackson, R.J.: Principles of sterilization and disinfection. In McGhee, J.R., Michalek, S.M., and Cassell, G.H., editors: Dental microbiology, New York, 1982, Harper & Row, Publishers, Inc.
19. Ernst, R.: Biohazards in dentistry. III. Procedures for clean vs. contaminated cases, Dent. Assist. **48**(3):31, 1979.
20. Evans, B.E.: Aseptic techniques for AIDS, J. Am. Dent. Assoc. **107**:706, 1983.
21. Fauci, A.S.: The acquired immune deficiency syndrome: the ever-broadening clinical spectrum, JAMA **249**:2375, 1983.
22. Francis, A.D., and Long, W.K.: Hepatitis and tumor viruses. In McGhee, J.R., Michalek, S.M., and Cassell, G.H., editors: Dental microbiology, New York, 1982, Harper & Row, Publishers, Inc.
23. Gitnick, G.L.: Hepatitis B immune globulin: a clinical guide, Chicago, 1979, Abbott Laboratories.
24. Gross, A., et al.: Microbial contamination of dental units and ultrasonic scalers, J. Periodontol. **47**:670, 1976.
25. Hargiss, C.O.: The patient's environment: haven or hazard, Nurs. Clin. North Am. **15**:671, 1980.
26. Hesselgren, S.: The spread of infection by dental suction devices, Quintessence Int. **10**(6):79, 1979.
27. Holbrook, W.P., et al.: Bacteriological investigation of the aerosol from ultrasonic scalers, Br. Dent. J. **144**:245, 1978.
28. Kolstad, R.: Asepsis in dental practice, Continuing education seminar, Williamsburg, Va., Jan. 31, 1981.
29. MacFarlane, R.W.: Sterilization in general dental practice, J. Dent. **8**:13, 1980.
30. Macrina, F.L., and Ranney, R.R.: Periodontal disease: microbiological and epidemiological aspects. In McGhee, J.R., Michalek, S.M., and Cassell, G.H., editors: Dental microbiology, New York, 1982, Harper & Row, Publishers, Inc.
31. McCracken, A.W., and Cawson, R.A.: Clinical and oral microbiology, Washington, D.C., Hemisphere Publishing Corp., 1983.
32. Micik, R.E., et al.: Studies on dental aerobiology. I. Bacterial aerosols generated during dental procedures, J. Dent. Res. **48**:49, 1969.
33. Micik, R.E., et al.: Studies on dental aerobiology. III. Efficacy of surgical masks in protecting dental personnel from airborne bacterial particles, J. Dent. Res. **50**:626, 1971.
34. Miller, R.L., et al.: Studies on dental aerobiology. II. Microbial splatter discharge from the oral cavity of dental patients, J. Dent. Res. **50**:621, 1971.
35. Muir, R.F.: Reduction of microbial contamination from ultrasonic scalers, Br. Dent. J. **145**:76, 1978.
36. Nakamura, M., et al.: Aminopeptidase activity of Capnocytophaga, J. Periodont. Res. **6**:597, 1982.

37. Oleski, J., et al.: Immune deficiency syndrome in children, JAMA **249:**2345, 1983.

38. Perkins, J.J.: Principles and methods of sterilization in health sciences, ed. 2, Springfield, Ill., 1978, Charles C Thomas, Publisher.

39. Pollok, A.L., et al.: Laminar air purge of microorganisms in dental aerosols, J. Am. Dent. Assoc. **81:**1131, 1970.

40. Ratcliffe, R.: Hepatitis and the dental hygienist, Dent. Hyg. **51:**493, 1977.

41. Roberts, M.W., and Henderson, D.K.: Dental considerations in acquired immune deficiency syndrome, J. Acad. Gen. Dent. **31:**444, 1983.

42. Runnells, R.R.: The need to monitor use and function of sterilizers, Dent. Surv. **56**(10):20, 1980.

43. Rytel, M.W.: Viral infections in hospital and dental clinic. In Viral infections in oral medicine, New York, 1982, Elsevier Science Publishing Co., Inc.

44. Sawyer, D.R., et al.: Bacterial contamination and disinfection of the high speed dental handpiece and the water it delivers, Va. Dent. J. **53**(6):14, 1976.

45. Slots, J., et al.: Actinobacillus actinomycetemcomitans in human periodontal disease: association, serology, leukotoxicity, and treatment, J. Periodont. Res. **17:**447, 1982.

46. Suggested guidelines for asepsis in the dental office environment, N.C. Dent. J. **63**(1):insert, 1980.

47. Taichman, N.S., et al.: Pathobiology of oral spirochetes in periodontal disease, J. Periodont. Res. **17:**449, 1982.

48. Tullman, M.J., et al.: Past infection with hepatitis B virus in patients at a dental school, J. Am. Dent. Assoc. **97:**477, 1978.

49. Tullman, M.J., et al.: The threat of hepatitis B from dental school patients, Oral Surg. **49:**214, 1980.

50. Van Palenstein Helderman, W.H.: Microbial etiology of periodontal disease, J. Clin. Periodontol. **8:**261, 1981.

51. Viera, J., and others: Acquired immune deficiency in Haitians: opportunistic infections in previously healthy immigrants, N. Engl. J. Med. **308:**125, 1983.

52. Wilkins, E.M.: Clinical practice of the dental hygienist, ed. 5, Philadelphia, 1983, Lea & Febiger.

53. Wistreich, G.A., and Lechtman, M.D.: Microbiology, Encino, Calif., 1980, Glencoe Publishing Co.

Review Questions

1 Your new patient is an 8-year-old girl. When conducting the oral examination, you notice that she is caries free. The community water is fluoridated. You would attribute the absence of tooth decay to
1. High salivary flow
2. Systemic fluoride
3. Proper nutrition
4. Good oral hygiene
5. Genetic consequence

2 *Streptococcus mutans* disappears from the oral cavity when
1. *Streptococcus sanguis* is present
2. Dentures are inserted
3. Full-mouth extractions occur
4. Broad-spectrum antibiotics are taken
5. Antiseptic mouthwash is used

3 Extracellular glucans are produced by
1. *Lactobacillus acidophilus* alone
2. *Streptococcus mutans* alone
3. Several species
4. *Streptococcus sanguis* alone
5. *S. mutans* and *S. sanguis*

4 The *most* strongly cariogenic bacteria in animals are
1. *Streptococcus sanguis*
2. *Streptococcus mutans*
3. *Actinomycetes* organisms
4. *Lactobacillus* organisms
5. *Streptococcus mitis*

5 The cariogenicity of *Streptococcus mutans* appears to be related to its ability to produce
1. Fructans
2. Glucans
3. Glycogen
4. Sucrose
5. Levans

6 Which of the following foods is *most* cariogenic?
1. Dried apricots
2. Apples
3. Bananas
4. Cake
5. Soda

7 In periodontal disease, a major pathogenic mechanism of bacteria is the production of
1. Lactic acid
2. Exotoxins
3. Interferon
4. Lymphocytes
5. Endotoxins

8 Your patient is complaining that his "upper right side hurts." Viewing the radiographs, you note that the maxillary second molar has caries and a radiolucent area around the apices of the roots. If you were to sample the bacteria from this radiolucent area and view it under a microscope, you would see a predominance of
1. *Streptococcus pyogenes*
2. *Actinomyces* organisms
3. *Staphylococcus aureus*
4. *Capnocytophaga* organisms
5. *Bacteroides* organisms

9 Hepatitis B virus is communicable
1. Only during the presence of clinical symptoms
2. Before and during the presence of clinical symptoms
3. During and after the presence of clinical symptoms
4. Only before the presence of clinical symptoms
5. Before, during, and after the presence of clinical symptoms

10 Which of the following is an example of an autogenous infection?
1. Bacteremia after scaling
2. Acute necrotizing ulcerative gingivitis (ANUG)
3. Herpes labialis
4. Periodontal abscess
5. Pericoronitis

11 Disinfection is defined as any process, chemical or physical, that
1. Destroys all forms of life, including bacterial spores and viruses
2. Destroys pathogenic organisms but not necessarily spores
3. Reduces microbial populations to safe levels
4. Prevents growth of microbial populations
5. Destroys all pathogenic bacteria and viruses

12 You have the opportunity to plan a new operatory to prevent disease transmission. What should you plan to have in the operatory?
(a) Foot-operated soap dispensers
(b) Vinyl flooring
(c) Carpeted walls
(d) Small autoclave
(e) Cuspidor
1. a and b
2. a, b, and d
3. a, b, and e
4. b, c, and d
5. a and d

Situation: You are a dental hygienist employed in a general dental practice that has six operatories, two dentists, four assistants, and two dental hygienists. You have been assigned the responsibility of planning the office's surface disinfection procedures. Questions 13 to 15 refer to this situation.

13 For the first step in planning the disinfection procedure, you decide to
1. Distribute a list to all personnel of surfaces they should disinfect
2. Recommend that all personnel wear gloves
3. Order 4 × 4 inch sponges and a supply of glutaraldehyde
4. Ask all personnel to make lists of surfaces they routinely touch
5. Conduct a short in-service session at the next staff meeting

14 Effective use of a surface disinfectant relies heavily on
1. The size of gauze used
2. Spraying over all surfaces
3. Saturation of the gauze with the disinfectant
4. Vigorous scrubbing action
5. Chemical components of the disinfectant

15 In a busy dental practice gauze for surface disinfection should be saturated with the chemical disinfectant
1. At the beginning of each day
2. One hour before use
3. In the morning and again at noon
4. Just before each use
5. At the end of each day

---

16 Dental unit waterlines should be flushed
1. At the end of each day
2. At the beginning of each day
3. At the beginning and end of each day
4. At the beginning of each day and between patients
5. At the beginning of each day and at noon

17 One recommendation to reduce aerosol production is to
1. Flush the air-water syringe between patients
2. Test the water spray for contamination
3. Pass detergent through suction systems
4. Use hand scaling instead of ultrasonic scaling
5. Use high-volume suction

18 After use, the preferred method of cleaning instruments is by
1. Placing instruments in an ultrasonic cleaning unit
2. Scrubbing instruments with a stiff brush
3. Soaking instruments in a blood solvent
4. Holding instruments under a hard spray of water
5. Placing instruments directly in an autoclave

19 Before sterilizing the prophylaxis angle, it must be
1. Soaked in a grease solvent
2. Disassembled and soaked in a disinfectant
3. Soaked in a disinfectant
4. Disassembled and scrubbed
5. Disassembled and soaked in a grease solvent

20 If instruments are sterilized without being wrapped, they should be transferred to storage areas with
1. Gloved hands
2. Cotton pliers
3. Central forceps
4. Sterile forceps
5. Clean hands

21 Most plastics can be sterilized by
1. Steam autoclaving
2. Soaking in glutaraldehyde
3. Dry heat
4. Chemical vapor
5. Ethylene oxide

22 In the autoclave, wrapped instrument packs should be arranged loosely and placed as upright as possible so that
1. Steam can penetrate
2. Instruments will not be bent or broken
3. Moisture will not collect and cause rust
4. A vacuum can be created
5. The temperature reaches the correct range

23 You are using a dry-heat oven to sterilize your instruments. The oven is preheated, and you have just placed your instruments in the oven. Approximately how long will it take until sterilization is achieved? (Include the time required for preheating to the appropriate temperature.)
1. 30 minutes
2. 90 minutes
3. 15 minutes
4. 2 hours
5. 3 hours

24 What is one disadvantage of chemical vapor pressure sterilization?
1. Materials must be aerated
2. Rusting can occur
3. Adequate ventilation is necessary
4. Instruments are wet at the end of the cycle
5. The process is too long

25 Your employer dentist, in an attempt to update office procedures, has asked you to recommend the *best* method for verifying that sterilization has occurred. Your recommendation should be to
1. Use spore strips daily
2. Use indicator strips in each load and color-change tape on each package
3. Use indicator strips daily and spore strips weekly
4. Use color-change tape daily and spore strips monthly
5. Use color-change tape in each load and spore strips weekly

26 The dental office staff use a steam autoclave for sterilization. If you are responsible for ordering spore strips to test sterility, which of the following would you order?
1. *Clostridium botulinum*
2. *Bacillus stearothermophilus*
3. *Clostridium tetani*
4. *Bacillus anthracis*
5. *Bacillus subtilis*

27 The patient you just dismissed has a history of hepatitis B virus. The supply of styrofoam film holders was exhausted, and you used plastic film holders on the patient. The office does not have an ethylene oxide sterilizer. Which of the following would you use to disinfect the plastic film holders?
1. Glutaraldehyde for 30 minutes
2. Sodium hypochlorite solution, 0.05%, for 30 minutes
3. Iodine surgical scrub and 70% isopropyl alcohol for 30 minutes (1:20 solution)
4. Fresh 0.5% sodium hypochlorite solution for 30 minutes
5. Glutaraldehyde for 1 hour

28 What is one reason for selecting a chemical disinfectant for instruments?
1. It is faster than heat sterilization
2. Verification of disinfection is possible
3. For use as a backup method if sterilization devices break down
4. It is inexpensive
5. The good penetrating ability when instruments are soaked

29 In designing a sterilization area, what is the most crucial requirement?
1. Availability of glutaraldehyde
2. Allowance for adequate counter space
3. Availability of instrument storage areas
4. Separation of sterile and nonsterile areas
5. Purchase of a dry-heat oven

30 You have taken radiographs on a patient. After dismissing the patient, your *first* step should be to
1. Develop the radiographs
2. Disinfect the radiographic unit
3. Label the radiographic mount
4. Reassemble the Rinn equipment
5. Wipe the Rinn equipment with Clorox

31 Dental personnel should be routinely tested for
1. Hepatitis A, hepatitis B, and non A/non B hepatitis
2. Hepatitis B
3. Tuberculosis and hepatitis A
4. Hepatitis B and non A/non B hepatitis
5. Hepatitis B and tuberculosis

32 The personnel in the office where you have just accepted employment do not wear uniforms, but instead wear regular street clothing. Your action should be to
1. Soak and wash clothes worn at the office in bleach
2. Refuse to conform, and wear uniforms
3. Launder clothes worn at the office with your other street clothing
4. Use specific clothing only in the clinical setting
5. Try to convince other office personnel to purchase uniforms

33 When considering factors to prevent disease transmission, which of the following is *most* acceptable?
1. Wristwatches
2. Bracelets that do not dangle
3. Small earrings
4. Wedding bands
5. Other rings

34 How often should face masks be changed?
1. After each patient
2. Three to four times a day
3. At noon
4. When damp
5. At midmorning and midafternoon

35 The dental hygienist is about to perform a prophylaxis examination on a patient who has no medical complications as indicated by the medical history and interview. For this appointment the dental hygienist should wear
1. Glasses
2. Glasses and a face mask
3. Glasses and gloves
4. Glasses and gloves for the initial examination
5. Glasses, gloves, and a face mask

36 You wear gloves routinely for all patients and are trying not to be wasteful with office supplies. What is the *best* alternative to changing gloves for each patient?
1. Wash and rinse gloved hands one time between patients
2. Perform a short scrub on the gloved hands between patients
3. Perform a surgical scrub before gloving
4. Lather and rinse gloved hands two to three times between patients
5. Hold gloved hands under a hard stream of water between patients

37 Which of the following behaviors associated with hand washing is recommended?
1. Use cloth towels for drying
2. Use a brush on hands two times a day
3. Perform a short scrub at the beginning of each day
4. Disinfect the scrub brush
5. Perform a surgical scrub at the beginning of each day

38 Which of the following is a *priority* in the selection of a hand cleanser?
1. Gentleness
2. Viricidal ability
3. Bacteriostatic ability
4. Bactericidal ability
5. Cost

39 Which of the following forms of hand cleansers is *least* likely to contribute to disease transmission?
1. Liquid or powdered
2. Bar or liquid
3. Liquid only
4. Powdered or bar
5. Powdered only

40 Your patient has a maxillary denture. To disinfect the denture, your first step should be to
1. Soak it in alcohol
2. Place it in an ultrasonic cleaner with an appropriate solution
3. Use scalers on the denture
4. Place it in a self-sealing bag with an appropriate solution
5. Brush it in the operatory sink

41 After a known carrier of hepatitis B has been treated, dental instruments should be
1. Soaked in sodium hypochlorite
2. Placed directly in the sterilizer
3. Handled with two pairs of household rubber gloves
4. Scrubbed with iodine surgical scrub
5. Sterilized twice as long

42 After a known carrier of hepatitis B has been treated, any surfaces touched that were not draped should be disinfected with
1. Iodine surgical scrub and isopropyl alcohol in 1:20 solution for 30 minutes
2. Iodine surgical scrub and isopropyl alcohol in 1:1 solution for 30 minutes
3. Iodine surgical scrub and isopropyl alcohol in 1:1 solution for 3 minutes
4. Sodium hypochlorite solution, 500 to 5000 parts per million (ppm) (0.05% to 0.5%), for 3 minutes
5. Sodium hypochlorite solution, 200 ppm, for 30 minutes

43 You are performing a prophylaxis on a patient whose medical history is negative. As you pick up your anterior scaler you accidentally puncture your index finger. You should
1. Arrange to receive hepatitis B immune globin (HBIg) after work
2. Request that the patient have a blood test for hepatitis B surface antigen (HB_sAg)
3. Proceed with scaling, since the medical history is negative
4. Have your blood tested for HB_sAg
5. Request that the patient have a blood test for antibody to HB_sAg (anti-HB_s)

44 One of the most important human disease barriers for the protection of the dental hygienist is the
1. Phagocytic mechanism
2. Normal oral flora
3. Coughing reflex
4. Inflammatory response
5. Intact skin

45 Classic immediate hypersensitivity is exemplified by
1. Poison ivy
2. Rheumatoid arthritis
3. Anaphylactic shock
4. Contact dermatitis
5. Rh incompatibility between mother and infant

46 The mature virus particle is called a
1. Bacteriophage
2. Capsid
3. Genome
4. Prophage
5. Virion

47 Causative agents of chickenpox and infectious mononucleosis are members of which virus group?
1. Picornavirus
2. Coronavirus
3. Paramyxovirus
4. Herpetovirus
5. Poxvirus

48 When an infection is present without symptoms, it is termed
1. Chronic
2. Subclinical
3. Localized
4. Secondary
5. Pathogenic

49 The virulence of many gram-negative bacteria is enhanced by their
1. Endotoxin production
2. Invasiveness
3. Lysogenic action
4. Interferon production
5. Capsule formation

50 Deuteromycetes include the
1. Common bread mold
2. Agents of ringworm
3. Mushrooms
4. Yeasts that ferment
5. Agents of plant diseases

51 Human diseases caused by protozoans include
1. Malaria and toxoplasmosis
2. Amoebic dysentery and ringworm
3. Toxoplasmosis and botulism
4. Malaria and diptheria
5. Amoebic dysentery and thrush

52 Which of the following groups of bacteria is considered medically significant?
1. *Treponema, Escherichia,* and *Lactobacillus* organisms
2. *Salmonella, Neisseria,* and *Peptococcus* organisms
3. *Staphylococcus, Pseudomonas,* and *Lactobacillus* organisms
4. *Streptococcus, Neisseria,* and *Escherichia* organisms
5. *Rickettsia, Mycoplasma,* and *Streptomyces* organisms

53 Streptococci and staphylococci are
1. Gram-negative aerobic cocci
2. Gram-positive cocci
3. Endospore-forming cocci
4. Gram-negative anaerobic cocci
5. Acid-fast aerobic cocci

54 The relationship of *Candida albicans* to the human host during oral moniliasis is called
1. Competition
2. Parasitism
3. Opportunistic
4. Commensalism
5. Predation

55 The relationship of normal oral bacteria to the human host is termed
1. Commensalism
2. Mutualism
3. Parasitism
4. Competition
5. Syntrophism

56 The transfer of genetic material by a bacteriophage is termed
1. Lysogenic conversion
2. Sexduction
3. Conjugation
4. Tranduction
5. Transformation

57 Viable counts of bacteria are expressed as
1. Colony-forming units
2. Viable cell units
3. Plaque-forming units
4. Stationary cell units
5. In vitro–forming units

58 The set of chemical reactions by which cells maintain life describes
1. Catabolism
2. Respiration
3. Glycolysis
4. Metabolism
5. Anabolism

59 The type of media generally used to show streptococcal hemolysis is
1. Selective
2. Anaerobic
3. Reducing
4. Differential
5. Selective and differential

60 Viruses are hypotrophic organisms, which means they
1. Require oxygen to survive
2. Grow only within a living host cell
3. Use inorganic compounds as sources of energy
4. Grow best near a neutral pH
5. Grow best between 0° and 20° C (32° to 68° F)

61 Of the following structures, the *most* important for the maintenance of the virulence of *Streptococcus mutans* is the
1. Capsule
2. Flagellum
3. Endospore
4. Cell wall
5. Genome

62 A major distinction between the procaryotic cell and the eucaryotic cell is that the eucaryotic cell has a
1. Cell wall
2. Distinct nucleus
3. Chromosome
4. Flagellum
5. Cell membrane

63 Bacteria are members of the Kingdom
1. Protista
2. Animalia
3. Procaryotae
4. Plantae
5. Mycetidae

64 Procaryotic cellular structure is typical of
1. Mammals
2. Fungi
3. Helminths
4. Bacteria
5. Protozoa

65 Clusters of spherical-shaped bacteria are referred to as
1. Streptococci
2. Streptobacilli
3. Coccobacilli
4. Spirilla
5. Staphylococci

66 The Gram stain is useful in
1. Grouping bacteria
2. Showing spore-formers
3. Identifying mycobacteria
4. Demonstrating bacterial size
5. Viewing dental plaque

67 The main agent of skin infections causing acute suppurative inflammation is
1. *Clostridium tetani*
2. *Mycobacterium leprae*
3. *Staphylococcus aureus*
4. *Streptococcus pyogenes*
5. *Haemophilus influenzae*

68 Of the following bacteria, which multiplies in standing water, including the dental unit water, and can become pathogenic in debilitated patients?
1. *Staphylococcus aureus*
2. *Streptococcus pyogenes*
3. *Treponema pallidum*
4. *Streptococcus pneumoniae*
5. *Pseudomonas aeruginosa*

69 An unwanted complication of a streptococcal sore throat infection could be
1. Scarlet fever
2. Rheumatic fever
3. Infectious mononucleosis
4. Influenza
5. Tuberculosis

70 An elderly, diabetic patient is scheduled for a morning appointment. When updating her medical history, you learn she has been taking penicillin for 7 to 10 days as a result of "strep" throat. During the oral examination, you note white areas on the patient's buccal mucosa and soft palate. The patient probably has
1. Diptheria
2. Another streptococcal infection
3. Pale tissues, common for her age
4. Oral moniliasis
5. Rheumatic fever

71 While seating a 40-year-old woman, you notice a lesion on the patient's lips. It appears as several discrete vesicles; some have ulcerated. When questioned, the patient says she always gets a sore like that before she gets a cold. You suspect the patient has
1. A chancre
2. Perlèche
3. An apthous ulcer
4. Herpes labialis
5. Basal cell carcinoma

72 Which of the following two diseases represents different forms of infection with the same agent?
1. Measles and German measles
2. Chickenpox and smallpox
3. Bacterial pneumonia and croup
4. Shingles and chickenpox
5. Infectious mononucleosis and cytomegalovirus (CMV)

73 The greatest possibility of contracting herpetic whitlow would be by touching an infected patient's
1. Vesicular lesions and blood
2. Clothing and saliva
3. Blood and saliva
4. Blood and clothing
5. Saliva and vesicular lesions

74 One of the *most* frequent agents of the common cold is
1. *Streptococcus pyogenes*
2. *Staphylococcus aureus*
3. Rhinovirus
4. *Haemophilus influenzae*
5. Influenza virus

Situation: Mr. Williams, an elderly patient, indicates on the health history form that he has night sweats and a cough that does not go away. You notice he looks somewhat thinner than at his last 6-month recall appointment. Questions 75 and 76 refer to this situation.

75 The dental hygienist suspects the possibility of what disease?
1. Hepatitis
2. Syphilis
3. Pneumonia
4. Infectious mononucleosis
5. Tuberculosis

76 What decision would be *most* appropriate for the dental hygienist regarding the patient?
1. Refer the patient to a physician and reschedule when the physician releases the patient
2. Perform an intraoral and extraoral examination and postpone the prophylaxis until the patient is checked by a physician
3. Wear gloves, perform an intraoral and extraoral examination, and postpone the prophylaxis until the patient is checked by a physician
4. Wear gloves and perform an intraoral and extraoral examination and prophylaxis
5. Refer the patient to a hospital equipped to treat the patient dentally with maximal precautions

77 Which of the following is a rickettsial infection?
1. Malaria
2. Psittacosis
3. Rocky Mountain spotted fever
4. Tularemia
5. Meningitis

78 A disease of special concern to pregnant women that may be contracted by handling cat litter is
1. Toxoplasmosis
2. Histoplasmosis
3. Cryptococcosis
4. Trichinosis
5. Rubella

79 Food poisoning resulting in an active infection, not associated with toxin production, is caused by
1. *Shigella* species
2. *Salmonella* species
3. *Clostridium botulinum*
4. Staphylococci
5. *Clostridium perfringens*

80 Which one of the following lists of diseases may develop into a carrier state?
1. Hepatitis B, hepatitis A, and herpes simplex
2. Hepatitis B, herpes simplex, and *Streptococcus pyogenes*
3. *S. pyogenes*, hepatitis A, and hepatitis B
4. Herpes simplex, *Staphylococcus aureus*, and hepatitis A
5. *S. aureus*, hepatitis A, and *S. pyogenes*

Situation: Your patient is a 40-year-old man who has worked in a blood bank for 15 years. He is scheduled for a 6-month recall prophylaxis. As you are seating the patient, he mentions he is just recovering from influenza. You now notice his eyes are somewhat yellowish. Questions 81 and 82 refer to this situation.

81 What disease might this patient have?
1. Hepatitis A
2. Influenza
3. Infectious hepatitis
4. Hepatitis B
5. Infectious mononucleosis

82 The *best* choice of treatment for this patient at this appointment would be to
1. Wear gloves and a face mask and perform an intraoral and extraoral examination
2. Refer to a physician and reschedule in 6 months
3. Refer to a hospital equipped to treat the patient dentally with maximal precautions
4. Wear gloves and a face mask and perform a prophylaxis examination
5. Refer to a physician and reschedule when appropriate tests are negative

83 Before receiving dental hygiene services, a patient with a prosthetic heart valve should be premedicated to prevent
1. Rheumatic fever
2. Subacute infectious endocarditis
3. "Strep" throat
4. Rheumatic heart disease
5. Toxemia

84 Most of the bacterial agents of subacute bacterial endocarditis (SBE) are oral
1. Fusobacteria
2. Streptococci
3. Lactobacilli
4. Staphylococci
5. *Actinomyces* organisms

85 Blood in the urine is a symptom of
1. Gonorrhea
2. Pinworm infection
3. Syphilis
4. Hookworm infection
5. Urinary tract infection

86 Infections affecting the nervous system include
1. Conjunctivitis and meningitis
2. Encephalitis and poliomyelitis
3. Rabies and herpes
4. Encephalitis and conjunctivitis
5. Meningitis and herpes

87 Viral encephalitis is spread by
1. Droplets
2. Dust
3. Contaminated food
4. Arthropods
5. Pigeon excreta

88 The agent of acute mucopurulent conjunctivitis is
1. *Staphylococcus aureus*
2. *Streptococcus pneumoniae*
3. Adenovirus
4. *Haemophilus aegyptius*
5. Newcastle disease virus

89 A 30-year-old patient calls and complains of sudden swelling in both sides of his neck, which seems to be getting bigger. Looking at his record, you note that he has cancelled two times recently. He needs to have restorative work done on the mandibular second molars, which have extensive decay. You suspect he may have
1. Actinomycosis
2. Mumps
3. Syphilis
4. Ludwig's angina
5. Pericoronitis

90 Wearing glasses during dental treatment helps prevent
1. Conjunctivitis and hepatitis A
2. Hepatitis B and ophthalmia neonatorum
3. Herpes and injury
4. Ophthalmia neonatorum and herpes
5. Injury and hepatitis A

91 Nutrient sources for oral microbes include
1. Exogenous and endogenous sources
2. Exogenous sources
3. The host's dietary sugar and starch
4. Endogenous sources
5. The host's saliva

92 Strains of *Streptococcus mutans* are described as
1. Anaerobic and acidogenic
2. Acidogenic
3. Anaerobic and aciduric
4. Aciduric
5. Aciduric and acidogenic

Answers and Rationales

1. (2) Systemic fluoride is the only proven means of reducing decay.
   (1) High salivary flow may contribute to lowering decay.
   (3) Proper nutrition may contribute to lowering decay.
   (4) Good oral hygiene contributes to reduced decay, but systemic fluoride, even with lax home care, reduces decay.
   (5) Genetic consequence may affect resistance to decay.
2. (3) *S. mutans* requires a hard tooth surface to attach to and disappears in edentulous mouths.
   (1) *S. sanguis* is antagonistic, but *S. sanguis* does not make *S. mutans* disappear.
   (2) When dentures are inserted, *S. mutans* reappears and adheres to the dentures.
   (4) Broad-spectrum antibiotics do not cause *S. mutans* to disappear from the oral cavity.
   (5) Although an antiseptic mouthwash may reduce the microbe population, it does not eliminate them.
3. (3) Extracellular glucans are produced by *S. mutans, S. sanguis, S. salivarius, L. casei, L. acidophilus,* and *Neisseria* organisms.
   (1) *L. acidophilis* alone does not produce extracellular glucans.
   (2) *S. mutans* alone does not produce extracellular glucans.
   (4) *S. sanguis* alone does not produce extracellular glucans.
   (5) *S. mutans* and *S. sanguis* are only two of several species that produce glucans.
4. (2) *S. mutans* is the most strongly cariogenic bacteria found in animals, according to research.
   (1) Although cariogenic in animals, *S. sanguis* is not as strongly cariogenic as *S. mutans.*
   (3) Although cariogenic in animals, *Actinomycetes* organisms are not as strongly cariogenic as *S. mutans.*
   (4) Although cariogenic in animals, *Lactobacillus* organisms are not as strongly cariogenic as *S. mutans.*
   (5) Although cariogenic in animals, *S. mitis* is not as strongly cariogenic as *S. mutans.*
5. (2) The cariogenicity of *S. mutans* appears related to its ability to produce glucans by aiding in adherence.
   (1) *S. mutans* produces fructosans, but they are reserve nutrients and are not used in adherence.
   (3) Glycogen, a reserve carbohydrate and intracellular polysaccharide, is not related to cariogenicity.
   (4) Sucrose is used by *S. mutans* to produce glucans.
   (5) *S. mutans* produces levans, but they are reserve nutrients and are not used in adherence.

6. (1) Dried apricots have the most retentive, high sucrose content of the foods listed.
   (2) Apples are used by cariogenic bacteria but do not have sucrose, which is the main substrate of cariogenic bacteria.
   (3) Bananas are used by cariogenic bacteria but do not have sucrose, which is the main substrate of cariogenic bacteria.
   (4) Cake, containing starch with sugar, is adhesive but not as retentive as dried fruit.
   (5) Soda has a high sucrose content but is not retentive.
7. (5) Bacteria do not invade tissue themselves, but endotoxins produced do so and destroy tissue.
   (1) Lactic acid is produced by cariogenic bacteria.
   (2) Exotoxins are not pathogenic mechanisms of bacteria associated with periodontal destruction.
   (3) Interferon might be stimulated as part of the immunologic response to bacterial activity but is not a mechanism of the bacteria themselves.
   (4) Lymphocytes also might be stimulated as part of the immunologic response to bacterial activity, but they are not a mechanism of the bacteria themselves.
8. (5) The patient's radiographs and symptoms suggest a periapical abscess. The predominant organisms found in the periapical area would be *Bacteroides* organisms.
   (1) *S. pyogenes* is not predominant in periapical infections.
   (2) *Actinomyces* organisms are not present in periapical infections but are present in root caries.
   (3) *S. aureus* is not predominant in periapical infections.
   (4) *Capnocytophaga* organisms are not present in periapical infections but are present in destructive periodontal disease.
9. (5) Hepatitis B can be transmitted before, during, and after the presence of clinical symptoms and even if the infected person never shows clinical symptoms.
   (1) Transmittal of hepatitis B can occur not only during the presence of clinical symptoms, but also before and after the clinical systems appear.
   (2) Hepatitis B can also be transmitted after the symptoms disappear.
   (3) Hepatitis B can also be transmitted before the symptoms appear.
   (4) Hepatitis B can also be transmitted during and after the presence of clinical symptoms.
10. (1) Bacteremia after scaling is an example of an autogenous infection, since it would be caused by introducing the patient's own oral flora into the injured tissue site.
    (2) ANUG is not a posttreatment infection caused by introducing the patient's microflora into an injured tissue.
    (3) Herpes labialis is not a posttreatment infection caused by introducing the patient's microflora into an injured tissue.
    (4) A periodontal abscess is not a posttreatment infection caused by introducing the patient's microflora into an injured tissue.

For each question the correct answer and rationale are listed first. The other alternatives are presented in order with the reasons why they are not correct.

(5) Pericoronitis is not a posttreatment infection caused by introducing the patient's microflora into an injured tissue.

11. (2) Disinfection destroys pathogenic organisms but not necessarily spores.

   (1) Sterilization destroys all forms of life including bacterial spores and viruses.

   (3) Sanitization is a cleaning process that reduces microbal populations to safe levels.

   (4) Disinfection not only prevents the growth of many organisms, it kills many organisms.

   (5) Disinfection does not destroy *all* pathogenic bacteria and viruses.

12. (1) Foot-operated soap dispensers prevent handling soap dispensers with their accumulation of bacteria. Vinyl flooring allows easy cleaning without collecting aerosols, as does carpeting.

   (2) The sterilizing area should not be in the same area as the operatory to prevent easy contamination.

   (3) The cuspidor is very difficult to disinfect, and it is difficult to keep the drain clean. High-speed suction with disposable or sterilizable tips are better.

   (4) Carpeted walls reduce the noise level, but they accumulate infectious aerosols and cannot be disinfected.

   (5) The sterilizing area should not be in the same area as the operatory to prevent easy contamination.

13. (4) Until you know the type of surfaces being touched in each operatory, you cannot make choices of the disinfectant to use or recommendations for the easiest routine to follow in each operatory.

   (1) Each operatory may be different or have specialized equipment; therefore one list of surfaces to disinfect might not include all surfaces in some operatories.

   (2) Wearing gloves while disinfecting surfaces helps the hands but is not directly related to the task you have been assigned.

   (3) A check of supplies in stock should be made before ordering more. Glutaraldehyde may not be the best choice for surface disinfection because of its cost.

   (5) Some prior assessment and planning are needed before an in-service staff meeting is called.

14. (4) Without vigorous scrubbing action, the penetration and removal of organisms and infectious agents are not achieved.

   (1) The size of gauze used is important so that infected gauze is not wiped over new areas or the cleaned area, but even with the use of large gauze, if the area is not vigorously scrubbed, the effectiveness of the procedure is reduced.

   (2) Spraying surfaces alone does not help a disinfectant penetrate infectious agents.

   (3) Although it is important that the gauze be saturated, if the surface is not scrubbed vigorously, the effectiveness is reduced.

   (5) Although the chemical components of the disinfectant are an important consideration, if the area is not scrubbed vigorously, the effectiveness of the disinfectant is reduced.

15. (4) For maximum effectiveness, the gauze and chemical should be stored in separate containers and the gauze should be wetted just before each use.

   (1) The gauze for surface disinfection should be wetted just before each use rather than at the beginning of the day.

   (2) The gauze for surface disinfection should be wetted just before each use, not 1 hour before use.

   (3) The gauze for surface disinfection should be wetted just before each use, not at various times during the day.

   (5) The gauze for surface disinfection should be wetted just before each use, not at the end of each day.

16. (4) According to the current recommendation for reducing bacterial contamination of water in the dental office, the dental unit waterlines should be flushed at the beginning of each day and between patients.

   (1) Dental unit waterlines should be flushed at the beginning of each day and between patients, not just at the end of each day.

   (2) Dental unit waterlines should be flushed between patients, as well as at the beginning of each day.

   (3) If dental unit waterlines are flushed at the beginning of each day and between patients, it is not necessary to flush them at the end of each day.

   (5) If there are appointments all day, dental unit waterlines should be flushed at the beginning of the day and between patients.

17. (5) The use of high-volume suction will reduce aerosol production.

   (1) Flushing the air-water syringe between patients helps reduce bacterial contamination of water but does not reduce aerosol production.

   (2) Testing the water spray for contamination will not reduce aerosol production.

   (3) Passing a detergent through the suction systems will help reduce bacterial buildup but will not reduce aerosol production.

   (4) Ultrasonic scaling, rather than hand scaling, is recommended for many patients. However, it is also recommended that high-volume suction accompany the use of ultrasonic scalers.

18. (1) An ultrasonic cleaner more thoroughly cleans instruments in less time, with less chance of injury, with less splatter, and penetrates grooves more thoroughly.

   (2) Scrubbing instruments with a sterile brush is *not* preferred. Disadvantages of this technique include the length of time necessary to clean instruments, a greater chance of injury, and increased splatter.

   (3) Instruments should be soaked in a blood solvent if there is a time lapse before using an ultrasonic cleaner.

   (4) Too much splatter is produced when holding instruments under a hard spray of water.

   (5) Organic debris acts as a barrier, so instruments should be cleaned first before placing them in an autoclave. (This step is recommended for patients with hepatitis and AIDS.)

19. (5) If the prophylaxis angle is not disassembled before sterilizing, steam may not penetrate all areas. If grease is not removed first, the sterilant cannot penetrate and the grease becomes caked on.
    (1) The prophylaxis angle should be soaked in a grease solvent, but it also must be disassembled for proper sterilizing.
    (2) It is not necessary to soak a prophylaxis angle in a disinfectant, but it is necessary to disassemble it and remove accumulated grease.
    (3) Merely soaking a prophylaxis angle in a disinfectant will not allow proper sterilization.
    (4) A prophylaxis angle should be disassembled and placed in a grease solvent before sterilizing. Scrubbing the prophylaxis angle is not sufficient to remove grease.
20. (4) Sterile forceps must be used to transfer unwrapped sterile instruments to avoid recontamination.
    (1) Gloved hands do not prevent recontamination when used to transfer unwrapped sterile instruments.
    (2) Cotton pliers are not sterile and therefore will allow recontamination when used to transfer unwrapped sterile instruments.
    (3) Central forceps are not sterile and therefore will allow recontamination when used to transfer unwrapped sterile instruments.
    (5) Clean hands are not sterile and therefore will allow recontamination when used to transfer unwrapped sterile instruments.
21. (5) Ethylene oxide is the only sterilization agent applicable to almost any material including plastics.
    (1) Most plastics cannot withstand steam autoclaving.
    (2) Soaking in glutaraldehyde is a disinfection procedure, not a sterilization procedure.
    (3) Most plastics cannot withstand dry-heat sterilizing.
    (4) Most plastics cannot withstand a chemical vapor.
22. (1) Moist heat travels vertically and coagulates protein. It must be able to reach all items for sterilization to take place. Therefore items must be arranged within the autoclave to accomplish this.
    (2) Properly wrapped and arranged instrument packs may prevent bent and broken instruments, but this is secondary to accomplishing proper sterilization.
    (3) Moisture can collect even if the instrument packs are in an upright position.
    (4) A vacuum is not created in an autoclave.
    (5) If the autoclave is operating properly, the correct temperature range should occur whether instrument packs are vertical or horizontal.
23. (2) It may take 15 to 60 minutes for the instruments to reach the sterilization temperature, and another 30 minutes (a total of 90 minutes) is required for sterilization to occur. The presence of a thermocouple and pyrometer on the oven would help determine when the proper sterilization temperature has been reached.

(1) After the instruments have actually reached the sterilization temperature, it takes 30 minutes for sterilization to take place. However, since it is uncertain exactly how long it will take the instruments to reach the sterilization temperature, a total time of 90 minutes would ensure sterilization.
(3) Even after the instruments have reached the sterilization temperature, 30 minutes are required for sterilization to be achieved.
(4) If the dry oven was not preheated, more than 90 minutes would be required to reach sterilization, but 2 hours would not necessarily guarantee that sterilization was achieved.
(5) Even without preheating the oven, a total of 3 hours would probably be a waste of time.
24. (3) Chemical vapors should not be inhaled; therefore adequate ventilation is required when chemical vapor pressure sterilization is used.
    (1) Materials must be aerated when ethylene oxide is used but not when chemical vapors are used.
    (2) Rusting instruments can occur when a steam autoclave is used, but this is not true for chemical vapor pressure sterilization.
    (4) When a steam autoclave is used, instruments are sometimes wet at the end of the cycle, but this is not true for chemical vapor pressure sterilization.
    (5) Since it requires only 20 minutes for chemical vapor pressure sterilization, the time required is not a disadvantage of this method.
25. (5) Color-change tape or indicator strips should be used in each load to provide evidence that instruments have been in the sterilizer or to provide warning of a gross malfunction. Spore strips are the most reliable test of sterilization, and their weekly use is recommended in the dental office.
    (1) Spore strips are somewhat inconvenient and expensive to use daily; however, some type of indicator is needed in *each* load.
    (2) The use of both indicator strips and color-change tape in each load would be a duplication of effort.
    (3) The use of indicator strips on a daily basis is not sufficient, since they must be used in each load. Spore strips are used weekly.
    (4) The use of color-change tape daily and spore strips monthly is *not* sufficient. Color-change tape must be used in each load, and it is recommended that spore strips be changed weekly.
26. (2) The spores of *B. stearothermophilus* are extremely resistant to moist heat, so they are used for testing steam autoclave sterilizers.
    (1) The spores of *C. botulinum* and *not* recommended for use in testing sterilization devices.
    (3) The spores of *C. tetani* are *not* recommended for use in testing sterilizing devices.
    (4) The spores of *B. anthracis* are *not* recommended for use in testing sterilizing devices.
    (5) The spores of *B. subtilis* are recommended for use in testing dry heat and ethylene oxide sterilizers.

27. (4) The strong solution of 0.5% sodium hypochlorite for 30 minutes is recommended for patients with hepatitis and is mixed fresh, since it deteriorates on standing.
    (1) Glutaraldehyde is sporicidal and is probably effective against hepatitis B after 10 hours.
    (2) The 0.05% dilution of sodium hypochlorite is recommended for normal usage but the sodium hypochlorite must be a freshly mixed 0.5% solution to be effective on patients with hepatitis.
    (3) A stronger solution (1:1) of iodine surgical scrub and isopropyl for 30 minutes is recommended for patients with hepatitis.
    (5) The use of glutaraldehyde for 1 hour may not be sufficient time to be effective against hepatitis B virus; 10 hours is recommended.

28. (3) There are only two reasons given in the literature for using disinfectants on dental instruments: (1) in an emergency situation if the sterilization equipment fails or (2) as a stopgap measure until sterilization devices are obtained.
    (1) Chemical disinfection is *not* faster than heat sterilization. Instruments require at least 30 minutes, usually more, to dry. Steam autoclaves can sterilize in 3 to 7 minutes, and sterile packages are produced. Additional time is required after soaking instruments in a disinfectant to rinse, dry, and place in storage areas with sterile forceps.
    (2) Verification of disinfection is *not* possible.
    (4) Noncorrosive disinfectants *are* expensive.
    (5) Chemical disinfectants cannot penetrate debris and crevices as well as steam heat, chemical vapor, dry heat, or ethylene oxide sterilization.

29. (4) The most important consideration in designing the sterilization area is preventing contamination or routes of cross-infection by separating sterile and nonsterile areas.
    (1) The availability of glutaraldehyde is a factor depending on the dental instruments and equipment used for instrument disinfection.
    (2) Although adequate counter space is important, it is not the first priority in designing a sterilization area.
    (3) Instrument storage areas may or may not be located in the sterilization area, since their location depends on individual office instrument flow patterns.
    (5) Although a dry-heat oven may be needed, it depends on the individual office—what equipment must be sterilized.

30. (2) Any part of the radiographic unit that has been touched by saliva coated hands has the potential for disease transmission and should be disinfected before the next patient is seated.
    (1) Before developing the radiographs, the radiographic unit must be disinfected before the next patient is seated.
    (3) Labeling the radiographic mount can be done later. The unit should be disinfected so other patients can use the x-ray room.
    (4) The Rinn equipment must be disassembled and sterilized or disinfected before it is reassembled.

(5) The Rinn equipment should be sterilized or *soaked* in a recommended disinfectant, not merely wiped.

31. (5) It is recommended that dental personnel be routinely tested for both hepatitis B and tuberculosis, since they are at risk of contracting both diseases.
    (1) Dental personnel are not at great risk of contracting hepatitis A. There are no tests for non A/non B hepatitis.
    (2) Dental personnel should be tested for both hepatitis B and tuberculosis.
    (3) It is not recommended to test dental personnel for hepatitis A.
    (4) There are no tests for non A/non B hepatitis.

32. (4) Uniforms or street clothing, whichever are worn in the clinical setting, should not be worn outside the clinical setting, because the office contamination could then be spread. If errands need to be done before a change of clothing can be made, a lab coat should be worn over the clothes and closed.
    (1) Colored uniforms or colored street clothes cannot be put in regular bleach. However, launder any clothes possible in bleach.
    (2) Wearing uniforms is no guarantee of more aseptic dress and care of clothing.
    (3) Launder any dental office clothing separate from regular clothes.
    (5) Wearing uniforms is no guarantee of more aseptic dress and care of clothing.

33. (3) It is recommended to not wear any jewelry on the hands or wrists, but small earrings are not in an operating zone in dental procedures.
    (1) Wristwatches are worn on the wrist and are therefore not acceptable.
    (2) Bracelets are worn on the wrist and are not acceptable.
    (4) Wedding bands are worn on the fingers and are not acceptable.
    (5) Rings are worn on the fingers and are not acceptable.

34. (4) Face masks should be changed whenever they become damp because they are not effective when damp.
    (1) There is no set time schedule to change face masks, only when they become damp.
    (2) There is no set time schedule to change face masks, only when they become damp.
    (3) There is no set time schedule to change face masks, only when they become damp.
    (5) There is no set time schedule to change face masks, only when they become damp.

35. (5) Wearing glasses, gloves, and a face mask is recommended for all patient treatments. It is impossible to detect from a medical history all patients who have tuberculosis, hepatitis, or AIDS or who are in the incubation stage or carrier state of a disease.
    (1) Wearing gloves and a face mask is also recommended.
    (2) Wearing gloves is also recommended.
    (3) Wearing a face mask is also recommended.
    (4) Wearing a face mask, glasses, and gloves is recommended for the initial examination and also for the rest of the treatment.

36. (4) If gloves cannot be changed between patients, the recommended procedure is to lather and rinse two to three times between patients. The friction of rubbing and rinsing is the most important action of hand washing to remove microbes. Gloves can be washed cleaner than bare hands.
    (1) Washing and rinsing more than one time is more effective in removing microbes.
    (2) One does want to use a brush to scrub if gloves are on, and it is impractical to remove gloves to scrub. The need is to remove germs from the gloves.
    (3) It is recommended to perform a short scrub at the beginning of the day whether gloves are worn or not. A surgical scrub is not necessary, but one must remove germs from the gloves after each patient.
    (5) The friction of rubbing and rinsing is the most important action to remove microbes, so holding hands under a stream of water is not sufficient.

37. (3) The recommended procedure is to perform a short scrub at the beginning of the day. It is too time consuming and harsh on the hands to scrub between patients.
    (1) Cloth towels can be used for drying instead of paper towels *if* a new towel is used for each patient.
    (2) Using a brush on the hands more than once a day is too irritating to the skin.
    (4) Scrub brushes need to be sterilized, not disinfected.
    (5) Only before surgery is a surgical scrub required at the beginning of the day.

38. (1) Gentleness in a hand cleanser must be a high priority because the intact skin is a natural defense.
    (2) A hand cleanser will never sterilize the hands, so it is important to choose one that is nonirritating and nonallergenic. Friction in cleaning is the most important factor in reducing microbes.
    (3) A hand cleanser will never sterilize the hands, so it is important to choose one that is nonirritating and nonallergenic. Friction in cleaning is the most important factor in reducing microbes.
    (4) A hand cleanser will never sterilize the hands, so it is important to choose one that is nonirritating and nonallergenic. Friction in cleaning is the most important factor in reducing microbes.
    (5) Although cost is important, preserving the intact skin is the first priority.

39. (3) A liquid hand cleanser is the fastest and least likely to become contaminated.
    (1) Powdered hand cleansers take longer to form a liquid, soapy state.
    (2) Bar hand cleansers accumulate microorganisms and are not recommended.
    (4) Powdered hand cleansers take longer to form a liquid, soapy state, and bar hand cleansers accumulate microbes.
    (5) Powdered hand cleansers take longer to form a liquid, soapy state.

40. (4) To disinfect a denture, it should first be placed in a self-sealing bag containing a disinfectant so that it does not contaminate the ultrasonic solution. It is then placed in an ultrasonic cleaner to clean and disinfect.
    (1) Use of an ultrasonic cleanser is preferred. Alcohol evaporates too quickly.
    (2) If the denture is placed directly in an ultrasonic cleaner, it will contaminate the ultrasonic solution.
    (3) Cleaning dentures with scaling instruments may scratch the dentures.
    (5) Brushing a denture in the sink spreads splatter and is an unnecessary step.

41. (2) Dental instruments used on a known carrier of hepatitis B should be placed directly in the sterilizer, then cleaned and resterilized.
    (1) Sodium hypochlorite is corrosive to metals.
    (3) One pair of heavy household rubber gloves is adequate for protection.
    (4) Instruments used on a known carrier of hepatitis B should not be handled except to place in a sterilizer.
    (5) It is not recommended that instruments used on known carriers of hepatitis B be sterilized twice as long as normal for added protection.

42. (2) After a known carrier of hepatitis B has been treated, any surfaces touched that are not draped should be disinfected with an iodine surgical scrub and isopropyl alcohol in a 1:1 solution for 30 minutes.
    (1) A 1:20 solution is not strong enough following treatment of a patient with hepatitis B.
    (3) A 3-minute scrub is not long enough. The recommended procedure is to keep the surface wet for 30 minutes and then rinse with alcohol.
    (4) A dilution of 500 to 5000 ppm of sodium hypochlorite solution is satisfactory, but 3 minutes is too short a time.
    (5) A 200 ppm sodium hypochlorite solution is not strong enough.

43. (2) Since it is impossible to know undetected carriers of hepatitis B virus by medical history, the only way to know if you have been accidentally exposed is to request that the patient have a blood test for hepatitis B surface antigen (HB_sAg).
    (1) It is not necessary to receive hepatitis B immune globulin (HBIg) if you are immune to hepatitis B virus or if the patient is not a carrier.
    (3) Since a negative medical history does not preclude a patient being a carrier, all precautions should be taken when a finger is accidentally punctured.
    (4) Dental personnel should not wait until an accidental puncture to verify the presence of HB_sAg.
    (5) You want to know if the patient has the hepatitis B antigen. If the patient has the antibody, he or she may or may not also have the antigen, which is the infective portion.

44. (5) Without considering artificial protective measures, intact skin of the hands is the first line of defense.
    (1) Phagocytic mechanisms are human disease barriers but not the first line of defense for a dental hygienist's most vulnerable area, the hands.

(2) The normal oral flora is a human disease barrier but not the first line of defense against disease.

(3) The coughing reflex is a human disease barrier but not the body's first line of defense against disease.

(4) The inflammatory response is a human disease barrier, but not the first line of defense against disease.

45. (3) Anaphylactic shock is an example of classic immediate hypersensitivity.

    (1) Poison ivy is a type IV, delayed, cell-mediated hypersensitivity.

    (2) Rheumatoid arthritis is an autoimmune disease or may be type IV.

    (4) Contact dermatitis is a type IV hypersensitivity.

    (5) Rh incompatibility between mother and infant is an example of a type II cytotoxic hypersensitivity.

46. (5) A virion is a mature virus particle.

    (1) A bacteriophage is a bacterial virus.

    (2) A capsid is a protein outer coat of virus.

    (3) A genome is genetic viral material.

    (4) Prophage is the integration of a temperate bacteriophage into the host cell.

47. (4) Herpetovirus is a causative agent of chickenpox and infectious mononucleosis.

    (1) Picornavirus is not a causative agent of chickenpox or infectious mononucleosis.

    (2) Coronavirus is not a causative agent of chickenpox or infectious mononucleosis.

    (3) Paramyxovirus is not a causative agent of chickenpox or infectious mononucleosis.

    (5) Poxvirus is not a causative agent of chickenpox or infectious mononucleosis.

48. (2) An infection present without symptoms is termed subclinical.

    (1) A chronic infection is a long-term infection, which could be sublinical.

    (3) A localized infection is one in which infectious organisms remain in one area.

    (4) A secondary infection is an infection following the original or primary infection.

    (5) *Pathogenic* refers to an organism that is capable of causing disease.

49. (1) The virulence of gram-negative bacteria is enhanced by their endotoxin production. Endotoxin has a direct pathologic effect on human tissues.

    (2) Many gram-negative bacteria that produce endotoxins do not directly invade tissue.

    (3) Lysogenic action applies to viruses and their destructive effects.

    (4) Interferon production is a protective mechanism and induces a state of resistance to viruses.

    (5) Capsule formation maintains virulence of some bacteria but not gram-negative bacteria as a group.

50. (2) Deuteromycetes include the agents of ringworm.

    (1) The common bread mold is a member of Zygomycetes.

    (3) Mushrooms are members of Basidiomycetes.

    (4) Yeasts that ferment are members of Ascomycetes.

    (5) Agents of plant diseases are members of Oomycetes or Myxomycetes.

51. (1) Malaria and toxoplasmosis are both caused by protozoans.

    (2) Ringworm is caused by a fungus.

    (3) Toxoplasmosis and botulism are both caused by bacteria.

    (4) Diptheria is caused by bacteria.

    (5) Thrush is caused by a fungus.

52. (4) *Streptococcus, Neisseria,* and *Escherichia* organisms all cause disease in humans.

    (1) *Lactobacillus* organisms are not considered of great medical importance. Evidence linking *Lactobacillus* to human caries is not strong.

    (2) *Peptococcus* organisms are not pathogenic to humans.

    (3) *Lactobacillus* organisms are not considered of great medical importance.

    (5) *Streptomyces* organisms are not medically significant.

53. (2) Streptococci and staphylococci are gram-positive cocci.

    (1) Streptococci and staphylococci are not gram negative.

    (3) Streptococci and staphylococci do not form spores.

    (4) Streptococci and staphylococci are not gram negative.

    (5) Streptococci and staphylococci are not acid fast.

54. (3) In this situation a normal commensal relationship has become pathogenic. *C. albicans,* a normal inhabitant of the oral cavity, has become pathogenic and is termed an opportunist.

    (1) The term *competition* does not describe this relationship.

    (2) The term *parasitism* does not describe this relationship.

    (4) The term *commensalism* does not describe this relationship.

    (5) The term *predation* does not describe this relationship.

55. (1) Commensalism is a form of symbiosis in which one organism benefits and the other neither benefits nor is harmed.

    (2) Mutualism is a relationship in which both members benefit.

    (3) In parasitism, one member benefits at the expense of the other.

    (4) Competition is an interaction between organisms as a result of the demand for nutrients that exceeds the supply.

    (5) In syntrophism, the organisms are not intimately associated with each other but benefit from each other.

56. (4) Transduction is the transfer of genetic material by a bacteriophage.

    (1) Lysogenic conversion occurs as a result of viral infections.

    (2) Sexduction involves transfer by an F particle.

    (3) Conjugation requires two living bacteria in physical contact.

    (5) Transformation is caused by soluble extracts of DNA.

57. (1) Viable counts of bacteria are expressed as colony-forming units.

    (2) There is no such unit of measurement.

    (3) Plaque-forming units are used to count viruses.

    (4) There is no such unit of measurement.

    (5) There is no such unit of measurement.

58. (4) The set of chemical reactions by which cells maintain life describes metabolism.
    (1) Catabolism is the breaking down phase of the life maintenance process.
    (2) Respiration is aerobic oxidation, one portion of the process of metabolism.
    (3) Glycolysis is a process of carbohydrate metabolism, one metabolic pathway.
    (5) Anabolism is the constructive phase of life maintenance.

59. (4) Differential media support the growth of different organisms while providing the environment to distinguish among them. Blood agar is the one usually used to show streptococcal hemolysis.
    (1) Selective media interfere with the growth of certain microorganisms and are not usually used to show streptococcal hemolysis.
    (2) Anaerobic media are not used for streptococci.
    (3) Reducing is an anaerobic medium.
    (5) Selective and differential media are not usually used to show streptococcal hemolysis.

60. (2) Hypotrophic organisms grow only within a living host cell.
    (1) Aerobes are organisms that require oxygen to survive.
    (3) Autotrophic organisms use inorganic compounds as sources of energy.
    (4) An hypotrophic organism does not grow best near a neutral pH.
    (5) A psychrophile grows best between 0° and 20° C (32° to 68° F).

61. (1) A capsule composed of polysaccharides is essential for adherence of *S. mutans*.
    (2) The flagellum does not maintain virulence and is used for motility.
    (3) Endospores are not formed by *S. mutans*.
    (4) The cell wall can *aid* in the maintenance of virulence.
    (5) Genome does not directly maintain virulence and is a genetic material.

62. (2) A distinct nucleus is not present in the procaryotic cell and is the major distinguishing factor between the two cell types.
    (1) Both cell types have a cell wall.
    (3) The procaryotic cells have one chromosome, whereas the eucaryotic cells have more than one chromosome.
    (4) Both types of cells can have flagella.
    (5) Both types of cells have cell membranes.

63. (3) The Procaryotae Kingdom includes bacteria.
    (1) The Protista Kingdom includes protozoa, not bacteria.
    (2) The Animalia Kingdom includes helminths and mammals.
    (4) The Plantae Kingdom includes plants.
    (5) The Mycetidae Kingdom includes fungi.

64. (4) Procaryotic cellular structure is typical of bacteria.
    (1) Mammals have eucaryotic cell structure.
    (2) Fungi have eucaryotic cell structure.
    (3) Helminths have eucaryotic cell structure.
    (5) Protozoa have eucaryotic cell structure.

65. (5) Clusters of spherical shaped bacteria are referred to as staphylococci.
    (1) Streptococci are chains of spherical bacteria.
    (2) Streptobacilli are chains of rodlike bacteria.
    (3) Coccobacilli are rounded rods.
    (4) Spirilla are spiral shaped bacteria.

66. (1) The Gram stain is a differential staining procedure that allows preliminary grouping by reaction to the dyes.
    (2) The spore stain identifies spore-producing bacteria.
    (3) The acid-fast stain identifies mycobacteria.
    (4) Simple staining procedures can show size, so there is no need to do a Gram stain.
    (5) The Gram stain is not used for viewing living organisms.

67. (3) *S. aureus* is the main agent of skin infections causing acute suppurative inflammation.
    (1) *C. tetani* is the agent causing tetanus.
    (2) *M. leprae* is the agent causing leprosy.
    (4) *S. pyogenes* is the agent causing ''strep'' throat.
    (5) *H. influenzae* is the agent in otitis media and also causes secondary infections after influenza.

68. (5) *P. aeruginosa* is a water parasite not normally pathogenic except in immunosuppressed patients and others with altered resistance.
    (1) *S. aureus* is a normal inhabitant of the skin and is not usually found in water.
    (2) *S. pyogenes* is not a normal inhabitant of water; it inhabits the skin and oropharynx.
    (3) *T. pallidum* does not survive outside the body very well.
    (4) *S. pneumoniae* is a normal inhabitant of the oropharynx.

69. (2) Streptococcal infections by β-hemolytic group A streptococci can lead to rheumatic fever.
    (1) Scarlet fever is a streptococcal infection with a generalized rash and therefore is not a consequence of streptococcal infection.
    (3) Infectious mononucleosis is caused by a viral agent, Epstein-Barr virus.
    (4) Influenza is caused by viruses, but streptococci can cause a secondary infection.
    (5) Tuberculosis is caused by *Mycobacterium tuberculosis*.

70. (4) Oral moniliasis is common in the elderly and in patients with diabetes after the use of broad-spectrum antibiotics and occurs on the buccal mucosa and soft palate.
    (1) A patient having diphtheria would be very ill.
    (2) Another streptococcal infection would cause the patient to be ill; the throat would be whitish gray, with no white patches found on the buccal mucosa.
    (3) Pale tissues might be common, but white patches must be differentiated from an overall pale tissue.
    (5) Rheumatic fever is usually a result of untreated streptococcal infections; no white patches are found on the buccal mucosa.

71. (4) The description of the lesion and patient history indicates the patient has recurrent herpes labialis.
    (1) A chancre is usually a red elevated lesion and does not recur.
    (2) Perlèche occurs in the corners of the mouth with cracking, not vesicular lesions.
    (3) An apthous ulcer is usually found in the mouth and as a single lesion.
    (5) Basal cell carcinoma does not recur before colds or heal.

72. (4) Shingles and chickenpox are both caused by varicella-zoster virus.
    (1) Measles and German measles are caused by two different viral agents.
    (2) Chickenpox and smallpox are caused by two different viral agents.
    (3) Bacterial pneumonia has a bacterial etiology; croup is caused by a virus.
    (5) Mononucleosis is caused by Epstein-Barr virus; CMV is caused by a different viral agent.

73. (5) Saliva and vesicular lesions are the known routes of transmission for herpetic whitlow and are where the highest counts of virus are available.
    (1) Blood is not a route of transmission for herpetic whitlow.
    (2) Whitlow is not likely to be transmitted by touching clothing, since the virus survives only seconds to minutes on surfaces.
    (3) Blood is not a route of transmission for herpetic whitlow.
    (4) Blood and contact with clothing are not routes of transmission for herpetic whitlow.

74. (3) The rhinovirus is the most frequent agent of the common cold.
    (1) A cold is a viral disease; S. pyogenes is a bacterium.
    (2) S. aureus is a bacterium.
    (4) H. influenzae is a bacterial agent, often in sinusitis or otitis media.
    (5) Influenza virus is the cause of influenza.

75. (5) Persistent coughing, weight loss, and night sweats are symptoms of tuberculosis.
    (1) Sweats and coughing are not common symptoms of hepatitis.
    (2) Sweats and coughing are not common symptoms of syphilis.
    (3) Pneumonia usually has a sudden onset with chest pains, high fever, and chills.
    (4) Infectious mononucleosis is more common in young adults; night sweats and persistent coughing are not common symptoms.

76. (1) A patient suspected of having tuberculosis should be referred to a physician and tested to rule out tuberculosis; rescheduling the dental appointment should wait until the treatment is finished, tests are negative, and the patient has been released by the physician.
    (2) Tuberculosis may be transmitted by saliva, droplets, and contaminated dust; it is not recommended to work in the oral cavity in such cases.
    (3) Gloves are not foolproof, so there is a risk of contracting tuberculosis; the pathogen survives days to weeks on surfaces, which could cause cross-contamination in clean-up procedures.
    (4) Gloves are not foolproof, so there is a risk of contracting tuberculosis.
    (5) It cannot be assumed that the patient has tuberculosis, so referring directly to a hospital is not appropriate.

77. (3) Rocky Mountain spotted fever is caused by Rickettsia.
    (1) Malaria is caused by a protozoan agent.
    (2) Psittacosis is caused by Chlamydia psittaci, which is not a part of Rickettsia.
    (4) The agent for tularemia is Francisella tularenisis, which is not a part of Rickettsia.
    (5) Meningitis may be a viral or bacterial disease but is not caused by Rickettsia.

78. (1) Toxoplasmosis is transmitted through infected cat feces; it may cause central nervous system damage to the fetus.
    (2) Histoplasmosis is transmitted by excreta of wild birds.
    (3) Cryptococcosis is transmitted by pigeon excreta.
    (4) Trichinosis is transmitted by eating improperly cooked or processed pork.
    (5) Rubella is of special concern to pregnant women, but transmission is not related to cat feces.

79. (2) Salmonella species cause a type of food poisoning that is an active infection not associated with toxin production.
    (1) Shigella species cause dysentery, not food poisoning.
    (3) C. botulinum causes botulism and results from toxins.
    (4) Staphylococcal food poisoning produces its effects from toxins.
    (5) Perfringens food poisoning produces its effects from toxins.

80. (2) Hepatitis B, herpes simplex, and S. pyogenes may develop into a carrier state.
    (1) Hepatitis A does not develop into a carrier state.
    (3) Hepatitis A does not develop into a carrier state.
    (4) Hepatitis A does not develop into a carrier state.
    (5) Hepatitis A does not develop into a carrier state.

81. (4) Persons working with blood are in a high-risk group; hepatitis B often is transmitted through blood. The longer a person works around blood products, the greater the chance of contracting hepatitis B. A yellowish tint to the eyes is suggestive of hepatitis symptoms; other symptoms can be similar to influenza.
    (1) Hepatitis A is not usually transmitted through blood products but is usually transmitted in unsanitary conditions.
    (2) Influenza is a possible choice, but the yellow color of the eyes is suggestive of hepatitis.
    (3) Infectious hepatitis is hepatitis A, but the occupation noted suggests hepatitis B.
    (5) Infectious mononucleosis is a possible choice, but the yellow color of the eyes suggests hepatitis B.

82. (5) Hepatitis B can be transmitted by all body fluids with the risk of contracting the disease or passing it on to other patients.
    (1) The disease is transmitted through all body secretions; gloves are not foolproof, and hepatitis B virus survives months on surfaces. It is also very resistant to chemical disinfectants.
    (2) Rescheduling should not be done until the status of blood tests is known.
    (3) It cannot be assumed that the patient has hepatitis B.
    (4) Gloves and a face mask are not foolproof against contracting the disease.

83. (2) Prosthetic heart valves are one of the predisposing factors to subacute infectious endocarditis and can be acquired by bacteria entering the bloodstream and lodging in the heart valve as a result of dental procedures.
    (1) Rheumatic fever occurs after a streptococcal infection that predisposes to rheumatic heart disease and subacute bacterial endocarditis; there is little risk of developing it as a result of dental treatment.
    (3) "Strep" throat may lead to rheumatic fever, but premedication is not given as a preventive measure before dental treatment.
    (4) Rheumatic heart disease results from rheumatic fever and is not a result of dental treatment; premedication is not given to a dental patient.
    (5) Toxemia is caused by toxins in the blood and is not a usual risk from dental treatments.

84. (2) Streptococci are the bacterial agents most often isolated from patients with SBE.
    (1) Fusobacteria are only sometimes isolated from patients with SBE.
    (3) Lactobacilli are not isolated from patients with SBE.
    (4) Staphylococci are sometimes isolated from patients with SBE.
    (5) *Actinomyces* organisms are not isolated from patients with SBE.

85. (5) Blood in the urine is a symptom of urinary tract infection.
    (1) Blood in the urine is not a symptom of gonorrhea; women are often asymptomatic; men have a discharge containing pus.
    (2) Blood in the urine is not a symptom of pinworm infection; itching is a symptom.
    (3) Blood in the urine is not a symptom of syphilis; symptoms include chancre, mucous patches, and gumma.
    (4) Blood in the urine is not a symptom of hookworm infection; symptoms include abdominal pain.

86. (2) Encephalitis and poliomyelitis both affect the central nervous system.
    (1) Conjunctivitis affects the eye.
    (3) Herpes resides in nerve cells but damages the skin or mucous membranes.
    (4) Conjunctivitis affects the eye.
    (5) Herpes resides in nerve cells but damages the skin or mucous membranes.

87. (4) Viral encephalitis is usually spread by arthropods, ticks, or mosquitoes.
    (1) Droplets are a method of spreading some diseases but not encephalitis.
    (2) Dust is a method of spreading some diseases but not encephalitis.
    (3) Contaminated food is a method of spreading some diseases but not encephalitis.
    (5) Pigeon droppings are a method of spreading some diseases but not encephalitis.

88. (4) *H. aegyptius* is the agent causing acute mucopurulent conjunctivitis (pink eye).
    (1) *S. aureus* causes another type of conjunctivitis.
    (2) *S. pneumoniae* causes another type of conjunctivitis.
    (3) Adenovirus causes another type of conjunctivitis.
    (5) Newcastle disease virus causes another type of conjunctivitis.

89. (4) Ludwig's angina is a bilateral, rapidly spreading swelling, with cellulitis in the floor of the mouth and neck; it often results from infected mandibular molars.
    (1) Actinomycosis usually occurs after trauma and on one side only.
    (2) The patient is somewhat old to have mumps, although it is not impossible to get mumps at his age; mumps do not produce a sudden, rapidly spreading swelling.
    (3) The gumma of syphilis does not develop suddenly.
    (5) Pericoronitis produces more pain in the mouth; it is not usually a rapid swelling and creates difficulty in opening the jaw.

90. (3) Wearing glasses during dental treatment helps prevent herpes and injury. Herpes is present in saliva even without clinical infections.
    (1) Conjunctivitis could be caused by splatter, but the eyes are not a likely route for contracting hepatitis A.
    (2) The eyes are not a likely route for hepatitis B transmission; ophthalmia neonatorum is acquired congenitally.
    (4) Ophthalmia neonatorum is acquired congenitally.
    (5) The eyes are not a likely route for hepatitis A transmission.

91. (1) Exogenous and endogenous sources are both sources of nutrients for bacteria. Bacteria can exist in the oral cavity when humans are fed by a stomach tube.
    (2) Exogenous sources are not the only nutrient sources for bacteria.
    (3) The host's dietary sugar and starch intake is not the only nutrient source for bacteria.
    (4) Endogenous sources are not the only nutrient sources for bacteria.
    (5) The host's saliva is not the only nutrient source for bacteria.

92. (5) Aciduric and acidogenic both describe *S. mutans*: acidogenic bacteria produce acid; aciduric bacteria tolerate a low pH.
    (1) *S. mutans* is not anaerobic.
    (2) *S. mutans* is acidogenic but also is aciduric.
    (3) *S. mutans* is not anaerobic.
    (4) *S. mutans* is aciduric but also acidogenic.

CHAPTER 8

Pharmacology

BARBARA REQUA-CLARK

The dental hygienist, as the individual who frequently takes the medical history, needs to have an understanding of the drugs a patient may be taking and the conditions for which these drugs are used. The medical history is the basis on which decisions regarding patient care rest; therefore, before any treatment is planned, the patient's medical conditions and the medications for them should be recorded in the patient's chart. Any medications whose use or whose contraindications or cautions to dental treatment are not known should be looked up in an appropriate reference.

Knowing the patient's medical condition is important because some patients may need prophylactic antibiotics or altered appointment times. Also, by being aware of any previous condition that a patient has, one may prevent foreseeable emergencies. Even if an emergency does occur, by being prepared, the dental office staff can act appropriately.

This chapter reviews the effects of a wide variety of drugs, including their pharmacologic effects, adverse drug reactions, and their usual indications and contraindications. When special dental implications or considerations are applicable, they too are listed.

GENERAL CONSIDERATIONS ■■■■■■

Definitions

A. Pharmacology-knowledge of various properties of drugs
B. Drugs
   1. Drug—substance used in prevention, diagnosis, alleviation, treatment, or cure of disease
   2. Nomenclature (names)—one drug always has several names
      a. Chemical—name based on the drug's chemical formula
      b. Trade (proprietary) name—each drug company producing a drug makes up its own trade name; there can be as many trade names as there are companies making a particular drug (e.g., Xylocaine, Octocaine)

c. Brand name—technically the name of the drug company itself, but often used interchangeably with the trade name (e.g., either Astra [company that makes Xylocaine] or Xylocaine can be considered the brand name)
d. Generic name—one name chosen by the U.S. Adopted Name Council that is used by all manufacturers of a particular drug (e.g., lidocaine)

References

A. *Physicians Desk Reference (PDR)*[4]—organized by drug manufacturers; entries prepared by each manufacturer; includes colored pictures of common drugs; updated yearly; most commonly found reference in a dental office
B. *Facts and Comparisons: Drug Information Compendium*[3]—organized by pharmacologic classes; prepared by independent editors; updated monthly
C. *Applied Pharmacology for the Dental Hygienist*[5]— specifically designed for the dental hygienist; more detailed than this review
D. *Goodman and Gilman's The Pharmacological Basis of Therapeutics*[1]—"the bible"; very detailed; difficult reading; good for reference
E. *Clinical Pharmacology in Dental Practice*[2]— review of pharmacology in the dental office; useful as a reference

Common Medical Terminology

See Appendix A.

Agencies/Legislation

A. Food and Drug Administration (FDA)—determines what drugs can be marketed in the United States; requires proof of both safety and efficacy
B. Drug Enforcement Administration (DEA)—branch of the Department of Justice; determines levels of degree of control for substances that have abuse potential; Schedules I through V are given in Table 8-1

Table 8-1 Drug Enforcement Administration Schedules I through V

Schedule	Abuse potential	Examples	Handling
I	Most	Heroin, marijuana	Experimental use; only in research
II	Great	Morphine, meperidine, amphetamine, secobarbital	Prescription must be written, no refills
III	Some	Codeine mixtures, "weaker" stimulants and sedatives	Prescriptions may be telephoned to pharmacy; may be refilled with limits
IV	A little	Diazepam (Valium), dextropropoxyphene (Darvon)	Prescription may be telephoned to pharmacy; may be refilled with limits
V	Least	Some codeine-containing cough syrups	Can be bought over the counter (OTC) in some states (many states now require prescription)

Drug Action

A. *Log dose-effect curve*—as the dose of a drug increases (x axis), the percent of maximum response rises (y axis) until increasing the dose further produces no increase in the percent of response (it plateaus) (Fig. 8-1)

B. Definitions
   1. Structure-activity relationships (SAR)—drugs with similar structures frequently exert similar actions (e.g., antihistamines have a structure similar to that of the local anesthetics; they possess some local anesthetic action also)
   2. Effective dose $(ED)_{50}$—dose that produces 50% of the maximum response; dose of a drug that produces a specified intensity of response in 50% of the subjects
   3. Lethal dose $(LD)_{50}$—dose that is lethal (kills) for 50% of the subjects; laboratory animals are used
   4. Onset—time required for a drug's effect to begin; very short if given intravenously, longer if administered by mouth
   5. Duration—length of time a drug's effect lasts; often related to a drug's half-life
   6. Half-life $(t_{1/2})$—time required for the serum concentration of the drug to be halved (fall to one half) after absorption is completed (e.g., if the $t_{1/2}$ of a drug is 2 hours, the blood level of the drug will fall to one half of what it was in 2 hours [after allowing time for absorption])
   7. Potency—amount it takes (e.g., in milligrams) to get an effect
   8. Efficacy—maximum effect one can expect

C. Routes of administration
   1. Oral (PO)—by mouth; easiest to use; good patient acceptance
   2. Rectal—suppository, enema; for either local or systemic effect

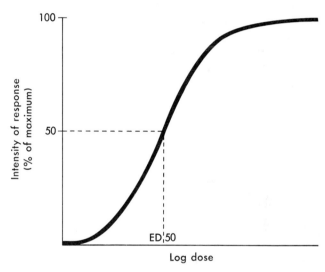

Fig. 8-1 Log dose-effect curve. (From Requa, B.S., and Holroyd, S.V.: Applied pharmacology for the dental hygienist, St. Louis, 1982, The C.V. Mosby Co.)

   3. Intravenous (IV)—into the vein; shortest onset of action; most dangerous
   4. Intramuscular (IM)—into the muscle; sometimes painful
   5. Subcutaneous (SC, SQ)—beneath the skin (e.g., insulin)
   6. Intradermal—into the dermis (e.g., skin test for tuberculosis—makes a bleb [bump])
   7. Intrathecal—into the spinal fluid (e.g., for meningitis)
   8. Intraperitoneal—into the peritoneal cavity (abdomen)
   9. Inhalation—into the lungs; particles, volatile liquids, or gas; all inhaled
   10. Topical—applied to the skin or mucous membranes; ointments or creams

11. Sublingual—dissolved under the tongue (for a systemic effect)
12. Parenteral—other than an oral route; usually refers to an injection

D. Dosage forms
 1. Capsule—gelatin shell
 2. Tablet—compressed or molded
 3. Ointment or cream—semisolid for topical application
 4. Suppository—rectal or vaginal; conical or ovoid solid
 5. Solution—one-phase system of more than one thing
 6. Suspension—insoluble particles in a liquid (e.g., milk of magnesia)
 7. Emulsion—two immiscible (not mixable) liquids (e.g., oil and water)
 8. Elixir—sweetened and hydroalcoholic (water and alcohol mixture)
 9. Tincture—highly alcoholic

E. Calculation of dosage
 1. Varies depending on the patient's
    a. Age
    b. Weight
    c. Condition (disease)
 2. Child's dose
    a. Less than the adult dose
    b. Based on
       (1) Surface area—good
       (2) Weight—OK
       (3) Age—very poor
       (4) Manufacturer's specific recommendations—best

Adverse Reactions

A. Manifestations
 1. Exaggerated effect on the target organ—more than the desired effect (e.g., an antianxiety agent producing too much sleepiness)
 2. Effect on a nontarget organ—some effect on an organ not intended to be altered (e.g., insomnia [inability to sleep] from a bronchodilator)
 3. Teratogenic effect—adverse effect on a fetus (e.g., thalidomide produced phocomelia [flipper arms and legs])
 4. Allergic reaction—varies from a mild rash to anaphylaxis; involves an antigen-antibody reaction (e.g., rash from penicillin)
 5. Idiosyncrasy—unexpected reaction to a drug; not predictable
 6. Interference with natural defense mechanisms—body is less able to fight infection (e.g., steroids)

B. Toxicity

$$\text{Therapeutic index} = \frac{LD_{50}}{ED_{50}}$$

A measure of safety—the bigger the ratio, the better

Prescription Writing

A. Measurement
 1. Apothecary—uses antiquated measures of weights and volumes such as grains (gr) and ounces (℥)

    1 ℥ ≅ 30 ml
    1 gr ≅ 60 mg

 2. Metric—based on the system of tens

    1 kg = 1000 g
    1 gm = 1000 mg
    1 mg = 1000 μg

 3. Other measures

    1 tsp = 5 ml
    1 kg = 2.2 lb
    1 qt ≅ 1000 ml

 4. Roman numbers

    ss = ½
    i/I = 1
    X = 10
    L = 50
    C = 100

    Examples

    iss = 1½
    XX = 20

B. Latin abreviations—directions to the patient used in prescriptions

ac	before meals	prn	as needed
bid	twice a day	q	every
c̄	with	qid	four times a day
d	day	s̄	without
h	hour	stat	immediately, now
hs	at bedtime	tid	three times a day
pc	after meals		

C. Examples

   Sig: 1 qid pc and hs—take 1 four times a day (after meals and at bedtime)
   Sig: 1-2 q 4-6h prn pain—take 1 or 2 every 4 to 6 hours if needed for pain

Biopharmaceutics

How the body handles drugs (body handling)
A. Absorption depends on
 1. Degree of ionization—the more ionized, the less absorbed; with weak acids or bases this is a function of pH
 2. Lipid solubility—the more lipid soluble, the more absorbed; the less lipid soluble, the less absorbed orally

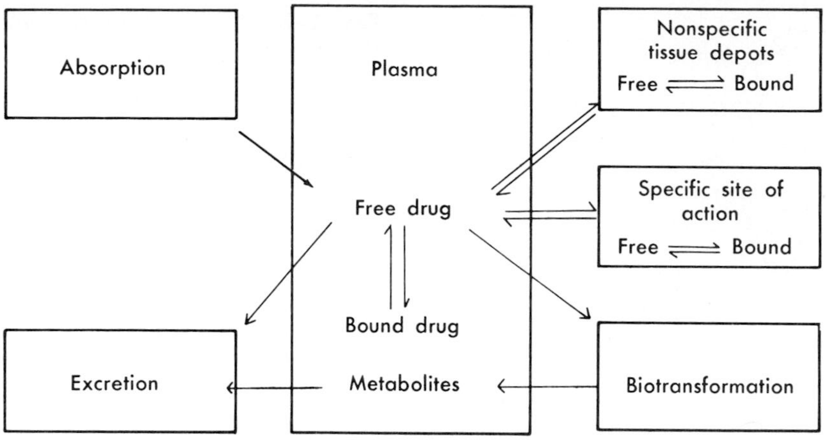

Fig. 8-2 Absorption and fate of drug. (From Holroyd, S.V.: Clinical pharmacology in dental practice, ed. 3, St. Louis, 1983, The C.V. Mosby Co.)

B. Distribution of the drug (Fig. 8-2)
1. Gets the drug to the site of action
2. Only the free drug can cross membranes *(arrows between boxes)*
3. In each compartment an equilibrium between the bound and unbound (free) drug occurs
4. Redistribution—moves from one tissue (there first) to another tissue (there later); one method of terminating a drug's effect
C. Metabolism (biotransformation)—takes place in the liver by hepatic microsomal enzymes; metabolites are more polar and less protein bound, more easily excreted
D. Excretion—usually via the kidneys (urine); can also be via the feces (enterohepatic circulation), sweat, or tears

Receptors

Areas in the body where a drug may bind
A. Agonists—binding causes an effect (e.g., narcotic analgesic agent)
B. Antagonist—binding produces no effect; may block the effect of an agonist (e.g., narcotic antagonist [blocks the effect of the agonist])

AUTONOMIC NERVOUS SYSTEM AGENTS

Cholinergic (Parasympathomimetic) Agents

"Mimic" the action of the parasympathetic autonomic nervous system (PANS)
A. Receptors—Fig. 8-3 illustrates a typical cholinergic nerve
1. *"Muscarinic"*—like the compound found in the poisonous mushroom *Amanita muscaria* (Fig. 8-3, *A*)

a. Areas affected *(A)*
(1) Smooth muscle
(2) Cardiac muscle
(3) Gland cells
b. Neurotransmitter—acetylcholine (ACh)
c. Location—postganglionic to the neuroeffector organ
d. Stimulated by muscarine
e. Blocked by atropine
2. "Nicotinic"—action resulting from nicotine; found in cigarettes (Fig. 8-3, *B* and *C*)
a. Areas affected
(1) Postganglionic neurons *(B)*
(2) Skeletal muscle end-plates *(C)*
b. Neurotransmitter—acetylcholine (ACh)
c. Location—autonomic ganglia *(B)* and neuromuscular junction *(C)*
d. Stimulated by nicotine
e. Blocked by hexamethonium (autonomic, *B*) and *d*-tubocurarine (neuromuscular junction, *C*)
B. Acetylcholine—synthesis and inactivation

$$
\begin{array}{ccc}
& & \text{Choline} \\
A \qquad \text{Ch} & \text{acetyltransferase} & \text{ACh} \\
\text{Acetyl + Choline} & \xrightleftharpoons{\qquad\qquad} & \text{Acetylcholine} \\
\text{(CoA)} & \text{Acetylcholinesterase} & \\
& \text{(AChE)} &
\end{array}
$$

C. Classification/mechanism of action
1. Direct acting—drug acts at the receptor just like acetylcholine
a. Choline derivatives
b. Pilocarpine
2. Indirect acting—drug indirectly increases the amount of acetylcholine; blocks acetylcholine inactivation by inhibiting acetylcholinesterase (AChE, enzyme that normally destroys acetylcholine)

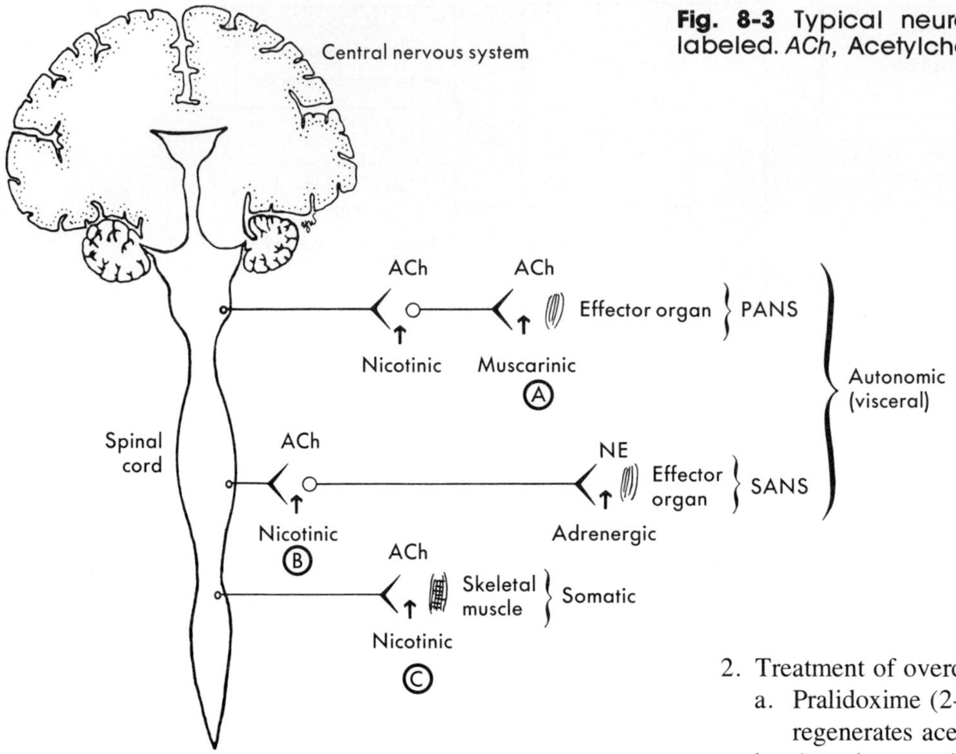

Fig. 8-3 Typical neurons with neurotransmitters labeled. *ACh*, Acetylcholine; *NE*, norepinephrine.

a. Reversible cholinesterase inhibitors—drugs can "come off" the acetylcholinesterase
   (1) Edrophonium (Tensilon)
   (2) Physostigmine (Eserine)
   (3) Neostigmine (Prostigmin)
b. "Irreversible" cholinesterase inhibitors—drugs do not "come off" the acetylcholinesterase once they are attached (at least only with great difficulty)
   (1) Organophosphorus inhibitors
   (2) Insecticides—malathion, parathion
D. Pharmacologic effects—similar to PANS stimulation
   1. Smooth muscle stimulation
      a. Increase in gastrointestinal (GI) motility—diarrhea may result; used to treat postoperative ileus (GI/GU—gastrointestinal/genitourinary)
      b. Bronchoconstriction
   2. Glands—increased secretion of saliva; used to treat xerostomia (dry mouth)
   3. Eye—decreased intraocular pressure; used to treat glaucoma
E. Adverse reactions (toxicity)—extension of the pharmacologic effects; "too much" effect
   1. SLUD—salivation, lacrimation (tearing), urination, and defecation (bowel movement)

2. Treatment of overdose
   a. Pralidoxime (2-PAM, Protopam)—regenerates acetylcholinesterase somewhat
   b. Atropine—antimuscarinic; blocks the muscarinic effects of acetylcholine excess (not the nicotinic effects)
F. Dental use—treatment of xerostomia
   1. Pilocarpine eye drops used orally
   2. May increase salivation

Anticholinergic (Parasympatholytic, Cholinergic Blocking) Agents

Block some actions (muscarinic) of the PANS
A. Basic principles
   1. Used to dry up saliva
   2. Know contraindications!
   3. Block the muscarinic receptors
B. Pharmacologic effects
   1. Heart—tachycardia (increased heart rate [HR]); useful during general anesthesia when the HR may fall too low
   2. Eye
      a. Mydriasis (dilation of the pupils; results in photophobia)
      b. Cycloplegia (paralysis for distant vision)
      c. Avoid repeated doses in narrow-angle glaucoma
   3. Decreased secretions—saliva flow reduced; useful in dentistry (Table 8-2 lists several drug groups producing dry mouth)
   4. Central nervous system (CNS)—sedation or excitation

Table 8-2 Xerostomia–producing drug groups with examples

Drug group	Examples
Anticholinergics*	Atropine, Donnatal, Artane
Antihypertensives*	Aldomet, guanethidine
Antipsychotics, phenothiazines*	Thorazine, Mellaril, Stelazine
Tricyclic antide-pressants*	Elavil, Tofranil
Antihistamines	Benadryl, Chlor-Trimeton
Adrenergic agents	Amphetamine, Preludin
Diuretics	Hydrochlorothiazide, Dyazide
Benzodiazepines	Valium, Librium

*More likely to produce xerostomia; effect still dose related.

C. Adverse reactions and toxicity; contraindications to use
   1. Dry mouth/skin/eyes; caution in patients wearing contact lenses; agent reduces milk flow in nursing mothers
   2. Eye—blurred vision; avoid in narrow-angle glaucoma; treated wide-angle glaucoma usually no problem
   3. Urinary retention—avoid in patients with prostatic hypertrophy (enlarged prostate)
   4. Dizziness/fatigue—delirium, hallucinations, coma, and convulsions (toxicity)
   5. Tachycardia (increased HR)—watch with cardiovascular patients
   6. Reduced GI motility—avoid in patients with gastric retention or intestinal obstruction
D. Clinical uses
   1. Gastrointestinal—agent has "antispasmodic" activity (reduces overactivity) and reduces secretions (e.g., stomach acid)
   2. Ophthalmology—agent dilates the eyes and paralyzes the muscles of accommodation (patient can see far away only)
   3. Dental
      a. Used before administration of a general anesthetic to dry up saliva and prevent vagal slowing of the heart
      b. Used to prepare the mouth for impressions or equilibrations to decrease secretions; agent produces a "drier field"
E. Examples

Atropine   } Natural, tertiary
Propantheline (Pro-Banthine)   ⎫
Methantheline (Banthine)   ⎬ Synthetic, quaternary
Glycopyrrolate (Robinul)   ⎭

Adrenergic (Sympathomimetic) Agents

"Mimic" the action of the sympathetic autonomic nervous system (SANS); act like norepinephrine (NE) in the SANS (Fig. 8-3)
A. Basic principles
   1. SANS is activated by fear; "fight or flight" response
   2. Catecholamine is a specific chemical structure possessed by some adrenergic agents
   3. Receptors (SANS)
      a. α-Receptors produce constriction of the skin, mucosa, and skeletal muscle blood vessels (vasoconstriction)
      b. β-Receptors
         (1) β_2—relaxes smooth muscles; produces
            (a) Dilation of the skeletal muscle blood vessels (vasodilation)
            (b) Bronchodilation
         (2) β_1—stimulates the heart; increases the HR, contractility, and conduction velocity
B. Pharmacologic effects/adverse reactions
   1. Central nervous system—increased alertness; anorexia (loss of appetite) (e.g., the amphetamines)
   2. Stimulation of the heart
      a. Direct effect—isolated heart would respond this way to all adrenergic agents
         (1) Positive chronotropic effect (increased HR)
         (2) Positive intropic effect (increased strength of contraction of the heart)
         (3) Predisposition to arrhythmias if higher doses are administered
      b. Indirect (reflex vagal) effect—total peripheral resistance determines the indirect effect
         (1) α-Receptor stimulation—decreased HR
         (2) β-Receptor stimulation—increased HR
         (3) $\alpha\beta$-Receptor stimulation—decreased HR
      c. Net effect on the HR—in the body the HR is determined by both direct and indirect effects
         (1) α—unpredictable
         (2) β—increased HR
         (3) $\alpha\beta$ (e.g., epinephrine)—unpredictable
   3. Vascular effects (effects on the arterial tree)
      a. α-Receptors—vasoconstriction; skin, mucosa, skeletal muscle blood vessels
      b. β-Receptors—vasodilation; skeletal muscle blood vessels

c. Total peripheral resistance (TPR)
  (1) α-Receptors—increased TPR
  (2) β-Receptors—decreased TPR
  (3) $\alpha\beta$-Receptors—decreased TPR
4. Mydriasis and reduced intraocular pressure; useful in treating glaucoma
5. Bronchodilation (β_2 effect); useful in treating asthmatic patients
6. Alterations in the blood glucose level; watch diabetic patients
7. Production of thick, viscid saliva

C. Drug interactions—reasonable quantities, administered carefully to patients taking the drugs listed below should not cause problems; adrenergic agents plus
1. Tricyclic antidepressants (e.g., Elavil, Tofranil)—increase blood pressure; produce dysrhythmias
2. Antidiabetic agents (e.g., insulin, Orinase, Diabinese)—increase blood glucose level
3. β-Blockers (e.g., Inderal)—produce hypertension and bradycardia (slowed HR)
4. Monoamine oxidase inhibitors (MAOI)—no problem with epinephrine; indirect-acting amines (e.g., pseudoephedrine) *must* be avoided
5. General anesthetics (halogenated hydrocarbons, e.g., halothane [Fluothane]) sensitize the myocardium to catecholamines; epinephrine is a catecholamine; increase the chance of arrhythmias

D. Therapeutic uses
1. Medical—treatment of
  a. Anaphylaxis
  b. Cardiac arrest
  c. Nasal congestion
  d. Asthma
  e. Narcolepsy
  f. Hyperkinesis in children
  g. Glaucoma
2. Dental
  a. Local anesthetic additive
  b. Hemostatic to reduce bleeding; provide adequate tissue retraction

E. Examples

Adrenergic agent	Receptor stimulated	Comments
Epinephrine (Adrenalin)	$\alpha\beta$	Endogenous catecholamine; local anesthetic additive
Isoproterenol (Isuprel)	β	Endogenous catecholamine
Phenylephrine (Neo-Synephrine)	α	Nasal decongestant
Levonordefrin (Neo-Cobefrin)	$\alpha > \beta$	Local anesthetic additive
Amphetamine	$\alpha\beta$	Diet pill (abused)
Ephedrine	$\alpha\beta$	Orally active nasal decongestant

F. Adrenergics as vasoconstrictors in local anesthetic solutions
1. Examples

  Epinephrine (Adrenalin)
  Levonordefrin (Neo-Cobefrin)

2. Advantages
  a. Prolong anesthesia
  b. Reduce systemic toxicity
  c. Provide hemostasis
3. Disadvantages
  a. Systemic toxicity occurs when an excess is administered
  b. Cardiovascular patients
    (1) Can use reasonable amounts as local anesthetic additives in stable cardiovascular patients
    (2) Avoid use of an epinephrine—impregnated retraction cord
    (3) Maximum safe dose for normal and cardiovascular patients
      (a) Epinephrine—normal patient, 0.2 mg; cardiovascular patient, 0.04 mg
      (b) Levonordefrin (Neo-Cobefrin)—normal patient, 0.5 to 1 mg; cardiovascular patient, 0.2 to 0.4 mg
  c. Hyperthyroid patients—avoid vasoconstrictors in untreated hyperthyroid patients or those receiving drug therapy; may produce a thyroid storm
  d. Minimize toxicity by injecting slowly, calming the patient (fear releases epinephrine)

β-Adrenergic Blockers (β-Blockers)

A. Mechanism of action—drug blocks SANS action (β-receptors); some β-blockers are more selective for the β_1-receptor than nonselective agents
B. Used to treat hypertension, angina, arrhythmias, and glaucoma; used to prevent migraine and myocardial infarction (MI, heart attack)
C. Examples (note ''olol'' ending with generic names)

  Propranolol (Inderal)
  Metoprolol (Lopressor)
  Atenolol (Tenormin)

NEUROMUSCULAR BLOCKING AGENTS ▬

A. Pharmacologic effects—paralysis of voluntary muscles; can include muscles of respiration; not autonomic nervous system (ANS) agents
B. Therapeutic use—agent produces paralysis during general anesthesia for intubation (passing an orotracheal or nasotracheal tube for anesthesia or to control pulmonary ventilation)
C. Examples

Tubocurarine ("curare")
Succinylcholine (Anectine)

LOCAL ANESTHETIC AGENTS ▬

A. Properties of the ideal local anesthetic
   1. Potent local anesthesia
   2. Reversible local anesthesia
   3. Absence of local reactions
   4. Absence of systemic reactions
   5. Absence of allergic reactions
   6. Rapid onset
   7. Satisfactory duration
   8. Adequate tissue penetration
   9. Low cost
   10. Stability in solution (long shelf life)
   11. Sterilization by autoclave
   12. Ease of metabolism and excretion
B. Chemistry
   1. Three components common to local anesthetic agents
      a. Aromatic lipophilic group—contains a benzene ring
      b. Intermediate chain—may be either esters or amides
      c. Hydrophilic amino group—secondary or tertiary amine
   2. Intermediate chain
      a. Esters
         (1) Cocaine
         (2) Ethyl aminobenzoate (Benzocaine)
         (3) Tetracaine (Pontocaine)
         (4) Procaine (Novocain)
         (5) Propoxycaine (in Ravocaine)
      b. Amides
         (1) Lidocaine (Xylocaine)
         (2) Mepivacaine (Carbocaine)
         (3) Prilocaine (Citanest)
         (4) Bupivacaine (Marcaine)
         (5) Etidocaine (Duranest)

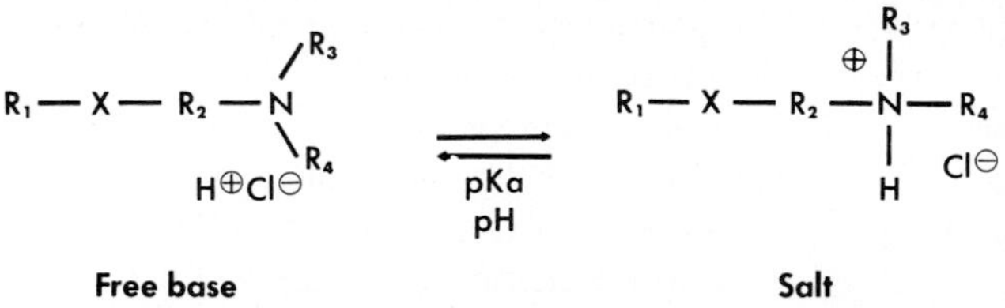

Fig. 8-4 Properties of base and salt forms of local anesthetics. *X*, Ester or amide. (From Requa, B.S., and Holroyd, S.V.: Applied pharmacology for the dental hygienist, St. Louis, 1982, The C.V. Mosby Co.)

C. Mechanism of action
   1. Base and salt forms of local anesthetics (Fig. 8-4)

Free base	Salt
Viscid liquids or amorphous solids	Crystalline solids
Fat soluble (lipophilic)	Water soluble (hydrophilic)
Unstable	Stable
Alkaline	Acidic
Uncharged, unionized	Charged, cation (ionized)
Penetrates nerve tissue	Active form at site of action
Form present in tissue (pH 7.4)	Form present in dental cartridge (pH 4.5-6.0)

   2. Inflammation
      a. pH of normal tissues is 7.4; pH in inflammation is 5.5; acid environment increases proportion in ionized form and reduces absorption
      b. Edema—dilutes the local anesthetic solution because of an increase in fluids present in the tissues
      c. Increased tissue vascularity—increased blood supply carries away the local anesthetic; duration of action is shortened
   3. Nerve fiber susceptibility varies; nerves generally affected in this order: automonic, cold, warmth, pain, touch, pressure, vibration, proprioception, and motor; regain function in reverse order
   4. Nerve impulse propagation is blocked by blocking the increased permeability to sodium (Na)
D. Pharmacokinetics (body handling)
   1. Absorption
      a. Effect on the vasculature
         (1) Most local anesthetics produce vasodilation; vasoconstrictors are added to counteract this
         (2) Cocaine is the only local anesthetic that consistently produces vasoconstriction
      b. Solubility
         (1) Lipid soluble—nonionized form penetrates tissue

(2) Water soluble—ionized form exerts the effect at the nerve
  c. Rate of absorption
    (1) The faster the rate of absorption, the greater the chance of systemic toxicity and the shorter the duration of action
    (2) Route of administration alters the rate of absorption; topical anesthetic can be absorbed quickly
2. Distribution—level of local anesthetic in the blood is determined by
  a. How fast it is absorbed
  b. How quickly it is distributed to other tissues
  c. How fast it is metabolized and/or excreted
3. Metabolism (biotransformation)
  a. Esters—hydrolyzed by plasma pseudocholinesterases
    (1) Procaine and other esters are metabolized by plasma esterases and cholinesterases to para-aminobenzoic acid (PABA), which is responsible for the allergic reactions not uncommonly occurring with the esters
    (2) Congenital cholinesterase deficiency is a congenital abnormality of pseudocholinesterase (atypical); hereditary; incidence of 1 in 3000; ester local anesthetics are absolutely contraindicated
  b. Amides—metabolized in the liver
    (1) Metabolized primarily in the liver— patients with liver dysfunction should be given amide local anesthetics cautiously because they may metabolize them more slowly, allowing toxic levels to build up
    (2) Prilocaine is metabolized to a product that can produce methemoglobinemia (increased levels of methemoglobin, which is less effective in carrying oxygen in the blood)
4. Excretion
  a. Esters are almost completely metabolized before being excreted
  b. Amides are mostly metabolized before being excreted
  c. Significant renal disease can cause local anesthetic metabolites to accumulate
  d. Avoid mepivacaine with renal dysfunction
E. Adverse reactions
  1. Factors influencing toxicity
    a. Drug
    b. Concentration
    c. Route
    d. Vascularity
    e. Vasoconstrictor
    f. Weight
    g. Rate of metabolism and excretion
  2. Symptoms of local anesthetic toxicity—central nervous system (CNS) and cardiovascular system (CVS) are affected most; severity of effects is related to blood levels
    a. Central nervous system—stimulation followed by depression
      (1) CNS stimulation (excitatory)— restlessness, shivering, tremors, convulsions
      (2) CNS depression—sedation, drowsiness, respiratory and cardiovascular depression, coma; lidocaine and procaine often produce CNS depression without previous excitation
    b. Cardiovascular system
      (1) Antiarrhythmic action—lidocaine and procainamide (which contains procaine) are used intravenously to treat arrhythmias (antiarrhythmics)
      (2) Vasodilation produces hypotension secondary to its direct effect on vascular smooth muscle
  3. Toxicity—the higher the number, the more likely it is that a local anesthetic agent is toxic; "absolute" considers only the drug, whereas "relative" considers the concentration available (%)

| | Toxicity | |
Drug	Absolute	Relative
Procaine (Novocaine)	1	1
Lidocaine (Xylocaine, Octocaine)	2	2
Mepivacaine (Carbocaine, Isocaine)	1.5	1.5
Prilocaine (Citanest)	1+	2+
Tetracaine (Pontocaine-topical)	10	5
Propoxycaine (in Ravocaine)	10	2
Bupivacaine (Marcaine)	4	3+
Etidocaine (Duranest)	4	3+

  4. Malignant hyperthermia—fever to 108° F, muscular rigidity, high mortality, familial; amides may be associated with precipitating this event
  5. Allergic reactions—caused not only by the local anesthetic agent, but also by other components in the solution (e.g., preservatives)
    a. Range of reactions—mild rash to anaphylaxis

Table 8-3 Selected local anesthetic agents available in dental cartridges

Agent	Concentration (%)	Vasoconstrictor	
ESTER			
Propoxycaine (Ravocaine mixed with 2% procaine) (Novocain)	0.4 0.4	Levonordefrin Levoarterenol	1 : 20,000 1 : 30,000
AMIDES			
Lidocaine (Xylocaine, Octocaine)	2 2 2	Epinephrine Epinephrine None	1 : 50,000 1 : 100,000
Mepivacaine (Carbocaine, Isocaine)	2 3	Levonordefrin None	1 : 20,000
Prilocaine (Citanest, Citanest Forte)	4 4	Epinephrine None	1 : 200,000
Bupivacaine (Marcaine)	0.5	Epinephrine	1 : 200,000

b. Esters—much more allergenic than amides; presence of true allergic reactions to the amides in question; few documented allergies to amides have been reported in the literature
c. Skin testing—poor; false-positive and false-negative results; last resort; need emergency equipment and trained personnel on hand; never should be done without the ability to give intravenous drugs and intubate to support respiration (hospital setting)
d. Other ingredients may produce allergic reactions

F. Drug interactions
  1. Esters plus sulfonamides—sulfonamides interfere with bacterial PABA; esters are metabolized to PABA, so they may interfere with the sulfonamides' (antibacterial agents') local antiinfective action
  2. Cimetidine (Tagamet)—prolongs liver metabolism of lidocaine; increases lidocaine blood levels

G. Composition of local anesthetic solutions
  1. Other ingredients
    a. Vasoconstrictor—epinephrine (Adrenalin), levonordefrin (Neo-Cobefrin)
    b. Preservatives (antiseptics)—methylparabens and propylparabens (dental cartridges formerly contained these); no longer present
    c. Antioxidant—sodium bisulfite or sodium metabisulfite; only present if the local anesthetic agent contains a vasoconstrictor; may precipitate asthma attacks in susceptible patients

d. Alkalinizing agent—sodium hydroxide; adjusts pH
    e. Sodium chloride—makes solution isotonic
  2. For selected products available in dental cartridges see Table 8-3

H. Topical local anesthetics
  1. Cocaine—CNS effects and abuse potential limit usefulness of this product; it is *never* indicated for dental use
  2. Ethyl aminobenzoate—good to use topically because it cannot be used systemically; some sensitization to esters occurs, especially in clinicians
  3. Lidocaine—topically active; use least soluble form
  4. Tetracaine—avoid topical use because of toxicity and slow onset of action

I. Dosage calculation—local anesthetic (LA)

$$\text{LA } 2\% = \frac{2 \text{ g}}{100 \text{ ml}} = \frac{2000 \text{ mg}}{100 \text{ ml}} = \frac{20 \text{ mg}}{1 \text{ ml}}$$

If cartridge is 1.8 ml, then 1 cartridge of 2% LA would contain

$$\frac{20 \text{ mg}}{1 \text{ ml}} \times \frac{1.8 \text{ ml}}{1 \text{ cartridge}} = 36 \text{ mg/cartridge}$$

J. Other local anesthetic—diphenhydramine (Benadryl) 1%
  1. Antihistamines have weak local anesthetic action
  2. Only used as a last resort (e.g., if the patient is allergic to all other local anesthetic agents)

GENERAL ANESTHETICS
General Considerations

A. Dental use—uncooperative patients with multiple dental procedures; usually patients hospitalized
B. History—dentists have played an important role in attempting to identify drugs that would alleviate pain
   1. Horace Wells—recognized nitrous oxide's use
   2. William P.G. Morton—recognized ether's usefulness
C. Stages and planes of anesthesia

> Stage I   Analgesia, three planes; nitrous oxide alone
> Stage II   Excitement, delirium; avoid if possible
> Stage III Surgical anesthesia, four planes
> Stage IV   Respiratory paralysis (medullary paralysis); death without treatment

D. Adverse reactions (Table 8-4)
   1. Cardiovascular system
      a. Cardiac arrest usually occurs in stage IV after respiration ceases
      b. Arrhythmias most commonly occur with the halogenated hydrocarbons, especially if catecholamines such as epinephrine are administered concomitantly
      c. Hypertension is common during excitement—stage II
      d. Hypotension is common in planes 3 and 4 of stage III and in stage IV
   2. Respiratory system
      a. Respiratory arrest is associated with stage IV
      b. Laryngospasm occurs in conjunction with the ultrashort-acting barbiturates, such as thiopental (Pentothal)
      c. Boardlike chest occurs with the combination of fentanyl and droperidol (Innovar), a neuroleptanalgesic

3. Physical problems
   a. Explosions—cyclopropane and ether are notorious for explosions; they are not used any more for this reason
   b. Flammability—some agents support combustion (nitrous oxide) and some can produce it
4. Teratogenicity (fetal abnormalities) and/or spontaneous abortions have been associated with clinician exposures as well as with spouses of those exposed
5. Hepatotoxicity is associated with the halogenated hydrocarbons such as halothane (Fluothane)

E. Routes of administration
   1. Intravenous anesthetics; fixed anesthetics (cannot be easily removed by respiration)
      a. Barbiturates (e.g., Thiopental [Pentothal])
      b. Dissociative—ketamine (Ketalar, Ketaject)
      c. Neuroleptanalgesic—fentanyl (Sublimaze) plus droperidol (Inapsine) combination (Innovar)
   2. Inhalation gases
      a. Nitrous oxide
      b. Cyclopropane
   3. Inhalation volatile liquids
      a. Diethyl ether (ether)
      b. Halogenated hydrocarbons (e.g., Halothane [Fluothane])

Specific Agents

A. Nitrous oxide (N_2O)
   1. Incomplete anesthetic unless anoxia is produced; used alone cannot reach stage III
   2. Usual concentration used—30% to 50%

Table 8-4 Drug interactions with general anesthetics

Drug class	Examples	Effect
Anticholinergics	Atropine, propantheline	Reduce respiratory secretions, block vagus nerve, slow heart
Narcotics	Meperidine, morphine	Potentiate respiratory depression
Catecholamines	Epinephrine, norepinephrine, isoproterenol	Cause arrhythmias with cyclopropane and halogenated hydrocarbons
Neuromuscular blocking agents	Tubocurarine, pancuronium, gallamine	Augment neuromuscular blockade of ether, cyclopropane, halothane, and methoxyflurane; potentiated by aminoglycoside antibiotics
Adrenergic blocking agents	Propranolol	Cause hypotension

From Requa, B.S., and Holroyd, S.V.: Applied pharmacology for the dental hygienist, St. Louis, 1982, The C.V. Mosby Co.

3. Advantages
   a. Rapid onset and recovery
   b. Least toxic; safe when used appropriately
   c. May be used in children
   d. Nonflammable
   e. Nonirritating to the GI tract
   f. Good analgesia
4. Disadvantages
   a. "Misuse" potential with both patients and dental workers
   b. Teratogenicity question unanswered
   c. Proper use of nitrous oxide is to produce analgesia or reduce anxiety; it is *not* a complete pain reliever; local anesthetic still required
   d. Nausea is the most common complaint; secondary to rapid changes in concentration in inspired air
   e. Diffusion hypoxia rarely occurs; give oxygen to prevent it
5. Contraindications
   a. Respiratory problems
      (1) Upper respiratory tract infection (URI) such as a cold—adequate exchange of air often cannot occur when the nasal passages are congested
      (2) Chronic obstructive pulmonary disease (COPD) such as emphysema or bronchitis—administering oxygen in the concentration normally used in conjunction with nitrous oxide could produce apnea (cessation of respiration), since the patient's respiration is driven by carbon dioxide
   b. Cardiac condition—only a potential problem if severe cardiac disease is present
   c. Pregnancy—questions are unanswered; first trimester is the most critical; greater number of spontaneous abortions
   d. Lack of communication
      (1) Psychologic—patients with psychologic problems may respond inappropriately
      (2) Language—patient cannot comprehend your language; speaks a foreign language
   e. Contagious disease—tuberculosis, hepatitis
B. Diethyl ether—unpopular because
   1. Explosive
   2. Slow induction and recovery
   3. Gastrointestinal—nausea and vomiting common

C. Halogenated hydrocarbons
   1. Examples

      Halothane (Fluothane)
      Enflurane (Ethrane)
      Isoflurane (Forane)

   2. No mucous membrane irritation; not explosive; poor muscle relaxation; no analgesia; little nausea or vomiting
   3. Sensitize the myocardium to catecholamines
   4. Hepatotoxic; related to exposures
D. Ultrashort-acting barbiturates
   1. Examples

      Thiopental (Pentothal)
      Methohexital (Brevital)
      Thiamylal (Surital)

   2. Rapid onset; short duration is secondary to redistribution
   3. Used to induce general anesthesia; advances to stage III rapidly
   4. Laryngospasm is adverse reaction
   5. Contraindicated in porphyria
E. Ketamine (Ketalar, Ketaject) produces dissociative anesthesia
   1. *Not* a complete anesthetic
   2. Can produce a trance
   3. Emergence—bad dreams, "bad trip"; more likely in adults; related to phencyclohexylpiperidine (PCP, angel dust)
   4. Can produce hyperactive reflexes such as cough, gag, or tongue movement
F. Innovar produces neuroleptanalgesia
   1. Fentanyl (narcotic) plus droperidol (major tranquilizer)
   2. Produces "lead pipe" chest as an adverse reaction

Balanced Anesthesia

Requires a careful mixing of a variety of pharmacologic agents working in concert
A. Premedication includes a narcotic to allay pain and apprehension; an anticholinergic to reduce secretions (saliva) and counteract the slowing of the heart produced by general anesthetics; an antihistamine and/or phenothiazine to also dry secretions and reduce nausea and vomiting; and finally a sedative-hypnotic or minor tranquilizer to allay apprehension
B. Induction is produced by an ultrashort-acting barbiturate while nitrous oxide–oxygen is being administered to reduce apprehension

C. Neuromuscular blocking agent paralyzes respiration momentarily so that intubation may be accomplished to support respiration

D. Surgical anesthesia is then maintained by administering a halogenated hydrocarbon along with the nitrous oxide–oxygen mixture

CENTRAL NERVOUS SYSTEM DEPRESSANTS

General Considerations

A. Several pharmacologic groups possess antianxiety properties: sedative-hypnotic agents, minor tranquilizers, nitrous oxide, narcotic analgesic agents and antihistamines

B. Definitions
   1. Sedative—provides relaxation during daytime hours
   2. Hypnotic—promotes sleep at bedtime
   3. Tranquilizers—major versus minor
      a. Minor tranquilizers (e.g., benzodiazepines) produce the following effects
         (1) Anxiety relief
         (2) Sedation and disinhibition
         (3) Anesthesia and death
         (4) Anticonvulsant effect
         (5) Voluntary muscle relaxation
         (6) Physical dependence and addiction
      b. Major tranquilizers (e.g., phenothiazines) produce the following effects
         (1) Control of psychotic behavior
         (2) Easy arousal
         (3) Convulsions
         (4) Extrapyramidal effects (parkinsonian)
         (5) Anticholinergic effect
         (6) *No* addiction

Sedative-Hypnotics (Barbiturates and Nonbarbiturates)

A. Pharmacologic effects
   1. Sedation and anxiety relief, sleep, anesthesia—a continuum as the dose increases
   2. Anticonvulsant—long-acting agents are usually the most useful
   3. Muscle relaxation—questionable whether this action is separate from CNS (sedation) effects
   4. *No* analgesic action—agitation may result if an analgesic is not also given in the presence of pain

B. Adverse reactions
   1. CNS depression—drowsiness, impaired performance and judgment; caution required when driving a car (see box)
   2. Abuse—euphoria, habituation, withdrawal, tolerance

SELECTED PHARMACOLOGIC GROUPS PRODUCING SEDATION

"Tranquilizers"
Barbiturates
Nonbarbiturate sedative-hypnotics
Benzodiazepines
Ethyl alcohol
Antihistamines
Narcotic analgesic agents
Nonsteroidal antiinflammatory agents
Phenothiazines
Tricyclic antidepressants
Centrally acting muscle relaxants

---

   3. Acute overdose—suicidal attempt produces respiratory arrest
   4. Barbiturates—contraindicated in porphyria

C. Therapeutic uses
   1. Medical—treatment of insomnia, anxiety, epilepsy
   2. Dental
      a. Preoperative anxiety reduction—oral or intramuscular injections
      b. Induction of general anesthesia—intravenous barbiturates

D. Examples
   1. Barbiturates
      a. Ultrashort acting—used for induction of general anesthesia

         Thiopental (Pentothal)
         Thiamylal (Surital)
         Methohexital (Brevital)

      b. Short acting—used for insomnia; most abused

         Pentobarbital (Nembutal)
         Secobarbital (Seconal)

      c. Intermediate acting—used for insomnia and daytime sedation

         Amobarbital (Amytal)
         Butabarbital (Butisol)

      d. Long acting—used for daytime sedation and as an anticonvulsant

         Phenobarbital (Luminal)
         Mephobarbital (Mebaral)
         Primidone (Mysoline)

   2. Other sedative-hypnotic agents
      a. Chloral hydrate (Noctec)
         (1) Produces GI irritation
         (2) Used historically for children
      b. Meprobamate (Equanil, Miltown)—tranquilizer

Benzodiazepines

A. Mechanism of action—drug has more specific anxiolytic (antianxiety) action than the barbiturates
B. Wide therapeutic index when ingested alone; much safer than the barbiturates
C. Adverse reactions
   1. Sedation—warn patients about driving a car while ingesting
   2. Addiction potential present
   3. Not uniformly safe in porphyria
   4. Teratogenicity—increased incidence of birth defects if taken during the first trimester
   5. Thrombophlebitis can occur with intravenous use
D. Specific agents
   1. Examples

Drug	Usual dose (mg)
Triazolam (Halcion)	0.25-0.5
Oxazepam (Serax)	15-30
Lorazepam (Antivan)	2-4
Temazepam (Restoril)	15-30
Alprazolam (Xanax)	0.25-0.5
Chlordiazepoxide (Librium)	5-20
Diazepam (Valium)	2-10
Clonazepam (Clonopin)	Anticonvulsant
Halazepam (Paxipam)	20-40
Chlorazepate (Tranxene)	7.5
Prazepam (Centrax)	10-20
Flurazepam (Dalmane)	15-30

   2. Differences
     a. Equivalent dose—different products require different doses; usual dose varies depending on the specific agent
     b. Duration varies between a few hours and a few days; shorter-acting agents are listed first under examples
     c. Metabolism—some are metabolized extensively, some hardly at all
     d. Excretion—some as metabolites, some unchanged

Antihistamines/Ataractics/Phenothiazines

A. Pharmacologic effects
   1. Antihistaminic action (H₁ blocker)—antiemetic (reduces vomiting); antisialagogue (reduces salivation)
   2. "Phenothiazinic" action (see also section on antipsychotic agents)
     a. Extrapyramidal (involves CNS functions outside the pyramidal tracts in the CNS)—tongue movements, lip smacking
     b. Xerostomia (dry mouth)—anticholinergic effect
   3. Potentiation of narcotics and/or sedative-hypnotics; must reduce the doses of other agents if used together

B. Therapeutic usefulness—not too useful alone for predental anxiety; drug provides some potentiation when added to other agents; helps reduce secretions and reduces the risk of vomiting (useful during and after surgery)
C. Examples

   Hydroxyzine (Vistaril, Atarax)
   Promethazine (Phenergan)

Antihistamines

A. Antihistamines are H₁-receptor antagonists
B. Pharmacologic effects—reduction of allergic symptoms; counteraction of some actions of histamine (increased capillary permeability and edema, flare, and itch)
C. Adverse reactions
   1. Sedation—CNS depression, drowsiness; all over-the-counter (OTC) sleep aids contain them; 50% of children exhibit excitation
   2. Xerostomia—weak anticholinergic effect
   3. Other—nausea, vomiting, constipation
D. Examples—vary in incidence of adverse reactions (e.g., sedation is high with Benadryl)

   Diphenhydramine (Benadryl)
   Chlorpheniramine maleate (Chlor-Trimeton)
   Tripelnnamine (Pyribenzamine)
   Triprolidine (Actidil, in Actifed)

ANALGESICS (Table 8-5)

General Considerations

A. Pain
   1. Perception—uniform
   2. Reaction—varies greatly from patient to patient
B. Variables—patient's age, sex, race, ethnic group, fatigue, fear
C. Placebo effect notable—all clinical trials must include a placebo; confidence expressed in medication often makes it more effective

Aspirin and the Salicylates

A. Mechanism of action—primarily peripheral; prostaglandin inhibitor (inhibits cyclooxygenase or prostaglandin synthetase)
B. Pharmacologic effects—"the three A's"
   1. Analgesic—reduces pain
   2. Antipyretic—therapeutic dose reduces an elevated body temperature
   3. Antiinflammatory—higher dose reduces inflammation
C. Adverse reactions
   1. Gastrointestinal—minimize by ingesting with food, ingesting with a full glass of water, or taking liquid antacids

Table 8-5 Analgesic summary

	Aspirin	Nonsteroidal antiinflammatory agents	Acetaminophen	Narcotics
Analgesic	+	++	+	+++
Antipyretic	+	+	+	−
Antiinflammatory	+	+	−	−
CNS effects	−	++	+	+++
GI effects	+	+	−	+
Alters bleeding	++	+	−	−
Hepatotoxic	?	+	+[a]	−
Nephrotoxic	+[b]	+	+[b]	−

a, Overdose; *b,* in combination.

2. Bleeding altered
   a. Hypoprothrombinemia—reduced prothrombin levels; requires several doses
   b. Platelet adhesiveness—reduced platelet adhesiveness for the life of the platelets (4 to 7 days); requires only a single small dose
3. Salicylate toxicity (''salicylism'') causes tinnitus, hyperthermia (increased body temperature), electrolyte problems, and an altered sensorium
4. Allergies—true allergy is rare; if the patient is allergic, there is some cross-reactivity with other agents. (e.g., nonsteroidal antiinflammatory agents [NSAIAs]), especially in asthmatic patients with nasal polyps
5. Reye's syndrome—children with chickenpox or influenza should *not* be given aspirin
D. Drug interactions—aspirin plus
   1. Warfarin (Coumadin) (used as an anticoagulant)—may result in bleeding or hemorrhage
   2. Probenecid (Benemid) (used to treat gout)—may result in an acute attack of gout
   3. Tolbutamide (Orinase) (used to control diabetes)—may result in an altered blood glucose level

Nonsteroidal Antiinflammatory Agents

A. Pharmacologic effects—''the three *A*'s'' (like aspirin)
   1. Analgesic
   2. Antipyretic
   3. Antiinflammatory
B. Adverse reactions
   1. Gastrointestinal—like those with aspirin; most common adverse reaction; from discomfort to frank ulcers
   2. Central nervous system—dizziness, sedation; caution required when driving a car

3. Blood coagulation—reduction in platelet aggregation and possible prolongation of bleeding time; alteration is less than with aspirin (reversible; with aspirin, effect is not reversible)
   4. Teratogenic effects—contraindicated if the patient is pregnant or nursing
C. Therapeutic uses
   1. Pain control—analgesic; some stronger than aspirin
   2. For arthritis—antiinflammatory
   3. For dysmenorrhea (painful menstruation)—very effective, since specific for disease; excess prostaglandins responsible for excessive uterine contractions
D. Mechanism of action—like aspirin, drug inhibits prostaglandin synthesis (cyclooxygenase)
E. Examples

   Ibuprofen (Motrin, Rufen, Nuprin,* Advil*)
   Naproxen (Naprosyn)
   Naproxen sodium (Anaprox)
   Diflusinal (Dolobid)†

Acetaminophen (N-Acetyl-p-aminophenol; Tylenol, Datril)

A. Pharmacologic effects
   1. Analgesic
   2. Antipyretic
   3. NOT antiinflammatory
B. Adverse reactions
   1. Analgesic nephropathy—adversely affects the kidneys; may be more likely to occur if acetaminophen is taken with aspirin
   2. Hepatotoxicity—with acute overdose; delayed reaction; treated with *N*-acetylcysteine

---
*Available without a prescription.
†Not actually classified as a nonsteroidal antiinflammatory agent but has very similar actions; a very long acting salicylate.

C. Therapeutic uses
1. Analgesic
2. Antipyretic
3. Not useful for inflammatory conditions

Narcotic Analgesic Agents

A. Pharmacologic effects—proportional to the ''strength'' of the narcotic
1. Analgesia
2. Sedation (anxiety relief)
B. Adverse reactions—proportional to the ''strength'' of the narcotic
1. Sedation/euphoria—may lead to abuse
2. Respiratory depression—dose related; cause of death in overdose
3. Gastrointestinal—nausea, vomiting, constipation
4. Abuse—can occur with *all* narcotic analgesics; tolerance develops to all the effects except miosis (pupillary constriction) and constipation
C. Therapeutic uses
1. Pain relief—central mechanism; agent affects patient's perception of pain; some can relieve severe pain
2. Sedation and anxiety relief—used preoperatively
3. Cough suppression—agents have antitussive action (suppress cough); only a small dose is needed
4. For diarrhea—symptomatic relief only; reduce GI motility by causing increased tone and spasm
D. Examples

Drug	Usual dose (mg)	"Strength"
Morphine	10	Stronger
Hydromorphone (Dilaudid)	2-4	
Meperidine (Demerol)	50-100	
Alphaprodine (Nisentil)	30	
Oxycodone (in Percodan)	5	
Hydrocodone (in Vicodin)	5	
Codeine (in Tylenol 3, Empirin 3)	30-60	
Dihydrocodeine (in Synalgos-DC)	16-32	Weaker

E. Narcotic antagonists—antagonize most actions of the narcotics
1. Naloxone (Narcan)
a. Therapeutic uses
(1) Counteracts respiratory depression caused by narcotic overdose
(2) Combined with a narcotic to reduce abuse potential (e.g., Talwin-NX—pentazocine plus naloxone)
b. Emergency kit should include naloxone

2. Butorphanol (Stadol)—used as an agonist for pain relief; has an analgesic effect; less addiction potential

ANTIINFECTIVES (ANTIBIOTICS)
General Considerations

A. Prevention of infection (see Chapter 7)
1. Sterilization measures such as autoclaving instruments should be used to prevent infection
2. Many infections can be handled with local measures (i.e., incision and drainage) instead of antibiotics; host (patient) resistance must be considered
3. Antibiotic administration is not without risk
4. Prophylaxis is rarely indicated except for prevention of infectious endocarditis
B. Definitions
1. Antimicrobial—against microbes
2. Antiinfective—against organisms causing infections
3. Antibacterial—against bacteria
a. Bactericidal—kills bacteria irreversibly
b. Bacteriostatic—retards or incapacitates bacteria (reversible); if bacteria are removed from the environment, they can grow or multiply again
4. Antiviral—against viruses
5. Antifungal—against fungi
6. Antibiotic—produced by microorganisms; suppresses growth of other organisms; effective in low concentrations
7. Spectrum—range of an antibiotic's antiinfective properties; may be narrow (few organisms) to wide or broad (many organisms)
8. Resistance—ability of an organism to be unaffected by an antiinfective agent; may be either natural (always has been resistant) or acquired (the resistance developed)
9. Suprainfection (superinfection)—appearance of a new infection by other than the original organism while the patient is taking an antimicrobial agent; new infection is usually more difficult to treat; most common when the spectrum is widest
10. Synergism—more than additive (1 + 1 > 2)
11. Antagonism—less than additive (1 + 1 < 2)
C. Treatment versus prophylaxis
1. Treatment—antiinfective is used to treat an infection present
2. Prophylaxis (to prevent)—antiinfective is used to prevent some future infection; not generally very useful

Table 8-6 Prevention of bacterial endocarditis (before and after a dental procedure)

	Standard regimen (rheumatic heart disease, congenital heart disease)	High risk (prosthetic heart values, history of bacterial endocarditis)
No penicillin allergy	Penicillin V 2 g 1 hr before and 1 g 6 hr later	Ampicillin 1-2 g and gentamicin 1.5 mg/kg (IM or IV) ½ hr before and penicillin V 1 g 6 hr later
Penicillin allergy	Erythromycin 1 g 1 hr before and 500 mg 6 hr later	Vancomycin 1 g IV over 1 hr, starting 1 hr before (nothing more)

D. See Appendix B for the American Heart Association's recommendation for the prevention of infectious (bacterial) endocarditis in dentistry (see also Table 8-6)

Penicillins

A. Mechanism of action—drug inhibits cell wall synthesis; bactericidal
B. Spectrum—three penicillin subgroups
 1. Penicillin G/penicillin V
 2. Penicillinase-resistant penicillins
 3. Extended-spectrum penicillins
  a. Ampicillin-like
  b. Carbenicillin-like
C. Stability
 1. Acid labile—degrade in stomach acid; therefore must be used parenterally (e.g., penicillin G, methacillin, carbenicillin)
 2. Acid stable—may be used orally (e.g., penicillin VK, amoxicillin)
D. Pharmacokinetics (body handling)
 1. Peak—blood levels peak in less than 30 minutes by oral or intramuscular route; peak immediately when used intravenously
 2. Half-life ($t_{1/2}$)—between 30 minutes and 1 hour
 3. Excretion is very rapid because penicillins are actively secreted; duration prolonged by concomitant probenecid (Benemid) administration
E. Adverse effects
 1. Relatively nontoxic except for allergic potential
 2. Convulsions occur only with very high parenteral doses
 3. Allergic reactions range from a mild rash to a severe anaphylactic reaction
 4. Nephrotoxicity (kidney damage) occurs occasionally; more likely with broader-spectrum penicillins

Penicillin G/Penicillin V

A. Spectrum—works against many gram-positive organisms; most active against gram-positive organisms (versus other penicillins) if organism is sensitive, not resistant, to penicillinase
B. Penicillin G—primarily parenteral; procaine and benzathine salts available for intramuscular use; longer acting than sodium or potassium forms
C. Penicillin V—more acid stable than penicillin G; potassium salt (K) is better absorbed; therefore penicillin VK is used most in dentistry

Penicillinase (β-lactamase) – Resistant Penicillins

A. Examples

Methicillin (Staphcillin)
Nafcillin (Unipen, Nafcil)
Oxacillin (Prostaphilin, Bactocill)
Cloxacillin (Tegopen, Cloxapen)
Dicloxacillin (Dynapen, Pathocil)

B. Therapeutic use—very limited; used against penicillinase-producing staphylococci or as prophylactic coverage for a hip prosthesis

Extended-Spectrum ("Broader" or "Wider" Spectrum) Penicillins

A. Ampicillin-like
 1. Examples

Ampicillin (Omnipen, Totacillin, Polycillin)
Amoxicillin (Amoxil, Larotid, Polymox)

 2. Spectrum—work against many gram-positive organisms and also some gram-negative bacteria such as *Haemophilus influenzae,* some *Escherichia coli,* and *Proteus mirabilis*
 3. *Not* penicillinase resistant
B. Carbenicillin-like
 1. Examples

Ticarcillin (Ticar)
Carbenicillin (Geopen, Pyopen)

 2. Spectrum—gram-negative coverage such as against *Pseudomonas aeruginosa* and *Proteus* species resistant to ampicillin-like drugs
 3. Used parenterally (in hospitalized patients) for systemic action

Erythromycins

A. Mechanisms of action—drug interferes with protein synthesis (binds to the 50S ribosomal subunit); bacteriostatic
B. Spectrum
   1. Work primarily against gram-positive microorganisms (like penicillin V)
   2. Also used against certain strains of *Rickettsia*, *Chlamydia*, and *Actinomyces*, as well as the drug of choice for *Mycoplasma pneumoniae* and *Legionella pneumophila*
C. Pharmacokinetics (body handling)
   1. Because of acid lability (instability), are enteric coated (do not dissolve in the stomach; dissolve in the intestine) or are prepared as esters to protect against stomach acid
   2. Effect peaks in 2 to 4 hours
D. Adverse effects
   1. GI upset is *very* common; can be taken with food if GI upset occurs
   2. Cholestatic jaundice is primarily associated with the estolate ester
E. Examples

   Erythromycin base (E-mycin)
   Erythromycin stearate (Erythrocin)
   Erythromycin ethylsuccinate (EES, Pediamycin)
   Erythromycin estolate (Ilosone)

F. Therapeutic use—treatment of dental infections in patients allergic to penicillin or for specific suspected infections (see spectrum)

Cephalosporins

A. Mechanisms of action—like that of the penicillins; drug inhibits cell wall synthesis; bactericidal
B. Chemistry is similar to that of the penicillins
C. Spectrum—work against many gram-positive and gram-negative organisms; the newest *third-generation* cephalosporins have the *widest* spectrum of action
D. Adverse reactions
   1. GI upset common (33%)
   2. Other—like those of the broader-spectrum penicillins (e.g., nephrotoxicity, suprainfection)
   3. Allergy—some cross-sensitivity (10%) with the penicillins, since they possess a similar structure
E. Examples

   Cephalexin (Keflex)
   Cephradine (Velosef, Anspor)

Clindamycin (Cleocin)

A. Mechanism of action—drug inhibits protein synthesis (binds to the 50S ribosomal subunit); generally bacteriostatic
B. Spectrum—works primarily against gram-positive organisms and some anaerobes such as *Bacteroides fragilis*
C. Adverse reactions
   1. Gastrointestinal—diarrhea common; pseudomembranous colitis (PMC) may have an incidence of up to 10%; drug should be discontinued if bloody stools with mucus occur
   2. Food and Drug Administration says "reserved for serious anaerobic infections"

Tetracyclines

A. Mechanism of action—drug inhibits protein synthesis (binds to the 30S ribosome); bacteriostatic
B. Spectrum—truly broad spectrum; work against many gram-positive and many gram-negative organisms
C. Pharmacokinetics
   1. Tetracyclines—divalent and trivalent cations (e.g., Ca^{++}, Mg^{++}, Fe^{++}, Al^{+++}) inhibit absorption
   2. Minocycline (Minocin) and doxycycline (Vibramycin) are less affected by food or dairy products than plain tetracycline
D. Resistance—cross-transference can occur (one microorganism tells another microorganism how to be resistant without the second microorganism being exposed to the drug at all)
E. Adverse effects
   1. GI upset is relatively common
   2. Suprainfection is very common because of the wide spectrum of action; drug alters the normal flora (e.g., vaginal candidiasis)
   3. *Photosensitivity*—exaggerated sunburn with exposure to sunlight (watch tanning booths)
   4. Teeth—both hypoplasia and discoloration can occur if given during enamel development; primary teeth are affected from the last half of the pregnancy to age 4 to 6 months; permanent teeth are affected from age 2 months to 7 to 12 years
F. Examples

   Tetracycline (Achromycin-V)
   Demeclocycline (Declomycin)
   Doxycycline (Vibramycin)
   Minocycline (Minocin)

G. Therapeutic uses
   1. Medical—treatment of acne, respiratory tract infections in patients with COPD (emphysema or bronchitis)

2. Dental—"shotgun" approach to treat an unknown infection or to "help" periodontal problems (no evidence that the drug works in either situation); new research is attempting to place the drug locally into the periodontal pocket by incorporating it into a variety of dosage forms (e.g., impregnated rods)

Aminoglycosides

A. Mechanism of action—drug inhibits protein synthesis (binds to the 30S ribosomal subunit); bactericidal
B. Spectrum—works against some gram-positive and many gram-negative organisms
C. Pharmacokinetics—not effective systemically if given orally; must be given parenterally
D. Adverse reactions—toxicity usually results from blood levels that are too high
   1. Ototoxicity—drug adversely affects cranial nerve VIII; affects both the vestibular (balance) and the auditory (hearing) functions
   2. Nephrotoxicity—drug adversely affects the kidney
E. Examples

    Neomycin (Mycifradin)
    Streptomycin (Streptomycin)
    Kanamycin (Kantrex)
    Gentamicin (Garamycin)
    Tobramycin (Nebcin)
    Amikacin (Amikin)

Other Antiinfectives

Vancomycin (Vancocin)

A. Mechanism of action—drug inhibits cell wall synthesis; bactericidal
B. Spectrum—primarily effective against gram-positive organisms
C. Has a chemical structure entirely different from that of any other antibiotic—no cross-resistance or cross-allergenicity
D. Only administered intravenously—not well absorbed orally; intramuscular route too irritating; used orally for local effect on the intestines to treat PMC
E. Dental use—infectious endocarditis prophylaxis in patients with a valvular prosthesis and an allergy to penicillin

Sulfonamides ("Sulfa" Drugs)

A. Mechanism of action—competitive antagonist of PABA; drug prevents use of PABA to make folic acid
B. Ester local anesthetics may inhibit sulfonamides' antibacterial action; esters are metabolized to PABA

C. Drug is not an antibiotic, because it is not *made* by an organism but is produced by a chemical reaction
D. Examples

    Sulfisoxazole (Gantrisin)
    Trimethoprim-sulfamethoxazole (Bactrim, Septra)

E. Used to treat urinary tract infections and otitis media (children's ear infections); dental use is presently unclear

Metronidazole (Flagyl)

A. Spectrum
   1. Trichomonocidal (works against *Trichomonas vaginalis*)
   2. Bactericidal (works against anerobes such as *Bacteroides* species)
B. Adverse reactions
   1. Nausea, vomiting, headache
   2. Disulfiram-like (Antabuse-like) reaction—alcohol ingestion during therapy can produce nausea and vomiting
   3. Carcinogenic in animals; mutagenic in organisms
C. Dental use—periodontal patients; proper place awaits controlled clinical trials

Antituberculosis Agents

A. Tuberculosis (TB)—a chronic disease
   1. Resistant organisms easily develop
   2. Treatment is difficult, and drug combinations are frequently required
   3. Duration of therapy is a minimum of 9 months
B. Drugs
   1. Ioniazid (INH)—used alone as prophylaxis; used in combination with rifampin to treat tuberculosis
   2. Rifampin (Rifadin, Rimactane)
   3. Ethambutol (Myambutol)
   4. Streptomycin—aminoglycoside used parenterally
C. Dental implications—take recommended precautions for contagious disease; patients appropriately treated for 6 weeks to 2 months should not be contagious

Antifungal Agents

A. Nystatin (Mycostatin, Nilstat)
   1. Useful against *Candida albicans* (candidiasis, thrush)
   2. Available as an oral suspension or a vaginal tablet (used as lozenge)
B. Clotrimazole (Mycelex)—lozenges available
C. Ketoconazole (Nizoral)
   1. Used orally for candidiasis

2. Acid environment in the stomach is required for adequate absorption
3. Adverse reactions include nausea and vomiting, hepatocellular dysfunction, and teratogenic potential

Antiviral Agents – Acyclovir (Zovirax)

A. Topical and intravenous—indicated for initial genital herpes in the nonimmunocompromised patient and for initial and recurrent mucocutaneous herpes in the immunocompromised patient
B. Oral—indicated for treatment and prophylaxis of initial and recurrent genital herpes

HEMOSTATICS
General Considerations

A. Definition—locally applied substances to reduce excessive bleeding
B. Useful only for bleeding from small blood vessels
C. Classification
   1. Adrenergic agents (vasoconstrictors)
   2. Styptics and astringents
   3. Mechanical agents
   4. Thrombin (clotting factor)

Adrenergic Agents (Vasoconstrictors)

See section on autonomic nervous system agents
A. Pharmacologic effects—α-receptors are stimulated to cause vasoconstriction of the arterioles and capillaries
B. Adverse reactions—systemic absorption may produce tachycardia or hypertension; a potential problem in patients with severe cardiac disease
C. Dosage forms
   1. Gingival retraction cord—amount of epinephrine in different products varies; need to check product's label
   2. Epinephrine 1:50,000 in a local anesthetic solution
   3. Epinephrine 1:1000—string or cotton pledgets are dipped into this solution and "wrung" out; actual amount administered is poorly controlled

Styptics and Astringents

A. Definition—agents that promote hemostasis by precipitating proteins; styptic is a more concentrated form of astringent
B. Agents
   1. Zinc chloride ($ZnCl_2$)
   2. Aluminum chloride ($AlCl_3$)
C. Advantages—no cardiovascular effects as with epinephrine; agent also shrinks tissue
D. Disadvantages—tissue irritation and necrosis; more likely in higher concentrations

E. Product examples
   Gingi-Aid
   Hemodent

Mechanical Agents

A. Act as matrices for blood cells and/or fibrin; absorbed into surrounding tissue
B. Useful for bleeding not controlled by the above means, but not enough for surgical intervention
C. Examples
   Oxidized cellulose (Oxycel)
   Oxidized regenerated cellulose (Surgicel)
   Absorbable gelatin sponge (Gelfoam)

Thrombin

A. Natural component of blood for coagulation
B. Used alone or in conjunction with the mechanical methods

DENTIFRICES AND MOUTHWASHES
Dentifrices

A. Effect—enhance the cleaning power of toothbrushing; control bacterial plaque
   1. Children—reduce decay
   2. Adult—reduce gum diseases
   3. Available as pastes, gels, and powders
B. Ingredients
   1. Abrasive—removes debris and stain; polishes the tooth surface; primarily insoluble salts
   2. Humectant—prevents water loss (e.g., sorbitol, glycerol, propylene glycol)
   3. Preservative—prevents the growth of microorganisms
   4. Thickening agent/binder—prevents separation and increases viscosity
   5. Foaming agent—detergent such as sodium lauryl sulfate
   6. Flavoring agent—important for patient acceptance
C. Therapeutic additives
   1. Reduce dental caries—fluoride
   2. Claim to reduce tooth sensitivity—formaldehyde, potassium nitrate, sodium citrate, strontium chloride, stannous fluoride
   3. Claim to reduce plaque formation—chlorhexidine, sanguinarine (Viadent), essential oils (Listerine), amyloglucosidase plus glucose oxidase (Zendium)
D. Ingestable dentifrice—for use with special-needs patients (e.g., NASAdent)

Mouthwashes

A. Definition—liquid with a pleasant taste and odor used to rinse the mouth
B. Potential benefits
1. Most claims are unsubstantiated—even control of bad breath is controversial
2. Germicide—questionable value
3. Surface-active agent—questionable value
4. "Therapeutic" ingredients
   a. Fluoride rinses—claim to reduce caries and tooth sensitivity
   b. Sanguinarine (Viadent)—claims to reduce plaque
   c. Chlorhexidine gluconate—experimental in the United States; claims to reduce plaque; stains teeth/oral structures; produces an aftertaste
   d. Amyloglucosidase plus glucose oxidase (Zendium)—claims to reduce plaque
   e. Quaternary ammonium compounds (Cepacol, Scope, Colgate 100)
   f. Essential oils (Listerine)
   g. Zinc chloride (Lavoris)

CARDIOVASCULAR AGENTS

See Chapters 7 and 14 for contraindications and cautions involving dental treatment in patients with cardiovascular disease

Digitalis Glycosides

A. Pharmacologic effects—heart beats more strongly (positive chronotropic effect), usually more slowly (bradycardia), and more efficiently
B. Adverse reactions—GI disturbances (nausea, vomiting); arrhythmias; altered vision (yellow-green vision, halos around lights)
C. Therapeutic uses—treatment of congestive heart failure, certain arrhythmias
D. Dental considerations—hypokalemia (low potassium) caused by a diuretic may exacerbate the arrhythmias (adverse effect of digitalis); epinephrine may make them worse
E. Examples

   Digoxin (Lanoxin)
   Digitoxin (Crystodigin, Purodigin)

Antiarrhythmics

A. Pharmacologic effects—arrhythmias are suppressed
B. Dental considerations—patients taking antiarrhythmics have cardiac problems

C. Examples

Quinidine	Propranolol (Inderal)*
Procainamide	Lidocaine (Xylocaine)†

Antianginal Agents

A. Pharmacologic effects—reduced oxygen consumption and reduced "work" of the heart
B. Adverse reactions—hypotension and severe headache are common; patient should sit, but not lie down, to take medication
C. Therapeutic use—for angina pectoris (for prophylaxis [to prevent] and to treat an acute attack)
D. Dental considerations
1. Storage—unstable products; must be stored properly; heat, light, and moisture degrade them more rapidly; opened container should be discarded after 2 months
2. Acute anginal attack—treated with sublingual nitroglycerin
3. Other routes of nitroglycerin
   a. Transmucosal—incorporated into pads and applied to the gums
   b. Transdermal—incorporated into pads and applied to the chest or arm
   c. Ointment—incorporated into an ointment; dose prescribed in inches
E. Examples

   Nitroglycerin (Nitrostat)
   Isosorbide dinitrate (Isordil)

Antihypertensives

A. Pharmacologic effects—elevated blood pressure is lowered
B. Adverse reactions—dry mouth, CNS depression, orthostatic hypotension (blood pressure falls on rapid rising from a supine position)
C. Therapeutic use—treatment of hypertension
D. Dental considerations
1. Take the patient's blood pressure to ensure that it is within normal limits
2. Check for dry mouth and question the patient as to self-treatment (lemon drop candy?)
E. Examples—patient is often taking a combination of several agents; agent is often combined with a diuretic

Aldomet	Minipres
Catapres	Aldactazide
Apresoline	Inderal ⎱ β-Blockers
Aldoril	Lopressor ⎰

*See β-blocker discussion in section on autonomic nervous system agents.
†Local anesthetic used parenterally as an antiarrhythmic agent.

Diuretics

A. Pharmacologic effects—removal of excess water and sodium via the kidneys; direct action on blood vessels to lower blood pressure
B. Adverse reactions—hypokalemia (low potassium); patient may be taking potassium replacement
C. Therapeutic uses—treatment of congestive heart failure, edema
D. Dental considerations
   1. Hypokalemia potentiates epinephrine-induced arrhythmias
   2. Patient may need to urinate more frequently after ingesting medicine (usually in the morning)
E. Examples

Dyazide*
Lasix†
Hygroton
Hydrochlorothiazide (HydroDiuril, Esidrix, Oretic)‡

Anticoagulants

A. Mechanism of action—drug interferes with vitamin K-dependent clotting factors, (II, VII, IX, X)
B. Pharmacologic effects—ability of blood to clot is inhibited; latent time required before full effect is seen (several days); conversely, comparable time required for effect to subside after discontinuing treatment
C. Adverse reactions—bleeding, hemorrhage
D. Therapeutic uses—after myocardial infarction, thrombophlebitis, emboli, valve replacement (any condition where too much blood clotting occurs)
E. Dental considerations
   1. Excessive bleeding may result from minor procedures; obtain a good history (every appointment)
   2. Monitor prothrombin time (PT)
F. Examples

Warfarin (Coumadin)
Dicumarol, bishydroxycoumarin

G. Drug interactions—anticoagulant plus
   1. Aspirin—potentiates bleeding problems; do not use concomitantly; alternatives—acetaminophen, narcotics, NSAIAs cautiously
   2. Vitamin K—helps the patient to clot more; used to treat an overdose or reduce the latent period for improving the clotting status; antibiotics may reduce the amount of vitamin K available to the patient by altering the intestinal flora; this would potentiate the anticoagulant's effect

---

*Most popular combination; combines thiazide diuretic with potassium-sparing diuretic; less hypokalemia.
†Very potent diuretic; hypokalemia is common.
‡Most common single-entity diuretic.

PSYCHOTHERAPEUTIC AGENTS

Antipsychotic Agents

A. Pharmacologic effects
   1. Antipsychotic—calms an agitated patient; reduces the response to external stimuli; watch what you say around the patient, who may perceive any comments as threats (paranoia)
   2. Sedation/drowsiness—additive CNS depression with other CNS depressants
   3. Antiemetic—depresses the chemoreceptor trigger zone (CTZ) to reduce nausea and/or vomiting
B. Adverse reactions
   1. Orthostatic hypotension—patient may faint on arising from a supine position too fast
   2. Extrapyramidal (areas in the brain affecting bodily movements) effects
      a. Dyskinesia—bizarre movements of the tongue or face that may become irreversible over years of use (tardive dyskinesia)
      b. Parkinsonian—tremors and rigidity like the disease parkinsonism
      c. Akathisia—motor restlessness (e.g., swinging legs)
      d. Difficulty in opening the mouth (jaw); jaw muscles are contracted; dislocation possible
   3. Anticholinergic—dry mouth may produce a high caries rate
C. Drug interaction—antipsychotic agent plus
   1. CNS depressants—results in additive CNS depression
   2. Anticholinergic—results in additive anticholinergic toxicity
   3. Epinephrine—α-blocking action of phenothiazine leaves the β-action of epinephrine unopposed; patients taking phenothiazines who are given intravenous epinephrine to treat hypotension could exhibit more hypotension; usual dental dose used as an additive to a local anesthesic can be given safely
D. Therapeutic uses
   1. Antipsychotic—treat psychosis (e.g., schizophrenia)
   2. Antiemetic—prevent and treat nausea or vomiting
   3. Narcotic potentiation—used with a narcotic to potentiate analgesia and sedation; dose of the narcotic must be reduced by one half if an antipsychotic is added
E. Examples

Chloropromazine (Thorazine)
Trifluoperazine (Stelazine) } Phenothiazines
Thioridazine (Mellaril)

Haloperidol (Haldol) } Not a phenothiazine; acts in a similar fashion

Antidepressants

A. Pharmacologic effects and adverse reactions—because of a similar structure to the phenothiazines, they have similar properties plus
   1. Antidepressant—reduces endogenous (no known cause) depression; onset of this effect is slow (days)
   2. Cardiac toxicity in overdose—arrhythmias; usual cause of death when used in a suicidal attempt
B. Drug interactions—antidepressant plus
   1. Epinephrine—results in hypertension (increased vasopressor response); usual doses contained in local anesthetic solutions can be used safely in normotensive patients (patients with normal blood pressure)
   2. Anticholinergic—results in additive anticholinergic action
C. Therapeutic uses—treatment of
   1. Endogenous depression—main use
   2. Nocturnal enuresis (bed-wetting) in children
D. Drugs
   1. Tricyclic antidepressants (TCA)
      a. Amitriptyline (Elavil)
      b. Imipramine (Tofranil)
   2. Trazodone (Desyrel)—new antidepressant (not tricyclic); lacks anticholinergic side effects of tricyclic antidepressants

Other Psychotherapeutic Agents

A. Lithium—for bipolar affective disorder; level difficult to maintain; poor control not uncommon
B. Monoamine oxidase inhibitors (MAOI)
   1. Last resort for depression
   2. Potential for *numerous severe* drug and food interactions (e.g., wine, sausage, cheese; indirect-acting adrenergic agents, meperidine)

Anticonvulsants

A. Pharmacologic effects—reduction or elimination of seizures (Table 8-7)
B. Dental considerations (see Chapter 18 for more information on seizures)
   1. Phenytoin (Dilantin)—gingival hyperplasia; scrupulous oral hygiene reduces gingival hyperplasia
   2. Several anticonvulsants
      a. Teratogenic potential (question of teratogenic association with seizures also unanswered)
      b. Sedation—tolerance often develops to this effect
      c. Blood dyscrasias can be serious; laboratory monitoring important
   3. Carbamazepine (Tegretol)—very toxic; close laboratory monitoring important; blood dyscrasias
   4. Benzodiazepines
      a. Clonazepam (Clonopin)—long-acting benzodiazepine; used orally for absence seizures
      b. Diazepam (Valium)—drug of choice for status epilepticus and emergency treatment of nonspecific seizures

ENDOCRINE AGENTS
Adrenocorticosteroids (Steroids)

A. Classification
   1. Glucocorticoids—regulate metabolism of glucose
   2. Mineralocorticoids—regulate sodium (minerals) and water
B. Pharmacologic effects of the glucocorticoids—antiinflammatory

Table 8-7 Anticonvulsant agents of choice for seizures

Seizures		Drugs	
Type	Comments	First choice	Alternatives
Absence (petit mal) or psychomotor	Consciousness lost	Ethosuximide (Zarontin)	Clonazepam (Clonopin), Trimethadione (Tridione)
Tonic-clonic (grand mal)	Consciousness lost	Phenytoin (Dilantin)	Phenobarbital (Luminal), Primidone (Mysoline), Carbamazepine (Tegretol)
Status epilepticus	Emergency situation	Diazepam (Valium)	Phenytoin (Dilantin), Phenobarbital (Luminal)
Trigeminal neuralgia (tic douloureux)	Not seizure type	Carbamazepine (Tegretol)	

C. Adverse reactions
1. Cushing's syndrome—long-term administration of high doses can produce symptoms of glucocorticoid excess, including
   a. Metabolic effects—"moon face," "buffalo hump," truncal obesity
   b. Peptic ulcers—excerbation and/or stimulation of stomach acid secretion
   c. Skin—bruising, striae, delay in healing
   d. Mental changes—euphoria when patient is taking medication; depression when dose is being tapered (reduced)
   e. Infection—masking of symptoms; watch closely and treat aggressively if symptoms occur; suppression of immunity
   f. Osteoporosis (reduced bone density)—bones break more easily
   g. Hypertension—water and sodium retention (mineralocorticoid action)
   h. Hyperglycemia (elevated blood pressure)— exacerbation of diabetes
2. Adrenal crisis—abrupt withdrawal of a steroid or stress (such as a dental appointment) can precipitate a crisis; prevent by premedicating with additional steroids; potentially serious situation
D. Therapeutic uses
1. Medical—treatment of many inflammatory conditions (e.g., arthritis, asthma, dermatitis)
2. Dental
   a. Aphthous lesions—palliative treatment; topical or intralesional (into the lesion) therapy
   b. Oral lesions secondary to collagen vascular diseases—topical, intralesional, or systemic therapy
   c. Temporomandibular joint (TMJ) pain— intraarticular injection (into the joint)
E. Examples—many more than these; differ primarily in potency and duration

Steroid	Comments
Hydrocortisone	Some mineralocorticoid action
Prednisone	Most commonly used orally
Triamcinolone (Kenalog)	Used primarily topically
Dexamethasone (Decadron)	More potent, so lower dose used

Agents for Diabetes Mellitus

See also Chapter 14, section on diabetes mellitus
A. Disease
1. Symptoms
   a. Polyuria—increased urination
   b. Polydipsia—increased thirst
   c. Polyphagia—increased hunger

2. Classification
   a. Insulinopenic—β-cells of the pancreas lack ability to secrete insulin; called juvenile onset; requires insulin
   b. Insulin insensitive—tissues lack sensitivity; called adult onset; sometimes controlled by diet and/or oral hypoglycemic agents
3. Complications—disease involves not only disorders of carbohydrate metabolism, but also many small blood vessels throughout the body, causing
   a. Retinopathy—vision problems, blindness
   b. Cardiovascular problems—circulation problems, heart problems, myocardial infarction, stroke
   c. Reduced ability to fight infections
   d. Neuropathy—reduced sensations in the extremities
   e. Nephropathy—kidney problems
   f. Slower, delayed healing
   g. Oral manifestations—reduced immunity (ability to fight infections), reduced vascular supply (small vessel disease), or other unknown functions predispose the patient to periodontal disease; alveolar bone loss occurs
B. Drugs
1. Insulin preparations

	Activity (hr)	
	Peak	Duration
Rapid acting: regular (crystalline)	½-3	5-7
Intermediate acting		
Isophane (NPH)	8-12	18-24
Lente	8-12	18-24

   a. Combine regular plus either NPH or Lente—once-a-day injection
   b. Human insulin now available from gene splicing (*E. coli* makes it)
2. Oral hypoglycemic agents (sulfonylureas)

	t½ (hr)	Duration (hr)
Tolbutamide (Orinase)	4-5	6-12
Tolazamide (Tolinase)	7	10-16
Acetohexamide (Dymelor)	6-8	12-24
Chlorpropamide (Diabinese)	36	60
Glyburide (DiaBeta, Micronase)	10	24
Glipizide (Glucotrol)	3	10-24

3. Adverse reaction—hypoglycemia
   a. Note the peak effect and the patient's eating pattern before the appointment
   b. Symptoms—nervousness, sweating, talking
   c. Treatment—"sugar" (glucose) is given orally if the patient is conscious; intravenous dextrose is given only if the patient is unconscious

Thyroid Gland Agents

A. Hypothyroidism
   1. Patient takes thyroid replacements to become euthyroid (normal thyroid)
   2. Examples

      Levothyroxine (Synthroid, Levothroid)
      Thyroglobulin (Proloid)
      Liothyronine (Cytomel)
      Liotrix (Euthroid, Thyrolar)

   3. No special handling required
B. Hyperthyroidism
   1. Partial thyroidectomy or radioactive iodine—ablates part of the thyroid function; patient often requires supplemental thyroid to be euthyroid; no unusual considerations
   2. Patients awaiting surgery or poor surgical candidates may be maintained on a regimen of thyroid suppressants
   3. Drugs
      a. Suppress thyroid function
      b. Examples

         Propylthiouracil (PTU)
         Methimazole (Tapazole)

      c. β-Blockers are given to reduce the elevated HR
   4. Dental implications—avoid epinephrine because it can trigger a thyroid storm

Agents for Gout

The drug treatment of gout is presented in Table 8-8; note that agents used to prevent gout are different from those used to treat an acute attack of gout

RESPIRATORY SYSTEM AGENTS

Agents for Asthma

A. Disease—extrinsic and intrinsic forms have different situations
B. Drugs
   1. Adrenergic agents (sympathomimetics)—see section on autonomic nervous system agents
      a. Used orally and by inhalation
      b. Examples

         Metaproterenol (Alupent, Metaprel)
         Albuterol (Proventil, Ventolin)

   2. Methylxanthines
      a. Examples

         Theophylline (Theo-Dur)
         Aminophylline (theophylline ethylenediamine)
         Caffeine (in coffee)*

      b. Pharmacologic effects
         (1) Bronchodilation (smooth muscle relaxation)—helpful in asthma
         (2) CNS stimulation—alertness, insomnia
         (3) Diuresis—increased urination
   3. Cromolyn sodium (Intal, Nasalcrom)—used for asthma prophylaxis by inhalation of powder; newly approved for allergic rhinitis
   4. Adrenocorticosteroids—see section on adrenocorticosteroids
C. Dental considerations
   1. Disease considerations
      a. Degree of control—avoid elective treatment if the condition is poorly controlled
      b. Patient's anxiety level during the dental appointment—preoperative sedation may be helpful (e.g., benzodiazepine)

---

*Not used clinically for bronchodilation.

Table 8-8   Drugs used for gout

	Drug	Mechanism	Comments
Prevention	Probenecid (Benemid)	Uricosuric (promotes uric acid excretion)	Aspirin interferes with uricosuric effect
	Allopurinol (Zyloprim)	Xanthine oxidase inhibitor; inhibits uric acid synthesis	Also used in cancer patients receiving chemotherapy or radiation therapy
Treatment	NSAIAs (e.g., indomethacin [Indocin], phenylbutazone [Butazolidin])	Antiinflammatory	See discussion on NSAIAs under analgesics
	Colchicine	Binds with microtubules in granulocytes; prevents granulocyte migration	GI toxicity—nausea, vomiting, diarrhea; sometimes given with probenecid

2. Analgesic choice—there is no easy answer
   a. Avoid aspirin-containing compounds; may precipitate an asthma attack
   b. Caution with NSAIAs—if aspirin causes bronchospasm, the NSAIAs are contraindicated
   c. Narcotics produce bronchoconstriction (histamine release) or respiratory depression
   d. Acetaminophen alone or mixed with a weak narcotic may be a reasonable choice

GASTROINTESTINAL AGENTS ▬▬▬
Agents Affecting GI Motility

A. Laxatives—increase GI motility; symptomatically treat constipation (e.g., milk of magnesia)
B. Antidiarrheals—reduce GI motility; symptomatically treat diarrhea (e.g., Lomotil, any narcotic agent)

Agent for Ulcers – Histamine (H₂) Blocker

A. Mechanism of action—agent blocks secretion of stomach acid
B. Examples

> Cimetidine (Tagamet)
> Ranitidine (Zantac)

C. Dental considerations
   1. Interferes with absorption with some drugs that need acid for absorption (e.g., ketoconazole [Nizoral]).
   2. Avoid ulcerogenic medications (e.g., aspirin, nonsteroidal antiinflammatory agents, and glucocorticoids)

Emetics and Antiemetics

A. Emetics—induce vomiting; used to treat most poisonings (e.g., syrup of ipecac—available without a prescription)
B. Antiemetics
   1. Reduce nausea or vomiting
   2. Examples

> Prochlorperazine (Compazine)
> Trimethobenzamide (Tigan)
> Benzquinamide (Emete-Con)

ANTINEOPLASTIC AGENTS ▬▬▬

A. Mechanism of action—drug interferes with metabolism or the reproductive cycle of malignant cells; also affects host cells
B. Drugs
   1. Alkylating agents
      a. Nitrogen mustards

> Mechlorethamine (Mustargen)
> Cyclophosphamide (Cytoxan)
> Chlorambucil (Leukeran)
> Melphalan (Alkeran)

b. Nitrosoureas

> Carmustine (BiCNU)
> Lomustine (CeeNU)
> Semustine (Methyl-CeeNU)

c. Bisulfan (Myleran)
   2. Antimetabolites
      a. Folic acid analog

> Methotrexate (MTX)

b. Pyrimidine analogs

> 5-Fluorouracil (5-FU)
> Floxuridine (FUDR)
> Cytosine arabinoside (Cytosar-U)

   3. Other antineoplastics
      a. Natural

> Vinblastine (Velban)
> Vincristine (Oncovin)

b. Antibiotics

> Dactinomycin (Actinomycin D)
> Doxorubicin (Adriamycin)
> Bleomycin sulfate (Blenoxane)
> Mitomycin (Mutamycin)

c. Hormones

> Adrenocorticosteroids
> Androgens/estrogens
> Progestins

d. Other

> L-Asparaginase
> Cisplatin (Platinol)

C. Adverse reactions
   1. Lack of specificity against tumor cells; some normal cells are destroyed
   2. Bone marrow suppression—leukopenia (lowered white blood cell count), thrombocytopenia (lowered platelets), anemia
   3. Gastrointestinal—stomatitis, mucosal sloughing
   4. Infection—reduced immunity
   5. Skin/hair—rash, alopecia (baldness)
   6. Oral effects
      a. Symptoms—pain, ulcers, dryness, impaired taste, gingival hemorrhage, sensitivity of teeth and gums
      b. Treatment—avoid oral mouthwashes; substitute saline or sodium bicarbonate instead of other mouthwashes
      c. Candidiasis—use antifungal agents (e.g., nystatin, clotrimazole, ketoconazole)
      d. Xerostomia—artificial saliva (Xero-lube)

D. Dental considerations
1. Improve oral hygiene before chemotherapy, if possible
2. Avoid elective procedures during chemotherapy; timing is important
3. Check coagulation status before emergency surgery
4. Prophylactic antibiotic coverage is controversial

REFERENCES

1. Gilman, A.G., Goodman, L.S., and Gilman, A.: Goodman and Gilman's the pharmacological basis of therapeutics, ed. 2, New York, 1980, Macmillan Publishing Co., Inc.
2. Holroyd, S.V., and Wynn, R.L.: Clinical pharmacology in dental practice, ed. 3, St. Louis, 1983, The C.V. Mosby Co.
3. Kastrup, E.K., editor: Facts and comparisons: drug information compendium, St. Louis, Facts and Comparisons, Inc.
4. Physician's desk reference, ed. 39 Oradell, N.J., 1985, Medical Economics Co.
5. Requa, B.S., and Holroyd, S.V.: Applied pharmacology for the dental hygienist, St. Louis, 1982, The C.V. Mosby Co.

Review Questions

1 A patient gives a history of an "allergic" reaction to aspirin. She describes the onset of stomach cramps with nausea one-half hour after swallowing three aspirin tablets. This reaction is *most* likely categorized as
(a) An allergic reaction
(b) A toxicity reaction
(c) Predictable
(d) Unpredictable
1. a and c
2. a and d
3. b and c
4. b and d
5. a, b, and c

2 When a drug is administered intravenously, which of the following is avoided?
1. Excretion
2. Nonspecific tissue depots
3. Plasma
4. Absorption
5. Biotransformation

3 The *most* common site of biotransformation of a drug is the
1. Plasma
2. Adipose tissue
3. Kidneys
4. Liver
5. Spleen

4 Which drug name must be used by all manufacturers even though each manufacturer may also give a drug a different name?
1. Generic
2. Brand
3. Trade
4. Chemical
5. Proprietary

5 Which of the following routes of administration produces the fastest onset of action?
1. Intravenous (IV)
2. Topical
3. Oral
4. Rectal
5. Intramuscular (IM)

6 Which of the following terminates a drug's effect without either biotransformation or excretion having occurred?
1. Hydrolysis
2. Tachyphylaxis
3. Tolerance
4. Redistribution
5. Metabolism

7 A patient who complains of dizziness, blurred vision, very hot, dry skin, and dry mouth is *most* likely suffering from toxicity associated with an overdose of the
1. Anticholinergic agents
2. Cholinergic agents
3. β-Adrenergic agonists
4. β-Blockers
5. α-Adrenergic agonists

8 A fear reaction produces activation of the sympathetic autonomic nervous system, causing
1. Miosis
2. Bradycardia
3. Hypertension
4. Profuse, watery saliva
5. Diarrhea

9 An anticholinergic agent is used preoperatively before general anesthesia to
1. Reduce the heart rate
2. Reduce salivation
3. Increase the blood pressure
4. Provide hemostasis
5. Provide anxiety relief

10 In dentistry a cholinergic drug is used to
1. Produce a dry field for taking impressions
2. Calm an anxious patient before a dental procedure
3. Increase a patient's salivary flow to treat dry mouth
4. Reduce the chance of a patient's getting an infection
5. Potentiate a local anesthetic agent

11 The *most* common symptom associated with hypertension is
1. None
2. Headaches
3. Blurred vision
4. Mental depression
5. Gastrointestinal distress

12 The medical uses of the adrenergic agents include treating
1. Anxiety
2. Hypertension
3. Anaphylaxis
4. Narrow-angle glaucoma
5. Angina pectoris

13 The neuromuscular blocking agents are used to
1. Reduce apprehension in an anxious patient
2. Provide relaxation and reduce spasms caused by muscular overexertion
3. Provide paralysis before intubation during general anesthesia
4. Provide an increase in the heart rate during general anesthesia
5. Prevent infections in diabetic patients undergoing surgery

14 Patients with which of the following conditions might experience the greatest problems if given an agent designed to dry their mouth?
1. Enlarged prostate
2. Diarrhea
3. Wide-angle glaucoma
4. Controlled angina pectoris
5. Mild high blood pressure

15 Adrenergic agents must be used with the greatest caution in patients who have
1. Hyperthyroidism
2. Addison's disease
3. Hypotension
4. Asthma
5. Prostate enlargement

16 A patient has a documented allergy to lidocaine (positive skin test). Which local anesthetic agent would be *least* likely to produce an allergic reaction in this patient?
1. Mepivacaine (Carbocaine)
2. Prilocaine (Citanest)
3. Procaine/propoxycaine (Ravocaine)
4. Bupivacaine (Marcaine)
5. Etidocaine (Duranest)

17 What agent may be used to provide some local anesthetic action to a patient with a history of an allergy to all of the local anesthetics?
1. Carbamazepine (Tegretol)
2. Acetaminophen (Tylenol)
3. Diphenhydramine (Benadryl)
4. Phenytoin (Dilantin)
5. Ibuprofen (Motrin)

18 Which of the following agents would be *best* to administer, if one were to anticipate both severe and prolonged postoperative dental pain?
1. Mepivacaine (Carbocaine)
2. Lidocaine with epinephrine (Xylocaine)
3. Prilocaine (Citanest)
4. Prilocaine with epinephrine (Citanest Forte)
5. Bupivacaine with epinephrine (Marcaine)

Situation: A patient needs local-infiltration anesthesia before deep subgingival scaling. Lidocaine 2% with 1:100,000 epinephrine is administered. Questions 19 and 20 refer to this situation.

19 Because the patient complains of inadequate ''numbing,'' eight more cartridges of lidocaine 2% with epinephrine 1:100,000 vasoconstrictor are injected. The patient then begins talking incessantly, exhibiting restlessness and fasciculations of the extremities, and then becomes sleepy and suffers a convulsion. These symptoms are *most* likely caused by
1. A toxicity reaction to the local anesthetic agent
2. A toxicity reaction to the vasoconstrictor
3. A fear reaction
4. The fact that the patient is epileptic
5. A synergistic effect between the local anesthetic and the vasoconstrictor

20 The *best* treatment for this patient's convulsions is
1. Awaiting their cessation
2. Intravenous diazepam (Valium)
3. Intravenous secobarbital (Seconal)
4. Intravenous thiopental (Pentothal)
5. Inhalation nitrous oxide

---

21 When considering Guedel's classification of general anesthetics, stage II includes
1. Regular respiration
2. Bradycardia
3. Loss of the vomiting reflex
4. Hypotension
5. Unconsciousness

Situation: A patient who is being given agents for general anesthesia is often given a variety of agents concomitantly. A typical combination might include thiopental (Pentothal), nitrous oxide, enflurane (Ethrane), succinylcholine (Anectine), and glycopyrrolate (Robinul). Questions 22 to 25 refer to this situation.

22 Thiopental is
1. Used for inducing a patient into stage III anesthesia
2. A long-acting inhalation anesthetic
3. An incomplete general anesthetic
4. Both flammable and explosive
5. Associated with hepatotoxicity

23 Nitrous oxide
1. Is an incomplete general anesthetic
2. Is used to induce stage III anesthesia quickly
3. Is both flammable and explosive
4. Is associated with cardiac arrhythmias
5. Requires a long time for recovery

24 Enflurane can be associated with cardiac arrhythmias. These are exacerbated by
1. The benzodiazepines
2. The sympathomimetic amines
3. The anticholinergic agents
4. Nitrous oxide
5. The neuromuscular blocking agents

25 The use of succinylcholine, a neuromuscular blocking agent, is to
1. Dry up secretions
2. Stimulate the heart
3. Induce respiratory paralysis
4. Potentiate the halogenated hydrocarbons
5. Maintain adequate blood pressure

---

26 A patient explains that she has difficulty relaxing before a dental appointment and is very nervous. Assuming that a pharmacologic agent were appropriate, which of the following medications would be the *best* to allay anxiety in a dental setting?
1. Secobarbital (Seconal)
2. Diazapam (Valium)
3. Chlorpromazine (Thorazine)
4. Amitriptyline (Elavil)
5. Penicillin (Pen-Vee-K)

27 All of the following pharmacologic groups produce central nervous system (CNS) depression *except*
1. Antihistamines
2. Adrenergic agents
3. Sedative-hypnotic agents
4. Nonsteroidal antiinflammatory agents
5. Narcotic analgesic agents

28 What is chloral hydrate's (Noctec's) major disadvantage in being used for dental anxiety in a child?
1. It is not approved for use in children
2. It produces nausea and vomiting
3. It has potential for addiction
4. It has a slow onset of action
5. It has no analgesic effect

29 One advantage of the benzodiazepines over the barbiturates is that they
1. Are not addicting
2. Have a wider therapeutic index
3. Are safe in a patient with porphyria
4. Are safe to use in a pregnant woman
5. Do not produce sedation

30 The barbiturates possess all of the following properties *except*
1. Anticonvulsant
2. Addicting
3. Extrapyramidal
4. Anesthetic
5. Muscle relaxant

31 A patient is given 100 mg of meperidine (Demerol) intramuscularly before a dental procedure. The patient's respiration ceases. What should be administered?
1. Naloxone (Narcan)
2. Pralidoxime (Protopam)
3. Physostigmine (Eserine)
4. Methylphenidate (Ritalin)
5. Diphenhydramine (Benadryl)

32 A patient with a history of a peptic ulcer may *most* safely be given
1. Aspirin
2. Codeine
3. Ibuprofen (Motrin)
4. Naproxen (Naprosyn)
5. Empirin 4

33 Which of the following should be avoided in a narcotic addict because it has the potential to precipitate withdrawal, since it has antagonist as well as agonist properties?
1. Hydromorphone (Dilaudid)
2. Meperidine (Demerol)
3. Methadone (Dolophine)
4. Pentazocine (Talwin)
5. Morphine

34 A patient exhibiting a white patchy lesion that is easily scraped off, leaving an erythematous or bleeding area, would *most* likely respond to treatment with
1. Isoniazid (INH)
2. Metronidazole (Flagyl)
3. Nystatin (Mycostatin)
4. Sulfisoxazole (Gantrisin)
5. Acyclovir (Zovirax)

35 Although many drugs have been associated with cholestatic jaundice, which antibiotic group seems to be more closely associated with this adverse reaction?
1. Sulfonamides
2. Cephalosporins
3. Tetracyclines
4. Erythromycins
5. Aminoglycosides

36 Penicillin V is *most* commonly used in dentistry because it
1. Is more acid stable than penicillin G
2. Has a wider spectrum of action than ampicillin
3. Has a longer duration of action than dicloxacillin
4. Is more resistant to penicillinase than dicloxacillin
5. Is less allergenic than penicillin G

37 Which agent is approved by the Food and Drug Administration (FDA) in the United States for the treatment of recurrent herpes labialis in the normal (nonimmunocompromised) host?
1. Idoxuridine (Herplex)
2. Acyclovir (Zovirax)
3. Nystatin (Mycostatin)
4. Lysine
5. None of the above

38 The cephalosporins are similar to the penicillins in all of the following respects *except* their
1. Mechanism of action
2. Bactericidal action
3. Propensity for allergic reactions
4. Spectrum of action
5. Relative lack of toxicity

39 Which adverse effect tends to limit the usefulness of clindamycin (Cleocin) in dental practice?
1. Its spectrum of action is too broad
2. It produces pseudomembranous colitis
3. It is not orally effective
4. It is associated with cholestatic jauandice
5. It produces ototoxicity

40 The therapeutic use of the β-adrenergic blockers includes all of the following *except*
1. Treatment of hypertension
2. Prevention of myocardial infarction
3. Angina pectoris
4. Prophylaxis of migraine headaches
5. Prophylaxis of status asthmaticus

Situation: A patient gives a history of taking warfarin (Coumadin), digoxin (Lanoxin), and hydrochlorothiazide (HydroDiuril). Questions 41 to 43 refer to this situation.

41 Which analgesic agent would be *least* desirable to administer to the patient for dental pain?
1. Acetaminophen (Tylenol)
2. Ibuprofen (Motrin)
3. Aspirin (Bayer)
4. Codeine
5. Meperidine (Demerol)

42 Which adverse reaction is *most* likely produced by this patient's warfarin?
1. Gum bleeding
2. Leg swelling
3. Excessive urination
4. Blurred vision
5. Water retention

43 Which of the following diseases does this patient *most* likely have?
1. Congestive heart failure
2. Arrhythmias
3. Angina pectoris
4. Hyperthyroidism
5. Cushing's syndrome

44 If given in overdose, the tricyclic antidepressants produce toxicity to the
1. Heart
2. Lungs
3. Liver
4. Kidneys
5. Spleen

45 The drug of choice for trigeminal neuralgia (tic douloureux) is
1. Ethosuximide (Zarontin)
2. Carbamazepine (Tegretol)
3. Phenobarbital (Luminal)
4. Phenytoin (Dilantin)
5. Diazepam (Valium)

Situation: A patient has been taking a combination of phenobarbital (Luminal) and phenytoin (Dilantin). Questions 46 to 49 refer to this situation.

46 This patient *most* likely has
1. Grand mal seizures
2. Cushing's syndrome
3. Tic douloureux (trigeminal neuralgia)
4. Myasthenia gravis
5. Narcolepsy

47 Which of the following "patient complaints" would *most* likely be related to one of this patient's medications?
1. "I feel sleepy"
2. "My hair is thinning"
3. "I have a sore throat"
4. "My gums are red and enlarged"
5. "I feel very nervous"

48 In order to minimize this patient's major complaint, the dental hygienist might suggest that the patient
1. Maintain scrupulous oral hygiene
2. Drink several cups of coffee daily
3. Increase daily exercise to enhance relaxation
4. Use a local anesthetic lozenge
5. Use a fluoride mouth rinse

49 A patient taking both phenytoin and phenobarbital *most* likely has
1. Absence seizures
2. Diabetes
3. Cushing's syndrome
4. Tonic-clonic seizures
5. Osteoporosis

50 Patients who are receiving tolbutamide (Orinase) may experience all of the following problems *except*
1. They may heal more slowly
2. They should be given aspirin cautiously
3. Their chance of infection may be greater
4. They may experience hypoglycemic reactions
5. They may have an increased incidence of peptic ulcers

Situation: A patient comes to the dental office giving a history of long-term high-dose adrenocorticoid administration (prednisone 50 mg every day for 3 years). Questions 51 to 53 refer to this situation.

51 This patient may exhibit all of the following side effects associated with steroids except
1. Osteoporosis
2. Frequent infections
3. Moon face
4. Peptic ulcer
5. Hypotension

52 If this patient is to be treated in the dental office and will experience stress, what would be the *most* important consideration? The patient
1. May become hypoglycemic during the procedure
2. May become hypotensive during the procedure
3. May exhibit an adrenal crisis during the procedure
4. Should not be given epinephrine
5. Will have a dry mouth

53 Which of the following is *not* a consideration in this patient?
1. Healing may be prolonged
2. Infections may be more likely
3. The redness of the gums may not be commensurate with the degree of periodontitis
4. Ulcerogenic medication should be avoided in this patient
5. The patient may have a thyroid storm

---

54 Colchicine
1. Is a uricosuric
2. Is a xanthine oxidase inhibitor
3. Commonly causes nausea, vomiting, and diarrhea
4. Is rendered ineffective by aspirin
5. Is rendered ineffective by acetaminophen

55 Probenecid (Benemid)
(a) Is a uricosuric
(b) Is a xanthine oxidase inhibitor
(c) Is rendered ineffective by aspirin
(d) Is rendered ineffective by acetaminophen
1. a only
2. b only
3. a and c
4. b and d
5. a, c, and d

56 Allopurinol (Zyloprim)
(a) Is a uricosuric
(b) Is a xanthine oxidase inhibitor
(c) Commonly causes nausea, vomiting, and diarrhea
(d) Is rendered ineffective by aspirin
1. a only
2. b only
3. a and d
4. b and c
5. b, c, and d

Answers and Rationales

1. (3) The gastrointestinal distress described by the patient is most likely a result of toxicity secondary to aspirin; since this is an adverse reaction, it is predictable.
   (1) Stomach cramps are not an allergic reaction.
   (2) Gastrointestinal distress with aspirin is predictable, not unpredictable.
   (4) Gastrointestinal distress with aspirin is predictable.
   (5) Stomach cramps are not an allergic reaction.
2. (4) When drugs are given intravenously, the absorption phase in body handling is avoided.
   (1) Drugs given intravenously are still excreted normally through the kidneys.
   (2) Drugs given intravenously can go to either or both specific and nonspecific tissue depots.
   (3) Drugs administered intravenously have the drug deposited in the plasma (blood).
   (5) Drugs given intravenously are still metabolized or biotransformed by the liver.
3. (4) The metabolism (biotransformation) of most drugs occurs in the liver (hepatic microsomal enzymes).
   (1) Metabolism of drugs only occasionally occurs in the plasma (e.g., ester local anesthetic agents).
   (2) Adipose tissue is not usually involved in metabolism.
   (3) Metabolism of drugs only occasionally occurs in the kidneys.
   (5) The spleen is not involved in metabolism.
4. (1) The generic name is the name that all manufacturers must include, even though they may give the drug their own name also.
   (2) The brand name is the name of the drug company itself or the name given by the manufacturer to a drug.
   (3) The trade name is the drug name given by the manufacturer to a drug; it is synonymous with brand name.
   (4) The chemical name is the name given to a compound based on its chemical structure.
   (5) The proprietary name is the name given by the manufacturer to a drug; it is synonymous with brand and trade names.
5. (1) Because the absorption phase is bypassed, a drug given IV acts fastest.
   (2) Although some absorption can occur through the skin, drug action with this route is usually much slower than with the IV route.
   (3) A drug must be absorbed from the gastrointestinal tract before systemic action can take place.
   (4) Drug action with the rectal route is slower than with the IV route.
   (5) Drug action with the IM route is slower than with the IV route.

For each question the correct answer and rationale are listed first. The other choices are presented in order with the reasons why they are not correct.

6. (4) Redistribution involves a drug's moving from the specific tissue depot to the nonspecific tissue depot without either biotransformation (metabolism) or excretion having occurred.
   (1) Hydrolysis is one means of biotransformation.
   (2) Tachyphylxis is when a patient becomes used to a drug that is administered repeatedly and more is needed for the same effect.
   (3) Tolerance is when a patient becomes used to a drug's effect.
   (5) *Metabolism* is another word for biotransformation.

7. (1) Anticholinergic agents produce hot, dry skin, dry mouth, and blurred vision.
   (2) Cholinergic agents produce sweating and increased salivation.
   (3) β-Adrenergic agonists produce tachycardia and hypertension.
   (4) β-Blockers primarily affect the cardiovascular system (CVS).
   (5) α-Adrenergic agonists primarily affect the CVS. They also produce vasoconstriction.

8. (3) An increase in blood pressure is a common effect when the sympathetic autonomic nervous system is stimulated in response to fear.
   (1) Patients with sympathetic nervous system discharge exhibit mydriasis (pupillary dilation), not miosis (pupillary constriction).
   (2) Sympathetic autonomic nervous system activation normally produces tachycardia (increased heart rate) rather than bradycardia (slower heart rate).
   (4) Sympathetic autonomic nervous system discharge produces thick, viscid saliva, not the profuse, watery saliva produced by stimulation of the parasympathetic autonomic nervous system.
   (5) Innervation of the gastrointestinal tract is primarily parasympathetic. Sympathetic discharge generally has little effect.

9. (2) Anticholinergic agents produce xerostoma, which is helpful during general anesthesia.
   (1) An increase in the heart rate sometimes occurs with these agents, since they block the vagal slowing of the heart.
   (3) The adrenergic agents are used to raise the blood pressure.
   (4) Hemostasis is provided by the adrenergic agents (sympathomimetics).
   (5) The anticholinergic drugs are neither as effective nor as reliable as the antianxiety agents for relief of anxiety.

10. (3) Cholinergic agents increase salivary flow and may be helpful in treating xerostomia.
    (1) Anticholinergic agents are used to produce a dry mouth.
    (2) In normal therapeutic doses the cholinergic agents produce little effect on the central nervous system.
    (4) Cholinergic drugs have no effect on infection.
    (5) Cholinergic drugs do not potentiate local anesthetic agents.

11. (1) Hypertension most commonly produces no symptoms.
    (2) Although commonly thought to be associated with high blood pressure, headaches are infrequently experienced.
    (3) Although blurred vision may occasionally be associated with hypertensive episodes, hypertension usually does not produce any side effects.
    (4) Some antihypertensive medications can produce mental depression, although high blood pressure does not.
    (5) High blood pressure does not produce gastrointestinal distress.

12. (3) Adrenergics produce bronchodilation that is helpful in treating anaphylaxis. Epinephrine is a physiologic antagonist to histamine.
    (1) Adrenergics make patients feel nervous.
    (2) Adrenergics generally elevate the blood pressure.
    (4) Narrow-angle glaucoma is treated surgically. Wide-angle glaucoma can be treated with adrenergics.
    (5) Angina pectoris can be exacerbated by the adrenergics.

13. (3) Neuromuscular blocking agents such as *d*-tubocurarine and succinylcholine are used to provide total skeletal muscle paralysis before intubation during general anesthesia.
    (1) Neuromuscular blocking agents are not effective in reducing apprehension.
    (2) Relaxing spasms caused by overexertion of muscles usually requires a centrally acting muscle relaxant, or "tranquilizer."
    (4) The heart rate is increased during general anesthesia by the administration of anticholinergic drugs.
    (5) Antiinfective agents are used to prevent infections in diabetic patients undergoing surgery.

14. (1) Patients who have an enlarged prostate may experience urinary retention or hesitancy if given anticholinergic agents.
    (2) Anticholinergics reduce gastrointestinal motility and would not be contraindicated in diarrhea.
    (3) Anticholinergics are contraindicated in narrow-angle, not wide-angle, glaucoma.
    (4) Patients with controlled angina pectoris may be given a single dose of an anticholinergic agent cautiously.
    (5) Patients with controlled high blood pressure may be given anticholinergic agents.

15. (1) A thyroid storm may be precipitated if patients who are hyperthyroid are given adrenergic agents.
    (2) Patients with Addison's disease require glucocorticoid and mineralocorticoid replacement.
    (3) Adrenergic agents generally raise the blood pressure and would not cause problems with a patient with hypotension.
    (4) Adrenergic agents are used to treat asthma.
    (5) Anticholinergics, not adrenergic agents, are contraindicated in prostatic hypertrophy.

16. (3) Procaine/propoxycaine is an ester combination chemically dissimilar to the amides (lidocaine is an amide).
    (1) Mepivacaine is an amide similar in structure to lidocaine.
    (2) Prilocaine is an amide similar in structure to lidocaine.
    (4) Bupivacaine is an amide similar in structure to lidocaine.
    (5) Etidocaine is an amide similar in structure to lidocaine.

17. (3) Diphenhydramine has some local anesthetic action.
    (1) Carbamazepine has no usable local anesthetic action.
    (2) Acetaminophen has no usable local anesthetic action.
    (4) Phenytoin has no usable local anesthetic action.
    (5) Ibuprofen has no usable local anesthetic action.

18. (5) Of the local anesthetic agents listed, bupivacaine with epinephrine has the longest duration of action (greater than 180 minutes, may be up to 10 hours).
    (1) The duration of action of mepivacaine without epinephrine may be less than 30 minutes.
    (2) Lidocaine with epinephrine has a duration of action of 45 to 75 minutes.
    (3) Prilocaine has a duration of action of 45 to 75 minutes.
    (4) Prilocaine with epinephrine has a duration of action of between 90 and 150 minutes.

19. (1) A patient who becomes hyperactive and then hypoactive is probably exhibiting a toxicity reaction to a local anesthetic agent.
    (2) Toxicity to the vasoconstrictor would be exhibited primarily by hyperactivity.
    (3) A fear reaction usually does not include sleepiness.
    (4) An epileptic patient would not become sleepy before a convulsion.
    (5) There is no synergistic effect between a local anesthetic and a vasoconstrictor in terms of producing convulsions.

20. (1) Since seizures secondary to local anesthetic agents are generally short lived, awaiting their cessation is preferable to treatment with other agents.
    (2) Intravenous diazepam is the drug of choice if the convulsions do not cease spontaneously.
    (3) Intravenous secobarbital is not the drug of choice for nonspecific convulsions.
    (4) Although intravenous thiopental can produce paralysis of the muscles, this is not the drug of choice for nonspecific convulsions.
    (5) Nitrous oxide used by inhalation is not the drug of choice for convulsions.

21. (5) The beginning of stage II is marked by the loss of consciousness.
    (1) Stage II is characterized by irregular respiration.
    (2) Tachycardia occurs during stage II.
    (3) The vomiting reflex is maintained during stage II.
    (4) Stage II is characterized by hypertension (increased blood pressure) rather than hypotension.

22. (1) Thiopental is used to induce general anesthesia to the surgical plane (stage III).
    (2) Thiopental is an ultrashort-acting barbiturate whose pharmacologic effects are terminated by redistribution.
    (3) Thiopental is a complete anesthetic.
    (4) Thiopental is neither flammable nor explosive.
    (5) Thiopental is not associated with hepatotoxicity.

23. (1) Nitrous oxide is an incomplete general anesthetic.
    (2) Nitrous oxide does not produce stage III anesthesia at all.
    (3) Nitrous oxide supports combustion but is not explosive.
    (4) Nitrous oxide does not produce cardiac arrhythmias.
    (5) Recovery from nitrous oxide is rapid.

24. (2) The halogenated hydrocarbons (e.g., enflurane) sensitize the myocardium to catecholamine (sympathomimetic)–induced arrhythmias.
    (1) The benzodiazepines are not arrhythmogenic.
    (3) The anticholinergic agents may produce tachycardia.
    (4) Nitrous oxide is not arrhythmogenic as long as adequate oxygenation is maintained.
    (5) The neuromuscular blocking agents produce respiratory paralysis.

25. (3) Succinylcholine is used to produce paralysis for intubation.
    (1) Succinylcholine is not used to dry up secretions.
    (2) Succinylcholine is not used to stimulate the heart.
    (4) Succinylcholine does not potentiate the halogenated hydrocarbons.
    (5) Succinylcholine is not used to maintain adequate blood pressure.

26. (2) A benzodiazepine is a good choice because of its anxiolytic effects.
    (1) The barbiturates would also reduce anxiety but are not as specific as the benzodiazepines.
    (3) The phenothiazines are used to treat other types of agitation.
    (4) The tricyclic antidepressants are used for endogenous depression.
    (5) An antibiotic has no antianxiety properties.

27. (2) Adrenergic agents normally produce CNS excitation.
    (1) Antihistamines produce sedation as a side effect.
    (3) Sedative-hypnotic agents commonly produce sedation.
    (4) Nonsteroidal antiinflammatory agents produce sedation as a side effect.
    (5) Narcotic analgesic agents produce sedation as a side effect.

28. (2) Chloral hydrate has a relatively high incidence of nausea and vomiting.
    (1) It is approved for use in children.
    (3) Although it has an addiction potential, this is not a problem for single-dose use in a child.
    (4) The onset of action of chloral hydrate is relatively rapid, especially if given in liquid form.
    (5) Although chloral hydrate possesses no analgesic action, that is not the effect for which it is being used. In fact, none of the sedative-hypnotics possess analgesic action.

29. (2) The benzodiazepines have a wider therapeutic index and are therefore safer than the barbiturates if accidentally given in overdose.
    (1) Both are addicting.
    (3) Both can cause problems if a patient has porphyria.
    (4) Benzodiazepines are contraindicated in pregnancy.
    (5) Both can cause sedation.

30. (3) Extrapyramidal side effects are associated with the phenothiazines (major tranquilizers) rather than with the barbiturates.
    (1) The barbiturates have anticonvulsant properties.
    (2) All of the barbiturates are addicting.
    (4) Given in high-enough doses, the barbiturates can produce general anesthesia. In fact, the ultrashort-acting barbiturates are used for induction of general anesthesia.
    (5) Although probably central in action, the barbiturates produce muscle relaxation.

31. (1) Naloxone, the "purest" narcotic antagonist available, would reverse the respiratory depression secondary to the narcotic.
    (2) Pralidoxime is useful in treating an overdose from an "irreversible" cholinesterase inhibitor.
    (3) Physostigmine has been used to treat an overdose of the benzodiazepines.
    (4) Methylphenidate or other "stimulants" are not helpful in treating respiratory depression secondary to either a narcotic overdose or a sedative-hypnotic agent.
    (5) Diphenhydramine, an antihistamine, is used for mild allergic reactions.

32. (2) Codeine's effect on the gastrointestinal tract produces constipation but does not adversely affect an ulcer.
    (1) Aspirin is ulcerogenic.
    (3) Ibuprofen, a nonsteroidal antiinflammatory agent (NSAIA), is ulcerogenic.
    (4) Naproxen, an NSAIA, is ulcerogenic.
    (5) Empirin 4 contains aspirin (ulcerogenic) and codeine.

33. (4) Pentazocine has both antagonist as well as agonist properties.
    (1) Hydromorphone has mainly agonist properties.
    (2) Meperidine has mainly agonist properties.
    (3) Methadone has mainly agonist properties.
    (5) Morphine has mainly agonist properties.

34. (3) Nystatin is the most logical treatment for candidiasis *(Candida albicans)* infection.
    (1) Isoniazid is used alone to prevent or in combination with other agents to treat, tuberculosis.
    (2) Metronidazole is used primarily to treat *Trichomonas* infection as well as certain other anerobes (*Bacteroides* species).
    (4) Sulfisoxazole is a broad-spectrum sulfonamide useful in treating a variety of infections.
    (5) Acyclovir has specific activity versus the herpesvirus.

35. (4) Erythromycin estolate is most closely associated with cholestatic jaundice.
    (1) Sulfonamides have been associated with Stevens-Johnson syndrome.
    (2) Cephalosporins have been associated with mild and reversible alterations of liver function tests.
    (3) Tetracyclines have been associated with hepatoxicity (usually large doses given to pregnant women).
    (5) Aminoglycosides are ototoxic and nephrotoxic.

36. (1) Because penicillin V is more acid stable than penicillin G, it is the most common penicillin used in dentistry. Its spectrum of action covers primarily gram-positive organisms, which are involved in oral infections.
    (2) The spectrum of action of penicillin V is not broader than that of ampicillin.
    (3) The duration of action of penicillin V and dicloxacillin are about the same.
    (4) Penicillin V is not penicillinase resistant, whereas dicloxacillin is. This resistance is useful in the treatment of penicillinase-producing staphylococci.
    (5) Penicillin V and penicillin G are equally allergenic.

37. (5) No medication is currently FDA approved for treatment of herpes labialis in the nonimmunocompromised patient.
    (1) Idoxuridine is approved for use topically in an eye solution for herpes simplex keratitis.
    (2) Acyclovir is approved for use topically in the treatment of recurrent genital (type 2) herpes in immunocompromised patients.
    (3) Nystatin is used for fungal infections (e.g., candidiasis).
    (4) Lysine is not approved for any use by the FDA.

38. (4) The spectrum of action of the cephalosporins generally is wider or broader than that of the penicillins and includes many gram-negative infections.
    (1) The mechanism of action of both cephalosporins and the penicillins involves cell wall synthesis inhibition.
    (2) Both cephalosporins and penicillins are bactericidal.
    (3) Both cephalosporins and penicillins have a tendency to produce allergic reactions ranging from a rash to anaphylaxis.
    (5) Both cephalosporins and penicillins tend to be relatively nontoxic (other than allergies).

39. (2) Pseudomembranous colitis has been associated with clindamycin (also other antibiotics). The FDA has currently limited its use to "severe anerobic infections."
    (1) The spectrum of action of clindamycin is primarily gram positive, as is that of both penicillin and erythromycin.
    (3) Clindamycin is orally effective.
    (4) The estolate salt of erythromycin has primarily been associated with cholestatic jaundice, although other antibiotics can also cause it.
    (5) The aminoglycosides are antiinfectives commonly associated with ototoxicity.

40. (5) β-Adrenergic blockers are contraindicated in patients with asthma because they can produce bronchoconstriction.
    (1) β-Adrenergic blockers are used in treatment of hypertension.
    (2) Several β-adrenergic blockers are approved for prevention of myocardial infarction.
    (3) β-Adrenergic blockers are used in treatment of angina pectoris.
    (4) β-Adrenergic blockers are used in prophylaxis of migraine headaches.

41. (3) Aspirin is absolutely contraindicated in patients taking warfarin unless it is prescribed concomitantly and titrated by prothrombin time (PT) under a physician's orders. (There is no good reason to do this.)
    (1) Acetaminophen would be acceptable to give this patient for mild dental pain.
    (2) Ibuprofen, although affecting blood coagulation in a reversible manner, can be used cautiously in patients receiving warfarin.
    (4) Codeine, a weak narcotic analgesic, can be used in this patient. Also, codeine mixtures can be used (e.g., Tylenol 3).
    (5) Meperidine, a stronger narcotic analgesic, can also be used in this patient.

42. (1) Because warfarin is an anticoagulant, bleeding gums are commonly observed in patients who are overmedicated.
    (2) Leg swelling, unless associated with a hematoma, is not commonly produced by warfarin.
    (3) Excessive urination is not a side effect of warfarin.
    (4) Blurred vision is not a side effect of warfarin.
    (5) Water retention is not a side effect of warfarin.

43. (1) The combination of digoxin and hydrochlorothiazide is commonly given to patients with congestive heart failure.
    (2) This patient is not receiving any antiarrhythmic other than digitalis, which can occasionally be used for arrhythmias (e.g., artial fibrillation).
    (3) No medication to treat angina pectoris (nitroglycerin-like) is being administered to this patient.
    (4) This patient's medical history does not indicate hyperthyroidism.
    (5) This patient is not taking any medication associated with or causing Cushing's syndrome (glucocorticoids).

44. (1) Tricyclic antidepressants can produce arrhythmias if given in overdose.
    (2) Toxicity in overdose to the lungs is not as significant as that of the heart.
    (3) Toxicity in overdose to the liver is not as significant as that of the heart.
    (4) Toxicity in overdose to the kidneys is not as significant as that of the heart.
    (5) Toxicity in overdose to the spleen is not as significant as that of the heart.

45. (2) Carbamazepine is the drug of choice for trigeminal neuralgia.
    (1) Ethosuximide is the drug of choice for absence seizures.
    (3) Phenobarbital is an alternative drug for tonic-clonic seizures. It is often combined with phenytoin.
    (4) Phenytoin is the drug of choice for tonic-clonic seizures.
    (5) Diazepam given intravenously is the drug of choice for nonspecific seizures.

46. (1) Treatment of grand mal seizures frequently involves combining both phenobarbital and phenytoin.
    (2) Cushing's syndrome is caused by excessive adrenocorticoids either from the adrenal gland or from exogenously administered adrenocorticoids.
    (3) Carbamazepine is the treatment of choice for tic douloureux (trigeminal neuralgia).
    (4) Myasthenia gravis, a weakness in the muscles, is treated by administering cholinesterase inhibitors to increase acetylcholine levels.
    (5) Narcolepsy, a disease where patients fall asleep spontaneously, is treated with adrenergic agents such as the amphetamines.

47. (4) Gingival hyperplasia, producing enlarged and sore gums, is a common side effect of phenytoin.
    (1) Tolerance usually develops to the central nervous system depression that is commonly produced by both phenobarbital and phenytoin.
    (2) Alopecia has not been associated with the anticonvulsants.
    (3) A sore throat may be indicative of agranulocytosis, an adverse effect rarely produced by phenytoin.
    (5) A nervous feeling is not usually associated with either phenobarbital or phenytoin.

48. (1) Scrupulous oral hygiene may reduce the gingival hyperplasia associated with phenytoin.
    (2) Drinking several cups of coffee may increase central nervous system excitation in cases of drowsiness.
    (3) Although increasing exercise may be beneficial to anyone, it would not be specific to this patient's complaint.
    (4) A local anesthetic lozenge may reduce local tenderness or soreness, but a more definitive treatment, including gingivectomy, may be required.
    (5) A fluoride mouth rinse may reduce the caries rate, but this is not usually the major problem with these patients.

49. (4) Phenytoin and phenobarbital are often used together to treat tonic-clonic seizures.
    (1) Absence seizures are treated with trimethadione.
    (2) Diabetes is treated with insulin or an oral hypoglycemic agent.
    (3) Cushing's syndrome is usually a result of administering excessive glucocorticoids.
    (5) Osteoporosis, a thinning of the bones, is treated wth estrogens and calcium.

50. (5) Diabetic patients who are taking oral hypoglycemic agents have no change in the incidence of peptic ulcers.
    (1) Patients who are diabetic may heal more slowly.
    (2) There is a potential for interaction between tolbutamide and aspirin, causing alterations in the blood glucose level.
    (3) Diabetic patients have a chance of more frequent infections because of their suppressed immunity.
    (4) Diabetic patients have a greater chance of exhibiting a hypoglycemic reaction with an overdose of their oral agent.

51. (5) Corticosteroids, because of their mineralocorticoid activity, usually produce hypertension (if the blood pressure is affected). Mineralocorticoid activity causes sodium and water retention, resulting in an elevated blood pressure.
    (1) Osteoporosis, or thinning of the bones, can be associated with long-term administration of steroids.
    (2) Infections, because of decreased immunity, are more frequent in patients taking steroids on a long-term basis.
    (3) The moon face exhibited by patients taking steroids on a long-term basis is secondary to their metabolic effects.
    (4) Because of an increase in stomach acid secretion, peptic ulcers may be exacerbated by adrenocorticoids.

52. (3) An adrenal crisis in the presence of stress may occur in a patient on long-term corticosteroid therapy. Additional steroids should be administered to prevent this possibility.
    (1) Hyperglycemia is most common in response to steroid therapy.
    (2) Hypertension usually results from steroids.
    (4) Epinephrine may be used in normotensive patients on long-term corticosteroid therapy. Even patients with a mild elevation of blood pressure may be given epinephrine cautiously.
    (5) Steroids have little effect on secretions in the mouth.

53. (5) A thyroid storm is associated with patients who are stressed and have hyperthyroidism.
    (1) Patients who are on long-term corticosteroid therapy may have prolonged healing.
    (2) Patients who are on long-term corticosteroid therapy may be more likely to get infections.
    (3) Potential erythema of the gums secondary to periodontitis may be suppressed by the antiinflammatory action of the steroids.
    (4) Because of the ulcerogenic potential of the steroids, additional ulcerogenic medication should be avoided.

54. (3) Colchicine commonly causes nausea, vomiting, and diarrhea.
    (1) Colchicine is not uricosuric.
    (2) Colchicine is not a xanthine oxidase inhibitor.
    (4) Aspirin does not interfere with colchicine's effectiveness.
    (5) Acetaminophen does not interfere with colchicine's effectiveness.

55. (3) Probenecid is uricosuric. Aspirin interferes with its effectiveness.
    (1) This is not a complete answer.
    (2) Probenecid is not a xanthine oxidase inhibitor.
    (4) Both of these are untrue.
    (5) Probenecid's action is unaffected by acetaminophen.

56. (4) Allopurinol is a xanthine oxidase inhibitor. It commonly causes nausea and vomiting.
    (1) Allopurinol is not uricosuric.
    (2) This is not a complete answer.
    (3) Probenecid is a uricosuric affected by aspirin administration.
    (5) Aspirin administration does not affect allopurinol's action.

CHAPTER 9

Biochemistry and Nutrition

MARY M. LEE

DIANNE M. FRAZIER

Humans are multicellular organisms who require an intake of specific chemicals or nutrients from food to grow and maintain homeostasis and optimal health. An understanding of cellular biochemistry and nutrition is essential for all health professionals actively involved in preventing and treating disease in patients. The science of nutrition includes the intake of food and all the processes involved in the digestion, absorption, transportation, metabolism, and excretion of nutrients in food. Nutrition is also an applied science that involves counseling patients to adapt food patterns to nutritional needs within the framework of a particular cultural, economic, and psychosocial environment. Nutritional counseling can be done effectively in the practice setting to motivate patients in modifying food habits so that better oral and general health can be achieved.

This chapter covers the six major nutrient groups and their metabolic activities in mammalian cells, dietary modifications for diseases, nutritional diseases and disorders, and oral manifestations of nutritional deficiencies and toxicities. Also described are the effects of nutrients on oral tissues and the dietary assessment tools and techniques available for counseling dental patients with various types of oral diseases. Since nutritional problems in the U.S. population are a result of overeating as well as undereating, the chapter includes a review of energy balances and weight control.

Cellular biochemistry is fundamental in studying nutrition; therefore the reader is referred first to Chapter 2, section on general histology and Chapter 3, section on cellular structures and organelles, for a review of the structural and functional similarities in cells.

SIX MAJOR CLASSES OF ESSENTIAL NUTRIENTS

Carbohydrates (CHO)

A. Definition—polyhydroxy aldehydes or ketones that serve as the body's primary source of quick energy; they are composed of basic units, monosaccharides, which contain carbon, hydrogen, and oxygen

B. Basic chemical structure
   1. Ratio of carbon, hydrogen, and oxygen is $1:2:1$
   2. Reactive portion of the molecule may be in a ketose or aldose form

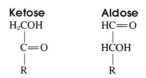

   3. Position of the hydroxyl (—OH) groups determines properties such as sweetness and absorbability

C. Classification
   1. Simple carbohydrates
      a. Monosaccharides
         (1) Trioses (C_3) and tetroses (C_4)—usually formed during intermediary metabolism and are not important dietary components
         (2) Pentoses (C_5)—important in nucleic acids and coenzymes, do not occur free (uncombined), and are not important dietary components (e.g., ribose)
         (3) Hexoses (C_6)—most important group physiologically
            (a) Glucose—blood sugar; primary energy source
            (b) Galactose—seldom found free but found in lactose
            (c) Fructose—fruit sugar; sweetest sugar; found in honey and fruits

b. Disaccharides—composed of two monosaccharide units
   (1) Sucrose—glucose plus fructose (cane and beet sugar)
   (2) Lactose—glucose plus galactose (milk sugar)
   (3) Maltose—glucose plus glucose (intermediate of starch hydrolysis [digestion])
c. Oligosaccharides—composed of two to six monosaccharide units

2. Complex carbohydrates
   a. Homopolysaccharides—made up of more than six identical monosaccharide units
      (1) Starch—plant storage form of glucose; source of half of dietary carbohydrates
         (a) Amylose—straight chain
         (b) Amylopectin—branched chain
      (2) Glycogen—animal storage form of glucose; found in the liver and muscle of living animals; insignificant source of dietary carbohydrates
      (3) Cellulose—chief constituent of the framework of plants; glucose units are in β-linkages, not capable of being hydrolyzed by human digestive enzymes; provides bulk and fiber to the diet
      (4) Inulin—''starch'' made up of fructose units used in kidney function tests
   b. Heteropolysaccharides—carbohydrates associated with noncarbohydrate molecules

   (1) Pectin, lignin—important contributors to fiber in the diet
   (2) Glycoproteins—carbohydrate and protein in a specific, functional arrangement (e.g., blood group substances and many hormones)
   (3) Glycolipids—carbohydrate and lipid, as in gangliosides
   (4) Mucopolysaccharides—protein and carbohydrate in a loose binding
      (a) Hyaluronic acid—vitreous humor and joint lubricant
      (b) Heparin—anticoagulant
      (c) Chondroitin sulfate—cartilage, skin, bone, and teeth
      (d) Keratin sulfate—nails and teeth

D. Digestion, absorption, and transport
   1. Digestion (Table 9-1)
      a. Mouth
         (1) Teeth and tongue—mechanical breakdown and mixing of food
         (2) Saliva—hydration and lubrication of food
         (3) Amylase (ptyalin)—initial enzymatic hydrolysis of starch
      b. Stomach—no digestive enzymes for carbohydrates; initial enzymatic hydrolysis of starch by amylase may continue
      c. Small intestines
         (1) Pancreatic juices—amylases

Table 9-1 Digestive action at various points along the gastrointestinal tract

	Carbohydrates	Proteins	Fats
Mouth	Salivary amylase: starch → maltose	No action	No action
Stomach	Salivary amylase*: starch → maltose	Pepsin: proteins → smaller peptides HCl: activates pepsin and denatures proteins	Gastric lipase†: short- and medium-chain triglycerides → fatty acids + monoglycerides
Small intestine Pancreatic enzymes	Pancreatic amylase: starch → maltose	Trypsin, chymotrypsin, carboxypeptidase: proteins, polypeptides → dipeptides, amino acids	Pancreatic lipase: triglycerides → fatty acids + monoglycerides
Bile salts	No action	No action	Bile salts: emulsification of fats
Brush border enzymes	Disaccharidases: disaccharides → monosaccharides	Aminopeptidases, dipeptidases: dipeptides → amino acids	Lecithinase: lecithin → monoglyceride + fatty acid + PO_4 + choline
Large intestine	Some fermentation of undigested nutrients but with negligible absorption of the fermentation products		

*A small amount of action within the bolus of swallowed food.
†A minor role in total fat digestion.

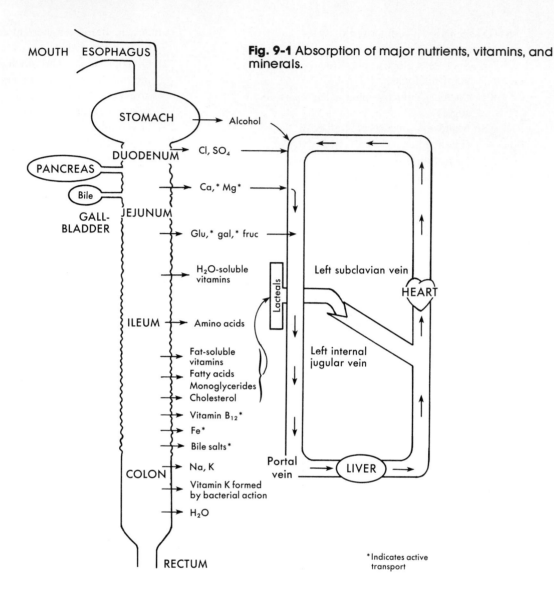

Fig. 9-1 Absorption of major nutrients, vitamins, and minerals.

*Indicates active transport

(2) Intestinal villi (brush border) enzymes—
disaccharidases
   (a) Sucrase—converts sucrose to
      glucose and fructose
   (b) Lactase—converts lactose to
      glucose and galactose
   (c) Maltase—converts maltose to
      glucose
 d. Large intestine—bacterial "fermentation"
of some undigested carbohydrates
   (1) No significant contribution to absorbable
carbohydrates
   (2) May be the cause of gas production and
bloating during primary or secondary
disaccharidase deficiency

2. Absorption (Fig. 9-1)
  a. Factors affecting absorption
    (1) Intestinal motility
    (2) Type of food mixture
    (3) Integrity of intestinal mucosa
    (4) Endocrine activity
  b. Mechanism
    (1) Passive diffusion along the osmotic
gradient (when the intestinal
concentration of carbohydrates is greater
than the blood level)
    (2) Active transport with the aid of a
sodium carrier at the brush border

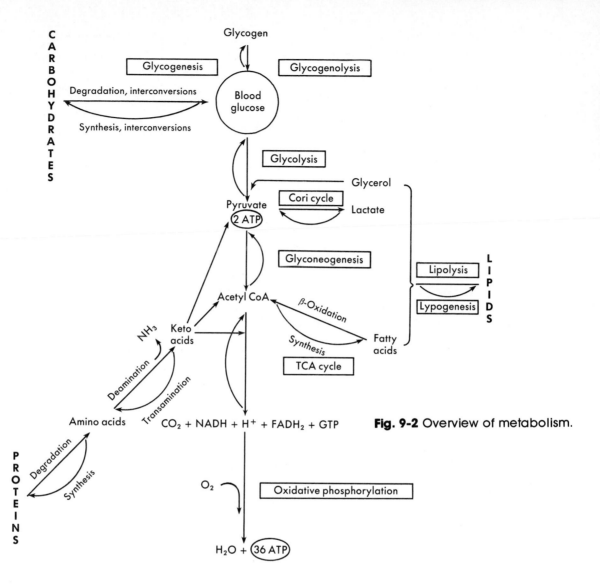

Fig. 9-2 Overview of metabolism.

c. Route
   (1) Carbohydrates are water soluble and are absorbed directly into the capillaries of the intestinal mucosa
   (2) Carried via the portal circulation to the liver
E. Metabolism—glucose is the main immediate source of energy for the body; a glucose level of 80 to 120 mg/100 ml blood is maintained by most healthy persons (Fig. 9-2)
   1. Sources of blood glucose
      a. Dietary carbohydrates—sugars, starches
      b. Stored liver glycogen breakdown—glycogenolysis
      c. Synthesis from intermediary metabolites such as pyruvic acid—glyconeogenesis
      d. Synthesis from noncarbohydrate sources by glyconeogenesis
         (1) Deaminated (glucogenic) amino acids
         (2) Glycerol portion of lipids

   2. Reactions of blood glucose—"burned" for energy
      a. Glycolysis—end product is pyruvate or lactic acid in the absence of oxygen (anerobic conditions) or acetylcoenzyme A (acetyl-CoA) in the presence of oxygen (aerobic conditions)
      b. Tricarboxylic acid cycle (TCA) or Krebs cycle—burning of acetyl-CoA with the release of carbon dioxide (CO_2)
      c. Oxidative phosphorylation and electron transport—production of adenosine triphosphate (ATP) (a high-energy molecule) and water (H_2O)

3. Storage for reserve use
   a. Glycogenesis—glycogen in the short-term shortage form of glucose (6 to 18 hours)
   b. Lipogenesis—excess carbohydrate in the diet is converted to fat to be stored in adipose tissue as a long-term energy storage form
4. Conversion to other molecules
   a. To other carbohydrates needed for structural or functional molecules
   b. To ketoacids to be used in the synthesis of amino acids for protein synthesis
F. Metabolic regulators
   1. Anabolic hormones (lower the blood glucose level)—insulin
      a. Increases entry of glucose into cells
      b. Increases glycogenesis
      c. Increases lipogenesis
   2. Catabolic hormones (raise the blood glucose level)
      a. Glucagon—stimulates glycogenolysis
      b. Steroid hormones—stimulate glyconeogenesis
      c. Epinephrine—stimulates glycogenolysis
      d. Growth hormone and adrenocorticotropic hormone (ACTH)—act as insulin antagonists
      e. Thyroxine—increases insulin breakdown, glucose intestinal absorption, and epinephrine release
   3. Coenzymes—B-complex vitamins are important precursors of the coenzymes involved in the metabolism of carbohydrates
G. Biologic role and functions
   1. Provide precursors of structural and functional molecules (e.g., gangliosides)
   2. Energy source (4 kcal/g)
   3. Spare protein
   4. Provide bulk and palatability to the diet
H. Oral biology
   1. Preeruptive effect on teeth
      a. Energy source for growth and development
      b. Protein-sparing nutrient
   2. Posteruptive effect on teeth (Fig. 9-3)
      a. Energy source for oral cariogenic bacteria (e.g., *Streptococcus mutans*)
      b. Acidogenic bacteria metabolize monosaccharides and disaccharides, particularly sucrose, for the production of energy through glycolysis that results in the formation of lactic acid and other acids
      c. *S. mutans* synthesizes polysaccharides (glucans, levans, and glycogen) from sucrose

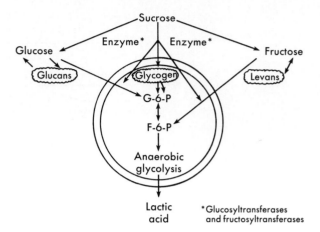

Fig. 9-3 Streptococcal cell. (From Lee, M., Stanmeyer, W., and Wight, A.: Nutrition and dental health, Part II, Diet and dental bacteriology, Carrboro, N.C., 1982, Health Sciences Consortium, Inc.)

         (1) Polysaccharides are used for energy when sucrose is unavailable
         (2) Glucans form insoluble complexes with *S. mutans* and have a strong affinity for enamel, thus enhancing plaque formation
      d. Firm texture of some complex carbohydrates, like raw fruits and vegetables, can help to remove food debris retained between teeth; chewing action can also stimulate salivary flow
   3. Dietary sweeteners (Table 9-2)
      a. Nutritive sweeteners are used by the body as an energy source; they provide calories
         (1) Sugar alcohols (xylitol, sorbitol, and mannitol) are noncariogenic nutritive sweeteners that are slowly fermented through anaerobic metabolism by oral bacteria; excessive intakes of these polyols can cause diarrhea because of the osmotic transfer of water into the bowel
         (2) Aspartame is a noncariogenic nutritive sweetener consisting of two amino acids: aspartic acid and phenylalanine; because it is at least 100 times sweeter than sucrose, the amount needed as a sugar substitute provides negligible calories; it has a large margin of safety for human consumption; since it is unstable and loses its sweetening power in low-pH and high-temperature environments, it is not used in frying and baking

Table 9-2 Dietary sweeteners

Type	Nutritive (N)/ Nonnutritive (NN)	Sweetener	Relative sweetness*	Relative acid production (cariogenicity)*
Sugars	N	Sucrose	1.0	1.0
		Glucose (dextrose)	0.7	†
		Fructose	1.1 to 1.7	0.8 to 1.0
		Lactose	0.4	0.4 to 0.6
		Maltose	0.5	†
		Galactose	0.6	†
Sugar alcohols	N	Sorbitol	0.5	0.1 to 0.3
		Mannitol	0.7	0
		Xylitol	0.9	0
Natural	N	Honey (fructose and glucose)	0.7 to 0.9	1.0
		Molasses (sucrose and invert sugar)	1.0	1.0
		Brown sugar (sugar and molasses)	1.0	1.0
Others	N	Glucose syrups	0.3 to 0.6	1.0
		High-fructose corn syrups	1.0 to 1.5	1.0
		Corn sweetners	1.0	1.0
Dipeptides	N	Aspartame	120 to 280	0
Artificial	NN	Sodium saccharin	200 to 700	0

From Lee, M., Stanmeyer, W., and Wight, A.: Nutrition and dental health, Part II, Diet and dental bacteriology, Carrboro, N.C., 1982, Health Sciences Consortium, Inc.
*Relative to sucrose = 1.0.
†Information not available.

(3) All other natural and synthetic nutritive sweeteners are cariogenic
   b. Nonnutritive sweeteners are calorie free and have no nutritive value; saccharin is the only nonnutritive sweetener approved by the Food and Drug Administration (FDA); it is noncariogenic
4. Cariogenicity factors of diet habits (in order of importance)
   a. Frequency of sugar intake—the more frequent the exposure to sugar, the more cariogenic the diet; six candy bars eaten at six different times during the day are more harmful in terms of acid and plaque formation than if the six candy bars were consumed at one time
   b. Form of sugar (liquid or retentive)—liquid sweets clear the oral cavity faster than solid or retentive sweets and therefore are less cariogenic
   c. Time of sugar ingestion—combining sweets with liquids and other noncariogenic foods during a meal is less cariogenic than a concentrated exposure to sweets between meals as a snack

   d. Total sugar intake—annual consumption of sugar for each American is over 100 pounds; 60% of the sugar intake is from processed foods (e.g., cereal), which are often called "hidden sugars"
   e. Combining cariogenic foods with noncariogenic foods—recent studies indicate that certain cariogenic foods (e.g., canned pears in syrup) are less cariogenic when combined with a particular noncariogenic food (e.g., cheese)
5. Carbohydrate importance in periodontal health
   a. Energy source for the growth and repair of periodontal tissues
   b. Protein-sparing nutrient
   c. Dietary monosaccharides and disaccharides enhance supragingival bacterial growth and plaque formation; these bacteria set the stage for the growth and development of subgingival bacteria and plaque that are responsible for the destructive effects of advanced periodontitis
   d. Firm texture of complex carbohydrates can promote circulation in gingival tissue

I. Requirements
  1. Minimum adult intakes (60 to 100 g) prevent use of body protein as an energy source; children and infants need additional carbohydrates to provide energy and spare protein for growth and development
  2. Recommendations
    a. Calories from simple carbohydrates (monosaccharides and disaccharides)—10% or less of the total caloric intake
    b. Calories from complex carbohydrates (including fiber)—48% or more of the total caloric intake
J. Dietary modifications for disease
  1. Obesity—cut total calories and percentage of simple carbohydrates (concentrated sweets) to increase the nutrient density of a lower-calorie diet
  2. Genetic defects
    a. Lactose intolerance (inability to hydrolyze lactose)—eat fewer milk products, use fermented products, or add a commercial lactase enzyme to milk
      (1) Primary—congenital absence of the lactase enzyme
      (2) Secondary—temporary or permanent loss of lactase activity resulting from intestinal injury or disease
    b. Galactosemia (congenital inability to metabolize galactose)—remove lactose and milk products from the diet
    c. Fructose intolerance (congenital inability to metabolize fructose)—remove fructose from the diet
  3. Dental caries and periodontal disease—protective diet
    a. Eat a diet that is low in retentive carbohydrates
    b. Do not eat cariogenic snacks
    c. Eat a diet that is adequate in all nutrients
    d. Include foods of firm or hard texture
  4. Diabetes (inability to metabolize glucose because of insufficient production of insulin)—dietary treatment
    a. Eat a high-fiber diet
    b. Eat a high-carbohydrate diet (50% to 60% of calories)
    c. Regulate carbohydrate intake and meal spacing during the day
    d. Coordinate food intake with medication
    e. Control weight—80% of patients with type II diabetes are overweight
  5. Reactive hypoglycemia—rare; symptoms of dizziness, hunger, and heart palpitations are lessened with a low-carbohydrate diet
  6. Dumping syndrome—after gastric surgery; postprandial symptoms of nausea, dizziness, cramping, and diarrhea are lessened by a low-carbohydrate diet
  7. Alcoholism—overconsumption of alcohol may cause malnutrition
    a. Depresses the appetite
    b. Empty-calorie food
    c. Causes vitamin B depletion because the liver needs niacin and thiamin to metabolize alcohol
    d. Causes folate and iron deficiency
    e. Depresses the antidiuretic hormone, causing loss of magnesium, potassium, and zinc in the urine
  8. Carbohydrate regulation in hyperlipoproteinemias—in types IIb, III, IV, and V, total carbohydrate and alcohol intake is controlled and concentrated sweets are restricted

Proteins

A. Definition—complex biologic compounds of high molecular weight containing nitrogen, hydrogen, oxygen, carbon, and small amounts of sulfur; each protein (PRO) has a specific size and is made up of amino acid building blocks linked through peptide bonds in a specific arrangement
B. Classifications
  1. Chemical
    a. Simple proteins—contain amino acids only
    b. Compound proteins (conjugated)—contain simple proteins and a nonprotein group
      (1) Nucleoproteins
      (2) Metalloproteins
      (3) Phosphoproteins
      (4) Lipoproteins
    c. Derived—fragments produced during digestion or hydrolysis (e.g., peptides, peptones, and proteoses)
  2. Biologic
    a. Complete proteins contain sufficient amounts of the essential amino acids for normal metabolic reactions; found in foods of animal origin
      (1) Essential amino acids cannot be synthesized by humans and must be provided in the diet in sufficient amounts to meet needs
        (a) Adult—isoleucine, leucine, lysine, methionine, phenylalanine, threonine, tryptophan, and valine
        (b) Infant—all of the above plus histidine
        (c) Premature infant—all of the above plus cysteine

(2) Nonessential amino acids can be synthesized by the body and need not be provided by the diet but are necessary for normal metabolic reactions

b. Incomplete proteins have insufficient quantities of one or more essential amino acids; plant proteins are often incomplete (e.g., corn protein is low in lysine; legume protein is low in methionine)

c. Complementary proteins are proteins that, when ingested singly, are incomplete but, when combined, provide sufficient essential amino acids

(1) In a vegan (or strict vegetarian) diet, the complementarity of plant proteins can be accomplished by combining appropriate incomplete proteins in the same meal; vegetarians often develop deficiencies in vitamin B_{12}, iron, and essential amino acids; major foods for these nutrients are from animal sources

(2) In an ovolacto vegetarian diet, milk and egg proteins can provide the essential amino acids that are inadequate in incomplete plant proteins

d. Protein quality is a measure of a protein's ability to support protein synthesis; it is measured by comparing the test protein with a reference protein, usually egg protein

(1) Amino acid or protein chemical score—compares proteins by their essential amino acid content

(2) Protein efficiency ratio (PER)—measures a protein's ability to support growth

(3) Biologic value (BV)—expression of the percentage of nitrogen retained for maintenance and growth compared with the amount absorbed

(4) Net protein utilization (NPU)—expression of the percentage of nitrogen retained compared with the amount ingested; differs from BV because it takes into account the protein's digestibility

C. Structure

1. Primary—linear sequence of the component amino acids

2. Secondary—steric relationship of amino acids that are close to one another in the linear sequence (e.g., the α-helix and the collagen helix)

3. Tertiary—steric relationship between amino acids far apart in the linear sequence that causes folding and the ultimate functional structure of the protein (e.g., globular, fibrous, and pleated sheet)

4. Quaternary—steric interaction between subunits of proteins with more than one polypeptide chain (e.g., hemoglobin; this is also a functional form)

D. Digestion, absorption, and transport (see Table 9-1 and Fig. 9-1)

1. Mouth—mechanical breakdown and moistening

2. Stomach

a. Hydrochloric acid from the parietal cells denatures or unfolds proteins and activates pepsinogen to give pepsin

b. Pepsin begins the hydrolysis of the peptide bonds of proteins to form peptides and proteoses

3. Small intestine

a. Pancreas secretes bicarbonate into the duodenum to neutralize the acidic products from the stomach and proteolytic enzymes in an inactive form; enzymes, activated by trypsin through a hormonal feedback mechanism, are chymotrysin, aminopeptidase, carboxypeptidase, and trypsin; each hydrolyzes peptide bonds formed by different classes of amino acids

b. Enzymes of the brush border are dipeptidases that hydrolyze dipeptides to amino acids

4. Absorption—at the brush border of the microvilli of the small intestine, absorption occurs by both simple diffusion along a concentration gradient and by active transport at specific amino acid sites involving carrier enzymes, a sodium-ATP pump, and vitamin B_6

5. Transport—absorbed amino acids are collected by the portal blood system and transported to the liver

E. Metabolism (see Fig. 9-2)

1. Amino acid pool—collection of amino acids in a dynamic equilibrium in the liver, blood, and other cells that provides the raw material for the body's protein and amino acid needs

a. Input into the pool comes from proteins in the diet, breakdown of body proteins, and synthesis of nonessential amino acids

b. Output from the pool is for synthesis of body structures, specialized substances (e.g., melanin from tyrosine), and energy as needed

2. Anabolism
   a. De novo synthesis—deoxyribonucleic acid (DNA), messenger ribonucleic acid (mRNA), and ribosomal ribonucleic acid (rRNA)
      (1) In the nucleus the DNA carries the genetic information in groups of three bases that make up the code for the individual amino acids
      (2) mRNA transports a copy of the code from the DNA into the cytoplasm
      (3) mRNA attaches to a ribosome and acts as a template for the alignment of amino acids that are attached to transfer RNA (tRNA)
      (4) If the proper amino acids are in the correct proportions and the synthetic enzymes and energy are available, the polypeptide chain is synthesized
   b. Transamination
      (1) Nonessential amino acids can be synthesized from the corresponding α-keto acids, an α-amino acid (as the NH_3^+ donor), a specific transaminase enzyme, and the coenzyme pyridoxal phosphate (vitamin B_6)
      (2) Intermediate complex formed in this reaction is called a Schiff base
3. Catabolism—amino acids in excess of those needed for the synthesis of proteins and other biomolecules cannot be stored or excreted; they may, however, be deaminated and the α-keto acid used as a metabolic fuel for immediate energy needs or for long-term energy storage as fat
   a. Amino group
      (1) Deamination—loss of the α-amino group, usually in the liver, through transfer to α-ketoglutarate to form glutamate; glutamate is then oxidatively deaminated to yield ammonia (NH_3)
      (2) Urea cycle—series of steps whereby the ammonia produced during deamination is converted to urea for excretion
   b. α-Keto acid
      (1) Ketogenic amino acids are those whose carbon skeleton, after deamination, yields acetyl-CoA or acetoacetyl-CoA, which then yields ketone bodies; high concentrations of ketone bodies lead to some of the undesirable side effects of high protein–low carbohydrate diets

      (2) Glycogenic amino acids are those that yield pyruvate, α-ketoglutarate, and other intermediates of the citric acid cycle that can, if needed, be converted to glucose
4. Nitrogen balance—comparison of the amount of nitrogen ingested with the amount excreted (e.g., urinary nitrogen plus about 1 g/day for nail, hair, skin, and perspiration losses) to determine whether there is net protein catabolism, anabolism, or equilibrium
   a. Positive balance—intake is greater than output; indicates net protein synthesis and is the normal situation for anyone building protein-containing tissue such as during childhood, pregnancy, and recovery from undernutrition, surgery, or illness
   b. Negative balance—intake is less than output; indicates net protein breakdown, when the body must break down its own protein to meet energy or metabolic needs; can result from insufficient protein or energy intake or from fever, infection, anxiety, or prolonged stress
F. Metabolic regulation
   1. Hormones
      a. Anabolic—growth hormone, insulin, normal thyroid hormone, and sex hormones
      b. Catabolic—adrenocortical hormones and large amounts of thyroid hormone
   2. Vitamins—pyridoxine and riboflavin are necessary for protein synthesis; when they are deficient in the diet, synthesis may be limited
G. Functions
   1. Structural
      a. Collagen and elastin
      b. Bone and tooth matrix
      c. Myosin fibrils
      d. Keratin
   2. Dynamic
      a. Transport of nutrients
         (1) Lipids and fat-soluble vitamins
         (2) Iron—transferrin
         (3) Oxygen—hemoglobin and myoglobin
         (4) Protein-bound molecules
         (5) Membrane transport
      b. Regulation and control
         (1) Immunoglobulins
         (2) Buffers
         (3) Hormones
         (4) Enzymes
         (5) Blood coagulation—fibrin
         (6) Muscle contraction—actin and myosin

3. Energy source (4 kcal/g)
4. Oral biology
   a. Preeruptive effects on teeth—essential for all cells and therefore necessary for normal tooth bud and pulp formation and synthesis of protein matrix for enamel and dentin
   b. Posteruptive effects on teeth
      (1) Essential for maintaining the integrity of pulpal tissue throughout life
      (2) Chemical nature of protein foods can neutralize acids produced by oral bacteria
   c. Periodontal health and disease
      (1) Essential for all cells in growth, development, and maintenance of the periodontium
      (2) Essential for the normal function of cellular defenses against subgingival bacteria and toxins
      (3) Necessary in the healing and repair of injured tissues from periodontitis or periodontal surgery

H. Requirements
   1. Determination and estimates of protein requirements
      a. Nitrogen-balance studies are used to determine the lowest protein intake that will support homeostasis
      b. Factoral method estimates maintenance requirements for adults on a protein-free diet (0.45 g/kg body weight)
      c. Estimates for growth needs in infants are based on the amount of protein provided by that quantity of milk that ensures a satisfactory growth rate
   2. Recommended Dietary Allowances (RDAs) developed by the National Research Council; based on the factoral method, with an added factor to allow for the 75% efficiency with which proteins are used and 30% more for the variation among individual needs (0.8 g protein/kg body weight); these allowances assume ingestion of a good-quality protein in a mixed diet; adjustments are made for growth, pregnancy, and lactation (Table 9-3)
   3. Food sources—protein needs of an average adult can be met by choosing two or more servings per day from any of the following groups: meats, poultry, fish, eggs, milk and dairy products, dried beans and peas, and nuts

I. Dietary modifications for disease
   1. Genetic disorders
      a. Phenylketonuria (PKU)—inherited enzyme defect in which individuals cannot metabolize the phenylalanine found in nearly all proteins; prescribed diet provides only enough phenylalanine to meet growth needs; dietary protein is restricted, but amino acids are provided by a synthetic, milklike formula from which most of the phenylalanine has been removed
      b. Maple syrup urine disease, homocystinuria, histidinemia, and tyrosinemia—other genetic disorders in which amino acid metabolism is altered, and patients are treated with low-protein diets and synthetic amino acid formulas
      c. Gout—characterized by excessive uric acid production leading to the formation of urate crystals deposited in the joints; treatment often includes restriction of protein to limit purine (and uric acid) production
   2. Protein needs are increased during fever and after severe injury, surgery, intestinal malabsorption, increased protein loss from the kidneys, or diminished protein synthesis by the liver
   3. Dietary protein must be restricted when the kidneys can no longer remove nitrogenous wastes from the body or in severe liver disease when the nitrogenous by-products of protein catabolism can no longer be synthesized
   4. Protein-energy (calorie) malnutrition
      a. Kwashiorkor (classical)—failure of the young child to grow because of an insufficient protein intake (usually because of weaning from the mother's milk); often edema masks muscle wasting
      b. Marasmus (classical)—failure of the infant or young child to grow because of partial starvation; total caloric intake, as well as protein intake, is insufficient

Lipids (Fats)

A. Definition—biochemical compounds composed of carbon, hydrogen, oxygen, and small amounts of phosphorus; they are insoluble in water and soluble in fatty substances and organic solvents
B. Classification
   1. Simple lipids

Table 9-3 Food and Nutrition Board, National Academy of Sciences — National Research
of good nutrition of practically

	Age (years)	Weight		Height		Protein (g)	Fat-soluble vitamins		
		(kg)	(lb)	(cm)	(in)		Vitamin A (μ RE)†	Vitamin D (μ g)‡	Vitamin E (mg α-TE)§
Infants	0.0-0.5	6	13	60	24	kg × 2.2	420	10	3
	0.5-1.0	9	20	71	28	kg × 2.0	400	10	4
Children	1-3	13	29	90	35	23	400	10	5
	4-6	20	44	112	44	30	500	10	6
	7-10	28	62	132	52	34	700	10	7
Males	11-14	45	99	157	62	45	1000	10	8
	15-18	66	145	176	69	56	1000	10	10
	19-22	70	154	177	70	56	1000	7.5	10
	23-50	70	154	178	70	56	1000	5	10
	51+	70	154	178	70	56	1000	5	10
Females	11-14	46	101	157	62	46	800	10	8
	15-18	55	120	163	64	46	800	10	8
	19-22	55	120	163	64	44	800	7.5	8
	23-50	55	120	163	64	44	800	5	8
	51+	55	120	163	44	44	800	5	8
Pregnant						+30	+200	+5	+2
Lactating						+20	+400	+5	+3

From Recommended dietary allowances, ed. 9, Washington, D.C., 1980, National Academy Press.
*The allowances are intended to provide for individual variations among most normal persons as they live in the United States under usual
ments have been less well defined.
†Retinol equivalents. 1 retinol equivalent = 1 μg retinol or 6 μg β-carotene.
‡As cholecalciterol. 10 μg cholecalciferol = 400 IU of vitamin D.
§α-Tocopherol equivalents. 1 mg d-α tocopherol = 1 α-TE.
‖ NE (niacin equivalent) is equal to 1 mg of niacin or 60 mg of dietary tryptophan.
¶ The folacin allowances refer to dietary sources as detemined by *Lactobacillus casei* assay after treatment with enzymes (conjugases) to
**The recommended dietary allowance for vitamin B-12 in infants is based on average concentration of the vitamin in human milk. The
other factors, such as intestinal absorption.
††The increased requirement during pregnancy cannot be met by the iron content of habitual American diets nor by the existing iron
tially different from those of nonpregnant women, but continued supplementation of the mother for 2-3 months after parturition is advisable

a. True fats—contain fatty acids attached to glycerol (a trihydroxy alcohol) through an ester linkage; these may be monoglycerides, diglycerides, or triglycerides, depending on the number of glycerol-hydroxyl groups esterified; chemical and biochemical characteristics of the glycerides depend on the number, order, and kind of fatty acids attached
  (1) Saturated fatty acids—contain no double bonds and are found in lipids from animal sources; are solids at room temperature (high melting point)
  (2) Unsaturated fatty acids—contain one or more double bonds and come from plant sources; are usually liquids at room temperature (low melting point)
  (3) Hydrogenation—addition of hydrogen to some or all of the double bonds; this is done in making margarine or butter substitutes from vegetable oils
  (4) Rancidity—addition of oxygen to some of the double bonds of fatty acids that contributes to spoilage; occurs spontaneously in foods and can be lessened by the addition of antioxidants such as butylated hydroxytoluene (BHT)
  (5) Iodine number—chemical indication of the degree of unsaturation of a fatty acid; the more molecules of iodine bound by the fatty acid, the more unsaturated and the higher the iodine number
b. Waxes—esters of a fatty acid and an alcohol other than glycerol; body is unable to use waxes because digestive enzymes do not hydrolyze their ester linkage
2. Compound lipids contain compounds added to the glycerol and fatty acids
  a. Phospholipids

  Glycerol + 2 Fatty acids + Phosphate group + R group

Council recommended daily dietary allowances, revised 1980 (designed for the maintenance all healthy people in the USA)*

Water-soluble vitamins							Minerals					
Vitamin C (mg)	Thia-min (mg)	Ribo-flavin (mg)	Niacin (mg NE)‖	Vitamin B-6 (mg)	Fola-cin¶ (µg)	Vitamin B-12 (µg)	Cal-cium (mg)	Phos-phorus (mg)	Mag-nesium (mg)	Iron (mg)	Zinc (mg)	Iodine (µg)
35	0.3	0.4	6	0.3	30	0.5**	360	240	50	10	3	40
35	0.5	0.6	8	0.6	45	1.5	540	360	70	15	5	50
45	0.7	0.8	9	0.9	100	2.0	800	800	150	15	10	70
45	0.9	1.0	11	1.3	200	2.5	800	800	200	10	10	90
45	1.2	1.4	16	1.6	300	3.0	800	800	250	10	10	120
50	1.4	1.6	18	1.8	400	3.0	1200	1200	350	18	15	150
60	1.4	1.7	18	2.0	400	3.0	1200	1200	400	18	15	150
60	1.5	1.7	19	2.2	400	3.0	800	800	350	10	15	150
60	1.4	1.6	18	2.2	400	3.0	800	800	350	10	15	150
60	1.2	1.4	16	2.2	400	3.0	800	800	350	10	15	150
50	1.1	1.3	15	1.8	400	3.0	1200	1200	300	18	15	150
60	1.1	1.3	14	2.0	400	3.0	1200	1200	300	18	15	150
60	1.1	1.3	14	2.0	400	3.0	800	800	300	18	15	150
60	1.0	1.2	13	2.0	400	3.0	800	800	300	18	15	150
60	1.0	1.2	13	2.0	400	3.0	800	800	300	10	15	150
+20	+0.4	+0.3	+2	+0.6	+400	+1.0	+400	+400	+150	††	+5	+25
+40	+0.5	+0.5	+5	+0.5	+100	+1.0	+400	+400	150††	††	+10	+50

environmental stresses. Diets should be based on a variety of common foods in order to provide other nutrients for which human require-

make polyglutamyl forms of the vitamin available to the test organism.
allowances after weaning are based on energy intake (as recommended by the American Academy of Pediatrics) and consideration of

stores of many women; therefore the use of 30-60 mg of supplemental iron is recommended. Iron needs during lactation are not substan-
in order to replenish stores depleted by pregnancy.

(1) Water-soluble emulsifiers (e.g., lecithin, where the R group is choline)
(2) Membrane constituents (e.g., sphingomyelin)
(3) Active intermediates in metabolism of lipid compound (e.g., coA)
b. Glycolipids—contain a carbohydrate component and are found in the brain and nervous tissue (e.g., cerebrosides)
c. Lipoproteins—are water soluble and are responsible for carrying lipids throughout the body
(1) Chylomicrons—about 2% protein; carry exogenous (absorbed from the diet) triglycerides around the body
(2) Very low density lipoproteins (VLDLs)—9% protein; carry endogenous triglycerides around the body
(3) Low-density lipoproteins (LDLs)—21% protein; carry mostly cholesterol from the liver to peripheral sites
(4) High-density lipoproteins (HDLs)—50% protein; carry cholesterol back to the liver; can be elevated by exercise
3. Derived lipids are compounds whose synthesis begins like that of fatty acid synthesis with acetyl groups added on one at a time
a. Sterols—all have a polycyclic nucleus as shown below

Cholesterol (chol) is a precursor for the synthesis of many steroid compounds and a constituent of cell membranes
(1) Sources
(a) Exogenous—average dietary intake is 600 mg from foods of animal origin
(b) Endogenous—average synthesis in the body is 1 to 2 g/day

(2) Regulation of cholesterol synthesis depends on total body cholesterol, dietary cholesterol, and percentage of fat in the diet

b. Steroids—similar to sterols but with side-chain modification (e.g., bile acids, sex hormones, adrenocortical hormones, and vitamin D)

C. Digestion, absorption, and transportation (see Table 9-1 and Fig. 9-1)

1. Digestion
   a. Mouth—no enzymatic action; mechanical and moistening action only
   b. Stomach—gastric lipase hydrolyzes some short- and medium-chain fatty acids from triglycerides
   c. Small intestine
      (1) Gallbladder—bile salts emulsify fats before digestion
      (2) Pancreas—pancreatic lipase (steapsin) hydrolyzes fatty acids from triglycerides to form diglycerides and monoglycerides
      (3) Intestinal mucosa—lecithinase converts lecithin to fatty acids, monoglyceride, phosphate, and choline

2. Absorption and transport
   a. Short-chain fatty acids can be absorbed into the portal system
   b. Medium- and long-chain fatty acids are water insoluble, require bile as a carrier (emulsifier), and are absorbed in stages
      (1) Bile separated out at the intestinal wall and recirculated
      (2) Complete breakdown of triglycerides within the mucosal cells by mucosal lipase
      (3) Resynthesis of new triglycerides that combine with protein carriers to form chylomicrons
      (4) Passage into the lymph system (lacteals) and the blood via the thoracic duct
      (5) At its destination, lipoprotein lipase hydrolyzes the triglycerides, clearing chylomicrons from the blood
      (6) Lipoprotein carriers (VLDLs, LDLs, and HDLs) carry endogenous lipids and cholesterol

D. Metabolism (occurs in liver and adipose tissue; see Fig. 9-2)

1. Anabolism
   a. Lipogenesis—synthesis of triglycerides for long-term storage of energy; starting material is acetyl-CoA, which can come from glucogenic amino acids, carbohydrates, or breakdown of dietary lipids; lipogenesis takes places in nearly all cells but is most active in adipose cells
   b. Synthesis of steroids occurs in all cells
   c. Synthesis of lipoproteins occurs mainly in the liver

2. Catabolism
   a. β-Oxidation—fatty acids are broken down in a stepwise manner to yield one molecule of acetyl-CoA for every two carbon atoms; acetyl-CoA can be catabolized further via the TCA and oxidative phosphorylation
   b. Ketone production—when the body's supply of carbohydrates is low, the TCA is depressed and acetyl-CoA from β-oxidation accumulates; alternate route for acetyl-CoA is ketone production; acetoacetone, acetone, and β-hydroxyl butyrate are the ketone bodies; excess ketone production can cause ketosis, ketonuria, and ketoacidosis (a sometimes fatal condition)

E. Metabolic regulators

1. Vitamins as coenzymes precursors
   a. Anabolism—biotin, riboflavin (in flavin adenine dinucleotide [FAD]) niacin (in nicotinamide-adenine dinucleotide [NAD]) and pantothenic acid (in CoA) (see Fig. 9-2)
   b. Catabolism—riboflavin, niacin, and pantothenic acid

2. Hormones
   a. Anabolism—insulin
   b. Catabolism—ACTH, thyroid-stimulating hormone (TSH), epinephrine, and glucagon

3. Enzymes necessary for the metabolism of lipids are synthesized or inhibited in response to the relative amounts of substrates and products available

F. Biologic role and functions

1. Structural components of cell membranes
2. Energy source
   a. Provides 9 kcal/g (compared with 4 kcal/g for protein or carbohydrates)
   b. Long-term storage form of energy
3. Carrier of fat-soluble vitamins
4. Protective padding for body organs
5. Insulation for the maintenance of body temperature
6. Oral biology
   a. Cariostatic properties
      (1) Oils in fats provide a coating on the tooth's surface and prevent retention of food particles

(2) Oils provide a fatty protective layer over plaque and prevent fermentable sugars from entering plaque or acids from leaving plaque
    b. No fat-periodontal relationship
G. Requirements
    1. Essential fatty acids (EFAs)—cannot be synthesized in sufficient amounts to meet needs; must be supplied in the diet; for humans the only EFA is linoleic acid; requirement is 1% to 2% of total kilocarlories for adults and 3% for infants
        a. Function—necessary for the synthesis of membranes and prostaglandins (local hormone)
        b. Deficiency symptoms—seen in infants on low–polyunsaturated fatty acid (PUFA) diets and adults receiving total parenteral nutrition feedings without lipids; characterized by slow growth and eczema
    2. Recommendations (U.S. dietary goals)
        a. Total fats less than or equal to 30% of total kilocalories
        b. Cholesterol less than or equal to 300 mg/day
        c. Saturated fats less than or equal to 10% of total kilocalories, with an approximately equal amount of polyunsaturated and monounsaturated fats
    3. Prudent diet from the New York City Anti-Coronary Club
        a. Reduced intake of foods high in cholesterol, saturated fats, and simple carbohydrates
        b. Increased intake of foods rich in PUFA and complex carbohydrates (cereals, grains, fruits, and vegetables)
    4. Fast foods may contain 38% to 48% of kilocalories as fat because of the type of preparation; one should make judicious choices to keep the total daily intake of lipids within the recommendations
H. Dietary modifications for disease
    1. Cardiovascular disease (CVD)—blood vessel lumens become narrower and sometimes completely blocked because of the accumulation of fatty substances, cellular debris, and calcium; blood pressure and the work required of the heart is increased; formation of clots is increased, and the result may be a heart attack (myocardial infarction) or stroke

a. Hyperlipoproteinemias—elevation of serum VLDL, LDL, and chylomycron levels is a diagnostic tool that indicates a patient is at risk for CVD; there is a genetic predisposition for certain hyperlipoproteinemias; elevated HDL levels may exert a protective effect against CVD; routine exercise elevates HDL levels in most people
        b. Dietary factors that may increase serum lipids—high intakes of cholesterol, saturated fats, total fats, sucrose, fructose and ethanol (alcohol)
        c. Dietary factors that may decrease serum lipids—PUFAs, vitamin D, and pectin; ethanol in moderate amounts may have a protective effect by increasing HDL levels; unidentified substances in garlic, yeast, onions, and some wines may also have a protective effect
    2. Obesity—because fats are a concentrated source of calories (9 kcal/g), most reducing diets recommend a decrease in fat intake; fat should not be too severely restricted, because it adds to the palatability and satiety of the diet
    3. Gallbladder disease and chronic pancreatitis—often cause pain after lipid ingestion; diet may have to be restricted in fats until the conditions are corrected.
    4. Cystic fibrosis and malabsorption disorders—often treated by using synthetic medium-chain triglyceride formulas that are more easily absorbed
    5. Dumping syndrome and gastric ulcers—often treated by increasing fat in the diet to delay gastric emptying
    6. Epilepsy—children with some types of epilepsy may be effectively treated with a ketogenic diet that is high in fats, low in carbohydrates, and causes a ketotic condition

Vitamins

A. Definition—organic substances that are essential to life and are needed in very small amounts; serve regulatory functions and often act as coenzymes or precursors of coenzymes; vitamins are present in food, but some can be produced in precursor form or activated in the body
B. Classification
    1. Water-soluble vitamins
        a. Vitamin C
        b. B-complex vitamins

2. Fat-soluble vitamins
   a. Vitamin A
   b. Vitamin D
   c. Vitamin E
   d. Vitamin K
C. Chemistry and general properties
   1. Water-soluble vitamins
      a. Soluble in water
      b. Sensitive to heat, light, and oxygen
      c. Contain the elements carbon, hydrogen, oxygen, and nitrogen and in some cases other elements such as cobalt or sulfur
      d. Absorbed into the blood by both active and passive transport from the upper portion of the digestive tract (see Fig. 9-1); vitamin B_{12} requires intrinsic factor for absorption
      e. Transported free and unbound to cells in the blood

   f. Minimal storage of dietary excesses except for
      (1) Vitamin C—stores may last 30 to 90 days
      (2) Vitamin B_{12}—stores may last 6 years
      (3) Folic acid—stores may last 4 to 5 months
   g. Excreted in urine
   h. Should be supplied in the diet nearly every day
   i. Deficiency symptoms often develop rapidly
   j. Relatively nontoxic with excessive dietary intakes, although the increased use of over-the-counter megavitamin preparations has caused the appearance of toxic symptoms
   2. Fat-soluble vitamins
      a. Soluble in fat and fat solvents (some water-soluble derivates are available)

Table 9-4 Estimated safe and adequate daily dietary intakes of selected vitamins and minerals*

| | Age (years) | Vitamins | | |
		Vitamin K (μg)	Biotin (μg)	Pantothenic acid (mg)
Infants	0-0.5	12	35	2
	0.5-1	10-20	50	3
Children	1-3	15-30	65	3
and	4-6	20-40	85	3-4
adolescents	7-10	30-60	120	4-5
	11+	50-100	100-200	4-7
Adults		70-140	100-200	4-7

| | Age (years) | Trace elements† | | | | | |
		Copper (mg)	Manganese (mg)	Fluoride (mg)	Chromium (mg)	Selenium (mg)	Molybdenum (mg)
Infants	0-0.5	0.5-0.7	0.5-0.7	0.1-0.5	0.01-0.04	0.01-0.04	0.03-0.06
	0.5-1	0.7-1.0	0.7-1.0	0.2-1.0	0.02-0.06	0.02-0.06	0.04-0.08
Children	1-3	1.0-1.5	1.0-1.5	0.5-1.5	0.02-0.08	0.02-0.08	0.05-0.1
and	4-6	1.5-2.0	1.5-2.0	1.0-2.5	0.03-0.12	0.03-0.12	0.06-0.15
adolescents	7-10	2.0-2.5	2.0-3.0	1.5-2.5	0.05-0.2	0.05-0.2	0.10-0.3
	11+	2.0-3.0	2.5-5.0	1.5-2.5	0.05-0.2	0.05-0.2	0.15-0.5
Adults		2.0-3.0	2.5-5.0	1.5-4.0	0.05-0.2	0.05-0.2	0.15-0.5

| | Age (years) | Electrolytes | | |
		Sodium (mg)	Potassium (mg)	Chloride (mg)
Infants	0-0.5	115-350	350-952	275-700
	0.5-1	250-750	425-1275	400-1200
Children	1-3	325-975	550-1650	500-1500
and	4-6	450-1350	775-2325	700-2100
adolescents	7-10	600-1800	1000-3000	925-2775
	11+	900-2700	1525-4575	1400-4200
Adults		1100-3300	1875-5625	1700-5100

From Recommended dietary allowances, ed. 9, Washington, D.C., 1980, National Academy Press.
*Because there is less information on which to base allowances, these figures are provided here in the form of ranges of recommended intakes.
†Since the toxic levels for many trace elements may be only several times usual intakes, the upper levels for the trace elements given in this table should not be habitually exceeded.

b. More stable in light, heat, and oxygen than water-soluble vitamins

c. Contain only elements of carbon, hydrogen, and oxygen

d. Must be emulsified and carried across the membranes of the intestinal cells in the presence of fat and bile (see Fig. 9-1); any conditions that decrease the digestion, absorption, or transport of lipids will lower the usable amount of fat-soluble vitamins

e. Absorbed into the lymphatic system and transported by attachment to protein carriers

f. Intake in excess of the daily need is stored in the body

g. Not readily excreted

h. Not absolutely necessary in the diet every day

i. Deficiency symptoms slow to develop

j. Toxic with chronic excessive intake

D. General functions

  1. Water-soluble vitamins

    a. Coenzymes for energy metabolism

    b. Synthesis of red blood cells and DNA

  2. Fat-soluble vitamins

    a. Vision

    b. Maintenance of the body's mucosal linings and epithelial cells

    c. Integrity of mineralized tissues of bone and teeth by regulating calcium and phosphorus levels in the body

    d. Cellular antioxidant

    e. Normal blood clotting

E. Requirements (Tables 9-3 and 9-4)

F. Dietary sources, specific body functions, and symptoms of deficiencies and toxicities (Table 9-5)

Table 9-5 Dietary sources and functions of vitamins

Vitamin	Dietary sources	Major body functions	Deficiency	Excess
WATER-SOLUBLE				
Vitamin B₁ (thiamine)	Meat (especially pork and organ meats), grains, dry beans and peas, fish, poultry.	Coenzyme (thiamine pyrophosphate) in reactions involving the removal of carbon dioxide in carbohydrate metabolism.	Beriberi (peripheral nerve changes, edema, heart failure).	None reported.
Vitamin B₂ (riboflavin)	Widely distributed in both animal and vegetable foods.	Constituent of two flavin nucleotide coenzymes involved in energy metabolism (FAD and FMN).	Cracks at corner of mouth (cheilosis), inflammation of lips, glossitis.	None reported.
Niacin (can be formed from tryptophan)	Liver, meat, fish, grains, legumes, poultry, peanut butter.	Constituent of two coenzymes involved in oxidation-reduction reactions (NAD and NADP).	Pellagra (skin and gastrointestinal lesions, nervous, mental disorders).	Flushing, burning and tingling around neck, face and hands.
Vitamin B₆ (pyridoxine)	Meats (liver), vegetables, whole-grain cereals, egg yolks.	Coenzyme (pyridoxal phosphate) involved in amino acid metabolism.	Irritability, convulsions, muscular twitching, kidney stones, microcytic hypochromic anemia.	None reported.
Pantothenic acid	Widely distributed in all foods; organ meats and whole-grain cereals.	Constituent of coenzyme A, which plays a central role in energy metabolism.	Fatigue, sleep disturbances, impaired coordination, nausea (rare in man).	None reported.
Folacin	Liver, kidney, yeast, mushrooms, green vegetables.	Coenzyme (reduced form) involved in transfer of single-carbon units in nucleic acid and amino acid metabolism.	Anemia, gastrointestinal disturbances, diarrhea, glossitis.	None reported.

From Lee, M., Stanmeyer, W., and Wight, A.: Nutrition and dental health, Part I, Assessment of human nutrition requirements, Carrboro, N.C., 1982, Health Sciences Consortium, Inc.

Continued.

Table 9-5 Dietary sources and functions of vitamins—cont'd

Vitamin	Dietary sources	Major body functions	Deficiency	Excess
WATER-SOLUBLE				
Vitamin B_{12} (cobalamin)	Muscle and organ meats, eggs, dairy products (not present in plant foods).	Coenzyme involved in synthesis of single-carbon units in nucleic acid metabolism.	Pernicious anemia, neurological disorders.	None reported.
Biotin	Liver, kidney, milk, egg yolk, yeast.	Coenzymes required for synthesis and oxidation of fats, carbohydrates and deamination.	Fatigue, depression, nausea, dermatitis, muscular pains, loss of hair.	Not reported.
Vitamin C (ascorbic acid)	Citrus fruits, tomatoes, green peppers, broccoli, spinach, strawberries, melon.	Maintains intercellular matrix of cartilage, bone and dentin. Important in collagen synthesis, utilization of iron, calcium and folic acid.	Scurvy (degeneration of skin, teeth, blood vessels, epithelial hemorrhages), delayed wound healing, anemia.	Relatively nontoxic, possibility of kidney stones.
FAT-SOLUBLE				
Vitamin A (retinol)	Provitamin A (beta-carotene) widely distributed in green and yellow vegetables and fruits. Retinol present in milk, butter, cheese, fortified margarine, egg yolk.	Constituent of rhodopsin (visual pigment). Maintenance of epithelial tissues. Role in mucopolysaccharide synthesis, bone growth and remodeling.	Xerophthalmia (keratinization of ocular tissue), night blindness, folliculosis, respiratory infections.	Headache, vomiting, peeling of skin, anorexia, swelling of long bones, resorption of bones.
Vitamin D	Fish-liver oil, eggs, dairy products, fortified milk and margarine.	Promotes growth and mineralization of bones and teeth, increases absorption of calcium at intestines.	Rickets (bone deformities) in children. Osteomalacia in adults.	Vomiting, diarrhea, loss of weight, kidney damage, hypercalcemia.
Vitamin E (tocopherol)	Vegetable oils and seeds, green leafy vegetables, margarines, shortenings.	Functions as an antitoxidant, in cellular respiration, synthesis of body compounds.	Possibly anemia.	Relatively nontoxic.
Vitamin K (phylloquinone)	Green and yellow vegetables. Small amount in cereals, fruits and meats.	Important in blood clotting (involved in formation of active prothrombin).	Conditioned deficiencies associated with severe bleeding, internal hemorrhages.	Relatively nontoxic. Synthetic forms at high doses may cause jaundice.

Table 9-6 Nutrients and their preeruptive effects on oral health

Nutrient	Role in tooth formation	Deficiencies*
Vitamin A	1. Normal growth of dentin and enamel.	1. Hypoplastic enamel formation. 2. Atrophy of odontoblasts with abnormal dentin tubular arrangement.
Vitamin C	1. Integrity of blood vessels. 2. Hydoxylation of proline and lysine in collagen synthesis.	1. Atrophy of odontoblasts. 2. Dentin laid down irregularly and at a greatly reduced rate. 3. Fragility of vessels in pulpal tissue.
Protein	1. Major organic substance in enamel and dentin. 2. Collagen formation.	1. Small size teeth. 2. Late eruption of third molars. 3. Altered cuspid patterns. 4. Increased susceptibility to carious lesions. 5. Poorly calcified dentinal matrix.
Calcium-phosphorus ratio	1. Normal tooth mineralization.	1. Decreased molar size. 2. Decreased mineralization of enamel and dentin.
Vitamin D	1. Control of calcification of dentin and enamel by regulating calcium absorption at intestines.	1. Non-functioning ameloblasts with poor enamel mineralization. 2. Disturbances in calcification of dentin and cementum. 3. Delays in tooth eruption. 4. Small size molars.
Fluoride	1. Forms strong dentin and enamel apatite crystals through a systemic action.	1. Increases solubility of enamel and dentin.
Selenium	1. Excessive intake during tooth formation changes protein components of enamel and makes it more prone to caries attack.	
Magnesium	1. Cofactor for enzymes involved with the transfer of phosphate groups.	1. Atrophy of ameloblasts and odontoblasts. 2. Retardation of dentin formation and hypoplastic enamel.

From Lee, M., Stanmeyer, W., and Wight, A.: Nutrition and dental health, Part III, Diet and teeth, Carrboro, N.C., 1982, Health Sciences Consortium, Inc.
*Many of these deficiencies have been demonstrated in animal research only.

G. Oral biology
  1. Functions
    a. Tooth formation (Table 9-6)
    b. Periodontium (Table 9-7)
  2. Oral manifestations of deficiencies and toxicities (Table 9-8)

Minerals

A. Definition—inorganic elements that are essential to life; serve both structural and regulatory functions
B. Classification (Table 9-9)
  1. Macrominerals—present in relatively high amounts in body tissues
  2. Microminerals or trace elements—present at less than 0.005% of body weight
C. Chemistry and general functions
  1. Exist as inorganic ions
  2. Chemical identity not altered in the body or food
  3. Indestructable
  4. Soluble in water and tend to form acidic or basic solutions
  5. Vary in amounts absorbed and in pathways of excretion (see Fig. 9-1)
  6. Some readily absorbed into the blood and transported freely
  7. Some require carriers for absorption and transportation
  8. Excessive intakes can be toxic
D. General functions
  1. Maintenance of acid-base balance
  2. Coenzymes or catalysts for biologic reactions
  3. Components of essential body compounds
  4. Maintenance of water balance
  5. Transmission of nerve impulses
  6. Regulation of muscle contraction
  7. Growth of oral and other body tissues

Table 9-7 Nutrients and their effects on oral soft and hard tissues

Nutrient	Function
Proteins (amino acids)	1. Synthesis of epithelial and connective tissues. 2. Synthesis of collagen. Essential for integrity of connective tissue fibers in soft tissues and the protein matrix in mineralized tissues. 3. Synthesis of antibodies and leukocytes. Essential for tissues to defend against bacterial irritants. 4. Synthesis of new epithelial and connective tissue in the healing process.
Vitamin A	1. Synthesis and function of epithelial cells. 2. Maintenance of the integrity of sulcus, an important part of the epithelial barrier. 3. Normal growth and function of salivary glands. 4. Essential for activity of epiphyseal cartilage cells and normal endochondral bone growth. 5. Release of proteolytic enzymes (lysosomes) in bone remodeling.
Vitamin C	1. Synthesis of connective tissue. Essential for hydroxylation of lysine and proline in collagen synthesis. 2. Essential for integrity of capillaries and oral mucosa. 3. Needed for normal bone matrix formation. 4. Needed for normal phagocytic function and antibody synthesis in host defense system.
B-complex	1. Function as coenzymes for essential metabolic reactions in epithelial and connective tissues. 2. Essential for integrity of gingiva, tongue, buccal mucosa, hard and soft palate. 3. Needed for normal phagocytic function and antibody synthesis in host defense system.
Iron	1. Synthesis of hemoglobin. Essential for the transport of oxygen to cells for metabolic activity. 2. Essential for normal antibody formation and healing. 3. Essential part of many enzymes.
Calcium	1. Functions in mineralization of protein matrix in oral hard tissues. 2. Essential for normal blood clotting, cell membrane function, muscle contraction and nerve impulse transmission.
Vitamin D	Essential for absorption and utilization of calcium and phosphorus.
Retentive sugars	1. Enhances growth of acidogenic bacteria. 2. Results in increased formation of bacterial irritants, such as acids, enzymes and endotoxins. 3. Enhances plaque formation and adherence.

From Lee, M., et al.: Nutrition and dental health, Part IV, Diet and periodontics, Carrboro, N.C., 1982, Health Sciences Consortium, Inc.

Table 9-8 Oral manifestations of nutritional deficiences and toxicities

Tissue	Nutrient	Deficiency symptoms	Toxicity symptoms
Oral mucosa	Vitamin A	Keratinizing of epithelium (squamous metaplasia) with hyperketatotic white patches; generalized gingivitis.	Thinning of epithelium resulting in inflamed, hemorrhagic membranes. Reddened gingiva.
	Vitamin C	Deep red to purple inflamed gingiva with edema, hyperplasia, spontaneous hemorrhaging, ulceration and necrosis.	None
	Thiamin (B_1)	Hypersensitivity and burning sensations.	None
	Riboflavin (B_2)	Occasional bluish to purple mucosa.	None
	Niacin	Thin and parakeratotic epithelium. Inflammation of mucosa (stomatitis). Reddened and inflamed marginal and attached gingiva. Nonspecific burning sensation.	None
	Pyridoxine (B_6)	Stomatitis.	None
	Vitamin B_{12}	Stomatitis. Pale or tinged-yellow mucosa.	None
	Folic acid	Inflamed gingiva. Erosion and ulcerations on mucosa. Pale mucosa with anemia.	None
	Iron	Painful, sore mouth. Stomatitis. Thinned buccal mucosa with ulcerations and pale to ashen gray color.	None
	Zinc	Thickening of epithelium.	None

From Lee, M., et al.: Nutrition and dental health, Part IV, Diet and periodontics, Carrboro, N.C., 1982, Health Sciences Consortium, Inc.

Table 9-8 Oral manifestations of nutritional deficiences and toxicities—cont'd

Tissue	Nutrient	Deficiency symptoms	Toxicity symptoms
Tongue and lips	Vitamin A	None	Cracking and bleeding of lips.
	Thiamin (B$_1$)	Painful or burning tongue. Loss of taste acuity.	None
	Riboflavin (B$_2$)	Inflammation, fissures and ulcers at the corner of the lips (angular cheilitis); dry, scaly lips. Red to purple color tongue. Atropy and inflammation of tongue papillae. Enlarged fungiform papillae giving the tongue surface a pebbly appearance.	None
	Niacin	Atrophy of tongue papillae resulting in a fiery, red, smooth, shiny surface. Edematous or enlarged tongue. Ulcerations of tongue on central surface. Angular cheilitis. Loss of appetite.	None
	Pyridoxine (B$_6$)	Inflamed and atrophic tongue with a red, smooth appearance. Angular cheilitis.	None
	Vitamin B$_{12}$	Atrophy and inflammation of tongue. Bright red, painful, edematous tongue with glossy appearance. Altered taste sensations and decreased appetite.	None
	Folic acid	Smooth, bright red tongue. Patchy surface of tongue as papillae atrophy. Ulcerations along edges of tongue. Angular cheilitis.	None
	Iron	Angular cheilitis. Burning, painful tongue with atrophy of papillae. Reddening at tip and around margins of tongue. Ulcerations of tongue. Pallor to ashen grey color of lips and tongue.	None
	Zinc	Impaired taste. Thickening and parakeratotic tongue with underlying muscle atrophy.	None
	Protein	Red, smooth, edematous tongue. Angular cheilitis. Fissures on lower lip. Depigmentation along buccal border of lips.	None
Skin, eyes, salivary glands	Vitamin A	Drying of conjuctiva and cornea of eyes. Decreased salivary flow.	Dry, scaly skin lesion. A high carotene intake results in a yellow color skin.
	Riboflavin (B$_2$)	Greasy, scaly dermatitis of nasolabial folds. Keratinizing of corneal surface of eyes resulting in opacities and ulcerations.	None
	Niacin	Scaly and inflamed skin. Skin thickening with dark pigmentation of sunlight-exposed skin.	None
	Pyridoxine (B$_6$)	Seborrheic lesions of face.	None
Bone	Vitamin D and calcium	Failure to mineralize bone matrix resulting in soft, fragile bones with pathological fractures and skeletal deformities. Thinning of cortical bone, resorption of cancellous bone, and enlargement of medullary cavity resulting in overall bone loss. Osteomalacia manifested in loss of lamina dura around roots of tooth and increased width of cortical bone.	Calcium deposits in bone.
	Vitamin C	Defect in collagen formation of osteoid matrix resulting in resorption of alveolar bone.	None
Teeth	Fluoride	Less resistant tooth structure to oral irritants.	Fluorosis
	Refined carbohydrate	None	Dental caries Plaque formation
	Vitamin A	Abnormal formation of ameleoblasts and odontoblasts during early stages of tooth formation; results in hypoplastic enamel and dentin.	None
	Vitamin D, calcium	Abnormal calcification of enamel and dentin.	None

Table 9-9 Dietary sources and functions of minerals

Mineral	Dietary sources	Major body functions	Deficiency	Excess
MACROMINERALS				
Calcium	Milk, cheese, dark-green vegetables, dried legumes, bread.	Bone and tooth formation, blood clotting, nerve transmission, muscle contraction.	Stunted growth, rickets, osteoporosis, convulsions.	Not reported in man.
Phosphorus	Milk, cheese, meat. poultry, grains, eggs.	Bone and tooth formation, acid-base balance, release of energy (ADP, ATP).	Weakness, demineralization of bone, loss of calcium.	Erosion of jaw (fossy jaw).
Sulfur	Sulfur amino acids (methionine and cystine) in dietary proteins.	Constituent of active tissue compounds, cartilage and tendon.	Related to intake and deficiency of sulfur amino acids.	Excess sulfur amino acid intake leads to poor growth.
Potassium	Meats, milk, many fruits, fish, eggs.	Acid-base balance, body water balance, nerve function, muscle relaxant.	Muscular weakness, paralysis, heart abnormalities.	Muscular weakness, death.
Chlorine	Table salt, cured and pickled foods, broth.	Formation of gastric juice, acid-base balance.	Muscle cramps, mental apathy, reduced appetite.	Vomiting.
Sodium	Table salt, cured and pickled foods, broth, canned foods.	Acid-base balance, body water balance, nerve function.	Muscle cramps, mental apathy, reduced appetite.	Possibly high blood pressure.
Magnesium	Whole grains, green leafy vegetables, cocoa, nuts, soybeans.	Activates enzymes, involved in protein synthesis.	Growth failure, muscle tremors and convulsions.	Diarrhea.
MICROMINERALS				
Iron	Eggs, lean meats, liver, legumes, whole grains, green leafy vegetables, dried fruit.	Constituent of hemoglobin and enzymes involved in energy metabolism.	Iron-deficiency anemia (weakness, reduced resistance to infection).	Siderosis, cirrhosis of liver.
Fluorine	Drinking water, tea, seafood.	May be important in maintenance of bone structure, forms strong apatite crystals during tooth formation.	More susceptible to tooth decay.	Mottling of teeth, increased bone density, neurological disturbances.
Zinc	High protein foods, whole grains.	Constituent of enzymes involved in digestion and metabolism.	Growth failure, small sex glands.	Loss of iron and copper, anemia.
Copper	Meats, drinking water, shellfish, nuts, whole grains.	Constituent of enzymes associated with iron metabolism and nerve function.	Anemia, bone changes (rare in man).	Rare metabolic condition (Wilson's disease).
Selenium	Seafood, meat, grains.	Functions in close association with vitamin E as an antioxidant.	Anemia (rare).	Gastrointestinal disorders, lung irritation, increased tooth decay.
Manganese	Whole grains, legumes, nuts, tea, green leafy vegetables.	Normal skeletal development; involved in fat synthesis, urea formation, energy release.	In animals: poor growth, disturbances of nervous system, reproductive abnormalities.	Poisoning in manganese mines: generalized disease of nervous system, abnormal iron metabolism.

From Lee, M., Stanmeyer, W., and Wight, A.: Nutrition and dental health, Part I, Assessment of human nutrition requirements, Carrboro, N.C., 1982, Health Sciences Consortium, Inc.

Table 9-9   Dietary sources and functions of minerals—cont'd

Mineral	Dietary sources	Major body functions	Deficiency	Excess
		MACROMINERALS		
Iodine	Marine fish and shell-fish, dairy products, table salt, eggs.	Constituent of thyroid hormones, regulates energy metabolism.	Goiter (enlarged thyroid), cretinism, myxedema.	Very high intakes depress thyroid activity.
Molybdenum	Legumes, cereals, organ meats.	Constituent of enzymes involved in uric acid formation and oxidation of aldehydes.	Not reported in man.	Inhibition of enzymes, bone abnormalities.
Chromium	Vegetables, grains and cereals, fruit.	Involved in glucose and energy metabolism, protein synthesis.	Impaired ability to metabolize glucose.	Occupational exposures: skin and kidney damage.
Cobalt	Organ and muscle meats, milk, poultry, shellfish.	Constituent of vitamin B_{12}.	Not reported in man.	Enlarged thyroid gland, hyperplasia of bone marrow, polycythemia.

Table 9-10   Nutrients and their posteruptive effect on oral health

Nutrient	Effect on caries	Mode of action
Carbohydrates	Cariogenic (sucrose)	1. Substrate for glycolytic organisms to form complex organic acids. 2. Substrate for bacterial synthesis of intra and extra cellular polysaccharides (glucan, levan, glycogen). 3. Predisposes implantation of caries-inducing streptococci. 4. Predisposes formation and attachment of dental plaque on tooth's surface.
Fluoride	Cariostatic	1. Favors formation of fluorapatite crystal structure during remineralization of enamel. 2. Antimicrobial action. 3. Increases rate of maturation of enamel surface. 4. Reduces enamel solubility.
Phosphate	Cariostatic	1. Iso-ionic exchange of phosphate in oral environment. 2. Acts as a buffer. 3. Complexes calcium.
Other mineral elements	Cariostatic	1. Reduces enamel solubility. 2. Enhances maturation process.
Fats	Cariostatic	1. Produces a protective oily film on enamel. 2. Antimicrobial action.
All nutrients and firm textured foods	Salivary glands	1. Normal development. 2. Increases flow rate by mastication. 3. Influences composition of saliva.

From Lee, M., Stanmeyer, W., and Wight, A.: Nutrition and dental health, Part III, Diet and teeth, Carrboro, N.C., 1982, Health Sciences Consortium, Inc.

E. Requirements (see Tables 9-3 and 9-4)
F. Dietary sources, specific body functions, and symptoms of deficiencies and toxicities (see Table 9-9)
G. Oral biology
   1. Function

    a. Tooth formation (Table 9-10; see also Table 9-6)
    b. Periodontium (see Table 9-7)
  2. Oral manifestations of deficiencies and toxicities (see Table 9-8)

Water

A. Definition—essential nutrient abundantly found in foods and beverages; makes up 50% to 60% of the total body weight; survival without water is limited to 2 or 3 days

B. Total body water
1. Body water as a percentage of body weight decreases with age, ranging from 69% in newborn infants to 49% in women
2. Distribution
   a. Intracellular compartment
      (1) Enclosed inside the cell membrane of each cell
      (2) Accounts for two thirds of the total body water
      (3) Increases with increased body cell mass
   b. Extracellular compartment
      (1) Intravascular
         (a) Approximately 3 L
         (b) Includes water in blood vessels
      (2) Intercellular
         (a) Approximately 12 L
         (b) Fluids that leave blood vessels
         (c) Fluids present in spaces between and surrounding each cell

C. Biologic role and functions
1. Medium in which most of the body's reactions take place
2. Means for transporting vital materials to cells and waste products away from cells
3. Regulates a constant body temperature
4. Maintains a constant composition of elements in body fluids (e.g., calcium, sodium, and fluoride)
5. Part of the chemical structure of compounds that form cells (e.g., proteins)
6. Active in many chemical reactions (e.g., digestion of a disaccharide)
7. Serves as a solvent (e.g., amino acids dissolve in water, and this permits their transport to body cells)
8. Lubricates and protects sensitive tissue around joints and mucosal linings

D. Water balance
1. Intake—controlled by thirst sensations; total daily intake ranges from 1500 to 3000 ml
   a. Sources
      (1) Ingested beverages and foods
      (2) Metabolic water from the oxidation of foods
   b. Amounts
      (1) Between 1200 and 2000 ml daily for adults from beverages and foods
      (2) Between 200 and 300 ml daily from oxidation of foods
2. Elimination—total water output is 1500 to 3000 ml daily
   a. Sensible or measurable losses though the kidneys as urine and through the bowel as feces; constant daily losses amount to 650 to 1800 ml
   b. Insensible or unmeasurable losses through the lungs with expired air and skin as perspiration; daily losses vary considerably with an average of 850 to 1200 ml

E. Regulation
1. Potassium (K) and sodium (Na) concentrations are responsible for maintaining the water balance; when extracellular sodium equals intracellular potassium, water will not move into or out of the cell
2. Mechanisms of regulation
   a. Thirst response—when the sodium increases, it stimulates the hypothalamus and induces drinking behavior
   b. Excretion regulation
      (1) Increased sodium causes release of the antidiuretic hormone (ADH), and water is reabsorbed in the kidney tubules
      (2) Decreased sodium causes the release of aldosterone, which causes a reabsorption of sodium at the kidney tubules

F. Requirements
1. Adults—1000 ml/1000 calories
2. Infants—1500 ml/1000 calories

G. Etiology of deficiency and toxicity conditions
1. Dehydration
   a. Malfunction of kidneys
   b. Blood loss
   c. Vomiting
   d. Diarrhea
   e. No water supply
2. Water intoxication
   a. Edema
   b. Hypertension
   c. Sodium retention

SPECIALIZED CELLS OF ORAL TISSUES — EFFECTS OF NUTRIENTS

A. Epithelial cells
   1. Important in tooth formation during the embryonic period
   2. Make up the outer layers of tissue in the oral mucosa
      a. Rapid cell renewal, especially in the sulcus area
      b. Cell renewal more frequent as age increases
   3. Important in the normal development of salivary glands
   4. Vitamin A and protein are essential for the normal proliferation of epithelial cells
B. Fibroblasts
   1. Synthesize collagen fibrils in connective tissues of the gingiva, periodontal ligament, and pulp
   2. Throughout life, fibroblasts maintain a rate of collagen synthesis equal to that of collagen breakdown; nutrient deficiencies can interfere with this equilibrium and cause a net loss of collagen tissue
   3. Vitamin C, zinc, copper, and protein are important in collagen formation
C. Cementoblasts and cementocytes
   1. Synthesize the protein matrix for cementum; vitamin C, zinc, copper, and protein are essential
   2. Calcify the protein matrix; protein, calcium, phosphorus, and vitamin D are essential
   3. Cementum is avascular and part acellular
   4. Cellular cementum consists of cementocytes that depend on diffusion from the periodontal ligament for their nutrient supply
D. Ameleoblasts
   1. Synthesize the protein matrix for enamel; vitamins A and C, zinc, copper, and protein are essential
   2. Calcify the protein matrix; protein, calcium, phosphorus, and vitamin D are essential; fluoride improves the quality of the apatite crystals formed
   3. Once enamel is formed, no metabolic cells are present
E. Odontoblasts
   1. Synthesize the protein matrix for dentin; vitamins A and C, zinc, copper, and protein are essential
   2. Calcify the protein matrix; protein, calcium, phosphorus, and vitamin D are essential; fluoride improves the quality of the apatite crystals formed
   3. Once dentin is formed, no metabolic cells are present, except in reaction to trauma; with trauma, new odontoblasts can form (possibly from pulpal tissue) and secondary dentin can be laid down
F. Osteocytes—osteoblasts and osteoclasts
   1. Function in the synthesis of the alveolus
   2. Function in the lifelong process of bone apposition (osteoblasts) and resorption (osteoclasts) in the alveolus
   3. Nutrients important in the formation and maintenance of the alveolus are protein, vitamin C and D, zinc, copper, calcium, and phosphorus

ENERGY BALANCES AND WEIGHT CONTROL

A. Definition—energy balance is a dynamic state in which the energy or calories from food is equal to the energy needs of the body; changes or disturbances in energy balance result in a relative gain or loss in body weight
B. Measurement of energy
   1. By calorimetry—food sample is burned in oxygen in an enclosed vessel surrounded by water; 1 kcal is the amount of heat produced sufficient to raise the temperature of 1 kg of water 1° C; (the term *calorie* as commonly used has the same definition)
   2. In the body—carbon, hydrogen, and oxygen (from protein, carbohydrates, or fats) are converted to carbon dioxide, water, and energy; energy (kilocalories) produced is "stored" in ATP until needed; when needed, each ATP molecule loses a high-energy phosphate bond and becomes adenosine diphosphate (ADP) with a release of approximately 7.3 kcal/mole
C. Energy-producing systems
   1. Blood glucose—immediate and preferred source of energy for cellular metabolism; glycogen stores provide glucose through glycogenolysis during the short periods of fasting between meals and in response to hormonal signals during sudden movement or intense exercise
      a. Protein—can be used as an energy source when the blood glucose level falls; glucogenic amino acids are converted into glucose by gluconeogenesis; in starvation, body proteins are used for energy, and this may cause irreversible damage if the essential protein components of the body are catabolized

b. Fat—mobilized from adipose tissue; triglycerides are broken down into glycerol and fatty acids in the liver; fatty acids are catabolized by β-oxidation to acetyl-CoA

c. Ethanol (alcohol)—can be oxidized to acetaldehyde, which is then converted into acetyl-CoA

2. Acetyl-CoA—enters the TCA from all sources

3. ATP—made during the process of oxidative phosphorylation in the mitochondria; because of their difference in molecular structure, proteins, carbohydrates, and fats do not all yield the same number of ATP molecules per molecule of starting material; the following can be used as a general guide when estimating the potential energy of foods: protein, 4 kcal/g; carbohydrate, 4 kcal/g; fat, 9 kcal/g; and ethanol, 7 kcal/g

D. Energy-using systems—ATP produced during catabolism is used by the body for biosynthetic activities, muscle contraction, ion transport, nerve conduction, and maintenance of body temperature

1. Energy for basal metabolism—basal metabolic rate (BMR) is a measure of the energy required to maintain a living state while at rest and without food; includes respiration, circulation, maintenance of body temperature, muscle tone, glandular activities, and cellular metabolism

a. Conditions for BMR measurement—postabsorptive state, muscles totally relaxed, awake, environmental temperature between 20° and 25° C (68° and 77° F), free of emotional stress, and not during ovulation

b. Factors influencing the BMR—age, gender, body size, nutritional state, muscular training, pathologic conditions, climate, and altitude

2. Energy for activity—activity component of the energy requirement is for voluntary physical activity and varies from 20% of the BMR for sedentary activity to 50% or more of the BMR for heavy activity; factors influencing energy needs for the activity component include the size of the individual and the intensity and duration of the activity

3. Energy for metabolizing food, or the specific dynamic energy (SDE), is the energy required to "gear up" to digest, absorb, and metabolize food; also called "nonshivering thermogenesis" because there is a slight elevation in body temperature after eating; not a clearly defined phenomenon; believed to include the energy needed to increase muscular contractions of the digestive tract, increase synthesis of digestive enzymes, and transport molecules; amounts to about 10% of the BMR and activity energy components

E. Requirements

1. Determination—by an intake of food energy that allows maintenance of ideal weight; data have been gathered from animal studies, balance studies, and intake surveys

a. Recommendations represent average needs of people in each age group and within a given activity category (Tables 9-11 and 9-12)

b. Recommendations are influenced by body size, gender, climate, age, and activity level

2. Empty-calorie foods—provide energy but few other nutrients (e.g., concentrated sweets, alcohol, and fats); index of nutrient density or nutrient quality (INQ)

$$\frac{\text{Percent U.S. RDA for a nutrient}}{\text{Percent energy requirement}}$$

F. Weight-reduction programs

1. Calculation of caloric intake needs

a. Determine the ideal body weight (IBW) from published tables (see Table 9-11) or by using the following rule of thumb

(1) Males IBW = 106 + (6 × inches over 5 feet tall)

(2) Females IBW = 100 + (5 × inches over 5 feet tall)

b. Determine the caloric requirement (kilocalories/pound)

	Activity level		
	Sedentary	Moderate	Very active
Overweight	10	11	12
Normal	13	14	15
Underweight	16	17	18

c. Alternate method—decrease in usual caloric intake by 500 kcal/day usually allows a 1 pound/week weight loss; this loss may plateau as the body adjusts to a new BMR

Table 9-11 Suggested desirable weights for heights and ranges for adult males and females

Height*		Weight†					
		Men			Women		
in	cm	lb		kg		lb		kg	
58	147	—		—		102	(92-119)	46	(42-54)
60	152	—		—		107	(96-125)	49	(44-57)
62	158	123	(112-141)	56	(51-64)	113	(102-131)	51	(46-59)
64	163	130	(118-148)	59	(54-67)	120	(108-138)	55	(49-63)
66	168	136	(124-156)	62	(56-71)	128	(114-146)	58	(52-66)
68	173	145	(132-166)	66	(60-75)	136	(122-154)	62	(55-70)
70	178	154	(140-174)	70	(64-79)	144	(130-163)	65	(59-74)
72	183	162	(148-184)	74	(67-84)	152	(138-173)	69	(63-79)
74	188	171	(156-194)	78	(71-88)	—		—	
76	193	181	(164-204)	82	(74-93)	—		—	

From Recommended dietary allowances, ed. 9, Washington, D.C., 1980, National Academy Press.
*Without shoes
†Without clothes. Average weight ranges in parentheses.

Table 9-12 Mean heights and weights and recommended energy intake*

Category	Age (years)	Weight (kg)	Weight (lb)	Height (cm)	Height (in)	Energy needs (kcal)	Energy needs (with range)	Energy needs (MJ)
Infants	0.0-0.5	6	13	60	24	kg × 115	(95-145)	kg × 0.48
	0.5-1.0	9	20	71	28	kg × 105	(80-135)	kg × 0.44
Children	1-3	13	29	90	35	1300	(900-1800)	5.5
	4-6	20	44	112	44	1700	(1300-2300)	7.1
	7-10	28	62	132	52	2400	(1650-3300)	10.1
Males	11-14	45	99	157	62	2700	(2000-3700)	11.3
	15-18	66	145	176	69	2800	(2100-3900)	11.8
	19-22	70	154	177	70	2900	(2500-3300)	12.2
	23-50	70	154	178	70	2700	(2300-3100)	11.3
	51-75	70	154	178	70	2400	(2000-2800)	10.1
	76+	70	154	178	70	2050	(1650-2450)	8.6
Females	11-14	46	101	157	62	2200	(1500-3000)	9.2
	15-18	55	120	163	64	2100	(1200-3000)	8.8
	19-22	55	120	163	64	2100	(1700-2500)	8.8
	23-50	55	120	163	64	2000	(1600-2400)	8.4
	51-75	55	120	163	64	1800	(1400-2200)	7.6
	76+	55	120	163	64	1600	(1200-2000)	6.7
Pregnancy						+300		
Lactation						+500		

From Recommended dietary allowances, ed. 9, Washington, D.C., 1980, National Academy Press.
*The data in this table have been assembled from the observed median heights and weights of children, together with desirable weights for adults for the mean heights of men (70 inches) and women (64 inches) between the ages of 18 and 34 years as surveyed in the U.S. population (HEW/NCHS data). The energy allowances for the young adults are for men and women doing light work. The allowances for the two older age groups represent mean energy needs over these age spans, allowing for a 2% decrease in basal (resting) metabolic rate per decade and a reduction in activity of 200 kcal/day for men and women between 51 and 75 years, 500 kcal for men over 75 years, and 400 kcal for women over 75 years. The customary range of daily energy output is shown in parentheses for adults and is based on a variation in energy needs of ±400 kcal at any one age, emphasizing the wide range of energy intakes appropriate for any group of people. Energy allowances for children through age 18 are based on median energy intakes of children of these ages followed in longitudinal growth studies. The values in parentheses are tenth and ninetieth percentiles of energy intake, to indicate the range of energy consumption among children of these ages. *MJ*, Megajoule.

2. Types of diet modifications
   a. Balanced, low calorie—if calories are about 1000 kcal/day and the intake is balanced and varied, this is the safest and healthiest reducing diet (e.g., Weight Watchers Diet)
   b. Low carbohydrate—may risk developing ketosis (e.g., Stillman's Diet)
   c. Low fat—may deprive the individual of essential fatty acids and fat-soluble vitamins; causes rapid emptying of the stomach (low satiety) and may make food seem flavorless; most individuals can decrease their usual fat intake without any harmful effects
   d. High fiber—increases fiber and bulk in the diet and allows a more rapid transit time for food in the gastrointestinal tract; fiber also binds other nutrients so they are not completely absorbed; moderate increases in the fiber content of the diet (such as in well-designed vegetarian diets) appear to be helpful in treating diabetes, diverticulosis, and hypercholesterolemia, as well as decreasing the total calorie intake in reducing diets; very high fiber diets cause gastrointestinal discomfort and may induce mineral deficiencies (e.g., Beverly Hills Diet)
   e. Single food (monotonous)—no one food by itself can provide a balance of nutrients; one must eat a variety of foods from the Basic Four food groups; diets that promote a single food with unrealistic claims are not recommended (e.g., the grapefruit diet)
   f. Liquid formulas (protein)—are very low calorie diets, and although they have been successfully used in treating very obese patients in a carefully monitored hospital setting, they are not recommended for the individual (e.g., Cambridge Diet)
3. Activity in weight management—even moderate activity such as walking will increase caloric expenditure and should be considered in every weight-loss program; moderate exercise also improves muscle tone, stimulates circulation, and often creates a sense of well-being
4. Behavior modification—often eating habits and attitudes need to be changed to prevent weight regain; many successful diet programs combine decreased food intake and increased activity with an analysis and modification of eating behaviors; group programs such as Weight Watchers help provide behavioral changes

5. Dietary aids—represent a multimillion dollar business, and although they may help cause an initial rapid weight loss, they are no more effective than mere calorie cutting in long-term weight maintenance; moreover, most diet drugs have the potential for serious side effects if used habitually over a long period or by persons with certain medical conditions; types most often used are appetite suppressants, stimulants, laxatives, diuretics, and bulk-producing agents
6. Long-term success in weight reduction by any plan is poor, with an estimated average success rate of only 5%

G. Underweight conditions
   1. Treatment
      a. Correct any underlying physiologic causes of weight loss
      b. Increase caloric intake with foods that are concentrated sources of energy and with several small meals per day
      c. Limit weight-gain goals to 1 to 2 pounds/week
   2. Anorexia nervosa—state of emaciation brought on by voluntary starvation (and usually with the use of diet aids, intense exercise, and self-induced vomiting); seen most often in middle- and upper-income adolescent females who are typically described as perfectionists, overachievers, and models of good behavior; they may begin dieting because they feel they are obese when actually they are either of normal weight or only slightly overweight; treatment usually includes psychiatric or psychologic counseling and hospitalization before voluntary weight gain is possible
   3. Bulimia—condition of alternate food gorging and purging by vomiting and/or use of laxatives to maintain weight; most often found in adolescent females who appear to be of normal weight; treatment involves counseling; self-induced vomiting can cause swelling of the salivary glands and esophagus and acid-destruction of tooth enamel

NUTRITIONAL COUNSELING ▄▄▄▄▄▄
Malnutrition

A. Overconsumption of nutrients
   1. Fat—can result in excess calories and weight; associated with coronary heart disease (CHD), obesity, and breast cancer
   2. Sugar—can result in excess calories and weight; associated with obesity, dental caries, and plaque-induced gingivitis

3. Salt or sodium—can result in excess body fluid retention; associated with high blood pressure
4. Calories—can result in excess weight and obesity; associated with CHD, hypertension, and diabetes mellitis type II
5. Vitamin and mineral supplementation—megadoses (500% to 1000% of U.S. RDAs) can result in toxicity of one or many nutrients

B. Nutrient deficiencies—health of a patient is at risk because of the unavailability of nutrients for cellular activities; end result of deficiencies is the same, but the multiple causes can be classified as primary or secondary
   1. Primary deficiency is a result of an inadequate food intake and can result from the following conditions
      a. Fad diets—low calorie or imbalanced diet plans
      b. Economics—inadequate food-purchasing power
      c. Illness—loss of appetite
      d. Improper food preparation—destruction of nutrients because of delayed storage and overcooking of foods
      e. Accessibility to food—nutritious foods unavailable because of patient transportation problems or market supplies
      f. Ignorance—lack of nutritional knowledge
      g. Flavor preferences—palatability of sweets and fats can lead to a diet high in empty-calorie foods
      h. Time constraints—inadequate time for food preparation can lead to the use of highly processed convenience foods, which have a lower nutrient density than the basic foods
      i. Poor oral health—inability to masticate food because of edentulism or oral disease; altered taste perceptions result from oral disease
   2. Secondary deficiency is a result of an inability to digest, absorb, and use foods consumed; patient may eat a balanced diet, but other factors interfere with the use of nutrients in foods; examples of these conditioning factors include
      a. Disease—any gastrointestinal or metabolic disease can interfere with the digestion and use of foods and nutrients (e.g., ulcers, lactase deficiency, partial obstruction of the gastrointestinal tract, and inborn errors or metabolism)
      b. Drug-nutrient interactions—certain drugs can interfere with and reduce the absorption, transportation, and metabolism of nutrients

      c. Allergies—sensitivity to certain foods or chemicals in foods can lead to malabsorption syndromes (e.g., gluten sensitivity such as in celiac disease)
   3. Manifestations of primary and secondary deficiencies
      a. Gradual decreases in the tissue level of nutrients
         (1) Earliest sign of malnutrition
         (2) Determined by blood and urine analysis for each nutrient
      b. Biochemical disturbances
         (1) Duration of deficiency is long enough to deplete body stores and interfere with cellular metabolism
         (2) Determined by blood and urine analysis for alterations in cellular levels of enzymes and metabolites
      c. Anatomic lesions
         (1) Signs of chronic and severe malnutrition, leading to destruction of body tissues
         (2) Determined by clinical examination of body tissues

Nutritional Assessment

A. Medical history
   1. Factors that influence food intake
      a. Socioeconomic conditions—food-purchasing power
      b. Home environment—family values and eating practices
      c. Patient motivation and education—interest and awareness of the principles for eating a nutritious diet
   2. Factors that influence food use
      a. Oral health—ability to masticate, saliva production, and presence of oral disease
      b. Medical health—ability to digest, absorb, and metabolize nutrients in food; therapeutic diets for disease control

B. Assessment of dietary intakes
   1. Collection of objective data on what a patient eats
      a. Assessment tools—screening questionnaire, 24-hour recall method, and food record or diary
      b. Specific amounts or quantities of foods eaten must be recorded to use assessment tools
   2. Analysis and evaluation of food intake
      a. Methods of analysis—Basic Four food groups, computer analysis for specific nutrients

Table 9-13 Some laboratory tests of blood and urine used in the evaluation of nutritional status*

Body fluid	General level of nutrient or metabolite tested	Nutrient imbalance suggested†
Whole blood	Low ascorbate	↓ Ascorbate
	Low hemoglobin	
	Low erythrocytes (hematocrit)	↓ Iron
Erythrocytes	Low folate	↓ Folate
Blood serum	High cholesterol	
	High triglycerides	↑ Lipids
	High lipoproteins	↑ Kcal
	Low albumin	↓ Protein
	Low total protein	
	Low vitamin B_{12}	↓ Vitamin B_{12}
	Low thymidylate synthetase	
	Low vitamin A	
	Low carotene	↓ Vitamin A
	Low 25-OH cholecalciferol	
	Low alkaline phosphatase	↓ Vitamin D
	Low-calcium and phosphorus	
Blood plasma	Low amino acids	↓ Protein
Urine	Low urea/creatinine	↓ Protein
	Low thiamin	
	Low erythrocyte transketolase	↓ Thiamin
	Low riboflavin	
	Low erythrocyte glutathione reductase	↓ Riboflavin
	Low methylmalonic acid	↓ Vitamin B_{12}
	Low iodine	↓ Iodine
	High FIGLU	↓ Folate
	High xanthurenic acid	↓ Vitamin B_6

From Reed, P.: Nutrition: an applied science, Edinburgh, 1980, Churchill Livingstone.
*The type of imbalance suggested by the general level of the nutrient or metabolite is included.
†↓ Indicates an undersupply of the nutrient; ↑ indicates an oversupply.

b. Methods of evaluation—comparing results of diet analysis with standards of adequacy (e.g., Basic Four recommendations and RDAs)
3. Diet modifications
a. Adding foods to the diet to correct for nutrient deficiencies
b. Eliminating or reducing excessive nutrient intakes for disease control and prevention (e.g., sugar, fat, or sodium)
C. Biochemical evaluation (Table 9-13)
1. Blood and urine analysis
a. Most objective and precise assessment data
b. Determines marginal nutritional deficiencies before overt clinical signs appear by measuring either the concentration of a nutrient or the functional activity of the nutrient
2. Delayed cutaneous hypersensitivity skin tests
a. Assessment of the host defense mechanisms by evaluating the patient's reaction to common skin test antigens as a nonspecific indicator of malnutrition

b. Most useful for evaluating the critically ill patient's ability to withstand the stresses of surgery
3. Multielemental hair analysis
a. Chemical analysis of hair for mineral status
b. Questionable usefulness as a reliable and accurate assessment
(1) Lack of information correlating hair mineral concentrations with body levels of minerals
(2) Lack of information on normal ranges for mineral concentration in hair
(3) Lack of control for hair changes because of environmental factors (e.g., shampoos and air pollution)
D. Clinical examination of body tissues—indicator of general health and nutritional status (Table 9-14; see also Table 9-8)
1. Oral tissues
a. Dental caries—excessive sugar exposure
b. Gingivitis and periodontal disease— excessive sugar intake and nutritional deficiencies

Table 9-14 Some classical symptoms of poor nutritional status and the nutrient imbalances they indicate

Area examined	Symptom	Nutrient imbalance suggested*
Skin	Follicular hyperkeratosis	↓ Vitamin A
	Petechiae	↓ Vitamin C
	Dark dermatitis in areas exposed to sunlight	↓ Niacin
	Flaky dermatitis	↓ Protein-energy (kwashiorkor)
	Pallor	↓ Iron, folate, vitamin B$_{12}$ copper
Eyes	Xerosis	↓ Vitamin A
	Keratomalacia	
	Bitot's spot	
	Inflamed conjunctiva	↓ Vitamin A, riboflavin
Mouth and tongue	Cheilosis	↓ Riboflavin
	Glossitis (magenta tongue)	
	Glossitis (red, raw tongue)	↓ Niacin, folacin, iron
	Gingivitis (bleeding, spongy gums)	↓ Vitamin C
	Carious teeth	↓ Fluoride
		↑ Sugar
Hair	Depigmentation	↓ Protein-energy
	Thin, sparse, poor texture	↓ Protein-energy
Nails	Koilonychia (spoon nails)	↓ Iron
Subcutaneous fat	Little fat	↓ Protein-energy (marasmus, starvation)
	Excessive fat	↑ Energy nutrients
	Edema	↓ Protein-energy (kwashiorkor), thiamin
Musculature	Wasted muscles	↓ Protein-energy (marasmus, starvation)
	Paralysis at extremities	↓ Thiamin, B$_{12}$
Skeletal structure	Bowed legs, knock-knees	↓ Vitamin D
	Rosary beading of ribs	↓ Vitamin C

From Reed, P.: Nutrition: an applied science, Edinburgh, 1980, Churchill Livingstone.
*↓ indicates an undersupply of the nutrient; ↑ indicates an oversupply.

c. Glossitis—nutritional deficiencies affecting tongue papillae and color
d. Stomatitis—nutritional deficiencies affecting oral soft tissues
e. Cheilosis—nutritional deficiencies affecting the lips and corners of the mouth
f. Acute necrotizing ulcerative gingivitis— excessive sugar and caffeine intakes combined with nutritional deficiencies result in stress and lowered tissue resistance to plaque and bacteria insults
2. Anthropometric analysis—determines the body structure, form, and composition (e.g., content of lean body mass and fat tissue); the following tools are useful, but each has its limitations
a. Height and weight standards based on body frame size

b. Skinfold thickness measurements
(1) Obtained by using skinfold calipers to measure subcutaneous fat in millimeters in selected areas (e.g., triceps and subscapular region)
(2) Measurements are compared with standards to estimate total body fat composition
c. Arm muscle circumference
(1) Sensitive indicator of the muscle mass that reflects protein stores
(2) Determined by measuring the arm circumference at the midpoint of the upper arm and triceps skinfold measurements
3. Other body tissues (Table 9-14)

Assessment of Dietary Intake

A. Dietary intake standards
1. RDAs (see Table 9-3)
   a. "The levels of intake of essential nutrients considered, in the judgment of the Committee on Dietary Allowances of The Food and Nutrition Board on the basis of available scientific knowledge, to be adequate to meet the known nutritional needs of practically all healthy persons"[1]
   b. Appropriate use
      (1) Planning and evaluating food supplies for groups
      (2) Standards for evaluating food-consumption records
      (3) Guidelines for new food products
      (4) Basis for regulatory standards of nutritional quality
      (5) Standards for nutritional labeling; U.S. RDAs use the highest value for any nutrient (males over age 4 and nonpregnant, nonlactating females over age 4); FDA requires that the processor of food, who states any nutritional information regarding the product or who adds any nutrient to the food, make a nutritional declaration using the U.S. RDAs.
2. Basic Four food groups
   a. Simple guide for the selection of foods to meet the daily recommended levels of nutrients; suggests the number of daily servings, serving size (based on age), and examples of foods for each of the four food groups: milk, meat, vegetable-fruit, and bread-cereal
   b. Foods and nutrient composition of the groups (Table 9-15)
   c. To fully meet the caloric needs and add palatability to the diet, additional foods may be selected from a "fifth group," containing fats and sweets; these provide few nutrients beyond calories
3. U.S. dietary goals—recommendations made by the U.S. Senate Select Committee on Nutrition and Human Needs in 1977 to modify the intake of those foods associated with the leading causes of mortality and morbidity in the United States
   a. Consume only enough calories to balance energy expenditures
   b. Increase the consumption of complex carbohydrates to 48% of the total energy intake
   c. Reduce the intake of refined and processed sugars to 10% of the total energy intake
   d. Reduce fat consumption to 30% of the total energy intake
   e. Reduce saturated-fat consumption to 10%, and balance it with equal amounts of polyunsaturated and monounsaturated fats
   f. Reduce cholesterol to 300 mg/day
   g. Limit sodium intake (salt or sodium chloride [NaCl]) to 5 g/day
4. U.S. RDA guidelines
   a. Eat a variety of foods
   b. Maintain an ideal weight
   c. Avoid too much fat, saturated fat, and cholesterol
   d. Eat foods with adequate starch and fiber
   e. Avoid too much sugar and sodium
   f. If you drink alcohol, do so in moderation
5. Food and Nutrition Board's recommendations for healthy adult Americans
   a. "Adjust dietary energy intake and energy expenditure so as to maintain appropriate weight for height; if overweight, achieve appropriate weight reduction by decreasing total food and fat intake and by increasing physical activity"[1]
   b. If the requirement for energy is low (e.g., reducing diet), reduce the consumption of foods such as alcohol, sugars, fats, and oils, which provide calories but few other essential nutrients
   c. Use salt in moderation; adequate salt intakes are considered to range between 3 and 8 g of sodium chloride daily
   d. Select a nutritionally adequate diet from the foods available by each day consuming appropriate servings of dairy products, meats or legumes, vegetables and fruits, and cereals and breads
   e. Select as wide a variety of foods in each of the major food groups as is practicable to ensure a high probability of consuming adequate quantities of all essential nutrients

B. Methods for collecting data on food intakes
1. Nutritional screening questionnaire (see box on p. 380)
   a. Description—patient indicates frequency of sugar and food-group intake over a day or week
   b. Advantages
      (1) Can be filled out by the patient while waiting in the dental office
      (2) Requires 15 to 20 minutes to complete

Table 9-15 Basic Four food plan

Food group	Daily recommended servings			Foods and portion sizes for one serving	Nutrient contribution
	Child	Adolescent	Adult		
Milk	3+	4+	2+ (Pregnancy = 4+) (Lactation = 4+)	Milk (skim, whole, low fat, buttermilk)— 1 cup Cheddar cheese—1½ inch cube or 1-1½ oz Cottage cheese—1 cup; sour cream—1 cup Ice cream—1½ cups Yogurt—1 cup; cream cheese—16 tbsp Pudding or custard—1 cup	Calcium Riboflavin Protein Phosphorus Vitamin D Vitamin A

Meat	2+	2+	2+ (Pregnancy = 3+)	Meat, fish, poultry—lean 2 oz; with fat: 3-4 oz
				Hot dogs—2; bacon—12 slices; sausage—6 oz
				Luncheon meats—3 slices or 3 oz
				Protein equivalents:
				  Eggs—2; peanut butter—4 tbs
				  Dry beans, peas (cooked)—1 cup
				  Nuts—2 oz or 8 tbsp
					Protein
					Niacin
					Iron
					Thiamin
					Vitamin A

Fruits and vegetables	4+	4+	4+	Cooked fruit or vegetable—½ cup Raw or fresh fruit or vegetable—1 cup Fresh fruit—1 medium size Juice—½ cup Grapefruit—½ medium Cantaloupe—¼ medium Raisins—¼ cup	Vitamin A Vitamin C Fiber Iron (dried fruits)
Bread and cereals	4+	4+	4+	Bread—1 slice Corn bread—2 inch square Hamburger/frankfurter roll—½ of the roll Cooked cereal—½ cup; dry cereal—1 cup (¾ oz) Crackers—4 to 6 Biscuits—1 (2 inch diameter) Rice, pastas—½ cup; pancake—1 (4 inch diameter)	Economical source of energy Thiamin Niacin Riboflavin Fiber Iron

From Lee, M., Stanmeyer, W., and Wight, A.: Nutrition and dental health, Part V, Nutrition counseling, Carrboro, N.C., 1982, Health Sciences Consortium, Inc.

(3) Allows analysis of food-group consumption

(4) Allows sugar-intake evaluation

c. Limitations

  (1) No nutrient analysis

  (2) Relies on the patient's memory

2. Twenty-four-hour dietary recall

a. Description—interviewer collects data from the patient on all food consumed over a 24-hour period

b. Advantages

  (1) Requires 20 minutes for the interview

  (2) Allows nutrient analysis

  (3) Allows analysis of food-group consumption

(4) Allows sugar-intake evaluation

c. Limitations

  (1) Requires a trained interviewer

  (2) Relies on the patient's memory

  (3) Represents only 1 day of food consumption

  (4) Requires a nutrient data file on foods to analyze nutrients

3. Three- to seven-day food record or diary

a. Description—patient keeps a record of food and eating times for 3 to 7 days

b. Advantages

  (1) No interviewer required except to give directions on how to fill out the record

NUTRITIONAL SCREENING QUESTIONNAIRE

Name _____ Date _____

Chart No. _____

1. How many meals do you have a day? _____
   About what times are these eaten? _____
2. Would you consider your appetite to be:
   Good _____
   Fair _____
   Poor _____
3. How often do you eat between meals?
   Never _____
   Occasionally _____
   Often _____
   What foods do you usually eat between meals? _____
   _____
4. How often do you drink soft drinks, fruit drinks, or any other sweetened beverages?
   Never _____
   Occasionally _____
   Often _____ (times/day)
   When do you drink these beverages?
   With meals _____
   Between meals _____
   At both/either time(s) _____
5. How often do you drink coffee and/or tea?
   Never _____
   Occasionally _____
   Often _____ (cups/day)
   How do you drink your coffee/tea? With:
   Milk/cream _____
   Cremora _____
   Sweetener _____
     (Specify the kind)
6. How often do you use gum and/or mints?
   Never _____
   Occasionally _____
   Often _____
   What brand do you use?
   _____
7. How often do you use cough drops, throat lozenges, and/or antacid tablets? (Please circle which ones)
   Never _____
   Occasionally _____
   Often _____
8. How often do you take vitamin or mineral supplements?
   Never _____
   Occasionally _____
   Daily _____
   What is in your supplement? _____
     (Specify the type of vitamins or minerals)

Modified from DePaola, D., and Cheney, H.: Preventive dentistry, Littleton, Mass., 1979, PSG/Wright Publishing Co., Inc.

NUTRITIONAL SCREENING QUESTIONNAIRE — cont'd

9. Are you presently on any special or restricted diet? Yes ____ No. ____
   If so, what kind?

	Never	Times/day	Times/week
10. a. How often do you eat/drink milk, cheese, yogurt, or other dairy foods?	_____	_____	_____
b. How often do you eat whole-grain or enriched breads, cereals, or pasta?	_____	_____	_____
c. How often do you eat cooked or raw vegetables?	_____	_____	_____
d. How often do you eat/drink citrus fruit or juice (orange, grapefruit, tomato)?	_____	_____	_____
e. How often do you eat one of the following: carrots, pumpkin, sweet potatoes, greens, broccoli, spinach (or other dark yellow or green vegetable or fruit)?	_____	_____	_____
f. How often do you eat meat, fish, poultry, or eggs?	_____	_____	_____
g. How often do you eat peanut butter, nuts, dried peas or beans, or soybean products?	_____	_____	_____
h. How often do you eat your meals in restaurants or fast-food places?	_____	_____	_____

---

(2) Allows for both nutrient and food-group analysis
(3) Allows for sugar-intake evaluation
(4) An average intake of several days may be more representative of the patient's food intake than 1 day
  c. Limitations
     (1) Represents the food consumption of only the days included in the record
     (2) Relies on the cooperation and ability of the patient to keep the record
     (3) Requires a nutrient data file for nutrient analysis
C. Methods for evaluating food intakes
  1. Basic Four food groups (Table 9-15)
     a. Nutrient contributions (Table 9-16)
        (1) Role in general health
        (2) Role in dental health

  b. Advantages for use in counseling
     (1) Patient participation
     (2) Simple
     (3) Inexpensive
     (4) Fairly accurate
     (5) Patient can use at home after a session for self and for family
  c. Limitations
     (1) No provisions made for combination foods (e.g., pizza or casseroles); need to break down into ingredients that correspond to the four food groups
     (2) No nutrient analysis
  2. Computer diet analysis
     a. Definition—foods are individually entered into a computer, and the specific amounts of each nutrient for each food consumed are calculated
     b. Nutrient data file (software)—contains foods with their nutrients

Table 9-16 Nutrient contribution and functions of the food groups

Food group	Nutrient contribution	Function in the body	Function in oral health
Milk	Proteins	4 Kcal per gram. Constituent of every cell. Builds and repairs tissues and forms antibodies to resist infection.	Collagen formation. Formation of the matrix of dentin and enamel. Maintains the integrity of periodontal tissues.
	Calcium and phosphorus	Calcification of the body's hard tissues. Involved in blood clotting, muscle and nerve activity.	Normal tooth and bone mineralization.
	B_{12} (B-complex)	Coenzyme involved in synthesis of single-carbon units in nucleic acid metabolism.	Integrity of nerve tissue and normal red blood cell formation in oral tissues.
	Riboflavin (B-complex)	Constituent of two flavin nucleotide coenzymes (FAD, FMN) in energy metabolism.	Energy metabolism of oral tissues.
	Vitamin D	Necessary for the absorption of calcium from the intestines; regulation of calcium and phosphorus homeostasis.	Needed for calcium absorption which is important for tooth and bone mineralization.
Meat	Proteins	(See milk group)	(See milk group)
	Pyridoxine (B-complex)	Coenzyme in carbohydrate and amino acid metabolism. Cofactor in formation of porphyrin in hemoglobin synthesis.	Normal carbohydrate and protein metabolism and hemoglobin synthesis in oral tissues.
	Niacin (B-complex)	Constituents of two coenzymes involved in oxidation-reduction reactions (NAD, NADP).	Integrity of oral tissues.
	Folacin (B-complex)	Coenzyme involved in transfer of single-carbon units in nucleic acid and amino acid metabolism.	Normal synthesis of protein compounds in oral tissues (e.g., enzymes, hemoglobin).
	Thiamin (B-complex)	Coenzyme (thiamine pyrophosphate) in reactions involving the removal of carbon dioxide.	Normal energy metabolism during development and maintenance of oral tissues.
	B_{12} (B-complex)	(See milk group)	(See milk group)
	Iron	Combines with protein to form hemoglobin. Constituent of enzymes involved in energy metabolism.	Normal hemoglobin formation and oxygen transportation to oral tissues.
	Vitamin A	Integrity of epithelial tissues. Synthesis of mucopolysaccharides and rhodopsin (visual purple).	Normal growth of enamel and dentin. Normal growth of periodontal tissues and maintenance of epithelium.
Fruits and vegetables	Vitamin A	(See meat group)	(See meat group)
	Vitamin C	Hydroxylation of lysine and proline in collagen formation. Wound healing and resisting infection.	Collagen formation. Integrity of blood vessels in gingival and pulpal tissues. Normal formation of dentin.
	Folacin (B-complex)	(See meat group)	(See meat group)
	Pyridoxine (B-complex)	(See meat group)	(See meat group)
	Fiber (indigestible carbohydrate)	Adds bulk to diet.	Stimulates salivary flow. Integrity of periodontal tissues.
Bread and cereal	Thiamin	(See meat group)	(See meat group)
	Riboflavin	(See milk group)	(See milk group)
	Niacin	(See meat group)	(See meat group)
	Iron	(See meat group)	(See meat group)
	Fiber	(See fruit and vegetable group)	(See fruit and vegetable group)

From Lee, M., Stanmeyer, W., and Wight, A.: Nutrition and Dental Health, Part V, Nutrition Counseling, Carrboro, N.C., 1982, Health Sciences Consortium, Inc.

c. RDAs—used as a standard for comparison with the patient's daily nutrient intake (see Table 9-3)
d. Advantages
(1) Accurate
(2) Specific
(3) Cost-efficient when hardware available
(a) Microcomputers in dental offices
(b) Services available outside the dental office for a fee
e. Limitations
(1) Limited patient participation and home use
(2) Hardware and software availability
(3) Expensive
3. Sugar analysis and evaluation
a. Dental caries and periodontal disease are multifactoral diseases that result from the interaction of the resistance of oral tissues (host factor) to the destructive effects of bacterial plaque and acids (agent factor) produced from metabolism of dietary sugars (diet factor); dental disease occurs when all three factors exist simultaneously and is often called the "triad" of dental disease; nutritional assessment of sugar exposure is an essential part of nutritional counseling in preventive dentistry programs and can be conducted using precise or simplified methods
(1) Precise analysis—computer analysis of the diet for carbohydrate content: total carbohydrate in grams, monosaccharides and disaccharides in grams (e.g., grams of sucrose), and fiber in grams; percentage of the total daily calorie intake from simple and complex carbohydrates can be calculated and compared with the recommendations: 48% complex, 10% simple
(2) Simplified analysis—dietary sugars (sweets and food processed with sugars; see Table 9-2) are circled on the food record or recall; cariogenicity of the diet is assessed based on the frequency and form of sugar exposure; frequent exposure to retentive solid sugars, especially between meals, is harmful; acid production potential of the diet can be calculated by using the following formula

Total daily solid sugar exposures × 40 minutes + Total daily liquid sugar exposures × 20 minutes = Total minutes of acid exposure to oral tissues from dietary sugars

Formula is based on research that shows glucose rinses result in a drop of oral pH below the critical level (5.5pH—where acids decalcify enamel) and that it takes 20 minutes for saliva to neutralize acids and raise the pH to a safe level; solid sugars adhere to teeth and have approximately double the acid production potential
b. Caries-activity tests—often involve counting the number of acidogenic bacteria or measuring the acids produced by these bacteria; provide information about the current oral environment and help to detect dental caries activity; are valuable adjuncts in patients' plaque control programs and can be used to monitor a patient's progress in oral home care and diet modifications; Table 9-17 summarizes the more widely used tests, the type of sample or basis used for testing, the method of analysis, and the test validity and reliability (clinical correlation)

Nutritional Counseling Techniques

A. Direct approach—counseling technique that focuses on the dietary problem
1. Role of the patient—patient provides information on the diet; is passive and listens to the counselor
2. Role of the counselor—counselor controls the session; analyzes and evaluates the patient's diet and makes recommendations for improvement
3. Advantages—easier for the counselor and often requires less time than a more patient-oriented approach
4. Limitations—fosters patient dependence; little chance of success if the patient is not committed to dietary changes
B. Nondirect or behavior modification approach—counseling technique that focuses on the patient
1. Role of the patient—patient actively participates in the diet analysis, evaluation, and modification program
2. Role of the counselor—counselor provides information on the etiology of dental disease, the role of the diet, and the use of dietary assessment tools
3. Method
a. Assumption—dietary habits are learned behaviors and can be "unlearned" and replaced with new behaviors
b. Collection of baseline data
c. Patient takes ownership of the dietary problem and is committed to change

Table 9-17 Caries activity tests—their basis, method, and clinical correlation

Test	Basis	Method	Clinical correlation
Lactobacillus count	Aciduric organisms (salivary)	Quantitative (count/ml) Plate culture	Group correlation, unsatisfactory for individuals
Snyder	Aciduric organisms (salivary)	Qualitative (rate > pH 3.8) Colorimetric tube culture	Group correlation, unsatisfactory for individuals
Swab	Aciduric organisms (plaque)	Qualitative (pH) Colorimetric tube culture	Unsatisfactory
Fosdick	Total organisms (salivary) Buffering capacity	Quantitative Ca dissolved from enamel powder	Not established
Dewar	Total organisms (salivary) Buffering capacity	Quantitative (pH) Modified Fosdick	Unsatisfactory
Rickles	Total organisms (salivary) Buffering capacity	Quantitative (pH)	Unsatisfactory
Reductase	Total organisms (salivary) Oxidation-reduction potential	Qualitative Dye color change	Group correlation, unsatisfactory for individuals
Amylase	Ability to hydrolyse starch	Qualitative or quantitative Reducing sugar or starch—12 color	Unsatisfactory
Buffer capacity	Buffer capacity	Quantitative titration	Correlation of extreme deviation
Streptococcus mutans screening	*S. mutans* (plaque)	Semiquantitative (size of plaque sample uncontrolled) Uses a selective medium	Best correlation for high caries activity group

From Newbrun, E.: Cariology, ed. 2, Baltimore, 1983, Williams & Wilkins.

    d. Patient determines the behavior changes and goals; develops own reward system to use when goals are met

    e. Changes are gradually made in small steps; appropriate changes are rewarded and failures ignored

    f. Close monitoring of progress until new behaviors become self-reinforcing

  4. Advantages—fosters patient independence; success more likely, since the patient is in control of the change process

  5. Limitations—more time and effort needed to arrive at appropriate solutions to dietary problems and rewards for behavior modification

C. Factors that influence the patient's food intake—any combination of the following influences affects food choices and needs to be addressed in a modification program

  1. Environmental influences—economics, lifestyle, geography, seasons, markets

  2. Social influences—family, culture, religion, social pressures, marketing strategies

  3. Psychologic influences—self-image, emotions, stresses, values

D. Determinants for dental patient selection

  1. High-risk patients—patients with conditions that would benefit most from nutritional counseling

    a. Pregnancy—nutrient needs are high; hormonal changes may lead to exaggerated responses to plaque and bacterial toxins; maternal diet affects the formation of fetal oral tissues

    b. Adolescence—nutrient needs are high; vulnerable to nutritional problems from fad diets for weight loss and muscle building; frequent snacking on empty-calorie foods; problems of anorexia and bulimia can lead to enamel erosion (permolysis), irritation to oral mucosa, and infected or swollen salivary glands with possible xerostomia

    c. Rampant caries—high plaque and calculus and/or a positive caries-activity test may indicate a frequent sugar-exposure problem

    d. Periodontal disease or necrotic ulcerated gingivitis—frequent exposure to sugar and nutritional deficiencies can contribute to the development and progression of these conditions

    e. Oral surgery—nutritional counseling before and after surgery is important for optimal surgical recovery; postsurgical nutrient needs are high because of blood loss, tissue repair, and host defense activities; modifications in food texture (e.g., soft foods) are made according to the ability to masticate

f. Edentulism—inability to masticate can result in nutrient deficiencies because of the limited nutrient content in soft and liquid foods
g. Oral cancer—nutrient needs are high because of host defense activities and tissue repair from cancer and its treatment; cancer or treatment may result in inadequate food intake because of decreased appetite, altered taste perceptions, irritated oral tissues, and xerostomia
2. Office resources—availability of trained personnel, time, and facilities to conduct nutrition counseling services
3. Patient factors—level of patient motivation to use and benefit from nutritional counseling and patient financial and intellectual capabilities for using nutritional counseling services

Dietary Modifications for Specific Dental Conditions

A. Dental caries (see Tables 9-6 and 9-10)
1. Role of nutrients in tooth formation
a. Preeruptive effects—nutrients are used systemically for enamel, dentin, and pulp formation; tooth bud formation begins at 6 weeks in utero, and calcification is completed at 13 years
b. Posteruptive effects—fluoride aids in the remineralization of small enamel lesions; there is evidence that specific minerals or combinations of minerals and fats have local cariostatic properties
2. Local effect of dietary carbohydrates on bacteria growth and plaque formation (see pp. 352-353)
3. Role of diet and nutrients in salivary gland function
a. Nutrients are used systemically for the normal development and secretory function of salivary glands
b. Foods of firm texture (e.g., raw vegetables) enhance mastication, stimulate the salivary flow rate, and modify the concentration of constituents in saliva, possibly improving antibacterial properties and the buffering capacity to neutralize decalcifying acids
B. Periodontal disease (see Table 9-7)
1. Role of nutrients in the formation of periodontal tissues
a. Nutrients are used systemically for the normal development of the gingiva, periodontal ligament, cementum, and alveolus

b. Periodontal tissues are metabolically active throughout the patient's life, and nutrients are constantly needed for maintenance (e.g., the cell population of the sulcular epithelium completely renews itself within 3 to 6 days)
2. Local effect of dietary carbohydrates on bacteria growth and plaque formation (see pp. 352-353)
3. Role of nutrients in the host defense system
a. During the initial stages of periodontitis the nutritional status of the patient is important in cellular immunocompetence for combating bacterial insults to the periodontium
b. After periodontal surgery, cellular immunocompetence is important for optimal healing and preventing infection
C. Oral surgery
1. Presurgical nutritional counseling
a. Adequate nutrient intake is needed to build up nutrient reserves in tissues to cope with postsurgical nutrient demands and complications
b. Counseling is helpful for advising the patient to plan and purchase appropriate food products before surgery for the convalescent period
2. Postsurgical nutritional counseling
a. Nutrient requirements are high because of blood loss, increased catabolism, tissue repair, and host defense activities
b. Dietary intakes will be influenced by surgical complications of anorexia, dysphagia, and oral discomfort; a liquid diet should be used initially for the first few days, followed by a soft diet until the patient can eat normally; during convalescence, high-protein liquid products fortified with vitamins and minerals (e.g., Ensure, Sustacal, and Instant Breakfast) are helpful but contain cariogenic sweeteners; safe levels of vitamin and mineral supplements (100% to 200% of U.S. RDAs) can also be used
D. Prosthodontics
1. Nutritional counseling in the preparation of the mouth for a prosthesis
a. Nutrients—systemically important for the health of oral soft tissues and the alveolar ridge
(1) Surgery—if surgery is necessary, nutrient requirements will be higher for postsurgical healing

(2) Tissue state—if any inflamed or soft tissue injuries and bone resorption conditions exist, nutrient requirements will be higher for repair and host defense activities

b. Dietary sugars—condition of the remaining dentition is important for maintaining the use of a new prosthesis; cariogenic sugars need to be restricted to control bacterial growth, acid production, and plaque formation

c. Texture of foods—partial or fully edentulous patients will often need to eat chopped, soft foods; if nutrient intake is compromised, fortified liquid products or nutrient supplements are helpful

2. Nutritional counseling after prosthesis insertion

a. Food texture—liquid foods for the first 24 hours, followed by soft foods and chopped or cut-up foods; this minimizes biting and chewing and allows time for the muscles and tongue to adjust to the new prosthesis

b. Counter-dislodgement forces—for every bite of food, food should be evenly divided in the right and left sides of the mouth before chewing to equalize occlusal forces

c. Nutrients—adequate intake for the integrity of the oral mucosa and alveolar ridge

d. Dietary sugars—restrict to prevent bacterial growth, acid production, and plaque formation on the remaining dentition and prosthesis

e. Food flavors—initially, flavors of foods will be altered because of the new prosthesis, but this side effect will eventually disappear with denture use

E. Orthodontics

1. Role of nutrients—systemically important for the integrity of periodontal tissues; requirements are higher as stresses of tooth movement result in more bone apposition and the synthesis of a new periodontal ligament; nutrients are needed for the healing and repair of gingival injuries and irritations from orthodontic bands

2. Role of sugars—to prevent enamel erosion and decay; dietary sugars (especially retentive sweets) must be restricted during the wearing of appliances

3. Role of food texture—when appliances or bands are tightened, chewing hard-textured foods may be painful, and liquid and soft foods should be eaten temporarily; retentive and sticky foods should be avoided, since they become trapped in appliances and are difficult to remove

F. Oral cancer

1. Nutritional support for healing and cellular immunocompetence

a. Compromised nutritional status—weight loss and nutrient deficiencies increase the risk of not withstanding the physiologic stresses of cancer and anticancer therapies

b. Surgical treatment—primary method in treating cancer; nutrient requirements are higher as a result of the increased catabolic activities, tissue repair, and host defense activities

c. Chemotherapy and radiation treatment— nutrient needs are higher because of the destruction of healthy cells and tissues that occurs during these types of treatments

2. Diet modifications useful in treating complications from cancer and/or cancer treatments

a. Patient unable to ingest or digest food

(1) Home enteral feedings can furnish nutrients (e.g., nasogastric tube feedings)

(2) Home parenteral feedings can furnish nutrients (e.g., intravenous feedings)

b. Eating problems arising from complications or side effects of anticancer therapies

(1) Nausea and vomiting—suck on ice chips; eat frequently; eat dry, bland foods; eat and drink slowly; avoid highly spiced and fatty foods

(2) Loss of appetite—use foods and recipes that are appealing; make up nutrient requirements at times when the appetite is good; use foods with a high nutrient density

(3) Food aversions and alterations in taste and smell—eliminate offending foods; use highly spiced and distinctive textures to improve taste perceptions; cook and serve food with plastic rather than metal utensils

(4) Dry mouth or xerostomia—chew sugar-free gum, suck on ice chips, or use synthetic saliva; drink liquids with meals; use cold-temperature foods rather than hot-temperature foods; concentrate on highly nutritious liquids

(5) Radiation caries—restrict cariogenic foods

(6) Glossitis and stomatitis—eat a variety of soft, easy-to-chew foods; use stewed foods rather than broiled and fried foods; avoid highly spiced or acidic foods; use moderate-temperature foods; use straws if swallowing is difficult

G. Special-needs patient (see Chapter 14)

  1. Dental problems—unmet needs of dental care for this population significantly exceeds that of the general population

    a. Caries rate similar to that of the general population because of poor oral hygiene and cariogenic food habits

    b. Increased periodontal disease as compared with the general population because of the following

      (1) Poor oral hygiene

      (2) Diets consisting of soft-textured foods

      (3) Frequent exposures to sweets

      (4) Metabolic disturbances affecting disease resistance and the reparative process

      (5) Nutritional deficiencies associated with diet or metabolic disturbance

      (6) Malocclusion and developmental defects

  2. Nutritional problems—slow growth, excessive weight loss or gain, and nutrient deficiencies can occur in the following situations

    a. Inability to consume an adequate diet

      (1) Absence or weak sucking response (e.g, cleft lip and palate)

      (2) Poor arm and head control (e.g., cerebral palsy)

      (3) Inadequate jaw, lip, and tongue control (e.g., tongue thrust and tonic bite)

      (4) Short attention span (e.g., mental retardation and hyperactivity)

    b. Impaired nutrient use

      (1) Malabsorption conditions (e.g., cystic fibrosis)

      (2) Inborn errors of metabolism (e.g., phenylketonuria)

      (3) Drug-nutrient interactions (e.g., anticonvulsant medications can interfere with calcium and phosphorus use)

      (4) Poor muscle control (e.g., constipation)

    c. Excessive intake of foods, calories, and sweets

      (1) Food, especially sweets, used as a reinforcer for good behavior

      (2) Overfeeding because of parental guilt

      (3) Overemphasis on feeding because it is the major time for parent-child interaction

      (4) Excessive calorie intake resulting from inactivity and the pleasurable aspects of eating

REFERENCE

1. Committee on Dietary Allowances: Recommended dietary allowances, ed. 9, Washington, D.C., 1980, National Academy of Sciences.

SUGGESTED READINGS

Alpers, D., Clouse, R., and Stenson, W.: Manual of nutritional therapeutics, Boston, 1983, Little, Brown & Co.

Christakis, G.: Nutritional assessment in health programs, Washington, D.C., 1973, American Public Health Association.

Curricular guidelines on biochemistry and nutrition for dental hygienists, J. Dent. Educ. **48:**318, 1984.

Guthrie, H.: Introductory nutrition, ed. 5, St. Louis, 1983, The C.V. Mosby Co.

Martin, D., Mayes, P., and Rodwell, V.: Harper's review of biochemistry, ed. 18, Los Altos, Calif., 1981, Lange Medical Publications.

Nizel, A.: Nutrition in preventive dentistry, ed. 2, Philadelphia, 1981, W.B. Saunders Co.

Randolph, P.M., and Dennison, C.I.: Diet, nutrition, and dentistry, St. Louis, 1981, The C.V. Mosby Co.

Reed, P.: Nutrition: an applied science, St. Paul, 1980, West Publishing Co.

Schneider, H., Anderson, C., and Coursin, D.: Nutritional support of medical practice, ed. 2, New York, 1983, Harper & Row, Publishers, Inc.

Whitney, E., and Hamilton, E.: Understanding nutrition, ed. 3, St. Paul, 1984, West Publishing Co.

Wilkins, E.: Clinical practice of the dental hygienist, ed. 5, Philadelphia, 1983, Lea & Febiger.

Review Questions

1 The monosaccharide that is the primary source of energy in the body is
1. Galactose
2. Fructose
3. Glucose
4. Sucrose
5. Disaccharide

2 Cellulose is an important constituent of the diet because
1. It adds fiber and bulk to the diet
2. It can be stored in the body for use when energy demands are high
3. It is made up of glucose units that are readily available as an energy source
4. Its glucose units are made available by the action of bacterial enzymes in the small intestine
5. It is easily digestible by humans

3 In which of the following ways can glucose be used in the body? It can be converted to
(a) Carbon dioxide, water, and adenosine triphosphate (ATP)
(b) Liver glycogen
(c) Acetylcoenzyme A (acetyl-CoA) and fat
(d) Amino acids and protein
1. b only
2. a and c
3. b and d
4. a, b, and c
5. c only

4 Even with a low intake of carbohydrates, normal blood levels of glucose can be maintained from
(a) Glycerol
(b) Liver glycogen
(c) Amino acids
(d) Muscle glycogen
1. b only
2. a and c
3. b and d
4. a, b, and c
5. c only

5 The element found in proteins but not in carbohydrates and fats is
1. Iron
2. Carbon
3. Calcium
4. Oxygen
5. Nitrogen

6 Gluconeogenesis is the conversion of
1. Glucose to glycogen
2. Amino acids to glucose
3. Glycogen to glucose
4. Glucose to fatty acids
5. Glucose to amino acids

7 A person who eats 100 excess kilocalories per day will gain 1 pound in about
1. One day
2. One week
3. Two weeks
4. One month
5. Two months

8 The minimum energy needed to carry on vital body processes is known as
1. Kilocalorie
2. Specific dynamic energy
3. Coefficient of digestibility
4. Basal metabolic energy
5. Heat of combustion

9 There is a positive correlation between obesity and which of the following?
(a) Diabetes mellitus type II
(b) Hyperthyroidism
(c) Hypertension
(d) Life span
1. a only
2. a and c
3. b and d
4. a, b, and c
5. d only

10 The nutritive value of a food protein is ultimately dependent on its
1. Molecular weight
2. Nitrogen content
3. Amino acid content
4. Ability to be converted to glucose
5. Tertiary structure

11 Which of the following foods has the best assortment of essential amino acids for the human body?
1. Cow's milk
2. Rice
3. Eggs
4. Gelatin
5. Corn

12 A person is in positive nitrogen balance during
(a) Growth
(b) Inadequate protein ingestion
(c) Pregnancy
(d) Old age
(e) A febrile illness (fever)
1. a, b, and c
2. a and c
3. a, c, and e
4. b and d
5. c and e

13 In an ideally planned daily menu, protein should contribute approximately
1. 10% to 15% of the total kilocalories
2. 20% to 25% of the total kilocalories
3. 30% to 35% of the total kilocalories
4. 40% to 45% of the total kilocalories
5. 50% to 55% of the total kilocalories

14 The nitrogen from excess protein in the diet is
  1. Stored as amino acids
  2. Converted and stored as fat
  3. Excreted by the kidneys in the urine
  4. Oxidized by the same process as for carbohydrates
  5. Converted to urea and stored in the liver

15 Kwashiorkor
  (a) Occurs most commonly in impoverished areas after children have been weaned
  (b) Refers to a condition where too few calories are consumed
  (c) Occurs when protein intake is lower than growth and maintenance needs
  (d) May be present in a child even though his muscles do not appear wasted
  1. a only
  2. a and b
  3. a, c, and d
  4. c and d
  5. b and d

16 Ninety-five percent of the lipids in the diet are
  1. Cholesterol
  2. Phospholipids
  3. Polyunsaturated fatty acids
  4. Triglycerides
  5. Lipoproteins

17 Which of the following are important properties or characteritics of dietary lipids?
  (a) Prevent scurvy
  (b) Carry riboflavin and thiamin
  (c) Provide satiety to the diet
  (d) Aid in absorption of minerals
  (e) Provide essential fatty acids
  1. a and b
  2. b and c
  3. a, b, and c
  4. b and d
  5. c and e

18 Saturated fatty acids
  (a) Are found in oils from plant food sources
  (b) Are found in fats from animal food sources
  (c) Have a high iodine number
  (d) Are usually solids at room temperature
  1. a only
  2. b only
  3. a and c
  4. b and d
  5. a, c, and d

19 Which of the following lipids is required in the diet?
  1. Cholesterol
  2. Lecithin
  3. Butyric acid
  4. Linoleic acid
  5. Steric acid

20 Cholesterol
  1. Should be completely eliminated from the diet
  2. Serves no useful function in the body
  3. Can be synthesized by the body
  4. Is present at a level of 600 g/day in the average U.S. diet
  5. Is negatively correlated with cardiovascular disease

21 The lipoproteins thought to be a protective factor against cardiovascular disease are
  1. Low-density lipoproteins (LDLs)
  2. Very low density lipoproteins (VLDLs)
  3. Very high density lipoproteins (VHDLs)
  4. High-density lipoproteins (HDLs)
  5. Chylomicrons

22 Lipid material, cellular debris, and calcium complexed within the artery walls are
  1. Aortas
  2. Plaques
  3. Embolisms
  4. Aneurysms
  5. Infarctions

23 Which of the following is considered an unhealthy or ineffective characteristic of a weight-loss plan?
  1. Weight loss of 1 to 2 pounds per week
  2. Negative energy (calorie) balance
  3. Increased exercise
  4. Eliminating fat from the diet
  5. Eating foods you like

24 Thiamin is essential for
  1. Formation of red blood cells
  2. Blood coagulation
  3. Enzymatic reactions involving production of energy
  4. Collagen formation
  5. Prevention of night blindness

25 Which of the following properties accurately describes the role of microminerals in the body?
  (a) Provide energy
  (b) Regulate body processes
  (c) Help maintain the acid-base balance
  (d) Give teeth and bones their rigidity and strength
  1. a, b, and c
  2. b, c, and d
  3. a, c, and d
  4. a, b, and d
  5. b and d

26 Which of the following pairs of vitamins can cause a macrocytic anemia if *either* one is deficient in the diet?
  1. Pantothenic acid and biotin
  2. Pyridoxine and vitamin B_{12}
  3. Vitamin B_{12} and folacin
  4. Thiamin and riboflavin
  5. Riboflavin and niacin

27 Sufficient niacin in the diet is related to protein intake because the body can synthesize some of its niacin from
1. Valine
2. Lysine
3. Tyrosine
4. Tryptophan
5. Phenylalanine

28 Which of the following describes the role(s) of vitamin A in the body?
(a) Maintains healthy epithelial tissue
(b) Maintains healthy eye tissues
(c) Promotes normal jaw development
(d) Promotes the laying down of new bone
1. a and b
2. a, b, and c
3. b and d
4. b, c, and d
5. a, b, c, and d

29 Good sources of vitamin A include servings of which of the following?
(a) Bread
(b) Apricots
(c) Legumes
(d) Pumpkin pie
(e) Vegetable oil
(f) Baked potatoes
(g) Liver
(h) Sweet potatoes
1. a, c, e, and g
2. b, d, g, and h
3. b, c, e , and h
4. a, c, f, and h
5. b, c, f, and h

30 Which of the following substances is converted to vitamin A in the body?
1. Tryptophan
2. Carotene
3. Xanthophyll
4. Chlorophyll
5. Cholesterol

31 Which of the following lists the daily recommended servings for adolescents from each of the Basic Four food groups?
1. Milk, three or more; meats, two or more; fruits and vegetables, four or more; breads and cereals, four or more
2. Milk, two or more; meats, two or more; fruits and vegetables, four or more; breads and cereals, four or more
3. Milk, four or more; meats, two or more; fruits and vegetables, four or more; breads and cereals, four or more
4. Milk, three or more; meats, two or more; fruits and vegetables, four or more; breads and cereals, four or more
5. Milk, four or more; meats, three or more; fruits and vegetables, four or more; breads and cereals, four or more

32 An 18-year-old female dental patient, weighing 115 pounds and 5 feet 4 inches tall, had enamel erosion on the lingual surfaces of most of her teeth. A dietary history revealed that she was subject to eating binges and sometimes consumed 5000 to 7000 kcal/day. What might be her problem?
1. Alcoholism
2. Drug abuse
3. Bulimia
4. Excessive smoking
5. Diabetes mellitus, type I

33 If you were doing a diet analysis on a patient following a pure vegetarian or strict vegetarian diet, which of the following nutrients are most likely to be deficient?
1. Vitamins A and C and essential amino acids
2. Vitamin B_{12}, essential amino acids, and iron
3. Magnesium, zinc, and essential amino acids
4. Pyridoxine, pantothenic acid, and vitamin B_{12}
5. Selenium, copper, and nonessential amino acids

34 Which of the following nutrients are essential in regulating water balance in the body?
1. Calcium and phosphorus
2. Chloride and sulfur
3. Sodium and potassium
4. Chloride and iodine
5. Sodium only

35 Dehydration can result from
(a) Blood loss
(b) Vomiting
(c) Diarrhea
(d) Edema
(e) Sodium retention
1. a, b, c, and d
2. a, b, c, and e
3. b and c only
4. a, b, and c
5. a, c, and e

36 Which of the following conditions would lead you to believe that your patient has a problem with malnutrition?
(a) Excessive fat intake
(b) Inadequate iron and protein intake
(c) Excessive sodium intake
(d) Inadequate calorie intake
1. b and d
2. a and c
3. a, b, c, and d
4. a, b, and d
5. b, c, and d

37 A primary nutritional deficiency can occur from
(a) A lactase deficiency
(b) A low-calorie fad diet
(c) Inadequate food-purchasing power
(d) Poor oral health
(e) A drug-nutrient reaction
1. a, b, c, d, and e
2. a, b, and c
3. b, d, and e
4. b, c, and d
5. c, d, and e

38 A secondary nutritional deficiency can result from
(a) Inborn errors of metabolism
(b) Improper preparation of food
(c) Food allergies
(d) Obstruction of the gastrointestinal tract
(e) Loss of appetite
1. a, b, c, and d
2. a, c, and d
3. b, c, d, and e
4. c, d, and e
5. b, d, and e

39 All of the following are examples of biochemical tests that are used determine nutritional status except
1. Blood analysis
2. Delayed cutaneous hypersensitivity skin tests
3. Hair analysis
4. Skinfold calipers
5. Urine analysis

40 Which of the following body tissues are valuable in determining the nutritional status of patients in a clinical examination?
(a) Oral tissues
(b) Height and weight
(c) Eyes
(d) Skin
(e) Nails
1. a, b, c, d, and e
2. a, c, and d
3. b, c, d, and e
4. b, d, and e
5. c, d, and e

41 Which of the following are useful assessment tools for obtaining objective data on "what" patients eat?
(a) Nutritional screening questionnaires
(b) Skinfold calipers
(c) Five-day food diaries
(d) Twenty-four-hour recall
(e) Blood tests
1. a, b, c, and d
2. b, c, d, and e
3. c, d, and e
4. a, c, and d
5. c and d

42 A nutritional screening questionnaire is one option available for collecting information on the eating patterns of dental patients. Which of the following is *not* true of this dietary assessment method?
1. The patient can fill out the questionnaire while waiting for the dental appointment
2. This is a good method to screen patients who need more dietary counseling
3. This is a good method to assess the caloric and iron intakes of patients
4. This method can be used to get a "feel" of the sugar habits of patients
5. This method gives information about the patient's use of vitamin and mineral supplements

43 All of the following analyses can be made about the patient's diet using a 24-hour recall or food diary *except*
1. Analysis of individual nutrients
2. Sugar analysis
3. Consumption of food groups
4. Analysis of nonnutritive food additives
5. Analysis of calorie intake

44 A major advantage in using the Basic Four food groups for evaluating a patient's diet is
(a) It is simple, easy, and relatively inexpensive
(b) The patient can actively participate in the diet analysis and evaluation
(c) Calorie estimates can be made
(d) Accurate calculation for vitamins can be made
(e) The patient can learn the method and use it at home
1. a, b, c, and e
2. a, b, and e
3. c and e only
4. b, c, d, and e
5. b, d, and e

45 A major advantage in using a computer diet analysis for dental patients is
1. The patient can learn the method and use it after leaving the dental office
2. It is a more accurate and specific analysis of a diet
3. The cost for computers and a nutrient data bank is inexpensive
4. The patient can actively participate in the diet analysis
5. The patient can easily interpret the results

46 Which of the following statements *most accurately* describes the nondirective or behavior modification approach in diet counseling?
1. The patient actively participates in the diet analysis and evaluation; the counselor makes the decisions for a diet-modification program for the patient
2. The patient actively participates in the diet analysis and evaluation and the diet-modification program; the counselor provides an explanation and rationale for the assessment tools used
3. The counselor provides an explanation on how to use the diet assessment tools and analyzes the patient's diet while the patient observes
4. The counselor provides an explanation of the assessment tools and analyzes and evaluates the patient's diet; the patient approves of the counselor's decisions on the diet-modification program
5. The patient cooperates in filling out a diet diary and by following the counselor's recommendations; the counselor analyzes and evaluates the patient's diary and gives the patient a summary report

47 All of the following are high-risk patients who would benefit from nutritional counseling *except*
1. Oral surgery patients
2. Periodontal patients
3. Adult recall patients
4. Patients with rampant caries
5. Patients with acute necrotic ulcerated gingivitis

48 Which of the following are determinants in selecting patients for nutritional counseling in the dental office?
(a) The patient's level of risk for nutritional problems (e.g., pregnancy or adolescence)
(b) The patient's level of interest and motivation in preventive dentistry
(c) Office personnel and their training in nutritional counseling
(d) The patient's educational background
(e) Office time and facilities to conduct nutritional counseling
1. a, b, d, and e
2. b, c, d, and e
3. a, b, c, and e
4. c, d, and e
5. b, d, and e

49 Dental disease is a multifactorial disease that occurs when three basic factors (frequently called the triad of dental disease) exist simultaneously. Which of the following is *not* considered a part of the triad of dental disease?
1. Periodontal tissues
2. Plaque bacteria
3. Saliva
4. Refined carbohydrates or sugars
5. Tooth

50 On examining the oral soft tissues of a patient, a dentist observes fiery red mucous membranes and a tongue that is a magenta color, with a smooth, dry, glazed appearance. The patient's gingiva is swollen and bleeds easily. There is also vertical fissuring and redness along the line of closure of the lips. After doing a dietary history and evaluation, the dentist concludes that this abnormal condition of the oral soft tissues is a result of nutritional deficiencies of
1. Vitamins C and D
2. B-complex vitamins and vitamin C
3. Calcium and phosphorus
4. Magnesium and zinc
5. Vitamin A and zinc

51 Dietary sugars are often used by oral acidogenic bacteria for all of the following *except*
1. Energy production
2. Urea formation
3. Acid production
4. Plaque formation
5. Polysaccharide synthesis

52 Which of the following polysaccharides are formed by *Streptococcus mutans* from sucrose and result in the formation of a sticky, insoluble starch that helps plaque bacteria adhere to the tooth's surface?
1. Levans
2. Glycogen
3. Cellulose
4. Glucans
5. Pectins

53 Saccharin is
1. A nutritive sweetener and is noncariogenic
2. A nutritive sweetener and is cariogenic
3. A nonnutritive sweetener and is noncariogenic
4. A nonnutritive sweetener and is cariogenic
5. Not a dietary sweetener

54 Lactose is
1. A nutritive sweetener and is noncariogenic
2. A nutritive sweetener and is cariogenic
3. A nonnutritive sweetener and is noncariogenic
4. A nonnutritive sweetener and is carioigenic
5. Not a dietary sweetener

55 Aspartame is
1. A nutritive sweetener and is noncariogenic
2. A nutritive sweetener and is cariogenic
3. A nonnutritive sweetener and is noncariogenic
4. A nonnutritive sweetener and is cariogenic
5. Not a dietary sweetener

56 Sorbitol is
1. A nutritive sweetener and is noncariogenic
2. A nutritive sweetener and is cariogenic
3. A nonnutritive sweetener and is noncariogenic
4. A nonnutritive sweetener and is cariogenic
5. Not a dietary sweetener

57 Sugar substitutes are protective against dental disease because oral bacteria cannot metabolize them. Which of the following sweeteners is *not* a caries-protective sugar substitute?
1. Sorbitol
2. Aspartame
3. Fructose
4. Saccharin
5. Xylitol

58 Which of the following statements most accurately describes the effect of pregnancy on the health of the mother's oral tissues?
1. Pregnancy gingivitis is caused by hormonal changes, and there is nothing that can be done about it
2. Most pregnant women experience the growth of tumors in the mouth that disappear after the baby is born
3. Hormonal changes during pregnancy result in increased gingival sensitivity to local irritants such as plaque and calculus, but pregnancy does not cause gingivitis
4. Pregnancy results in hormonal changes, but these changes do not affect the mother's oral tissues
5. Pregnancy results in hormonal changes that lead to decalcification of enamel

59 The presurgical nutritional status of oral surgery patients is important because of all of the following physiologic consequences of trauma *except*
1. Increased nutrient losses from tissue injury and blood loss
2. Increased nutrient needs for cellular defense and tissue repair
3. Decreased appetite and ability to chew
4. Hypermetabolic state
5. Increased liver glycogenesis

60 If a handicapped patient does not eat an adequate diet, the *least* likely reason for this problem would be
1. Availability of foods
2. Absence of sucking response
3. Poor arm and head control
4. Inadequate jaw, lip, and tongue control
5. Short attention span

Answers and Rationales

1. (3) Glucose is the primary energy source for all cells of the body. Other dietary monosaccharides and disaccharides are converted to glucose by the liver.
   (1) Galactose is part of the disaccharide lactose found in milk.
   (2) Fructose may be used as an energy source by some cells but is not the primary energy source for the body.
   (4) Sucrose is a disaccharide of glucose and fructose that is hydrolyzed before it is absorbed.
   (5) Disaccharides are formed by the condensation of two monosaccharides.

2. (1) Cellulose contains glucose units in a β-linkage that cannot be hydrolyzed by human digestive enzymes; however, cellulose, hemicellulose, pectin, and other complex carbohydrates found in plants are important in the diet because they provide bulk and fiber.
   (2) Cellulose is not absorbed from the digestive tract and therefore cannot be stored for energy.
   (3) Although cellulose is made up of glucose units, they are not able to be used by the body.
   (4) Bacterial hydrolysis of cellulose is possible for ruminants but not humans.
   (5) Cellulose is generally not digestible by humans but does provide fiber and bulk.

3. (4) Glucose can be used directly for energy, and the reaction products would be carbon dioxide, water, and ATP; it may be stored as glycogen for later use, or it may be converted to acetyl-CoA and then to fat for long-term energy storage.
   (1) Carbon dioxide, water, and ATP are the reaction products of glucose for energy, or glucose may be converted to acetyl-CoA and fat.
   (2) Glucose also may be stored as liver glycogen.
   (3) Glucose cannot be converted to amino acids without a nitrogen source to provide the amino group.
   (5) Glucose can be used directly for energy with the reaction products of carbon dioxide, water, and ATP, or it can be stored as glycogen for later use.

4. (4) The glycerol portion of triglycerides, liver glycogen (by glycogenolysis), and glucogenic amino acids can all provide glucose to maintain normal blood levels.
   (1) The glycerol portion of triglycerides and glucogenic amino acids, as well as liver glycogen, can provide glucose to maintain normal blood levels.
   (2) Liver glycogen can also provide glucose to maintain normal blood levels.
   (3) Muscle glycogen is used almost exclusively by the muscles themselves and does not contribute to the blood glucose concentration.
   (5) The glycerol portion of triglycerides and liver glycogen can also provide glucose to maintain normal blood levels.

5. (5) Nitrogen is found in all amino acids and proteins, and measurement of the nitrogen content is often the chemical method used to determine the protein concentration of materials.
   (1) Iron is bound with certain proteins such as hemoglobin but is not a component of all proteins.
   (2) Carbon is found in proteins, carbohydrates, and fats.
   (3) Calcium may be associated with certain proteins, such as in the enzymes involved in the blood-clotting mechanism, but is not a component of all proteins.
   (4) Oxygen is found in proteins, carbohydrates, and fats.

6. (2) Gluconeogenesis is the series of enzymatic reactions whereby glucose is synthesized from noncarbohydrate precursors.
   (1) Glycogenesis is the synthesis of glycogen from glucose.
   (3) Glycogenolysis is the conversion of glycogen to glucose.
   (4) The processes that convert glucose to fatty acids include glycolysis, the tricarboxylic acid cycle, and lipogenesis.
   (5) Glucose can be converted to amino acids by the processes of glycolysis, the tricarboxylic acid cycle, and transamination.

7. (4) A person who eats an excess of 100 kcal/day should gain 1 pound when the excess totals 3600 kcal, or in about 36 days.
   (1) In 1 day, the gain would be $^1/_{36}$ of a pound.
   (2) In 1 week, the gain would be $^7/_{36}$ of a pound.
   (3) In 2 weeks, the gain would be $^{14}/_{36}$ of a pound.
   (5) In 2 months, the gain would be almost 2 pounds.

8. (4) The basal metabolic energy is the energy required to maintain a living state while at rest and without food. It includes respiration, circulation, maintenance of the body temperature, muscle tone, glandular activities, and cellular metabolism.
   (1) A kilocalorie is a unit of energy; 1 kcal represents the amount of heat produced when a food sample is burned in oxygen sufficient to raise the temperature of 1 kg of water 1° C.
   (2) Specific dynamic energy is the extra energy needed to metabolize ingested food.
   (3) The coefficient of digestibility is a measure of the amount of food actually absorbed compared with the total amount ingested.
   (5) The heat of combustion is the quantity of heat liberated per mole when a substance undergoes complete oxidation.

9. (2) Diabetes mellitus type II (adult onset) and hypertension are both positively correlated with obesity. In most cases patients with type II diabetes and patients with hypertension improve dramatically on achieving their ideal body weight. Hyperthyroidism causes an increase in the basal metabolic rate and hence a person's caloric needs. Most patients with hyperthyroidism are underweight. Obesity tends to shorten one's life span because of its positive correlation with some of the major causes of death (i.e., cardiovascular disease).

For each question the correct answer and rationale are listed first. The other choices are presented in order with the reasons why they are not correct.

(1) Diabetes mellitus type II and hypertension are both positively correlated with obesity.

(3) Hyperthyroidism causes an increase in the basal metabolic rate and hence a person's caloric needs, and in most cases patients with hyperthyroidism are underweight. Also, obesity tends to shorten one's life span because of its positive correlation with some of the major causes of death (i.e., cardiovascular disease).

(4) Hyperthyroidism causes an increase in the basal metabolic rate and hence a person's caloric needs; also, in most cases patients with hyperthyroidism are underweight.

(5) Obesity tends to shorten one's life span because of its positive correlation with some of the major causes of death.

10. (3) The nutritive value of a protein is dependent on whether the amount and ratio of essential amino acids meet the body's needs.

(1) The molecular weight of a protein does not affect its nutritive value.

(2) The nitrogen content of all proteins is fairly constant at about 16% of the total weight of the protein.

(4) The amino acids of proteins are not converted to glucose unless there is inadequate dietary carbohydrate.

(5) The tertiary structure of a protein does not affect its nutritive value, because the protein is unfolded, denatured, and hydrolyzed during the digestive process.

11. (3) Eggs contain very high quality protein, have all the essential amino acids in the right proportions for human protein synthesis, and have been chosen as the standard against which to evaluate all other proteins.

(1) Cow's milk contains all the essential amino acids, but when compared with egg protein, it does not score as high in biologic value.

(2) Rice is low in the essential amino acids lysine and isoleucine.

(4) Gelatin is an animal protein, but it is an incomplete protein because it lacks tryptophan.

(5) Corn is low in the essential amino acids tryptophan and lysine.

12. (2) A positive nitrogen balance represents a condition in which a person is taking in more nitrogen (as protein) than is being excreted. This occurs during periods in which the body is synthesizing new tissue such as during childhood, pregnancy, and recovery from an illness or surgery.

(1) With inadequate protein ingestion, there is breakdown of the body's own protein tissue such as muscle to provide amino acids for essential protein molecules. This results in a net loss of nitrogen by excretion.

(3) During febrile illnesses protein tissue is often broken down to provide energy, and there is a net loss of nitrogen.

(4) Old age itself will not cause either a positive or negative nitrogen balance. The nitrogen balance will depend on the health and diet of the older person.

(5) During febrile illnesses protein tissue is often broken down to provide energy, and there is a net loss of nitrogen.

13. (1) On the basis of the recommendations for (and the usual intake of) healthy Americans, 10% to 15% of the total kilocalories of the diet should come from protein.

(2) Between 20% and 25% of the total kilocalories is more than recommended.

(3) Between 30% and 35% of the total kilocalories is more than recommended.

(4) Between 40% and 45% of the total kilocalories is more than recommended.

(5) Between 50% and 55% of the total kilocalories is more than recommended.

14. (3) Excess amino acids are deaminated. The resulting keto acid can be converted to and stored as fat, and the amino group is converted to urea and excreted in the urine.

(1) Amino acids are not stored.

(2) Fat contains no nitrogen.

(4) Animals cannot oxidize nitrogen.

(5) Urea is not stored in healthy persons.

15. (3) When a small child is weaned from breast milk in a population too poor to provide another good source of protein to meet growth and maintenance needs, the child often develops kwashiorkor. Although there is muscle wasting, this is often masked by edema that occurs because there are insufficient serum proteins being synthesized to maintain osmotic balance.

(1) Kwashiorkor also occurs when protein intake is lower than growth and maintenance needs and may be present in a child even though the muscles do not appear wasted.

(2) Although protein and caloric malnutrition often are closely associated, *kwashiorkor* refers specifically to a protein deficiency in the presence of adequate or nearly adequate calories. *Marasmus* refers to the condition in which proteins and calories may be in correct proportion to each other, but total calories are insufficient.

(4) Kwashiorkor also occurs commonly in impoverished areas after children have been weaned.

(5) See 2.

16. (4) The majority of the fat in a normal diet is in the form of triglycerides.

(1) Cholesterol accounts for approximately 0.6 g out of the 100 g fats consumed.

(2) Phospholipids such as lecithin in eggs account for a very small percentage of the total fat intake.

(3) Of the fatty acids in dietary triglycerides, less than one third are consumed as polyunsaturated fatty acids.

(5) Lipoproteins constitute a very small percentage of the total fat intake. Their importance lies in their role in transporting lipids in the circulatory system.

17. (5) Dietary lipids provide the essential fatty acids (linoleic, linolenic, and arachidonic acids) and slow the stomach's emptying time, which provides satiety to the diet.

(1) Scurvy is prevented by providing adequate amounts of water-soluble vitamin C; the water-soluble vitamins riboflavin and thiamin are not found in fats.

(2) The water-soluble vitamins riboflavin and thiamin are not found in fats.

(3) Scurvy is prevented by providing adequate amounts of water soluble vitamin C; riboflavin and thiamin are not found in fats.

(4) Fats do not aid in the absorption of minerals; a very high-fat diet can cause formation of mineral-fat complexes, called soaps, that will inhibit both mineral and fat absorption.

18. (4) Saturation of the double bonds of a fatty acid changes the physical (and chemical) properties so that they have a higher melting point and are solids at room temperature. Saturated fats are more often found in animal fats than in fats from plant sources.

(1) Oils have a lower melting point than solid fats because of the greater number of double bonds in the oils.

(2) Saturated fatty acids are also usually solids at room temperature.

(3) Oils have a lower melting point than solid fats, and the iodine number is directly related to the number of double bonds or the degree of unsaturation.

(5) The iodine number is directly related to the number of double bonds or the degree of unsaturation.

19. (4) Linoleic acid is the only essential fatty acid in the list. The amount of dietary linoleic acid found to prevent both biochemical and clinical evidence of deficiency in humans is 1% to 2% of the total daily kilocalories. The average diet has about 6%.

(1) Cholesterol, although necessary for many body functions, need not be supplied in the diet, because it can be synthesized in vivo (in the body).

(2) Lecithin is a phospholipid important for its ability to act as an emulsifier.

(3) Butyric acid is a short, four-carbon fatty acid.

(5) Stearic acid, an 18-carbon fatty acid, is one of the most abundant fatty acids found in animal fats.

20. (3) The body synthesizes 1 to 2 g of cholesterol each day.

(1) If cholesterol is completely eliminated from the diet in those individuals who have high serum cholesterol levels, de novo cholesterol synthesis will still occur.

(2) Cholesterol is a precursor in the synthesis of bile and many hormones.

(4) The average cholesterol intake in the U.S. diet is approximately 600 mg.

(5) There is a positive correlation between serum cholesterol levels and cardiovascular disease.

21. (4) HDLs are believed to carry cholesterol away from the peripheral vessels to the liver for degradation. A higher HDL fraction would be expected to prevent the deposition of cholesterol in vascular plaques. HDL levels may be increased by exercise.

(1) LDLs are the main carrier of cholesterol from the liver to all parts of the body. High blood cholesterol levels usually reflect high LDL levels.

(2) VLDLs carry mainly triglycerides to all parts of the body.

(3) VHDLs is a nonsense term.

(5) Chylomicrons carry lipids from the gastrointestinal tract to the liver via the lymphatic system.

22. (2) Plaques are the combination of lipid material, mostly cholesterol, smooth muscle cells, and calcium that become lodged in the walls of arteries. (*Plaque* also refers to the accumulation of other kinds of materials on teeth.)

(1) The aorta is a large artery coming from the heart.

(3) An embolism is a blockage of a blood vessel by a blood clot that has become dislodged.

(4) An aneurysm is a ballooning out of the wall of an artery.

(5) An infarction is a sudden cutting off of the blood flow to the heart (heart attack).

23. (4) Complete elimination of all fats from the diet is extremely difficult to do without eating an artificially formulated diet or cutting out certain food groups entirely. If a fat-free diet is consumed for any length of time, one would run the risk of essential fatty acid deficiency and deficiencies of water-soluble vitamins. Furthermore, fats lend aroma and satiety to foods, whereas their absence makes foods less pleasing.

(1) A 1- to 2-pound weight loss per week is safe and sufficient for a steady loss over a period of time.

(2) A negative calorie balance forces the body to use the stored calories in adipose tissue.

(3) Increased exercise is a good way to help achieve a negative energy balance.

(5) Eating favorite foods, but cutting down on quantities, is a good incentive for sticking to a diet.

24. (3) Thiamin becomes part of the coenzyme thiamine pyrophosphate (TPP), which is involved in many of the reactions in the catabolism (or breakdown for energy) of carbohydrates, fats, and amino acids.

(1) Formation of the components of red blood cells requires many vitamins as coenzymes; however, one of the most significant is the role played by folic acid.

(2) Blood coagulation requires vitamin K.

(4) Collagen formation requires vitamin C.

(5) Prevention of night blindness requires vitamin A.

25. (2) Among the many and varied properties of minerals are the ability to regulate body processes (e.g., calcium and the regulation of nerve impulses), help maintain acid-base balance (e.g., phosphorus and phosphoric acid), and give rigidity and strength to bones and teeth (e.g., calcium, phosphorus, and fluoride).

(1) Minerals are not ''burned'' by the body for energy.

(3) Minerals are not ''burned'' by the body for energy.

(4) Minerals are not ''burned'' by the body for energy.

(5) Minerals also help maintain acid-base balance.

26. (3) Folacin is required for the synthesis of deoxyribonucleic acid (DNA) that must be present for the formation of new cells. Since vitamin B_{12} is necessary to convert folacin (folic acid) to its active form, both folacin *and* vitamin B_{12} are necessary for the synthesis and maturation of red blood cells. If there is a shortage of DNA, the red blood cells will remain in the immature macrocytic stage and not mature and divide.

(1) Pantothenic acid is a part of CoA; biotin is necessary in reactions in which there is a transfer of carbon dioxide groups.

(2) Pyridoxine is part of the coenzyme pyridoxal phosphate; vitamin B_{12} is necessary for the formation of the active form of folacin.

(4) Thiamin is part of the coenzyme thiamine pyrophosphate; riboflavin is part of the coenzyme flavin adenine dinucleotide (FAD).

(5) Niacin is part of the coenzyme nicotinamide-adenine dinucleotide.

27. (4) For each 60 mg of tryptophan ingested, approximately 1 mg is converted to niacin. The average U.S. diet supplies 500 to 1000 mg or more of tryptophan daily and 8 to 17 mg of niacin, for a total of 16 to 34 mg of niacin equivalents.

(1) Valine cannot be converted to niacin.

(2) Lysine cannot be converted to niacin.

(3) Tyrosine cannot be converted to niacin.

(5) Phenylalanine cannot be converted to niacin.

28. (5) Vitamin A plays a role in all the given functions.

(1) Vitamin A also plays a role in promoting normal jaw development and in promoting the laying down of new bone.

(2) Vitamin A also plays a role in promoting the laying down of new bone.

(3) Vitamin A also plays a role in maintaining healthy epithelial tissue and in promoting normal jaw development.

(4) Vitamin A also plays a role in maintaining healthy epithelial tissue.

29. (2) Apricots (225 retinol equivalents [RE]), pumpkin pie (700 RE), liver (7000 RE), and sweet potatoes (900 RE) are all good sources of vitamin A.

(1) Bread, vegetable oil, and legumes are poor sources of vitamin A.

(3) Vegetable oil and legumes are poor sources of vitamin A.

(4) Bread, legumes, and baked potatoes are poor sources of vitamin A.

(5) Legumes and baked potatoes are poor sources of vitamin A.

30. (2) β-Carotene is enzymatically converted to retinol; 6 μg of β-carotene will yield 1 μg of retinol (one of the active forms of vitamin A).

(1) Tryptophan is not converted to vitamin A in the body.

(3) Xanthophyll is not converted to vitamin A in the body.

(4) Chlorophyll is not converted to vitamin A in the body.

(5) Cholesterol is not converted to vitamin A in the body.

31. (3) These are the recommended servings from the Basic Four food groups for adolescents.

(1) These are the recommended daily servings for children.

(2) These are the recommended daily servings for adults.

(4) These are the recommended daily servings during pregnancy.

(5) These are the recommended daily servings during lactation.

32. (3) Bulimia is a condition occurring most often in young women who have eating binges that can result in daily calorie intake of 5000 to 10,000; normal body weight is maintained by self-induced vomiting. The acidic nature of the stomach contents erodes the tooth enamel, especially on lingual surfaces.

(1) Alcoholism may increase the energy input to maintain weight but does not cause decalcification of tooth enamel.

(2) Drug abuse may cause an increased energy input to maintain weight but does not cause decalcification of tooth enamel.

(4) Excessive smoking may cause an increased energy input to maintain weight but does not cause decalcification of tooth enamel. It usually causes staining of the enamel.

(5) Diabetes mellitus type I may cause an increased energy input but does not cause decalcification of tooth enamel.

33. (2) Meats and dairy products are a major source of vitamin B_{12}, essential amino acids, and iron, and pure vegetarians eliminate these foods from their diets.

(1) Pure vegetarians include fruits and vegetables in their diet, which are good sources of vitamins A and C.

(3) Magnesium, zinc, and essential amino acids are found in green leafy vegetables, grains, and legumes, which are included in a pure vegetarians diet.

(4) Pyridoxine, pantothenic acid, and vitamin B_{12} are found in vegetables, whole grains, and legumes.

(5) Selenium, copper, and nonessential amino acids are found in grains and a variety of vegetables.

34. (3) Sodium regulates extracellular water; potassium regulates intracellular water.

(1) Calcium and phosphorus maintain the integrity of mineralized tissues.

(2) Chloride and sulfur function in acid-base balance and maintenance of cartilage and muscle.

(4) Chloride and iodine function in acid-base balance and energy metabolism

(5) Potassium also functions in acid-base balance and maintenance of cartilage and muscle.

35. (4) Blood loss, vomiting, and diarrhea lead to excessive loss of body water.

(1) A condition characterized by water retention is called edema.

(2) Sodium retention leads to excessive water retention.

(3) Diarrhea can also lead to dehydration.

(5) Sodium retention leads to excessive water retention.

36. (3) Malnutrition can result from overconsumption of fat, sodium, and other nutrients in addition to underconsumption of all the essential nutrients.

(1) Inadequate intake of essential nutrients can lead to disease.

(2) Excessive intake of fat can lead to excessive calorie intake and weight gain; excessive intake of sodium can lead to excessive fluid retention.

(4) Excessive intake of sodium can lead to excessive fluid retention.

(5) Inadequate calorie intake is a nutritional problem.

37. (4) A low-calorie fad diet, inadequate food-purchasing power, and poor oral health all lead to an inadequate food intake and are causes of a primary nutritional deficiency.
    (1) A lactase deficiency and drug-nutrient reactions affect nutrient use and are classified as secondary nutritional deficiencies.
    (2) A lactase deficiency affects nutrient use.
    (3) Drug-nutrient reactions affect nutrient use.
    (5) Drug-nutrient reactions affect nutrient use.
38. (2) Inborn errors of metabolism, food allergies, and obstruction of the gastrointestinal tract interfere with the ability to digest, absorb, and use nutrients even if food intake is adequate and are classified as secondary nutritional deficiencies.
    (1) Improper food preparation is a cause of primary nutritional deficiencies.
    (3) Improper food preparation and loss of appetite are causes of primary nutritional deficiencies.
    (4) Loss of appetite is a cause of primary nutritional deficiencies.
    (5) Improper food preparation and loss of appetite are causes of primary nutritional deficiencies.
39. (4) Skinfold calipers measure fat and lean body tissues without invasive biochemical testing.
    (1) Biochemical analysis reveals the level of nutrients and their function in the body.
    (2) With the use of common antigens, the patient's immunocompetence is assessed.
    (3) Chemical analysis of hair is used to determine mineral status.
    (5) Urine analysis reveals the level of nutrients and their function in the body.
40. (1) Oral tissues, height, weight, eyes, skin, and nails all provide information about the nutritional status.
    (2) Height, weight, and nails also provide information about the nutritional status.
    (3) Oral tissues also provide information about the nutritional status.
    (4) Oral tissues and eyes also provide information about the nutritional status.
    (5) Oral tissues, height, and weight also provide information about the nutritional status.
41. (4) Nutritional screening questionnaires, 5-day food diaries, and 24-hour recall are useful in finding out what the patient eats.
    (1) Skinfold calipers provide information on fat and lean body tissues.
    (2) Blood tests determine nutritional status, not food intake.
    (3) Blood tests determine nutritional status, not food intake.
    (5) Nutritional screening questionnaires are also useful in finding out what the patient eats.
42. (3) A nutritional screening questionnaire does not provide information on serving sizes of food consumed and therefore no nutrient analysis (e.g., calories or iron) can be made.

(1) A nutritional screening questionnaire can be filled out while waiting for a dental appointment.
(2) A nutritional screening questionnaire is a good method to screen patients who need more dietary counseling.
(4) A nutritional screening questionnaire can be used to get a "feel" about the patient's sugar intake.
(5) A nutritional screening questionnaire gives information about the patient's use of vitamin and mineral supplements.
43. (4) An analysis of nonnutritive food additives can be obtained only if brand names for food products are known; this type of analysis is usually done by industry and chemical laboratories.
    (1) An analysis of individual nutrients can be done with the use of a computer and nutrient data banks.
    (2) An analysis of the total amount of sugars in grams can be done by computers; assessment of the form and frequency of sugar exposure can be done from the diet forms.
    (3) An analysis of the diet using the four food groups can be done directly from the diet forms.
    (5) An analysis of caloric intake can be done with the use of a computer and nutrient data banks.
44. (2) Simplicity, cost, patient participation, and ease of learning are advantages in using the Basic Four food groups for dental patients.
    (1) The caloric content of diets cannot be determined using the Basic Four food groups.
    (3) The caloric content of diets cannot be determined using the Basic Four food groups.
    (4) There are no specific or accurate calculations for any nutrient; the Basic Four is a method to determine general adequacy of the diet.
    (5) There are no specific or accurate calculations for vitamins.
45. (2) A computer diet analysis is a specific measure of individual nutrients from food consumed.
    (1) Current methodology does not involve patient participation, and patients cannot use it at home unless they have the necessary hardware and software.
    (3) Hardware and software are expensive.
    (4) Patients are provided with the results and are not involved in the analysis.
    (5) A trained counselor is needed to interpret the results for the patient.
46. (2) The patient becomes actively involved in analyzing his or her diet and developing a realistic modification program.
    (1) The counselor is in control.
    (3) The patient is passive.
    (4) The counselor is in control.
    (5) The counselor is in control.
47. (3) Adult recall patients could benefit from nutritional counseling but are not at risk because of disease.
    (1) Nutrient needs are higher because of tissue repair and host defense activities; appetite and mastication may be adversely affected by surgery.
    (2) Nutrient needs are higher because of tissue repair and gingival inflammation.

(4) Dietary sugars may be involved in the problem.

(5) Poor dietary intake and excessive sugar and caffeine may aggrevate acute necrotic ulcerated gingitivitis.

48. (3) The patient's level of risk for nutritional problems and level of interest and motivation in preventive dentistry, as well as office personnel and their training in nutritional counseling, office time, and facilities, are determinants in selecting patients for counseling.

(1) For counseling to be valuable to a patient, the counselor needs to be trained in the science of nutrition and behavior modification technique.

(2) A patient with high nutritional needs or with disease is at risk for nutritional deficiencies and would benefit from counseling.

(4) Educational background should not be a determinant unless it is accompanied by poor motivation.

(5) The patient's educational background is not a determinant unless accompanied by poor motivation.

49. (3) The presence of saliva is protective against dental disease.

(1) The host factor is part of the triad of dental disease.

(2) The agent factor is part of the triad of dental disease.

(4) The substrate factor is needed by oral bacteria for growth.

(5) The host factor is part of the triad of dental disease.

50. (2) Deficiencies in the water-soluble vitamins result in the following alterations of oral tissues: vitamic C deficiency results in inadequate collagen formation and integrity of blood vessels, leading to edematous and bleeding gingiva; water-soluble vitamins are needed for the integrity of the oral mucosa and lips.

(1) Vitamin D is important in calcium absorption, and deficiencies affect mineralized tissues.

(3) Calcium and phosphorus do not play an important role in oral soft tissue health.

(4) Zinc deficiency leads to thickness of the epithelium.

(5) Zinc deficiency leads to thickness of the epithelium.

51. (2) Sugar does not contain nitrogen and therefore cannot be converted to urea.

(1) Energy production results from the metabolism of sugars.

(3) Acid production is an end product of glycolysis.

(4) Plaque formation results from the synthesis of glucans from dietary sugars.

(5) Polysaccharides are synthesized from dietary sugars.

52. (4) Glucans are insoluble polysaccharides synthesized from glucose and give the sticky, retentive nature to plaque.

(1) Levans are soluble polysaccharides synthesized from fructose and do not have some qualities of glucans.

(2) Glycogen is a polysaccharide synthesized from fructose and glucose and stored intracellularly to be readily used for energy.

(3) Cellulose is not formed by *S. mutans*.

(5) Pectins are not formed by *S. mutans*.

53. (3) The body cannot use saccharin for energy; bacteria cannot use it for energy.

(1) Saccharin is not a nutritive sweetener.

(2) Saccharin does not lead to dental decay.

(4) Saccharin does not lead to dental decay.

(5) Saccharin is a dietary sweetener used in many food products (e.g., Sweet n' Low sugar substitute).

54. (2) The body uses lactose for calories; bacteria can use lactose for energy, thus resulting in acid production and decay.

(1) Lactose can lead to dental decay and is cariogenic.

(3) Lactose is both a nutritive and cariogenic sweetener.

(4) Lactose is a nutritive sweetener.

(5) Lactose is a nutritive sweetener found in milk and milk products.

55. (1) Aspartame is made up of two amino acids and therefore used by the body; bacteria do not metabolize aspartame for energy.

(2) Aspartame does not lead to dental decay.

(3) Aspartame is a nutritive sweetener.

(4) Aspartame is a nutritive sweetener.

(5) Aspartame is a dietary sweetener and is used in industry. NutraSweet and Equal are product names.

56. (1) Sorbitol is a sugar alcohol that provides calories; it is noncariogenic because acidogenic bacteria can only minimally use it for energy.

(2) Sorbitol is not cariogenic.

(3) Sorbitol is a nutritive sweetener.

(4) Sorbitol is a nutritive sweetener and noncariogenic.

(5) Sorbitol is a dietary sweetener and is used in diabetic products and sugarless gum.

57. (3) Fructose is a nutritive sweetener readily used by acidogenic bacteria, resulting in acid production and plaque formation.

(1) Sorbitol is a sugar alcohol and is minimally used by acidogenic bacteria.

(2) Aspartame is a sugar substitute consisting of two amino acids.

(4) Saccharin is a sugar substitute and is not used by acidogenic bacteria.

(5) Xyletol is a sugar alcohol and is minimally used by acidogenic bacteria.

58. (3) Hormonal changes during pregnancy result in increased gingival sensitivity to local irritants such as plaque and calculus, but pregnancy does not cause gingivitis.

(1) Good oral hygiene will control pregnancy gingivitis.

(2) Oral pregnancy tumors occur infrequently.

(4) Hormonal changes during pregnancy do alter tissue resistance.

(5) Bacteria acids, not hormones, cause enamel decalcification.

59. (5) Trauma often results in liver glycogenolysis (glycogen breakdown) to meet caloric and energy needs rather than glycogenesis (glycogen synthesis).
    (1) Nutrient losses from tissue injury and blood loss are physiologic consequences of oral surgery.
    (2) Increased nutrient needs for cellular defense and tissue repair are physiologic consequences of oral surgery.
    (3) Decreased appetite and ability to chew are physiologic consequences of oral surgery.
    (4) A hypermetabolic state is a physiologic consequence of oral surgery.

60. (1) Often the food is available to handicapped patients, but they do not have the ability to feed themselves or eat it.
    (2) Absence of the sucking response can lead to inadequate food intake.
    (3) Poor arm and head control can lead to inadequate food intake.
    (4) Inadequate jaw, lip, and tongue control can lead to inadequate food intake.
    (5) A short attention span can lead to inadequate food intake.

CHAPTER 10

Dental Materials

JOHN M. POWERS

STEPHEN C. BAYNE

An understanding of the vast array of dental materials and their application is important for rendering quality dental hygiene services, for implementing dental disease control concepts, and for answering patient questions about oral health care. The dental hygienist, knowledgeable about dental materials theory and practice, can participate competently in these areas and manipulate dental materials when necessary. The subject of dental materials has advanced with recent developments in new materials, as well as alterations in the manipulation of materials and in the techniques and procedures for using them. This chapter focuses on the properties of dental materials; cements, bases, liners, and varnishes; metallic and other restorative materials; preventive agents; gypsum products; impression materials, models, and dies; waxes; materials for dental prostheses; and finishing, polishing, and cleansing materials.

PROPERTIES OF MATERIALS ▰▰▰▰▰

General Considerations

A. Types of properties
   1. Physical
   2. Electrical
   3. Mechanical
B. Importance of understanding properties
   1. Materials used to replace teeth are exposed to attack by the oral environment and subjected to biting forces
   2. Properties are used as the basis for selection of materials
   3. Establishment of critical properties has resulted in American Dental Association specifications
      a. Helpful in the selection of materials
      b. Assurance of quality control of certified materials

Dimensional Change

A. Changes caused by the setting reaction
   1. Examples include the setting of dental amalgam, composites, and rubber impression materials
   2. Calculation of the rate of change is

   $$\frac{(l_1 - l_0)}{l_0} \times 100$$

   where l_1 is the length at 24 hours and l_0 is the original length
B. Changes caused by a change in temperature
   1. Thermal expansion of restorative material does not usually match that of the tooth structure
   2. Calculation of the rate of change is

   $$\left(\frac{l_2 - l_1}{l_1}\right) \div (t_2 - t_1)$$

   with values typically reported in units of $10^{-6}/°C$
   3. Values of linear coefficient of thermal expansion range from $10 \times 10^{-6}/°C$ for human teeth to $300 \times 10^{-6}/°C$ for waxes
   4. Percolation results when fluids penetrate the space between the restoration and tooth during cyclic heating and cooling

Thermal Conductivity

A. Importance
   1. Tooth with a metal restoration may be sensitive temporarily to hot and cold foods and liquids
   2. Individuals wearing acrylic complete dentures may experience temperature effects different from those experienced by dentulous patients
B. Comparison of materials
   1. Human enamel and dentin, dental cements, and plastic restorative materials are good thermal insulators compared with dental amalgam and gold alloys

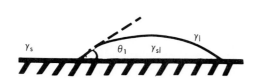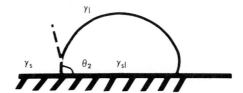

Fig. 10-1 Contact angles of water on hydrophilic *(left)* and hydrophobic *(right)* surfaces. (From Craig, R.G., O'Brien, W.J., and Powers, J.M.: Dental materials: properties and manipulation, ed. 3, St. Louis, 1983, The C.V. Mosby Co.)

  2. To be an effective insulator, the remaining tooth structure or the cement layer must be at least 0.5 mm thick

Electrical Properties

A. Galvinism
  1. Results from the presence of dissimilar metals in the mouth
  2. Contact of dissimilar metals can result in a flow of current that can cause pain
  3. Temporary plastic crowns are used to prevent this problem
B. Corrosion (tarnish)
  1. May be caused by galvanic action or chemical attack by foods
  2. Metal goes into solution; roughness and pitting result

Solubility and Sorption

A. Solubility
  1. Dissolution of material in distilled water or acid may not completely describe clinical observations, but the ranking is usually valid
  2. Dissolution may be followed by disintegration, as in dental cements
  3. Calculated as weight percent or weight per square centimeter
B. Sorption
  1. Absorption—uptake of liquid by the bulk solid (e.g., water absorbed in a denture resin)
  2. Adsorption—concentration of molecules at the surface of a solid or liquid (e.g., saliva adsorbed to tooth structure)
  3. Calculated as weight percent or weight per square centimeter

Wettability

A. Definition
  1. Wetting depends on the surface tension of the liquid-solid interface and the surface energy of the solid

  2. Good wetting occurs when the surface tension of the liquid is low and that of the solid is high
    a. Cleanliness of the solid is important
    b. Surface-active agents (detergents) in the liquid improve wetting
    c. Increased temperature of the liquid improves wetting
B. Examples
  1. Wetting of denture plastics by saliva
  2. Wetting of tooth enamel by pit and fissure sealants
C. Measurement
  1. Shape of a drop of liquid on the solid surface is observed (Fig. 10-1)
  2. Contact angles are defined by the solid surface and a line through the periphery of the drop and tangent to the surface of the liquid
    a. Hydrophilic surface has a low contact angle with water and is easily wet
    b. Hydrophobic surface has a high contact angle (greater than 90 degrees) and is poorly wet

Mechanical Properties

A. Biting forces
  1. Decrease from molars (130 pounds) to incisors (40 pounds)
  2. Decrease with restorations—molar area of a fixed bridge can exert 50 pounds, whereas molar area of a denture can exert 25 pounds
B. Stress
  1. Resistance in a material when force is applied to it
  2. Calculated by force/area; units are in pounds per square inch (lb/in^2) or meganewtons per square meter (MN/m^2)
  3. Types
    a. Compressive
    b. Tensile
    c. Shear

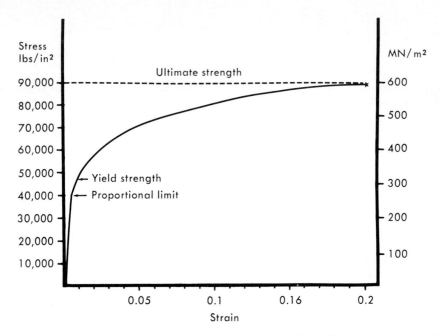

Fig. 10-2 Stress-strain curve in tension for dental gold alloy. (From Craig, R.G., O'Brien, W.J., and Powers, J.M.: Dental materials: properties and manipulation, ed. 3, St. Louis, 1983, The C.V. Mosby Co.)

C. Strain
1. Change in length per unit of length when a material is subjected to a force
2. Calculated by deformation/length; units are dimensionless

D. Stress-strain curve
1. Plot of stress versus strain allows convenient comparison of mechanical properties of materials (Fig. 10-2)
2. Determined in compression, tension, or shear

E. Elastic modulus
1. Measure of the stiffness of a material
2. Equal to the ratio of stress to strain in the linear portion of the stress-strain curve; units are in pounds per square inch or meganewtons per square meter (Fig. 10-2)
3. Gold alloy and human enamel have similar stiffness—12×10^6 lb/in^2—followed by human dentin and zinc phosphate cement—3×10^6 lb/in^2—followed by polysulfide rubber—400 lb/in^2

F. Proportional limit (yield strength)
1. Stress at which a material no longer functions as an elastic solid
2. Measured at a small amount of permanent strain, such as 0.002; units are in pounds per square inch (Fig. 10-2)

3. Materials are elastic below the proportional limit and plastic above it

G. Ultimate strength
1. Stress at which a material eventually fractures in tension or compression (Fig. 10-2)
2. Compressive strength is usually greater than tensile strength for brittle dental materials such as human enamel, amalgam, and cements

H. Elongation and compression
1. Percent of elongation (or compression) is the amount of deformation a material can withstand before fracture (Fig. 10-2)
2. Determined as strain at fracture times 100%
3. Measure of ductility and malleability
a. Materials with elongation of less than 5% are brittle
b. Materials with elongation of more than 5% are ductile

I. Resilience and toughness
1. Resilience (Fig. 10-3, *A*)—measure of energy required to deform a material permanently
2. Toughness (Fig. 10-3, *B*)—measure of energy required to fracture a material

J. Hardness
1. Measure of resistance of a material to indentation

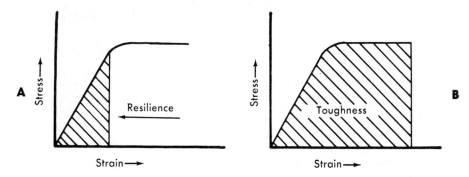

Fig. 10-3 Stress-strain curves illustrating areas that measure resilience, **A,** and toughness, **B.** (From Craig, R.G., O'Brien, W.J., and Powers, J.M.: Dental materials: properties and manipulation, ed. 3, St. Louis, 1983, The C.V. Mosby Co.)

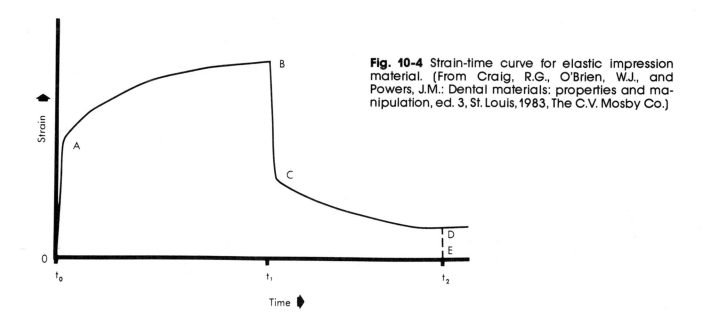

Fig. 10-4 Strain-time curve for elastic impression material. (From Craig, R.G., O'Brien, W.J., and Powers, J.M.: Dental materials: properties and manipulation, ed. 3, St. Louis, 1983, The C.V. Mosby Co.)

2. Types
    a. Knoop hardness—varies from 460 kg/mm² for porcelain to 40 kg/mm² for human cementum and zinc phosphate cement
    b. Rockwell hardness—used for composites and plastics
    c. Shore A—used for elastomeric materials such as mouth protectors

K. Strain-time curve
  1. Important for materials in which strain is dependent on the time the load is maintained—describes viscoelastic materials
  2. Characteristics (Fig. 10-4)
    a. Line *OA*—load applied at t_0 results in elastic strain

    b. Line *AB*—load maintained until t_1; strain results from viscoelastic strain (time dependent but recoverable) and viscous flow (time dependent but not recoverable)
    c. Line *BC*—elastic recovery when the load is removed
    d. Line *CD*—gradual recovery of viscoelastic strain
    e. Segment *DE*—magnitude of permanent strain

L. Dynamic properties
  1. Result from an extremely high rate of application of the load
  2. Dynamic modulus—measure of stiffness at a high rate of strain
  3. Dynamic resilience—measure of energy absorbed at high rates of strain

Color

A. Definition
1. Perception of color is a physiologic response to a physical stimulus
2. Eye can distinguish three parameters of color
   a. Dominant wavelength—blue, green, yellow, orange, and red
   b. Luminance—lightness of color from black to white
   c. Excitation purity—saturation of light
B. Measurement
1. Visual technique by the Munsell Color System (Fig. 10-5)
   a. Hue—family of colors including red *(R)*, yellow-red *(YR)*, yellow *(Y)*, green-yellow *(GY)*, green *(G)*, blue-green *(BG)*, blue *(B)*, purple-blue *(PB)*, purple *(P)*, and red-purple *(RP)*
   b. Value—measures lightness and ranges from black (0/) to white (10/)
   c. Chroma—measures saturation of color and ranges from achromatic or gray (/0) to highly saturated color (/18)
   d. Example of measurement—color of attached gingiva of a healthy patient is 5R 6/4
2. Instrumental technique
   a. Curves of spectral reflectance versus wavelength from 405 to 700 nm are used to determine the dominant wavelength, excitation purity, and luminous reflectance
   b. Reflectance values are used with color-matching functions to calculate tristimulus values relative to a particular light source, from which chromaticity coordinates are determined with a chromaticity diagram (Fig. 10-6)
C. Metamerism
1. Metameric colors are color stimuli of identical tristimulus values under a particular light source but with different spectral energy distributions
2. Quality and intensity of light must be controlled in matching colors
D. Fluorescence
1. Emission of luminous energy by a material when a beam of light is shown on it
2. Blue or ultraviolet light typically produces fluorescent light that is in the visible range
3. Sound human teeth and some composites and porcelains emit blue fluorescent light when excited by ultraviolet light
E. Opacity, translucency, and transparency
1. Opacity—property that prevents the passage of light through a material
2. Translucency—property that permits the passage of light but disperses it to such an extent that objects cannot be seen through the material
3. Transparency—property that allows the passage of light with little distortion
4. Measurement of these properties is done instrumentally or visually by determination of the contrast ratio, which ranges from 0 (translucent) to 1 (opaque); composites range from 0.55 to 0.70

CEMENTS, BASES, LINERS, AND VARNISHES

Zinc Phosphate Cement

A. General considerations
1. Used primarily for final cementation when high strength is necessary
2. Pulpal protection required
B. Composition and reaction
1. Powder—composed of zinc oxide with some magnesium oxide and pigments
2. Liquid—phosphoric acid in water buffered by aluminum and zinc ions
3. Reaction
   a. Surface of alkaline powder is dissolved by acidic liquid; powder and liquid are matched by the manufacturer to control the setting time
   b. Exothermic reaction—heat given off
   c. Set cement—porous, hydrated network of zinc phosphate that surrounds incompletely dissolved powder particles
   d. Factors that accelerate setting reaction
      (1) Heat
      (2) Moisture
      (3) Higher powder/liquid ratio
      (4) Faster incorporation of powder into liquid
C. Properties
1. Setting time—normally 5 to 9 mintues
2. Strength (Table 10-1)
   a. Compressive strength is 20 times tensile strength—brittle
   b. Adversely affected by a low powder/liquid ratio, improper mixing, and premature exposure to oral fluids
   c. Develops rapidly—two thirds within first hour
3. Retention—mechanical interlocking of cement with the tooth and restoration
4. Film thickness—25 μm maximum; within clinically acceptable limits

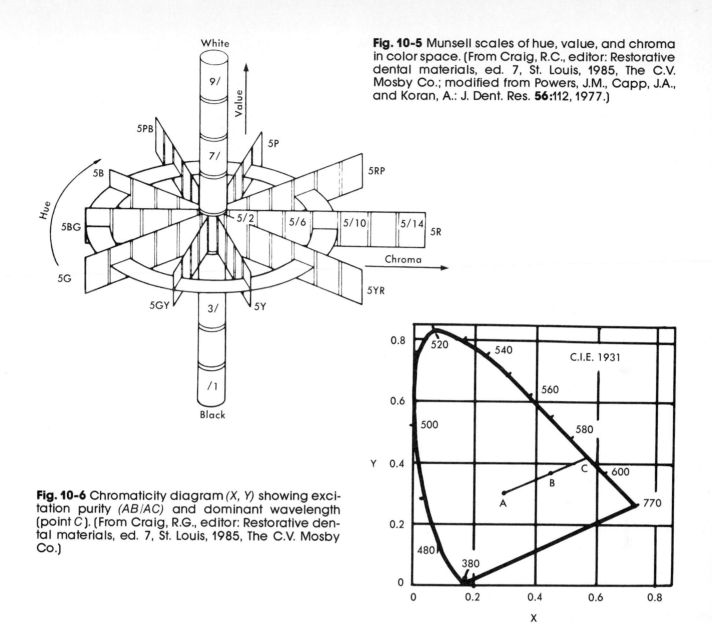

Fig. 10-5 Munsell scales of hue, value, and chroma in color space. (From Craig, R.C., editor: Restorative dental materials, ed. 7, St. Louis, 1985, The C.V. Mosby Co.; modified from Powers, J.M., Capp, J.A., and Koran, A.: J. Dent. Res. **56**:112, 1977.)

Fig. 10-6 Chromaticity diagram *(X, Y)* showing excitation purity *(AB/AC)* and dominant wavelength (point *C*). (From Craig, R.G., editor: Restorative dental materials, ed. 7, St. Louis, 1985, The C.V. Mosby Co.)

Table 10-1   Mechanical properties of cements for final and temporary cementation*

Cement	Compressive strength (psi [MN/m²])	Tensile strength (psi [MN/m²])	Modulus of elasticity (10⁶ psi [GN/m²])†
Cements for final cementation			
Zinc phosphate	13,000-17,000 (90-115)	600-1200 (4-8)	2.0 (13)
Zinc silicophosphate	19,000-25,000 (130-170)	—	—
Zinc oxide–eugenol (type II)			
Polymer reinforced	7000 (50)	600 (4)	0.4 (3.0)
EBA-alumina reinforced	9000 (64)	1000 (7)	0.8 (5.4)
Zinc polycarboxylate	8000-11,000 (55-76)	700-1400 (5-10)	0.6 (4.4)
Glass ionomer	17,000 (115)	1100 (8)	—
Cements for temporary cementation			
Zinc oxide–eugenol (type I)	200-3000 (1-20)	—	—
Noneugenol zinc oxide	580 (4)	160 (1.1)	0.03 (0.18)

From Craig, R.G., O'Brien, W.J., and Powers, J.M.: Dental materials: properties and manipulation, ed. 3, St. Louis, 1983, The C.V. Mosby Co.
*Properties measured at 24 hours.
†10⁶ psi = 1,000,000 psi, and giganewtons per square meter (GN/m²) = 1000 MN/m².

5. Solubility—within clinically acceptable limits
6. Acidity
    a. pH increases from 4.2 to 7 within 48 hours
    b. Pulpal protection recommended
D. Manipulation
    1. Normal technique
        a. Powder/liquid ratio is normally 2.6 g to 1.0 ml
        b. Slab is cooled to about 21° C but above the dew point
        c. Powder is incorporated into liquid in four to six 15-second increments within 60 to 90 seconds
        d. Mixing occurs over a large area of the slab to dissipate heat
        e. Luting consistency strings about 1 inch above the slab
        f. Properties are affected by manipulative variables (Table 10-2)
    2. Frozen slab technique—provides longer working times and a shorter setting time in the mouth
        a. Slab is cooled at 6° or −10° C
        b. Condensed moisture is incorporated into cement with 50% to 75% additional powder
        c. Powder is added to liquid within 30 seconds to achieve the correct consistency

Zinc Silicophosphate Cement

A. General considerations
    1. Used primarily for final cementation of porcelain jacket crowns
    2. Excellent translucency and high strength
    3. Pulpal protection required
B. Composition and reaction
    1. Powder—acid-soluble silicates, zinc oxide, magnesium oxide, and fluorides
    2. Liquid—buffered phosphoric acid in water
    3. Reaction—matrix of fluorides and insoluble phosphates surround partially reacted powder particles

C. Properties
    1. Strength (see Table 10-1)—50% stronger than zinc phosphate cement
    2. Retention—mechanical interlocking of cement with the tooth and restoration
    3. Acidity
        a. pH initially more acidic than zinc phosphate, but pH of 7 after 48 hours
        b. Pulpal protection recommended
    4. Translucency—contributes to esthetics of porcelain restorations
    5. Fluoride content—provides anticariogenic action
D. Manipulation
    1. Technique is similar to that with zinc phosphate
    2. Cooled slab is used to increase the working time

Zinc Oxide–Eugenol Cement

A. General considerations
    1. Used for final cementation on teeth with exposed dentinal tubules
    2. Temporary cements are not strong but are useful for short-term cementation
B. Composition and reaction
    1. Powder
        a. Type I—zinc oxide (70%) and rosin (30%) with zinc acetate
        b. Type II—zinc oxide (80%) and acrylic resin (20%)
        c. EBA-alumina type—zinc oxide (70%) and alumina (30%)
    2. Liquid
        a. Types I and II—eugenol or a mixture of eugenol and other oils
        b. EBA-alumina type—ethoxybenzoic acid (62%) and eugenol (38%)
    3. Reaction
        a. Types I and II—powder reacts with liquid in the presence of moisture to form an amorphous chelate of zinc eugenolate

Table 10-2 Effects of manipulative variables on selected properties of zinc phosphate cement

Manipulative variables	Property				
	Compressive strength	Film thickness	Solubility	Initial acidity	Setting time
Decreased powder/liquid ratio	Decrease	Decrease	Increase	Increase	Lengthen
Increased rate of powder incorporation	Decrease	Increase	Increase	Increase	Shorten
Increased mixing temperature	Decrease	Increase	Increase	Increase	Shorten
Water contamination*	Decrease	Increase	Increase	Increase	Shorten

From Craig, R.G., O'Brien, W.J., and Powers, J.M.: Dental materials: properties and manipulation, St. Louis, 1983, The C.V. Mosby Co.
*Water contamination should not be confused with water incorporated in the frozen slab method.

   b. EBA-alumina type—stronger, crystalline matrix
   c. Factors that accelerate the setting reaction—heat and moisture
C. Properties
   1. Setting time—EBA-alumina type has a long working time but sets on exposure to oral conditions
   2. Strength (see Table 10-1)
      a. Compressive strength not as high as that of zinc phosphate
      b. Type I—low strength allows easy removal of temporary restorations
      c. Type II and EBA-alumina type—successful clinically for final cementation of crowns and bridges with good retention
   3. Retention—mechanical interlocking of cement with the tooth and restoration
   4. Film thickness—25 μm maximum; within clinically acceptable limits
   5. Solubility—within clinically acceptable limits
   6. Acidity—neutral; pulpal protection not required
D. Manipulation
   1. Type I
      a. Equal lengths of two pastes are dispensed onto a paper pad
      b. Mixing continues until a uniform color is obtained
      c. Patient's lips and adjacent teeth should be coated with a silicone grease to allow easy cleanup
      d. Oil of orange is a useful solvent for cleaning spatulas and slabs
   2. Type II
      a. Powder and liquid are dispensed onto a glass slab
      b. Powder is incorporated into liquid all at once and mixed for 30 seconds
   3. EBA-alumina type—mixed like type II, but stropped for 60 seconds after incorporation of powder

Zinc Polycarboxylate Cement

A. General considerations
   1. Used primarily for final cementation of crowns and bridges
   2. Not as strong as zinc phosphate but less irritating to the pulp
B. Composition and reaction
   1. Powder
      a. Powder-liquid type—composed of zinc oxide
      b. Anhydrous type—composed of zinc oxide coated with solid polyacrylic acid

   2. Liquid
      a. Powder-liquid type—viscous solution of polyacrylic acid in water
      b. Anhydrous type—water or solution of tartaric acid in water
   3. Reaction
      a. Surface of alkaline powder is dissolved by acidic liquid
      b. Set cement—zinc polyacrylate matrix that surrounds partially reacted zinc oxide particles
      c. Reaction less affected by heat than zinc phosphate
C. Properties
   1. Setting time—normally 5 to 9 minutes
   2. Strength (see Table 10-1)
      a. Compressive strength less than that of zinc phosphate; similar to that of type II zinc oxide–eugenol
      b. Sufficient for retention of well-fitting restorations
   3. Retention
      a. Mechanical interlocking of cement with the tooth and restoration
      b. Chemical bonding to properly prepared enamel, but clinical significance not demonstrated
   4. Film thickness—25 μm maximum; within clinically acceptable limits
   5. Solubility—within clinically acceptable limits
   6. Acidity—acid is weakly dissociated; histologic reactions are similar to those with zinc oxide–eugenol
D. Manipulation
   1. Powder/liquid ratio is normally 1.5 to 1 g
   2. About 90% of the powder is added to the liquid and mixed for 20 to 30 seconds
   3. Glass mixing slab and powder may be cooled to increase the working time
   4. Cement is no longer usable when its luster is lost and cobwebs form

Glass Ionomer Cement

A. General considerations
   1. Used for final cementation of crowns and bridges
   2. Consistency is thinner than that of glass ionomer restorative material
B. Composition and reaction
   1. Powder
      a. Powder-liquid type—finely ground aluminosilicate glass

b. Anhydrous type—finely ground aluminosilicate glass coated with a solid polycarboxylate copolymer
2. Liquid
  a. Powder-liquid type—polycarboxylate copolymer in water
  b. Anhydrous type—water or solution of tartaric acid in water
3. Reaction
  a. Surface of glass is dissolved by acidic liquid
  b. Set cement—cross-linked gel matrix surrounds partially reacted particles
  c. Chelation between polycarboxylate molecules and calcium on the surface of the tooth
C. Properties
1. Setting time—normally 5 to 9 minutes
2. Strength (see Table 10-1)—initially similar to that of zinc phosphate but continues to increase with time by about 50%
3. Retention—mechanical interlocking of cement with the tooth and restoration and adhesion to tooth structure (bonding to enamel is greater than to dentin)
4. Film thickness—25 μm maximum; within clinically acceptable limits
5. Acidity—pulpal protection with calcium hydroxide is recommended in a deep cavity
6. Solubility
  a. Early solubility is high—margins must be protected during the first 24 hours
  b. After 24 hours solubility is within clinically acceptable limits
D. Manipulation
1. Powder/liquid ratio is normally 1.25 to 1.0 g
2. Power is incorporated into liquid in four portions within 45 seconds on paper or a glass mixing surface
3. End of working time is characterized by a thicker consistency or the formation of ''skin''
4. Contact with water must be avoided during early life
  a. Field must be completely isolated
  b. Margins must be coated with an agent supplied with the cement

Resin Cement

A. General considerations
1. Used for cementation of conventional crowns and bridges and bonding of acid-etched bridges and direct-bonded orthodontic brackets
2. Strong, insoluble cement
3. Types
  a. Unfilled—powder-liquid type used for orthodontic bonding
  b. Filled—powder-liquid, two-paste, no-mix (self-cured), and light-cured types used for cementation and bonding
B. Composition and reaction
1. Unfilled
  a. Components—acrylic monomers, polymer particles, initiators, and accelerators
  b. Reaction—amine-accelerated polymerization of the monomer with polymer particles
2. Filled
  a. Components—diacrylate monomers with diluent monomers, treated filler particles, initiators, and accelerators or light absorbers
  b. Reaction—filler particles bonded to a resin matrix
    (1) Powder-liquid and two-paste types—set after components are mixed
    (2) No-mix type—sets as a result of diffusion of components when paste and primer come into contact
    (3) Light-cured type—sets on exposure to the appropriate curing light
C. Properties
1. Mechanical properties are much higher than those of zinc phosphate cement
2. Film thickness of crown and bridge resin cement is high
3. Bond strength with orthodontic brackets
  a. Adequate bonding to properly etched enamel
  b. Failures occur at the bracket-cement interface with metal brackets
D. Manipulation
1. Isolation and acid-etching of the enamel is a critical step for bonding
2. Acrylic cements—applied by a brush technique
3. Two-paste cements—equal volumes of each paste are combined
4. No-mix cements—primer is applied to the enamel, and paste is applied to the bracket
5. Light-cured cements—single paste is polymerized by light

Temporary Filling Materials

A. General considerations
1. Provide pulpal protection
2. Reduce pulpal inflammation
3. Maintain the tooth position with an esthetic restoration

B. Types
1. Unmodified zinc oxide–eugenol cement—mixed with cotton fibers
2. Polymer-modified zinc oxide–eugenol cement
3. Zinc silicophosphate and zinc polycarboxylate cements—used less frequently

High-Strength Bases

A. General considerations
1. Provide mechanical support for the restoration
2. Provide thermal protection for the pulp
3. Thicker consistency of zinc phosphate, zinc polycarboxylate, and zinc oxide–eugenol cements

B. Properties
1. Strength (Table 10-3)—stronger than cements of luting consistency
2. Modulus of elasticity—higher values correlate with better support of restoration
3. Thermal conductivity—similar to that of tooth structure, but thickness is important

C. Manipulation
1. Luting consistency is attained first
2. Final powder/liquid ratio for zinc phosphate is 4.8 g to 1 ml

Low-Strength Bases

A. General considerations
1. Low-strength cements that harden when mixed
2. Provide a barrier to irritating chemicals
3. Provide a therapeutic benefit to the pulp

4. Used in non-stress-bearing areas of the cavity base

B. Composition
1. Zinc oxide–eugenol type—unmodified zinc oxide and eugenol
2. Calcium hydroxide type
   a. Base paste—calcium tungstate, calcium phosphate, and zinc oxide in glycol salicylate
   b. Catalyst paste—calcium hydroxide, zinc oxide, and zinc stearate in ethylene toluene sulfonamide

C. Properties
1. Zinc oxide–eugenol type
   a. Retards penetration of acids
   b. Obtundent to the pulp in a deep but nonexposed cavity
   c. Strength—inferior to that of the calcium hydroxide type
   d. Thermal insulation—thin layer provides little protection
2. Calcium hydroxide type
   a. Strength—superior to that of nonsetting calcium hydroxide liners
   b. Stimulates formation of reparative dentin under an indirect pulp cap or at the site of a direct pulp cap

D. Manipulation
1. Both types are two-paste systems
2. Both types are mixed to a uniform color on a paper pad

Liners and Varnishes

A. General considerations
1. Function as a protective barrier between dentin and the restorative material
2. Applied as a thin film

Table 10-3 Mechanical properties of cements for high- and low-strength bases*

Cement	Compressive strength (psi [MN/m²])	Tensile strength (psi [MN/m²])	Modulus of elasticity (10^6 psi [GN/m²])†
High-strength bases			
Zinc phosphate	19,000-23,000 (130-160)	1200 (8)	3.0 (22)
Zinc polycarboxylate	12,000 (80)	2400 (16)	0.7 (5.0)
Polymer-reinforced zinc oxide–eugenol (type III)	5500 (38)	500 (3.4)	0.3 (2.1)
Low-strength bases			
Zinc oxide–eugenol (type IV)	800 (5.5)	60 (0.4)	0.04 (0.3)
Calcium hydroxide	1200 (8.3)	150 (1.0)	0.06 (0.4)

From Craig, R.G., O'Brien, W.J., and Powers, J.M.: Dental materials: properties and manipulation, St. Louis, 1983, The C.V. Mosby Co.
*Properties measured at 24 hours
†10^6 psi = 1,000,000 psi, and GN/m² = 1000 MN/m².

B. Composition
1. Varnishes—solutions of resin in organic liquids (chloroform or alcohol)
2. Liners—suspensions of calcium hydroxide in water or an organic solvent
C. Properties
1. No mechanical strength
2. Too thin to provide thermal insulation
3. May be disrupted by monomers in resin or composite restorations
4. Some liners are susceptible to solubility and disintegration in oral fluids
D. Manipulation
1. Varnishes
a. Apply a thin layer with a saturated cotton pledget
b. Dry with a gentle stream of air
c. Use multiple layers to provide more protection
d. Keep the bottle closed to minimize evaporation of the solvent
2. Liners—restrict usage to coverage of dentin

Special Applications of Cement

A. Root canal sealers
1. Uses
a. Cementation of a silver cone or gutta-percha point
b. Paste filling material
2. Types
a. Zinc oxide–eugenol cement
b. Cement other than zinc oxide–eugenol
c. Therapeutic cement
3. Properties include flow, film thickness, strength, solubility, radiopacity, and biologic properties
B. Gingival tissue packs
1. Provide temporary displacement of gingival tissues
2. Slow-setting zinc oxide–eugenol cement mixed with cotton twills
C. Surgical dressings
1. Applied to gingiva following surgical periodontal procedures
2. Contain zinc oxide, eugenol, tannic acid, rosin, and various oils
D. Cementation of orthodontic bands
1. Zinc phosphate cement used most frequently
2. Routinely mixed on a cold or frozen slab to extend the working time
E. Cementation of orthodontic brackets
1. Acrylic or composite resin cements used (see section on resin cement)

2. Applied to acid-etched enamel
3. Removal of brackets and cement after treatment requires care

METALLIC RESTORATIVE MATERIALS ▬▬▬
Mercury

A. General considerations
1. Dense liquid that can be toxic
2. Combines with amalgam alloy to form dental amalgam
B. Properties
1. High density (13.6 g/cm^3)—bulk package is deceptively heavy
2. High vapor pressure when pure—increased by increased temperature; decreased by contamination
3. Easily contaminated, as evidenced by a dull film on the surface
C. Precautions
1. Potential health hazard
a. Systemic absorption of liquid mercury through the skin
b. Inhalation of mercury vapor
c. Inhalation of airborne particles
2. Simple precautions
a. Do not handle liquid mercury in the palm or with the fingers
b. Clean up spills to minimize vaporization of mercury
c. Minimize inhalation of airborne particles by using properly sealed amalgam capsules and a covered amalgamator

Dental Amalgam

A. General considerations
1. Alloy that results from reaction of mercury with amalgam alloy; combination of silver, tin, copper, and sometimes zinc
2. Amalgam alloy is marketed as small spherical, comminuted, or blended particles
3. Freshly mixed mass can be condensed in the cavity
4. Used usually in posterior teeth
B. Amalgamation
1. Amalgam alloys
a. Shapes—comminuted, spherical, and blends
b. Types
(1) Low copper—silver (70%), tin (26%), copper (4%)
(2) High copper
(a) Silver (60%), tin (27%), copper (13%)
(b) Silver (40%), tin (30%), copper (30%)

(3) Admixed—low-copper alloy mixed with eutectic particles of silver (72%) and copper (28%)

2. Reaction
   a. Low-copper alloy

   Mercury + Silver-tin alloy → Silver-tin phase +
        Silver-mercury phase + Tin-mercury phase

   b. Admixed alloy

   Mercury + Silver-tin alloy + Silver-copper alloy →
       Silver-tin phase + Silver-copper phase +
         Copper-tin phase + Silver-mercury phase

   c. High-copper alloy

   Mercury + Silver-tin-copper alloy →
      Silver-tin-copper phase + Copper-tin phase +
         Silver-mercury phase

   d. Hardening is the result of solution and crystallization

3. Phases in set amalgam
   a. γ-Phase—unreacted silver-tin alloy particle
      (1) Strongest
      (2) Resistant to corrosion
   b. γ_1-Phase—silver-mercury compound
      (1) Matrix that joins unreacted particles
      (2) Less resistant to corrosion
   c. γ_2-Phase—tin-mercury compound
      (1) Weakest
      (2) Least resistant to corrosion
      (3) Eliminated in admixed and high-copper amalgams
   d. Silver-copper unreacted particle—reacts with the γ_2-phase to form a copper-tin phase
   e. Copper-tin phase—has better properties than the tin-mercury phase

C. Properties
   1. Dimensional change
      a. Solution (contraction) and crystallization (expansion) occur at the same time to produce an overall change of normally less than 20 μm/cm total
      b. Excessive expansion can cause postoperative sensitivity
      c. Excessive contraction can allow leakage to occur
   2. Strength
      a. Enamel support needed for resistance to normal masticatory forces
      b. Insufficient strength characterized by gross fracture or marginal breakdown
      c. Phases present affect strength—γ-phase strongest; γ_2-phase weakest
      d. Tensile strength (7500 lb/in^2) substantially less than compressive strength (33,000 to 64,000 lb/in^2)

   e. Spherical high-copper alloys develop tensile strength much faster than other alloys—permits early polish
   3. Creep
      a. Viscoelastic dimensional change under load
      b. Excessive creep is associated with the γ_2-phase (tin-mercury phase) and early marginal failure
   4. Tarnish and corrosion
      a. Leads to loss of esthetics and reduced mechanical properties
      b. Most susceptible phase is tin-mercury
      c. Corrosion product—tin hydroxychloride
   5. Marginal failure
      a. Correlated with high creep and poor resistance to corrosion
      b. Observed more frequently with comminuted and spherical low-copper amalgams

D. Manipulation
   1. Selection of the product
      a. Determine clinical requirements such as high occlusal forces
      b. Determine the type of packaging
         (1) Powder or tablets
         (2) Bulk or precapsulated
   2. Proportioning of mercury and alloy
      a. Unique characteristic of each alloy is dependent on the composition, surface condition, and particle size and shape
      b. Ranges from 43% mercury for spherical high-copper alloy to 54% for others
      c. Mercury is dispensed by volume
      d. Alloy powder is dispensed by volume (from a dispenser unique to the alloy) or by weight
      e. Average restoration needs 800 mg of alloy with the proper amount of mercury
         (1) Avoid mixing too much or too little
         (2) Store scrap amalgam under water in a covered container
   3. Methods of mixing
      a. Mechanical amalgamators
         (1) Medium-, high-, and variable-speed units
         (2) Each alloy requires characteristic settings for time and speed
      b. Replace reusable capsules when worn
   4. Factors in mixing
      a. Trituration affected by
         (1) Time
            (a) Spherical high-copper alloy requires 6 to 10 seconds
            (b) Low-copper alloys requires 10 to 20 seconds

(2) Speed—changes as the amalgamator ages

(3) Force—usually applied by a 0.2 to 1 g pestle

b. Mulling—mixing for several seconds with no pestle to collect the mass

c. Overmixed or undermixed mass

(1) Overmixed mass is difficult to remove from the capsule

(2) Undermixed mass is crumbly and difficult to manipulate—poor properties

5. Condensation—goals

a. Adaptation of amalgam to prepared cavity walls

(1) Spherical alloys require a condenser with a larger diameter tip than that needed for comminuted or admixed alloys

(2) Force of 8 to 10 pounds should be applied to the condenser

b. Development of a uniform, compact mass

(1) Condense in small increments

(2) Overpack the restoration, since the surface layer contains excess mercury

(3) Avoid delays in condensation and contamination by saliva

c. Reduction of excess mercury content

(1) Excess mercury in the restoration causes excessive dimensional change, higher creep, and a decrease in strength

(2) Spherical high-copper alloys are less sensitive because they are mixed with less mercury

6. Finishing

a. Carve within a few minutes after condensation

b. Avoid burnishing over margins

c. Final finishing requires 24 hours except for spherical high-copper alloys, which can be finished at the same appointment

(1) Initial reduction with green stones, burs, and abrasive disks

(2) Final polish with silex and tin oxide slurry in water

Gold Alloys

A. General considerations

1. Gold foil—original metallic restorative material largely replaced by amalgam and cast gold inlays

2. High gold content alloy—main material for cast crowns and bridges; now being replaced by low gold content, palladium-silver, and nickel alloys

B. Gold content

1. Karat (K)—karat/24 × 100 = percent gold

2. Fineness (F)—percent gold × 10 = fineness

Gold Foil

A. Used for fabrication of direct restorations

B. Types—gold foil, sponge gold, mat gold, fibrous foil, and powdered gold-calcium alloy

C. Properties

1. Tarnish resistance is high

2. Ductility is high enough to allow compaction in layers into the cavity

3. Capable of welding to itself during compaction

D. Manipulation

1. Foil is made cohesive by degassing the surface—process called annealing

a. Heat is applied by an oven (tray method)— 10 minutes at 454° C or

b. Heat is applied by an alcohol flame

2. Force is applied to the foil by striking a condenser with a mallet or by use of an automatic mechanical condenser

Gold Casting Alloys

A. Alloys with high and low noble metal content

1. Type I—simple inlays (83% minimum noble metal content)

2. Type II—large two- or three-surface inlays (78% minimum noble metal content)

3. Type III—crown and bridge applications (78% minimum noble metal content)

4. Type IV—partial dentures (75% minimum noble metal content)

5. Low gold—alloy of gold (46% noble metal content with 54% copper and silver)

B. Ingredients and function

1. Gold—contributes to ductility, color, and tarnish resistance

2. Copper and silver—contribute to hardness and strength but lower tarnish resistance

3. Platinum and palladium—contribute to strength and raise the melting temperature

4. Zinc—deoxidizing element

C. Heat treatment

1. Softening treatment

a. Casting is heated at 705° C for 15 minutes, then cooled to room temperature in water

b. Entire mold is quenched in water shortly after the metal is cast

2. Hardening treatment

a. Casting is heated at 370° C for 15 minutes, then cooled in air

b. Entire mold is cooled to room temperature in air after the metal is cast

OTHER RESTORATIVE MATERIALS ▬▬▬
Composite Restorative Materials

A. General considerations
1. Recommended for Class III to V restorations with adequate pins or acid etching and for Class I restorations with low occlusal stress
2. Types—conventional, microfilled, and blended
3. Systems—two-paste, powder and liquid (predispensed capsules or bulk), and one-paste (packaged in a syringe and activated by visible light)
4. Properties are improved compared with unfilled acrylics by the addition of a filler
   a. Polymerization shrinkage and abrasive wear reduced
   b. Hardness and bonding to etched enamel increased
B. Composition and reaction
1. Introduction
   a. Monomer—dimethacrylate (BIS-GMA) with lower molecular weight diluents that copolymerize
   b. Filler—particles of colloidal silica, quartz, glass, or silicates of various sizes ranging from 0.04 to 20 μm in diameter and from 35% to 77% by weight
   c. Coupling agent—silane that bonds the polymer and filler
   d. Polymerization involves

   BIS-GMA + Initiator + Accelerator +
                   Treated particles → Composite

   (1) Self-cured material accelerated by organic amine
   (2) Light-cured material accelerated by diketone and visible light
2. Conventional composite
   a. Characterized by quartz, silicate, or glass particles about 8 to 15 μm in diameter and about 77% by weight
   b. Accelerated by organic amine or light
3. Microfilled composite
   a. Characterized by colloidal silica 0.04 μm in diameter and 33% to 50% by weight
   b. Accelerated by organic amine or light
4. Blended composite
   a. Characterized by quartz, silicate, or glass particles 5 μm in diameter and colloidal silica
   b. Accelerated by organic amine or light
C. Properties
1. Radiopacity—composites with sufficient barium glass particles are radiopaque

2. Abrasive wear—resistance to wear is improved by filler particles
3. Bond strength—increases with increased filler content
4. Thermal coefficient of expansion—lowest for conventional composites, followed by blended and microfilled composites and unfilled acrylics
5. Marginal penetration controlled by
   a. Acid etching of the enamel
   b. Penetration of the composite into etched areas of the tooth
   c. Appropriate cavity design
6. Strength—has lower compressive strength, higher tensile strength, and lower elastic modulus that human enamel
7. Toughness—less than that of unfilled acrylic
8. Anatomic form—inadequate after 2 years in posterior restorations
D. Manipulation
1. Acid etching of enamel—1 minute with phosphoric acid supplied by the manufacturer, followed by rinsing and drying
2. Two-paste system
   a. Mixing
      (1) Use one end of the stick to dispense the universal shade and the other end to dispense the catalyst
      (2) Dispense equal amounts of the pastes by volume
      (3) Mix for 20 to 30 seconds
      (4) Tint the universal shade before mixing with the catalyst
      (5) Working time—1 to 1½ minutes
   b. Place the material in the cavity with a plastic instrument or syringe
   c. Finishing
      (1) Use a matrix strip to achieve the best finish
      (2) Use diamonds, carbide finishing burs, or green stones for gross reduction
      (3) Use aluminum oxide disks for final finishing
3. Mixing of the powder-liquid system in predispensed capsules
   a. Rupture the plastic diaphragm of the capsule
   b. Use a high-speed mixer for 10 to 15 seconds or a low-speed mixer for 30 seconds
4. Single-paste systems
   a. Dispense the proper amount of paste into the cavity

b. Use visible light source to activate polymerization
   (1) Exposure time of 20 to 60 seconds required for 2 mm deep cure, depending on the shade of the conventional composite
   (2) Microfilled composites require more exposure to light

E. Other applications
1. Bonding agents
   a. Mechanical and possibly chemical bonding of a composite to enamel and dentin
   b. Made from low molecular weight dimethacrylates to decrease viscosity with adhesion-promoting agents
2. Core buildups—used as the foundation for a gold restoration
3. Acid-etched bridge—used to cement a bridge to etched enamel
4. Repair of composites and porcelain—bonding is adequate if thin areas are avoided

Unfilled Plastic Restorative Materials

A. General considerations
1. Used successfully to repair fractured anterior teeth, for Class III restorations, and in pedodontic practices
2. Used alone or with metal pins to provide improved retention
3. Susceptible to wear but can be built up periodically

B. Composition and reaction
1. Powder—poly(methyl methacrylate) polymer with an initiator and coloring agents
2. Liquid—methyl methacrylate monomer with an accelerator and inhibitor
3. Reaction
   a. Monomer polymerizes by a free-radical reaction and bonds to polymer particles
   b. Reaction inhibited by water and air but accelerated by increases in temperature

C. Properties
1. Thermal coefficient of expansion—$90 \times 10^{-6}/°C$
   a. Nine times greater than that of tooth structure
   b. Temperature changes in the mouth can cause percolation
2. Volumetric contraction
   a. Free volumetric dimensional change of -5%
   b. Controlled by proper technique to -0.1% to -0.3%

3. Strength—substantially weaker and more flexible than tooth structure
4. Knoop hardness—value of $19\ kg/mm^2$ is much lower than that of enamel ($340\ kg/mm^2$)
5. Bonding to tooth structure
   a. Mechanical retention required in the cavity preparation
   b. Enamel etched by organic acid improves retention
6. Pulpal response
   a. Calcium hydroxide bases required
   b. Zinc oxide–eugenol bases inhibit setting reaction

D. Manipulation
1. Bulk technique
   a. Liquid is dispensed and powder added
   b. Excess powder is removed and the mass stirred for 15 seconds
   c. Cavity is slightly overfilled and protected by a matrix until set (4 minutes)
   d. Finishing is done with a finishing bur or disk followed by polishing with silex and tin oxide
2. Brush technique
   a. Liquid is placed in a Dappen dish
   b. Small brush is moistened with liquid and dipped into powder (in another dish)
   c. Cavity is overfilled with acrylic in increments
   d. Acrylic is protected from moisture and air, allowed to set, and finished

Glass Ionomer Restorative Materials

A. General considerations
1. Used for erosion lesions
2. Retained better than composites in cervical areas

B. Composition and reaction
1. Powder—aluminosilicate glass
2. Liquid—water solution of polymers and copolymers of acrylic acid
3. Setting reaction
   a. Formation of metallic salt bridges between aluminum and calcium ions and acid groups on polymers
   b. Protection from saliva necessary during setting

C. Properties
1. Increased inorganic content, bonding to dentin, and opacity than with composites
2. Lower mechanical strength and coefficient of thermal expansion than with composites

D. Manipulation
1. Powder and liquid are dispensed onto a paper pad
2. Powder is added in two increments within 30 to 40 seconds
3. Setting occurs after 4 minutes
4. Restoration should be protected with varnish and finished after 24 hours

Silicate Restorative Materials

A. General considerations
1. Used in non-load-bearing areas in which esthetics are important
2. Placed directly into a cavity preparation in a plastic condition
3. Considered short-term restorations with moderate strength and resistance to solubility and disintegration
B. Composition and reaction
1. Powder—acid-soluble, alumina-silica glass containing fluoride
2. Liquid—buffered solution of phosphoric acid
3. Reaction
   a. Acid reacts with the surface of the glass to form a matrix of alumina-silica gel bonded to unreacted glass particles
   b. Reaction accelerated by increases in temperature and humidity
C. Manipulation
1. Material is mixed on a glass slab with 90% of the powder added to the liquid immediately; mixing is confined to a small area of the slab; remaining powder is added and mixed within 1 minute
2. Pulpal protection by a varnish is required
3. Final finishing is done after 24 hours

PREVENTIVE AGENTS

Fluoride Gels

See Chapter 12, section on professionally administered topical fluoride treatments
A. General considerations
1. Used to prevent smooth-surface caries
2. Applied to teeth in a tray after a dental prophylaxis
B. Composition
1. Ingredients include 2% sodium fluoride, 0.34% hydrogen fluoride, and 0.98% orthophosphoric acid with thickening, flavoring, and coloring agents in a aqueous gel
2. Fluoride ion concentration ranges from 1.22% to 1.32% in commercial gels

C. Properties
1. Clinical effectiveness
   a. Reduction in caries depends on the method and frequency of application
   b. Reductions range from 26% to 80% over 2 to 3 years
2. pH ranges from 3 to 4 but is difficult to measure
3. Viscosity must allow ease of handling during loading and insertion of the tray but must permit flow to gain efficient contact with the teeth
D. Manipulation
1. Gels are applied in soft, spongy trays after a prophylaxis
2. Teeth should be free from saliva
3. Maxillary and mandibular trays are loaded, placed in position, and squeezed to mold the tray tightly around the teeth
4. Tray is held in position for 4 minutes
5. Patient should not eat for 30 minutes

Pit and Fissure Sealants

See Chapter 12, section on dental sealants
A. General considerations
1. Reduction of smooth-surface caries is accomplished by
   a. Fluoridation of community water
   b. Topical application of fluoride during enamel development
   c. Individual plaque-control program
2. Reduction of pit and fissure caries is accomplished by
   a. Prophylactic odontotomy with dental amalgam
   b. Application of pit and fissure sealants
3. Pits and fissures are the result of noncoalescence of enamel during tooth formation
B. Composition and reaction
1. Types of sealants
   a. Amine accelerated
   b. Visible light activated
2. Components
   a. Dimethacrylate resin (BIS-GMA) with resin diluents (methyl methacrylate monomer, MMA) to permit flow before polymerization of the resin
   b. Initiator (benzoyl peroxide) and accelerator (organic amine) in an amine-accelerated sealant
   c. Activator is a diketone in a visible light–cured sealant

d. Some products contain an inorganic filler to improve strength and wear resistance

e. Reaction is

$$BIS\text{-}GMA + MMA + Accelerator \rightarrow Sealant$$

C. Properties
1. Retention is the result of mechanical bonding
    a. Improved by acid etching, which results in
        (1) Cleaning the area to be sealed
        (2) Increasing the surface area of the enamel
        (3) Forming spaces into which the resin can penetrate
    b. Affected by the penetration coefficient of the resin, which depends on
        (1) Surface tension and viscosity of the sealant
        (2) Contact angle of the sealant on enamel
2. Efficacy
    a. Retention varies from 79% after 1 year to 31% after 5 years
    b. Effectiveness varies from 83% after 1 year to 40% after 5 years
    c. Affected by materials and techniques used, teeth studied, and clinical criteria chosen for evaluation
3. Other properties
    a. Setting time varies from 60 seconds for amine-cured sealants to 20 seconds for light-cured sealants
    b. Compressive strength varies from 13,000 to 22,000 lb/in^2
    c. Knoop hardness varies from 16 to 25 kg/mm^2
    d. Water sorption varies from 1.3 to 2.0 mg/cm^2 after 7 days
D. Manipulation
1. Cleanse and etch the occlusal surfaces
    a. Etching agent is 37% to 50% phosphoric acid and may be a liquid or gel
    b. Etching agent is applied liberally for 60 seconds to the occlusal surfaces
2. Wash the occlusal surfaces for 20 seconds
    a. If contamination by saliva occurs, reetching is necessary
    b. Residual etching agent will interfere with bonding
3. Mix the sealant components (if necessary) for 15 seconds
4. Apply the sealant with small tube (cannula) or ball applicators
    a. Apply promptly to improve penetration into etched areas
    b. Avoid application to unetched areas
    c. Avoid brushes—they introduce air bubbles

5. Allow polymerization to occur
    a. Amine-cured sealants set within 1 minute
    b. Light-cured sealants require exposure to light for 20 seconds with the tip of the light source 1 to 2 mm from the surface of the tooth
6. Finish
    a. Use a cotton pellet to remove unpolymerized sealant
    b. Use a sharp explorer to examine the hardness of the sealant
    c. Follow the sealant with a fluoride treatment

Mouth Protectors

A. General considerations
1. Causes of dental injury (broken teeth or concussion) in football and other contact sports are
    a. Blows under the chin
    b. Blows that slip past the face guard
    c. Gritting the teeth or snapping the jaws shut
    d. Blows on top of the head that snap the jaws shut
2. Injuries are prevented by use of any type of mouth protector
B. Types and composition
1. Stock protectors
    a. Made from thermoplastic polyvinyl acetate–polyethylene copolymer
    b. Least desirable because of poor fit
2. Mouth-formed protectors
    a. Made from thermoplastic copolymer
    b. Improved fit compared with stock type
3. Custom-made protectors
    a. Made from thermoplastic copolymer, rubber, or polyurethane
    b. Preferred because of durability, low speech impairment, and comfort
C. Properties
1. Laboratory studies
    a. Properties measured include tensile strength, elongation, tear strength, hardness, water sorption and solubility, and dynamic modulus and resilience
    b. Mouth protectors fabricated from polyvinyl acetate–polyethylene copolymers seem to have adequate properties
    c. After exposure to the oral environment, mouth protectors become more flexible and better able to absorb energy but are less strong

2. Clinical studies
   a. Properties measured include gagging, taste, irritation, impairment of speech, feel, durability, staining, deformation, and changes in the mouth
   b. Properly fabricated custom-made protector eliminates problems associated with gagging, taste, irritation, and impairment of speech
   c. Clinical failure results from "bite-through" and chewing, both of which are affected by the emotional involvement of the athlete
     (1) Mouth protectors should be evaluated for deterioration on a regular basis
     (2) Mouth protectors should be protected from heat and pressure during storage
     (3) Chewing can be minimized by selection of a softer material

D. Fabrication
  1. Four basic steps for fabrication of a custom-made mouth protector
   a. Making an impression of the arch
     (1) An alginate impression is made of the maxillary arch—use a disposable tray for convenience
     (2) Removable appliances should be removed, and fixed orthodontic appliances should be blocked out on the model
   b. Pouring a model
     (1) Model should be poured immediately in high-strength stone for durability
     (2) Do not pour the palate
   c. Forming the thermoplastic material
     (1) Vacuum method reproduces occlusal anatomy better than hand forming
     (2) Material can be heated in boiling water or by a forming device with an electrical heater
     (3) Material should be vacuumed for 2 minutes and then cooled for 1 minute
   d. Finishing the mouth protector
     (1) Mouth protector should be trimmed ⅛ inch short of the labial fold, and clearance should be provided for buccal and labial frena
     (2) Edges should be flamed and smoothed

E. Instructions to give the athlete
  1. Rinse the protector under cold water
  2. Clean the protector occasionally with soap and cool water
  3. Store the protector in a rigid container

GYPSUM PRODUCTS — PLASTER AND STONE

A. General considerations
  1. Model plaster—used for study models
  2. Dental stone—stronger; used for casts of full-arch impressions
  3. High-strength dental stone—most accurate; used for dies

B. Chemical and physical nature
  1. Physical form
   a. Plaster
     (1) Produced by heating gypsum ($CaSO_4$ 2 H_2O) in an open kettle
     (2) Hemihydrate particles ($CaSO_4$ ½ H_2O) are porous and irregularly shaped
   b. Dental stone
     (1) Produced by heating gypsum under pressure at 125° C in the presence of water vapor
     (2) Hemihydrate particles are less porous and more uniform in shape
   c. High-strength dental stone
     (1) Produced by boiling gypsum in a 30% solution of calcium chloride
     (2) Hemihydrate particles are least porous and most uniform in shape
  2. Setting reaction
   a. Reaction is

$$CaSO_4 \cdot \tfrac{1}{2} H_2O + 1\tfrac{1}{2} H_2O \rightarrow CaSO_4 \cdot 2 H_2O + Heat$$

   b. For chemical reaction, 100 g powder requires 18.6 g water
   c. Mechanism of setting
     (1) Difference in solubility between the hemihydrate and dihydrate
     (2) Solution followed by growth and interlocking of crystals
   d. Reaction affected by temperature and chemical accelerators and retarders
  3. Excess water
   a. Additional water is necessary to wet and mix the powder
   b. Amount depends on the size, shape, and porosity of the hemihydrate particles
     (1) Plaster requires most—about 30 ml
     (2) Stone—about 13 ml
     (3) High-strength stone—about 4 ml
   c. Does not react chemically and is replaced by voids during evaporation

C. Properties
  1. Initial setting time
   a. Time at which the gypsum mass should no longer be manipulated

b. Occurs within 8 to 16 minutes from the start of mixing

c. Detected by loss of gloss

2. Final setting time
   a. Time at which the material can be separated from the impression
   b. Occurs within 20 minutes, but often the model is allowed to set for an additional 40 minutes

3. Reproduction of detail—adequate but not as good as electroplated or epoxy dies

4. Compressive strength
   a. Related to the density of the set mass
   b. High-strength stone (5000 psi) > stone > plaster (1300 psi)
   c. Dry strength at 7 days is twice the wet strength at 1 hour

5. Tensile strength—much lower than compressive strength

6. Hardness and abrasion resistance
   a. Higher compressive strength yields greater hardness and abrasion resistance
   b. High-strength stone > stone > plaster
   c. Improvements attempted by impregnation of resin have not been successful
   d. Hardening solutions increase the hardness of some products

7. Dimensional accuracy
   a. All gypsum products expand on setting
      (1) Plaster—0.2% to 0.3%
      (2) Stone—0.08% to 0.1%
      (3) High-strength stone—0.05% to 0.07%
   b. Gypsum dies are more accurate than other die materials
   c. Expansion is controlled by manipulative variables and chemicals
   d. Hygroscopic expansion—increased setting expansion if gypsum sets when immersed in water; about twice the normal expansion

D. Manipulation
   1. Water/powder ratio
      a. Plaster—45 to 55 ml water per 100 g powder
      b. Stone—30 ml water per 100 g powder
      c. High-strength stone—19 to 24 ml water per 100 g powder
      d. Increasing the amount of water during mixing results in
         (1) Longer setting time
         (2) Lower strength because of additional excess water
         (3) Decreased expansion

2. Hardening solutions
   a. Composed of 30% colloidal silica, water, and modifiers
   b. Used in place of mixing water
   c. Increases in hardness depend on the impression material against which the gypsum product is poured
   d. Slightly higher expansion results

3. Spatulation
   a. Water is dispensed first, then powder
   b. Powder is allowed to settle for 30 seconds before spatulation for 1 minute by hand
   c. Vacuum mixing results in
      (1) Decreased setting time and setting expansion
      (2) Increased consistency

4. Accelerators
   a. Chemicals that increase the rate of reaction and reduce the setting time
   b. Examples—2% solution of potassium sulfate and calcium dihydrate crystals

5. Retarders
   a. Chemicals that decrease the rate of reaction and increase the setting time
   b. Examples—2% solution of borax and colloidal systems such as blood, saliva, and hydrocolloids

6. Temperature and humidity
   a. Increases in temperature between 23° and 37° C shorten the setting time
   b. Increases in temperature between 37° and 100° C lengthen the setting time
   c. Hemihydrate crystals absorb moisture and convert to dihydrate, lengthening the setting time

7. Construction of a model or cast
   a. Boxing wax method
      (1) Wax is wrapped around the impression extending ½ inch beyond the tissue side to form the base
      (2) Teeth are poured in stone, and the base is poured in plaster
      (3) Gypsum is allowed to harden for 45 to 60 minutes
   b. Glass plate method—impression is filled with stone and inverted onto a mass of plaster resting on a glass plate
   c. Model former method—impression is filled with stone and placed in a mass of plaster in the model former

IMPRESSION MATERIALS, MODELS, AND DIES

A. General considerations
  1. Function
    a. Record dimensions of oral tissues
    b. Record spatial relationships
  2. Negative reproduction—impression
  3. Positive reproduction—model, cast, or die
B. Requirements of impression materials
  1. Ease of manipulation and reasonable cost
  2. Adequate flow properties
  3. Appropriate setting time
  4. Sufficient mechanical strength to not tear or permanently deform on removal
  5. Good dimensional accuracy
  6. Acceptability to patients
  7. Safety (nontoxic or nonirritating)
  8. Compatibility with die and cast materials
  9. Good shelf life

Impression Materials

Dental Impression Compound

A. General considerations
  1. Tray compound
    a. Used to prepare the custom-made preliminary impression or tray that will later hold the final impression material (wash)
    b. Supplied in larger pieces in the shape of a tray
  2. Impression compound
    a. Low fusing—used to prepare the final impression of a tooth preparation
    b. High fusing—used to stabilize rubber dam clamps
    c. Supplied in sticks and other shapes
  3. Rigid materials—used in nonundercut areas
B. Composition
  1. Resins and wax—provide thermoplastic properties
  2. Stearic acid and filler—control flow properties
C. Properties
  1. Thermoplasticity—material softens on heating and hardens on cooling; reversible
  2. Flow
    a. Tray compound—less than 2% at 37° C
    b. Impression compound (low fusing)—less than 6% at 37° C
  3. Thermal conductivity—poor heat transfer in the material affects manipulation
  4. Residual stress—causes dimensional change when released on heating or storage of the tray or impression

  5. Thermal contraction—shrinks 0.3% from mouth to room temperature
D. Manipulation
  1. Tray compound
    a. Soften in a thermostatically controlled water bath
    b. Adapt the compound to the dental stone cast to form a custom tray
    c. Final impression material—zinc oxide–eugenol or light-bodied impression rubber
  2. Impression compound
    a. Soften over a flame, ensuring that the inside is soft
    b. Place in a suitably adapted copper band
    c. Cool in the mouth with a water spray (16° to 18° C)
    d. Prepare the stone or copper die

Impression Plaster

A. General considerations
  1. Used for impressions of nonundercut areas when excess saliva is present
  2. Used for mounting casts on articulators
B. Composition and reaction
  1. Powder—calcium sulfate hemihydrate with inorganic salts to modify the setting time and dimensional change
  2. Reaction—powder mixed with water forms calcium sulfate dihydrate (see section on gypsum products)
C. Properties
  1. Setting time—3 to 5 minutes
  2. Dimensional change during setting—expansion of 0.06%
  3. Compressive strength—400 lb/in² after 1 hour; adequate
  4. Properties affected by storage—humid conditions cause deterioration
D. Manipulation
  1. Water/powder ratio—55 to 60 ml/100 g
  2. Mixed in a rubber bowl with a stiff spatula for 30 seconds or less
  3. Used with a custom tray
  4. Die material—stone (separator required)

Zinc Oxide–Eugenol Impression Material

A. General considerations
  1. Used as a wash in combination with a custom-made tray to record impressions of partially or completely edentulous arches

2. Limited to nonundercut areas
3. Supplied as two-paste or powder-liquid systems
4. Available as hard and soft set

B. Composition and reaction
1. Two-paste system
   a. One paste—zinc oxide, oils, and additives
   b. Second paste—eugenol, oils, resin, and additives
2. Powder-liquid system
   a. Powder—zinc oxide plus additives
   b. Liquid—eugenol plus additives
3. Reaction
   a. Reaction is

   Zinc oxide + Eugenol → Zinc eugenolate +
   Unreacted zinc oxide

   b. Contact with water or a higher temperature accelerates the reaction

C. Properties
1. Toughness—soft-set not as brittle as hard-set
2. Consistency—hard-set more fluid than soft-set (described as buttery)
3. Initial setting time—3 to 5 minutes
4. Final setting time—soft-set, 15 minutes; hard-set, 10 minutes
5. Dimensional change on setting—contraction of 0.1%

D. Manipulation
1. Two-paste system
   a. Equal lengths are extruded from tubes onto an oil-resistant pad
   b. Mixed to a uniform color with broad strokes in 30 to 45 seconds
      (1) Setting can be accelerated by mixing in a drop of water
      (2) Setting can be slowed by incorporating a drop of glycerin in the mix
   c. Removed from the face and lips with oil of orange
   d. Stored in a cool, dry area to maintain the shelf life
2. Powder-liquid system
   a. Ratio of 1 teaspoon of liquid to 2 teaspoons of powder
   b. Liquid
      (1) Fast setting for cold, dry conditions (humidity less than 50%)
      (2) Slow setting for warm, humid conditions
3. Die material—stone model material (no separator needed)

Agar Hydrocolloid Impression Material

A. General considerations
1. Flexibility allows impressions of undercut areas
2. Used for fully dentulous impressions of the entire arch
3. Reversible material—can be reused several times
4. Supplied as a gel—collapsible tube, small glass cartridges, or cylinders in a glass jar
5. Used in a water-cooled tray or applied with a syringe for tray or copper-band techniques

B. Composition and liquefaction-solidification
1. Tray material
   a. Agar (12% to 15%)—forms a gel with water
   b. Borax (0.2%)—improves strength
   c. Potassium sulfate (1% to 2%)—accelerates the setting of gypsum poured against the agar impression
   d. Water (85%)
2. Syringe material—same components but less agar (6% to 8%)
3. Liquefaction—when heated at 100° C, the gel network breaks up to form agar particles dispersed in water (sol)
4. Solidification—when the sol is cooled to 43° C, agar particles agglomerate to form a gel
5. Hysteresis—liquefaction temperature of the gel is different from the solidification temperature of the sol
6. Syneresis—continued agglomeration of agar particles causes water to be exuded to the surface of the impression, resulting in shrinkage

C. Properties
1. Accuracy—highly accurate on removal from the mouth but shrinkage occurs when the material is stored in air or 100% relative humidity; expansion occurs when the material is stored in water
2. Flexibility—4% to 15% under standard conditions
3. Permanent deformation—1% under standard conditions
4. Tear strength—4 lb/in
5. Compressive strength—116 lb/in²

D. Manipulation
1. Important temperatures
   a. 100° C—material is heated for 10 to 12 minutes to liquify
   b. 60° to 66° C—material is stored as a sol during office hours

c. 43° to 46° C—material is tempered to a lower temperature before placement in the mouth

d. <43° C—material gels in the mouth when cooled with water at 13° C

2. Material is placed in the mouth in a water-cooled tray

3. After gelation the impression is removed with a single stroke

4. Impression is rinsed with water, and excess water is removed

5. Storage—1 hour in 100% relative humidity or no storage at all

6. Die material—gypsum model material

Alginate Impression Material

A. General considerations
  1. Most widely used impression material
    a. Ease of manipulation
    b. Minimal equipment required
    c. Flexibility of set material
    d. Accurate if properly handled
    e. Low cost
  2. Used to prepare study models of either the entire arch or a segment of it
  3. Used to prepare a cast for construction of an athletic mouth protector
  4. Packaging—bulk containers or preweighed individual containers

B. Composition and reaction
  1. Components
    a. Sodium alginate—reacts with calcium ions to form insoluble calcium alginate
    b. Calcium sulfate—provides calcium ions for precipitation reaction
    c. Sodium phosphate—retarder to provide working time
    d. Water—forms hydrogel
  2. Reaction
    a. Reaction is

    Sodium alginate + $CaSO_4$ + H_2O →
      Calcium alginate + H_2O + Sodium and sulfate ions
    (Paste → Gel)

    b. Precipitation reaction with calcium alginate forms a network with water in the capillary spaces (hydrogel)
    c. Irreversible reaction—cannot be reversed by heat like agar
    d. Reaction accelerated by warmer water and thicker mix (more powder)

C. Properties
  1. Mixing and setting times
    a. Normal-set product—1-minute mixing time; setting within 4.5 minutes
    b. Fast-set product—30-second mixing time; setting within 1 to 2 minutes
  2. Permanent deformation—1.5% under standard conditions; slightly greater than that of agar
  3. Flexibility—11% to 15% under standard conditions; slightly more flexible than agar
  4. Tear strength—2 to 4 lb/in; slightly less than that of agar
  5. Compressive strength—not as strong as agar
  6. Factors that affect properties
    a. Thicker mix (if usable)—lowers permanent deformation and flexibility, increases strength, and shortens the working and setting times
    b. Warmer water—shortens the working and setting times
    c. Rate of removal of the impression from the mouth (rate of deformation)—more rapid removal of the impression over undercut areas increases strength and decreases permanent deformation
    d. Time of removal of the impression from the mouth—increased time in the mouth increases strength and decreases permanent deformation
  7. Accuracy
    a. Slightly less accurate than agar or polysulfide rubber impressions
    b. Affected by storage
      (1) Shrinks on storage in air—not recommended
      (2) Swells on storage in water—not recommended
      (3) Shrinks on storage in 100% relative humidity as a result of syneresis— recommended storage if needed

D. Manipulation
  1. Equipment needed—powder-dispensing cup, water-dispensing cup, rubber mixing bowl, and spatula with a wide, flexible blade
  2. Dispensing
    a. Powder in a bulk container is fluffed and dispensed in the measuring cup provided, or powder is dispensed from a prepackaged envelope
    b. Water at 21° C is dispensed in a cup

3. Mixing
   a. Powder is added to water in a rubber bowl to minimize bubbles
   b. Mixture is stirred to wet the powder, then stropped for 1 minute (or 30 seconds for fast-set material)
4. Loading of the impression tray
   a. Tray should be selected to allow 6 mm between the tissues and the tray
   b. Alginate is added to the posterior part of the tray, then to the anterior part
   c. Alginate is smoothed with a wet finger
5. Making the impression
   a. Posterior part of the tray is seated first, followed by the anterior part
   b. Impression is allowed to remain in the mouth for an additional 2 minutes to gain improved strength
6. Removal of the impression
   a. Impression seal is broken
   b. Impression and tray are removed with a single firm motion
7. Preparing the impression for the model or die material
   a. Impression is rinsed to remove blood or saliva—colloidal substances retard the setting of gypsum materials
   b. Excess water is removed
8. Storage of the impression
   a. Tray, not impression, is placed on the bench to minimize distortion
   b. Unsupported alginate is cut away to minimize distortion
   c. Die material is poured immediately or stored for short periods in a humidor
9. Die material—gypsum products only

Polysulfide Rubber Impression Material

A. General considerations
   1. Flexible but stable during storage compared with agar and alginate
   2. Can be electroplated to form metal dies
   3. Used to produce accurate impressions for crowns, bridges, and complete dentures
   4. Packaged as a two-paste system in various consistencies (light, regular, heavy, and single)
B. Composition and reaction
   1. Catalyst or accelerator paste
      a. Accelerator—lead dioxide (brown color), copper hydroxide (green color), or peroxides (variety of colors)
      b. Inert oil—carrier

2. Base paste
   a. Low molecular weight organic polymer with reactive mercaptan groups (80%)
   b. Reinforcing agent (20%)—titanium dioxide, zinc sulfate, or silica
3. Reaction
   a. Reaction is

$$\text{Mercaptan} + \text{Lead dioxide} \rightarrow \text{Polysulfide} + H_2O$$

   b. Mercaptan groups are oxidized to form disulfide groups with water as a by-product
   c. Reaction accelerated by increases in temperature and humidity
C. Properties
   1. Working time—5 to 7 minutes (Table 10-4)
   2. Consistency—stiffer consistency associated with a shorter working time
   3. Permanent deformation during removal—2% to 3%
   4. Dimensional stability
      a. Shrinkage is 0.1% to 0.3% during the first 24 hours
      b. Less shrinkage with light-consistency materials than with heavy-consistency materials
   5. Flow after setting
      a. Flow of 0.3% to 0.9% at 15 minutes after setting
      b. Distortion can occur if the impression is wrapped tightly or stored with the impression on the bench
   6. Flexibility—varies between 2% and 20%, with values for heavy-consistency materials being lower than values for other consistencies
   7. Shelf life
      a. Excellent, but the material should not be stored in a warm location
      b. Can be extended by storage in a refrigerator
D. Manipulation
   1. Mixing
      a. Equal lengths of the base and accelerator are extruded onto a paper pad
      b. Tapered, stiff-bladed spatula is used to stir for 10 seconds, then strop for 35 seconds to attain a uniform color without streaks
      c. Material is loaded into a tray or syringe
      d. Tray
         (1) Requires retention with holes or an adhesive
         (2) Should be rigid to minimize distortion of the impression

Table 10-4 Typical physical and mechanical properties of polysulfide, silicone, and polyether rubber impression materials

Material	Physical properties			Mechanical properties		
	Working time (min)	Consistency (mm)	Dimensional change, 24 hr (%)	Permanent deformation (%)	Flow (%)	Flexibility (%)
Polysulfide						
Light	7	39	−0.13	2.7	0.9	10
Regular	5	33	−0.25	2.1	0.5	7
Heavy	5	28	−0.22	3.0	0.3	5
Silicone (condensation type)						
Light	4	35	−0.52	0.9	0.1	7
Regular	3	28	−0.58	0.5	0.09	5
Heavy	3	24	−0.58	0.4	0.09	4
Putty	—	14	−0.28	2.2	0.07	2
Silicone (addition type)						
Light	4	39	−0.05	0.16	<0.04	3
Regular	5	37	−0.05	0.07	<0.03	3
Heavy	5	29	−0.06	0.07	<0.05	3
Polyether						
Regular	2	27	−0.10	1.1	0.03	2
Plus thinner	4	—	−0.07	1.1	<0.05	4

From Craig, R.G., O'Brien, W.J., and Powers, J.M.: Dental materials: properties and manipulation, St. Louis, 1983, The C.V. Mosby Co.)

2. Techniques
   a. Light-bodied–heavy-bodied technique
      (1) Light material is injected into the cavity preparation
      (2) Heavy material in the tray is placed over the light material
      (3) Both set together to give a single impression
   b. Single-mix technique
      (1) Regular material in the tray is placed in the area of the impression
      (2) Single-consistency material is used in both the syringe and the tray
3. Removal of the impression
   a. Steady force is used
   b. Tearing is minimized by leaving the impression in the mouth longer
   c. Impression is thoroughly rinsed and gently dried
   d. Die should be prepared immediately to minimize dimensional changes
4. Die materials
   a. Gypsum products
   b. Electroplated silver
   c. Epoxy—requires separator

Silicone Rubber Impression Material

A. General considerations
   1. Flexible but stable during storage
   2. Can be electroplated (copper) to form metal dies
   3. Used to produce accurate impressions for crowns, bridges, and complete dentures
   4. Packaging
      a. Two-paste system in various consistencies (light, regular, heavy, and putty)
      b. Catalyst may be supplied as a tube of liquid
   5. Types—condensation and addition
B. Composition and reaction
   1. Condensation type
      a. Catalyst or accelerator paste (or liquid)
         (1) Tin octoate suspension
         (2) Ortho-ethyl silicate—provides cross-linking
      b. Base paste
         (1) Low molecular weight silicone liquid (dimethylsiloxane) with reactive OH groups
         (2) Reinforcing agents—silica (35% for light consistency to 75% for putty)
      c. Reaction
         (1) Reaction is

Dimethylsiloxane + Ortho-ethyl silicate + Tin octoate → Silicone rubber + Ethyl alcohol

(2) Ethyl alcohol (by-product) evaporates, causing shrinkage

(3) Reaction accelerated by increases in temperature and humidity

2. Addition type
   a. Catalyst paste
      (1) Low molecular weight silicone with terminal vinyl groups
      (2) Filler—for reinforcement
      (3) Chloroplatinic acid—catalyst
   b. Base paste
      (1) Low molecular weight silicone with terminal hydrogen
      (2) Filler—for reinforcement
   c. Reaction
      (1) Reaction is

> Silane-terminated siloxane +
> Vinyl-terminated siloxane +
> Chloroplatinic acid → Silicone rubber

      (2) No volatile by-product—minimal shrinkage on polymerization
      (3) Reaction accelerated by increases in temperature and humidity

C. Properties
   1. Condensation type (Table 10-4)
      a. Working time—3 to 4 minutes; shorter than that of polysulfides
      b. Consistency—silicones are more fluid than comparable polysulfides but set faster, resulting in lower values of consistency
      c. Permanent deformation during removal— 0.4% to 2.2%; less than that of polysulfides
      d. Dimensional stability
         (1) Shrinkage is 0.3% to 0.6% during the first 24 hours, with most occurring in the first hour
         (2) More shrinkage than occurs with polysulfide material
      e. Flow after setting
         (1) Less than 0.1% at 15 minutes after setting
         (2) Much lower than that of polysulfides
      f. Flexibility—varies between 2% and 7%; stiffer than polysulfides
      g. Tear strength—25 lb/in; lower than that of polysulfides
      h. Shelf life—reasonable but shorter than that of polysulfides
   2. Addition type (Table 10-4)
      a. Working time—4 to 5 minutes
      b. Permanent deformation during removal— 0.2%; lowest of all rubber impression materials

      c. Dimensional stability—0.5% shrinkage; lowest of all rubber impression materials
      d. Flow after setting—similar to that of condensation silicones
      e. Flexibility—stiffer than condensation silicones
      f. Shelf life—reasonable but shorter than that of polysulfides

D. Manipulation
   1. Mixing
      a. Technique similar to that for polysulfides
      b. Tray—mechanical retention recommended for the addition type, since adhesives not effective
   2. Techniques
      a. Double-mix and single-mix procedures similar to those used with polysulfides
      b. Putty-wash technique is used with the condensation type to minimize dimensional changes
   3. Die materials
      a. Gypsum products
      b. Electroplated copper
      c. Epoxy—may require a separator

Polyether Rubber Impression Material

A. General considerations
   1. Flexible but stable during storage
   2. Can be electroplated to form metal dies
   3. Used to produce accurate impressions for crowns and bridges
   4. Packaged as a two-paste system in regular consistency with a thinner available

B. Composition and reaction
   1. Catalyst paste—aromatic sulfonic acid ester
   2. Base paste—low molecular weight polyether with ethylene imine terminal groups
   3. Reaction
      a. Reaction is

> Polyether + Sulfonic ester → Cross-linked rubber

      b. Reaction accelerated by increases in temperature and humidity

C. Properties
   1. Working time—2 minutes; 4 minutes with a thinner (Table 10-4)
   2. Consistency—stiffer consistency compared with that of other regular materials
   3. Permanent deformation during removal—1%; less than that of polysulfide but greater than that of silicones
   4. Dimensional stability—lower than that of all rubber materials except addition silicone

5. Flow after setting—lower than that of all rubber materials except addition silicone
6. Flexibility—about 2%; 4% with a thinner

D. Manipulation
   1. Mixing
      a. Equal lengths of base, accelerator, and thinner are extruded onto a paper pad
      b. Mixing is accomplished as with other rubber impression materials
      c. Material is loaded into a tray or syringe (if mixed with a thinner)
      d. Tray—thickness of 4 mm should be allowed between the tray and teeth for greater flexibility
   2. Removal of the impression
      a. Steady force is used
      b. Impression is immediately rinsed and the model prepared
      c. Care should be used in removal of the model from the impression to avoid breakage of teeth
   3. Die materials
      a. Gypsum products
      b. Electroplated silver

Model and Die Materials

A. General considerations
   1. Model, cast, or die—replica of hard or soft tissues
      a. Model—replica used primarily for observation
      b. Cast—working replica on which is fabricated an appliance or restoration
      c. Die—working replica of a single tooth or several teeth
   2. Relationship between a replica and an impression
      a. Low points of the impression are high points of the replica
      b. Right side of the impression becomes left side of the replica
      c. Flaws that exist in the impression will be reproduced in the replica

B. Types and selection
   1. Types
      a. Gypsum products—model plaster, dental stone, and high-strength dental stone
      b. Metal—electroplated copper and electroplated silver
      c. Resin—epoxy
   2. Selection
      a. Gypsum products—dental compound, zinc oxide–eugenol, agar or alginate, plaster (with a separator), or rubber impression materials
      b. Electroplated copper—dental compound or silicone rubber
      c. Electroplated silver—rubber impression materials except condensation silicones
      d. Epoxy resin—rubber impression materials (some require separators)

C. Desirable qualities
   1. Accuracy
   2. Dimensional stability
   3. Ability to reproduce fine detail
   4. Strength and resistance to abrasion
   5. Ease of adaptation to the impression
   6. Color
   7. Safety
   8. Economy of time

Electroplated Dies

A. General considerations
   1. Copperplating of compound and silicone impressions
   2. Silverplating of rubber impressions (except condensation silicones)
   3. Metal die is somewhat less accurate but tougher, harder, and more resistant to abrasion

B. Theory of electroplating
   1. Electrolysis—ions move to an electrode of opposite change under the influence of the electrical field
   2. Cathode
      a. Attracts positively charged ions (cations)
      b. Impression made conductive serves as the cathode
   3. Anode
      a. Attracts negatively charged ions (anions)
      b. Bar of pure silver or copper

C. Copperplating
   1. Apparatus—transformer and rectifier to convert AC current to DC current
   2. Electroplating solution—acidic solution of copper sulfate
   3. Impression—coated with a conductor of electricity such as a colloidal solution of graphite
   4. Current
      a. Initial current for a single tooth—15 mA
      b. Current maintained for 12 to 15 hours—30 to 45 mA

D. Silverplating
1. Process—similar to copperplating but smaller currents (5 mA initially, then 10 to 15 mA) are used
2. Electroplating solution—basic solution of silver cyanide
   a. Solution and vapors are toxic
   b. Solution must be kept basic in pH to minimize cyanide gas formation

Epoxy Dies

A. General considerations
1. Used in fabrication of crowns, bridges, and inlays
2. Separators required with some impression materials
3. Epoxy dies are tougher and more abrasion resistant than gypsum but are not as accurate or dimensionally stable
B. Composition and reaction
1. Two component system
   a. Resin—difunctional epoxy with filler
   b. Hardener—polyamine
2. Polymerization involves

$$Resin + Hardener \rightarrow Epoxy$$

C. Properties
1. Working time—15 minutes
2. Setting time—2 to 12 hours
3. Knoop hardness—less than that of gypsum
4. Abrasion resistance—superior to that of gypsum
5. Dimensional change—shrinkage of 0.03% to 0.3%; continues for several days

WAXES ■■■■■■■■■■■■■■

Inlay Pattern Waxes

A. General considerations
1. Pattern duplicates the shape and contour of the desired restoration
2. Used with lost wax pattern technique
3. Types
   a. Direct wax (type I)—used to prepare patterns in the mouth
   b. Indirect wax (type II)—used to prepare patterns on a die
4. Supplied as rods, cones, and in small jars
B. Composition
1. Principal waxes—paraffin, carnauba, ceresin, and beeswax
2. Modified by additions of higher-melting paraffins and more carnauba

C. Properties
1. Excess residue
   a. Residue can cause incomplete casting of inlay margins
   b. Nonvolatile residue is limited to less than 0.1%
2. Flow
   a. Slippage of molecules affected by
      (1) Temperature
      (2) Composition of the wax
      (3) Force causing deformation
      (4) Length of time force is applied
   b. Type I waxes—low flow (less than 1%) at mouth temperature to minimize distortion on removal from the mouth
   c. Type II waxes—softer wax allows greater ease of carving
3. Thermal expansion
   a. High value of coefficient of thermal expansion—$323 \times 10^{-6}/°C$
   b. Temperature changes can cause inaccuracies in the pattern that must be compensated for in the investing procedure
   c. Maximum allowable expansion between 25° and 37° C is 0.6%
4. Mechanical properties
   a. Low values of elastic modulus, proportional limit, and compressive strength compared with those of other dental materials
   b. Properties decrease greatly with increases in temperature
5. Residual stress
   a. Caused by cooling the wax under tensile or compressive forces and by manipulating the wax at temperatures below the melting range
   b. Release of stress causes nonuniform dimensional change or distortion
   c. Release results from effects of time and temperature
D. Manipulation
1. Temperature of the wax at the moment of contact with the die must be above 50° C to record detail
2. Minimize the development of residual stress
   a. Soften the wax uniformly at 50° C for 15 minutes
   b. Add the wax to the die in small increments to minimize changes caused by solidification and thermal contraction
   c. Use a warmed die and carving instruments

3. Minimize the release of residual stress
   a. Greater warpage results at higher storage temperatures and at longer storage times
   b. Invest the pattern immediately or within 30 minutes
   c. Store the pattern in a refrigerator but warm it to room temperature before investing
   d. Readapt margins if the pattern is stored

Other Pattern, Processing, and Impression Waxes

Baseplate Wax

A. Establishes the vertical dimension, plane of occlusion, and initial arch form of a complete denture
B. Types
   1. Type I—soft wax used for building contours and veneers
   2. Type II—medium wax used for patterns to be tried in the mouth
   3. Type III—hard wax used for try-ins in warmer climates
C. Supplied as sheets
D. Composition—ceresin, beeswax, carnauba, and other waxes
E. Properties
   1. Flow at 37° C
      a. Type I—5% to 80%
      b. Type II—2.5% maximum
      c. Type III—1.2% maximum
      d. Excessive flow causes changes in vertical dimensions and occlusion
   2. Thermal coefficient of expansion—200 to 400 × 10^{-6}/°C
F. Manipulation
   1. Avoid pooling the wax with a hot spatula
   2. Avoid manipulation of the wax below its working temperature
   3. Avoid storage of the pattern for long periods of time

Casting Wax

A. Pattern for the metallic framework of a removable partial denture
B. Available in sheets, ready-made shapes, and in bulk
C. Composition—similar to that of inlay waxes
D. Properties
   1. Slightly tacky
   2. Must vaporize with minimal residue

Boxing Wax

A. Used to form a box around the impression before pouring the model
B. Wax should be readily adaptable to the impression at room temperature

Utility Wax

A. Soft, pliable adhesive wax
B. Used for customizing alginate impression trays
C. Composition—mostly beeswax and other soft waxes

Sticky Wax

A. Used to assemble metallic or resin pieces in a fixed temporary position
B. Sticky when melted, adheres closely to surfaces to which it is applied
C. Brittle at room temperature; breaks if distorted

Corrective Impression Wax

A. Forms a wax veneer over an original impression to register detail of soft tissue
B. Formulated from hydrocarbon waxes and may contain metallic particles
C. Flow of 100% at 37° C

Bite Registration Wax

A. Used to articulate accurately certain models of opposing quadrants
B. Formulated from beeswax and hydrocarbon waxes
C. Flow ranges from 2.5% to 22% at 37° C
D. Susceptible to distortion on removal from the mouth

MATERIALS FOR DENTAL PROSTHESES ▄▄▄

Solders

A. Method of joining metal components together by fusion of a lower-melting alloy
   1. Brazing—joining alloy melts at temperatures above 500° C
   2. Soldering—joining components with low-melting lead-tin alloys
B. Types—different solders are needed for cast gold alloys, porcelain-substrate alloys, and orthodontic wires
   1. Gold solder must be completely molten at a temperature 80° C below the melting temperature of the cast alloy
      a. Composition—lower gold content than that of the cast alloy, with additional zinc and tin
      b. Designation—16-650 solder is solder with 650 fineness used with 16 K alloy

2. Gold solder for porcelain-substrate alloys must not soften during firing of the porcelain
3. Silver solder—alloy of gold and silver used with stainless steel, nickel, and gold alloy wires

C. Fluxes
1. Prevent oxidation of parts being soldered
2. Composed of borax (for gold alloys) or fluoride (for stainless alloys)

Alloys for Bonding to Porcelain

A. Cast as substructures for porcelain-fused-to-metal crowns and bridges
B. Coefficient of thermal expansion matched to porcelain (13 to 14 × 10^{-6}/°C)

High-Gold Alloys

A. Composition—98% gold, platinum, and palladium
B. Oxide layer and hardening are produced by a small amount of tin, iron, and indium
C. Replaced by alloys with 80% noble metal—lower in cost and stronger

Palladium-Silver Alloys

A. Composition—50% to 60% palladium, 30% to 40% silver, and some base metals
B. Properties—lower density and cost; potential greening of porcelain caused by silver is bad

Nickel-Chromium Alloys

A. Composition—70% to 80% nickel, 15% chromium, and other metals
B. Properties—less dense and costly; harder, stiffer, and more difficult to cast and finish
C. Nickel sensitivity—10% of females and 1% of males are allergic to nickel

Cobalt-Chromium Alloys for Partial Dentures

A. General considerations
1. Used to cast a partial denture framework
2. Types—cobalt-chromium, nickel-chromium, and cobalt-chromium-nickel alloys
B. Compsition
1. Nickel—increases the ductility of the alloy
2. Chromium—increases tarnish resistance
3. Cobalt—increases the rigidity of the alloy
4. Other metals—increase strength; improve castability
C. Properties
1. Strength comparable to that of type IV gold alloys but harder

2. Density less than that of gold alloys; more difficult to cast
3. More difficult to finish
4. Casting procedure
   a. Higher melting temperature than that of gold alloys
   b. Special casting equipment needed
5. Investment—special investments needed

Dental Casting

A. General considerations
1. Lost wax process is used for casting inlays, crowns, and partial dentures
2. Accuracies of 0.05% dimensional variation are possible
B. Wax pattern
1. Pattern is formed in the mouth (direct method) or on a die (indirect method)
2. Pattern can change dimensions because of its high coefficient of thermal expansion or its release of residual stress
3. Pattern should be invested immediately
C. Spruing
1. Sprue forms a channel for molten metal to flow into the cavity of the investment mold
2. Wax pattern is attached to a short pin called a sprue
   a. Sprue is attached at the thickest part of the pattern
   b. Pin should be short and 2.1 to 2.6 mm in diameter
D. Investing
1. Investment—forms a mold for casting
2. Types—gypsum bonded or phosphate bonded
3. Composed of a refractory (quartz or cristobalite) and binder (calcium sulfate hemihydrate or a phosphate) mixed with water or a silica solution
4. Slurry of investment is painted and vibrated around the wax pattern and allowed to set
E. Wax elimination
1. Investment is heated to 482° to 650° C
   a. To burn away wax
   b. To provide increased expansion of the mold cavity
2. Compensation—wax shrinkage plus gold shrinkage equals wax expansion plus setting expansion plus hygroscopic expansion plus thermal expansion
F. Casting the alloy
1. Alloy is melted by a gas-air blowtorch or in an electric casting machine

2. Alloy is cast when fully fluid in a centrifugal casting machine
3. Mold is broken away
4. Casting is finished by being pickled in acid and polished with abrasive wheels, rubber wheels, pumice, tripoli, and rouge

Plastics in Prosthodontics

A. General considerations
  1. Acrylic plastics are used for a variety of applications
  2. Characteristics—rigid and brittle or soft and flexible
B. Polymerization process
  1. Process in which low molecular weight ingredients react to form high molecular weight ingredients
  2. Monomer—one repeat unit of an organic molecule with one or more reactive groups (e.g., methyl methacrylate)
     a. Low molecular weight (100)
     b. Volatile liquid; boils at 100° C
     c. Low density
  3. Polymer—number of monomer units bonded together in a regular way (e.g., poly[methyl methacrylate])
     a. High molecular weight (10,000)
     b. Increase in density to form a solid
  4. Other ingredients
     a. Initiator—organic peroxide provides free radicals
     b. Accelerator—heat or organic amine
  5. Reaction is

Monomer + Initiator + Accelerator → Polymer

C. Types of polymers
  1. Cross-linked polymers
     a. Polymer molecules linked together to form a network
     b. Polymer is more resistant to surface cracking (crazing)
  2. Copolymers
     a. Monomers that react with methyl methacrylate to form polymers containing both monomer units
     b. Copolymer has different values of impact resistance, hardness, and water sorption
  3. Modified polymers
     a. Polymers with compounds added that do not polymerize, such as oily organic esters, rubbers, and inorganic fillers
     b. Properties such as impact resistance and hardness are changed

Acrylic Denture Base Plastics

A. General considerations
  1. Used to support artificial teeth
  2. Supplied in powder-liquid form, gels, or sheets
  3. Types—heat-cured and self-cured systems
B. Composition
  1. Powder
     a. Polymer—poly(methyl methacrylate); reduces shrinkage during polymerization
     b. Initiator—organic peroxide; provides free radicals to start polymerization
     c. Pigments—provide color and opacity
  2. Liquid
     a. Monomer—methyl methacrylate; polymerizes
     b. Inhibitor—hydroquinone; provides shelf life
     c. Cross-linking agent—minimizes surface cracking
     d. Accelerator—organic amine (in self-cured systems)
C. Properties
  1. Strength—low in strength, fairly flexible, brittle, soft, and highly resistant to failure in fatigue
  2. Thermal conductivity—low value
     a. Affects processing conditions and residual stress in the denture
     b. Results in a substantial decrease in thermal stimulation of oral tissues under the denture
  3. Heat distortion temperature—residual stresses are released at temperatures above 94° C
  4. Polymerization shrinkage—linear shrinkage of 2% can be reduced to 0.5% by proper processing techniques
  5. Water sorption—0.6 mg/cm^2; fairly high value permits the denture to expand slightly and offset polymerization shrinkage somewhat
  6. Bonding to metal and porcelain—mechanical retention required
  7. Color stability—good
  8. Biologic compatibility—good; instances of allergic reactions related to residual monomer in processed dentures have been reported
D. Manipulation and processing
  1. Most common technique—dough molding of the powder-liquid system
  2. Mixing
     a. Powder/liquid ratio—3:1 ratio by volume reduces polymerization shrinkage and temperature rise during processing
     b. Powder is added to liquid until liquid is absorbed

c. Dough consistency is reached after several minutes
   (1) Involves wetting, solution, and absorption
   (2) No chemical reaction occurs until heat is applied (except in self-cured systems)
3. Packing the denture flask
   a. Denture mold is constructed with a clinically acceptable waxed-up denture on a stone cast
   b. Waxed-up denture and cast are invested in a split denture flask
   c. Wax is removed with boiling water
   d. Excess amount of acrylic dough is packed in the mold under pressure several times (trial packing)
   e. Flask is finally closed and clamped under pressure
4. Processing the acrylic
   a. Heat-cured material—cured in a water bath at 73° C for 8 hours
   b. Self-cured material—cured at room temperature for 8 hours
5. Finishing the denture
   a. Denture is separated from the plaster mold and cast
   b. Denture is finished with acrylic burs
   c. Denture is polished under wet conditions with pumice

E. Retention
   1. Based on the fit of the tissue-bearing surface
   2. Factors—surface tension of saliva, surface area of the denture, wettability of the denture by saliva, and viscosity of saliva
   3. Denture adhesives are not needed for a properly fitting denture

F. Care of dentures (see Chapter 12, section on removable appliance maintenance)
   1. Dentures should be kept moist when not in the mouth to retain dimensions
   2. Dentures should not be cleaned with abrasive pastes
   3. Tissue-bearing surface of the denture should be cleaned carefully with a soft brush
   4. Some denture cleaning solutions will corrode the metal framework of a partial denture
   5. Dentures should not be cleaned in hot water; distortion occurs

Other Applications of Plastics

A. Soft liners
   1. Types—long-term and short-term materials
      a. Long-term materials—used over a period of months for patients with severe undercuts or with continually sore residual ridges
      b. Short-term materials (treatment materials or tissue conditioners)—used to initiate healing of tissues over several days
   2. Composition
      a. Long-term materials—acrylic copolymers plus plasticizers or silicone rubbers
      b. Short term materials—poly(ethyl methacrylate), ethanol, and aromatic esters
   3. Properties
      a. Low initial hardness, which increases as plasticizers are leached from the material
      b. Tissue conditioners flow under static load to conform to the shape of the tissues but are rigid under chewing (dynamic) forces
      c. Some silicone rubbers support the growth of yeasts—causing hard spots

B. Prosthetic teeth
   1. Plastic teeth
      a. Used for patients with poor ridges and to oppose natural teeth
      b. Composed of acrylic polymer with different pigments in layers to provide more natural esthetics
      c. Bond chemically to acrylic dentures and are easy to grind
   2. Porcelain teeth
      a. Used when patients have good ridge support and enough room between the arches
      b. Do not bond chemically to acrylic; require mechanical retention and are difficult to grind

C. Plastic-metal combinations
   1. Plastics combined with metals as bases in partial dentures, facings in crown and bridge construction, and orthodontic appliances
   2. Plastic must be mechanically bonded to metal
   3. Wear resistance of plastic facings is not as good as that of porcelain, but the worn plastic can be repaired
   4. Acrylics are processed under heat and pressure to reduce porosity

D. Maxillofacial materials
   1. Used for replacement of tissues of the face
   2. Types—silicones (most common), plasticized acrylics, and urethanes
   3. Desired properties—readily cleaned, remain soft with changes in temperature of the environment, readily colored to match skin tones, and high resistance to tearing

E. Temporary crown and bridge materials
   1. Serve as a temporary restoration until a permanent restoration is fabricated
   2. Composition—acrylic plastics

3. Properties
   a. Hardness—low value compared with that of plastic teeth
   b. Color stability—fair to good
   c. Wear resistance—adequate
4. Manipulation
   a. Powder and liquid are mixed to a creamy consistency
   b. Restoration is formed using the mix and a crown form or alginate impression of the tooth before preparation of the tooth
   c. Material is placed in hot water (57° C) to harden
   d. Restoration is cemented with low-strength zinc oxide–eugenol material

F. Tray materials
   1. Used to form a custom tray for an impression
   2. Composition—highly filled powder-liquid acrylic
   3. Manipulation
      a. Powder and liquid are mixed for 1 minute
      b. Patty is prepared with a roller and wooden block
      c. Patty is placed on the palatal area of a moist maxillary model and adapted
      d. Excess material is trimmed
      e. Material is allowed to polymerize for 6 minutes at room temperature
      f. Tray is finished with acrylic finishing instruments, and retention holes are drilled if rubber impression material to be used

Dental Porcelain

A. General considerations
   1. Used for jacket crowns, porcelain-fused-to-metal bridgework, and denture teeth
   2. Classification—high, medium, and low fusing
   3. Desirable properties include excellent esthetics, tissue tolerance, and wear resistance
B. Composition
   1. Feldspathic porcelains—raw materials of silica, feldspar, and alumina manufactured to form glass
   2. Aluminous porcelains—40% crystalline alumina in the core material to improve strength
C. Properties
   1. Coefficient of thermal expansion—similar to or lower than that of tooth structure
   2. Strength—low in tension but high in compression; brittle
   3. Hardness—harder than human enamel

4. Shrinkage
   a. Nearly 14% shrinkage occurs on sintering
   b. Restoration must be oversized initially to accommodate this change
D. Manipulation
   1. Jacket crown
      a. Porcelain powder is mixed with water to form a paste
      b. Paste is applied to a platinum foil matrix on a die made from an impression of the prepared tooth
      c. Paste is condensed to remove excess water
      d. Porcelain is sintered (partially melted and bonded) in layers to form a uniform, esthetic mass
      e. Restoration is finished, glazed, and cemented in place
   2. Porcelain-fused-to-metal crown
      a. Porcelain is fired directly on a crown constructed from a special porcelain-substrate alloy
      b. Porcelain is fired in layers to provide bonding and esthetics

FINISHING, POLISHING, AND CLEANSING MATERIALS

Abrasion

A. General considerations
   1. Action of hard, irregularly shaped particles cutting a softer material to remove the material from the surface
   2. Process affected by the hardness, strength, ductility, and thermal conductivity of the substrate being abraded
B. Rate of abrasion depends on
   1. Size of the abrasive particle—larger particles cause deeper scratches
   2. Pressure of the abrasive against the surface—heavier pressure causes more rapid removal of the material
   3. Speed with which the abrasive travels across the material—higher speed increases the rate
C. Types of abrasives
   1. Finishing—hard, coarse abrasives are used for developing contour and removing material quickly
   2. Polishing—used to smooth surfaces roughened by finishing abrasives
   3. Cleansing—soft abrasives with small particle sizes
   4. Commonly used agents—aluminum oxide, cuttle, diamond, garnet, sand, silicon carbide, calcite, kieselguhr, pumice, rouge, silex, tin oxide, tripoli, and zirconium silicate

5. Abrasives in prophylactic pastes—quartz, anatase, feldspar, montmorillonite, aluminum hydroxide, kaolinite, and talc
6. Abrasives in dentifrices—calcium carbonate, dibasic calcium phosphate dihydrate, anhydrous dibasic calcium phosphate, tricalcium phosphate, calcium pyrophosphate, sodium metaphosphate, hydrated alumina, and silica

Prophylactic Pastes

A. General considerations
  1. Used for removal of exogenous stains, pellicle, materia alba, and oral debris without causing undue abrasion to tooth structure
  2. Should precede application of a fluoride gel to make enamel more accessible and reactive
B. Composition
  1. Commercial pastes contain abrasives such as kaolinite, silicon dioxide, calcined magnesium silicate, diatomaceous silicon dioxide, pumice, sodium-potassium aluminum silicate, and zirconium silicate
  2. Some pastes contain sodium fluoride or stannous fluoride
C. Properties
  1. Abrasion and cleansing
    a. Products with pumice and quartz show higher cleansing values but also greater abrasion to enamel and dentin
    b. Zirconium silicate is an effective cleansing and polishing agent, but distribution of particle sizes is an important factor
    c. Coarse pumice is the most abrasive
    d. Abrasion of dentin is five to six times the abrasion of enamel regardless of the product
    e. Polymeric restorative materials such as denture base and artificial tooth resins, composites, and acrylic veneering materials can be abraded excessively
  2. Effect of fluoride—ranges from no benefit to 35% reduction in caries after 3 years

Denture Cleansers

A. General considerations
  1. Soft debris can be removed from dentures by light brushing and rinsing
  2. Hard deposits (stains and calculus) require
    a. Professional repolishing
    b. Soaking or brushing on a daily basis
B. Requirements
  1. Nontoxic and easy to remove from the denture
  2. Able to dissolve or attack organic and inorganic debris
  3. Harmless to materials used to fabricate the denture, including plastics, elastomers, and metals
  4. Harmless to eyes, skin, or clothing if accidentally spilled
  5. Stable during storage
  6. Preferably bactericidal and fungicidal
C. Types
  1. Alkaline perborates
    a. Do not easily remove heavy deposits
    b. May be harmful to soft liners
  2. Alkaline peroxides—harmful to soft liners
  3. Alkaline hypochlorites
    a. May cause bleaching
    b. Can corrode base metal alloys
    c. May leave an odor or taste on the denture
  4. Dilute acids—may corrode some alloys
  5. Abrasive powders and creams—can abrade denture plastics
D. Effectiveness
  1. Brushing—effective if done regularly
  2. Daily overnight immersion in alkaline peroxide —safe and effective
  3. Customary 15-minute soaking—no effect on mature plaque, stains, or deposits
  4. Denture cleansers containing enzymes— effective but still experimental
E. Recommended techniques and precautions
  1. Recommendations
    a. Immersion in a solution of one part 5% sodium hypochlorite in three parts water
    b. Immersion in a solution of 1 teaspoon of hypochlorite (Clorox) and 2 teaspoons of glassy phosphate (Calgon) in half a glass of water
    c. Clean the soft liner with a cotton swab and cold water and the denture with a soft brush

2. Precautions
   a. Soaking in hypochlorite solution is not recommended for appliances fabricated from base metals; causes discoloration
   b. Soaking in hot water is not recommended; causes distortion of the plastic
   c. Brushing with dentifrices is not recommended; causes scratching
   d. Cleansing with organic solvents is not recommended; may dissolve or craze the plastic
   e. Storage of the denture should be in water to maintain its dimensional stability
   f. Soaking may cause soft liners to change color or acquire an odor or taste

Dentifrices

See Chapters 8 and 12, sections on dentifrices

SUGGESTED READINGS ▬▬▬

Craig, R.G.: Dental materials: a problem-oriented approach, St. Louis, 1978, The C.V. Mosby Co.

Craig, R.G., editor: Restorative dental materials, ed. 7, St. Louis, 1985, The C.V. Mosby Co.

Craig, R.G., O'Brien, W.J., and Powers, J.M.: Dental materials: properties and manipulation, ed. 3, St. Louis, 1983, The C.V. Mosby Co.

Dentists' desk reference: materials, instruments and equipment, ed. 2, Chicago, 1983, American Dental Association.

Farah, J.W., and Powers, J.M.: The dental advisor: materials, instruments and equipment quarterly, Ann Arbor, 1984, Dental Consultants, Inc.

Leinfelder, K.F., Barton, R.E., and Taylor, D.F.: Dental assisting manual, VI, Dental materials and technical application, ed. 3, Chapel Hill, 1980, The University of North Carolina Press.

O'Brien, W.J., and Ryge, G.: An outline of dental materials and their selection, Philadelphia, 1978, W.B. Saunders Co.

Phillips, R.W.: Skinner's science of dental materials, ed. 8, Philadelphia, 1982, W.B. Saunders Co.

Phillips, R.W.: Elements of dental materials, ed. 4, Philadelphia, 1984, W.B. Saunders Co.

Review Questions

1 Coarse pumice is not recommended for prophylaxis because it
   1. Is too soft to remove calculus
   2. Is too abrasive to dental enamel
   3. Generates significant heat
   4. Will not polish dental amalgam
   5. Reacts with sodium fluoride

2 Which of the following restorative materials is relatively resistant to prophylactic procedures?
   1. Acrylic resin veneers
   2. Composite resins
   3. Denture base resins
   4. Artificial tooth resins
   5. Dental amalgam

3 Which of the following properties is the most troublesome for composite materials used for posterior restorations?
   1. Wear resistance
   2. Water sorption
   3. Coefficient of thermal expansion
   4. Compressive strength
   5. Solubility

4 Which of the following techniques is not proper in the acid-etching procedure for composite restorations?
   1. Etching permanent teeth for 60 seconds
   2. Etching with phosphoric acid solution
   3. Applying fluoride before etching
   4. Rinsing the etchant with water for 20 seconds
   5. Drying the etched area with an air stream for 20 seconds

5 The smoothest surface on a composite resin is produced by
   1. A mylar strip during setting
   2. Finishing with a 12-fluted carbide bur
   3. Finishing with a white stone
   4. Polishing with an aluminum oxide disk
   5. Polishing with pumice

6 Excessive expansion of dental amalgam will lead to
   1. Marginal percolation
   2. Postoperative sensitivity
   3. Electrical conductivity
   4. Increased tarnish
   5. Isthmus fracture

7 Marginal failure in dental amalgam restorations is attributed to
   1. Excessive creep
   2. Poor abrasion resistance
   3. Tarnish
   4. Loss of cavity varnish
   5. Low compressive strength

8 Tarnish of amalgam is most often caused by
   1. Crevice corrosion
   2. Concentration cell corrosion
   3. Sulfide formation
   4. Staining
   5. Phase changes

9 Which of the following cannot be removed by finishing or polishing an amalgam restoration?
1. Surface tarnish
2. Superficial plaque
3. Occlusal stain
4. Interfacial corrosion products
5. Corrosion crevices on the surface

10 Which of the following factors is least important in mixing dental amalgam?
1. Trituration time
2. Mercury/alloy ratio
3. Frequency of the amalgamator
4. Room temperature
5. Amplitude of the amalgamator

11 A poorly condensed amalgam exhibits all of the following properties except
1. Delayed expansion
2. Increased strength
3. Increased corrosion
4. Increased mercury content
5. Increased tin-mercury and silver-mercury phases

12 The principal application of zinc phosphate cement is
1. In final cementation
2. As temporary cementation
3. As a temporary filling material
4. As an obtundent base
5. As a permanent filling material

13 The main component in zinc phosphate cement liquid is
1. Eugenol
2. Ortho-ethoxybenzoic acid
3. Polyacrylic acid
4. Methyl salicylate ester
5. Phosphoric acid

14 Which of the following is incorrect for the manipulation of zinc phosphate cement?
1. Chill the glass slab to about 21° C
2. Dispense the liquid first
3. Incorporate the powder in four to six increments
4. Mix over a large area of the slab
5. Mix for 60 to 90 seconds depending on the product

15 Increasing the powder/liquid ratio of zinc phosphate cement
1. Decreases solubility
2. Decreases tensile strength
3. Decreases residual zinc oxide
4. Decreases compressive strength
5. Decreases the modulus of elasticity

16 The main component in zinc oxide–eugenol cement liquid is
1. Water
2. Phosphoric acid
3. Oil of cloves
4. Ortho-ethoxybenzoic acid
5. BIS-GMA

17 The principal advantage of zinc oxide–eugenol cement over zinc phosphate cement is its
1. Obtundent effect on the pulp
2. Higher strength
3. Lower intraoral solubility
4. Chemical reactivity with dentin
5. Higher modulus of elasticity

18 The principal reason for applying cavity varnish is to provide
1. Strength to cut dentinal tubules
2. Thermal insulation beneath an amalgam
3. A means of preventing percolation with an amalgam
4. Increased mechanical support of the amalgam
5. A temporary chemical barrier over dentin

19 Which of the following impression materials is rigid?
1. Zinc oxide–eugenol
2. Reversible hydrocolloid
3. Alginate
4. Polysulfide rubber
5. Silicone rubber

20 What is the major restriction for all rigid impression materials?
1. Insufficient tear resistance
2. Cannot be used in undercut areas
3. Hydrophobic toward dental stone
4. Insufficient accuracy
5. Insufficient dimensional stability

21 Agar hydrocolloid impression material is generally supplied as
1. Two pastes to be mixed
2. Powder and liquid to be mixed
3. Two powders to be mixed with water
4. Paste and powder to be mixed
5. Solid individual cylinders to be heated

22 The loss of water from hydrocolloids during continued reaction is called
1. Syneresis
2. Imbibition
3. Inhibition
4. Hysteresis
5. Adsorption

23 Which of the following impression materials does not undergo a chemical reaction during setting?
1. Zinc oxide–eugenol
2. Agar
3. Alginate
4. Polyether rubber
5. Silicone rubber

24 Rapid removal of rubber impressions with a single firm motion results in
1. Reduced dimensional instability
2. Improved adhesion of the impression to the tray
3. Minimal permanent deformation
4. Reduced contamination by saliva
5. Reduced flexing of the tray

25 A replica of oral tissues used primarily for observation is called a
1. Cast
2. Die
3. Replica
4. Duplicate
5. Model

26 Which of the following materials is not a gypsum product?
1. Model plaster
2. Dental stone
3. Epoxy die material
4. High-strength dental stone
5. Orthodontic stone

27 Before being mixed with water gypsum products have the chemical name
1. Calcium sulfate hemihydrate
2. Calcium sulfate monohydrate
3. Calcium sulfate dihydrate
4. Calcium phosphate
5. Calcium alginate

28 Which of the following factors is least important to the setting time of dental stone?
1. Water/powder ratio
2. Water temperature
3. Chemical accelerators
4. Chemical retarders
5. Method of spatulation

29 For which of the following materials does loss of gloss *not* indicate the end of the working time?
1. Polycarboxylate cement
2. Composite resin
3. Glass ionomer cement
4. Model plaster
5. Dental stone

30 Dies should be waxed in small increments to accommodate for which property of wax?
1. Residue on burnout
2. Thermal contraction
3. Modulus of elasticity
4. Compressive strength
5. Flow

31 Metallic frameworks for partial dentures are patterned with
1. Inlay wax
2. Baseplate wax
3. Boxing wax
4. Utility wax
5. Casting wax

32 Planes of occlusion are often established with
1. Inlay wax
2. Boxing wax
3. Baseplate wax
4. Utility wax
5. Casting wax

33 An alloy that is 65% gold is classified as
1. 28 karat
2. 24 karat
3. 18 karat
4. 16 karat
5. 12 karat

34 Which of the following alloying elements is primarily responsible for the corrosion resistance of type III gold alloys?
1. Gold
2. Copper
3. Silver
4. Palladium
5. Nickel

35 The joining of metal components by fusion with a lower-melting-point alloy that melts at a temperature below 500° C is called
1. Welding
2. Brazing
3. Sintering
4. Soldering
5. Fluxing

36 The pin added to a wax pattern before investing and casting is used to form a
1. Sprue
2. Vent
3. Crucible
4. Reservoir
5. Liner

37 Pickling solutions are composed primarily of
1. Citric acid
2. Phosphoric acid
3. Ortho-ethoxybenzoic acid
4. Inorganic acids
5. Polyacrylic acid

38 The major reason for pickling a casting is to
1. Create a coating of chemically adherent salts
2. Remove oxides or carbonaceous residues
3. Etch grain boundaries to enhance bonding of the cement
4. Polish the surface of the casting chemically
5. Remove investment material from the casting

39 Application of a sealant requires all of the following except
1. Reetching, rinsing, and drying if contamination by saliva occurs
2. Application of the sealant only to etched areas of the tooth
3. Etching by a 37% solution of phosphoric acid
4. Application of fluoride immediately before etching
5. Use of tube (cannula) or ball applicators

40 Mercury can be characterized by
1. Its low density
2. Its low vapor pressure
3. Its ability to absorb through the skin
4. Its high melting point
5. Its toxicity when combined with amalgam alloy

41 Which of the following is the most important factor in sealant retention?
1. Acid etching
2. Developmental groove depth
3. Abrasion resistance
4. Sealant compressive strength
5. Diet

42 The principal advantage of glass ionomer restorations over composites is
1. Better esthetic appearance
2. Better retention in cervical areas
3. Higher compressive strength
4. Lower solubility
5. Better thermal insulation

43 Glass ionomer restorations should be finished in a manner similar to
1. Dental amalgam
2. Dental composites
3. Gold casting alloys
4. Unfilled restorations
5. Silicate restorations

44 Setting of dental amalgam is caused by
1. Physical reaction
2. Cross-linking
3. Crystallization
4. Reprecipitation
5. Trituration

45 Polysulfide rubber impression material is mixed as
1. Powder and liquid onto a chilled glass slab
2. Two equal lengths of a base and accelerator pastes
3. Paste and liquid spatulated on a paper pad
4. Powder and water mixed on a pad
5. Powder and water mixed in a bowl

46 Which of the following accelerators (activators) is involved in denture base material polymerization?
1. Ultraviolet light
2. Amine
3. Visible light
4. X-rays
5. Heat

47 Before delivery, a denture should be stored in water to
1. Desorb unreacted components
2. Allow sorption to offset shrinkage
3. Stabilize the color
4. Prevent fungal growth
5. Prevent contact with air

48 Generalized soft tissue irritation in response to denture wearing after 2 to 3 days is most likely related to
1. Poor finishing techniques
2. Improper denture cleaning solutions
3. Hypersensitivity to residual monomer
4. Errors in dimensional accuracy during processing
5. Occlusal disharmonies

49 The active ingredient in a dentifrice paste that is responsible for cleaning and polishing teeth is
1. Water
2. Sorbitol
3. Stannous fluoride
4. Glycerin
5. An abrasive

50 Which of the following cleaning materials is acceptable for mouth protectors?
1. Toothpaste and a toothbrush
2. Slurry of baking soda in water
3. Alcohol-containing mouthwashes
4. Denture cleanser in warm water
5. Cool soap-and-water solutions

51 Which of the following is a problem even for a properly fabricated mouth protector?
1. Gagging
2. Deformation
3. Taste
4. Irritation
5. Speech impairment

52 Which of the following is *not* a step in the fabrication of a thermoplastic custom-made mouth protector?
1. Making an alginate impression of the arch
2. Pouring a gypsum cast
3. Forming the thermoplastic material over the cast
4. Finishing the mouth protector
5. Heat treating the mouth protector to increase its hardness

53 The energy required to deform a material to fracture is called its
1. Hardness
2. Toughness
3. Plasticity
4. Resilience
5. Viscoelasticity

54 The elastic modulus is a measure of
1. Toughness
2. Stiffness
3. Viscoelasticity
4. Plasticity
5. Hardness

55 Stress is defined as
1. Load per unit of area
2. Deformation per unit of length
3. Strength per unit of volume
4. Percent of elongation
5. Stiffness per unit of length

56 The uptake of water molecules into a restoration is called
1. Solubility
2. Disintegration
3. Absorption
4. Chemical reaction
5. Adsorption

57 Which one of the following pairs of restorations might cause galvanism to occur in a patient's mouth?
1. Porcelain crown and dental amalgam
2. Dental amalgam and dental amalgam
3. Gold crown and gold crown
4. Gold crown and composite resin
5. Gold crown and dental amalgam

58 Which one of the following categories of dental materials has the highest thermal conductivity?
1. Unfilled acrylic plastics
2. Gold alloys
3. Porcelains
4. Zinc phosphate cements
5. Zinc oxide–eugenol cements

Answers and Rationales

1. (2) Coarse pumice will cause rapid wear of enamel and dentin.
   (1) Coarse pumice will remove calclus, but is too abrasive to tooth structure.
   (3) Abrasives should be used with water and light pressure to minimize heat.
   (4) Coarse pumice is too abrasive for use with dental amalgam.
   (5) Coarse pumice does not react with sodium fluoride.

2. (5) Dental amalgam is hard enough to resist wear by most prophylactic procedures.
   (1) The acrylic resin veneers are soft and abrade easily.
   (2) The resin matrix of a composite abrades easily.
   (3) Acrylic resins are soft and abrade easily.
   (4) Artificial tooth resins abrade easily.

3. (1) Low wear resistance is a cause of clinical failure.
   (2) Water sorption does not directly cause clinical failure.
   (3) The coefficient of thermal expansion does not directly cause clinical failure.
   (4) The compressive strength is sufficient for a properly designed restoration.
   (5) The solubility is low and does not cause clinical failure.

4. (3) A fluoride treatment decreases the solubility of the enamel, making it more difficult to etch.
   (1) A 60-second etch is recommended for permanent teeth.
   (2) Etching with 37% phosphoric acid is recommended.
   (4) A 20-second rinse is necessary to remove the acid from the tooth.
   (5) Drying is necessary to remove excess water from the tooth.

5. (1) A mylar strip produces the smoothest surface because the surface is rich in resin.
   (2) A 12-fluted carbide bur roughens the surface by preferentially removing the resin matrix.
   (3) A white stone roughens the surface by preferentially removing the resin matrix.
   (4) An aluminum oxide disk roughens the surface by preferentially removing the resin matrix.
   (5) Pumice roughens the surface by preferentially removing the resin matrix and is not recommended for composites.

6. (2) Excessive expansion of amalgam exerts pressure on the tooth.
   (1) Marginal percolation is not caused by excessive expansion.
   (3) Electrical conductivity is not affected by the expansion of the amalgam.

   (4) Tarnish is not affected directly by the dimensional change of the amalgam.
   (5) Excessive expansion does not result in isthmus fracture.

7. (1) Amalgams with high values of creep exhibit more marginal failure clinically.
   (2) Amalgams have acceptable resistance to abrasion.
   (3) Tarnish is a surface phenomenon.
   (4) The absence of cavity varnish affects leakage and pulpal sensitivity.
   (5) Compressive strength is not directly related to marginal failure.

8. (3) The formation of sulfides produces a dark film on amalgam.
   (1) Tarnish is less severe than corrosion.
   (2) Tarnish is less severe than corrosion and is limited to the surface.
   (4) Staining is a result, not a cause, of tarnish.
   (5) Phase changes at the surface result from tarnish.

9. (4) Interfacial corrosion products are not removed.
   (1) Tarnish can be removed by polishing.
   (2) Superficial plaque can be removed by polishing.
   (3) Occlusal stain can be removed by polishing.
   (5) Corrosion crevices can be removed by finishing and polishing.

10. (4) The temperature of the room is normally not important.
    (1) The time of trituration affects amalgamation.
    (2) The mercury/alloy ratio affects amalgamation.
    (3) The frequency, amplitude, and path of the amalgamator affect amalgamation.
    (5) The frequency, amplitude, and path of the amalgamator affect amalgamation.

11. (2) Decreased strength results from the increased mercury content.
    (1) Expansion results from the increased mercury content.
    (3) Increased corrosion results from the increased mercury content.
    (4) The mercury content is increased.
    (5) Increased tin-mercury and silver-mercury phases result from the increased mercury content.

12. (1) Luting of crown and bridge restorations is the principal use of zinc phosphate cement.
    (2) Zinc phosphate cement is too strong for temporary cementation.
    (3) Zinc phosphate cement is too soluble for use as a temporary filling material.
    (4) Zinc phosphate cement is not obtundent, but is used as a base.
    (5) Zinc phosphate cement is not strong enough for use as a permanent filling material.

13. (5) Phosphoric acid and water are the main components of the liquid.
    (1) Eugenol is the principal component in zinc oxide–eugenol cements.
    (2) Ortho-ethoxybenzoic acid is a component in EBA-alumina zinc oxide–eugenol cements.

For each question the correct answer and rationale are listed first. The other choices are presented in order with the reasons why they are not correct.

(3) Polyacrylic acid is an important component in poly-carboxylate cements.

(4) Methyl salicylate ester is a component in calcium hydroxide bases.

14. (2) The powder is dispensed first.
    (1) Chilling the slab above the dew point allows more powder to be mixed.
    (3) The powder is incorporated into the liquid in increments.
    (4) A large area of the slab is used to dissipate the heat.
    (5) Mixing typically requires 60 to 90 seconds.

15. (1) The solubility is decreased with less zinc phosphate matrix.
    (2) The tensile strength is increased with less zinc phosphate matrix.
    (3) More residual zinc oxide results from a higher powder/liquid ratio.
    (4) The compressive strength is increased with less zinc phosphate matrix.
    (5) The modulus of elasticity is increased with less zinc phosphate.

16. (3) Eugenol is also called oil of cloves.
    (1) Water is required for setting but is not a main component in the liquid.
    (2) Zinc oxide–eugenol cement does not contain phosphoric acid.
    (4) Some modified zinc oxide–eugenol cements contain ortho-ethoxybenzoic acid in the liquid.
    (5) BIS-GMA is the major component in a composite resin.

17. (1) Zinc oxide–eugenol cements obtund the pulp.
    (2) Zinc oxide–eugenol cements are weaker.
    (3) Zinc oxide–eugenol cements are more soluble.
    (4) Neither cement reacts chemically with dentin.
    (5) Zinc oxide–eugenol cements have a lower modulus of elasticity.

18. (5) Varnish serves as a barrier to the passage of ions toward the pulp.
    (1) Varnish has no mechanical strength.
    (2) Varnish has no thermal insulation characteristics.
    (3) Varnish does not prevent microleakage.
    (4) Varnish provides no mechanical support to a restoration.

19. (1) Zinc oxide–eugenol impression pastes are rigid and must be used only in nonundercut areas.
    (2) Agar is a flexible impression material and may be used in undercut areas.
    (3) Alginate is a flexible impression material and may be used in undercut areas.
    (4) Polysulfide rubber is a flexible impression material and may be used in undercut areas.
    (5) Silicone rubber is a flexible impression material and may be used in undercut areas.

20. (2) Rigid impressions would lock over the undercut and be difficult to remove.
    (1) Rigid materials are not used in areas where tearing would be a problem.
    (3) Most impression materials (except silicones) are hydrophilic.

(4) The rigid impression materials have sufficient accuracy for the reproduction of soft tissues.

(5) The rigid impression materials have sufficient dimensional stability but should be poured immediately for best results.

21. (5) Agar is supplied as cylinders or in tubes in bulk and is heated for use.
    (1) Zinc oxide–eugenol impression materials may be supplied as two pastes.
    (2) Zinc oxide–eugenol impression materials may be supplied as a power-liquid system.
    (3) Such an impression material is not available.
    (4) Such an impression material is not available.

22. (1) The exuding of fluid from a hydrocolloid impression is termed syneresis and results in shrinkage.
    (2) Imbibition is the absorption of water and results in swelling.
    (3) Inhibition is the slowing of a chemical reaction.
    (4) Hysteresis refers to the different temperatures necessary to form a sol and a gel.
    (5) Adsorption is the attraction of water to the surface of an impression.

23. (2) Agar is heated and cooled during use.
    (1) Zinc oxide and eugenol react chemically.
    (3) Alginate reacts chemically with calcium sulfate to set.
    (4) The polymerization of polyether rubber is a chemical reaction.
    (5) The polymerization of silicone rubber is a chemical reaction.

24. (3) The increased loading rate minimizes the viscous component of the material and reduces the permanent deformation.
    (1) The dimensional stability of the impression is not affected by the rate of removal.
    (2) The adhesion of the impression to the tray is not affected by the rate of removal.
    (4) Saliva is easily rinsed from a rubber impression.
    (5) The rigidity of the tray is not affected by the removal of the impression.

25. (5) A model is made primarily for observation of dental symmetry.
    (1) A cast is a working model made of multiple teeth.
    (2) A die is a working model of a single tooth.
    (3) The term *replica* describes models, casts, and dies.
    (4) A duplicate is a second cast prepared from an original cast.

26. (3) Epoxy die material is a polymer.
    (1) Model plaster is a gypsum product.
    (2) Dental stone is a gypsum product.
    (4) High-strength dental stone is a gypsum product.
    (5) Orthodontic stone is a gypsum product.

27. (1) All gypsum products contain the hemihydrate form of calcium sulfate before being mixed with water.
    (2) This compound is not found in gypsum products.
    (3) This compound results when the hemihydrate reacts with water.
    (4) This compound is not a major component of gypsum products.
    (5) This compound forms alginate impression material.

28. (5) The method of spatulation will affect the setting time, but to a lesser extent than the other factors listed.
    (1) Increasing the water/powder ratio slows the setting.
    (2) Increasing the temperature from 23° to 37° C will cause the stone to set more quickly.
    (3) An accelerator causes the stone to set more quickly.
    (4) A retarder causes the stone to set more slowly.
29. (2) Composite resin becomes stiff at the end of its working time.
    (1) Polycarboxylate cement loses its gloss and forms cobwebs at the end of its working time.
    (3) Glass ionomer cement loses its gloss and forms a skin at the end of its working time.
    (4) Model plaster loses its gloss as water is drawn into the setting mass.
    (5) Dental stone loses its gloss as water is drawn into the setting mass.
30. (2) The high contraction caused by solidification and cooling of the wax requires incremental additions to maintain accuracy.
    (1) Residue on burnout is not affected by the waxing technique.
    (3) The modulus of elasticity is not affected by the waxing technique.
    (4) The compressive strength is not affected by the waxing technique.
    (5) The flow is not affected by the waxing technique.
31. (5) Casting wax has properties necessary for making a pattern of a partial denture framework.
    (1) Inlay wax is used for waxing inlays, crowns, and bridges.
    (2) Baseplate wax is used for waxing dentures.
    (3) Boxing wax is used in conjunction with pouring an impression.
    (4) Utility wax is used to extend an impression tray.
32. (3) Baseplate wax is used to establish bite relations.
    (1) Inlay wax is used for waxing inlays, crowns, and bridges.
    (2) Boxing wax is used in conjunction with pouring an impression.
    (4) Utility wax is used to extend an impression tray.
    (5) Casting wax is used to prepare patterns for partial denture frameworks.
33. (4) A 16-karat alloy would be about 65% gold.
    (1) This term does not make sense.
    (2) A 24-karat alloy would be 100% gold.
    (3) An 18-karat alloy would be 75% gold.
    (5) A 12-karat alloy would be 50% gold.
34. (1) Gold is a noble metal that is resistant to corrosion.
    (2) Copper is a component of gold alloy that can corrode.
    (3) Silver is a component of gold alloy that can corrode.
    (4) Palladium is a noble metal but not a primary component of type III gold alloy.
    (5) Nickel is a base metal that is not present in gold alloy.
35. (4) Soldering is when the joining alloy melts below 500° C.
    (1) Welding is a method of joining metals without the addition of another metal.
    (2) Brazing is when the joining alloy melts above 500° C.
    (3) Sintering is a joining of particles of metal or ceramic by diffusion at a temperature below the melting temperature.
    (5) Fluxing is a method of cleaning areas to be soldered.
36. (1) The wax pattern is attached to a short metal or wax pin called a sprue.
    (2) A vent may be attached to a wax pattern to allow gases to escape more easily during casting.
    (3) The casting alloy is melted in a crucible.
    (4) The sprue pin is mounted on a base that acts as a reservoir for the molten alloy during the casting procedure.
    (5) A heat-resistant liner is used to line the casting ring and allow some additional expansion for the investment.
37. (4) Commercial pickling solutions contain complex inorganic acids.
    (1) Citric acid is used as a mild etchant for dentin.
    (2) Phosphoric acid is used in zinc phosphate and zinc silicophosphate cements.
    (3) Ortho-ethoxybenzoic acid is used in a modified zinc oxide–eugenol cement.
    (5) Polyacrylic acid is used in zinc polycarboxylate cement.
38. (2) Pickling dissolves films of oxides and carbon.
    (1) The casting is rinsed carefully to remove any salts.
    (3) The internal surfaces of a casting are usually sufficiently rough to allow mechanical retention of a cement.
    (4) The surfaces of castings are polished mechanically.
    (5) Investment material is not easily dissolved by pickling solution, so it must be removed by sand blasting.
39. (4) The fluoride is applied after the sealant treatment is completed, because the fluoride interferes with the etching of the tooth.
    (1) If contamination occurs, the entire etching procedure must be repeated.
    (2) Application of the sealant to unetched areas may result in leakage and decay.
    (3) The etching solution is typically 37% to 50% phosphoric acid.
    (5) These tools control the application so sealant is not applied to unetched areas of the tooth.
40. (3) Mercury should not be handled with bare skin because it is easily absorbed.
    (1) Mercury has a high density, which makes a small bottle deceptively heavy.
    (2) Mercury has a high vapor pressure that increases with temperature.
    (4) Mercury is a liquid at room temperature.
    (5) Mercury in dental amalgam is combined with silver and is no longer toxic.
41. (1) Sealant retention depends primarily on continued micromechanical retention developed by bonding to acid-etched enamel.
    (2) Developmental groove depth is not important, even though it might provide some gross mechanical retention of sealant.

(3) Abrasion resistance of sealant is not critical, because sealants are not crucial on abrading surfaces that are self-cleaning.

(4) Sealant compressive strength is not a measure of retention to tooth structure or abrasion resistance.

(5) Diet may influence sealant abrasion but has not been shown to compromise sealant effectiveness in caries reduction.

42. (2) Glass ionomer restorations are chemically adhesive to tooth structure and therefore have a retention advantage over composites in cervical areas.

(1) Composites have a better esthetic appearance.

(3) Composites have a higher compressive strength.

(4) Composites have a lower intraoral solubility.

(5) Composites and glass ionomers are approximately equal in providing thermal insulation.

43. (5) Glass ionomers are remarkably similar to silicate restorations because of the composition of the glass powder. Therefore they require very similar finishing procedures and precautions.

(1) Dental amalgam is stronger than glass ionomer.

(2) Dental composite is stronger than glass ionomer.

(3) Cast gold alloys are much stronger and harder than glass ionomers.

(4) Unfilled restorations are approximately the same strength but are softer than silicates.

44. (3) Dental amalgam sets to a hard solid because of the crystallization of the reaction product phases.

(1) Physical reactions involve changes of state without chemical bonding changes.

(2) Cross-linking is the tying together of polymer molecules into an extended network.

(4) Reprecipitation is the precipitation of phases again.

(5) Trituration is the mixing of dental amalgam alloy with mercury.

45. (2) Polysulfide rubber impression materials are dispensed as equal lengths of catalyst paste and base paste for mixing on a paper pad.

(1) Zinc phosphate cement components are dispensed as a powder and liquid onto a chilled glass slab.

(3) Zinc oxide–eugenol cement components are dispensed as a powder and liquid to be spatulated on a paper pad.

(4) Anhydrous cements are mixed as powder with water on a paper pad.

(5) Alginate impression material is mixed as a powder with water in a bowl.

46. (5) Heat is used in combination with heating rate and pressure to control the polymerization reaction for processing heat-cured denture base materials.

(1) Ultraviolet light used to be a method of activating some composite resin materials.

(2) Amines are used to chemically accelerate self-curing acrylic resins.

(3) Visible light may be used to activate composite resins and sealants.

(4) X-rays are not used at the present time for activation but are a possible energy source.

47. (2) Denture base resin absorbs water and expands slightly. The absorption process requires approximately 17 days to reach equilibrium and should be started as soon as possible to ensure proper denture fit.

(1) Small amounts of unreacted components may slowly desorb, but that process occurs over months or years.

(3) Denture color should not visibly change.

(4) Fungal growth is prohibited by smooth acrylic surfaces and proper oral hygiene.

(5) Acrylic denture base materials are not affected by air exposure.

48. (3) If a patient experiences generalized tissue irritation in the first few days of wearing a new denture, it is often a hypersensitivity response to the release of residual monomer from an improperly processed denture.

(1) Poor finishing techniques generally result in increased staining on the top surface of the denture or in localized irritation.

(2) Improper denture cleaning solutions may cause the denture gloss or color to change.

(4) Errors in fit will cause patient discomfort because of local mechanical irritation at the site of mismatch.

(5) Occlusal disharmonies do not cause soft tissue problems.

49. (5) During cleaning and polishing, the abrasive in a dentifrice paste is the key ingredient involved in abrasion to remove unwanted intraoral adherents. Abrasives make up about 40% of the composition.

(1) Water is a solvent for fluoride salts in the dentifrice.

(2) Sorbitol is a humectant that keeps the dentifrice from drying.

(3) Stannous fluoride is for fluoride ion release into enamel.

(4) Glycerin is added to stabilize the suspension of the abrasive.

50. (5) Mouth protectors should be protected from heat or solvents that might contribute to their distortion. Therefore a cool soap-and-water solution is the mildest cleaning procedure.

(1) Cleaning with a toothbrush and toothpaste is abrasive to the mouth protector.

(2) Baking soda in water is not effective.

(3) Alcohol-containing mouthwashes can dissolve parts of the mouth protector or be absorbed by it.

(4) Denture cleansers in warm water will cause softening and flow of the mouth guard.

51. (2) Even a perfectly formed mouth protector will be subject to occlusal biting stresses and will permanently deform.

(1) Gagging is more common with the use of improperly formed mouth protectors.

(3) Taste is more of a problem with mouth-formed protectors.

(4) Irritation is more common with improperly formed mouth protectors.

(5) Speech impairment is more of a problem with improperly formed mouth protectors.

52. (5) After adaptation of the features of a mouth protector, it should be protected from heat, which will accelerate its unwanted deformation.
    (1) The first step in custom fabrication is to obtain an alginate impression of the arch to be protected.
    (2) A gypsum cast is prepared from the impression.
    (3) Thermoplastic material is adapted to the cast with the use of heat.
    (4) Excess material is trimmed away, and the edges of the mouth protector are smoothed as a finishing step.
53. (2) The toughness of a material is its ability to absorb energy before failure or the total energy under the stress-strain curve up to the point of fracture.
    (1) Hardness is the resistance to plastic deformation as measured by indentation.
    (3) Plasticity is the ease of plastic deformation.
    (4) Resilience is the ability of a material to absorb energy elastically before permanent deformation.
    (5) Viscoelasticity is the deformation and time-dependent elastic recovery of a material.
54. (2) The elastic modulus is a measure of the resistance to deformation in response to loading; therefore it represents the stiffness of a material.
    (1) Toughness is a measure of the total energy a material can absorb.
    (3) Viscoelasticity is the time-dependent elastic deformation and recovery of a material.
    (4) Plasticity is the ease of plastic deformation.
    (5) Hardness is the resistance to plastic deformation as measured by indentation.
55. (1) Stress is the normalization of load by dividing it by the cross-sectional area of the solid into which it is distributed.
    (2) Deformation per unit of length is strain.
    (3) Strength per unit of volume is a meaningless quantity.
    (4) Percent of elongation is the strain in terms of percent.
    (5) Stiffness per unit of length is a meaningless quantity.
56. (3) Absorption is the addition of external materials physically "into" the interior of a solid.
    (1) Solubility is the loss of components from the surface of a solid or from the interior into the surrounding fluid.
    (2) Disintegration is the physical destruction of a solid into smaller and smaller pieces.
    (4) Chemical reaction is the change in bonding patterns between components.
    (5) Adsorption is the addition of external material physically "onto" the surface of a solid.
57. (5) Galvanism results from the contact of mixed metals, which causes electrochemical corrosion. The opposition of a gold crown and dental amalgam restoration will cause galvanism.
    (1) Contact of a porcelain crown with dental amalgam does not cause galvanism, because the porcelain is not a metal.
    (2) Dental amalgam in contact with dental amalgam does not cause galvanism, because they are the same metal alloy.
    (3) A gold crown in contact with a gold crown does not cause galvanism, because they are the same metal alloy.
    (4) A gold crown in contact with a composite resin does not cause galvanism, because the composite is not a metal.
58. (2) As a class of materials, metals have the highest values of thermal conductivity because metallic bonding permits thermal conduction easily.
    (1) Unfilled acrylic plastics are polymers and have a low thermal conductivity.
    (3) Porcelains are ceramic materials and have a low thermal conductivity.
    (4) Zinc phosphate cements are ceramics and have a low thermal conductivity.
    (5) Zinc oxide–eugenol cements are principally ceramic and have a low thermal conductivity.

CHAPTER 11

Periodontics

CHARLOTTE HANGORSKY

A thorough understanding of periodontics is essential to the practice of dental hygiene and to the role of the dental hygienist as cotherapist with the dentist and patient. A plethora of research exists in the area of periodontics; however, knowledge and understanding of periodontal disease are changing rapidly. This chapter reflects today's standard level of knowledge and practice and provides an outline of the fundamentals of periodontics, including the anatomy and histology of the periodontium, the changes within the periodontium associated with disease (including etiologic and contributing factors), clinical assessment of the periodontium, common diseases of the periodontium, and clinical interventions in the treatment of periodontal disease.

BASIC FEATURES OF THE PERIODONTIUM

A. Periodontium (Fig. 11-1) is composed of
  1. Gingiva
  2. Periodontal ligament
  3. Root cementum
  4. Alveolar bone
B. Function of the periodontium is to attach the tooth to the alveolar bone tissues of the mandible and maxilla
C. Changes in the periodontium may be a result of
  1. Morphologic and functional alterations
  2. Changes in the oral environment
  3. Age

Gingiva

Definition
A. Part of the oral masticatory mucosa that surrounds the cervical portion of the teeth and covers the alveolar process of the jaws
  1. Apical border is the mucogingival junction that separates the gingiva from the adjacent lining mucosa
  2. On the palatal surface it blends into palatal masticatory mucosa

B. Components
  1. Marginal gingiva (unattached or free gingiva)
    a. Unattached cufflike tissue that surrounds the teeth facially, lingually, and interproximally
    b. Parts of marginal gingiva
      (1) Gingival margin—most coronal portion of the gingiva, which surrounds the teeth in a scalloped outline; located at or approximately 0.5 mm coronal to the cementoenamel junction
      (2) Gingival groove—only present in 30% to 40% of adults; when present, it is located 1.0 to 1.5 mm apical to the gingival margin
      (3) Gingival sulcus—space formed by the tooth and the sulcular epithelium laterally and by the coronal end of the junctional epithelium (base of the sulcus) apically; in absolute periodontal health, almost no gingival sulcus exists; however, a sulcular measurement of 1 to 2 mm facially and lingually and 1 to 3 mm interproximally is considered to be within the range of health
      (4) Interdental gingiva—that portion of the gingival margin that occupies the interdental space coronal to the alveolar crest (clinically, it fills the embrasure space)
        (a) Posterior teeth—gingiva consists of two interdental papillae (one buccal and one lingual) that are connected by the concave-shaped interdental col
        (b) Anterior teeth—col is usually not present, since the interdental papilla is formed by a single pyramid-shaped structure
        (c) Col is not present when teeth are not in contact

Fig. 11-1 Anatomy of periodontium.

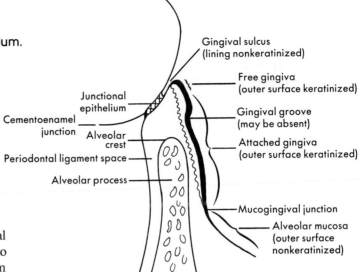

Gingival sulcus
(lining nonkeratinized)

Junctional epithelium

Cementoenamel junction

Alveolar crest

Periodontal ligament space

Alveolar process

Free gingiva
(outer surface keratinized)

Gingival groove
(may be absent)

Attached gingiva
(outer surface keratinized)

Mucogingival junction

Alveolar mucosa
(outer surface nonkeratinized)

(d) Interdental gingiva, like the facial and lingual gingiva, is attached to the tooth by junctional epithelium and connective tissue fibers

2. Attached gingiva
   a. That part of the gingiva that is attached to the underlying periosteum of the alveolar bone and to the cementum by connective tissue fibers and the epithelial attachment
   b. Boundaries
      (1) Apically demarcated by the mucogingival junction (demarcates attached gingiva from alveolar mucosa)
      (2) Coronally demarcated by the base of the gingival sulcus
   c. Width of attached gingiva varies
      (1) Generally widest in facial anterior maxillary areas and narrowest in mandibular premolar facial areas
      (2) Width of attached gingiva is not measured on the palate, since it cannot be clinically distinguished from palatal mucosa

Histologic Features

See Chapter 2, section on oral histology
A. Epithelium
   1. Epithelium on the outer surface of marginal and attached gingiva is parakeratinized or keratinized
   2. Sulcular epithelium—stratified squamous, nonkeratinized epithelium that is continuous with the oral epithelium; lines the peripheral surface of the sulcus extending to the coronal border of the junctional epithelium
   3. Junctional epithelium—stratified, nonkeratinized epithelium that surrounds and attaches to the tooth on one side and attaches

on the other side to the gingival connective tissue; new cells originate from the cells in the apical portion adjacent to the tooth and from the cells in contact with the connective tissue; epithelial cells are shed (desquamation) at the coronal end of the junctional epithelium, which forms the base of the gingival sulcus
   a. Junctional epithelium is more permeable to cells and fluids
   b. Serves as the preferred route for the passage of fluid and cells from the connective tissue into the sulcus and for the passage of bacterial products from the sulcus into the connective tissue
   c. Is easily penetrated by the periodontal probe; this penetration is increased in inflamed gingiva
   4. Epithelial attachment—refers to the basal lamina and hemidesmosomes that connect the junctional epithelium to the tooth surface
   5. Rete pegs—connective tissue projections that interweave with the gingival oral epithelium
B. Connective tissue (or lamina propria)—composed of gingival fibers (connective tissue fibers), intercellular ground substance, cells, and vessels and nerves
   1. Gingival fibers—composed of collagen fibers (60% of connective tissue volume), reticular fibers, oxytalan fibers, and elastic fibers; fiber bundle groups provide support for marginal gingiva, including the interdental papilla (Fig. 11-2; see also Figs. 2-27 and 2-28)

Fig. 11-2 Connective tissue fibers of gingiva. NOTE: Not shown are transseptal fibers that extend from cementum of one tooth through lamina propria to cementum of adjacent tooth (see also Figs. 2-27 and 2-28).

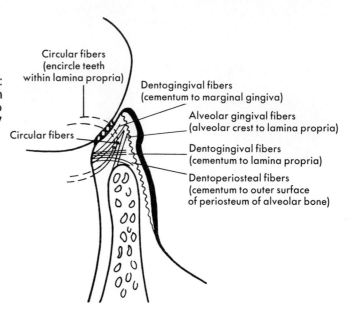

Circular fibers (encircle teeth within lamina propria)

Circular fibers

Dentogingival fibers (cementum to marginal gingiva)

Alveolar gingival fibers (alveolar crest to lamina propria)

Dentogingival fibers (cementum to lamina propria)

Dentoperiosteal fibers (cementum to outer surface of periosteum of alveolar bone)

  a. Circumferencial or circular fibers—encircle each tooth separately in a cufflike fashion within the free gingiva
  b. Dentogingival fibers—embedded in the cementum located between the cementoenamel junction and the crest of the alveolar bone; extend outward into the gingival margin tissues
  c. Dentoperiosteal fibers—embedded in the same portion of the cementum as the dentogingival fibers, but extend apically *over* the alveolar crest and terminate in the attached gingiva
  d. Transseptal fibers—embedded in the same portion of the cementum as dentogingival and dentoperiosteal fibers; run a horizontal path from adjacent teeth
 2. Intercellular ground substance (or matrix)
  a. Gel-like medium that surrounds connective tissue cells
  b. Essential for maintenance of normal function of connective tissue (e.g., transportation of water, electrolytes, nutrients)
  c. Composed of water, mucopolysaccharides, and hyaluronic acid
 3. Cells
  a. Fibroblasts (predominant cells)
   (1) Produce various types of fibers found in connective tissue
   (2) Instrumental in synthesis of intercellular ground substance
  b. Other connective tissue cells
   (1) Mast cells—participate in the early phase of inflammation
   (2) Macrophages—host defense and repair
   (3) Polymorphonuclear leukocytes—host defense
   (4) Lymphocytes—host defense
   (5) Plasma cells—host defense
 4. Vessels and nerves (see section on blood supply to the periodontium)

Normal Clinical Features

A. Color—in light-skinned individuals, pale or coral pink; in dark-skinned individuals, coral pink to brown (may vary depending on the degree of vascularity, amount of melanin, and epithelial keratinization)
B. Texture
 1. Gingival margin—dull, smooth surface
 2. Attached—stippled, "orange peel" surface present on facial surfaces (stippling may not always be present in healthy gingiva)
C. Consistency
 1. Gingival margin—firm; resists displacement
 2. Attached gingiva—firmly bound to the underlying alveolar bone and cementum
D. Papillary contour—pointed; papilla fills the interproximal space to the contact point
E. Marginal contour—most coronal edge should form a thin, knifelike edge with a scalloped configuration mesiodistally

Periodontal Ligament

Definition

A. Connective tissue that surrounds the root and connects it with the alveolar bone
B. Is continuous with the connective tissue of the gingiva
C. Contains collagen fibers, which are attached on one side to the alveolar bone and on the other side to the cementum; terminal portions of these fibers, which are embedded into the cementum and alveolar bone, are called Sharpey's fibers

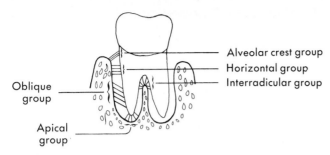

Oblique group

Apical group

Alveolar crest group
Horizontal group
Interradicular group

Fig. 11-3 Principal fiber bundles of periodontal ligament (see also Fig. 2-27).

D. Is organized into fiber groups called principal fiber bundles, which are distinguished by their location and direction

Principal Fiber Bundles (Fig. 11-3; see also Fig. 2-27)

A. Alveolar crest group—fibers extend from the cementum just below the junctional epithelium and extend obliquely to the alveolar crest
B. Horizontal group—fibers extend at right angles to the long axis of the tooth, from the cementum to the alveolar bone
C. Oblique group—fibers extend from the alveolar bone to the cementum in an apical direction, forming the most numerous fiber group and providing the main support to the tooth
D. Apical group—fibers extend from the alveolar bone to the cementum at the apex of the root
E. Interradicular group—fibers extend from the alveolar bone to the cementum in furcation areas

Functions

A. Physical—attachment of the tooth to the bone and absorption of occlusal forces
B. Formative—formation of connective tissue components by activities of connective tissue cells (cementoblasts, fibroblasts, osteoblasts)
C. Resorptive—by activities of connective tissue cells (fibroclasts, osteoclasts, cementoclasts)
D. Nutritive—nutrients carried through blood vessels to the cementum, bone, and gingiva
E. Sensory—proprioceptive and tactile sensitivity provided by innervation to the periodontal ligament

Clinical Considerations

A. Thickness varies from 0.1 to 0.4 mm (mean, 0.2 mm); ligament is thicker in functioning than in nonfunctioning teeth and thicker in areas of tension than in areas of compression
B. Periodontal ligament cells can remodel the ligament and adjacent bone when altered forces are applied (e.g., orthodontics)

C. Accidentally exfoliated teeth can be replanted if handling of the torn ligament is minimized before reimplantation

Cementum

See Chapter 2, section on cementum

Definition

A. Calcified mesenchymal tissue that covers the surface of the root
B. Main function is to attach the fibers of the periodontal ligament to the tooth
C. Features
 1. Does not contain blood or lymph vessels
 2. Has no innervation
 3. Does not resorb or remodel as does bone
 4. Is continuously deposited in the apical area of the root throughout life
D. Two different types (see Fig. 2-25)
 1. Acellular—forms in conjunction with root formation and tooth eruption
 2. Cellular—forms after the tooth is erupted in the apical one third of the root; contains cementoblasts, inactive cementocytes, fibroblasts from the periodontal ligament, and cementoclasts

Relationship to Enamel

A. Cementum overlaps enamel (60%)
B. Cementum and enamel meet (30%)
C. Cementum and enamel do not meet, leaving an area of dentin exposed (10%)

Clinical Considerations

A. Compensates for occlusal wear by apical deposition of cementum
B. Protects the root surface from resorption during tooth movement
C. Has a reparative function, which permits reestablishment of new connective tissue attachment following certain types of periodontal therapy
D. When enamel and cementum do not meet, cervical hypersensitivity and caries are more likely to develop

Alveolar Process

See Chapter 2, section on alveolar bone, and Fig. 2-26

Definition

A. Bone that forms and supports the tooth sockets (alveoli)

B. Consists of
1. Alveolar bone proper (or cribriform plate)
   a. Thin layer of compact bone that forms the inner socket wall; numerous perforations are present to permit vascular communication between marrow spaces of cancellous bone and the periodontal ligament
   b. Bundle bone—alveolar bone adjacent to the periodontal ligament (contains Sharpey's fibers)
   c. Lamina dura—radiographic image of the alveolar bone proper
   d. Alveolar crest—coronal rim of the alveolar bone; generally parallels adjacent cementoenamel junctions; is 1.5 to 2 mm apical to the cementoenamel junction
2. Supporting bone
   a. Surrounds and supports the alveolar bone proper
   b. Composed of two parts
      (1) Compact cortical plate (facial and lingual aspects)
      (2) Spongy or cancellous bone—located between the cortical plate and alveolar bone proper

Shape, Thickness, and Location

A. Contour of the alveolar bone follows the contour of the cementoenamel junctions and the arrangement of the dentition
B. Shape of the alveolar crest is generally parallel to the cementoenamel junctions of adjacent teeth; is approximately 1.5 to 2 mm apical to the cementoenamel junction
C. Cortical plates are generally thicker in the mandible
D. Posterior areas—bone is generally thick, and cancellous bone separates the cortical plate from the alveolar bone proper
E. Anterior areas—bone is thin, with little or no cancellous bone separating the cortical plate from the alveolar bone proper
F. Dehiscence—situation in which the marginal alveolar bone is apical to the normal level, exposing an abnormal amount of root surface
G. Fenestration—situation in which the margin of the alveolar bone is intact; however, there is an isolated lack of alveolar bone on the root surface (root surface area is covered only by gingiva)

Radiographic Features of the Normal Periodontium

A. Alveolar crest—thin, radiopaque line that is continuous with the lamina dura; shape is dependent on
1. Proximity of adjacent teeth and roots
2. Level of adjacent cementoenamel junctions
B. Periodontal ligament space—thin radiolucent line surrounding each root
C. Supporting bone—not actually seen; however, it will influence the radiopacity of the radiograph depending on the amount, pattern, and/or presence of cancellous and cortical bone
D. Limitations of radiographs
1. Do not show soft tissue–to–hard tissue relationships
2. Do not show early bone loss
3. May not show interproximal bony changes accurately
4. May not show bone changes on facial or lingual surfaces

Blood Supply to the Periodontium

A. To the gingiva via supraperiosteal arterioles
1. Supraperiosteal arterioles are vessels of the periodontal ligament that extend coronally into the gingiva
2. These arterioles are mainly along the facial and lingual surfaces of the cortical plate
3. These arterioles emerge from the alveolar crest
B. To the periodontal ligament via inferior and superior alveolar arteries, which reach the periodontal ligament via
1. Apical vessels
2. Penetrating vessels from the alveolar bone
3. Anastomosing (joining) vessels from the gingiva
C. To the alveolar process
1. To the alveolar bone proper via branches of the apical vessels in the ligaments and vessels in the interdental septum
2. To the cortical plate via branches of the supraperiosteal arterioles
3. To cancellous bone via the interdental septum vessels and vessels that also supply the cortical plate and alveolar bone proper

Innervation and Lymphatic Drainage of the Periodontium

Follows pathways similar to those of the vessels supplying blood to the periodontium

CHANGES WITHIN THE PERIODONTIUM ASSOCIATED WITH DISEASE ▬▬▬▬

A. Factors that influence periodontal health
   1. Extrinsic etiologic factors—microbial dental plaque (primary etiologic factor)
   2. Extrinsic contributing factors
      a. Other soft deposits associated with oral hygiene
      b. Tooth position and anatomy
      c. Condition of dental restorations, permanent or removable prostheses, and/or orthodontic appliances
      d. Oral (functional) habits that create excessive traumatic forces to the periodontium
   3. Intrinsic (systemic) contributing factors
      a. Immunologic defects
      b. Endocrine dysfunctions
      c. Nutritional disorders
      d. Genetically transmitted diseases
      e. Emotional disorders
      f. Drug intake
B. Response of the periodontium to these factors; basic inflammatory response produces
   1. Clinical changes
   2. Histologic changes
   3. Radiographic changes
C. Response within the soft tissue only (gingival inflammation)
   1. Stage I, or initial lesion—2 to 4 days following plaque accumulation
      a. Changes are not clinically visible
      b. Histologic changes
         (1) ''Widening'' of blood vessels
         (2) Increase in leukocytes, particularly polymorphonuclear leukocytes (PMNs), in the connective tissue, junctional epithelium, and gingival sulcus
         (3) Increase in flow of gingival fluid into the sulcus
   2. Stage II, or early lesion—4 to 7 days following plaque accumulation
      a. Changes are not clinically visible
      b. Histologic changes
         (1) Leukocyte infiltration into the connective tissue (especially lymphocytes)
         (2) Junctional epithelium is infiltrated with neutrophils and may begin to show development of rete pegs
         (3) Destruction of collagen fibers (especially circular and dentogingival)
         (4) PMNs found within the sulcular area
   3. Stage III, or established (chronic) lesion—2 to 3 weeks following plaque accumulation
      a. Clinical changes
         (1) Erythema (redness) of the gingiva as a result of proliferation of capillaries (begins in the papillary area) and/or a bluish hue superimposed over the reddened gingiva as a result of congested blood vessels and sluggish blood flow
         (2) Bleeding may occur on probing as a result of thinning and/or ulceration of the sulcular epithelium
         (3) Color changes begin in the papillary area, spread to the gingival margin, and then to attached gingiva
         (4) Consistency may be either soft, spongy, or firm and leathery; depends on whether destructive changes or reparative changes within the gingiva are dominant
         (5) Texture may be either
            (a) Smooth and shiny (destructive, exudative factors dominant) or
            (b) Stippled and nodular (reparative, fibrotic proliferation dominant)
         (6) Gingiva may be tender to touch by instruments and home care aids
         (7) Increase in depth of the gingival sulcus is caused by enlargement of the gingival tissue *only;* creates a gingival or pseudopocket
            (a) Begins with papillary enlargement
            (b) Extends into margins, producing rounded and bulbous gingival margins

(8) Progression of inflammation
   (a) May remain only within the gingival tissues (gingivitis)
   (b) May extend into the supporting periodontal tissues (periodontitis)
   NOTE: Periodontitis must be proceded by gingivitis, but gingivitis does not always progress into periodontitis

b. Histologic changes
   (1) Increase in number and predominance of plasma cells, which invade deep into the connective tissue
   (2) Widened intercellular spaces in the junctional epithelium contain lysosomes, lymphocytes, and monocytes
   (3) Junctional epithelium protrudes into the connective tissue, creating rete pegs
   (4) Collagenase actively breaking down connective tissue collagen
   (5) Simultaneous proliferation of collagen fibers and epithelium
   (6) Bone loss has *not* occurred

D. Pathway of inflammation from the gingiva to supporting periodontal tissues (transition from gingivitis to periodontitis)
   1. Generally follows the course of the blood vessels through soft tissues and into the alveolar bone
   2. Pattern of inflammatory pathway affects the pattern of bone destruction
   3. Initially, inflammation penetrates and destroys gingival fibers near the gingival fiber attachment to the cementum, then spreads
      a. Interproximally
         (1) Into the bone and periodontal ligament
         (2) From the bone to the periodontal ligament
      b. Facially and lingually
         (1) From the gingiva to the outer periosteum and periodontal ligament
         (2) From the periosteum into the bone

E. Formation of the periodontal pocket—persistent, chronic gingivitis may progress to periodontitis, which results in loss of connective tissue attachment, bone destruction, and periodontal pocket formation (see Chapter 13, sections on types of pockets and description of a pocket)
   1. Periodontal pocket—pathologic deepening of the gingival sulcus produced by destruction of the supporting tissues and apical proliferation of the epithelial attachment
   2. Classification
      a. Suprabony pocket—base of the pocket is coronal to the alveolar crest

      b. Infrabony pocket—base of the pocket is apical to the alveolar crest
3. Histopathology
   a. Gingival epithelium may show evidence of inflammatory changes
      (1) Epithelium proliferates into the connective tissue in fingerlike projections
      (2) Inflammatory cells are found in the epithelium
      (3) Epithelium lining the pocket may be ulcerated
   b. Connective tissue changes
      (1) Inflammatory cells (lymphocytes, plasma cells, and macrophages) infiltrate the connective tissue
      (2) Inflammatory infiltration proceeds through the loose connective tissue along vascular pathways
   c. Changes within the supporting bone as inflammatory processes progress
      (1) Osteoclastic cells become evident
      (2) Bone marrow component (fatty tissue) is replaced with inflammatory cell infiltrate, fibroblastic proliferation, and deposition of collagen fibers
      (3) Cortical plate of the interdental septum is the first area to be involved (central crestal area where blood and lymph vessels emerge)
      (4) Once this central breakthrough has occurred, the supporting bone is destroyed in a lateral direction

F. Common clinical changes associated with periodontitis
   1. Similar changes in the gingiva as seen in gingivitis, usually a more chronic appearance
   2. Areas of gingival recession
   3. Bleeding on probing
   4. Loose, extruded, or migrated teeth; diastemas may develop
   5. Exudate from the gingival margin in response to pressure
   6. Symptoms—patient may complain of itching gums, loose teeth, food impaction, and bad taste; relief is felt with pressure applied to the gums

G. Radiographic changes associated with periodontitis (usually follow this sequence)
   1. Fuzziness and discontinuity of the lamina dura at the proximal aspects of the crest of the interdental septum

2. Center of the crestal portion of the interdental septum also becomes fuzzy, and faint cup-shaped areas of alveolar crest bone loss appear
3. Progression of interdental bone loss
   a. Horizontal bone loss—reduction in height of the interdental septa; however, the crest is parallel to an imaginary line connecting adjacent cementoenamel junctions
   b. Angular or vertical bone loss—crest is reduced in a manner that creates angular defects

BACTERIAL DENTAL PLAQUE

See Chapter 7, section on bacterial dental plaque
A. Definition—dense, noncalcified, highly organized bacterial mass, firmly adherent to the teeth or other hard materials within the mouth; cannot be washed off by salivary or water flow
B. Stages in plaque formation
   1. Acquired pellicle
      a. Thin, amorphous bacteria-free membranous layer covers the clinical crown; consists of salivary glycoproteins
      b. Forms on a cleaned tooth within minutes
      c. Within hours bacteria begin to deposit on the surface of the pellicle and are surrounded by a matrix that differs from that of the acquired pellicle
      d. This bacteria and surrounding matrix make up dental plaque
   2. Microbial dental plaque
      a. Heterogenous, dense, noncalcified bacterial mass that develops on the acquired pellicle
      b. Rate of formation varies from person to person, tooth to tooth, and even in different areas on the same tooth
      c. Shifts in the types of microorganisms occur as plaque ages
         (1) Young plaque is composed of
            (a) Gram-positive cocci (40% to 50%)
            (b) Gram-positive rods (10% to 40%)
            (c) Gram-negative rods (10% to 15%)
            (d) Filaments (4% or less)
         (2) As plaque ages, the percentage of gram-positive organisms decreases (2-week-old plaque is 50% gram positive and 30% gram negative)
         (3) As plaque ages, the number of cocci decreases and the number of filaments (particularly actinomyces) increases
         (4) As plaque ages, aerobic bacteria decrease and anaerobic bacteria increase

C. Structure and composition
   1. Water (80%)
   2. Solids (20%; 95% of which is bacteria)
   3. Growth of bacteria (not deposition of salivary bacteria) accounts for the increase in plaque bulk with age
   4. Different organisms may be found in plaque (cocci, rods, filaments, and spiral forms), and their proportions change with time, diet, and location
   5. Extracellular microbial products (e.g., polysaccharides, endotoxins)
   6. Host-derived products such as salivary constituents and immunoglobulins (IgG, IgA)
D. Dental calculus—dental plaque that has mineralized (see Chapter 13, section on calculus)
   1. Mineralization can begin from 24 to 48 hours or up to 2 weeks after plaque deposition
   2. Earliest mineralization occurs along the inner surface of the plaque
   3. Composition
      a. Inorganic material (70% to 90%)
      b. Remainder is organic material and water
   4. Classification
      a. Supragingival (supramarginal, salivary)—derives its minerals from saliva
      b. Subgingival (submarginal, serumnal)—derives its minerals from gingival fluid
   5. Modes of attachment to teeth (see Chapter 13, section on modes of attachment)
      a. By acquired pellicle
      b. Directly to the tooth surface
      c. Mechanically locking into tooth surface irregularities, including penetration into cemental separations or defects
   6. Effect on the periodontium—since bacterial plaque always covers calculus, calculus plays a significant role as a contributing factor in the pathogenesis of periodontal disease
E. Pathogenic effect on the periodontium
   1. Microorganisms found in plaque generally *do not* penetrate the deeper gingival tissues
   2. Damage to tissues is caused by mediators such as enzymes and bacterial by-products (e.g., endotoxins)
      a. The enzyme collagenase causes dissolution of collagen within connective tissue
      b. The enzyme hyaluronidase affects the ground substance within connective tissue
      c. Endotoxins (cellular components of gram-negative bacteria) contribute to continuation of the inflammatory response

F. Summary—current knowledge of the effect of dental plaque on tissues is expanding; however, many questions remain unanswered; to maintain oral health, plaque must be
1. Removed or
2. Changed in composition from predominantly gram-negative, motile anaerobic bacteria associated with disease to predominantly gram-positive, nonmotile aerobic or facultative bacteria found in periodontal health

CLINICAL ASSESSMENT OF THE PERIODONTIUM ▰

A. Indices—system for documenting clinical observations to help patients become aware of their present status, demonstrate changes in health over a period of time, and survey large populations for present status and trends in health (see Table 15-3)
1. Periodontal Disease Index (Ramfjord's) (PDI) —assesses the prevalence and severity of periodontal disease of individuals or groups, using the following parameters
   a. Gingivitis index—assesses color, form, consistency, and bleeding to determine the presence or absence of inflammation
   b. Calculus index—assesses the presence or absence of calculus
   c. Crevice (sulcus) depth—measurement to determine the distance between the cementoenamel junction and the base of the sulcus (method to assess apical migration of the epithelial attachment)
2. Loe and Silness Gingival Index (GI)—assesses the presence, severity, or absence of gingival inflammation
3. Silness and Loe Plaque Index (PI)—assesses the quantity and location of plaque
4. Muhlemann Bleeding Index (BI)—assesses the presence, severity, or absence of bleeding on probing
B. Periodontal documentation
1. Uses—documentation of existing periodontal status; baseline for future reference
2. Updated periodically to determine changes in periodontal health
3. Necessary for treatment planning
4. Serves as a guide for the clinician during treatment
5. Serves as a legal document
C. Complete periodontal documentation includes
1. Recording missing or malpositioned teeth, existing restorations, crowns, bridges, caries, and findings of the extraoral and intraoral examinations

2. Complete description of gingival components using the four parameters: color, shape, consistency, and texture (may include indices)
3. Periodontal charting
   a. Recession—measures the amount of exposed root surface
   b. Sulcus/pocket measurement (probing depth)—measures the distance from the gingival margin to the base of the sulcus (see Chapter 13, section on the probe)
   c. Masticatory mucosa—distance from the mucogingival junction to the gingival margin; difference between the masticatory mucosa measurement and the probing depth demonstrates the amount of attached tissue present
   d. Furcation involvement—classifications
      (1) Class I (incipient)—furcation area detected but cannot be penetrated with an instrument
      (2) Class II (moderate)—bone loss is only partially penetrating into the furcation; instrument can enter the furcation but cannot pass entirely through the area
      (3) Class III (advanced)—"through and through"; furcation may be entered from two sides
   e. Mobility classifications
      (1) Grade 1—tooth is mobile approximately 1 mm horizontally
      (2) Grade 2—tooth is mobile more than 1 mm horizontally
      (3) Grade 3—tooth is mobile horizontally and is vertically compressible
   f. Open contacts—existing or potential areas of food impaction
   g. Overhanging restorations or defective restorations—potential areas of plaque and food retention
4. Radiographic evaluation—periodontal charting is done in conjunction with radiographic evaluation to assess
   a. Level of the alveolar crest in relation to the cementoenamel junction
   b. Interdental bone
   c. Furcation areas
   d. Width of the periodontal ligament space
   e. Existing dental restorations and caries
   f. Periapical disease
   g. Length and shape of roots

5. Documentation of oral habits
   a. Bruxing (grinding) or clenching of the teeth
   b. Chewing on fingernails or foreign objects
   c. Smoking habits
   d. Alcohol habits
   e. Movement of the temporomandibular joint (evidenced by crepitus, tenderness, or deviations)
6. Assessment of occlusion—includes
   a. Angle's classification and anterior relationships
   b. Degree of tooth mobility
   c. Excessive wear patterns (facets)
   d. Defective prematurities—isolated occlusal contacts that cause deflection in the pathway of physiologic mandibular movement
   e. Teeth, restorations, or prosthetic appliances that may interfere with normal movements of the mandible
   f. Temporomandibular joint discomfort
   g. Fremitus—vibration of root surufaces as the patient "taps" teeth together
   h. Tooth sensitivity to pressure and to hot and cold substances
7. Classification of occlusal trauma (NOTE: Occlusal trauma does not initiate periodontal disease; however, existing periodontal destruction can be aggravated by occlusal trauma)
   a. Primary occlusal trauma—normal, healthy periodontium is subjected to excessive occlusal forces (e.g., patient grinds on one or two opposing teeth, or a restoration is "high"), but the periodontium remains healthy; result could be mobility, excessive wear of a tooth or teeth, sensitivity of involved teeth, or fremitus
   b. Secondary occlusal trauma—supporting periodontium is not normal (some loss of supporting structures is present); tooth or teeth are not able to withstand even normal occlusal forces without trauma; could result in mobility or sensitivity
8. Additional information obtained through patient interview
   a. Complete documentation of the patient's past and current medical status
   b. Complete documentation of the patient's dental history
   c. Patient's daily oral hygiene routine
   d. Patient's attitude toward oral health
   e. Patient's oral health knowledge level

INFLAMMATORY DISEASES OF THE PERIODONTIUM ASSOCIATED WITH BACTERIAL DENTAL PLAQUE

Methods of Classification

A. Classification according to onset and duration
   1. Acute disease
      a. Gingivitis
      b. Periodontitis ("rapidly progressive")
      c. Acute necrotizing ulcerative gingivitis (ANUG)
      d. Pericoronitis
      e. Periodontal abscess
   2. Chronic disease
      a. Gingivitis
      b. Periodontitis ("adult")
      c. Juvenile periodontitis
      d. Dystrophies
      e. Gingival recession
B. American Dental Association's classification of periodontal disease

Case type	Periodontal findings
I	Gingivitis
IA	Gingivitis with complicating factors (systemic or physical disabilities)
II	Early periodontitis (moderate pockets, minor to moderate bone loss)
IIA	Early periodontitis with complicating factors
III	Moderate periodontitis (moderate to deep pockets, moderate to severe bone loss, slight mobility)
IIIA	Moderate periodontitis with complicating factors
IV	Advanced periodontitis (deep pockets, extensive bone loss, obvious mobility)
IVA	Advanced periodontitis with complicating factors

Diseases

A. Gingivitis—inflammation of the gingiva
   1. Clinical features (see section on changes in the periodontium associated with disease)
   2. Classification of gingivitis by
      a. Duration
         (1) Acute—sudden onset; short duration; usually some pain or tenderness noticed
         (2) Chronic—long duration; painless; may have periods of subacute or acute episodes
      b. Distribution
         (1) Localized—confined to a single tooth or specific groups of teeth
         (2) Generalized—involves the entire mouth
         (3) Papillary—involves interdental papillae only
         (4) Marginal—involves the gingival margins, including the papillae
         (5) Diffuse—involves the gingival margin, papilla, and attached gingiva

3. Treatment
   a. By clinician—removal of hard deposits and other contributing factors (e.g., overhanging restorations)
   b. By patient—daily removal of bacterial dental plaque
B. Periodontitis—disease resulting from the inflammatory process originating in the gingiva (gingivitis) and extending into the supporting periodontal structures; may progress slowly or rapidly with periods of remission or acceleration
   1. Clinical features (see section on changes in the periodontium associated with disease)
   2. Radiographic features (see section on changes in the periodontium associated with disease)
   3. Etiology—tissue response (inflammatory process) to bacterial plaque
   4. Treatment
      a. By clinician—removal of hard deposits and contributing factors, including reduction of the pocket depth through a surgical procedure
      b. By patient—daily removal of bacterial dental plaque
C. Juvenile periodontitis—a disease of the periodontium of the permanent dentition that occurs in otherwise healthy young individuals; characterized by rapid loss of connective tissue attachment and alveolar bone
   1. Localized juvenile periodontitis—only permanent first molars and incisors are affected
   2. Generalized juvenile periodontitis—most permanent teeth are affected
   3. Epidemiology
      a. Onset between 11 and 13 years of age
      b. Seems to affect females more than males
      c. May have familial tendencies
   4. Etiology—bacterial dental plaque with the following characteristics
      a. Coccoid and straight nonmotile rods dominate; few spirochetes present in contrast to adult periodontitis
      b. Predominantly gram-negative organisms (*Actinobacillus actinomycetem-comitans, Capnocytophaga sputigena*) have been found within the connective tissue
      c. Subgingival plaque is relatively thin and tends to not mineralize
   5. Clinical findings
      a. Gingiva around the affected area may appear normal
      b. Periodontal probing reveals deep pockets on one or more proximal surfaces of affected teeth

c. Bleeding occurs on probing in affected areas
d. Amount of soft and hard deposits is *not* commensurate with the amount of periodontal destruction
   6. Radiographic appearance
      a. If localized—angular bone loss around the first molars and incisors; usually bilateral ("mirror image")
      b. If generalized—fairly extensive bone loss throughout the dentition
   7. Treatment is the same as for periodontitis; may use short-term antibiotics in conjunction with initial therapy
D. Acute necrotizing ulcerative gingivitis (ANUG)—inflammatory destructive disease of the gingiva that has a sudden onset with periods of remission and exacerbation; predisposing conditions may be preexisting (e.g., gingivitis, smoking, period of severe stress, radical change in eating or sleeping habits)
   1. Clinical findings are characterized by craterlike depressions at the crest of the interdental papilla that progress into the marginal gingiva
      a. Surface of the lesion(s) is covered by a gray, necrotized slough surrounded by an obvious erythematous (red) zone
      b. Bleeding may be spontaneous and will also occur when necrotic tissue is gently removed
      c. Initially moderate pain increases as the disease advances
      d. Fetid odor and increased salivation are present
      e. Swelling and tenderness of regional lymph nodes (especially submandibular nodes) are present
      f. Fever and malaise may be present
   2. Radiographic findings—none unless the disease has not been treated and has led to destruction of supporting structures
   3. Etiology—predisposing factors are present, with spirochetes and fusiform bacteria found within the tissue; however, the primary etiologic factor is uncertain
   4. Treatment
      a. Plaque and debris removal—initially by the clinician and daily by the patient (may be difficult because of pain)
      b. Mouth rinses (twice daily for 2 weeks) of 3% hydrogen peroxide and warm water
      c. Soft nutritious diet
      d. Avoidance of spicy foods, alcohol, and smoking

e. After acute symptoms disappear, tissue may need to be recontoured surgically (gingivectomy or gingivoplasty) to remove shallow craters; deep defects may require periodontal flap surgery

E. Pericoronitis—inflammation of the tissue flap (operculum) surrounding the crown of a partially erupted tooth
   1. Most frequent in third molar areas
   2. May be acute, subacute, or chronic
   3. Clinical findings if acute
      a. Extremely red, swollen lesion with exudate is present
      b. Area is extremely tender, with pain radiating to the ear, throat, and floor of the mouth
      c. There is a foul taste in the mouth
      d. Inflammation may progress so that swelling, inability to close the jaw, fever, and malaise may be present; symptoms are less obvious as the situation becomes more chronic
   4. Etiology—accumulation of food debris and bacterial growth between the soft tissue flap and tooth; tissue inflammation may be compounded by trauma from the opposing tooth
   5. Treatment
      a. Give antibiotics if fever, swelling, or lymphadenopathy is present
      b. Cleanse the area (lavage and curettage) and create access for drainage of the exudate
      c. Have the patient rinse frequently with warm water; have the patient return for retreatment after 24 hours
      d. After pain subsides and the infection is controlled, either extract the involved tooth or remove (excise) the soft tissue flap

F. Periodontal (or lateral) abscess—localized, purulent area of inflammation within the periodontal tissue
   1. Clinical findings
      a. Abscess may be in the supporting periodontal tissues on the lateral aspect of the root, which results in a sinus (fistula) through the bone extending out to the external surface
      b. Abscess may develop in the soft tissue wall of a deep periodontal pocket
      c. Abscess may be acute or chronic
         (1) Acute—extreme pain, sensitivity, mobility, enlarged lymph nodes
            (a) Gingival area is edematous, red, and smooth with a shiny surface
            (b) Exudate may be expressed from the gingival margin on pressure

         (2) Chronic—usually asymptomatic or episodes of dull pain; elevation of the tooth; desire to grind on the tooth (may have acute episodes); usually has a sinus opening onto the gingival mucosa along the root
      2. Radiographic findings (many variations according to the location, stage, and extent of the lesion)—typical appearance is that of a discrete radiolucent area along the lateral aspect of the root.

G. Dystrophies—pathologic condition caused by abnormal cell biology and physiology
   1. Types
      a. Atrophy—diminished size of the organ or tissue
      b. Hyperplasia—abnormal increase in volume of the tissue or organ caused by the formation and growth of new normal cells
      c. Hypertrophy—increase in size of the tissue or organ caused by an increase in size of its cells; does not occur in gingiva; can occur in periodontal ligaments, cementum, and alveolar bone because of an increase in functional influences
   2. Gingival hyperplasia—overgrowth of gingiva caused by an increase in the fibrous tissue component of the gingiva
      a. Localized "fibroma"—etiology may be unknown or local irritation; treated by surgical removal and elimination of local irritating factors
      b. Generalized gingival fibrous hyperplasia— rare; etiology is unclear
      c. Idiopathic gingival hyperplasia (fibromatosis)—genetic; seems to involve a defect in collagen metabolism; treatment may include surgery; condition tends to recur
      d. Inflammatory hyperplasia—overgrowth that occurs in response to bacterial plaque
      e. Pyogenic granuloma—exaggerated tissue response possibly initiated by minor trauma; if it occurs in pregnant woman, it is called a pregnancy tumor; high incidence of recurrence
      f. Phenytoin (Dilantin) hyperplasia— hyperplastic reaction of epithelium and connective tissue to phenytoin, usually with inflammation being a secondary, complicating factor; treatment includes daily, thorough plaque control with or without surgery (gingivectomy); may also try changing the patient's drug to carbamazepine

3. Gingival recession (or gingival atrophy)—exposure of the root surface caused by an apical shift in the position of the epithelial attachment
   a. Severity of the recession is determined by the amount of apical migration
   b. Recession may be clinically visible if the gingival margin has also receded or may be hidden by marginal gingiva and only apparent by probing for the level of the epithelial attachment
   c. Recession may be partially clinically visible and partially hidden (covered by inflamed pocket wall); total amount of recession is the sum of the clinical and hidden recession (NOTE: ''Recession'' documented on periodontal charts is that which is clinically visible only)
   d. *Recession* refers only to the location of the gingiva, not the condition of the gingiva; may have recession of gingiva that is inflamed or noninflamed
   e. Etiology—the following factors have been implicated as possible etiologic factors
      (1) Gingival inflammation
      (2) Faulty toothbrushing (gingival abrasion)
      (3) Tooth position
          (a) In the arch
          (b) Mesiodistal curvature of the tooth
      (4) Location and amount of pull on the margin of the frenum attachment
      (5) Dehiscence
   f. Clinical significance
      (1) Exposed roots are susceptible to caries and abrasion
      (2) Wearing away of cementum on the exposed surface leaves exposed dentin, which may be sensitive to mechanical, chemical, or thermal stimuli
      (3) Interproximal recession creates space for accumulation of plaque and other debris
   g. Treatment
      (1) Removal of etiologic or contributing factors
      (2) Maintenance of daily thorough plaque control
      (3) Root desensitization if needed
      (4) Gingival graft may be performed to prevent further recession and loss of attached gingiva

TREATMENT

Initial Treatment Plan

A. Collection of data to assess the status of the periodontium (see section on clinical assessment of the periodontium)
B. Formulation of initial treatment plan based on data collected and assessment
   1. Determination of all etiologic and contributing factors
   2. Removal or control of factors in an organized, logical sequence to include
      a. Plaque removal and control
      b. Pocket reduction or elimination
      c. When possible, removal of contributing factors
   3. Order of treatment will depend on
      a. Severity of the patient's periodontal condition
      b. General health status of the patient
      c. Patient's motivation and cooperation
      d. Prognosis
C. Contributing factors influencing the prognosis
   1. Local factors
      a. Degree of periodontal destruction (amount of attachment lost)
      b. Rate of periodontal destruction (amount of attachment lost per unit of time)
      c. Presence of contributing local factors (e.g., malocclusion, parafunctional habits, position of teeth in alveoli, malalignment, root proximity, missing teeth)
      d. Quality of restorations present
   2. Systemic factors—patient's general health (presence or absence of systemic diseases)
   3. Personal considerations
      a. Patient's home care habits, motivation, and willingness to assume responsibility for oral hygiene
      b. Patient's ability to finance specific types of periodontal treatment and restorative/prosthetic needs

Scaling and Root Planing

A. Goal of the ''initial'' or ''phase I'' stage of periodontal treatment is to reduce or eliminate gingival inflammation by removing bacterial plaque, hard deposits, and other contributing factors that aid in retention of bacterial plaque; clinical procedures known as scaling and root planing are performed as one component of the initial therapy to try to attain the goal of reducing or eliminating gingival inflammation

B. Scaling—clinical procedure whereby calculus (which contains bacterial plaque) is removed with no deliberate attempt to remove any tooth substance (see Chapter 13, section on scaling—steps for calculus removal)
   1. Supragingival or supramarginal scaling—use of scaling instruments coronal to the gingival margin to remove supragingival deposits
   2. Subgingival or submarginal scaling—use of scaling instruments within the gingival sulcus or pocket to remove subgingival deposits (NOTE: Some soft tissue curettage (removal) of the sulcular lining may occur inadvertently during subgingival scaling; however, this incidental tissue removal is not to be confused with gingival curettage)

C. Root planing—clinical procedure whereby instrumentation occurs on the exposed root surface or within the periodontal pocket (see Chapter 13, section on root planing)
   1. During this process cementum (with endotoxins) and calculus that have permeated the root surface are removed
   2. To accomplish this, root cementum and possibly some dentin are removed during the root-planing procedure

D. Rationale for scaling and root planing
   1. Assists in removal of etiologic (plaque) and contributing factors (calculus, stain, endotoxins) of periodontal disease
   2. Permits gingival tissues to return to a healthier status
   3. Permits the clinician to later reevaluate the tissues to determine the need for additional periodontal treatment
   4. Assists the patient in performing required oral home care procedures

E. Clinical objectives
   1. Calculus-free tooth surface
   2. Smooth, firm root surface free of embedded calculus and endotoxins (NOTE: Need for root planing should be determined by the clinical status of the gingival tissues [e.g., if the root surface feels "rough" but the surrounding tissues show no clinical signs of inflammation, root planing is *not* indicated])

F. Evaluation
   1. Immediate evaluation is accomplished through visual and tactile inspection of tooth surfaces
   2. Healing of tissues for 10 to 14 days should be permitted; gingival tissues are then reevaluated for response to treatment

3. Reevaluation should include
   a. Evaluation of the patient's home care
   b. Updated periodontal chart to assess soft tissue changes
   c. Reassessment of the clinical health of tissues; if areas still show signs of inflammation, the cause should be determined
      (1) Dental plaque present—review or supplement home care
      (2) Deposits of calculus still present—rescale
      (3) No plaque or calculus noted—check the root surface to determine whether root planing is needed; root plane as indicated
      (4) Pocket depth still moderate to severe—surgical procedures might be warranted
      (5) Inflammation still severe and etiology and contributing factors cannot be identified—consider physical examination by a physician for a possible systemic factor

G. Limitations
   1. Ability to thoroughly remove all calculus and to root plane root surfaces as needed is limited by
      a. Pocket depth
      b. Location of deposit on the root surface in terms of access for thorough instrumentation (e.g., furcation); areas that are inaccessible may require periodontal flap surgery to gain adequate access to the root surface
   2. Long-term success of scaling and root planing therapy is dependent on
      a. Patient's diligence in plaque removal
      b. Accessibility of pocket areas to the patient's home care procedures; additional therapy may be needed in order to permit the patient to attain daily access to all areas requiring plaque removal

Gingival Curettage

A. Definition—procedure to remove the ulcerated, chronically inflamed tissue lining a pocket
B. Objectives
   1. Eliminate gingival inflammation
   2. Eradicate pockets through shrinkage and gingival reattachment
   3. Increase fibrotic tissue and increase healing
   4. Replace diseased pocket lining with new connective tissue and sulcular epithelium

5. Provide alternative in cases where extensive surgery is contraindicated (e.g., systemic impairment, financial limits, emotional resistance)
C. Contraindications
   1. Chronic, fibrotic marginal gingiva
   2. Infrabony pockets where the crestal bone prevents shrinkage to the base of the pocket
D. Procedure may be performed ''closed'' or ''open'' (tissue curetted after laying of a periodontal flap) (see Chapter 13, section on closed gingival curettage)

Additional Clinical Interventions

A. Treatment of occlusal problems
   1. Once diagnosed, occlusal trauma may be treated by
      a. Occlusal adjustment—selective grinding of teeth to equalize the distibution of occlusal forces
      b. Construction of occlusal appliances (e.g., night guard, removable orthodontic appliance) to minimize the effect of destructive forces and/or for minor tooth movement to improve tooth alignment
      c. Splinting of teeth for temporary or permanent stabilization
      d. Restorative dentistry to improve the occlusal plane and replace missing teeth
   2. Limitation of treatment—since occlusal trauma is not the primary etiologic factor of periodontal disease, treatment of occlusal trauma will only result in removal of a contributing factor and will not cure periodontal disease
B. Surgical procedures
   1. Rationale
      a. Render the periodontium more cleanable by the patient
         (1) Improvement in hard and soft tissue contours
         (2) Pocket elimination
      b. Replace damaged or destroyed periodontium
         (1) Soft tissue replacement (gingival grafts)
         (2) Hard tissue replacement (osseous grafts)
      c. Surgery is rarely performed to remove inflammation or infection, but rather to
         (1) Eliminate both hard and soft defects created by disease
         (2) Try to restore normal architecture
         (3) Try to gain new attachment of the supporting structures

2. Types
   a. Gingival curettage—procedure to remove the ulcerated, chronically inflamed tissue lining a pocket (see section on gingival curettage)
   b. Gingivectomy—surgical procedure for pocket reduction by complete removal of the soft tissue pocket wall
      (1) Indications
         (a) Gingival pockets composed of enlarged fibrotic tissue
         (b) Suprabony periodontal pockets with adequate zones of keratinized gingiva
      (2) Contraindications
         (a) Reduction of infrabony pockets
         (b) Reduction of pockets that extend to or into the alveolar mucosa
   c. Periodontal flaps—may be used as a method of open curettage or for pocket elimination by apically repositioning the soft tissue
      (1) Advantages (depends on the type of flap)
         (a) Better access to achieve thorough scaling and root planing
         (b) Thorough removal of the pocket lining (as compared with closed curettage)
         (c) Elimination of pockets
         (d) Means to obtain access to the alveolar bone to correct osseous defects
      (2) Indications
         (a) Deep periodontal pockets
         (b) Furcation involvements
         (c) Fibrotic tissue
         (d) Base of the pocket at or beyond the mucogingival junction
      (3) Contraindications—if situation correctable by a more conservative approach (scaling, root planing, and daily, thorough home care)
   d. Mucogingival surgery
      (1) Objectives
         (a) Prevent additional loss of keratinized gingiva and/or recession
         (b) Regain additional keratinized gingiva
      (2) Indications
         (a) Base of the pocket extending apically to the mucogingival junction

(b) Inadequate zone of keratinized
gingiva
(c) Frenum pull on the gingiva, causing
gingival recession
(d) Localized gingival recession
associated with inflammation
(3) Treatment options
(a) Apically positioned flap
(b) Soft tissue graft
(c) Partial or full frenectomy
e. Osseous surgery
(1) Objective—attempt to regenerate lost
periodontal supporting structures
(2) Indication—infrabony pocket
(3) Common grafting materials used—bone
marrow, osseous coagulum, freeze-dried
bone, alloplast, sclera

Sutures

A. Objectives
1. Used to hold soft tissues in place until the
healing process has progressed to the point
where tissue placement can be self-maintained
2. Stabilizing the soft tissue helps
a. Maintain the blood clot around the wound
b. Protect the wound area during the healing
process
B. Desired properties of a suture material
1. Easy to handle
2. Nonallergenic and does not create an
environment conducive to bacterial growth
3. Does not shrink after placement
4. Know holds securely and does not fray
5. Does not easily cut or tear through thin,
delicate tissue
6. If absorbable, does so with minimal tissue
reaction
C. Types of suture materials
1. Absorbable—gut (from intestines of sheep)
a. Difficult to manipulate
b. Does not hold knot well
c. Tends to harden and cause trauma around
the surrounding mucosa
d. Mild inflammatory reaction occurs during
the absorption process
2. Nonabsorbable
a. Surgical silk (twisted or braided)
(1) Most widely used material in
periodontal surgery
(2) Is a foreign protein and thus is treated
by tissues as a foreign body
(inflammatory reactions are usually
limited if sutures are removed within 7
days)

(3) Braided material tends to trap bacteria
within the material
(4) Relatively comfortable and easy to use
b. Surgical cotton and linen—weak material;
not used in periodontics
c. Synthetic fibers (polyester, nylon,
polypropylene)—strong and well tolerated
by tissue, but difficult to knot
D. Procedure for suture removal
1. Gently grasp the knotted end with
cotton/college pliers and pull it away from the
tissue
2. Insert the tip of scissors under the suture and
cut the suture material that had been in the
tissue
3. Gently pull the knotted end so that only suture
material that had previously been incorporated
within the tissue will pass through the tissue
during the removal process
4. Count and record the number of sutures
removed and compare this number with the
suture placement record
5. Gently cleanse the wound sites (may use an
oxygenating agent, warm water, and cotton
swabs)
6. Check for bleeding points and control with
gauze and pressure
7. Check for and gently remove any calculus or
granulation tissue

Periodontal Dressings

A. Rationale for use of a periodontal dressing to
promote wound healing is controversial, since it
has been demonstrated that wound healing
progresses at the same rate with or without a
dressing; however, periodontal dressings are used
for the following reasons
1. Patient comfort, especially if the surgical
procedure has left exposed connective tissue or
exposed root surfaces
2. Protection of the wound against trauma (e.g.,
from sharp, hard food or toothbrush bristles)
and prevention of the tongue from constantly
rubbing the area
3. Maintenance of the initial blood clot—dressing
may be helpful in preventing the initial blood
clot from being dislodged; dressing should be
applied only after bleeding has been controlled
4. Tissue placement—maintains the desired
location of the soft tissue flap position (if
performed)

B. Desired properties of a dressing material
   1. Soft and flexible to allow for proper adaptation
   2. Reasonable setting time
   3. After setting, should be rigid but not brittle
   4. Smooth dressing surface
C. Types
   1. Zinc oxide–eugenol dressing—eugenol is added, since it has a soothing (obtundent) effect on exposed root surfaces and connective tissue and has antiseptic properties; eugenol may have an irritating effect on bone; firm consistency of this dressing requires some pressure during placement
   2. Zinc oxide–noneugenol dressing—softer dressing than eugenol type; also more pleasant tasting
   NOTE: Research is controversial regarding healing properties of eugenol versus noneugenol dressings
D. Ingredients
   1. Eugenol type
      a. Powder
         (1) Zinc oxide—slightly astringent and/or antiseptic
         (2) Rosin—filler for strength (NOTE: Asbestos no longer used)
         (3) Tannic acid—hemostasis (need for this is questionable)
      b. Liquid
         (1) Eugenol—slightly anesthetic
         (2) Peanut oil—regulates the setting time
   2. Noneugenol type
      a. Paste 1
         (1) Zinc oxide—slightly astringent and/or antiseptic
         (2) Magnesium oxide and oils—regulate the setting time
      b. Paste 2
         (1) Rosin—strength
         (2) Chlorothymol—bacteriostatic
E. Procedure for dressing placement
   1. Explain the process to the patient
   2. Make sure bleeding has ceased
   3. Mix the dressing according to the directions
   4. Gently place the dressing, trying to establish retention in the embrasure spaces
   5. Make sure the dressing does not cover more than the cervical one third of the tooth, does not overextend into the mucobuccal fold, and does not interfere with muscle attachments or with the patient's occlusion
   6. Make sure the surface of the dressing is smooth and well contoured

7. Check the dressing to make sure it has not been forced between the soft tissue flap and the underlying tissue or root surface
   8. May place dry foil over the dressing until it has hardened (few hours); foil is then removed (not necessary to use foil)
   9. Give postsurgical instructions to the patient (see section on patient instructions and education
F. Removal of the periodontal dressing
   1. Remove the dressing within 7 days
   2. Gently tease the edges of the dressing away from the teeth with a curette or cotton/college pliers; be sure that sutures are not embedded in the dressing
   3. After the pack has been removed, gently cleanse the area (use *warm* water or dampened cotton tips)
   4. Check tissue healing (*do not probe sulcular areas*)
   5. Remove sutures
   6. Gently cleanse the area again (may use an oxygenating agent)
   7. Evaluate wound healing and determine if the area needs to have a new periodontal dressing

POSTOPERATIVE CARE
Patient Instructions and Education

A. Discomfort
   1. Expect discomfort after the anesthesia wears off
   2. Use the prescribed pain medication
   3. Rest and limit physical activities during the first few days to prevent excessive bleeding and promote healing
   4. Use an ice pack to prevent swelling
   5. Eliminate spicy, hot, cold, or hard, sticky foods/liquids and smoking to limit tissue irritants and protect the dressing
B. Care of the periodontal dressing
   1. Do not eat anything for the first few hours until the dressing hardens; may drink cool liquids
   2. During the week, pieces of the dressing may chip off; call the office if the area is extremely sensitive, the entire dressing is loose, or the chipped area is irritating the tongue or mucosa
C. Oral hygiene procedures
   1. Do not rinse the mouth on the first day, since it may disturb the blood clot
   2. After the first day, may rinse gently with lukewarm water and a small amount of mouthwash
   3. Brush and floss nonsurgical areas as usual
   4. Gently brush occlusal surfaces of the surgical area

5. Use a soft brush and water very gently to clean the surface of the dressing
6. Brush the tongue

D. Bleeding
1. Slight seepage of blood during the first few hours is normal
2. Any unusual, persistent bleeding should be reported

Follow-up Visit

A. Patient returns approximately 7 days after surgery
B. Dressing and sutures are removed; new dressing may or may not be applied
C. Tooth sensitivity may be experienced; fluoride rinses or gels may be prescribed
D. Home care procedures are provided for plaque control

MAINTENANCE OF THE PERIODONTAL PATIENT

A. Establish intervals of oral health maintenance (recall) appointments
B. Intervals of oral health maintenance appointments are based on
1. Status of periodontal health following therapy
2. Ability and compliance of the patient in removal of dental plaque
3. Rate of plaque and calculus formation; bacterial monitoring may be used
4. Presence of periodontal risk factors (e.g., furcation involvement, iatrogenic dentistry that cannot be replaced, malaligned teeth)
5. Tendency for development of gingivitis and destruction of tissue; host tissue resistance and pathogenicity of the host's bacterial dental plaque

SUGGESTED READINGS

American Academy of Periodontology: Guidelines for periodontal therapy, Chicago, 1983, The Academy.

Carranza, F.A.: Glickman's clinical periodontology, ed. 6, Philadelphia, 1984, W.B. Saunders Co.

Finley, C.W., et al.: Periodontal therapy: a summary status report, Chicago, 1983, American Academy of Periodontology.

Goldman, H.M., and Cohen, D.W.: Periodontal therapy, ed. 6, St. Louis, 1980, The C.V. Mosby Co.

Grant, D.A., Stern, I.B., and Everett, F.G.: Periodontics in the tradition of Orban and Gottlieb, ed. 5, St. Louis, 1979, The C.V. Mosby Co.

Lindhe, J.: Textbook of clinical periodontology, ed. 1, Copenhagen, 1983, Munksgaard.

Pawlak, G.A., and Hoag, P.M.: Essentials of periodontics, ed. 3, St. Louis, 1984, The C.V. Mosby Co.

Woodall, I.R., et al.: Comprehensive dental hygiene care, ed. 2, St. Louis, 1985, The C.V. Mosby Co.

Review Questions

1 The term *lamina dura* refers to the radiographic image of the
1. Periodontal ligament space
2. Alveolar bone proper
3. Cortical plates
4. Cancellous bone
5. Alveolar crest

2 On clinical examination, you recorded the following data on the facial surface of the tooth No 24:
Probings: Distal = 3 mm
Facial = 3 mm
Mesial = 4 mm
Width of masticatory mucosa: 6 mm
What is the width of the attached gingiva?
1. 3 mm
2. 2 mm
3. 4 mm
4. 1 mm
5. 6 mm

3 A pseudopocket (or gingival pocket) is formed by the
1. Coronal migration of the gingival margin
2. Coronal migration of the epithelial attachment
3. Apical migration of the gingival margin
4. Apical migration of the epithelial attachment
5. Apically directed resorption of the alveolar crest

4 Periodontal pockets can *best* be detected by
(a) Radiographic detection
(b) The color of the gingival tissues
(c) The contour of the gingival margin
(d) Probing the sulcular area
(e) Noting the presence or absence of bleeding on probing
1. a and d
2. b, c, and e
3. b, d, and e
4. d only
5. d and e

5 Gingival recession tends to occur in
(a) Areas where the roots are prominent
(b) Areas where the gingival tissues are thin
(c) The presence of frenum attachments that impinge on the gingival margins
(d) Areas exposed to vigorous toothbrushing methods
1. a, b, c, and d
2. c and d
3. a and b
4. b and c
5. d only

6 Periodontitis may *best* be described as
1. A chronic inflammatory disease with periods of remission and exacerbation
2. A chronic inflammatory disease that usually does not manifest itself clinically before the age of 40
3. A degenerative disease of the periodontium
4. An acute inflammatory disease of long duration
5. A chronic inflammatory disease that most often affects the entire dentition equally

7 In cases of periodontitis, the first area to be involved in bone resorption is the
1. Facial and lingual aspects of supporting bone
2. Cribriform plate
3. Cancellous bone
4. Cortical plate of the interdental septum
5. Bone surrounding the apical area of the tooth

8 Which of the following is *least* helpful in detecting subgingival calculus on the lingual aspects of the mandibular right first and second molars?
1. Air
2. Explorer
3. Radiographs
4. Appearance of adjacent soft tissues
5. Curette

9 Sharpey's fibers are
1. Collagen fibers
2. Elastic fibers
3. Gingival fibers
4. Oxytalan fibers
5. Transseptal fibers

10 *Tissue consistency* refers to
1. Thickness
2. Resiliency
3. Texture
4. The location of the margin
5. The presence or absence of stippling

11 All of the following are diagnostic of occlusal trauma *except*
1. Wear facets
2. Loss of alveolar bone
3. Increase in tooth mobility
4. Periodontal pocket formation
5. Increased width of the periodontal ligament space

12 Radiographs will show the
1. Relationships between soft and hard tissue
2. Degree of tooth mobility
3. Extent of all bone loss
4. Presence of calculus
5. None of the above

13 The radiographic findings of gingivitis will demonstrate a (an)
1. Vertical bone loss
2. Horizontal bone loss
3. Increase in bone density
4. Change in bone trabeculation
5. Normal bone pattern

14 The *primary* objective of closed gingival curettage is a (an)
(a) Reduction of edema of the gingival tissues
(b) Decrease in pocket depth
(c) Increase in length of the connective tissue attachment to the root surface
(d) Removal of necrotic cementum
1. a only
2. a and b
3. b and c
4. a, c, and d
5. b, c, and d

15 All of the following are contraindications for gingival curettage *except*
1. Extensive furcation involvement
2. A fibrous, thick gingival wall of the pocket
3. An extremely thin tissue wall of the pocket
4. Suprabony pockets with edema, pus, and granulomatous tissue
5. Deep periodontal pockets with very little change in gingival tissue color and almost no bleeding on probing

16 Root planing is performed to remove
1. The outer layer of cementum, which may contain endotoxins
2. The outer layer of cementum, which may contain exotoxins
3. The epithelial attachment
4. Granulation tissue
5. Calculus deposits

17 The mucogingival junction is located between the
1. Free gingiva and attached gingiva
2. Free gingiva and tooth
3. Attached gingiva and alveolar mucosa
4. Base of the sulcus and alveolar mucosa
5. Gingival groove and gingival margin

18 Which tissue(s) has (have) little or no keratinization?
(a) Attached gingiva
(b) Sulcular epithelium
(c) Alveolar mucosa
(d) Interdental papilla
1. b only
2. a and c
3. c only
4. a, b, and d
5. b and c

19 The first bacteria to deposit on the tooth in dental plaque formation are
1. Gram-negative rods
2. Gram-positive rods
3. Spirochetes
4. Gram-positive cocci
5. Gram-negative cocci

20 The fibers of the attached gingiva are mainly
1. Collagen
2. Elastic
3. Cellulose
4. Keratinized
5. Oxytalan

21 Systemic factors are important in the pathogenesis of periodontal disease because
1. They can be the direct cause of periodontal disease
2. They have a direct effect on pocket depth
3. If they are corrected, the periodontal disease can be eliminated
4. They usually determine the pattern of bone loss
5. They can intensify the response of the periodontium to the etiologic and local factors

22 The tissue lining of a healthy gingival sulcus consists of
1. Keratinized epithelium with rete pegs
2. Keratinized epithelium without rete pegs
3. Nonkeratinized epithelium with rete pegs
4. Nonkeratinized epithelium without rete pegs
5. Parakeratinized epithelium with rete pegs

23 The gingival fibers
1. Brace the marginal gingiva against the tooth
2. Help the tooth withstand horizontal forces
3. Keep the tooth from being forced into the bony socket
4. Form and resorb cementum
5. Transmit sensations of occlusal forces applied to the tooth

24 Which of the following is the first *clinical* feature of inflammatory periodontal disease?
1. Tooth mobility
2. Drifting of the anterior teeth
3. Periodontal pocket formation
4. Gingival recession
5. Change in gingival tissue consistency

25 A cuplike resorptive area at the crest of the alveolar bone is a radiographic finding of
1. Periodontal abscess
2. Gingivitis
3. Occlusal trauma
4. Acute necrotizing ulcerative gingivitis
5. Incipient periodontitis

26 The area within the periodontium *most* susceptible to tissue breakdown is the
1. Free gingiva
2. Gingival sulcus
3. Interdental col
4. Interdental papilla
5. Attached gingiva

27 The characteristics of gingivitis are
(a) Bone loss
(b) Swelling of the soft tissue
(c) Apical migration of the epithelial attachment
(d) Widening of the periodontal ligament space
(e) Bleeding on probing
1. a, b, and c
2. b, c, and e
3. a, c, d, and e
4. b and e
5. a, b, c, d, and e

28 Which is *not* a contributing factor of periodontal disease?
1. Open proximal contacts
2. Diet high in sucrose content
3. Mouth breathing
4. Blood dyscrasias
5. Hormonal imbalance

29 On completion of a patient's gingival assessment, you have noted that the gingivae are normal in appearance except on the facial area of teeth Nos. 28 and 29. In this area you noted inflammation on the gingival margin. All sulcular readings are between 1 and 3 mm, and the bases of the sulci are at the cementoenamel junctions. The most accurate description would be

1. Generalized marginal periodontitis
2. Localized marginal periodontitis
3. Generalized papillary gingivitis
4. Localized marginal gingivitis
5. Localized papillary gingivitis

30 During a periodontal examination a 6 mm pocket is detected on the direct facial surface of tooth No. 19. The gingival margin is located at the cementoenamel junction. What type of pocket is this?
1. Pseudopocket
2. Periodontal pocket
3. Gingival pocket
4. Combination pseudopocket and periodontal pocket
5. Combination gingival and periodontal pocket

31 Which situation would be an indication for a gingivectomy?
1. An edematous, 5 mm pseudopocket
2. A fibrotic area of free gingiva that covers part of the occlusal surface of tooth No. 32
3. An infrabony pocket of 6 mm on the distal aspect of tooth No. 30
4. A fibrotic periodontal pocket that extends into the alveolar mucosa
5. A localized area of acute necrotizing ulcerative gingivitis

32 The *specific* objective(s) of periodontal pocket elimination is (are) to
(a) Improve the esthetics of the patient
(b) Improve tissue contour
(c) Remove diseased tissue
(d) Assist the patient in daily plaque control
1. a and b
2. a, b, and c
3. c only
4. c and d
5. a, b, c, and d

33 A pyogenic granuloma
1. Is also referred to as a pregnancy tumor
2. Tends to occur frequently in cases of phenytoin hyperplasia
3. Is usually associated with gingival recession
4. Is frequently associated with juvenile periodontitis
5. Is usually treated with antibiotics

34 A gingivectomy is *primarily* employed to treat conditions in which
1. An infrabony pocket is present
2. The base of the pocket is apical to the mucogingival junction
3. There is an adequate zone of attached gingiva
4. The tissues are edematous
5. There is a gingival recession

35 A mucogingival problem exists when
1. The base of the pocket extends apically to the mucogingival junction
2. The base of the pocket is coronal to the mucogingival junction
3. There is less than 3 mm of attached gingiva
4. There is less than 5 mm of alveolar mucosa
5. There is significant bone loss

36 The purpose of placing sutures after periodontal flap surgery is to
   (a) Hold the soft tissues in place
   (b) Protect the wound
   (c) Maintain the blood clot
   (d) Prevent food impaction into the wound area
   1. a only
   2. a and b
   3. b and c
   4. a and c
   5. a, b, c, and d

37 The advantage of gut sutures is
   1. Their ease of manipulation
   2. They hold the knot well
   3. They do not cause an inflammatory reaction
   4. They dissolve
   5. They do not cause any trauma to the surrounding tissues

38 An advantage of silk braided sutures is that they
   1. Are dissolved by the surrounding tissues
   2. Have antibacterial properties
   3. Are relatively easy to manipulate
   4. Are not treated by the surrounding tissues as a foreign body
   5. Can remain in the tissues for up to 3 weeks without creating an inflammatory reaction

39 The reason(s) for using a periodontal dressing is (are) to
   (a) Minimize the patient's discomfort
   (b) Protect the wound from possible food impaction
   (c) Minimize the chance of hemorrhage
   (d) Help protect the teeth against root sensitivity
   (e) Help maintain tissue placement
   1. a, b, and c
   2. b, c, and d
   3. d and e
   4. b, c, and e
   5. a, b, c, d, and e

40 The purpose of using rosin in the periodontal dressing is to
   1. Provide an antibacterial property
   2. Provide a slight anesthetic action
   3. Serve as an astringent
   4. Improve the taste
   5. Act as a filler for strength

41 Following the completion of periodontal therapy, the patient should be placed on a recall interval of
   1. Every 12 months
   2. Every 6 months
   3. Every 4 months
   4. Every 2 months
   5. No standard time interval

Answers and Rationales

1. (2) Alveolar bone proper (or the cribriform plate) is referred to as lamina dura on a radiograph and is seen as a thin radiopaque line outlining the tooth socket.
   (1) The periodontal ligament space is a radiolucent space seen between the root and lamina dura.
   (3) Cortical plates are not identifiable on a full-mouth series of radiographs.
   (4) Cancellous bone is seen as a lacelike radiopaque image.
   (5) The alveolar crest is the interproximal extension of the alveolar bone proper (or lamina dura).

2. (1) The width of attached gingiva is calculated by subtracting the facial probing depth (3 mm) from the width of the masticatory mucosa.
   (2) The width of the attached gingiva is 3 mm, not 2 mm.
   (3) The width of the attached gingiva is 3 mm, not 4 mm.
   (4) The width of the attached gingiva is 3 mm, not 1 mm.
   (5) The width of the attached gingiva is 3 mm, not 6 mm.

3. (1) The enlargement of the gingival margin coronally (as an inflammatory reaction) is the process that creates a deeper gingival sulcus.
   (2) Coronal migration of the epithelial attachment would constitute a "new" attachment.
   (3) Apical migration of the gingival margin constitutes recession.
   (4) Apical migration of the epithelial attachment is the formation of a true pocket.
   (5) A pseudopocket does not involve any changes in the bone; the alveolar crest is located at its normal level, whereas it is the gingiva that enlarges to create the pocket depth.

4. (4) Measuring the sulcular areas (by probing) is the most accurate method of assessing the presence or absence of a pocket.
   (1) A radiograph does not illustrate the level of the soft tissues.
   (2) The color of the gingiva may be misleading in that it may appear "normal" even if a periodontal pocket is present, and the contour of the gingiva can be normal even if a periodontal pocket is present.
   (3) Bleeding on probing may not be readily detected in a chronic, fibrotic situation.
   (5) Bleeding on probing may not be readily detected in a chronic fibrotic situation.

For each question the correct answer and rationale are listed first. The other choices are presented in order with the reasons why they are not correct.

5. (1) Gingival recession tends to occur in all the areas listed.
   (2) Gingival recession also occurs in areas where roots are prominent and where gingival tissues are thin.
   (3) Gingival recession also occurs in the presence of frenum attachments and in areas exposed to vigorous toothbrushing.
   (4) Gingival recession also occurs where roots are prominent and in areas exposed to vigorous toothbrushing.
   (5) Gingival recession occurs in other areas besides those exposed to vigorous toothbrushing.

6. (1) Periodontitis is usually a long-standing disease that may have episodes of acute inflammatory signs and symptoms.
   (2) Periodontitis can start in adolescents and even in children.
   (3) Periodontitis is an inflammatory and not a degenerative disease.
   (4) The signs and symptoms of periodontitis are not consistent with those of acute inflammation.
   (5) Periodontitis is "site specific" (i.e., each area of the mouth is affected at a different rate).

7. (4) Following the pathway of inflammation through the periodontal structures, the cortical plate is the first bony area to be affected by periodontitis.
   (1) The facial and lingual aspects of supporting bone are not the first areas to be involved in bone resorption caused by periodontitis.
   (2) The cribriform plate is not the first bony area to be affected by periodontitis.
   (3) Cancellous bone is not the first bony area to be affected by periodontitis.
   (5) The bone surrounding the apical area of the tooth is not the first area to be affected by periodontitis.

8. (3) Calculus on the direct facial or lingual surfaces is not observable on a periapical or bitewing radiograph.
   (1) The use of air to detect the gingival margin could assist in identifying subgingival calculus.
   (2) An explorer assists in the tactile detection of calculus.
   (4) A localized, deep red or bluish inflamed appearance of soft tissue is often an indication of subgingival calculus.
   (5) A curette assists in the tactile detection of calculus.

9. (1) Sharpey's fibers are composed of collagen fibers.
   (2) Elastic fibers are not part of Sharpey's fibers.
   (3) Gingival fibers are found coronal to the periodontal ligament and are not part of Sharpey's fibers.
   (4) Oxytalan fibers are immature elastic fibers.
   (5) Transseptal fibers are part of the gingival fiber system.

10. (2) *Consistency* or *resiliency* refers to the response of the tissue to pressure; this response may change as a result of the presence or absence of edema or destruction of the underlying collagen fibers.
    (1) *Tissue consistency* does not refer to thickness of the tissue.
    (3) *Texture* refers to the visual characteristics of the outer surface of the tissue.
    (4) The location of the margin helps describe the overall architecture of this gingiva.
    (5) *Stippling* refers to the visual characteristics of the outer surface of the tissue.

11. (4) Periodontal pockets are soft tissue lesions that are not affected by occlusal trauma.
    (1) Wear facets are a symptom of occlusal trauma.
    (2) Loss of alveolar bone is a symptom of occlusal trauma.
    (3) Increase in tooth mobility is a symptom of occlusal trauma.
    (5) Increased width of the periodontal ligament space is a symptom of occlusal trauma.

12. (5) None of the answers is correct.
    (1) Soft tissue cannot be seen on a radiograph.
    (2) The presence or absence of mobility can be detected only clinically.
    (3) Bone level or loss cannot be accurately determined radiographically, since a radiograph cannot present a three-dimensional image.
    (4) Only large, dense pieces of calculus on proximal surfaces can be detected radiographically and then only if the angulation is correct (i.e., no overlap of proximal surfaces of teeth).

13. (5) The changes within the periodontium in cases of gingivitis are confined to the soft tissue.
    (1) Gingivitis does not affect alveolar bone, including vertical bone loss.
    (2) Gingivitis does not affect horizontal bone loss.
    (3) Gingivitis does not increase bone density.
    (4) Gingivitis does not change bone trabeculation.

14. (2) Curettage of the sulcular lining reduces the edema present, thereby decreasing the pocket depth.
    (1) Curettage decreases the pocket depth as a result of reducing edema.
    (3) Closed gingival curettage does not increase the amount of connective tissue attached to the root surface.
    (4) *Gingival curettage* refers to instrumentation applied only to the sulcular lining, not to the tooth surface; also, it does not refer to removing necrotic cementum.
    (5) See 4.

15. (4) Suprabony pockets with edema, pus, and granulomatous tissue are clinical conditions that respond favorably to curettage.
   (1) Closed curettage will not provide access to clean the furcation areas.
   (2) Fibrous conditions will not respond to curettage.
   (3) Curettage in extremely thin walls will result in the perforation of the soft tissue.
   (5) Closed curettage will not provide access to deep periodontal pockets.

16. (1) The embedded endotoxins prevent tissue healing and must be removed by root planing.
   (2) Exotoxins do not play a role in the pathogenesis of periodontal disease.
   (3) Epithelium removal is part of curettage.
   (4) Granulation tissue removal is part of curettage.
   (5) The procedure to remove calculus deposits is known as scaling.

17. (3) The attached gingiva and alveolar mucosa meet at the mucogingival junction.
   (1) The gingival groove demarcates the free gingiva and the attached gingiva.
   (2) The gingival margin demarcates the free gingiva and the tooth.
   (4) The space between the base of the sulcus and the alveolar mucosa is occupied by the epithelial attachment and the connective tissue.
   (5) The area between the gingival groove and the gingival margin is the free gingiva.

18. (5) The sulcular epithelium and alveolar mucosa are generally nonkeratinized.
   (1) The alveolar mucosa is also nonkeratinized.
   (2) The epithelial tissues of the attached gingiva are keratinized.
   (3) The sulcular epithelium is also nonkeratinized.
   (4) The epithelial tissues of the attached gingiva are keratinized; the interdental papilla is covered with keratinized epithelial tissues of the outer surface of the free gingiva.

19. (4) Gram-positive cocci are dominant in the initial formation of dental plaque.
   (1) Gram-negative rods are found in older dental plaque.
   (2) Gram-positive rods are found in older dental plaque.
   (3) Spirochetes are found in older dental plaque.
   (5) Gram-negative cocci are found in older dental plaque.

20. (1) The gingival fibers are composed of collagen.
   (2) Elastic fibers are predominantly found in the alveolar mucosa.
   (3) No such fibers exist in the gingival tissues.
   (4) This term is descriptive of a certain form of epithelial tissues, not connective tissue fibers.
   (5) Oxytalan fibers are an immature form of elastic fibers.

21. (5) Systemic factors are the so-called contributing factors to the pathogenesis of periodontal disease (i.e., they *cannot* initiate the disease process, but they can affect the severity of the tissue response).
   (1) Systemic factors cannot be the direct cause of periodontal disease.
   (2) Systemic factors do not have a direct effect on pocket depth.
   (3) Systemic factors alone cannot eliminate the periodontal disease.
   (4) Systemic factors do not determine the pattern of bone loss.

22. (4) The lining of a healthy gingival sulcus is composed of nonkeratinized epithelial tissues with no rete pegs present. The presence of rete pegs is indicative of the presence of inflammation.
   (1) Healthy gingival sulcus is lined with nonkeratinized epithelium without rete pegs.
   (2) Healthy gingival sulcus lining is composed of nonkeratinized epithelium.
   (3) Healthy gingival sulcus lining does not have rete pegs.
   (5) Healthy gingival sulcus lining is composed of nonkeratinized epithelium without rete pegs.

23. (1) The function of the gingival fibers is to support the margin of the gingiva up against the tooth.
   (2) The periodontal ligament is responsible for withstanding horizontal forces.
   (3) The periodontal ligament is responsible for preventing the tooth from being forced into the bony socket.
   (4) The periodontal ligament is responsible for the formation and resorption of cementum (by cementoblasts and cementoclasts).
   (5) The periodontal ligament is responsible for the transmission of sensations of occlusal forces.

24. (5) The initial inflammatory response occurs within the confines of the gingival tissues only, with one of the first changes being edematous gingiva.
   (1) Tooth mobility is indicative of the progression of the disease from gingivitis to periodontitis and is the result of loss of supporting structures of the periodontium.
   (2) Drifting of the anterior teeth indicates the progression of the disease and is a result of loss of supporting structures of the periodontium.
   (3) Periodontal pocket formation is indicative of the progression of the disease from gingivitis to periodontitis.
   (4) Gingival recession is indicative of the progression of the disease.

25. (5) The alveolar area that is initially altered by periodontal disease is the crest of the alveolar bone.
   (1) When a periodontal abscess does affect the alveolar bone, it usually results in a vertical bony defect.
   (2) Gingivitis does not affect the alveolar bone; it is confined to the gingival tissues.
   (3) Occlusal trauma is usually associated with a vertical pattern of bone loss.
   (4) Occlusal trauma in the absence of bacterial plaque will not cause soft tissue inflammation and therefore will not initiate periodontitis.

26. (3) The interdental col has the thinnest nonkeratinized epithelial layer. Furthermore, it is the most inaccessible area to plaque removal. Both situations cause this area to be the most susceptible to tissue breakdown and the area where gingival changes are first noticed.
    (1) The free gingiva is not the most susceptible to tissue breakdown.
    (2) The gingival sulcus is not the most susceptible to tissue breakdown.
    (4) The interdental papilla is not the most susceptible to tissue breakdown.
    (5) The attached gingiva is not the most susceptible to tissue breakdown.

27. (4) The changes associated with gingivitis are associated only with the soft tissue.
    (1) Bone loss and apical migration of the epithelial attachment are characteristics of periodontitis.
    (2) Apical migration of the epithelial attachment is a characteristic of periodontitis.
    (3) Gingivitis is inflammation that is confined to supracrestal soft tissue and does not therefore influence the width of the periodontal ligament; bone loss is a characteristic of periodontitis.
    (5) Gingivitis is associated only with soft tissue.

28. (2) The presence or absence of sucrose has no effect on the bacteria that are involved in the periodontal disease process.
    (1) Open contacts may result in food impaction and mechanical irritation of the tissues.
    (3) Mouth breathing causes desiccation of the anterior gingival tissues, which results in their irritation.
    (4) Some blood dyscrasias may result in altered cellular and/or hormonal immunity, thus rendering the person more susceptible to periodontal disease.
    (5) Hormonal imbalance may intensify the body's immunologic response to bacterial plaque.

29. (4) The inflammation is confined to a limited area of the mouth ("localized"), and the margin is inflamed ("marginal"), which includes papillary inflammation, since it is initiated in the papilla and spreads to the margins. Since the bases of all sulci are at their normal location, the disease is still confined only to the soft tissues ("gingivitis").
    (1) The disease is localized, and therefore not generalized, marginal periodontitis.
    (2) The disease is localized marginal gingivitis, not periodontitis.
    (3) The disease is localized and marginal, not generalized and papillary.
    (5) The disease is marginal gingivitis, not papillary gingivitis.

30. (2) Since the gingival margin is located at its normal level, the pocket depth is created by the "apical migration of the epithelial attachment" (which is the definition of a periodontal pocket).
    (1) A pseudopocket is created by the enlargement (coronally) of the gingival margin; the epithelial attachment is still located in its normal position.
    (3) A gingival pocket is a synonym for a pseudopocket.
    (4) The pocket is a periodontal pocket only.
    (5) The pocket is a periodontal pocket only.

31. (2) A gingivectomy is indicated in areas of fibrotic tissues that are forming pseudopockets, since this area needs total elimination of the excess tissue but does not need to have the level of the epithelial attachment repositioned.
    (1) This area would most likely respond to thorough scaling, root planing (if needed), and daily plaque removal. No surgical procedure is warranted.
    (3) A gingivectomy is contraindicated in the case of an infrabony pocket.
    (4) A gingivectomy is contraindicated in areas of little or no attached tissue or in cases where the base of the pocket extends into the alveolar mucosa.
    (5) Initially, no surgical procedure should be performed. Once the disease is no longer present, a gingivoplasty (recontouring of the gingival margin) may be needed.

32. (4) The rationale for pocket elimination is to reduce the pocket depth to one that can be adequately cleansed by the patient on a daily basis.
    (1) Periodontal disease may or may not have changed the patient's appearance; while tissue contours may be improved during periodontal surgery, this is not a *specific* objective of pocket elimination procedures.
    (2) See 1.
    (3) Periodontal pocket elimination may also assist the patient in daily plaque control.
    (5) See 1.

33. (1) A pyogenic granuloma is an exaggerated tissue response to local irritants and occurs frequently during hormonal changes such as those that take place during pregnancy. It is treated by thorough scaling, root planing (if needed), and plaque control. If the tissue is fibrotic, a gingivectomy is sometimes warranted.
    (2) A pyogenic granuloma is not related to phenytoin hyperplasia.
    (3) A pyogenic granuloma is not associated with gingival recession.
    (4) A pyogenic granuloma is not associated with juvenile periodontitis.
    (5) Pyogenic granulomas are treated by thorough scaling, root planing, and plaque control

34. (3) A gingivectomy results in a loss of attached gingiva. Therefore an adequate amount of attached gingiva must be present before the surgical procedure is done; otherwise the result will be an area with minimal or no attached gingiva.
    (1) A gingivectomy does not provide access to the osseous area, and therefore it is not useful in treating this type of periodontal pocket.
    (2) See 3.
    (4) A gingivectomy is most commonly used to treat areas of enlarged, fibrotic pseudopockets.
    (5) Since a gingivectomy results in loss of gingiva, this procedure will only exacerbate the preexisting condition.

35. (1) When this situation exists, all of the keratinized tissue is detached, thus creating a mucogingival problem (i.e., lack of any or an adequate amount of attached gingiva).
    (2) The base of the pocket is normally coronal to the mucogingival junction.
    (3) The minimal zone of attached gingiva is 1 to 2 mm; therefore a 3 mm zone is adequate.
    (4) The width of alveolar mucosa does not determine whether or not a mucogingival problem exists.
    (5) The amount of bone loss does not determine whether or not a mucogingival problem exists.

36. (5) The successful outcome of flap surgery is dependent to a great extent on the maintenance of the correct flap position after surgery, as well as on the wound-healing process. The placement of sutures helps in maintaining the correct flap position as well as allowing wound healing to progress with a minimal amount of trauma.
    (1) In addition to holding the soft tissues in place, sutures protect the wound, maintain the blood clot, and prevent food impaction.
    (2) Sutures also maintain the blood clot and prevent food impaction.
    (3) Sutures also hold the soft tissues in place and prevent food impaction.
    (4) Sutures also protect the wound and prevent food impaction.

37. (4) Gut sutures are dissolved by the inflammatory process that occurs in the surrounding tissues.
    (1) Gut sutures are rather difficult to manipulate, since they are stiff and break easily.
    (2) Gut sutures, being somewhat stiff, unravel easily.
    (3) An inflammatory reaction does occur around the gut sutures, and in fact it is this process that dissolves the gut sutures.
    (5) Any suture (being a foreign body) will cause trauma to the surrounding tissues.

38. (3) The silk material makes this type of suture extremely easy to manipulate through the tissues and to knot securely.
    (1) The silk cannot be dissolved.
    (2) The braided sutures readily trap bacteria and often cause bacterial contamination of the surrounding tissues.
    (4) Any type of suture is treated by the body as an antigen (foreign body).
    (5) Sutures should be removed within a week to 10 days. Leaving them in place for longer than this time will continue, and possibly exaggerate, the inflammatory response surrounding the sutures.

39. (5) While the routine use of a periodontal dressing following surgery has *not* been shown to enhance the healing *rate* of the tissues, the placement of a dressing does have all of the advantages listed.
    (1) In addition, a periodontal dressing helps protect the teeth against root sensitivity and helps maintain tissue placement.
    (2) In addition, a periodontal dressing minimizes patient discomfort and helps maintain tissue placement.
    (3) In addition, a periodontal dressing minimizes patient discomfort, protects the wound, and minimizes the chance of hemorrhage.
    (4) In addition, a periodontal dressing minimizes patient discomfort and helps protect the teeth against root sensitivity.

40. (5) The purpose of adding rosin to the dressing material is strictly to add strength to the dressing so that it can withstand the normal forces of eating and tongue movement.
    (1) A periodontal dressing does not provide an antibacterial property.
    (2) A periodontal dressing has no anesthetic action.
    (3) A periodontal dressing does not serve as an astringent.
    (4) A periodontal dressing does not improve the taste.

41. (5) The frequency of recall intervals must be established based on the individual needs of the patient: severity of the disease, microbial count, plaque control, general health of the patient, etc. There is no set standard of recall interval for all postoperative periodontal patients.
    (1) A 12-month recall interval might not be appropriate for some patients.
    (2) A 6-month recall interval might not be appropriate for some patients.
    (3) A 4-month recall interval might not be appropriate for some patients.
    (4) A 2-month recall interval might not be appropriate for some patients.

CHAPTER 12

Strategies and Techniques for Oral Health Maintenance and Disease Control

SUSAN SCHWARTZ MILLER

Promotion of oral health and prevention of dental disease have been the focus of dental hygiene practice since its inception. As the professional responsible for preventive services and education, the dental hygienist must have an understanding of the strategies and techniques that support and enable prevention-oriented practice. This chapter addresses the dental hygienist's role as a facilitator of behaviors directed toward health and as a clinician implementing the clinical modalities generally accepted as being effective for the prevention and control of dental disease. Topics include educational strategies, mechanical methods of plaque control (including toothbrushing and flossing), disease control for patients with fixed and/or removable appliances, oral irrigation, professionally administered fluoride treatments, sealant application, phase-contrast microscopy, oral cancer self-examination, desensitization procedures, pulpal vitality testing, and oral exfoliative cytology.

GENERAL CONSIDERATIONS

Historical Perspective

A. Dental disease has plagued humankind throughout history
B. Records of every ancient civilization contain descriptions of medications and implements used to prevent the loss of teeth, and evidence of tooth decay and periodontal disease has been found in fossilized human skulls of ancient populations
C. That oral hygiene was practiced in many ancient populations is evidenced in the earliest written records of civilization
D. The Hindus used frayed sticks to brush their teeth, the Chinese used a chew stick, and the Assyrians and Babylonians wrapped linen strips around their fingers to wipe tooth surfaces clean

Dental Hygiene Process of Care

A. Dental hygiene can be viewed as a method of care based on a process that involves the steps of assessment, planning, implementation, and evaluation
B. Inherent in the process model is a continuum of care that supports a logical system of deciding and expressing what care needs or problems exist within an individual

Components

A. Assessment—systematic collection of objective and subjective data that the dental hygienist then analyzes to determine the current or potential dental hygiene needs of the individual
   1. Data collection techniques should be appropriate to the nature of the information sought; data may be collected by interview, questionnaire, observation, measurement, and/or examination; information gathered is always documented and placed in a permanent record
   2. Dental hygiene data collection procedures may include any or all of the following
      a. Comprehensive health history
      b. General physical evaluation, including vital signs
      c. Extraoral evaluation
      d. Intraoral evaluation
      e. Examination of the teeth, including charting of carious lesions and restorations, occlusal evaluation, and deposit evaluation
      f. Examination of the periodontium, including sulcus and/or pocket measurement and mobility determination
      g. Bacterial evaluation using phase-contrast microscopy

    h. Exposure and reading of radiographs
    i. Health behavior evaluation, including the appropriateness and skill level of home care procedures and identification of psychosocial factors that might be influencing behaviors
    j. Intraoral photography
    k. Impressions for study models
    l. Oral exfoliative cytology
    m. Pulpal vitality testing
  3. Data analysis—once collected, the data must be coordinated and interpreted for significance; determination of the patient's status and identification of current and potential dental hygiene needs involve a decision-making process that procedes the design of a plan to meet the needs specified

B. Planning—act of determining what types of dental hygiene interventions can be implemented to facilitate meeting the patient's needs and solving the patient's problems; goals as well as the scope and sequence of care are based on an integration of assessment data; patient participation in this phase of the process of care increases the potential for active participation during the implementation phase

C. Implementation—initiation and completion of activities necessary to meet assessed needs; activities or strategies may be educational, motivational, or therapeutic

D. Evaluation—act of appraising the success of dental hygiene interventions (Were the goals established met? If not, why not? Was the initial assessment faulty? Were the initial goals possible and realistic? Did the patient receive the type of services necessary to meet specific needs?); it is in the evaluation phase that the dental hygienist determines the extent to which the plan for care and the interventions provided were effective

DISELASE CONTROL EDUCATION

Basic Concepts

A. Caries and the inflammatory periodontal diseases are complex disease states that require the colonization of bacteria; neither will occur in the absence of microbial plaque; thus control of plaque is an essential component of any program designed for the prevention of these dental diseases

B. Where once the focus in dentistry was on restorative procedures and surgical interventions, today the emphasis has shifted to preventing disease and maintaining oral health

C. Prevention of dental disease requires the participation of a patient with adequate knowledge of the disease process, sufficiently developed skills in implementing home care procedures, and the motivation to practice control procedures over time

D. Many different strategies can be used to facilitate changes in the health behaviors of others; an understanding of the basic concepts underlying educational, motivational, and behavioral theory is necessary to understand the forces influencing a person's oral health practices

Process

A. Assessing current status—comprehensive assessment of an individual's preventive needs requires collection and documentation of both clinical and behavioral data; clinical assessment areas are outlined in Chaper 11, section on clinical assessment of the periodontium; behavioral data are collected by interviewing the person to ascertain
  1. Entering levels of knowledge about the disease process and methods available for disease control and prevention
  2. Home care regimen currently used and the frequency with which it is implemented
  3. Attitudes toward prevention and self-care; having the patient demonstrate the home care regimen provides data on adequacy and effectiveness of plaque control skills

B. Determining educational needs—actual educational needs are identified by correlating and analyzing the assessed clinical and behavioral data; a precise determination of the person's needs is essential for focusing on an appropriate educational plan

C. Designing an appropriate program
  1. Design for disease control education should address needs, consider the comprehensive dental and dental hygiene treatment plans, and be based on sound educational and motivational principles
  2. Singular needs are more easily planned for than compound needs; the greater the extent and severity of disease, the more complex the modifying factors or deficiencies in knowledge, skill, or compliance, and the more important it becomes to develop a formal and specific plan for action

D. Implementing strategies
1. When implementing strategies, the dental hygienist should try to create an environment, both physical and psychologic, that supports and facilitates open communication and the behavioral changes necessary for optimal oral health
2. During the action-oriented implementation phase, educational, interpersonal, and technical strategies are employed and coordinated so that defined goals can be met
E. Evaluating effectiveness and continuing needs
1. Appraisals of changes in the person's behavior and clinical status as a result of dental hygiene actions should take place throughout the educational program
2. When needed change is not occurring, the dental hygienist must attempt to assess the reasons for the lack of progress and modify the educational plan accordingly
3. Patient conditions may make the attainment of all goals unlikely; this should, however, not result in the abandonment of objectives; these unmet needs can be identified and addressed at a later time

Sequence in Total Care – Options

A. Before instituting any dental treatment—rationale for choosing this sequence is that the patient will see positive changes resulting from his or her actions and that any treatment required will progress much more effectively and comfortably in an inflammation-free mouth; plan for dental interventions is not finalized until the patient's level of compliance is ascertained
B. Incorporated throughout comprehensive dental and/ or dental hygiene care—rationale for this sequence is based on the idea that spaced practice is more effective than amassed practice; patients need time to go through the stages involved in learning and habituation; evaluation can occur on a continuum and over time

Stages in Making a Commitment to a New Behavior

See Chapter 17, section on successful patient management

Basic Concepts

A. One approach to achieving the habit of plaque control is based on the concept that humans learn in a series of sequential steps referred to as the learning-ladder continuum or the decision-making continuum

B. Dental hygienist must first determine the patient's entering level on the ladder and then plan for moving up the steps in sequence

Learning-Ladder or Decision-Making Continuum

A. Step 1. Unawareness or ignorance—individual lacks information or has incorrect information about the problem
B. Step 2. Awareness—individual knows there is or can be a problem but does not act on this knowledge
C. Step 3. Self-interest—individual recognizes the problem and indicates a tentative inclination toward action
D. Step 4. Involvement—individual's attitudes and feelings are impacted, and desire for additional knowledge increases
E. Step 5. Action—new behaviors directed toward solving the problem are instituted
F. Step 6. Habit or commitment—new behavior is practiced over a period of time to become a part of the individual's life-style

Learning Domains

A. To be considered successful, disease control education must result in evident behavioral changes; once an individual's learning needs have been assessed, a plan for teaching can be designed
B. Three domains of learning have been classified in hierarchies and are used to specify learning objectives describing behaviors expected of the learner as the result of instruction
1. Cognitive domain—concerned with knowledge outcomes and intellectual abilities and skills; major hierarchical steps are knowledge, comprehension, application, analysis, synthesis, and evaluation
2. Affective domain—concerned with attitudes, interests, appreciation, and modes of interest; major hierarchical steps are receiving, responding, valuing, organization, and characterization
3. Psychomotor domain—concerned with levels of motor skill; major hierarchical steps are perception, set, guided response, mechanism, complex overt response, adaptation, and organization

Instructional Principles

A. A teacher must know how to direct and facilitate learning in order to help people make positive changes in their behavior
B. To maximize learning, the following principles can be applied to the design of an educational plan
   1. Small step size—present only what the person can assimilate in one session; provide conceptual or factual information when the "need to know" is evidenced
   2. Active participation—provide the time and opportunity for the person to ask questions; offer suggestions and practice new skills to enhance learning and increase retention
   3. Immediate feedback—provide the learner with early and frequent information regarding progress; make suggestions for improvement and use positive reinforcement to support and encourage learning
   4. Self-pacing—recognize that each person will progress at a different pace; recognize the learner's needs and establish an instructional pace tailored to each individual

Health Belief Model

A. Based on the concept that one's beliefs direct behavior; model is used to explain and predict health behaviors and acceptance of health recommendations; emphasis is placed on the *perceived* world of the individual, which may differ from the objective reality
B. Components
   1. Perceived susceptibility—individual must believe that he or she is susceptible to a particular disease or condition
   2. Perceived severity—individual must believe that if he or she gets the particular disease or condition, the consequences will be serious
   3. Perceived benefits versus barriers—individual must believe that there are effective means of preventing or controlling the potential or existing problem and that action on his or her part is worth any effort necessary
   4. Cues to action—once beliefs 1 to 3 are accepted, the individual will act on them when necessary; the stronger the beliefs regarding susceptibility, severity, and benefits, the greater the potential that appropriate action will occur; action can be stimulated by internal cues such as the physical symptoms of pain or bleeding or by external cues such as mass media communications advocating seat belts or warnings on the dangers of smoking

Maslow's Hierarchy of Needs

A. Definition—theory regarding human nature that is used to explain the motivational process; Maslow believed that inner forces, or needs, drive a person to action; he classified needs in a pyramid according to their importance to the individual, their ability to motivate, and the importance placed on their satisfaction; only when an individual's lower needs are met will the individual become concerned about higher-level needs
B. Hierarchy of needs
   1. Level 1. Physiologic needs—these survival needs are the most powerful and must be met before any others; they include the components necessary for body homeostasis such as food, water, oxygen, sleep, temperature regulation, and sex
   2. Level 2. Security and safety needs—these needs are required for protection against physical or psychologic damage and are more cognitive than physiologic in nature; they include shelter, a job for economic self-sufficiency, and a well-organized, stable environment
   3. Level 3. Social needs—once the physiologic and security needs have been met, then the needs for love and social belongingness become prime motivators; needs at this level include being accepted and loved, belonging to a group, and having the chance to give and receive friendship and love
   4. Level 4. Esteem or ego needs—two categories of needs exist at this level: one involves feelings of basic worth such as competence, achievement, mastery, and independence; the other involves gaining the esteem of others and triggers learning and acquiring status, power, skills, etc.
   5. Level 5. Self-actualization or self-realization needs—needs that drive the individual to reach the very top of his or her field; based on positive actions toward development, growth, and self-enhancement

PLAQUE DETECTION AND DISCLOSING

General Considerations

A. Because bacterial plaque is relatively invisible, teaching patients the skills necessary for disease control can be difficult
B. Agents that make supragingival plaque visible can enhance the teaching-learning process by
   1. Demonstrating a relationship between the presence of supragingival (supramarginal) plaque and the clinical signs of disease

2. Guiding skill development when applied before cleaning

3. Allowing evaluation of skill effectiveness when applied after cleaning

C. Presence of subgingival (submarginal) plaque cannot be demonstrated by the use of disclosing agents

D. Plan for disease control education should also include establishing the association between the presence of plaque and such clinical signs of disease as bleeding

E. Subgingival plaque detection by the patient is best managed when there is an understanding of the clinical changes that will occur when plaque removal is not effective

Agents in General Use

A. Erythrosin (FD & C Red No. 3)
1. Available in tablet or solution form; most widely used agent
2. Tablet form can be dissolved into a solution or chewed to dissolve in the mouth
3. Tends to stain soft tissues, making postapplication evaluation of the gingiva difficult

B. Fluorescing dye (FD & C Yellow No. 8)
1. Plaque stained with sodium fluorescein is visible only with the use of a special light source
2. More expensive to use but has the advantage of not interfering with gingival evaluation or leaving visible stain or oral tissues

C. Temporal dyes (FD & C Red No. 3 and Green No. 3)
1. Combination solution; has the advantage of differentiating mature from new plaque
2. Discloses plaque but will not stain gingival tissues

D. Others
1. Substances such as iodine, basic fuchsin, merbromin (Mercurochrome), and Bismarck Brown have been used in the past but are rarely used today
2. Iodine solutions were a particular problem, since they caused severe allergic reactions in sensitive individuals

Application Methods

A. Painting—dry the teeth, moisten a cotton pellet or tip with solution, retract the cheeks and lips, and paint on the facial and lingual surfaces of the crowns

B. Rinsing—place several drops of concentrated solution in a paper cup, add water, and instruct the patient to swish the solution around the mouth

C. Use of tablets or wafers—instruct the patient to chew a tablet or wafer, dissolving it in saliva, and then swish it around the mouth

D. Precautions
1. Avoid using iodine solutions, since they have an unpleasant taste and a high rate of allergic reactions
2. Avoid staining restorative materials that may be susceptible to permanent discoloration
3. Dispense the solution into a Dappen dish; do not contaminate the solution by introducing applicators into the container bottle
4. Erythrosin solutions contain alcohol, which can evaporate over time and alter the concentration of the solution
5. To avoid staining the lips, apply a light coat of petroleum jelly
6. Avoid using before a sealant application
7. Avoid the potential for staining clothing by providing appropriate protective drapes and using small amounts of solution

PLAQUE CONTROL ON FACIAL, LINGUAL, AND OCCLUSAL TOOTH SURFACES ▬▬

Basic Concepts

A. Products of plaque metabolism contribute to the initiation of both caries and periodontal disease

B. Mechanical disruption of organized plaque colonies is an effective and widely used means of preventing and controlling dental disease

C. Toothbrushing is the most widely used and effective means of controlling plaque on the facial, lingual, and occlusal surfaces of teeth

D. A wide variety of toothbrush shapes, sizes, and textures are available

E. Which particular brush should be used depends on the patient's needs and preferences

Manual Toothbrush

A. Description
1. Parts include the handle, head, and shank; head, or working end, holds clusters of bristles, called tufts, in a pattern
2. Design variables
   a. Handle can be in the same plane with the head or offset at an angle
   b. Total length varies with adult brushes; longer than those recommended for children
   c. Tuft placement can be in two to four rows with anywhere from 5 to 12 tufts per row
   d. Brushing planes are even, flat, or uneven

3. Bristle characteristics
   a. Natural bristles come from hog or boar hairs and are nonuniform in diameter, texture, or durability; hollow bristles may harbor bacteria and absorb water, making them soft and soggy with repeated use
   b. Nylon bristles, or filaments, are manufactured according to specifications that control for uniformity in texture, shape, and size; nonabsorbent nylon bristles are easily cleaned, dry quickly, and are more durable than natural bristles
   c. Relative stiffness—diameter and length of the bristle determine whether the brush will be termed hard or soft
   d. Bristle ends can be cut flat or polished to be rounded at the tip
B. Desirable characteristics—the American Dental Association (ADA) Council on Dental Therapeutics recommends that toothbrushes have the following desirable characteristics
   1. Conform to individual requirements in size, shape, and texture
   2. Be easily and efficiently manipulated
   3. Be readily cleaned and aerated
   4. Be impervious to moisture
   5. Be durable and inexpensive
C. Factors in toothbrush selection—the following factors will influence the recommendation of a particular toothbrush
   1. Oral health status
   2. Method of brushing recommended
   3. Configuration of hard and soft tissues
   4. Patient dexterity and ability to use a brush in an effective and nontraumatic manner
   5. Patient preference and motivation

Manual Toothbrushing Methods

NOTE: While some methods are no longer in general use because they are now recognized as being ineffective and/or destructive to hard or soft tissue, it is helpful to know about each of the major techniques
A. Bass method, or sulcular brushing method
   1. Bristle direction and placement—direct the bristles into the gingival sulcus at a 45-degree angle to the tooth surface
   2. Motion—with the bristle ends in the sulcus, vibrate the brush in short back-and-forth strokes; turn the brush the long way for lingual surfaces
   3. Advantages—disrupts plaque at and under the gingival margin; good gingival stimulation; some access into the interproximal area; moderate dexterity required

4. Problems—too much motion or pressure can result in tissue trauma; time consuming
B. Stillman method
   1. Bristle direction and placement—position the bristles on the attached gingiva and direct them apically at a 45-degree angle to the tooth
   2. Motion—use a firm but gentle vibration and rotary motion with the bristles stationary; position the brush the long way for lingual surfaces; scrub on occlusal surfaces
   3. Advantages—good gingival stimulation; moderate dexterity required
   4. Problems—bristles do not clean the gingival margin area adequately and do not enter the gingival sulcus;
C. Roll method
   1. Bristle direction and placement—place the side of the brush on the attached gingiva with the bristles directed apically
   2. Motion—apply inward pressure, then turn the wrist to roll, or sweep, the bristles over the gingiva and tooth surfaces; position the brush the long way for lingual surfaces and move toward the occlusal; scrub on occlusal surfaces
   3. Advantages—easy to learn; moderate dexterity needed; good gingival stimulation
   4. Problems—areas at and under the gingival margin are not adequately cleaned
D. Charters method
   1. Bristle direction and placement—position the brush tips toward the occlusal at a 45-degree angle to the occlusal plane; bristles make contact at the junction of the free margin and tooth surface and are flexed to force the tips interdentally; on lingual surfaces place the toe end of the brush head into each embrasure
   2. Motion—use a vibratory circular motion with the bristles stationary
   3. Advantage—cleans interdentally; good gingival stimulation
   4. Problems—bristles do not enter the gingival sulcus; placement is difficult, especially on lingual surfaces; requires a high level of manual dexterity
E. Fones method
   1. Bristle placement and direction—with teeth together, place the brush perpendicular to the tooth surfaces
   2. Motion—on buccal surfaces use a fast, wide circular motion covering the gingiva and tooth surfaces of both arches; on lingual surfaces use a back-and-forth horizontal motion

3. Advantages—easy to learn; minimal dexterity needed
4. Problems—too random; can traumatize soft tissues; bristles do not enter the sulcus

F. Circular scrub brush method
1. Bristle placement and direction—with the brush parallel to the occlusal plane, place the bristles in an apical direction at a 70- or 80-degree angle to the teeth; bristle tips contact the outer surfaces of the teeth, with some bristles extending onto the adjacent gingiva; position the brush the long way for lingual surfaces
2. Motion—use circular vibratory strokes with the tips of the bristles moving over the teeth and gingiva
3. Advantages—more effective in breaking up plaque than the stationary vibratory motion; cleans at and under the gingival margin; relatively easy to learn; good gingival stimulation
4. Problems—too vigorous scrubbing can result in gingival recession and tooth abrasion

G. Combination methods
1. Modified Bass method—combination of the Bass and rolling stroke methods; precede the roll, or sweep, with short back-and-forth vibratory strokes over the gingival and tooth surfaces; scrub on occlusal surfaces
2. Modified Stillman method—combination of the Stillman and rolling stroke methods; with the brush initially positioned at the junction of the gingiva and tooth, begin vibratory strokes and continue while turning the wrist and rolling the brush over the crown

Powered Toothbrushes

A. General description
1. Brush head and shank are separate from the handle, which contains the power source
2. Brush heads are smaller and handles are larger than manual brushes

B. Power sources
1. Direct—brush plugs into an electrical outlet for a consistent level of power
2. Batteries—replaceable or rechargeable batteries can be expensive and inconsistent in the level of power provided over time
3. Rechargeable—stand plugs into an electrical outlet; when the brush handle is replaced in the stand, the power unit in the handle is recharged; power level is relatively consistent

C. Motion—rapid, short strokes occur in one or a combination of the following basic motions
1. Back and forth—reciprocating
2. Circular—orbital
3. Up and down—arcuate
4. Vibratory

D. Speed
1. Model, power source, and brush type influence speed
2. Strokes vary from 1000 to 3600 motions per minute

E. Indications for use
1. When a person does not have the manual dexterity or discipline necessary to master an effective manual toothbrushing technique, the powered toothbrush should be considered
2. Many handicapped patients (or those responsible for their care) elect to use the powered brush

Powered Toothbrushing Methods

A. Patient variables and manufacturer instructions will determine the need for individualized modifications
B. General principles
1. Select soft-bristle brushes to avoid tissue trauma
2. Select a low-abrasive dentifrice to control the potential for tooth abrasion
3. Apply the dentifrice to the teeth before activating the brush to minimize splattering
4. Position the head and bristles for specific brushing needs and the specific method being used
5. Hold the brush in one location for a period of time; powered brushes are frequently used for too short a period of time
6. Gain access and visibility by retracting the lips and cheeks
7. Monitor pressure applied to avoid trauma to soft and hard tissues

Comparison of Powered and Manual Toothbrushes

A. Reported effectiveness—powered brushes compare favorably with manual brushes in their ability to remove plaque, keep tooth surfaces clean, and stimulate the gingiva
B. Instruction time—powered brushes tend to be easier to learn; because the motion is built in, the patient has only to properly position the brush head and hold it in place long enough to be effective
C. "Novelty effect" has been the reason suggested for reported increases in patient compliance when powered brushes are initially recommended; dental hygienist should monitor this potential for early, but short-lived success

Factors in Toothbrush Effectiveness

A. Sequence
   1. A methodical, systematic approach will minimize forgetting or skipping over an area
   2. Begin systematic overlapping strokes at the buccal aspect of the maxillary right or left terminal tooth and continue around the arch to the terminal tooth on the opposite side; switch to the lingual aspect and begin working back toward the starting side; use the same pattern for the mandible, then clean the occlusal surfaces
B. Duration
   1. Each time the brush is moved, the time spent in an area should be monitored by counting each stroke or counting seconds
   2. Stroke counting is more exact, since it is linked to patient needs and the specific brushing method used
C. Frequency
   1. Theoretically, thorough plaque removal once a day is the minimum requirement for maintaining periodontal health; it may not, however, be the optimum regimen for some individuals
   2. Frequency should be increased when gingival or periodontal conditions warrant it or when caries susceptibility or activity is high
   3. Brushing will remove residual sucrose as well as plaque and is one method for self-application of topical fluoride
D. Skill level
   1. Careful attention should be given to evaluating skill development in all components of brush manipulation, including grasp, placement, activation, wrist movement, and amount of pressure applied
   2. Control of the brush and brush motion are essential for effectiveness

Improper Toothbrushing

A. Need to assess
   1. Improper toothbrushing may be a result of a lack of education in proper technique or incorrect application following instruction
   2. The dental hygienist should plan to evaluate the brushing technique and monitor hard and soft tissue conditions at each recall visit
   3. Faulty placement, overvigorous motion and/or pressure, and use of a brush with frayed or broken bristles can lead to unwanted consequences

B. Acute consequences—soft tissue injuries such as denuded attached gingiva, lesions that appear punched out and red, and clusters of small ulcerations at the gingival margin
C. Chronic consequences
   1. Soft tissue—loss of gingival tissue or change in contour; malpositioned and/or prominent teeth and an inadequate band of attached gingiva are predisposing factors
   2. Hard tissue—loss of tooth structure and creation of wedge-shaped indentations at the cervical third of the tooth; malpositioned and/or prominent teeth and toothpastes with highly abrasive formulas contribute to the problem

Toothbrush Maintenance

A. Brushes should be rinsed clean after each use, then allowed to air dry in an upright position
B. Practice of using more than one brush at a time prolongs brush life
C. Brushes should be replaced when bristles splay or lose resiliency

TONGUE CLEANING

A. The tongue is a major focal point and harbor for bacteria that constitute the oral flora; instruction for the control of microorganisms should include methods for cleaning the tongue
B. Technique
   1. Brushing
      a. Place the sides of the brush on the dorsum of the tongue with the tips directed toward the throat
      b. Apply light pressure and move the brush forward and out; repeat to cover the entire surface
   2. Tongue-cleaning devices
      a. Tongue-cleaning devices are available in various designs, but all have some sort of flexible or rigid scraping surface or strip
      b. Device is placed toward the back of the tongue on the dorsal surface, then pulled forward while light pressure is applied
      c. Tongue-cleaning devices can be recommended for patients when they have elongated papillae, deep fissures, or surface coating

INTERDENTAL PLAQUE CONTROL ▰▰▰▰▰▰
Basic Concepts

A. While toothbrushes are effective in removing plaque from the facial, lingual, and occlusal surfaces of the teeth, they are relatively ineffective on the proximal surfaces
B. Devices designed for cleaning interproximal surfaces are essential for effective control of bacterial plaque
C. Interdental col area is a protected area that tends to harbor microorganisms, which can initiate disease
D. Anatomy of the interdental area is a significant factor in both disease initiation and control
E. Anatomic changes that result with loss of papillae, the presence of malpositioned teeth, or tooth loss may also contribute to interdental bacterial retention

Factors to Consider When Selecting Interdental Cleaning Methods

A. Soft tissue variables include the level of health or disease and the position and architecture of the gingiva and attachment
B. Hard tissue variables include tooth position, root anatomy, the status of restorations and/or prostheses, and the presence and degree of hard accretions
C. Patient variables include the level of compliance and skill development, as well as personal preferences

Flosses and Tapes

A. Dental floss is the most frequently recommended device for interdental cleaning
B. Flossing precedes brushing in a home care regimen, since it serves to deplaque proximal surfaces in preparation for optimal uptake of fluoride in toothpastes
C. Floss types—two types of floss, unwaxed and waxed, are in common use; clinical trials have failed to demonstrate one as being superior to the other
   1. Unwaxed—unbound filaments spread on the tooth and have more friction for cleaning; filaments hold plaque and debris for easier removal; floss, being less bulky, slips through contacts more easily
   2. Waxed—resists tearing and shredding on faulty restorations or when moved through very tight contacts

Flossing Technique

A. Floss length—varies with the holding technique; 10 to 15 inches when forming a loop; 12 to 24 inches when wrapping around fingers

B. Holding technique
   1. Ends may be tied together to form a loop, wrapped around the middle fingers, or tucked into the palm
   2. With equal tension in both hands, grasp with both thumbs or the thumb and forefinger for use on the maxilla or with both forefingers for use on the mandible; leave one-half to one-inch length between fingers
C. Insertion
   1. Approach the embrasure space obliquely and ease the floss past the contact using a back-and-forth motion
   2. Snapping through the contact can cause tissue injury
D. Adaptation and stroke
   1. Position the fingers so that the floss wraps securely against the proximal surface
   2. Slide beneath the gingival margin and move in an apicocoronal direction several times

Improper Flossing

A. Acute consequences—snapping through contacts, failure to curve the floss against proximal surfaces, and application of excessive pressure can result in floss cuts directly beside or at the midpoint of the papilla
B. Chronic consequences
   1. Soft tissue—excessive pressure applied submarginally can be destructive to the attachment fibers
   2. Hard tissue—repeated heavy sawing movements in a faciolingual direction will abrade proximal tooth structure

Floss Variations

A. Flexible filament floss
   1. Bulky spongelike segment supposedly acts like a brush against proximal surfaces and adapts into irregular surfaces and concavities
   2. Stiffened end aids access for patients with fixed prostheses or orthodontic appliances
B. Yarns
   1. When embrasure spaces are wide, teeth isolated, or pontics present, a thick synthetic knitting yarn may be more effective than a thin floss for removing supramarginal plaque
   2. Yarns are used with floss threaders for cleaning under pontics or to gain access to areas where the contacts are closed

Flossing Aids

A. Types of aids
   1. Floss holders
      a. General description—double-pronged plastic device onto which the floss is threaded and held, forming a span between the prongs
      b. Technique—prepared holder is positioned for insertion, then adapted and activated in much the same manner as hand-held floss; special care should be taken not to snap the floss through contacts
   2. Floss threaders
      a. General description—also known as carriers or caddies; firm but flexible devices for moving floss through closed contacts or under pontics; a variety of designs are available
      b. Technique—position the floss in the threader with even lengths on each side; pass the threader through the embrasure from the buccal to the lingual aspect, leaving sufficient length on the buccal aspect; remove the threader and use the floss in a normal manner
B. Indications for use—when an individual lacks the dexterity to floss properly or when tooth position or restorations prevent passing floss through contact areas

Interdental Brushes

A. General description
   1. Soft nylon filaments are twisted onto a stainless steel wire to form either a tapered or nontapered small brush
   2. Some brushes must be used with a special handle; others have wires long enough to use as handles
   3. Provide excellent access to root concavities
B. Technique
   1. Choose a brush of appropriate size, moisten the filaments, insert it interproximally, and use an in-and-out motion from the buccal to the lingual aspect or the lingual to the buccal aspect
   2. Filaments compress when moving through constricted areas and flare out to adapt to larger spaces
C. Precautions
   1. Avoid forcing through tight, tissue-filled areas, since serious trauma can result
   2. Unless properly adapted and activated, the stainless steel wire can puncture tissue
   3. Discard the tip when filaments lose their original shape

D. Indications for use—when access permits, for removing plaque from root concavities and proximal surfaces

AUXILIARY PLAQUE CONTROL DEVICES

Gauze Strips

A. Suggested use—to remove plaque from proximal surfaces when large diastemas are present, teeth are isolated, or there is no adjacent tooth
B. Technique—use one 1-inch width of bandage gauze cut into a 6-inch length and folded the long way into thirds; adapt to the open proximal surface and move back and forth several times

Pipe Cleaners

A. Suggested use—to remove plaque from exposed furcation areas and open interdental areas
B. Technique—cut the pipe cleaner to a manageable length, approximately 2 inches; attempt to round off the sharp wire edges and adapt the end to the space; move back and forth several times
C. Precautions—if not properly adapted, pipe wire can cause trauma to soft tissues

Wooden Devices

A. Toothpicks
   1. Suggested use—to remove plaque from proximal surfaces and concavities, furcation areas, and just under the gingival margin; also useful for cleaning fixed orthodontic bands
   2. Technique—toothpicks can be used alone in some areas or inserted into special holders angulated to enhance access; moisten the tip and adapt it to the surface to be cleaned; submarginally use a 45-degree angle to the tooth; move in and out several times for interproximal surfaces and follow the tooth contour on facial or lingual surfaces
   3. Precautions—rigid pointed tips can cause injury if forced into tight tissue areas; over time papillae will abrade if toothpicks are used improperly
B. Balsa wedges
   1. Suggested use—to remove plaque from proximal surfaces or just under the gingival margin; triangular in cross section; should be used interproximally only when there is adequate space for insertion
   2. Technique—moisten the tip, position the flat base of the triangle at the gingival border, insert with the tip angled slightly toward the occlusal, and move the wedge in and out with moderate pressure against the surface

3. Precautions—to avoid gingival splinters, discard tips as soon as splaying occurs; using a fulcrum increases control and reduces the risk of inserting with too much pressure

Single-tufted Brushes

A. Suggested use—to remove plaque from surfaces not accessible with larger brushes, including areas of crowded or malpositioned teeth, distal surfaces of terminal molars, around pontics, and lingual surfaces of molars; also useful for cleaning fixed orthodontic appliances
B. Technique—position the tuft at or just under the gingival margin and use a sulcular brushing stroke

Special Tips

A. Rubber tip
   1. Suggested use—cleaning proximal surfaces, in exposed furcations, and under gingival margins; authors differ on the rubber tip's ability to remove plaque or reshape gingiva after periodontal surgery
   2. Technique—place, but do not force, the tip into the interdental contour with the tip angled occlusally, press the side of the tip against the gingiva, and use a firm rotary motion to apply intermittent pressure
   3. Precaution—insertion perpendicular to the long axis of the tooth can result in flattened interdental papillae
B. Plastic tip
   1. Suggested use—to remove plaque from open furcation and interdental areas
   2. Technique—similar to that with the rubber tip
   3. Precautions—hard, rigid tip does not adapt easily and can cause discomfort if its edges are forced against tissue

DENTIFRICES

Basic Concepts

A. Definition—substance used with a toothbrush to clean accessible tooth surfaces; generally available in gel, paste, or powder form
B. Purposes
   1. Primarily cosmetic—tooth surfaces are cleaned and polished; breath is freshened
   2. Cosmetic-therapeutic—certain nondrug substances augment the efficiency of the brush in the removal of plaque, debris, and stain
   3. Therapeutic—vehicle for transporting biologically active ingredients to the tooth and its environment

C. Basic ingredients
   1. Detergents—lower surface tension to loosen debris for easier removal; provide the foaming characteristic
   2. Cleaning and polishing agents—abrasives that help remove stain, plaque, and debris from tooth surfaces and to give a luster to the tooth surface; should provide maximal cleaning benefit with minimal abrasion
   3. Humectants—retain moisture to ensure a chemically and physically stable product
   4. Binding agents—prevent separation by increasing the consistency of the mixture of liquid and solid ingredients
   5. Flavoring and sweetening agents—provide a pleasant and refreshing flavor and aftertaste and cover unpleasant flavors
   6. Coloring agents—contribute to the product's attractiveness and desirability
   7. Preservatives—prevent bacterial growth and prolong shelf life

Therapeutic Ingredients

A. Definition—biologically active ingredients that produce a beneficial effect on either the hard or soft tissues; dentifrices claiming therapeutic effects are eligible for evaluation by the ADA Council on Dental Therapeutics; most recent edition of *Accepted Dental Therapeutics* should be consulted for evaluation results
B. Fluoride agents—substantial data exist to show that approved fluoride dentifrices will reduce the incidence of caries; fluorides most commonly used are sodium fluoride, stannous fluoride, and sodium monfluorophosphate
C. Plaque-inhibiting agents—research has been, and continues to be, done on the formulation of dentifrices with agents that will reduce and/or prevent plaque formation; examples include sanguinarine and lactoperoxidase
D. Desensitizing agents—fluoride agents have been claimed to have desensitizing properties and are contained in specialized dentifrices; nonfluoride agents commonly used in desensitizing dentifrices include strontium chloride, potassium nitrate, and sodium citrate
E. Guidelines for dentifrice selection
   1. Avoid dentifrices with high abrasive quality, since they can cause alterations in natural and synthetic surfaces; patients with exposed root surfaces should use low or no abrasive substances when brushing

2. Dentifrices containing fluoride and that are "accepted" by the ADA Council on Dental Therapeutics should be recommended for most people, since caries control is a concern for patients of all ages
3. Desensitizing dentifrices can be recommended for patients with dentinal hypersensitivity

ORAL IRRIGATION

A. Definition—oral irrigation, also known as hydrotherapy, can be a valuable adjunct in helping to maintain oral cleanliness and health; oral irrigating devices force a steady or pulsating stream of water over the gingival tissue and teeth with the goal of removing unattached debris and reducing the concentration of bacteria and cellular end products that may be present; irrigators have also been used to flush gingival tissues with therapeutic solutions
B. Suggested use
1. Before brushing and flossing to remove debris or retained food particles
2. Debridement of recessed areas of fixed prosthetic or orthodontic appliances
3. Flushing of periodontal pockets with a controlled, low-intensity stream of water (not accepted by some authors)
C. General description
1. Power-driven device—unit with a water reservoir; plugs into an electrical outlet to create a pulsating jet of water; water pressure is regulated by an adjustable dial
2. Water pressure–driven devices—attaches directly to the water faucet to deliver a constant stream of water; pressure is controlled by regulating the faucet
D. Technique for use
1. Adjust the water stream to moderate the pressure
2. Lean over the washbasin
3. Direct the tip interproximally at a right angle to the tooth surfaces; stream should move in a horizontal direction through the gingival embrasure
E. Precautions
1. Patients should be educated in the proper use of irrigating devices and monitored for adverse effects
2. Tissue punctures or reductions in the height of papillae are potential outcomes if the pressure used is too great or application is too long in one area

3. Transient bacteremias may occur following oral irrigation, particularly when untreated disease is present; patients who are prophylactically premedicated for dental procedures should be advised against using these devices

DISEASE CONTROL FOR PATIENTS WITH FIXED AND/OR REMOVABLE APPLIANCES
Basic Concepts

A. Patients wearing fixed and/or removable dental appliances have unique disease control needs and must learn specific procedures for maintaining both the appliance and the involved natural teeth
B. Terms commonly used when describing appliances[1]
1. Appliance—in dentistry, general term referring to devices used to provide a function or therapeutic effect
2. Abutment—tooth or root used as anchorage for either a fixed or removable dental prosthesis
3. Clasp—retains and stabilizes denture by attaching it to the abutment teeth
4. Denture—artificial or prosthetic replacement for missing natural teeth and adjacent tissues
5. Pontic—artificial tooth on a fixed partial denture that replaces the lost natural tooth, restores its function, and usually occupies the space previously occupied by the natural crown
6. Prosthesis—artificial substitution for a missing organ or tissue; used for functional or cosmetic reasons, or both
7. Dental prosthesis—replacement for one or more of the teeth or other oral structures, ranging from a single tooth to a complete denture
8. Fixed prosthesis—dental prosthesis firmly attached to natural teeth, roots, or implants, usually by a cementing agent; normally not capable of removal by the patient and only with difficulty by the patient

Fixed Appliance Maintenance

A. Fixed appliances increase the potential for plaque and debris retention and accumulation and make access to proximal surfaces more difficult
B. Patients must learn to use devices that will
1. Move floss between pontics and abutments
2. Access interdental spaces above or beneath closed contacts
3. Move into and/or around orthodontic brackets, bands, and wires

4. Adapt to the area between orthodontic appliances and the gingival margin
   a. Special orthodontic brushes are available that are three rows wide with a trimmed, shorter middle row that fits over bands, brackets, and wires
   b. Two-row brushes that will adapt to the narrow area between bands and brackets and the gingiva are also available

Removable Appliance Maintenance

A. Patients with removable appliances must be educated to the need for conscientious cleaning and learn to do so without damage to the appliance body or clasps
B. Debris, stain, plaque, and calculus will collect on removable appliances if they are not routinely cleaned
C. Inadequate cleaning may also contribute to the development of lesions on the soft tissue underlying the appliance or to carious lesions on abutting tooth surfaces
D. Removable appliances can be maintained by
   1. Brushing with water and a mild detergent or dentifrice after each meal and before retiring
      a. Special denture brushes have two different arrangements of filaments to access both the inner curved surface and the outer and occlusal surfaces
      b. Special clasp brushes have a narrow, tapered cylindric design that can adapt to the inner surfaces of clasps, a prime site for plaque formation and retention
   2. Immersion in a solvent or detergent solution that chemically loosens or removes stains and deposits; appliance should always be brushed following soaking to clear residual debris material and chemicals; agents in common use are dilute sodium hypoclorite (bleach), alkaline peroxide, vinegar, and various enzymes that render proteins less adhesive
E. Procedures
   1. Hold the appliance securely to avoid dropping and breakage
   2. When brushing, hold the appliance over a sink that is partly filled with water or lined with a cushioning material
   3. Avoid overzealous brushing or the use of a strong abrasive, since the plastic resin material can be scratched or abraded to the extent that fit is compromised

4. Remove denture adhesive material from the appliance and underlying mucosa several times a day
5. Brush the underlying mucosa at least once a day with a soft toothbrush

PROFESSIONALLY ADMINISTERED TOPICAL FLUORIDE TREATMENTS
General Considerations

See Chapter 10, section on preventive agents
A. Topical fluoride treatments were developed soon after it was clearly established that waterborne fluoride is effective in reducing the incidence of caries; applied directly to erupted teeth, topical fluorides provide local protection at or near the tooth surface
B. Topical fluorides have been formulated as aqueous solutions, gels, pastes, and varnishes; most commonly used topical agents are neutral sodium fluoride, stannous fluoride, and acidulated phosphate fluoride
C. When properly implemented, fluoride treatments have been shown to have value for patients of all ages
D. Optimal preventive benefits are dependent on a clear understanding of the full range of fluoride treatments available, including types of agents, concentrations, routes of administration, levels of effectiveness, frequency of use, methods of delivery, and indications or contraindications for use

Profile of Fluoride Agents for Professional Application

A. Neutral sodium fluoride (NaF)
   1. Characteristics—first fluoride used for topical application; available as a powder or liquid; recommended for use in a 2% concentration
   2. Application intervals—series of four appointments at intervals that coincide with the eruption of primary and deciduous teeth; ages suggested are 3, 7, 10, and 13 years; single applications are applied at routine recall intervals
   3. Advantages—prepared solution is stable in plastic containers; relative absence of taste; does not stain teeth or irritate soft tissues
B. Stannous fluoride (SnF_2)
   1. Characteristics—available as a powder or gel; recommended for use at either 8% or 10% concentrations
   2. Application intervals—single applications at 6-month intervals beginning at age 3 years; more frequent applications are indicated when the caries activity or risk is high

3. Advantages—application intervals parallel typical recall patterns
4. Disadvantages and/or precautions—not stable in solution; must be freshly prepared just before application; astringent nature and disagreeable taste compromise patient acceptance; if spilled, can stain clothing; causes pigmentation associated with pellicle, carious lesions, demineralized areas, silicate restorations, and restoration margins; gingival reactions such as burning or sloughing have occurred; stannous ions can cause artifacts on radiographic films (radiographs should be taken before stannous fluoride procedures are implemented)
C. Acidulated phosphate fluoride (APF)
   1. Characteristics—available as aqueous solutions or gels; 1.23% sodium fluoride with orthophosphoric acid is the recommended concentration
   2. Application intervals—every 6 months or more frequently when indicated; as with most fluorides, levels of protection are influenced by the frequency of application
   3. Advantages—stable when kept in a plastic container; high level of patient acceptance; not irritating to soft tissues; does not discolor tooth structure

Fluoride Media

A. Solutions—aqueous solutions are compatible with all fluorides and were the first vehicles for topical application
B. Gels—all fluorides are now available in a gel vehicle; gel form is easily applied by either the tray or "paint-on" technique and is colored to enable visualization and better control; thixotropic gels have the additional advantage of flowing under pressure, which may increase their penetration into proximal areas
C. Pastes—fluoride was originally incorporated into pastes to allow cleansing and fluoride application in one time-saving step; formulation problems, however, compromised effectiveness; cleansing with a fluoride-containing dentifrice does not replace a topical treatment with high concentrations of fluoride
D. Varnishes—varnishes are applied using the paint-on technique and are then allowed to harden for 5 to 6 minutes; by adhering to the enamel for a long period and releasing fluoride slowly, they increase the total length of fluoride exposure time

Indications for Professional Application

A. Topical fluoride therapy by the dental hygienist is an accepted part of the prevention-oriented treatment plan
B. Assessment of the patient's status and identification of current or potential needs will determine an individualized plan for fluoride therapy
C. In many cases the therapy regimen will include application of both professionally applied and self-applied agents
D. Topical fluoride should be considered for inclusion in the treatment plan in the following situations
   1. For children and young adults—application should coincide with eruption patterns, and special attention should be given to monitoring for need during the "cavity-prone" years
   2. If caries activity is out of control
   3. Immediately following root instrumentation—dentin can be exposed, and dentinal tubules opened, as a result of root instrumentation; fluoride application contributes to prevention and/or control of the hypersensitivity that often follows instrumentation
   4. When gingival recession exposes root surfaces —fluoride application reduces the incidence of root caries and hypersensitivity
   5. When xerostomia is present—irradiation to the head and neck region, certain medications, and some medical conditions cause a decrease in the rate of saliva production; caries destruction occurs rapidly and is generalized when salivary production is minimal; multiple fluoride treatments are used to control the high caries risk for patients with xerostomia

Application Principles—General Guidelines

A. Patient preparation
   1. Explain the reason for the procedure, the steps involved, the time it will take, the need to control saliva and avoid ingestion, and the postapplication restriction of anything by mouth for 30 minutes
   2. Position the patient upright (facilitates salivary control and reduces the potential for gagging)
B. Preparation of tooth surfaces by polishing—there are differing opinions regarding the need to polish the teeth before professional fluoride application
   1. Rationale for polishing is that materia alba, plaque, and other accretions serve as a barrier to fluoride uptake, thus reducing effectiveness
   2. Rationale for *not* polishing is that the abrasive removes the fluoride-rich, highly protective, surface enamel and that neither fluoride uptake nor effectiveness is reduced by the presence of pellicle or plaque

Application Methods

Tray Systems

A. Designed to be used with fluoride gels; trays cover all the teeth in one arch, come in a variety of materials, shapes, and sizes, and can be used with or without paper or foam liners; tray systems are not appropriate for solutions, since they cannot be adequately retained within tray boundaries

B. Examples of trays
   1. Custom-fitted polyvinyl—relatively expensive; must be remade as the dentition matures; provides excellent coverage
   2. Reusable vinyl—comes in a limited number of sizes; difficult to adapt for good coverage; can be uncomfortable; more effective when used with liners that retain gel
   3. Air cushion system—used with liners; has its own portal for saliva suction; good adaptation and coverage; reusable; not autoclavable
   4. Wax—takes time to shape and adapt; poor retainer of gel; can leave a waxy residue
   5. Disposable styrofoam—available in a variety of sizes and shapes; soft, pliable, and comfortable; good retention of gel

C. Factors in tray selection—selection of an appropriate tray is important to the success of the procedure; the following criteria can be used to evaluate tray suitability
   1. Adapts to facial and lingual surfaces without extreme gapping
   2. Achieves complete coverage; depth is sufficient to reach the cervical third of the teeth
   3. Minimizes loss of the agent into the mouth
   4. Is comfortable for the patient
   5. Is cost-effective

D. Components of the application procedure
   1. Assemble armamentarium—this might include trays, inserts, fluoride gel, a saliva ejection device, cotton-tip applicators, gauze squares, and a timer or clock
   2. Prepare the patient
   3. Prepare the teeth
   4. Place a thin ribbon of gel in the tray and spread; to minimize ingestion of fluoride, minimize the amount of gel used
   5. Dry each arch; prevents dilution and controls for a potential salivary barrier
   6. Insert tray(s); one or two trays can be inserted at once; tray type, patient variables, and clinician preference will influence the method selected
   7. Insert the saliva ejection device; optimal suctioning methods reduce both the potential for ingestion and the incidence of nausea and vomiting
   8. Adapt tray(s); dental hygienist or patient can gently press on the trays to close any small anterior gaps that may exist
   9. Have the patient apply gentle biting pressure to force gel interproximally
   10. Begin timing; trays are left in position for at least 4 minutes
   11. Remove tray(s); if only one tray was inserted initially, insert the second tray at this point; do not allow the patient to rinse between insertions
   12. Clear excess agent from the mouth; instruct the patient to expectorate and/or swab the tongue, teeth, and soft tissues with gauze squares
   13. Do not allow the patient to rinse; remove the water cup from the unit before beginning the application
   14. Provide posttreatment instructions; patients are typically told not to eat, rinse, smoke, or put anything in their mouths for at least 30 minutes; this increases the total time fluoride will be in contact with the teeth

E. Advantages of the tray system
   1. Ease of application—fluoride agent is dispensed once
   2. Time efficient—both arches can be treated at once; preparation time is minimal
   3. Patient acceptance level is high—trays are comfortable and do not require that the mouth be kept open for long periods

Isolation and Continuous Application Systems

When fluoride agents are in solution, they must be applied using a technique that allows for small amounts to be continuously applied to properly prepared tooth surfaces; gels may also be applied using this technique

A. Components of the application procedure
   1. Assemble the armamentarium—long and short cotton rolls and cotton roll holders, fluoride solution and container, saliva ejection device, applicator (cotton pellets or tips, a brush, or special sponges), timing device
   2. Prepare the patient
   3. Prepare the teeth

4. Isolate the teeth on one side of the mouth using cotton rolls and a suitable holder; two cotton rolls, a long curved one placed on the buccal aspect and a short one placed on on the lingual aspect, are used to simultaneously isolate the maxillary and mandibular quadrants on one side
5. Insert the saliva ejection device
6. Dry the isolated teeth; use a systematic approach to avoid missing any teeth
7. Begin timing
8. Apply the prepared fluoride using a thoroughly moistened applicator; swab the teeth continuously for 4 minutes, being careful to cover all surfaces
9. Remove the cotton rolls and holders
10. Clear excess solution; use optimal evacuation methods and/or ask the patient to expectorate
11. Do not allow the patient to rinse
12. Provide posttreatment instructions

B. Advantages
1. Allows selective omission of an area or tooth; solution can be kept from surfaces where fluoride is contraindicated
2. Relatively inexpensive to use; cotton roll holders are autoclavable and reusable; eliminates the need for trays in multiple sizes and shapes
3. Allows direct observation of the solution or gel during application; dental hygienist can control the placement of the solution or gel and evaluate the status of salivary control, thus reducing the potential for ingestion

C. Disadvantages
1. Time consuming—cotton roll placement and adaptation should be precise for good results; each side of the mouth is treated independently for 4 minutes
2. Patient discomfort—mouth must remain open and the tongue controlled for a relatively long period of time

DENTAL SEALANTS

General Considerations

See Chapter 10, section on pit and fissure sealants

A. In the 1980s dental caries is a disease primarily of pits and fissures of the teeth; while systemic and topical fluorides provide increased resistance to decay, the pit and fissure surfaces do not benefit to the same degree as smooth surfaces
B. Placement of sealants is a safe and highly effective means of reducing or eliminating the carious process occurring in pits and fissures

C. Pits and fissures allow for accumulation and stagnation of fermentable substrates and serve as accumulation sites for acidogenic microorganisms capable of demineralizing tooth tissue
D. Effectiveness of dental sealants in prevention of tooth decay has been clearly demonstrated in a variety of research settings
E. Modern comprehensive primary prevention programs incorporate the complementary use of sealants and fluorides

Functions

A. Sealant technique is a primary preventive, noninvasive approach to retaining teeth in a caries-free state; sealant is a resin material resistant to chemomechanical breakdown that is bonded to the pit and fissure surfaces of a tooth; physical barrier that results functions to
1. Prevent bacteria, bacterial nutriments, and debris from entering pits and fissures
2. Plug pit and fissure depressions, thus minimizing stagnation and enhancing cleaning
B. Sealant systems are grouped by
1. Nature of the resin material used
a. Filled resin sealants
b. Nonfilled resin sealants
2. Method of polymerization or curing
a. Chemically cured or self-cured sealants
b. White light– or visible light–cured sealants

Protocol for Application

A. Seal all pits and fissures as the teeth erupt; this no-decision, no-criteria approach ensures that all susceptible pits and fissures are protected, but it is not cost-effective
B. Individual practitioners develop specific criteria to decide when and which teeth should be sealed; criteria suggested have included a range of the following factors
1. Age and oral hygiene status of the patient; to be truly preventive, the sealant is ideally applied shortly after tooth eruption
2. Familial and individual history of dental caries
3. History of fluoride exposure
4. Dietary patterns
5. Tooth type and morphology; pits and fissures that are sharp and deep are more likely to become carious than those that are shallow and well coalesced
NOTE: The criteria, while well conceived, are somewhat subjective; this multiple decision-making approach might result in some teeth not being sealed when they should have been, or unnecessary sealing of other teeth

C. Place patients in triage groups as they reach the age of eruption for primary and permanent molars and premolars and apply clinical judgment criteria suggested in the approach discussed in B; triage groups would be formed using the following guidelines
   1. Patients whose teeth are not carious and will probably not become carious
   2. Patients whose teeth, although presently diagnosed as caries free, will become carious if left unsealed
   3. Patients with rampant caries who will, in all likelihood, get interproximal caries as rapidly as pit and fissure caries
   NOTE: This is a very controversal protocol; the focus is on cost containment rather than ''pure'' prevention; only the patients in group 2 would routinely receive sealants

Contraindications to Sealant Application

A. Patient behavior does not allow for the maintenance of the dry field necessary for successful application
B. There is a frank carious lesion on the occlusal surface
C. There is a carious lesion on the smooth surface
D. Tooth has been previously restored

Application Guidelines

A. Mechanical cleansing of enamel
   1. Serves to remove plaque and surface debris, which interferes with the effectiveness of the conditioning agent
   2. Cleansing agent of choice is a watery slurry of flour of pumice; avoid using commercial pastes, since they may contain ingredients such as glycerin or fluoride, which will inhibit bonding
   3. Careful rinsing to remove pumice residue is important
B. Isolation
   1. Salivary contamination of etched enamel surfaces is thought to be a major reason for sealant failure
   2. Careful isolation using either a rubber dam or cotton rolls is essential for consistent success
C. Drying
   1. Dry the isolated tooth thoroughly in preparation for application of the conditioner
   2. Avoid water contamination if using syringes, which deliver combinations of water and air

D. Conditioning
   1. Acid conditioning to etch the enamel surface is an essential prerequisite to application of the resin material; acid solution removes a layer of enamel and increases the total surface area by rendering the deeper enamel regions porous; these micropores are penetrated by the resin monomer to produce a mechanical lock on polymerization
   2. Phosphoric acid in a concentration of from 30% to 50% is the current etching agent of choice
   3. Conditioning agents are available in either a solution or gel form
      a. Solution should be applied by gently dabbing the enamel surface with a saturated cotton pellet, sponge, or brush; avoid rubbing the surface, since it causes a breakdown of the latticelike micropores
      b. Gels are applied with a special applicator, brush, cotton tip, or cotton pellet
   4. Suggested etching time for permanent teeth is 1 minute; retention in primary teeth is thought to improve when the application time is increased to 2 minutes
E. Rinse the conditioned tooth
   1. Thoroughly rinse the etched enamel surfaces using a water syringe and high-speed evacuation system; do not let the patient swish; when the gel form is used, the rinsing time may need to be increased to ensure complete removal
   2. Salivary contamination at this point will result in a substantial reduction in bond strength
      a. Do not allow the patient to close, rinse, or touch the conditioned surface with the tongue
      b. When cotton rolls and/or absorbent pads are used, change as necessary, being careful to avoid salivary contamination
F. Dry the conditioned tooth
   1. Prepare the tooth for resin application by drying thoroughly; completely dry surface is essential
   2. Examine the conditioned surface; properly etched surfaces will appear dull and chalky; repeat the conditioning process when these changes are not seen
G. Apply the sealant material (procedure for applying the resin material differs with the method of polymerization)
   1. Chemical or self-cured sealants—catalyst and sealant are mixed and while still in the fluid, unpolymerized, state are applied to prepared surfaces with a brush or custom dispenser; working time from mixing to setting is 1 to 3 minutes

2. Ultraviolet or visible light–cured sealants—prepared sealant is applied to the conditioned surface in a fluid state; light is then directed over the entire sealant for a specified period; working time for application is flexible, since polymerization does not occur until the light is applied
3. Regardless of the polymerization method employed, the sealant material should be drawn into all the grooves; pits and all unetched and soft tissue areas should be avoided

H. Evaluate the results
1. Examine the placed sealant to determine the adequacy of the bond strength and the absence of voids, underextensions, overextensions, or undercuring
2. Sealed surface should feel completely smooth; sticky surface layer is not uncommon and should be wiped off

PHASE-CONTRAST MICROSCOPY
Use for Disease Control

A. Clinical assessment
1. Microscopic evaluations of plaque are employed to determine disease activity and to supplement conventional assessment and evaluation procedures
2. It has been postulated that specific bacterial species act as etiologic agents in the initiation and development of periodontal disease, that microorganisms found in periodontal lesions will seldom be found in healthy gingival crevices, and that these organisms are indicators of disease
3. Periodic microscopic evaluation of plaque samples lets the clinician determine the effectiveness of treatment modalities, aids in determining a prognosis, and directs planning for recalls

B. Patient education and motivation
1. When a microscope is linked with a television screen, patients are able to view a bacterial sample from their own mouths
2. Because the majority of organisms associated with periodontal disease are highly mobile, viewing a plaque sample is a graphic way of demonstrating the significance and role of bacteria in the disease process

Using the Microscope

A. Slide preparation
1. Hold the slide by its edges to avoid fingerprint marks
2. Place a drop of water on a slide
3. When multiple sites are being sampled, multiple separate drops may be used

B. Obtaining the sample
1. Based on clinical evaluation, select sites with potential or current problems (e.g., deep probe readings, malpositioned teeth, poorly contoured restorations)
2. Use a curette or other submarginal instrument to obtain a sample from the most apical portion of the site selected
3. Avoid contaminating the sample with calculus or supramarginal deposits
4. Dislodge the sample onto the drop of water
5. Gently disperse the sample; overmanipulation may disrupt the original organized colony
6. Place the cover slip on the slide

C. Mounting the slide
1. Place the prepared slide onto the microscope stage; most microscopes have a spring-loaded curved arm that secures the slide
2. Center the specimen over the light coming from below; the stage can be moved horizontally, from left to right, and vertically

D. Selecting the objective—most systems come with two objects (lenses): 40× and 100×; each requires a different condenser setting; 100× lens must always be used with immersion oil to eliminate optical interferences from air; one drop of oil is placed directly on the cover slip; 40× lens must never be used with oil

E. Focusing the sample
1. Adjust the interpupillary distance; position the eyes about 1 inch from the eyepieces and close or pull the eyepieces apart until a single circular viewing field is seen
2. Raise the stage until the lens seems to *almost* touch the cover slip
3. Use the fine-focus adjustment to bring the specimen into sharp focus

F. Viewing the sample
1. Sample can be viewed directly or on a video monitor; image seen on the video screen is a portion of the image seen through the eyepieces
2. Scan the slide by adjusting the fine focus with one hand while moving the specimen on the stage with the other hand

Evaluating the Sample

A. Many species and quantities of bacteria can be found in the gingival crevice; to date, there is no universally agreed-on reference pattern to use when classifying a patient's microscopic status

B. It has been suggested that the quantity and type of *motile* bacteria and white blood cells can be used as indicators of disease potential and/or severity

C. Organized and highly active masses of spirochetes, rods, and amebae are thought to be unique to periodontal disease states

D. Gingivitis is characterized by a wide variety of unorganized motile forms, mostly various rods, and some leukocytes but no amebae

E. In health, there is a distinctive relative absence of motile organisms; loosely organized bacterial complexes are present, as are leukocytes in low levels

Use of the Microscope in Keye's Technique — Rationale

A. Bacterial organizations associated with health are different from those associated with disease

B. Therapy should be directed toward elimination or suppression of bacterial populations not associated with health

C. Microscopic examinations of subgingival bacterial complexes should be employed to *monitor* the patient's status and to *modulate* the antibacterial therapy instituted to eliminate bacterial risk factors

ORAL CANCER SELF-EXAMINATION ▬▬

Basic Concepts

A. Many oral cancers are, unfortunately, not detected until they have invaded deep tissues and require radical surgical and/or extensive chemotherapy or irradiation

B. Early detection and early treatment are the best ways to manage oral cancer

C. While all patients can potentially benefit from self-examination skills, it is especially important that the dental hygienist educate individuals considered to be at high risk

Oral Cancer High-Risk Factors

A. Tobacco use
  1. Smokers are estimated to be two to four times at greater risk than nonsmokers
  2. Snuff users and tobacco chewers are prone to squamous cell carcinomas at or near the site where the material is held

B. Alcohol use
  1. There is a positive correlation between alcohol use and the incidence of oral cancer
  2. Evidence suggests a cocarcinogenesis of tobacco and alcohol

C. Sun exposure—individuals who work out-of-doors, especially those with fair complexions, seem to be at higher risk for basal cell tumors of the skin

Examination Technique

Materials Needed

A. Large mirror and adequate light source are essential for self-examination procedures

B. Use of a flashlight, mouth-sized mirror, and gauze or tissue squares enhances access to and visualization of intraoral structures

Systematic Approach

A. Face and neck
  1. Symmetry—one-sided irregularities should be questioned; right and left sides should have the same outline and shape
  2. Skin—remove eyeglasses; check for sores, bumps, and discolorations
  3. Neck—palpate lymph chains for lumps or tender areas

B. Lips and gums
  1. Remove full or partial dentures
  2. Retract the lips to look for sores or color changes
  3. Palpate the lips and run a finger over the gingiva to feel for irregularities, tenderness, or roughened areas

C. Cheek
  1. Retract the right, then the left side to visualize the inner surface; look for red, white, brown, or speckled patches
  2. Palpate for lumps or tenderness
  3. Run a finger over the inside surface to check for rough or raised places

D. Roof of the mouth
  1. Tilt the head back and use a flashlight to increase visualization
  2. Use a mouth-sized mirror to reflect the image in a larger mirror
  3. Look for sores, color changes, etc.; feel for lumps or areas of tenderness

E. Tongue
   1. Extend the tongue and look at the top surface
   2. Using a gauze square or tissue, grasp the tongue and pull it to the right, then the left side
   3. Look for sores, color changes, and irregularities
   4. Feel for lumps, areas of tenderness, or roughened surfaces
F. Floor of the mouth
   1. Place the tip of the tongue against the roof of the mouth
   2. Look for asymmetry, sores, color changes, etc.
   3. With the fingers of one hand under the jaw, use the index finger of the other hand to compress structures
   4. Check for lumps, tenderness, or irregularities

Teaching Factors

A. Several demonstrations of the self-assessment procedure will probably be necessary for mastery; pamphlets explaining and demonstrating techniques are extremely helpful
B. Introduce the concept of ''normal range'' and familiarize the patient with what is normal in his or her mouth
C. Provide criteria for determining significant deviations from normal
   1. Sores that fail to heal within 2 weeks
   2. Appearance of white, red, or dark-colored patches
   3. Presence of swellings, lumps, bumps, or growths
D. Reinforce the need for a systematic approach to ensure thoroughness
E. Define the dentist's roll in interpreting findings; patient should report, not diagnose, unusual findings
F. Establish the concept that self-examination is not meant to be a substitute for periodic regular professional evaluation

CONTROL OF DENTINAL HYPERSENSITIVITY
Definition

A. Dentinal hypersensitivity is an *abnormal* condition occurring when vital dentin is exposed to the environment of the oral cavity with the result that painful stimuli can reach the pulp and be translated as pain
B. Dental hygienists need to be concerned with this problem, since one of every seven persons over the age of 21 years who seek dental care has some degree of hypersensitivity

Etiology

A. Primary cause of hypersensitivity is exposed dentin and open dentinal tubules
B. Dentin exposure occurs
   1. In 10% of all teeth; during development the enamel and cementum do not join
   2. When cementum is lost through erosion, dental caries, or scaling and root-planing procedures
   3. When soft tissue is lost because of gingival recession, periodontal surgery, or improper toothbrushing habits

Pain Mechanism

A. There is no universally accepted theory of the pain transmission mechanism in dentinal hypersensitivity
B. The most widely accepted theories propose that
   1. Lymphatic fluid present in the dentinal tubules transmits stimuli
   2. Odontoblasts and their processes act as receptors and transmitters of sensory stimuli
   3. Stimuli create movement of tubular fluids, causing nerve endings at the pulpal wall to be stimulated

Pain Stimuli

A. Not all stimuli cause pain; each patient has a unique set of stimuli to which he or she is sensitive
B. Mechanical stimuli include instrumentation procedures, home care devices, eating utensils, and friction from removable prosthetic or orthodontic devices
C. Chemical stimuli include foods high in acid or sugars, plaque end products, and some topical medications
D. Thermal stimuli include foods and liquids at extreme temperatures, cold air, and too-rapid drying of a tooth surface, which causes a concurrent rapid drop in tooth temperature

Assessing Hypersensitivity

A. It is important to distinguish the pain reaction caused by dentinal hypersensitivity from the reaction caused by manipulation of the adjacent soft tissues; specific tooth or teeth involved must also be identified
B. Assessment techniques attempt to produce the pain response on suspect teeth
   1. Draw an explorer along areas of exposed dentin and along the cementoenamel junction
   2. Apply a cold solution or cold air to suspect areas

Treatment Goals

A. Reestablish an effective separation between the oral cavity and pulp by open dentinal tubules
B. Presence of plaque in areas of exposed dentin is directly linked to hypersensitive experiences; conscientious plaque control eliminates irritating plaque end products and provides a surface open to natural obturation of tubules by salivary salts

Desensitizing Agents

A. Modes of action—agents are thought to seal dentinal tubules by either surface precipitation of ions, subsurface incorporation of ions, or stimulation of secondary dentin
B. Optimal agent characteristics—professionally applied agents should ideally be rapidly acting, nontoxic, easy to apply, and have consistent outcomes and long-term effects

Types of Agents

A. To date, no single agent or form of treatment is effective for all patients
B. Numerous agents have been tried with varying degrees of success; they include
 1. Solutions or pastes of fluoride in varying compounds and percentages, calcium hydroxide, strontium chloride, potassium nitrate, sodium citrate, formaldehyde, etc.
 2. Adhesive, varnish, or bonding materials
 3. Iontophoretic devices—iontophoresis is the application of an electrical current to impregnate tissues with ions from dissolved salts; fluoride iontophoresis is thought to result in increased uptake and penetration of fluoride ions into dentin

Desensitization Methods

A. Home/self-care regimens
 1. Patient's performance of rigorous plaque control is critically important in gaining and maintaining control of hypersensitivity
 2. Toothpastes containing fluoride have been shown to be effective and have the added benefit of contributing to the control of root caries
 3. Specially formulated toothpastes should be adjuncts to, not replacements for, fluoride pastes
 4. Daily use of a fluoride gel or rinse is advisable when the problem is generalized or recurrent

B. Professionally delivered regimens should support and/or make possible home/self-care regimens; when sensitivity is severe enough to interfere with necessary home measures, professional application is necessary
 1. General guidelines
  a. Remove all accretions and necrotic cementum; involved surface must be free of barriers to the agent
  b. Local anesthesia is appropriate when scaling and root-planing procedures and/or application of the agent are too painful
  c. Isolate the sensitive tooth and control saliva
  d. Dry the tooth with cotton pellets or cotton rolls; avoid using the air syringe
  e. Apply the agent according to the manufacturer's instructions for the method and time required; pastes are usually burnished in with a wooden point, whereas solutions are bathed on; some patients may experience an acute pain reaction to the agent; immediately remove the agent, wait a few minutes, and then attempt reapplication
  f. Remove any excess agent to avoid ingestion
  g. Test for change in pain reaction; this will not be possible with anesthetized patients
  h. Plan for future reapplication if desensitization has not occurred
 2. Precaution—some agents have very high concentrations of fluoride; to prevent nausea, use good agent application and salivary control techniques

ELECTRICAL PULPAL VITALITY TESTING
Basic Concepts

A. Teeth may become nonvital as a result of bacterial invasion of the pulp or from injuries of a physical nature such as mechanical or thermal trauma
B. Any tooth suspected of being nonvital should be tested for pulpal vitality
C. Method that provides qualitative assessment is preferred
D. Use of thermal tests (applying hot or cold agents to a tooth surface) to observe the absence or presence of a pain response is highly subjective and lacks an adequate degree of consistency and reliability
E. Precaution—do not use electrical vitality testing procedures for patients with cardiac pacemakers or other electronic life-support devices

Testing Devices

A. Electrical pulp tester (also known as a vitalometer) is an instrument that uses gradations of electrical current to excite a response in pulpal tissues; pulp testers are either battery-operated portable instruments or have cords that plug into electrical outlets for a direct power source; all testers have rheostats with a scale (e.g., 1 to 10 or 1 to 50), which indicates the relative amount of current being applied

B. Procedure
   1. Armamentarium
      a. Testing device
      b. Cotton rolls
      c. Toothpaste or other conducting medium
   2. Patient preparation
      a. Avoid undue apprehension by explaining that the procedure is used to determine the minimal stimulation necessary to evoke a response
      b. Instruct the patient to raise a hand when the slightest warmth or tingling sensation is first felt
      c. To acquaint the patient with the type of sensation created and to determine a normal response pattern, first test the teeth adjacent and contralateral to the tooth in question
   3. Obtaining a reading
      a. Isolate and dry the teeth to be tested; this prevents the conduction of current into soft tissues
      b. Apply a small amount of toothpaste, or alternative conductor, to the tester tip
      c. Place the tip on sound tooth structure within the middle third of the crown for a single-rooted tooth and within the middle third of each cusp for a multirooted tooth
      d. Avoid contact with restorations and/or soft tissues
      e. Slowly advance the rheostat from zero to increasingly higher numbers until sensation is indicated; rheostat should not be moved above that point for that tooth
   4. Documentation
      a. Two readings should be taken for each tooth tested and the readings averaged
      b. Record for all teeth tested: the lowest average reading, the type of testing device and conductor used, and any patient actions or reactions that may have affected results

C. Variables affecting results
   1. Pulpal conditions may vary from early inflammation to complete necrosis; responses vary with each condition; pulp of a test tooth is considered to be degenerating when, compared with a control, much more current is required to gain a response
   2. Metallic restorations conduct electrical charges more rapidly than tooth structure and can produce false readings
   3. Teeth involved in splints or bridges or with proximal restorations may produce false-positive reactions, since the circuit can be transferred from adjacent vital teeth
   4. Multirooted teeth may have some combination of vital and nonvital canals and test falsely positive
   5. Pain reactions are influenced by attitudes, age, sex, emotions, fatigue, and medications

EXFOLIATIVE CYTOLOGY

Definition

A. Suspicious lesions in the mouth require microscopic evaluation before a definitive diagnosis can be made
B. Exfoliative cytology is a nonsurgical technique for collecting surface cells of a lesion for microscopic evaluation

Procedure

A. Armamentarium
   1. Glass microscope slides
   2. Collection instrument
   3. Fixative
   4. Gauze sponges
   5. Laboratory forms
B. Documentation
   1. Print the patient's name and the data on the glass slide
   2. Complete laboratory data forms; information usually includes name and address for patient and dentist, lesion history, and clinical description (location, size, color, and consistency)
C. Obtaining and preparing the sample
   1. Cleanse the lesion—remove surface debris by irrigating with water or gently wiping with wet gauze
   2. Collect the sample—using a flexible metal spatula or moistened wooden tongue blade, firmly scrape the entire surface of the lesion; move in one direction only
   3. Prepare the glass slide—holding the slide by its edges, evenly spread the sample material across the slide surface

4. Fix the sample—to prevent cell dehydration, quickly cover the sample surface with a layer of 70% alcohol; allow the sample to air dry in an area protected from airborne contamination
5. Prepare for transfer to the laboratory

Laboratory Findings

A. Classification categories
   1. Unsatisfactory—specimen is not adequate for diagnosis
   2. Class I. Normal—only normal cells are present
   3. Class II. Atypical—some cellular changes may be present, but there is no suggestion of malignancy
   4. Class III. Intermediate—changes may be suggestive of malignancy, but findings are not clear-cut; biopsy is recommended
   5. Class IV. Suggestive of cancer—cells with malignant characteristics are present; biopsy is mandatory
   6. Class V. Positive for cancer—cells are obviously malignant; biopsy is manditory
B. Follow-up needs
   1. Unsatisfactory—schedule for another smear to be taken
   2. Class III, IV, or V findings—patient should be referred for biopsy
   3. Class I or II findings—patient should be monitored for healing of the lesion or reevaluated if the lesion fails to resolve; false-negative reports are a possibility; healed lesion is the best reassurance for reports in categories I and II

Advantages

A. Nonsurgical, noninvasive procedure requiring minimal patient preparation and no postoperative care
B. Easily and efficiently implemented in any setting, making it ideal for mass screening or use in remote areas
C. Clinical laboratory and professional personnel costs are relatively low

Disadvantages

A. Lacks precision
   1. Only surface lesions can be evaluated; no matter how hard the lesion is scraped, only surface (not basal) cells are collected
   2. Heavily keratinized lesions will not yield adequate cells for examination

B. May delay definitive treatment
   1. Definitive treatment cannot be decided on smear results alone; valuable time may be lost obtaining and analyzing a biopsy specimen
   2. When clinical evidence clearly suggests a malignant lesion, the more precise biopsy is the first procedure of choice

REFERENCE

1. Joblonski, S.: Illustrated dictionary of dentistry, Philadelphia, 1982, W.B. Saunders Co.

SUGGESTED READINGS

American Dental Association, Council on Dental Therapeutics: Accepted dental therapeutics, ed. 39, Chicago, 1982, The Association.

The Baltimore College of Dental Surgery, Dental School, University of Maryland at Baltimore and the Maryland Division, Inc., of the American Cancer Society: Mouth cancer: finding it early may save your life (pamphlet).

Boundy, S.S., and Reynolds, N.J., editors: Current concepts in dental hygiene, vol. 2, St. Louis, 1979, The C.V. Mosby Co.

Brannstrom, M., Johnson, G., and Nordenvall, K.J.: Transmission and control of dentinal pain: resin impregnation for the desensitization of dentin, J. Am. Dent. Assoc. **99:**10, 1979.

Ciancio, S.G., and Bourgault, P.C.: Clinical pharmacology for dental professionals, New York, 1980, McGraw-Hill Book Co.

Ford, C.W., editor: Clinical education for the allied health professions, St. Louis, 1978, The C.V. Mosby Co.

Green, B.L., Green, M.L., and McFall, W.T.: Calcium hydroxide and potassium nitrate as desensitizing agents for hypersensitive root surfaces, J. Periodontol. **48:**10, 1977.

Harris, N.O., and Christen, A.G.: Primary preventive dentistry, Reston, Va., 1982, Reston Publishing Co., Inc.

Horowitz, A.M.: Health education and promotion to prevent dental caries: the opportunity and responsibility of dental hygienists, Dent. Hyg. **57:**5, 1983.

Horowitz, H.S.: Alternative methods of delivering fluorides: an update, Dent. Hyg. **57:**5, 1983.

Jablonski, S.: Illustrated dictionary of dentistry, Philadelphia, 1982, W.B. Saunders Co.

Katz, S., McDonald, J.L., and Stookey, G.K.: Preventive dentistry for the dental hygienist, for the dental assistant, Upper Montclair, N.J., 1977, D.C.P. Publishing.

Keyes, P.H., and Rams, T.E.: A rationale for management of periodontal diseases: rapid identification of microbial "therapeutic targets" with phase-contrast microscopy, J. Am. Dent. Assoc. **106:**6, 1983.

Lutins, N.D., Greco, G.W., and McFall, W.T.: Effectiveness of sodium fluoride on tooth hypersensitivity with and without iontophoresis, J. Periodontol. **55:**5, 1984.

Lynch, M.A., Brightman, V.J., and Greenberg, M.S., editors: Burket's oral medicine: diagnosis and treatment, ed. 8, Philadelphia, 1984, J.B. Lippincott Co.

National Institutes of Health Consensus Development Conference: Dental sealants in the prevention of tooth decay, Proceedings, J. Dent. Educ. **48**(suppl.):2, 1984.

Pipe, P., et al.: Developing a plaque control program: a motivational approach to involving patients in dental care, University of California, San Francisco, 1972, Praxis Publishing Co.

Ramfjord, S.P., and Ash, M.M., Jr.: Periodontology and periodontics, Philadelphia, 1979, W.B. Saunders Co.

Ripa, L.W.: Professionally (operator) applied topical fluoride therapy: a critique, Clin. Prevent. Dent. **4**:3, 1982.

Shafer, W.G., Hine, M.K., and Levy, B.M.: A textbook of oral pathology, ed. 4, Philadelphia, 1983, W.B. Saunders Co.

Silverstone, L.M.: The current status of adhesive sealants, Dent. Hyg. **57**:5, 1983.

Stallard, R.E.: A textbook of preventive dentistry, ed. 2, Philadelphia, 1982, W.B. Saunders Co.

Steele, P.F.: Dimensions of dental hygiene, ed. 3, Philadelphia, 1982, Lea & Febiger.

Swongo, P.A.: The use of topical fluorides to prevent dental caries in adults: a review of the literature, J. Am. Dent. Assoc. **107**:9, 1983.

Tarbet, W.J., et al.: Home treatment for dentinal hypersensitivity: a comparative study, J. Am. Dent. Assoc. **105**:8, 1982.

Weinstein, P., and Getz, T.: Changing human behavior: strategies for preventive dentistry, Chicago, 1978, Science Research Associates.

Wilkins, E.M.: Clinical practice of the dental hygienist, ed. 5, Philadelphia, 1983, Lea & Febiger.

Wilson, M.B.: The science and art of basic microscopy, Bellaire, Tex., 1976, American Society for Medical Technology.

Woodall, I.R., et al.: Comprehensive dental hygiene care, ed. 2, St. Louis, 1985, The C.V. Mosby Co.

Yura, H., and Walsh, M.B.: The nursing process, ed. 3, New York, 1978, Appleton-Century-Crofts.

Review Questions

1 Powered toothbrushes
1. Are less effective than manual toothbrushes
2. Require increased instruction time
3. Are contraindicated for patients with diabetes
4. Are often used for too little time to be effective
5. Can cause hypocalcification of cementum

2 The application of dental sealants is
1. Limited to the permanent dentition
2. Contraindicated for teeth with sclerotic dentin
3. Not effective for smooth surface caries control
4. Repeated every 6 months beginning at age 3 years
5. Still considered an experimental procedure

3 To be truly a primary preventive procedure, dental sealants should be applied
1. At the first clinical signs of decalcification
2. Shortly after teeth erupt
3. Before the first professional prophylaxis
4. Only to those teeth at high risk for decay
5. After disease control techniques are mastered

4 A major factor in the failure of a dental sealant application is
1. Omission of a postapplication fluoride treatment
2. Insufficient rinsing time after the resin hardens
3. Etching for 10 seconds longer than recommended
4. Salivary contamination of the etched surface
5. Drying the conditioned surface before placing the resin

5 When a dental sealant procedure is being implemented, the etching process is considered successful when the
1. Solution has been rubbed into the enamel
2. Tooth feels rough to the patient's tongue
3. Dried tooth appears dull and chalky
4. Surrounding soft tissues blanch easily
5. Height of contour is adequately reduced

6 Ultraviolet or visible light sealant systems
1. Require the careful mixing of a catalyst with the resin material
2. Allow for longer working times than self-cure systems
3. Are contraindicated for deciduous teeth
4. Achieve polymerization with heat
5. Do not require an acid to etch the tooth surface

7 An etiologic factor associated with a high risk of oral cancer is
1. A history of premature use of stannous fluoride
2. Failure to have routine oral prophylaxis
3. A pattern of loosely organized bacterial complexes
4. The presence of a fixed partial prosthesis
5. Habitual use of tobacco

8 The use of a hot or cold agent to test for pulpal vitality
1. Provides qualitative assessment data
2. Produces the most consistent results
3. Is recommended for patients over 40 years of age
4. Is contraindicated for patients with cardiac pacemakers
5. None of the above

9 The rheostat of an electrical vitality tester should be
1. Positioned at zero when testing begins
2. Removed when deciduous teeth are being tested
3. Advanced quickly to prevent false readings
4. Placed on sound tooth structure
5. Lubricated with a conducting agent

10 The results of electrical vitality testing may be affected by all of the following *except*
1. The level of plaque control achieved
2. The presence of a full crown on the tooth
3. Certain medications
4. The age of the patient
5. The condition of the pulp

11 Oral exfoliative cytology
1. Includes excision of connective tissue
2. Requires administration of a local anesthetic
3. Is a nonsurgical technique
4. Can cause localized scarring
5. Is diagnostically definitive for cancer

12 When oral exfoliative cytology laboratory findings are negative, the patient should be
1. Dismissed from care
2. Retested each week for 3 weeks
3. Referred for incisional biopsy
4. Monitored until the lesion resolves
5. Given a prescription for basic fuchsin

13 Exfoliative cytology is *not* an appropriate diagnostic technique for
1. Mass screening
2. Questionable surface lesions
3. Postmenopausal women
4. Lesions characteristic of cancer
5. Implementation in the private dental office

14 Which of the following can be used as *an initiator* in an autopolymerizing dental sealant?
1. Ultraviolet light
2. Cryanoacrylates
3. BIS-GMA
4. Monomer
5. Tertiary amines

15 When a tooth is being conditioned to receive dental sealant resin, the etching agent should be
1. Mixed with a catalyst
2. Exposed to ultraviolet light
3. Rubbed into the enamel
4. Flowed onto proximal surfaces
5. Gently dabbed on the tooth surface

16 Patients who do *not* believe that they are personally susceptible to dental disease are *not* likely to
1. Get a dental disease
2. Practice daily disease control
3. Develop psychomotor skills
4. Need immediate feedback
5. Require disease control education

17 Having patients chart the disclosed plaque in their mouths is an example of
1. Small step size
2. Self-actualization
3. Active participation
4. Attitudinal motivation
5. Approach-avoidance reaction

18 Which of the following is an acute consequence of improper flossing technique?
1. Abraded tooth structure
2. Enamel mottling
3. Laceration of papillae
4. Dilaceration of the root
5. Proximal amalgam fracture

Situation: A 34-year-old woman is a new patient in the practice where you work as a dental hygienist. Initial assessment reveals a medical history that is essentially negative, a pattern of sporadic dental care, lack of knowledge regarding dental disease, poor oral hygiene, significant amounts of supramarginal and submarginal deposits, generalized gingival recession, flattened or missing papilla in several areas, probe measurements ranging from 5 to 7 mm, Class III furcation involvement on tooth No. 30, and multiple carious lesions. Ten years ago teeth Nos. 3 and 18 were extracted because of caries, but no prostheses were made to replace them. The patient says she is very apprehensive about dental care but wants to have her teeth fixed to look better for an important job interview. During the initial visit she appears uncomfortable and has to go to the bathroom several times. Questions 19 to 23 refer to this situation.

19 Data collection techniques for this patient included all of the following *except*
1. Interview
2. Observation
3. Measurement
4. Examination
5. Implementation

20 Patients who lack knowledge about the process of dental disease often have poor oral hygiene *because* a learner is helped by early and frequent feedback regarding progress in learning.
1. Both the statement and the reason are correct and related
2. Both the statement and the reason are correct but are *not* related
3. The statement is correct, but the reason is *not*
4. The statement is *not* correct, but the reason is an accurate statement
5. *Neither* the statement nor the reason is correct

21 Given this patient's gingival architecture and probe measurements, toothbrushing and flossing
1. Are sufficient methods for controlling plaque
2. Alone are *not* sufficient methods for controlling plaque
3. Instruction should be delayed until caries control is achieved
4. Are contraindicated in the areas of gingival recession
5. Techniques are best taught by demonstration on a model

22 Topical fluoride therapy
1. Is useless for this patient
2. Should not be implemented before the bridges are seated
3. Is contraindicated for furcation exposures
4. Should be delivered before root instrumentation to prevent hypersensitivity
5. Is a valid part of the comprehensive treatment plan for this patient

23 Fixed prostheses are planned to replace teeth Nos. 3 and 18. The dental hygiene treatment plan should
1. Not be formalized until the bridges are cemented
2. Not be concerned with the dental treatment plan
3. Include instruction on the proper use of a denture brush
4. Include instruction in methods for cleaning pontics and abutments
5. None of the above

---

24 Patients with exposed root surfaces
1. Have dentinal hypersensitivity
2. Collect more calculus
3. Should avoid brushing those surfaces
4. Should use a low-abrasive dentifrice
5. Must eliminate grapefruit from their diets

25 The *least* effective means of preventing occlusal caries is
1. Applying dental sealants
2. Fluoridating community water supplies
3. Toothbrushing and flossing
4. Prescribing fluoride supplements in nonfluoridated areas
5. Daily fluoride rinses

26 Electrical pulp testers are also known as
1. Vitalometers
2. Pulp cappers
3. Pulp probes
4. Desensitizers
5. Rheostats

27 Clinical examination is not valid in assessing the effectiveness of plaque control procedures *because* erythrosin disclosing solutions stain gingival tissues.
1. Both the statement and the reason are correct and related
2. Both the statement and the reason are correct but are *not* related
3. The statement is correct, but the reason is *not*
4. The statement is *not* correct, but the reason is an accurate statement
5. *Neither* the statement nor the reason is correct

28 Which of the following is *least* significant for retention of dental sealants?
1. Etching for a sufficient period of time
2. Preventing salivary contamination after etching
3. Applying topical fluoride after the resin is placed
4. Removing surface debris before etching
5. Thorough drying of the etched surface

29 A plaque sample taken from a healthy mouth would show which of the following when viewed with a phase microscope?
1. Highly active masses of spirochetes
2. Numerous loosely organized amebae
3. Cementoblasts and rod forms
4. Relative absence of motile forms
5. Unorganized masses of spirochetes

30 The major benefit of using opaque dental sealant resins is that
1. They are retained longer
2. Etching is not required
3. They are easily visualized
4. Fluoride is incorporated
5. They are not abraded

31 Pulsating oral irrigators are contraindicated
1. For drug addicts
2. Before amalgam polishing
3. After brushing
4. For patients with rheumatic heart disease
5. For patients with fixed orthodontic appliances

32 Patients wearing fixed orthodontic bands are *not* usually advised to use
1. Dental floss
2. Oral irrigators
3. Topical fluorides
4. Interdental brushes
5. Floss threaders

33 Prevention of dental disease is
1. The primary purpose of patient education
2. Not possible
3. Solely achieved by mechanical methods
4. The goal of oral cancer self-examination
5. Achieved by topical fluoride application

34 Enamel is etched before placement of dental sealant resin to
1. Produce micropores that mechanically hold the resin material
2. Break down the calcium fluoride layer
3. Expose the more porous dentin
4. Produce a hard, lustrous surface
5. Increase the surface tension

35 Data collection procedures are
1. The same for all patients
2. Determined by patient conditions
3. Treatment planned after patient education
4. Performed during the implementation phase of care
5. Focused on solving the patient's identified problems

36 Determining the success of a plan for care is the purpose of
1. Disease control education
2. Influencing a person's oral health practices
3. The evaluation component of the dental hygiene process of care
4. The Periodontal Disease Index
5. Collecting behavioral data

37 Oral irrigating devices have been shown to
1. Reduce the incidence of juvenile periodontitis
2. Promote healing after periodontal surgery
3. Negate the effects of occlusal trauma
4. Initiate keratinization of sulcular epithelium
5. None of the above

38 Before patients will become concerned about oral health, they must believe that
1. Dental disease can be fatal
2. Dental disease can have serious consequences
3. Dental care is not too expensive
4. Dental care is accessible
5. Dental decay is limited to children

39 The incorporation of fluoride into a dentifrice has
1. Been proved to reduce decay
2. Questionable value in reducing decay
3. Cosmetic as well as therapeutic benefit
4. Never been researched properly
5. No benefit in water-fluoridated communities

40 The primary reason for using dental floss is to
1. Remove calculus
2. Stimulate the gingiva
3. Disrupt bacterial plaque
4. Remove impacted flood
5. Prevent cigarette stain

Answers and Rationales

1. (4) Powered toothbrushes must be held in one place long enough to be effective.
   (1) Powered toothbrushes compare favorably with manual toothbrushes in removing plaque.
   (2) Powered toothbrushes tend to be easier to learn, since the motion is built in.
   (3) Patients with diabetes can safely use powered toothbrushes.
   (5) Hypocalcification occurs during tooth formation, before eruption.

2. (3) Dental sealants are applied to pit and fissure surfaces.
   (1) Caries control for deciduous teeth includes the application of dental sealants.
   (2) Sclerotic dentin is not identifiable clinically.
   (4) Properly applied, dental sealants can be retained for years. The need for reapplication is determined by examination of the surfaces sealed and is not related to a schedule for application.
   (5) Research has shown sealants to be a safe and effective means of reducing the incidence of pit and fissure caries.

3. (2) Primary prevention measures are designed to prevent disease completely. Sealing teeth as soon as they are properly erupted is a primary prevention measure.
   (1) Providing treatment after the clinical signs of incipient disease have been recognized is a secondary preventive measure.
   (3) Sealing for primary prevention can occur before the first prophylaxis.
   (4) All, rather than selected, teeth are sealed in a primary prevention protocol.
   (5) Disease control techniques such as brushing are relatively ineffective for control of pit and fissure caries.

4. (4) Salivary contamination after etching reduces the bonding strength because the surface is contaminated by salivary constituents.
   (1) Sealant retention is related to tooth selection and technique during application.
   (2) Once polymerization has occurred, rinsing will not influence retention.
   (3) A slightly longer etching time will not in itself contribute to sealant failure. Care should be taken not to rub the solution onto the surface.
   (5) Proper technique includes drying the etched and washed surface before resin placement.

For each question the correct answer and rationale are listed first. The other choices are presented in order with the reasons why they are not correct.

5. (3) The clinical sign of a properly etched tooth is a dull, chalklike surface.
   (1) Rubbing the solution into the enamel will damage the enamel latticework necessary for retention; however, this fact cannot be determined by clinical examination.
   (2) Patients cannot feel a difference in surface character. Salivary contamination can occur if the tongue contacts the etched tooth surface.
   (4) Changes in hard tooth structure are evaluated in determining etching success.
   (5) *Height of contour* is a term used to describe the furthest extension of a tooth. The etching process does not alter this point.

6. (2) More time can be spent manipulating the resin material, since it will not harden until the light is applied.
   (1) Ultraviolet and visible light systems do not require a catalyst for polymerization.
   (3) Deciduous teeth are effectively sealed with light-cure systems.
   (4) Polymerization occurs on exposure to light, not heat.
   (5) Properly etched surfaces are necessary for sealant retention regardless of the system used.

7. (5) Smokers are estimated to be two to four times at greater risk than nonsmokers.
   (1) Fluoride therapy is not an etiologic factor in oral cancer.
   (2) Compliance or noncompliance with an oral prophylaxis schedule is not an etiologic factor in oral cancer.
   (3) The organization of bacterial complexes may impact on periodontal status, but not on oral cancer risk.
   (4) Properly designed and fabricated, fixed prostheses are nonirritating to tissues and not etiologic factors in oral cancer.

8. (5) None of the answers is correct.
   (1) Qualitative assessment involves measurements on a discrete scale.
   (2) Temperature variances are not easily measured or controlled.
   (3) Age is not the significant factor in selecting an agent to test for tooth vitality.
   (4) Electrical pulp testing is contraindicated for patients with cardiac pacemakers.

9. (1) The zero position indicates that no charge is being produced and is the proper beginning position.
   (2) The rheostat controls the charge produced and is an essential component of the vitality tester.
   (3) Advancing too quickly can produce false readings.
   (4) The tip of the instrument is placed on sound tooth structure.
   (5) A conducting agent is applied to the tester tip.

10. (1) Plaque control effectiveness or compliance will not alter electrical charges.
    (2) Metallic restorations conduct electrical charges more rapidly.
    (3) Certain medications can influence pain reactions.
    (4) Reactions to pain stimuli may vary with age.
    (5) A necrotic pulp will give no response. Acutely or chronically inflamed pulpal tissue will produce varying degrees of response.

11. (3) Only the surface cells of a lesion are collected for microscopic evaluation.
    (1) Underlying connective tissue is not collected.
    (2) Collection of surface cells does not require pain control procedures.
    (4) Scarring does not result unless deeper tissues are disturbed.
    (5) Biopsy is the definitive diagnostic test for cancer.

12. (4) The best indication that a negative finding was accurate is a healed lesion.
    (1) The lesion should be monitored for healing.
    (2) There is no standard schedule for retesting.
    (3) Biopsy is mandatory when laboratory findings reveal cells suggestive of, or having, malignant characteristics.
    (5) Once used as a disclosing agent, basic fuchsin is now thought to have carcinogenic potential.

13. (4) Biopsy is the appropriate diagnostic technique when a lesion is suggestive of cancer.
    (1) Exfoliative cytology is relatively inexpensive; it requires minimal patient preparation; implementation is simple; and it requires no postoperative care.
    (2) Surface cell collection and examination are appropriate for surface lesions.
    (3) The character of the lesion, not menopausal status, is the factor that guides selection of the diagnostic technique.
    (5) See 1.

14. (5) Polymerization occurs when a tertiary amine is mixed with the monomer.
    (1) Autopolymerizing systems do not require the use of ultraviolet light.
    (2) Cryanoacrylates are a plastic material.
    (3) BIS-GMA is the most routinely used sealant resin.
    (4) The unpolymerized resin is called a monomer.

15. (5) Gentle application prevents destruction of the fragile micropores into which the resin will flow and be held.
    (1) In self-cure sealant systems a catalyst is mixed with resin material to initiate polymerization.
    (2) Ultraviolet light is applied to resin material to initiate polymerization.
    (3) Rubbing will break down the lattice formed and result in poor retention.
    (4) Proximal surfaces are not sealed and therefore should not be etched.

16. (2) The Health Belief Model suggests that individuals will act to prevent disease only when they believe they are susceptible to it.
    (1) Belief alone will not control dental disease.
    (3) Skill development occurs with practice.
    (4) Immediate feedback reinforces learning and desired behaviors.
    (5) Education should be provided as a standard of care.

17. (3) Learning and retention are enhanced with patient participation in the learning process.
    (1) Small step size is an educational concept that information be limited to what can be assimilated in one session.
    (2) Self-actualization is the highest level in Maslow's Hierarchy of Needs.
    (4) Attitudes are formed, not motivated.
    (5) Approach-avoidance is a psychologic concept.
18. (3) Floss snapped through contacts or poorly adapted to surfaces can cut into papillary tissues.
    (1) Abrasion is a chronic consequence.
    (2) Enamel mottling is a developmental disturbance.
    (4) Root dilaceration occurs during tooth development.
    (5) Floss will not fracture amalgam material
19. (5) Implementation, the third step in a dental hygiene process of care, follows assessment and planning.
    (1) Medical history data include interview techniques.
    (2) Observations are made of general appearance, behaviors, etc.
    (3) Measuring techniques are used to determine sulci and/or pocket depths.
    (4) Determinations of oral hygiene status, gingival health, the location and extent of deposits, caries activity, etc., are made using examination techniques.
20. (2) *The statement is correct.* If a person does not know that plaque is a primary etiologic factor in dental disease, poor oral hygiene will not be seen as a problem. *The reason is correct.* Instructional theory suggests that early and frequent feedback maximizes learning. The statement and reason are *not* related.
    (1) Both the statement and the reason are correct but are not related.
    (3) The reason is correct.
    (4) The statement is correct.
    (5) Both the statement and the reason are correct.
21. (2) Neither a standard brush nor floss will access deep pockets, root concavities, or furcation surfaces. Access for plaque control may require surgical interventions and/or the use of additional mechanical devices.
    (1) See 2.
    (3) Caries activity does not contraindicate instruction in plaque control techniques.
    (4) If not kept clean, exposed root surfaces are at high risk for caries development.
    (5) Techniques are best demonstrated in the patient's mouth.
22. (5) Fluoride therapy is appropriate when caries activity is high and root surfaces are exposed.
    (1) This patient has a high caries rate and exposed root surfaces. The dental hygiene treatment would appropriately include fluoride therapy.
    (2) Fluoride therapy is not contraindicated before placement of a fixed prosthesis.
    (3) Exposed root surfaces would benefit from fluoride therapy.
    (4) Root instrumentation would remove any fluoride deposited at the end of open dentinal tubules.

23. (4) The dental hygiene treatment plan should address both current and potential, or future, needs. When the prostheses are placed, the patient should be scheduled for instruction in the specific procedures needed to maintain the appliance and the involved natural teeth.
    (1) The dental hygiene treatment plan is formalized after the assessment process.
    (2) A comprehensive dental hygiene treatment plan must be coordinated with the dental treatment plan.
    (3) A denture brush is used with removable, not fixed, prostheses.
    (5) The correct answer is 4.
24. (4) Exposed cementum and dentin are softer than enamel and more easily abraded.
    (1) Not all exposed root surfaces are hypersensitive.
    (2) Root exposure and calculus formation are not in a cause-effect relationship.
    (3) It is essential that these surfaces be kept clean. Proper brushing technique will not contribute to further exposure.
    (5) Acid foods in reasonable amounts can be consumed.
25. (3) Toothbrush bristles are too large to access deep pits and fissures. Floss is not used occlusally.
    (1) Sealants have been shown to significantly reduce the incidence of occlusal caries.
    (2) Water fluoridation significantly reduces caries incidence.
    (4) When water supplies are not fluoridated, supplemental fluorides are effective.
    (5) Daily fluoride rinsing reduces caries incidence.
26. (1) Pulpal vitality testers are sometimes called vitalometers.
    (2) Pulp capping is a therapeutic procedure used to maintain pulpal vitality.
    (3) "Pulp probe" is a fabricated term.
    (4) Desensitizing agents are used to control dentinal hypersensitivity.
    (5) A rheostat is a device for controlling electrical current.
27. (4) *The statement is not correct.* Examination of hard and soft tissues provides definitive information on plaque control effectiveness. *The reason is an accurate statement.* Gingival tissues are temporarily stained with erythrosin disclosing agents. The statement and reason are *not* related.
    (1) The statement is not correct.
    (2) The statement is not correct.
    (3) The statement is not correct.
    (5) The reason is correct.
28. (3) Sealant retention is negatively affected by improper techniques during the application process. Postapplication fluorides do not affect retention rates.
    (1) The etching agent must contact enamel surfaces long enough to create the micropores into which the resin will flow and be held.
    (2) Contamination of etched surfaces by saliva is the major reason for sealant failure.
    (4) Surface debris is a barrier to the etching agent.
    (5) Drying allows for evaluation of surface changes and removes fluid barriers.

29. (4) In health, there is a relative absence of motile bacteria.
    (1) Active masses of spirochetes are unique to disease states.
    (2) Amebae are found in periodontal disease states.
    (3) Cementoblasts are not seen in plaque samples.
    (5) Spirochetes are not typically found in healthy mouths.

30. (3) Opaque or colored sealants are easily visualized and evaluated for retention.
    (1) Sealant retention is not altered by opacifying or coloring agents.
    (2) Etching is essential for sealant retention.
    (4) Fluoride is not incorporated into sealant resins.
    (5) All sealant materials are abraded to some extent over time.

31. (4) Transient bacteremias may occur with oral irrigation. Patients who require prophylactic premedication for dental procedures are best advised not to use oral irrigating devices.
    (1) Irrigators do not endanger the health of drug addicts.
    (2) Amalgams are not altered by oral irrigators.
    (3) Oral irrigation preferably follows brushing to remove accessible debris and plaque.
    (5) Orthodontic brackets and bands are appropriately cleaned with oral irrigators.

32. (4) Orthodontic bands and brackets hender safe access to embrasure spaces.
    (1) Orthodontic patients must learn to use floss to maintain gingival health.
    (2) Oral irrigators effectively remove loosely adherent deposits from orthodontic appliances.
    (3) Topical fluoride therapy is standard for orthodontic patients.
    (5) Floss threaders are used to move floss around appliances and onto proximal surfaces.

33. (1) Patient education provides the information and skills necessary for prevention behaviors.
    (2) A range of strategies and techniques are successful in preventing dental disease.
    (3) Mechanical interventions are but one means of disease control.
    (4) Self-examination skills allow early detection of problems but not necessarily prevention.
    (5) Topical fluoride therapy achieves caries reduction but will not prevent periodontal disease.

34. (1) Resin flows into open micropores to be held in a mechanical bond.
    (2) The goal of etching is the creation of micropores.
    (3) Etching agents do not penetrate through enamel into dentin.
    (4) Etching creates a dull, chalklike surface.
    (5) Increased surface tension would impede resin flow.

35. (2) Data collection procedures are determined by patient conditions. The full-denture patient will not require periodontal pocket measurements.
    (1) While certain assessment procedures are indicated for all patients, the range of procedures will differ for each patient.
    (3) The plan for patient education is based on data collection and analysis.
    (4) Interventions are based on previous assessment of the patient's status.
    (5) Assessment focuses on the patient's current or potential problems. Interventions are focused on solving the problems.

36. (3) Evaluation is the act of appraising the success of planned interventions.
    (1) The purpose of disease control education is to provide the information and develop the skills necessary for health behaviors.
    (2) Influencing behavior differs from evaluating the outcomes of interventions.
    (4) Indices provide limited information on a patient's status and may not measure conditions or specific sites for which interventions were planned.
    (5) Behavioral changes are definitively evaluated by changes in tissue conditions.

37. (5) None of the answers is correct.
    (1) The etiology of juvenile periodontitis is multifactorial, and its incidence is not affected by oral irrigation.
    (2) Surgically treated tissues are fragile and should not be disturbed by pressurized irrigating devices.
    (3) Uncorrected, trauma from occlusion will continue regardless of the level of oral cleanliness.
    (4) Sulcular epithelium is not keratinized.

38. (2) According to the Health Belief Model, one's beliefs direct behavior. Before individuals initiate health behaviors, they must believe that if they get a particular disease, the consequences can be serious.
    (1) Dental diseases are not typically fatal.
    (3) Concern about oral health can exist independently of concern for cost of care.
    (4) Concern precedes consideration of accessibility.
    (5) Adults as well as children are susceptible to dental decay.

39. (1) Fluoridated dentifrices have been accepted as having a therapeutic benefit in the reduction of decay.
    (2) Sufficient research exists to support the therapeutic benefit of fluoridated dentifrices.
    (3) Fluoride provides therapeutic, not cosmetic, benefits.
    (4) See 2.
    (5) Research has shown that fluoridated dentifrices contribute to caries reduction even in water-fluoridated communities.

40. (3) The mechanical disruption of interdental plaque is the primary goal of flossing.
    (1) Floss will not remove hardened deposits.
    (2) Gingival stimulation is a secondary benefit.
    (4) The removal of impacted food is a flossing function but not the primary reason for its use.
    (5) Tobacco will stain tooth surfaces even if floss is used.

CHAPTER 13

Instrumentation for Patient Examination and Treatment

ESTHER M. WILKINS

As a health service provider, the dental hygienist participates in the patient's total oral care, using preventive, educational, and therapeutic methods. The dental hygienist is a cotherapist with the dentist and the patient and has responsibility during various phases of treatment.

Initially, the dental hygienist collects and records data for use by the dentist in making the dental diagnosis, and for formulation of the dental and dental hygiene treatment plans. The techniques required for preparation of the personal, health, and dental histories, the radiographic survey, study casts, photographs, records of extraoral and intraoral conditions observed, and chartings of dental and periodontal findings, are all part of the specialized skills of the dental hygienist.

As professional treatment is started, the patient participates by learning therapeutic disease control techniques for daily home treatments. Scaling and root planing, the basic initial treatment procedures performed by the dental hygienist, are difficult and exacting and require a high level of skill. This chapter has as its primary focus the dental hygienist's responsibilities in the use of instruments for assessment and periodontal therapy.

BASIC CONCEPTS ▄▄▄▄▄▄

A. Selection and use of instruments depend on knowledge of the characteristics of the area of operation in health and disease, namely, the anatomic and topographic features of the natural and restored tooth surfaces, and the anatomy and histopathology of the periodontium (gingiva, periodontal ligament, cementum, alveolar bone)
B. Periodontal examination and recording of findings provide the data for the diagnosis and treatment plan, which is the blueprint for instrumentation
C. Ultimate purpose of all treatment is to create an environment in which the periodontal tissues can first be restored to health and then be maintained in health without the recurrence of disease

D. Success of professional treatments depends on the control of bacterial plaque; therefore, instruction and supervision in plaque removal procedures for the daily participation of the patient precedes, continues simultaneously with, and follows instrumentation by the clinician

ENVIRONMENT OF INSTRUMENTATION ▄▄▄▄

Types of Pockets

See Chapter 11, section on changes within the periodontium associated with disease
A. Pocket—diseased sulcus or crevice; it is the presence or absence of disease and the level of attached periodontal fibers on the tooth that distinguish a pocket from a sulcus, not only the depth of the pocket as measured with a probe
B. Gingival pocket—pocket formed by gingival enlargement without change in the attachment level and without destruction of the underlying periodontal tissues
   1. Attachment level—at or above the cementoenamel junction
   2. Tooth pocket wall—enamel
   3. Instrumentation surfaces—enamel
C. Periodontal pocket—pocket formed by destruction of underlying periodontal tissues that resulted in migration of the soft tissue attachment; there may also be enlargement of the gingival tissue
   1. Attachment level—below the cementoenamel junction, along the root surface
   2. Tooth pocket wall—when the gingival margin is above the cementoenamel junction, the tooth wall may be partly enamel and partly cementum
   3. Instrumentation surface—may be cementum or both enamel and cementum
   4. Types of periodontal pockets (Fig. 13-1)
      a. Suprabony—base of the pocket is coronal to the crest of the alveolar bone; all gingival pockets are suprabony because no changes have occurred in the bone level or contour

Fig. 13-1 Types of pockets. (From Wilkins, E.M.: Clinical practice of the dental hygienist, ed. 5, Philadelphia, 1983, Lea & Febiger.)

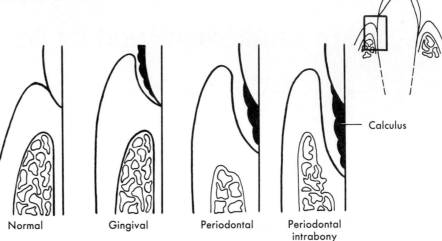

Normal   Gingival   Periodontal   Periodontal intrabony

Calculus

  b. Infrabony (intrabony)—base of the pocket is below or apical to the crest of the alveolar bone

Description of a Pocket

See Chapter 11, section on changes within the periodontium associated with disease

A. Description
 1. A pocket is formed by the tooth surface wall and the gingival wall
 2. At the base of the pocket the soft tissue is attached to the tooth by the epithelial attachment, which is the inner layer of cells of the junctional epithelium
 3. Location and nature of subgingival instrumentation is directly related to the anatomic and pathologic features of the pocket
B. Gingival wall of the pocket
 1. In health
  a. Lining of the sulcus is called sulcular epithelium, which is nonkeratinized stratified squamous epithelium
  b. Sulcular epithelium connects directly with the junctional epithelium
 2. In disease
  a. Lining of the pocket is called pocket epithelium
  b. Pocket is characterized by
   (1) Degenerative changes in the epithelium with varying degrees of destruction of the intercellular substance
   (2) Ulceration and proliferation of epithelium with increased rete ridges extending into the connective tissue
    (3) Enlargement, which may be either
     (a) Soft, spongy tissue—related to edema and local circulatory stasis
     (b) Hard, firm—with long-standing chronic inflammation, fibrosis results
C. Junctional epithelium
 1. In health—normal junctional epithelium is a collarlike band of stratified squamous epithelium 10 to 20 cells thick near the sulcus, and 2 to 3 cells thick at the apical end; it is 0.25 to 1.35 mm long
 2. In disease—migration of the junctional epithelium occurs, along with degeneration in the connective tissue under the attachment; as the junctional epithelium proliferates along the root surface, the coronal portion detaches
D. Tooth surface wall of the pocket
 1. Gingival pocket—tooth surface wall is enamel; calculus on the subgingival surface is attached to the enamel
 2. Periodontal pocket—tooth surface wall may be entirely cementum, or partly cementum and partly enamel; calculus is attached to cementum or partly to cementum and partly to enamel
 3. Root surface
  a. Thickness of cementum
   (1) Thickest near apex—may be 150 to 200 μm (0.15 to 0.2 mm)
   (2) Thinnest at cervical third—may be 20 to 50 μm (0.02 to 0.05 mm)
  b. Causes of surface roughness as detected by a probe or explorer may be
   (1) Diseased altered cementum

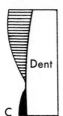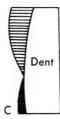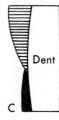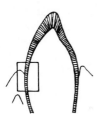

Fig. 13-2 Different configurations of cemento-enamel junction. *C,* Cementum; *Dent,* dentin. (Redrawn from Stone, S., and Kalis, P.J.: Periodontics, Module 6. In Dunn, M.J., editor: Dental auxiliary practice, Baltimore, 1975, Williams & Wilkins.)

(2) Cemental resorption

(3) Calculus

(4) Decalcification or caries

(5) Anomalies

(6) Abrasion

(7) Overhanging or deficient filling

(8) Previous instrumentation grooves or scratches

4. Diseased, altered cementum
   a. As the junctional epithelium migrates along the root surface, the pocket deepens and the periodontal ligament detaches
   b. Cementum is exposed to the pocket environment; the pocket contains many microorganisms, bacterial products, sulcus fluid, and white blood cells
   c. Cementum is altered, and its physical and chemical properties are changed; bacterial products become incorporated, especially endotoxin, which can interfere with healing of periodontal tissues
   d. Calculus subsequently forms on the exposed cementum
      (1) Rough surface of calculus harbors many microorganisms of subgingival plaque, which perpetuate inflammation in the pocket wall
      (2) Diseased cementum must be removed during instrumentation to create an environment for tissue healing and reattachment

5. Cementoenamel junction (Fig. 13-2)
   a. Cementum overlaps enamel—60% to 65%
   b. Cementum and enamel meet directly—30%
   c. Small zone of dentin between cementum and enamel—5% to 10%

Calculus

See Chapters 7 and 11, sections on bacterial dental plaque

A. Definition
   1. Calcified or mineralized bacterial plaque
   2. Hard tenacious mass that forms on the clinical crown* of natural teeth and on dentures and other dental appliances
   3. Surface is very rough and is covered by a layer of bacterial plaque
   4. Calculus is designated clinically as light, moderate, or heavy, based on quantity and hardness

B. Types, distribution, and shape
   1. Supragingival (supramarginal, salivary)
      a. Located above the gingival margin
      b. Rarely generalized
      c. Most frequent locations
         (1) Lingual mandibular anterior teeth
         (2) Facial maxillary molars
         (3) Teeth out of occlusion
      d. Subgingival calculus may become supragingival when the pocket wall shrinks and recession occurs
      e. Shape—determined by the anatomy of the teeth, contour of the gingival margin, and pressure of the tongue, lips, and cheeks
         (1) Generally amorphous, bulky
         (2) Gross deposits may form an interproximal bridge between adjacent teeth and/or extend over the margin of the free gingiva
   2. Subgingival (submarginal, serumal)
      a. Located below or beneath the gingival margin
      b. May be generalized or localized; heaviest on proximal surfaces
      c. Extends along the root surface nearly to the bottom of the pocket; the newest, less calcified calculus is at the most apical area, near the soft tissue attachment
      d. Shape—flattened to conform to pressure from the gingival pocket wall; forms of calculus on the tooth surface may include combinations of the following
         (1) Crusty, spiny, or nodular
         (2) Ledge or ringlike formations
         (3) Thin, smooth veneers
         (4) Finger and fernlike formations
         (5) Individual calculus islands

---

*The clinical crown is the part of the tooth above the attached periodontal tissues—the part of the tooth where clinical techniques and instrumentation are applied. The clinical root is the part of the tooth to which periodontal fibers are attached.

C. Modes of attachment—calculus is more readily removed from some tooth surfaces than others; difficulty is related to the manner in which the calculus is attached; on any one tooth more than one mode of attachment can be observed; attachment to hard, smooth enamel is different from attachment to the rough, porous, less hard cemental surface
   1. By an acquired pellicle
      a. Pellicle is a thin, homogeneous, acellular layer that occurs on all exposed tooth surfaces; it appears between the smooth tooth surface and the calculus deposit
      b. Calculus may be removed readily, since there is no interlocking or penetration; this is the most frequent mode of attachment to enamel
   2. By minute irregularities in the tooth surface that permit locking into undercuts
      a. Enamel irregularities—cracks, lamellae, carious defects
      b. Cemental irregularities—tiny spaces left where Sharpey's fibers were detached, resorption lacunae, scaling grooves, cemental tears, or fragmentation
      c. Difficult to detect complete removal, since the instrumentation may smooth the surface over an irregularity
   3. By direct attachment of the calcified calculus matrix to the tooth surface
      a. Interlocking of inorganic crystals of the tooth with the mineralizing plaque
      b. During removal distinction between calculus and cementum is difficult
D. Examination and identification of calculus
   1. Supragingival/supramarginal
      a. Direct observation using appropriate procedures of retraction and lighting; mouth mirror is used for indirect lighting and vision
      b. Compressed air—small amounts of calculus may be invisible when wet with saliva; retraction and drying with gentle air stream helps to make the calculus visible
      c. Explorer may be needed for areas not directly observable (see section on explorers)
   2. Subgingival/submarginal
      a. Visual—calculus within a pocket may be seen just within the edge of the pocket margin; for direct vision the margin may be moved away by a gentle air stream

b. Transillumination—light through teeth may reveal dark opaque areas; calculus can be confirmed by use of an explorer
      c. Tactile
         (1) Probe will reveal root surface roughness
         (2) Subgingival explorer can be adapted to all surfaces to detect calculus or other irregularities before treatment and at the end of treatment to verify completeness of calculus removal and tooth surface smoothness

PRINCIPLES FOR INSTRUMENTATION ▬▬▬
Basic concepts
A. Each instrument is designed for a particular purpose and is intended to be used for that purpose
B. Effective instrumentation is accomplished by certain general principles of patient and clinician positioning; visibility through adequate lighting and retraction of the patient's lips, cheeks, and tongue; and maintenance of a clean field
C. Stability during the application of an instrument depends on the grasp and the finger rest applied; stability is essential for controlled action of the instrument and to prevent trauma to the patient
D. Activation of an instrument is accomplished by adaptation, angulation, and stroke
E. Precise familiarity with the specific form, shape, and surface topography of each tooth and the relationship to other teeth in the permanent, mixed, and primary dentitions is essential to the understanding and use of the instruments

Parts of an Instrument
A. Working end—end of the instrument that contacts the tooth or soft tissue to perform the intended function; ends take a variety of shapes; some are sharp, some not sharp; examples include
   1. Blade
      a. Sharp—scaler, curette
      b. Dull—probe; the term *nib* is sometimes used to designate the working end of a nonsharp instrument, particularly in restorative dentistry
   2. Point—explorer
   3. Other—head of a mirror, spatula end
B. Shank—connects the working end with the handle; length, rigidity, and shape are designed to allow proper access of the working end to accomplish the intended instrumentation
   1. Straight—for an area with unrestricted access such as an anterior tooth
   2. Angled or curved—for an area of restricted access such as proximal surfaces of posterior teeth

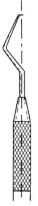

Fig. 13-3 Balanced instrument. Middle of tip (working end) should be centered over long axis of handle. (Modified from Wilkins, E.M.: Clinical practice of the dental hygienist, ed. 5, Philadelphia, 1983, Lea & Febiger.)

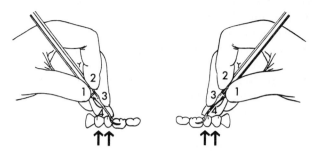

Fig. 13-4 Modified pen grasp. Thumb *(1)* and index finger *(2)* are held opposite each other near junction of handle and shank; middle finger *(3)* is placed on shank; ring finger *(4)* is used for rest or fulcrum point. (Modified from Wilkins, E.M.: Clinical practice of the dental hygienist, ed. 5, Philadelphia, 1983, Lea & Febiger.)

3. Lower shank—part of the shank next to the working end
4. Complex shank—curette designed for deep pockets in posterior interdental areas may have a complex shank with several angles

C. Handle—part of the instrument held or grasped during activation of the blade; there are a variety of shapes, weights, sizes, and surface serrations (smooth, ribbed, or knurled)
   1. Single end—with one working end
   2. Double end—may have paired (mirror image) or complementary working ends, one on each end; paired working ends are used for access to proximal surfaces, one for access from the lingual aspect and the opposite for access from the facial aspect
   3. Cone socket—working end and shank are separable from the handle to permit instrument exchanges and replacements

D. Balance of an instrument—balanced instrument has the working end centered in line with the long axis of the handle (Fig. 13-3)

Instrument Identification

A. Classification by purpose or use
   1. Examination (examples—probe, explorer)
   2. Treatment (examples—scalers, curettes)
B. Description on the instrument handle
   1. Design name (may be abbreviated); school or individual originally responsible for the design or development (e.g., TU-17, in which *TU* stands for Tufts University, School of Dental Medicine)
   2. Design number—traditional exact number; often an instrument may be manufactured by different companies but the same number is used (example—Gracey series 1-2, 3-4, etc.)

Stabilization During Instrumentation

The instrument grasp and finger rest provide stabilization for instrument control and for prevention of trauma to the patient's teeth and soft tissues
A. Grasp—manner in which an instrument is held
   1. Modified pen grasp (Fig. 13-4)
      a. Instrument is held by the thumb and index finger at the junction of the instrument shank and handle
      b. Pad of the middle finger is placed on the shank
         (1) To hold and guide the movement
         (2) To prevent the instrument handle from turning
      c. Ring finger is the finger rest and provides the fulcrum
      d. Tightness of grasp
         (1) Light grasp is needed for increased tactile sensitivity (example—use of an explorer or probe during pocket examination)
         (2) Firm grasp is needed during the stroke of a scaler or curette when calculus is being removed
      e. Uses—generalized use during all instrumentation except as suggested below for the palm grasp
   2. Palm grasp
      a. Handle of the instrument is held firmly in the palm by cupped index, middle, ring, and little fingers
      b. Thumb serves as the finger rest
      c. Uses—air syringe, rubber dam clamp holder, porte polisher on facial anterior surfaces

B. Fulcrum (finger rest)
1. Definitions
    a. Fulcrum—support, or point of rest, on which a lever turns in moving a body
    b. Finger rest—support, or point of rest, of the finger on the tooth surface, on which the hand turns in moving an instrument
2. Types of finger rests
    a. Conventional intraoral
        (1) Placed on a tooth adjacent to the area of instrumentation (Fig. 13-4, note finger numbered *4*).
        (2) Precaution—not placed in line of the stroke to prevent instrument stick of the clinician or the clinician's glove in case of an unexpected movement by the patient
        (3) Conventional intraoral finger rest is considered the most desirable because it provides the greatest stability
    b. Other intraoral—variations of the finger rest may be required for visibility and access; as the rest is moved farther from the work area, less stability may be evident
3. Pressure applied—pressure on the rest should provide an even balance with the grasp of the instrument and the amount of pressure needed for the particular instrument action; excess pressure decreases stability, tactile sensitivity, and instrument control
4. Objectives—grasp and finger rest
    a. Prevent laceration
    b. Control length of the stroke

Adaptation

A. Definition—relationship between the instrument and the surface of the tooth or soft tissue
B. Characteristics
1. Correct adaptation is when the working end of an instrument is positioned to conform to the morphology of the tooth surface
2. Adaptation for line angles
    a. Roll the handle of the instrument between the fingers of the grasp to maintain correct adaptation
    b. Only a small portion of the tip or toe of the blade of a scaler or curette can be used
    c. Side of the pointed tip of an explorer is adapted so the sharp tip is held carefully against the tooth (Fig. 13-5)
    d. Round, tapered probe adapts readily around a line angle; flat, rectangular probe must be removed and turned for adaptation at a line angle

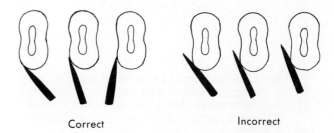

Correct   Incorrect

Fig. 13-5 Adaptation of explorer tip. Side of sharp tip is held carefully against tooth surface; at line angle correct adaptation is maintained by rolling handle between fingers of grasp. (Redrawn from Pattison, G.L., and Pattison, A.M.: Periodontal instrumentation, a clinical manual, Reston, Va., 1979, Reston Publishing Co., Inc.)

Angulation

A. Definition— angle formed by a working end of an instrument with the surface to which the instrument is applied; each instrument is applied to a surface in a specific manner for optimal action
B. Probe—usual adaptation of a probe is to maintain the side of the blade on the tooth with the long axis of the blade nearly parallel with the tooth surface
C. Explorer
1. Occlusal surface—tip is held at a right angle to detect occlusal pit or fissure caries
2. Smooth surface
    a. Side of the tip is held against the surface at no more than a 5-degree angle to detect surface irregularities; may require turning or rolling between the fingers depending on each type of explorer (see section on explorers)
    b. For a subgingival explorer, a close adaptation and a 5-degree angle prevent unnecessary trauma to the pocket or sulcus soft tissue
D. Scalers and curettes
1. Scaling and root planing—angle between 45 and 90 degrees is formed by the tooth surface with the face of the blade, with approximately 70 degrees a usual position; burnishing of the calculus may result with an angle of under 45 degrees
2. Closed gingival curettage—curette is angulated against the soft tissue pocket wall at less than 90 degrees but no less than 45 degrees

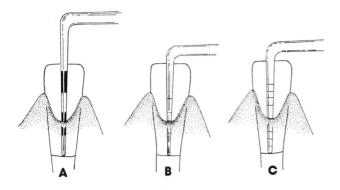

Fig. 13-6 Measurement of same 5 mm pocket with three different probes. **A,** Color coded. **B,** Michigan O. **C,** Williams. (From Wilkins, E.M.: Clinical practice of the dental hygienist, ed. 5, Philadelphia, 1983, Lea & Febiger.)

Lateral Pressure

A. Definition—pressure of the instrument against the tooth during activation; described as light, moderate, or heavy
B. Explorers and probe—for the detection instruments, a light touch but with definite contact with the tooth surface is needed for the maximum degree of tactile sensitivity
C. Scalers and curettes
  1. Exploratory stroke—light pressure until the instrument is positioned
  2. Working stroke
    a. For calculus removal—pressure varies with the type, hardness, and attachment of the deposit
    b. For root planing—pressure is progressively reduced until a light pressure is used as the root surface becomes smooth

Activation – Strokes

A. Definition (stroke)—unbroken movement made by an instrument; it is the action of an instrument in the performance of the task for which it was designed
B. Types of strokes
  1. Pull (e.g., scaler removing calculus)
  2. Push (e.g., exploratory stroke when a curette is being positioned; stroke of a chisel scaler on a proximal surface when moved from the facial to the lingual aspect)
  3. Combined push and pull (e.g., explorer in a walking stroke when the side of the instrument tip is held against the side of the tooth and moved up and down with equal pressure)
  4. Walking stroke (e.g., probe moved up and down, touching the bottom of the sulcus or pocket with each down stroke; Fig. 13-7)
C. Directions for strokes
  1. Vertical—parallel with the long axis of the tooth

2. Horizontal—perpendicular with the long axis of the tooth
3. Diagonal or oblique—diagonal to the long axis of the tooth
4. Circular—small (1 to 2 mm diameter) strokes (e.g., for a porte polisher when applying an agent such as a desensitizing agent or polishing paste)

INSTRUMENTATION FOR EXAMINATION ▬
Basic Concepts

A. Successful treatment depends on well-developed detection skills for the use of the instruments of examination
  1. Before treatment for assessment, analysis, and treatment planning
  2. After instrumentation for evaluation of the completeness of treatment
B. Complete examination involves all aspects of the periodontium and the teeth; emphasis on certain parts with omission of other parts may lead to overlooking items of importance to the total oral health of the patient
C. Patient preparation based on information from the personal, health, and dental histories is essential for safe instrumentation

Essentials for Effective Use of Examination Instruments

A. Accessibility
  1. Patient and clinician position
  2. Retraction
  3. Isolation and maintenance of a clean field
B. Visibility
  1. Adequate illumination
  2. Mouth mirror
    a. Purposes
      (1) Indirect vision
      (2) Indirect illumination
      (3) Transillumination
      (4) Retraction of the tongue and cheeks
    b. Technique for use—modified pen grasp with a finger rest placed to provide stability and to aid in retraction

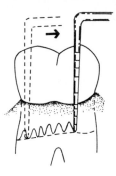

Fig. 13-7 Probe walking stroke. Side of tip of probe is held in contact with tooth. From base of pocket, probe is moved up and down in 1 to 2 mm strokes. Attached periodontal tissue is contacted on each downstroke to identify pocket depth in each area. (Redrawn from Wilkins, E.M.: Clinical practice of the dental hygienist, ed. 5, Philadelphia, 1983, Lea & Febiger.)

Probe

A. Characteristics
1. Straight blade
   a. Shape—slender, rodlike, with a smooth rounded end; may be tapered or straight; round, flat, or rectangular in cross section
   b. Calibrations—millimeter marks at intervals specific for each probe design; some are colored coded; examples of markings (Fig. 13-6) include
      (1) Williams—1-2-3-5-7-8-9-10 mm
      (2) Michigan 0—3-6-8 mm
      (3) Color coded—3-6-9-12 mm; 3-6-8-11 mm
2. Curved blade—noncalibrated furcation probe: curved, narrow, smooth probe with rounded blunt end for investigation of the topography within a furcation area; (e.g., Nabers probes)
B. Purposes and uses
1. Assess the periodontal status and prepare the treatment plan
   a. Aid in classifying the patient's disease as gingivitis or periodontitis by determining pocket depth, the level of periodontal attachment, and whether there is bone loss
   b. Determine the extent of inflammation in conjunction with the pocket depth and attachment level; bleeding on probing is an early sign of inflammation
2. Make a sulcus and pocket survey
   a. Examine the shape, topography, and dimensions of sulci and pockets
   b. Measure attachment levels
   c. Measure pocket depths

d. Evaluate the tooth surface pocket wall for calculus and other irregularities
3. Make a mucogingival examination
   a. Determine the relationship between the gingival margin position, mucogingival junction, and the level of attached periodontal tissue
   b. Measure the width of the attached gingiva
4. Evaluate bleeding
   a. Identify inflammation if present
   b. Prepare a gingival bleeding index
5. Determine the consistency of the gingival tissue by gently pressing on the free gingiva
   a. Firm—resists the probe, fibrotic
   b. Spongy—soft, smooth, shiny, edematous
6. Measure the extent of apparent (visible) gingival recession
7. Provide a guide to treatment
   a. Gingival characteristics, including pocket depth, bleeding, and consistency provide a basis for patient instruction
   b. Depth of the pocket defines the depth for scaling, root planing, and closed gingival curettage
   c. Anatomic configuration of tooth surfaces, shape of calculus deposits, and tooth anomalies and irregularities that complicate instrumentation may be defined by carefully probing before instrumentation
8. Evaluation of treatment outcomes
   a. Tissue response to the patient's self-treatment (therapeutic plaque control)
   b. Tissue response to professional treatment (e.g., scaling, root planing)
   c. Evidence of health determined by the probe
      (1) No bleeding on gentle probing
      (2) Reduced pocket depth
      (3) Firm tissue

Techniques for Use

A. Grasp and finger rest for all determinations
1. Grasp—modified pen
2. Finger rest—on tooth surface; fulcrum should be located near the area being probed, especially in the same arch, and where possible in the same quadrant
B. Examining pockets
1. Insertion
   a. Hold the side of the tip against the tooth with a firm but light lateral pressure
   b. Direct the tip toward the gingival margin; gently insert the probe

2. Activation
   a. Slide the probe along the tooth surface vertically; maintain contact with the tooth at all times.
      (1) Gingival pocket—side of the probe is held against the enamel surface
      (2) Periodontal pocket—probe is held against the enamel in the coronal part, and then against the root surface as the pocket extends beyond the cementoenamel junction
   b. Evaluate the nature and topography of the tooth surface as the probe passes into the pocket
   c. Interferences—any of the items listed as tooth surface irregularities may be noted; when a protrusion of calculus is felt, the probe should be passed over the surface of the calculus and guided back to the tooth apically
   d. Base of the pocket or sulcus (level of *actual* recession)
      (1) Will feel soft, resilient, and offer slight to moderate tissue resistance depending on the health of the tissue
      (2) Pressure to use—as little as possible to provide tactile sensitivity to the attached tissue; from 10 to 20 g is usually sufficient

C. Measuring pocket depth—reading the probe (Fig. 13-6)
   1. With the probe in vertical position and in contact with the attached tissue at the base of the pocket, count the millimeters that appear above the gingival margin
   2. Subtract the millimeters appearing above the margin from the total number of probe marks of the particular probe being used to obtain the pocket depth at that site
   3. When the gingival margin appears between the probe marks, use the higher number for the final reading

D. Circumferential probe strokes
   1. Pocket is continuous around a tooth, and pocket depth may vary considerably on different surfaces; circumferential probing is necessary for a complete evaluation
   2. Maintain the probe in the sulcus or pocket
      a. Proceed to examine the pocket around the tooth
      b. Repeated insertion and removal can cause trauma to the free gingival margin

3. Walking step (Fig. 13-7)
   a. Hold the probe with a moderate lateral pressure against the tooth
   b. Move the tip up and down in strokes of 1 to 2 mm, gently touching the attachment area on each downstroke while progressing in small 1 to 2 mm steps along the side of the tooth
   c. Observe probe measurements at the gingival margin with each step

E. Adaptation of probe—individual teeth
   1. Molars and premolars
      a. Insert the probe at a distal line angle (facial, then lingual) and probe in a distal direction, adapting the probe around the line angle, following the tooth contour across the distal surface
      b. Reinsert the probe at the distal line angle and proceed in a mesial direction, around the mesial line angle, toward the contact area
   2. Anterior teeth—initial insertion may be at the distal line angle or from the center of the facial and lingual surfaces
   3. Proximal surfaces
      a. Pocket depths are frequently deepest in the col area, the place where it may be most difficult to position and read the probe
      b. Advance the probe around the line angle and continue under the contact area, tipping the probe slightly as needed to ensure that the probe is applied half way, to overlap with the probe from the opposite side (Fig. 13-8)

F. Examining furcation areas
   1. Definition—bone loss extends apical to the level where the bifurcation or trifurcation begins and periodontal disease invades the area between and about the roots
   2. Types of furcations—probing of the three general classes may be described as follows
      Class I. Early, beginning involvement; probe can enter the furcation area; anatomy of the root surfaces can be felt by moving the probe from side to side, passing over the root, into the tip of the furcation area, and up the other side to the adjacent root
      Class II. Moderate involvement; bone has been destroyed to an extent that allows the probe to enter the furcation area but not to pass through
      Class III. Severe involvement; probe can be passed between the roots through the entire furcation

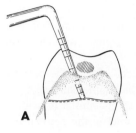 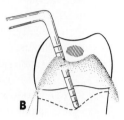

Fig. 13-8 Proximal surface probing. **A,** Probe must be applied more than halfway across from facial to overlap with probing from lingual. **B,** Probe in area of crater formation. Pocket is usually deeper on proximal under contact area than on facial or lingual. (From Wilkins, E.M.: Clinical practice of the dental hygienist, ed. 5, Philadelphia, 1983, Lea & Febiger.)

3. Anatomic features—probe insertion for furcation detection
   a. Bifurcation (teeth with two roots)
     (1) Mandibular molars—probe midfacial and midlingual aspects
     (2) Maxillary first premolars—probe from mesial and distal aspects, under the contact area
     (3) Primary mandibular molars—probe midfacial and midlingual aspects
   b. Trifurcation (teeth with three roots)
     (1) Maxillary molars—to examine around the palatal root and the two facial roots, probe midfacial, mesial, and distal aspects
     (2) Maxillary primary molars—probe midfacial, mesial, and distal aspects
4. Furcation accessibility
   a. Apparent gingival recession over the furcation; when the furcation entrance is visible, probing is facilitated
   b. Furcation covered by a soft tissue pocket wall—access with a straight probe may be hampered by firm tissue that resists distention outward when probing to gain access at the facial or lingual division of roots; specially designed, curved probe may be helpful
G. Measuring attachment level
  1. Definition—*attachment level* refers to the position of the periodontal attached tissue at the base of a sulcus or pocket as measured from a fixed point
  2. Rationale
   a. Pocket depth is changeable because of the variability of the position of the gingival margin as inflammation fluctuates
   b. Measuring from a fixed point provides a more significant indication of the level of the attached tissue

   c. More realistic evaluation can be made of the outcome of periodontal therapy and the stability of the tissue attachment during maintenance; when periodontal disease is active, pocket formation can continue and the attachment fibers migrate along the root surface; attachment level changes
  3. Fixed points from which measurement can be made—cementoenamel junction is usually used, or a margin of a permanent metallic restoration; in research studies a notch may be made on the tooth
  4. Area of apparent (visible) recession
   a. Measure directly from the cementoenamel junction to the base of the pocket
   b. Scale away calculus if the cementoenamel junction is obliterated
  5. Area where the cementoenamel junction is covered by a soft tissue pocket wall
   a. Scale as necessary to uncover the cementoenamel junction subgingivally
   b. Apply the probe and determine by tactile sensitivity the location of the cementoenamel junction; measure the distance from the gingival margin to the cementoenamel junction
   c. Subtract the distance from the gingival margin to the cementoenamel junction from the total pocket depth to obtain the attachment level
H. Measuring the amount of attached gingiva (Fig. 13-9)
  1. Measure the amount of total gingiva (free and attached) by placing the probe on the outside of the oral gingiva and measuring from the gingival margin to the mucogingival junction
  2. Measure the sulcus or pocket depth and subtract that amount from the amount of total gingiva to obtain the width of the attached gingiva
  3. When the pocket depth is equal to or greater than the amount of total gingiva, there is no attached gingiva; if the probe goes through the mucogingival junction, it means there is mucogingival involvement

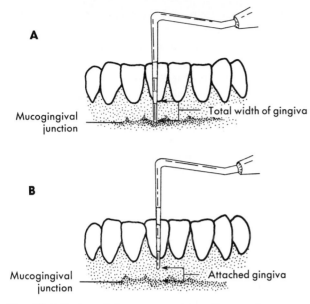

A

Mucogingival junction

Total width of gingiva

B

Mucogingival junction

Attached gingiva

Fig. 13-9 Determining amount of attached gingiva. **A,** On surface of gingiva, measure from gingival margin to mucogingival junction to find total width of gingiva. **B,** Measure pocket depth. Width of attached gingiva equals total width of gingiva minus pocket depth. (Modified from Nield, J.S., and O'Connor, G.H.: Fundamentals of dental hygiene instrumentation, Philadelphia, 1983, W.B. Saunders Co.)

I. Bleeding on probing
  1. Rationale
    a. Bleeding on probing is a significant indicator of the presence of inflammation and is an earlier clinical sign than the appearance of marginal redness
    b. Bleeding on probing correlates with increases in motile organisms, especially spirochetes, in the pocket
    c. No bleeding on probing is a criterion for healthy tissue
  2. Bleeding indices—several indices have been developed for use in clinical and research evaluation; scores can be helpful motivating devices for patient cooperation during therapeutic plaque control
  3. Procedure
    a. Insert the probe a few millimeters into the pocket
    b. Slide the probe horizontally along the pocket wall with light pressure
    c. Spongy tissue of a pocket wall will usually bleed near the orifice; firm chronic pocket linings do not usually bleed until the probe is in the deeper part of the pocket

Probing Factors Summarized

A. Characteristics of a satisfactory technique
  1. Minimal trauma to the tissues and minimal patient discomfort
  2. Time spent is minimal
  3. Findings are consistent; dependable for comparison so that tissue changes may be clearly evident
B. Influence of the severity of the periodontal disease
  1. Tissue resistance—with application of light pressure, the probe is passed to the attached tissue level; diseased tissue offers less resistance, so that with increased severity of periodontal disease the probe inserts to a deeper level
  2. Position of the probe tip
    a. Normal tissue—probe is stopped at the base of the sulcus (crevice), which is the coronal part of the junctional epithelium
    b. Gingivitis and early periodontitis—probe tip is within the junctional epithelium
    c. Advanced periodontitis—probe tip may penetrate through the junctional epithelium to reach the attached connective tissue fibers
C. Factors that affect accurate probe determinations
  1. Probe itself
    a. Calibration—must be accurately marked
    b. Thickness—a thinner probe may slip through the tissue more easily
    c. Readability—aided by clear markings, color coding, and technique
  2. Technique—control and stability
    a. Grasp—appropriate for maximal tactile sensitivity
    b. Finger rest—always on a firm tooth surface; contributes to uniform application
    c. Placement problems
      (1) Anatomic variations—tooth contours, furcations, contact areas.
      (2) Interferences—calculus, anomalies, irregular margins of restorations and others
      (3) Accessibility, visibility.
  3. Technique—pressure needed is only enough to detect by tactile means the level of attached tissue, whether that is the junctional epithelium or the deep connective tissue fibers; using a securely placed finger rest, a light pressure of 10 to 20 g should be sufficient

Explorers

A. Characteristics
  1. Flexible, thin wire, round in cross section, with angulated or straight shank for application of the sharp tip to the tooth surfaces; some are designed primarily for supragingival, others for subgingival, instrumentation
  2. Design
     a. Single—may be a universal tip or designed for specific application
     b. Paired—mirror images of each other, curved to provide access to contralateral tooth surfaces
  3. Shapes—many different explorers are available; general shapes with specific examples are as follows
     a. Orban-type explorer (e.g., TU-17, Orban 20)—balanced instrument with a short tip (less than 2 mm) for adaptation to narrow roots and configurations of the subgingival tooth surfaces (see Fig. 13-3); long straight lower shank permits use in deep pockets
     b. Curved No. 3 explorer—single-ended, tapered instrument applicable to varying degrees of depth in pockets depending on the anatomic interferences of tooth contours and flexibility of the soft tissue pocket wall
     c. Pigtail or cow-horn explorers—paired, double-ended, designed especially for proximal surfaces; limited to access in 4 to 5 mm pockets because of the wide curvature near the working end
     d. Shepherd's hook—sickle-shaped explorer usually of a thicker wire; useful for supragingival examinations for dental caries and irregular margins of restorations; difficult to adapt for fine determinations on proximal surfaces; not applicable in pockets
B. Purposes and uses
  1. Detect, by tactile sensitivity, the texture and character of tooth surfaces before (for treatment planning), during, and after treatment to assess the progress and completeness
  2. Examine supragingival tooth surfaces for
     a. Calculus
     b. Decalcified and carious lesions
     c. Defects in tooth surfaces and margins of restorations
     d. Anomalies
     e. Other irregularities not apparent to direct observation or that need confirmation by exploring after direct observation

  3. Examine subgingival surfaces for
     a. Calculus
     b. Decalcified and carious lesions
     c. Diseased, altered cementum
     d. Cemental changes that may have resulted from pocket formation
     e. Anomalies
     f. Anatomic grooves, curvatures, furcations, and other configurations where instrumentation may be required
  4. Define the extent of instrumentation for treatment procedures of the tooth surface, including
     a. Scaling and root planing
     b. Finishing of restorations
     c. Removal of overhanging margins
     d. Sealant placement
  5. Evaluate completeness of scaling and root planing by detection of smooth surfaces where instrumentation was performed
  6. Evaluation of tooth surfaces, restorations, and sealants at each recall follow-up

Techniques for Use

A. Basic instrumentation for all explorers
  1. Consistency of findings—it is important that a routine application that will relay consistent comparative information be used
  2. Grasp—modified pen grasp
  3. Finger rest—a definite finger rest on a tooth surface is necessary
     a. For complete control of the fine, sharp explorer
     b. For uniform tactile sensitivity
B. Supragingival adaptation
  1. Unnecessary exploring should be avoided; with adequate light and a source of air, direct vision or indirect vision with a mouth mirror can provide the necessary information; confirmation with gentle exploration can then be made
  2. Sensitivity—cervical third of the anatomic crown and the root surface apical to the cementoenamel junction are usually the most sensitive to air blasts and the touch of metal instruments
  3. Adapt the side of the explorer tip to the tooth surface with a light but definite lateral pressure
  4. Lead with the tip around line angles by rolling the handle to maintain adaptation of the tip

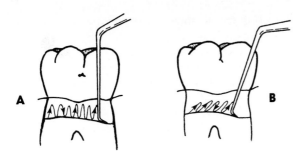

Fig. 13-10 Explorer walking stroke. With side of explorer tip in contact with tooth surface at all times, explorer is moved over surface in, **A**, vertical walking stroke or, **B**, diagonal or oblique walking stroke. Complete exploration of tooth surface is needed; therefore groups of strokes are overlapped. (Modified from Wilkins, E.M.: Clinical practice of the dental hygienist, ed. 5, Philadelphia, 1983, Lea & Febiger.)

5. Restorations—follow the margins of all restorations around with an explorer to detect margin irregularities; overhanging or deficient margins may or may not appear in radiographs depending on the angulation and tooth surface

C. Subgingival adaptation (single explorers No. 3 and No. TU-17)
   1. Hold the side of the sharp tip always against the tooth surface; position with the lower shank (part next to the tip) nearly parallel with the long axis of the tooth
   2. Slide the tip under the margin of the gingiva, down the tooth surface until the base of the pocket is felt with the back of the tip in a manner similar to that described for the probe; calculus and other rough areas of the root may be detected by using a light grasp with definite contact to enhance the tactile sensitivity transmitted to the fingers
   3. Strokes—vertical or diagonal walking stroke may be used (Fig. 13-10); for a very deep pocket, the root can be divided into two or more sections; great care is taken to overlap the strokes
   4. Proximal surfaces
      a. Lead with the tip into the proximal area; do not "back into" an area with the heel of the explorer
      b. As the walking step strokes are continued around a line angle, the instrument handle is rolled between the fingers of the grasp to ensure continued adaptation of the sharp tip
      c. Continue strokes under the contact area to provide careful examination of the entire exposed tooth surface; overlap the strokes from the lingual aspect with those from the facial aspect

INSTRUMENTATION FOR TREATMENT

Basic Concepts

A. Complete supragingival and subgingival scaling and root planing, accompanied by the patient's therapeutic daily bacterial plaque removal, are specific procedures in the treatment of inflammatory periodontal diseases

B. Basis for personalized patient care is *planned* rather than *intuitive* intervention; dental hygiene treatment plan is determined from the information collected during the initial questioning and clinical examinations

C. Instrumentation requirements as a part of the total treatment plan will vary with the severity of the disease, attachment levels, pocket depths, and the amount and distribution of calculus deposits

Definitions

A. Scaling—basic procedures by which calculus is removed from the surfaces of the teeth; scaling is divided into supragingival and subgingival scaling with reference to the location of the calculus

B. Root planing—procedures that follow calculus removal to include removal of residual calculus and altered cementum and the smoothing of the root surfaces; root planing may be supragingival when gingival recession or periodontal surgery has exposed the root surfaces; otherwise, root-planing procedures are subgingival

C. Overhang removal—recontouring procedures by which defective margins of restorations are corrected to provide a smooth tooth surface that will not harbor plaque deposits and will be cared for more readily by the patient

D. Closed gingival curettage—planned systematic procedure to remove the diseased pocket epithelial lining and underlying inflamed connective tissue to supplement other conservative procedures in the effort to return diseased gingiva to a healthy state that can be maintained by the patient

E. Phase I or initial therapy—series of treatment procedures employed to eliminate or at least reduce etiologic and inflammatory factors by therapeutic plaque control instruction and periodontal instrumentation including scaling for complete removal of calculus, root planing for root preparation, removal of overhanging fillings, and elimination of other plaque-retaining factors; also included in phase I therapy may be emergency dental care, endodontic requirements, removal of hopeless teeth, caries control, occlusal adjustment, and temporary stabilization; phase I is followed by a careful reevaluation; for many patients, phase I takes care of the total periodontal treatment needs and phase II is entirely for restorative therapy; for others, phase II includes periodontal surgical treatment; for all patients, the maintenance phase is the third essential phase.

F. Maintenance phase—series of recall appointments for routine examination and additional therapy as required to keep the periodontal tissues healthy without recurrence of disease; maintenance phase starts immediately following phase I and represents the long-term prevention and control program

Rationale for Scaling and Root Planing

A. Arrest the progress of disease

B. Induce positive changes in the subgingival bacterial flora (count and content)
   1. Before instrumentation the predominant characteristics of subgingival plaque are anaerobic, gram-negative, motile forms with many spirochetes and rods, very high counts of all microorganisms, and many white blood cells
   2. After scaling and root planing, the total number of microorganisms and white blood cells decreases and there is a shift to a predominance of aerobic, gram-positive, nonmotile, coccoid forms

C. Create an environment that permits the gingival tissue to heal, therefore eliminating inflammation
   1. Convert pocket (disease) to sulcus (health)
      a. Shrinkage of tissue
      b. Reduction of probed pocket depth
   2. Eliminate bleeding
   3. Change quality of tissue from spongy to firm; tissue regeneration
   4. Improve integrity of attachment

D. Make the patient's plaque control procedures more effective

E. Provide initial preparation (tissue conditioning) for complicated periodontal treatments such as surgery
   1. Reduce etiological and predisposing factors

2. Permit reevaluation: surgery may be lessened in extent and confined to specific areas, or, in certain instances, not needed

F. Prevent recurrence of disease through recall/maintenance evaluation and treatment

Rationale for Removal of Overhangs

A. Eliminate irregular surfaces where bacterial plaque can collect

B. Induce positive changes in the microflora of the pocket when the overhang extends subgingivally

C. Encourage resolution of inflammation

D. Facilitate interdental plaque removal and control by the patient

Preparation for Instrumentation

A. Dental hygiene responsibilities for patient safety during treatment
   1. Review the health history and patient's records for indications of special needs; prepare for a possible emergency
   2. Observe the patient; note signs of stress
   3. Make a blood pressure determination

B. Dental hygiene responsibilities for prevention of cross-contamination (see Chapter 7, section on clinical application of microbiology in dentistry)
   1. Postpone and reschedule the appointment for a patient with a communicable disease or open lesion
   2. Provide methods for lowering the bacterial count of the patient's oral surfaces
      a. Present instruction in bacterial plaque control using a brush, floss, and other aids *before* any instrumentation
      b. Provide an oral germicidal mouth rinse for the patient
   3. Prepare all instruments, materials, operating area, and environmental surfaces for conducting aseptic techniques
   4. Use personal barriers, including gloves, mask, and eyeglasses, for prevention of intercommunication of infective material between clinician and patient

Instruments

Scalers

A. Sickle
   1. Description
      a. Two cutting edges, formed by the face and the two lateral surfaces, converge to form the tip of the scaler, which is a sharp point
      b. Lateral surfaces meet to form a sharp, pointed back; some types are made with flattened backs

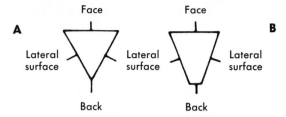

Fig. 13-11 Cross sections of two types of sickle scalers. **A,** Triangular. **B,** Trapezoidal. (Redrawn from Pattison, G.L., and Pattison, A.M.: Periodontal instrumentation: a clinical manual, Reston, Va., 1979, Reston Publishing Co., Inc.)

   c. Cross section—triangular or trapezoidal (Fig. 13-11)
   d. Internal angles of approximately 70 degrees are formed where the lateral surfaces meet the face at the cutting edges
2. Blade types
   a. Straight sickle—face between the cutting edges is flat
   b. Curved sickle—face between the cutting edges is curved lengthwise
3. Shank types
   a. Straight shank—primarily for anterior teeth
   b. Modified or contraangle—paired instruments that are mirror images of each other to provide access to the proximal surfaces, particularly of posterior teeth
4. Uses
   a. Primarily for removal of supragingival calculus
   b. May be helpful in the removal of gross deposits located just beneath the gingival margin
   c. Small sickle blades are especially adaptable beneath the contact area of anterior teeth when the interdental area is triangular and a curette may not be adaptable
5. Flat sides of a sickle cannot be adapted to the curved contours of the teeth
6. Application
   a. Angulation—face of the blade is adapted to the tooth surface at an angle of approximately 70 degrees (less than 90 degrees but more than 45 degrees)
   b. Stroke—pull stroke may be vertical or oblique
B. Hoe scaler
  1. Description
   a. Single straight cutting edge beveled at a 45-degree angle to the end of the blade

   b. Blade turned at a 99- to 100-degree angle to the shank
   c. Shank variously angulated for adaptation of the cutting edge to tooth surfaces; some hoes are paired, double-ended instruments
2. Uses
   a. Removal of gross supragingival deposits
   b. May be helpful for removal of gross calculus 2 to 3 mm below the gingival margin, provided the tissue is soft and flexible and can easily be displaced by the bulky hoe scaler
3. Contraindications and precautions
   a. Lack of adaptability of the wide straight cutting edge to the curved tooth surfaces
   b. Difficulty in use on cementum because of the ease of gouging the cemental surface with a sharp corner of the cutting edge; gouging may also occur because it is not possible to apply an even pressure with the whole cutting edge
   c. Impossible to reach the base of a pocket because of the size and shape of the blade without overextension and trauma to the soft tissue pocket wall
4. Application
   a. Place the blade under a deposit and use a pull vertical stroke
   b. Use a working angulation of approximately 90 degrees
   c. Balance the instrument by making a two-point contact (the cutting edge is on the deposit and the side of the shank is held against the crown of the tooth)
   d. Primarily for facial and lingual surfaces or on proximal surfaces adjacent to edentulous areas
C. Chisel scaler
  1. Description
   a. Single straight cutting edge beveled at 45 degrees
   b. Blade is continuous with a slightly curved shank
2. Uses
   a. Removal of gross supragingival calculus from exposed proximal surfaces of anterior teeth when interdental soft tissue is missing
   b. Appropriate for dislodgement of heavy calculus, such as a continuous bridge of calculus across several teeth
3. Precautions
   a. Straight cutting edge not readily adaptable to curved tooth surfaces

b. Sharp edges and ends of blade can nick and groove the tooth surface, particularly the cementum

4. Application
   a. Apply with a horizontal push stroke
   b. Do not direct a push stroke toward the sulcus or pocket to prevent calculus from becoming imbedded

D. File scaler
   1. Description
      a. Multiple cutting edges lined up as a series of hoes on a round, oval, or rectangular base
      b. Blades turned at a 90- or 105-degree angle to the shank
      c. Shanks are variously angulated similar to the hoes; some are paired and double ended; others are single ended
   2. Uses
      a. Supplementary instrument used selectively for gross calculus removal
      b. Useful for smoothing down overextended or rough amalgam restorations in sites where the file can be effectively applied, such as on certain proximal surfaces or with great care in a cervical area
   3. Precautions
      a. Blades are straight on a flat base, so are not readily adaptable to curved tooth surfaces
      b. Where a tooth surface is rounded, the file blade would have a tangential relationship
      c. Where the tooth surface is convex, the file blade would form a bridge over the dip
   4. Application
      a. Apply with a pull stroke
      b. Excessive pressure could lead to gouging

Curette

A. Description
   1. Two cutting edges that converge in a round toe on a curved spoon-shaped blade; cutting edge is continuous around the blade (Fig. 13-12)
   2. Face—inner surface between the cutting edges; flat in cross section and curved lengthwise
   3. Back is rounded, continuous with the lateral surfaces
   4. Internal angles of approximately 70 degrees are formed where the lateral surfaces meet the face at the cutting edges
   5. Shank is curved, with the shank, handle, and blade in a relatively flat plane in curettes designed for anterior instrumentation; for posterior teeth, the shank is contraangled for access

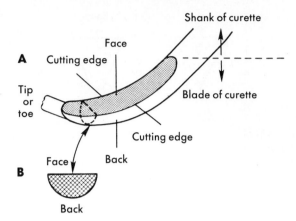

Fig. 13-12 Parts of a curette. **A,** Labeled diagram to show specific parts of curette blade. **B,** Cross section of blade. (Modified from Parr, R.W., et al.: Subgingival scaling and root planing, Berkeley, Calif., 1976, Praxis Publishing Co.)

B. Characteristics of a universal curette
   1. May be adapted for instrumentation on any tooth surface; with paired mirror-image ends, usually placed on a double-ended handle
   2. Both cutting edges are sharpened and used; proper angulation determines the side that fits a given surface to be treated

C. Characteristics of area-specific curettes (Gracey series; seven pairs)
   1. Only one cutting edge is used: the longer, outer cutting edge
   2. Blade is "offset" at an angle of approximately 60 degrees with the lower shank
   3. The curette pairs are designed for specific adaptation to certain teeth and certain surfaces

D. Uses
   1. Standard instrument for subgingival instrumentation, including scaling, root planing, and closed gingival curettage
   2. Used after ultrasonic scaling to complete the root planing
   3. Recommended for fine supragingival calculus, particularly near the free gingival margin where the triangular back of a scaler could lacerate
   4. Useful for obtaining a sample of subgingival plaque to place on a glass slide to observe with a phase microscope

E. Application
   1. Angulation—blade is applied so that the face forms an angle of approximately 70 degrees with the tooth surface (less than 90 degrees but no less than 45 degrees (Fig. 13-13)
   2. Strokes—pull stroke only is used, in a vertical or oblique direction

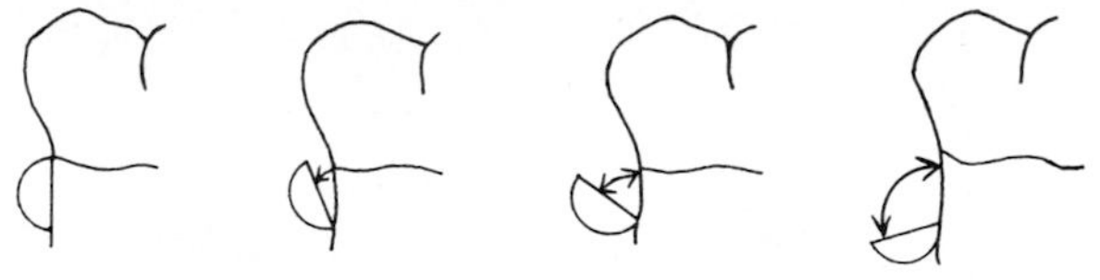

0°   <45°   45°-90°   >90°

Fig. 13-13 Curette blade in cross section positioned at various angulations against tooth surface: 0 degrees for insertion into pocket, less than 45 degrees ineffective for instrumentation, 45 to 90 degrees used for scaling and root planing, and greater than 90 degrees against soft tissue pocket wall for gingival curettage. (Redrawn from Pattison, G.L. and Pattison, A.M.: Periodontal instrumentation: a clinical manual, Reston, Va., 1979, Reston Publishing Co., Inc.)

3. Universal curettes are used initially to remove as much calculus as possible; smaller curettes and the area-specific Graceys are for fine scaling and root planing
4. Design features that make curettes the instruments of choice for subgingival instrumentation are
   a. Curved blade that can be adapted to curved tooth surfaces
   b. Rounded, smooth back that permits placement at the base of the pocket without irritation or trauma

Steps in a Treatment Appointment

A. Treatment plan—depends on the distribution and amount of calculus, depths of pockets, and characteristics of the soft tissue
   1. Single appointment—when it is expected that total scaling can be accomplished in one appointment, supragingival scaling may be completed first, followed by specific finer scaling systematically around each dental arch
   2. Planned multiple appointments—when supragingival and subgingival calculus deposits indicate extensive instrumentation, it is recommended that the dentition be divided into quadrant or sextant units and instrumentation divided among an appropriate number of appointments
B. Sequence for an individual appointment
   1. Patient disease control instruction
      a. Initial appointment—detailed introduction to instruction
      b. Subsequent appointments
         (1) Observe the tissue response
         (2) Apply a disclosing agent and record the plaque score
         (3) Reeducate the patient as needed to obtain patient dexterity, motivation, and disease control
      c. Immediate objectives for plaque check and instruction before instrumentation
         (1) Patient appreciation of importance of personal care
         (2) Removal of plaque and debris provides preoperative preparation for instrumentation in a clean environment
         (3) Removal of bacteria from teeth and mucosal surfaces lessens the contamination of aerosols
         (4) Professional time should not be spent removing loose bacteria and debris that are the important visual aids for patient instruction and can be removed best by the patient
   2. Selection of a segment or quadrant for instrumentation
      a. Probe to review pocket depths and plan strategies
      b. Explore to locate calculus and root roughness
   3. Administration of an anesthetic

Scaling

Steps for Calculus Removal
A. Technique objectives
   1. Complete calculus removal
   2. Smooth tooth surface
   3. Minimal soft tissue trauma
B. Retract and position the mouth mirror
C. Grasp the instrument
   1. Use a modified pen grasp
   2. Use a light grasp during positioning of the instrument
   3. Tighten the grasp for application of lateral pressure and strokes for calculus removal
   4. Use the thumb to roll the instrument for adaptation to tooth contours
D. Establish a finger rest
   1. Apply the finger rest—select the correct end of a paired instrument
   2. Apply the ring and little finger together for a firm fulcrum point on a tooth surface
   3. Location of the rest
      a. Near the site of instrumentation in the same dental arch
      b. Precise calculus removal with a carefully controlled stroke becomes increasingly difficult as the finger rest is moved farther away

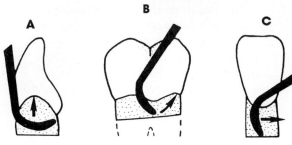

Fig. 13-14 Directions of strokes for scaling and root planing. **A,** Vertical. **B,** Diagonal. **C,** Horizontal. (Modified from Carranza, F.A.: Glickman's clinical periodontology, ed. 6, Philadelphia, 1984, W.B. Saunders Co.)

E. Adjust the grasp-hand-wrist-forearm unit
   1. Position the middle finger of the instrument grasp close to the ring finger of the finger rest to allow the hand to perform as a unit
   2. Rationale—hand and arm work together for instrument activation
     a. Control of instrument movement—less possibility of slipping
     b. Stroke length can be limited to the height of the calculus, which is the correct length of a stroke
F. Adapt the cutting edge
   1. Exploratory stroke—slide the blade lightly over the calculus to the base of the deposit
   2. Adapt the blade in keeping with the topography of the tooth surface
   3. Position the blade at proper angulation for the working stroke (approximately 70 degrees but not greater than 90 degrees or less than 45 degrees (Fig. 13-13)
G. Apply appropriate lateral pressure
   1. Grasp tenses; pressure adapts on the finger rest
   2. Nature of calculus deposit or root surface roughness defines the lateral pressure needed; lateral pressure for root planing is described in the section on root planing
   3. Pressure must be sufficient to prevent burnishing of the deposit, yet light enough to prevent gouging the tooth surface
     a. Burnishing can result from shaving the calculus by layers
     b. Burnished surface may be indistinguishable (when explored) from the tooth surface; removal may be difficult
H. Activation—strokes
   1. Direction—vertical and oblique strokes are most used; horizontal strokes may be applied selectively for otherwise inaccessible areas (Fig. 13-14)

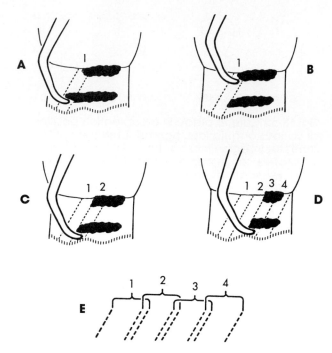

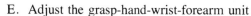

Fig. 13-15 Channel scaling. **A,** Curette inserted to bottom of pocket and positioned in contact with base of calculus deposit. **B,** Calculus removed from first channel. **C,** Curette lowered into pocket to be repositioned for scaling second channel. **D,** Curette in third channel. More than one stroke in each channel is needed to be sure tooth surface is smooth. **E,** Each channel should overlap previous one. (Modified from Parr, R.W., et al.: Subgingival scaling and root planing, Berkeley, Calif., 1976, Praxis Publishing Co.)

   2. Pull strokes in a coronal direction are used to prevent particles of calculus from being pushed into the soft tissue
   3. Length—short, smooth, even, controlled strokes for calculus removal; longer strokes for finishing and smoothing the surface
   4. Overlap—strokes should overlap to ensure complete coverage; long, large areas of deposits are treated in sections, from base to crest, with overlapping strokes; also called scaling in "channels" (Fig. 13-15)
   5. Hand-wrist-forearm unit action—strength and control are provided
     a. Movement is initiated at the fulcrum point
     b. Position of the fingers remains constant
     c. Wrist is activated back and forth or up and down (also called "wrist rock")
   6. Completion of stroke
     a. Grasp, finger rest, and lateral pressure are lightened

b. Blade is returned and positioned for another stroke

7. Circumferential instrumentation
   a. Calculus surrounding the tooth is removed section by section
   b. Blade is adapted at the line angle by rolling the handle between the thumb and fingers of the grasp
8. Area is checked frequently with a fine explorer to check progress and completion

Applications for Subgingival Scaling

A. Insertion of the instrument (exploratory stroke)
   1. After selection of the correct end of a double-ended curette and establishment of a definite finger rest, turn the blade for careful insertion into the pocket
   2. Close the face of the blade toward the tooth to insert the blade at an angle of 0 to 10 degrees
   3. Direct the toe under the gingival margin and pass the instrument over the tooth surface or calculus deposit until contact with the tissue attachment is felt; depth can be anticipated by checking the charted probe findings
   4. Adjust the blade to the correct angulation for scaling (approximately 70 degrees)
B. Strokes
   1. Vertical and oblique pull strokes, overlapped
   2. Lateral pressure—light pressure that could burnish the subgingival calculus should be avoided; heavy pressure that can diminish tactile sensitivity and decrease instrument control should also be avoided
   3. Length of strokes—will be determined by the depth of the pocket, the morphology of the tooth surface, and the nature of the deposit being removed; short, smooth, decisive strokes within the confines of the pocket will prevent the need for continued trauma to the gingival margin by repeated insertion and withdrawal
C. Characteristics of subgingival instrumentation
   1. Accessibility and visibility difficult; potential for trauma to soft tissue is greater than with supragingival instrumentation
   2. Keen tactile sensitivity required; most instrumentation will be covered and confined by the soft tissue pocket wall
   3. Adaptation of the curette at the base of the pocket can be difficult
   4. Root surface topography and tooth morphology present problem areas for instrument adaptation, including grooves, concave and convex surfaces, anomalies, narrowing of roots apically, and furcation areas

5. Pocket depths vary around the tooth; pocket narrows near the attachment
6. Subgingival calculus is harder, more condensed, and more tenacious
   a. Attachment to the tooth is primarily by underlocking in the minute irregularities or by direct apposition, which makes distinction and removal difficult
   b. Irregular deposits occur in nodular, ledge, or smooth veneer forms

Root Planing
Basic Concepts
A. Root planing is the continuation of subgingival scaling
B. Subgingival scaling without root planing can be inadequate because endotoxins and other bacterial products left within the cementum after instrumentation can provide continuing sources of irritation to the soft tissue and hence perpetuate inflammation

Procedures
A. Technique objectives
   1. Removal of all calculus
   2. Removal of diseased, altered cementum
   3. Smooth the tooth surface—no irregularities left when checked with a subgingival explorer
   4. Produce no undue trauma to soft tissue and no grooving of the root surface
B. Variations from subgingival scaling
   1. Lateral pressure—as the root surface becomes smoother with repeated strokes, the pressure is lightened to prevent grooving; even pressure is needed throughout the entire stroke
   2. Strokes
      a. Become longer as the thin layer of altered cementum is removed and the smoothing process continues
      b. Vertical, oblique, and horizontal strokes are used in an attempt to prevent or correct grooving
   3. Instrument sharpness—sharp curette is essential; use of sterile sharpening stone during the procedure is indicated

Posttreatment Procedures
A. Examination for completion of treatment
   1. Use a fine, sharp, subgingival explorer that can be adapted to the base of each pocket
   2. Adapt the strokes of the explorer in various directions (vertical, oblique, horizontal) to check for minute grooving of the cemental surface

B. Irrigate and suction—to remove particles of calculus and cementum
C. Apply pressure with sponge—to arrest bleeding, minimize the size of the blood clot in the pocket, and adapt the tissue to the tooth
D. Provide the patient with postoperative instructions

Ultrasonic Scaling

Basic Concepts

A. Ultrasonic scaling is an adjunct to manual scaling but not a substitute
B. Principal use is for gross calculus and stains during initial appointments for adult patients
C. Ultrasonic scaling must always be followed by use of an explorer for examination of treated surfaces and use of curettes to provide smooth surfaces, since tactile sensitivity with an ultrasonic device is greatly diminished or missing
D. Adverse effects on a tooth may be prevented by using low energy output from the machine, no pressure with the instrument against the tooth, a blunt, smooth insert tip applied at the correct angulation of 15 degrees with the tooth surface, and adequate water for cooling

Description

A. High-frequency electrical energy is converted by the machine into rapid vibrations of the instrument tip; vibrations approximating 25,000 cycles per second act to fracture and hence dislodge calculus from the tooth surface
B. Heat is produced, which must be dissipated by a steady water stream through the handpiece; machine is tuned to turn the exiting water into a fine spray near the tip, which helps to clear debris from the area being treated

Indications

A. Presence of gross calculus
B. Heavy tenacious deposits of calculus and stain, provided care is taken not to overheat the tooth
C. Initial debridement for a patient suffering from an acute condition such as necrotizing ulcerative gingivitis, provided loose debris and microorganisms are first removed by rinses, brushing, and flossing during patient instruction to prevent the creation of contaminated aerosols
D. Prescaling for oral surgery including tooth removal

Contraindications

A. Patient with a communicable disease that can be disseminated by aerosols
B. Compromised patient with outstanding susceptibility to infection that can be transmitted by contaminated water, aerosol, or other means (e.g., debilitated, uncontrolled diabetic, or immunosuppressed patients)
C. Patient with a cardiac pacemaker
D. Young, growing tissue
E. Primary and newly erupted teeth—danger of heat on the tissues in the large pulp chambers
F. Subgingival areas where lack of visibility and narrow pockets interfere with proper angulation of the insert tip
G. Maintenance care patients who are oriented to daily self-care, so that only small amounts of calculus accumulate between recall appointments
H. Cemental surfaces where ultrasonic scaling can remove tooth surface structure; calculus is harder than cementum
I. Porcelain jacket crowns that can be fractured by the vibration of the ultrasonic scaler

Preparation and Use

A. Operator and assistant—must wear protective eyeglasses and mask
B. Unit
   1. Run water through the tubing a full 2 minutes before use, particularly after overnight; use of contaminated water is a potential source for disease transmission
   2. Sterilized insert tip is adapted to the handpiece after the unit water has been cleared
   3. Follow the manufacturer's instructions carefully
   4. Use the lowest power setting—test by holding the tip loosely between the thumb and finger; if excessive heat can be felt, reset to a lower power setting
   5. Adjust the water flow to keep the tip constantly cool
C. Operation
   1. Apply the tip at 15-degree angle with the tooth surface
   2. Keep the tip in motion at all times with no pressure; use a light brush stroke to contact the area of calculus
   3. Provide suction with continual clearance for patient comfort
D. Completion of treatment
   1. Use manual instruments
   2. Check surfaces with an explorer for calculus removal and smoothness

Limitations

A. Visibility problem because of the water spray
B. Lack of tactile sensitivity
C. Water control difficult
D. Patient may experience sensitivity of the teeth
E. Heat produced may be threatening to the pulp tissue
F. Aerosols produced may be contaminated with pathogens
G. Hearing shifts have been reported; effect on the ears of a clinician who uses the ultrasonic scaler frequently has not been researched

Follow-up Evaluation after Scaling and Root Planing

A. Examine after soft tissue healing (10 days to 2 weeks)
B. Expected findings of clinical examination (signs of gingival health)
  1. Improved color, size, shape, consistency
  2. No bleeding on probing
  3. Shrinkage of edematous tissues—reduced pocket measurements
C. Reasons for lack of complete signs of health
  1. Inflammation from residual deposits or incomplete root planing
  2. Inadequate plaque removal procedures daily by the patient
D. Evaluation for continuing treatment plan
  1. Revision of original dental hygiene treatment plan based on effectiveness of and response to dental hygiene care to date
  2. Needs for additional periodontal therapy— recommendations and consultation
  3. Determination of recall frequency

Gingival Curettage

Basic Concepts

A. Gingival curettage is a selective procedure; when indicated, it is used to supplement the patient's disease control program (daily therapeutic plaque removal) and in conjunction with thorough professional scaling and root planing
B. Gingival curettage must be preceded by subgingival scaling and root planing to provide a smooth root surface that is free from diseased, altered cementum with irritants to the gingiva, if healing can be expected
C. Gingival curettage will promote healing by aiding the body in the removal of tissue debris from the pocket

Definitions

A. Closed gingival curettage (gingival curettage, soft tissue curettage)—planned, systematic procedure to remove the diseased lining of the soft tissue wall including pocket and junctional epithelium and the underlying inflamed connective tissue.
B. Closed subgingival curettage—planned, systematic procedure to remove the diseased lining of the soft tissue wall including pocket and junctional epithelium as well as the deep connective tissue attachment down to the crest of the bone, with the objective of producing reattachment.
C. Open subgingival curettage (surgical curettage, open-flap curettage, modified Widman flap, excisional new attachment procedure [ENAP])— surgical flap procedure in which the diseased pocket and junctional epithelium and the underlying inflamed connective tissue below the base of the pocket are removed down to the crest of the bone
D. Definitive curettage—in general, a definitive treatment is one that corrects the defect and eliminates the disease; purposeful curettage is expected to have a direct role in inflammation elimination and pocket reduction to maintainable levels
E. Nondefinitive curettage
  1. For reduction of inflammation and conditioning of gingival tissue as preparation for subsequent surgery
  2. For maintenance therapy when extensive surgery cannot be performed for various reasons such as systemic health problems, personal reasons, or emotional disturbances
F. Coincidental curettage (inadvertent, unintentional, unpremeditated)—debridement of a soft tissue pocket wall during scaling and root planing by the back and lateral side of the offset cutting edge of the curette during strokes for scaling and root planing (*Coincidental* contrasts with *deliberate,* which refers to open, closed, definitive, and nondefinitive; see above)

Treatment Objectives

In conjunction with the patient's therapeutic plaque control and the professional treatment through complete scaling and root planing, gingival curettage, as a definitive procedure, can contribute to
A. Elimination of inflammation by establishing drainage for fluids in the tissue (edema)
B. Reduction of pocket depth by shrinkage of the gingival pocket wall
C. Increased fibrosis and healing
D. Replacement of the diseased pocket lining by newly formed connective tissue and sulcular epithelium
E. Return of the gingiva to a normal, physiologic contour

Selection of Treatment Areas

A. Indications for definitive curettage
   1. Tissue—spongy, edematous
   2. Pockets—suprabony, relatively shallow
   3. Areas of persistent inflammation—after scaling and root planing has been completed and plaque control seems adequate, but tissue has not responded and there is bleeding on probing
B. Contraindications for definitive curettage
   1. Tissue—fibrotic, firm
   2. Pockets—deep, intrabony
   3. Mucogingival involvement
   4. Furcation involvement
   5. Acute periodontal inflammation such as necrotizing ulcerative gingivitis
   6. Thin, fragile pocket walls that might be punctured easily during instrumentation
C. Indications for nondefinitive curettage
   1. Preparation for pocket elimination by surgical methods
      a. Reduction of inflammation
      b. Encouragement of fibrosis
   2. Maintenance
      a. Complicated periodontal surgery is not possible because of systemic, age, or personal reasons
      b. For recall maintenance—to control recurrent areas of inflammation

Preparation for Instrumentation

A. Prerequisites
   1. Perfection of personal plaque control; without adequate daily plaque removal, benefits from gingival curettage can be expected to be short-lived
   2. Complete scaling and root planing
   3. Removal of overhanging fillings
B. Patient preparation
   1. Explanation to the patient concerning procedures, possible postoperative discomforts, expected results, and personal care responsibilities
   2. Review of the patient's history—antibiotic for prevention of bacteremia or other premedication may be needed
   3. Anesthesia
      a. Topical anesthesia may be adequate for isolated areas or for patients with a high pain threshold
      b. Infiltration is sufficient for some patients; block anesthesia may be preferred for quadrant treatment of deep pockets

   4. Root planing—when curettage is not performed at the same appointment as scaling and root planing, the tooth surfaces should be carefully checked and replaned in preparation for tissue adaptation and healing
C. Instruments
   1. Curettes for curettage should be kept separate from those used for scaling and root planing; marking tapes may prove helpful
   2. Curettes must be very sharp for efficient instrumentation to prevent undue pressure and excess numbers of strokes
   3. When it is necessary to use the same curettes that have just been used for subgingival scaling and root planing, the curettes must be carefully resharpened; a sterile sharpening stone is part of every instrument setup

Steps for Clinical Instrumentation

A. Technique objectives
   1. To remove the diseased pocket lining epithelium and underlying inflamed connective tissue
   2. To remove tissue debris and chronic granulation tissue
B. Arrange instruments and equipment
C. Isolate the area—use sterile sponges; place the saliva ejector
D. Reexamine—use a probe to review pocket depths and pocket contour
E. Select and apply a curette
   1. Select the appropriate supersharp curette from the instrument tray
      a. Use a modified pen grasp
      b. Establish a finger rest on a tooth near the area to be curetted; fulcrum finger (ring finger) is applied and maintained
      c. Identify the correct curette—face of the instrument will be readily seen (Fig. 13-16) (in contrast to the correct end for scaling and planing, when the back of the instrument is seen); remove from the area of the patient's face when necessary to reverse the ends of a double-ended instrument
F. Sequence—start with the most posterior tooth of a quadrant
   1. For convenient retraction and patient comfort
   2. For a systematic, time-saving, efficient procedure
G. Angulation and adaptation
   1. Position the blade on the tooth surface over the pocket to be treated: blade will be open and in relation to the tooth surface, at an angle over 90 degrees

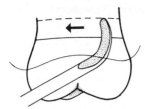

Fig. 13-16 Face of curette with instrument in position for gingival curettage. (Modified from Pattison, G.L., and Pattison, A.M.: Periodontal instrumentation: a clinical manual, Reston, Va., 1979, Reston Publishing Co., Inc.)

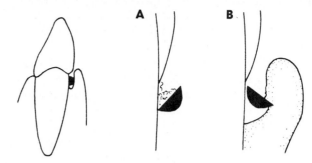

Fig. 13-17 Curette angulation during instrumentation. **A,** Scaling and root planing at approximately 70 degrees (less than 90, greater than 45 degrees) with tooth surface. **B,** Gingival curettage at approximately 70 degrees with soft tissue pocket wall. (Modified from Wilkins, E.M.: Clinical practice of the dental hygienist, ed. 5, Philadelphia, 1983, Lea & Febiger.)

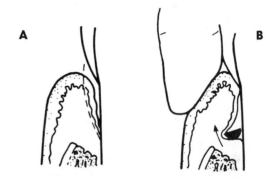

Fig. 13-18 Gingival curettage. **A,** Objective of soft tissue curettage is to remove diseased lining of pocket so that new healthy tissue can replace old. **B,** Curette positioned at bottom of pocket with cutting edge toward gingival wall. Pressure can be applied with thumb or finger to outside of pocket for support while curette is activated. (Modified from Wilkins, E.M.: Clinical practice of the dental hygienist, ed. 5, Philadelphia, 1983, Lea & Febiger.)

2. When inserted, the correct angle will be approximately 70 degrees (between 45 and 90 degrees), formed between the soft tissue and the face of the instrument (Fig. 13-17)
3. Note the relation of the handle, grasp, finger rest, and the angulation of the blade, so that after insertion the blade can be promptly positioned for action
4. Insertion
   a. Direct the toe of the curette toward the apex; open the blade for easy insertion under the gingival margin
   b. Slide the curette to the base of the pocket; use the rounded back of the curette to determine the bottom of the pocket
5. Position the blade to the correct angulation of approximately 70 degrees between the face and soft tissue
H. Activation of the curette to accomplish curettage
   1. Maintain a finger rest
   2. Tighten the grasp and finger rest slightly to allow definitive moderate pressure for tissue removal
   3. Support the pocket wall
      a. Facial and lingual aspects—apply a finger of the nonworking hand to the outside of the pocket wall to offset the pressure of the blade on the inner surface and make the cutting action effective (Fig. 13-18)
      b. Interdental papilla—apply pressure against the adjacent tooth on the opposite side of the interdental area
   4. Strokes (see Fig. 13-14)
      a. Vertical and oblique
         (1) Direct toward the gingival margin to treat the walls of the pocket
         (2) Use smooth, even strokes to include as much granulation tissue as possible

         (3) Overlap deep strokes with those positioned nearer to the margin when a pocket is too deep for a stroke to pass from the base to the margin
      b. Horizontal
         (1) Direct strokes circumferentially
         (2) Use a horizontal stroke to curette an entire facial or lingual surface
            (a) At the base of the pocket take care to follow above the probing depth to prevent deliberate detachment of attached fibers

(b) Near the margin at the pocket opening to finish off the ends of the vertical and oblique strokes

c. Removal of junctional epithelium—it has been shown that the attachment area is usually removed or at least disturbed during scaling and planing when no deliberate strokes are applied to the attachment area; therefore, only conservative strokes need be applied with intent to remove the attachment, and care should be taken not to gouge the connective tissue fibers below the junctional epithelium

d. Length of strokes
  (1) Longer, continuous strokes produce clean areas of debrided pocket wall
  (2) Length of strokes depends on the tooth contour and the ability to maintain adaptation of the cutting edge

e. Precaution—care must be taken not to pierce or tear the pocket wall

f. Completion—an experienced sense of touch can distinguish the soft, mushy granulation tissue from the underlying firm connective tissue; when the curette is sharp, only a few strokes are needed in each area

I. Irrigation
  1. Irrigate with sterile water to limit the possibility of bacteremia
  2. Use suction to remove debris from the pocket and to test for residual "tags" of tissue
  3. Remove tags by direct incision—place the curette blade at the root of the tag and press against the tooth to incise; avoid dulling the cutting edge by not moving the cutting edge over the tooth surface

J. Adapt the treated tissue; provide hemostasis
  1. Apply pressure over the area with a sponge to adapt the tissue closely and stop the bleeding
  2. Press to reduce the size of the blood clot; a small clot is beneficial during healing
  3. Place a dressing when indicated (see Chapter 11, section on periodontal dressings)
    a. To hold detached papillary epithelium in position covering the interdental area; dentist may choose to place a suture to position the papillary tissue
    b. To prevent trauma to the area that might cause additional bleeding and lengthen the healing time
    c. To minimize the clot size

K. Provide postoperative instructions (see Chapter 11, section on postoperative care)

Healing Following Curettage

A. Formation of a blood clot immediately after curettage; clot fills the pocket area, which is adapted against the tooth by pressure and a dressing

B. Initial reaction of inflammation, as with any wound

C. Proliferation of fibroblasts and new blood vessels to form granulation tissue

D. Migration of epithelial cells that arise from the epithelium at the edge of the gingival margin begins as early as 24 hours after curettage

E. New epithelium begins to cover the area within 2 to 3 days and is complete in 7 to 10 days; junctional epithelium is formed as early as 5 days

F. Connective tissue healing proceeds and is well organized by 2 weeks; immature collagen fibers appear within 21 days

G. Keratinization of outer oral epithelium may be observed as early as 2 weeks after curettage but does not reach normal thickness until 28 to 40 days

Postoperative Evaluation

A. Criteria
  1. Gingival appearance—tissue color and recession related to shrinkage progresses toward health from 4 to 8 days
  2. Probe—pocket depths and bleeding
    a. Probing should be withheld for 10 days to 2 weeks
    b. Pocket reduction and no bleeding on probing are evidences of healing
  3. Plaque deposits
    a. Effects of daily plaque removal
    b. Techniques used by the patient
  4. Residual or new calculus deposits

B. Causes of delayed healing
  1. Plaque accumulation leading to reinfection of the area; supervision of the patient's postoperative personal care is essential
  2. Trauma from external forces such as foods, misuse of toothbrush or other plaque removal devices.
  3. Smoking in excess
  4. Systemic factors that can influence healing (e.g., diseases and drugs that alter the healing ability, such as diabetes, immunosuppressive drugs)

DENTAL STAINS

Basic Concepts

A. Discolorations of the teeth and restorations occur in three general ways
   1. Stain adhering directly to the tooth surfaces
   2. Stain contained within calculus and soft deposits
   3. Stain incorporated within the tooth structure
B. Removal of unsightly stains may improve the overall appearance, but research has not shown that stain removal directly contributes to periodontal health or to the prevention of dental caries or any oral disease
C. No specific detrimental physical or pathologic effects have been shown to result from the presence of discolorations of the teeth; psychologic influences related to an individual's appearance can be significant both as regards the individual's self-esteem as well as how others respond toward the individual
D. Polishing should be considered a conservative, selective procedure because of potential deleterious effects of stain removal materials and devices on the general health and environment and on the teeth and gingival tissues
E. Decision to include polishing in an individual treatment plan can best be made after patient instruction in procedures for plaque removal daily and after complete scaling and root planing

Definitions of Types of Stains

A. Identified by location
   1. Intrinsic—stains occur within the tooth substance
   2. Extrinsic—stains occur on the external surface of the tooth
B. Identified by sources of the discoloration
   1. Endogenous—stain that originates from within the tooth
      a. Endogenous stains are always intrinsic and frequently are discolorations of the dentin reflecting through the enamel
      b. Examples of sources—drugs, changes in pulp tissue of pulpless teeth, imperfect tooth development
      c. Removal—bleaching techniques or jacket crown to cover the tooth as advised and carried out by the dentist
   2. Exogenous—stain that originates from an external source
      a. Exogenous intrinsic—becomes incorporated into the tooth structure
         (1) Examples of sources—restorative materials, dental caries

         (2) Removal—same as for endogenous intrinsic; by dental bleaching or prosthetic coverage
      b. Exogenous extrinsic—remains on the tooth surface
         (1) Modes of attachment to the tooth
            (a) Contained within bacterial plaque adhering to the tooth surface
            (b) Contained within calculus
            (c) Directly attached to the tooth surface
         (2) Examples of sources of color—drugs, foods, tobacco products, chromogenic bacteria
         (3) Removal—plaque removal by patient and scaling, planing, and polishing procedures by a professional

Rationale for Removal of Extrinsic Stain During Dental Hygiene Therapy

A. Removal of unsightly stains improves appearance
B. Removal of stains contributes to a patient's well-being and motivation to adhere to appropriate effective daily plaque removal for disease prevention

Contraindications and Precautions

The abrasiveness of the agent used, the extent of aerosols produced by a power-driven polishing device, and the integrity of the patient's tooth surfaces need particular consideration; the following are some of the specific cases where polishing is either contraindicated indefinitely or should be postponed

A. Immediate evaluation
   1. Patient susceptible to bacteremia—since bacteremia can be created during use of a rotating rubber cup polisher, the medical history must be prepared initially and reviewed and updated at recall appointments; antibiotic prophylaxis is needed by patients susceptible to bacteremia, including those with damaged or abnormal heart valves, prosthetic valves, total joint replacements, and rheumatic heart disease
   2. After instrumentation—polishing is not recommended immediately following subgingival instrumentation for scaling, root planing, and closed gingival curettage, because the abrasive agent and other constituents of the polishing paste can become embedded in the soft tissue pocket lining and, as an irritant, hinder the progress of healing; it is recommended that the use of a power-driven polishing cup be withheld until the tissue has healed

3. Enlarged, inflamed gingival tissue—polishing is not recommended at any age when the gingiva is enlarged, soft, spongy, and bleeds readily on slight provocation; irritants from the polishing paste can enter the gingival tissue, and the action of the rotating rubber cup can traumatize the gingiva; it is recommended that instruction in plaque control be given and polishing be withheld until the gingiva does not bleed on brushing or probing

B. Factors related to tooth surface—polishing with an abrasive agent has been shown to remove the surface layer of tooth structure where the fluoride content is the greatest and most protective; although protection against dental caries is essential for all patients of all ages, the following are special cases where the fluoride of the tooth surface has particular significance and polishing with an abrasive would be contraindicated

1. Caries-susceptible teeth
   a. Rampant caries
   b. Radiation therapy to the oral area
   c. Xerostomia from any cause, including medications for systemic conditions
   d. Handicapped patients with limited ability to practice personal plaque removal and who have difficulty managing a caries-preventive diet
   e. Areas of decalcification—white spots
2. Areas of thin or deficient enamel
   a. Amelogenesis imperfecta—enamel in this condition is poorly calcified and partially or completely missing; teeth may be easily abraded
   b. Dentinogenesis imperfecta—enamel may be of normal thickness but may be chipped and lost early through fracturing; attrition may be evident
   c. Enamel erosion
3. Cemental surfaces
   a. Exposed surface near cementoenamel junction has thin cementum or dentin surface that can be abraded or removed by polishing with an abrasive
   b. Root-planed cemental surface is clean, smooth, and free of deposits and stains; by definition, it is "glassy smooth" after root planing; polishing with an abrasive can create a rough, scratched root surface
4. Areas of hypersensitivity—application of fluoride is a treatment for tooth sensitivity; protective fluoride must be left undisturbed
5. Restored tooth surfaces—gold and other restorations may be scratched by a polishing abrasive

C. Use of power-driven polishing
1. Aerosol production
   a. Contaminated aerosols present a hazard to the clinician, other dental personnel, and other patients in the clinic or office
   b. Power-driven equipment should not be used for a patient with a known communicable condition
2. Splatter
   a. Protective eyeglasses are needed for patients and dental team members
   b. Constituents of commercial prophylaxis pastes may include various chemicals that can cause a severe inflammatory response in the eye
3. Heat production—care must be taken to use a wet polishing agent with minimal pressure and low speed to prevent overheating of a tooth, particularly the pulp tissues of small children

Technique Objectives

A. Patient selected for removal of unsightly exogenous extrinsic stains needs instruction in how the stains can be prevented in the future
B. When a polishing agent is used, it should be after plaque control procedures have been supervised and professional scaling and root planing completed
C. Objectives of stain removal are
1. Remove surface discolorations
2. Provide minimal removal or abrasion of tooth structure
3. Minimize trauma to the gingiva
4. Minimize heat production on the tooth surface
5. Leave no damage to restorations

Manual Polishing – the Porte Polisher

A. Description
1. Prophylactic instrument with a thick handle and an adjustable working end designed to hold a wood point at a contraangle
2. Wood points may be wedge shaped, spoon shaped, or cone shaped to fit various tooth surfaces; orangewood has proved to be the most satisfactory for polishing purposes
B. Technique
1. Grasp
   a. Modified pen grasp—for all surfaces except maxillary anterior
   b. Palm—for maxillary anterior using the thumb for the fulcrum finger

2. Activation—strokes
   a. Round—small circles $\frac{1}{16}$ to $\frac{1}{8}$ inch diameter; apply at the cervical third
   b. Vertical, oblique, and horizontal strokes may be applied to all other surfaces except near the gingival margin, depending on access
   c. Arm and wrist motion is applied with firm pressure, and slow, controlled strokes
C. Special uses
   1. Patients for whom a power-driven instrument cannot be used, such as a patient with a communicable disease; manual polishing can prevent contaminated aerosols
   2. Tooth surfaces that may be inaccessible for a prophylaxis angle, such as
      a. Long proximal surfaces exposed by gingival recession or periodontal surgery
      b. Lingual surfaces of lingually inclined mandibular posterior teeth
      c. Distal surfaces of maxillary molars
   3. Homebound or otherwise bedridden patients where portable power-driven equipment is not available
   4. Application of desensitizing agents

Power-driven Polishing

A. Description of instruments
   1. Straight handpiece—connected to a power source
   2. Prophylaxis angle—attaches to the handpiece; holds rubber cups and bristle brushes
   3. Attachments
      a. Rubber cups
         (1) Attached by a mandrel or threaded stem, or snap on
         (2) Use—stain removal from tooth surfaces and for polishing restorations
      b. Bristle brushes
         (1) Attached by a mandrel or threaded stem
         (2) Use—stain removal from deep pits and fissures and enamel surfaces away from the gingival margin
         (3) Contraindicated for use on cementum or dentin because of possible grooving and scratching
B. Procedure for use of the rubber cup
   1. Grasp—modified pen grasp to hold the handpiece; position the middle finger pad to provide support; rest the handpiece in the V between the thumb and index finger
   2. Finger rest—establish an intraoral rest on firm teeth (avoid mobile teeth or pontics)

3. Application of the agent
   a. Spread the wet agent over a group of teeth (or the rubber cup may be dipped repeatedly into a Dappen dish held closely)
   b. Keep the work area wet; use the least abrasive agent possible
4. Activate the rubber cup—after applying the grasp and establishing the finger rest, bring the cup almost in contact with the tooth surface before turning on the power
5. Use the lowest possible speed
6. Apply the cup to the tooth with a light, intermittent pressure
   a. Edges of the rubber cup should just barely flare
   b. Use continuous motion—avoid holding the cup in a single spot for long to prevent frictional heat
   c. Remember, there is a space in the middle of the cup, so the action on the stain is at the rim
7. Sequence
   a. From the posterior distal aspect to the mesial aspect; from the cervical aspect to the occlusal aspect
   b. *Apply only where needed to remove stain*
C. Bristle brush
   1. Indications
      a. Selective use—only when the rubber cup cannot accomplish the stain removal
      b. Occlusal pits
         (1) Use a pointed bristle brush
         (2) Recommended during preparation for a pit and fissure sealant (used with fine pumice and water with no additives)
   2. Contraindications
      a. Near the gingival margin where epithelium could easily be denuded
      b. Cemental surfaces—both the bristle brush and the abrasive can remove and groove cementum
   3. Procedure for use
      a. Soak a stiff brush in warm water
      b. Grasp, finger rest, and other techniques are similar to those described above for the rubber cup

Postoperative Procedures

A. Remove particles of abrasive at the contact areas by applying dental floss
B. Loosen and remove particles in pockets and sulci by irrigation and aspiration with central suction
C. Provide postoperative instruction

SUGGESTED READINGS ▬▬▬▬▬

American Dental Association: Dentist's desk reference: materials, instruments and equipment, ed. 2, Chicago, 1983, The Association.

Armitage, G.C.: Biologic basis of periodontal maintenance therapy, Berkeley, Calif., 1980, Praxis Publishing Co.

Canis, M.F., Kramer, G.M., and Pameijer, C.M.: Calculus attachment: review of the literature and new findings, J. Periodontol. **50:**406, 1979.

Carranza, F.A.: Glickman's clinical periodontology, ed. 6, Philadelphia, 1984, W.B. Saunders Co.

Goldman, H.M., and Cohen, D.W.: Periodontal therapy, ed. 6, St. Louis, 1980, The C.V. Mosby Co.

Grant, D.A., Stern, I.B., and Everett, F.G.: Periodontics, ed. 5, St. Louis, 1979, The C.V. Mosby Co.

Lang, N.P., Kiel, R.A., and Anderhalden, K.: Clinical and microbiological effects of subgingival restorations with overhanging or clinically perfect margins, J. Clin. Periodontol. **10:**563, 1983.

Listgarten, M.A.: Structure of the microbial flora associated with periodontal health and disease in man: a light and electron microscopic study, J. Periodontol. **47:**1, 1976.

Listgarten, M.A., and Helldén, L.: Relative distribution of bacteria at clinically healthy and periodontally diseased sites in humans, J. Clin. Periodontol. **5:**115, 1978.

Mousquès, T., Listgarten, M.A., and Phillips, R.W.: Effect of scaling and root planing on the composition of the human subgingival microbial flora, J. Periodont. Res. **15:**144, 1980.

Nield, J.S., and O'Connor, G.H.: Fundamentals of dental hygiene instrumentation, Philadelphia, 1983, W.B. Saunders Co.

Parr, R.W., Green, E., and Miller, S.R.: Hygienists in periodontal maintenance therapy, Berkeley, Calif., 1978, Praxis Publishing Co.

Parr, R.W., John, R., and Ratcliff, P.A.: Tooth preparation, Berkeley, Calif., 1974, Praxis Publishing Co.

Parr, R.W., et al.: Subgingival scaling and root planing, Berkeley, Calif., 1976, Praxis Publishing Co.

Pattison, G.L., and Pattison, A.M.: Periodontal instrumentation: a clinical manual, Reston, Va., 1979, Reston Publishing Co., Inc.

Ramfjord, S.P., and Ash, M.M.: Periodontology and periodontics, Philadelphia, 1979, W.B. Saunders Co.

Ramfjord, S., and Kiester, G.: The gingival sulcus and the periodontal pocket immediately following scaling of teeth, J. Periodontol. **25:**167, 1954.

Rosenberg, E.S., Evian, C.I., and Listgarten, M.A.: The composition of the subgingival microbiota after periodontal therapy, J. Periodontol. **52:**435, 1981.

Wilkins, E.M.: Clinical practice of the dental hygienist, ed. 5, Philadelphia, 1983, Lea & Febiger.

Woodall, I.R., et al.: and: Comprehensive dental hygiene care, ed. 2, St. Louis, 1985, The C.V. Mosby Co.

Review Questions

1 A curette may be inserted to the attached tissue with minimal tissue trauma because its blade
1. Has a rounded back
2. Is easy to sharpen
3. Has rounded cutting edges
4. Provides good tactile sensitivity
5. Has two cutting edges

2 The cutting edge of a scaler or curette is formed by the junction of the
1. Blade surface and shank
2. Lateral surface and face
3. Two lateral surfaces
4. Back, lateral surface, and face
5. Shank and lateral surface

3 In a 6 mm pocket in periodontitis, the subgingival flora is composed predominantly of organisms that are
1. Aerobic, gram positive, and nonmotile
2. Gram positive, anaerobic, and nonmotile
3. Nonmotile, gram negative, and aerobic
4. Anaerobic, motile, and gram positive
5. Gram negative, anaerobic, and motile

4 When the probe is in position to measure a periodontal pocket, the side of the tip of the probe is held against the
1. Cementum with or without calculus
2. Enamel with or without calculus
3. Connective tissue
4. Bone
5. Col

5 While probing, the end of the probe extends beyond the mucogingival junction. The end of the probe is in the
1. Junctional epithelium
2. Periodontal ligament
3. Pocket epithelium
4. Alveolar mucosa
5. Attached gingiva

6 During probing to the bottom of a pocket in severe periodontitis, the probe tip is likely to be
1. In the sulcular epithelium
2. Prevented from reaching the junctional epithelium because of calculus deposits
3. Touching the coronal end of the junctional epithelium
4. In the middle of the junctional epithelium
5. Into the connective tissue beyond the junctional epithelium

7 Bleeding is elicited when the probe is used subgingivally in a certain patient. Which of the following is true?
1. Unless there is bleeding when the patient brushes, bleeding while probing is nonsignificant
2. Bleeding indicates the presence of inflammation
3. The patient damaged the gingiva by brushing too vigorously
4. The probe is being used with too great a pressure
5. It is normal for gingiva to bleed a little

8 Of the following which is the earliest sign of inflammation?
1. Loss of stippling
2. Marginal redness
3. Bleeding on probing
4. Tooth mobility
5. Rolled, enlarged, bulbous margin

9 Probe pressure at the bottom of a sulcus or pocket should be no more than enough to
1. Feel the top of the crestal bone
2. Balance the pressure between the fulcrum and grasp
3. Define the location of the apical end of calculus deposits
4. Feel the coronal end of the attached tissue
5. Limit the lateral pressure

10 For pocket evaluation and measurement, the pressure of a probe at the base of a sulcus or pocket should be approximately
1. 50 to 70 ounces
2. 10 to 20 ounces
3. 1 ounce
4. 50 to 70 g
5. 10 to 20 g

11 To determine whether there is furcation involvement in the maxillary left first permanent molar, it is necessary to probe the
1. Mesial and distal aspects under contact areas
2. Midfacial and midlingual areas
3. Mesial, distal, and midlingual areas
4. Mesial, distal, and midfacial areas
5. Midfacial, midlingual, mesial, and distal areas

12 Which of the following is the *best* evidence that a patient who had previous periodontal treatment is being maintained adequately?
1. The patient faithfully keeps every 3-month recall appointment
2. There is no extrinsic stain
3. The patient spends a total of up to 30 minutes daily on plaque control
4. No mobility or fremitus is present
5. There is no bleeding on probing

13 Clinical examination shows the gingival margin to be 1 mm coronal to the cementoenamel junction. Without radiographs, which of the following makes it quite sure that the patient has periodontitis?
1. The patient is 55 years old
2. Medical history shows a history of rheumatic fever
3. There is bleeding on probing
4. A pocket measures 4 mm
5. Oral hygiene is fair to poor, with visible plaque

14 The patient has apparent (visual) recession. Using the periodontal probe, you measure 6 mm from the exposed cementoenamel junction to the bottom of the pocket. You are measuring
1. Apparent recession
2. Pocket depth
3. Amount of attached gingiva
4. Attachment level
5. Amount (millimeters) of total gingiva

15 Signs of inflammation with probing readings that do not extend beyond the cementoenamel junction establish a diagnosis of
1. Trauma from occlusion
2. Gingivitis
3. Periodontitis
4. Localized juvenile periodontitis
5. Periodontal abscess

16 For closed gingival curettage the curette should be angulated against the pocket wall at approximately
1. 35 degrees
2. 70 degrees
3. 90 degrees
4. 100 degrees
5. 110 degrees

17 If root planing is performed at one appointment and a decision to perform gingival curettage is made at a subsequent appointment, which of the following is true?
1. Tissue trauma will be reduced
2. The root surface must be replaned just before the curettage
3. Less shrinkage can be anticipated
4. Plaque and debris will be easier for the patient to remove
5. Anesthesia will not be necessary

18 The technique objective of closed gingival curettage is to remove diseased
1. Altered cementum
2. Sulcular epithelium
3. Pocket epithelium
4. Pocket epithelium and underlying inflamed connective tissue
5. Cementum, pocket epithelium, and underlying inflamed connective tissue

19 A periodontal dressing placed after closed gingival curettage may be for the purpose of
(a) Preventing plaque formation
(b) Adapting detached tissue closely
(c) Excluding saliva from the wound
(d) Minimizing the size of the blood clot
(e) Protecting the area from outside trauma
1. a, b, and c
2. a, c, and e
3. b, c, and d
4. b, d, and e
5. c, d, and e

20 Although the healing tissue after closed gingival curettage may appear healthy sooner, probing should be withheld until
1. 6 weeks
2. 1 month
3. 3 weeks
4. 10 days to 2 weeks
5. 5 to 7 days

21 Root planing contributes to a reduction of inflammation in the adjacent gingival soft tissue by
   (a) Elimination of calculus
   (b) Removal of altered cementum
   (c) Induction of change in pocket flora to gram-negative, motile anaerobes
   (d) Enhancement of the patient's plaque control
   (e) Removal of endotoxin
   1. a, b, c, d, and e
   2. a, b, c, and d
   3. a, b, d, and e
   4. a, c, d, and e
   5. b, c, d, and e

22 Which of the following are applied to minimize contamination of aerosols created by an ultrasonic scaler?
   (a) Run water through the tubing 2 minutes before each use
   (b) Wear safety glasses and a mask
   (c) Use high-power suction
   (d) Have the patient rinse with an antiseptic mouth rinse at the beginning of the procedure
   (e) Do not use the instrument for a patient with a known communicable disease.
   1. a and b
   2. a, b, and c
   3. a, b, c, and d
   4. b, c, d, and e
   5. a, c, d, and e

23 Which of the following are contraindications for use of an ultrasonic scaler for a 49-year-old obese woman?
   (a) Generalized apparent (visual) recession
   (b) "Cold sore" on her lip
   (c) Diabetes mellitus treated by diet
   (d) Thick calculus on the mandibular anterior
   (e) Moderate periodontitis
   1. a and b
   2. b and c
   3. c and d
   4. d and e
   5. a, b, c, and d

24 Which of the following is true about subgingival calculus?
   1. The surface is rough and covered with bacterial plaque
   2. The apical section is most dense and most calcified
   3. It is primarily attached by an acquired pellicle
   4. It is shaped by pressure of the lips and cheeks
   5. It is readily separated from the cementum during scaling

25 An open curettage procedure is one that requires
   1. Anesthesia
   2. A firm, collaginous tissue
   3. Gracey curettes
   4. A flap procedure
   5. A periodontal dressing

26 Endotoxin is deposited in altered cementum from
   1. Sulcus fluid
   2. Bacteria
   3. White blood cells
   4. Saliva
   5. Calculus

27 The most common relationship of the cementum and enamel at the cementoenamel junction is
   1. The cementum and enamel meet directly
   2. There is a small zone of dentin between the enamel and cementum
   3. The cementum overlaps the enamel
   4. The enamel overlaps the cementum
   5. The dentin overlaps the enamel

28 After closed gingival curettage the following can be expected
   (a) Increased amount of attached gingiva
   (b) Resolution of inflammation
   (c) Reduction of probed pocket depth
   (d) Regeneration of crestal bone
   (e) Improved attachment level
   1. a and b
   2. b and c
   3. c and d
   4. d and e
   5. a and e

29 Which of the following is true of "pocket" epithelium? It
   1. Forms during healing after gingival curettage
   2. Contains thick basal layer cells
   3. Forms the lining of the gingival sulcus
   4. Is transformed sulcular epithelium
   5. Is another name for long junctional epithelium

30 A gingival pocket results from
   1. Migration of junctional epithelium
   2. Enlargement of gingival tissue
   3. Changes in attachment level
   4. Loss of crestal bone in col
   5. Increased fibrosis

Answers and Rationales

1. (1) The back fits at the bottom of the pocket like a hammock.
   (2) Ease of sharpening has nothing to do with the question.
   (3) No cutting edges are rounded if they are sharp.
   (4) Tactile sensitivity is not really essential to the placement, but is used on the insertion.
   (5) All curettes have two cutting edges.

2. (2) The cutting edge is formed by the junction of the lateral surface and face.
   (1) The blade surface and lower (terminal) shank blend slightly; no edge is formed.
   (3) The two lateral surfaces are separated.
   (4) The back does not meet the face at any point.
   (5) The lateral surface blends into the shank.

3. (5) The subgingival flora in a periodontal pocket is composed mainly of gram-negative, anaerobic, and motile organisms.
   (1) Aerobic, gram-positive, nonmotile organisms are a healthy composition after scaling procedures.
   (2) Gram-positive and anaerobic organisms do not appear together predominantly in a periodontal pocket.
   (3) Nonmotile, gram-negative, aerobic organisms do not appear together.
   (4) Anaerobic, motile, gram-positive organisms do not appear together.

4. (1) Cementum forms the tooth wall in the deep part of a periodontal pocket.
   (2) The tip of the probe is held against the enamel for a *gingival* pocket with no bone loss.
   (3) The probe is held against the tooth, although the tip of the probe may be in connective tissue in very severe cases of periodontitis.
   (4) The tip of the probe is never held against the bone in routine examination.
   (5) Col, by definition, is the proximal soft tissue.

5. (4) The mucogingival junction is the divider between alveolar mucosa and the attached gingiva.
   (1) When the pocket extends beyond the mucogingival junction, there is no junctional epithelium at that spot.
   (2) The periodontal ligament is on the other side of the bone.
   (3) Pocket epithelium lines the pocket down to the mucogingival junction.
   (5) The attached gingiva has been destroyed.

6. (5) During probing to the bottom of a pocket in severe periodontitis, the probe tip is likely to be into the connective tissue beyond the junctional epithelium.
   (1) The probe tip is never into sulcular epithelium; it passes along the sulcular epithelium to reach into the bottom of the sulcus.
   (2) The probe can pass over the calculus down and under to the attachment.
   (3) The probe tip might be touching the coronal end of the junctional epithelium in a healthy condition or in very early gingivitis.
   (4) In moderate periodontitis, the probe goes into the junctional epithelium.

7. (2) Bleeding on probing is an earlier sign of inflammation than color change.
   (1) Both are very significant; healthy tissue does not bleed.
   (3) Rarely is bleeding a sign of too-vigorous brushing.
   (4) Only with extremely heavy pressure would the normal gingiva bleed.
   (5) Healthy tissue does not bleed.

8. (3) The earliest sign of inflammation is bleeding on probing.
   (1) Loss of stippling is a late change.
   (2) Marginal redness occurs later than bleeding.
   (4) Tooth mobility means there is inflammation in the periodontal ligament and occurs later.
   (5) Rolled, enlarged margins accompany redness.

9. (4) The coronal end of the junctional epithelium is felt in healthy gingiva or in cases of slight gingivitis. In severe periodontitis, the probe passes through to the connective tissue fibers.
   (1) Probe pressure should not be great enough to feel the top of the crestal bone.
   (2) By applying as light a pressure as possible, the grasp and finger rest pressure automatically lighten to give more tactile sensitivity.
   (3) Probe pressure should be only great enough to feel soft tissue attachment, not hard calculus.
   (5) Probe pressure at the bottom of a sulcus has little to do with limiting lateral pressure.

10. (5) Probe pressure should be no more than necessary to feel the top (coronal end) of the attached tissue, about 10 to 20 g.
    (1) Fifty to seventy ounces of pressure is too much pressure.
    (2) Ten to twenty ounces of pressure is too much pressure.
    (3) One ounce of pressure is too much pressure.
    (4) Fifty to seventy grams of pressure is too much pressure.

For each question the correct answer and rationale are listed first. The other choices are presented in order with the reasons why they are not correct.

11. (4) For furcation involvement in maxillary first permanent molars, it is necessary to probe between the mesiobuccal and distobuccal roots, then mesially and distally for either side of the palatal root.
    (1) Probing mesially and distally under contact areas would apply to the maxillary first premolars.
    (2) Probing in the midfacial and midlingual areas would apply to the mandibular first molars.
    (3) Probing mesially, distally, and in midlingual areas would apply to no particular tooth.
    (5) Probing in the midfacial, midlingual, mesial, and distal areas would apply to no particular tooth.

12. (5) Bleeding is a serious sign of inflammation. Every recall patient should be carefully and completely (circumferentially) probed.
    (1) Keeping a 3-month recall appointment does not guarantee periodontal maintenance.
    (2) Stain indicates very little; some stains are kept to a minimum by the patient's own home care.
    (3) Spending 30 minutes daily on plaque control is good as long as the technique touches every sulcus and surface.
    (4) Mobility and fremitus are different symbols than those being treated.

13. (4) Probing 4 mm from 1 mm above the cementoenamel junction brings the attachment level down on the cementum, which indicates loss of bone; thus it would be periodontitis, not gingivitis.
    (1) The age of the patient is not relevant; periodontal disease occurs from childhood through old age.
    (2) Rheumatic fever does not predispose a person to periodontal disease.
    (3) Bleeding on probing means inflammation but does not distinguish gingivitis from periodontitis.
    (5) Poor oral hygiene with visible plaque can also be present with gingivitis.

14. (4) A fixed point, such as the cementoenamel junction, is used to measure the attachment level.
    (1) Apparent recession is measured from the cementoenamel junction to the crest of the free gingiva.
    (2) Pocket depth is measured from the crest of the free gingiva to the bottom of the pocket.
    (3) The amount of attached gingiva is the total gingiva minus the free gingiva (pocket depth).
    (5) Total gingiva is measured from the free gingival margin to the mucogingival junction.

15. (2) Not probing beyond the cementoenamel junction means that there is no bone loss; therefore it is gingivitis, not periodontitis.
    (1) Probing is not a method of diagnosing trauma caused by occlusion.
    (3) If there is no bone loss, the diagnosis is gingivitis, not periodontitis.
    (4) Localized juvenile periodontitis shows bone loss; therefore the probe can extend beyond the cementoenamel junction.
    (5) Periodontal abscess occurs with other symptoms; it would probably extend beyond the cementoenamel junction.

16. (2) Many authors believe the angulation should be under 90 degrees but not under 45 degrees; however, the far ends of that range leave questions of effectiveness.
    (1) A 35-degree angle is really the insertion for scaling level.
    (3) Using a curette at a 90-degree angle would produce "chatter" if root planing is being done.
    (4) A 100-degree angle would be wide open.
    (5) A 110-degree angle also would be wide open, almost like the insertion for curettage.

17. (2) When a firm attachment is expected, new calculus, plaque, and any existing diseased or altered cementum should be removed.
    (1) Only the instrument grasp, finger rest, control, curette adaptation, and the condition of the tissue influence trauma.
    (3) More shrinkage could be anticipated after thorough planing.
    (4) Ease of removal of plaque and debris is not relevant to the question.
    (5) Anesthesia requirements are generally the same for both root planing and curettage.

18. (4) The technique objective of closed gingival curettage is to remove all diseased soft tissue, including junctional epithelium.
    (1) Cementum is removed during root planing.
    (2) Sulcular epithelium is healthy as it lines the sulcus.
    (3) Pocket epithelium should be removed, but to remove only the epithelium would be incomplete.
    (5) Cementum is not removed during gingival curettage.

19. (4) b, d, and e are all good reasons for placing a periodontal dressing after closed gingival curettage.
    (1) The dressing may even encourage plaque collection around and under, especially since the patient cannot get to the tissue during plaque removal. Saliva also flows under the dressing.
    (2) a and c are incorrect as described above.
    (3) c is incorrect as described above.
    (5) c is incorrect as described above.

20. (4) Research indicates the attachment area is intact in 10 to 14 days, although probing should continue to be gentle.
    (1) There is no need to wait 6 weeks for evaluation.
    (2) There is no need to wait 1 month for evaluation.
    (3) Probing could begin at the end of 2 weeks.
    (5) In 5 days the epithelial lining is usually covering the sulcular wall, but the attachment is not firm.

21. (3) The change is from gram negative, anaerobic, and motile to gram positive, aerobic, and nonmotile.
    (1) After scaling, subgingival calculus that is imbedded in undercuts may remain. Root planing may be required to remove it.
    (2) Root planing takes off the diseased cementum.
    (4) With a smooth surface, tissue shrinks and bleeding is reduced; all of the factors of healing enhance plaque control.
    (5) Endotoxin is removed with altered cementum but, if left, would be toxic to the soft tissue.

22. (5) All the items described are important, but wearing safety glasses and masks will not affect the aerosols.
    (1) Wearing safety glasses and masks will not affect the aerosols but will protect the operator.
    (2) Wearing safety glasses and masks will not affect the aerosols; also, d and e are important in minimizing contamination by the ultrasonic scaler.
    (3) Wearing safety glasses and masks will not affect the aerosols.
    (4) Wearing safety glasses and masks will not affect the aerosols.
23. (1) Ultrasonic cleaning is not recommended on cementum, since it is easily grooved; herpesvirus could be aerosolized.
    (2) Patients with controlled diabetes are treated the same as normal patients.
    (3) Thick calculus would be an indication, not a contraindication, for use of an ultrasonic scaler.
    (4) The severity of the disease does not determine the need for ultrasonic scalers, only the amount of calculus present.
    (5) See the reasons above why c and d are incorrect.
24. (1) Under a microscope the surface resembles a coral reef.
    (2) The apical section is the deepest, the newest, and the least calcified.
    (3) Attachment by an acquired pellicle usually occurs on enamel, but not on cementum.
    (4) Subgingival calculus is shaped mostly by the pocket wall, which in turn receives pressure by the tongue and facial musculature.
    (5) Subgingival calculus is difficult to remove and frequently is not completely removed even after root planing.
25. (4) By definition, open curettage is a flap procedure.
    (1) Any type of curettage may require anesthesia.
    (2) Firm collaginous tissue does not shrink; it may or may not be selected, depending on other factors.
    (3) Open curettage requires any type of curette, not only Gracey curettes.
    (5) A periodontal dressing can be required for any type of curettage.
26. (2) The endotoxin occurs in the cell wall of certain bacteria.
    (1) Sulcus fluid is a thin, serouslike fluid from the connective tissue; its flow is stimulated during inflammation.
    (3) The endotoxin is not deposited from white blood cells.
    (4) The endotoxin is not deposited from the saliva.
    (5) Calculus contains endotoxin in its surface but is not a source for the altered cementum.

27. (3) The cementum overlaps the enamel 60% to 65% of the time.
    (1) The cementum and enamel meet directly 30% of the time.
    (2) There is a small zone of dentin between the enamel and cementum 5% to 10% of the time.
    (4) The enamel cannot overlap the cementum, because the enamel forms first.
    (5) The dentin cannot overlap the enamel.
28. (2) Drainage of fluid permits lessening of inflammation. The removal of diseased pocket lining provides for the development of new healthy epithelium with a reduced pocket depth.
    (1) Rarely does conservative therapy affect the amount of attached gingiva except to arrest disease and prevent further apical migration of the attachment.
    (3) Regeneration of crestal bone is not an objective of closed gingival curettage.
    (4) An improved attachment level is not a predictable result.
    (5) a and e are not correct answers for the reasons stated above.
29. (4) As disease develops, sulcular epithelium is transformed and changed by the toxic products of invading bacteria.
    (1) Pocket epithelium is removed by gingival curettage, along with the underlying diseased connective tissue.
    (2) Pocket epithelium does not contain thick basal layer cells.
    (3) The sulcus in health is lined by sulcular epithelium.
    (5) Pocket epithelium is not another name for long junctional epithelium.
30. (2) A gingival pocket results from the enlargement of tissue covering a portion of enamel, without changes in deeper structures.
    (1) During *periodontal* pocket formation the junctional epithelium migrates.
    (3) Changes in the attachment level are related to a periodontal pocket.
    (4) Bone loss is associated with periodontal pocket formation.
    (5) Increased fibrosis could occur, but it does not mean that a gingival pocket was formed.

CHAPTER 14

Dental Hygiene Care for Special-Needs Patients

BEVERLY ENTWISTLE

Every patient is a unique individual with differing abilities and dental needs. Four out of ten patients may require a modified treatment plan at some point because of "special needs." These special needs may be transient, such as pregnancy, or lifelong, such as chronic kidney failure or mental retardation. With the recent national emphasis on improving access to care for underserved populations, dental hygienists encounter increased numbers of persons with special needs. The dental hygienist must be ready to meet the challenge of treating a wide range of patients with various problems in a number of settings.

Patient considerations covered in this chapter primarily relate to specific handicapping conditions and medical problems with special considerations for various life stages. The format for each section follows a similar pattern, including definition; incidence and prevalence; etiology and diagnostic information; signs, symptoms, and clinical manifestations; general treatment (nondental treatment); and oral manifestations. The contemporary dental hygienist should be familiar with all of this information.

GENERAL CONSIDERATIONS
Life Span Approach to Care

A. Principles of growth, development, and maturation
   1. Growth includes physical and functional maturation
   2. Growth is generally a continuous and orderly process, but can be modified by numerous factors (e.g., nutritional deficiencies)
   3. Different parts of the body grow and mature at different rates
   4. Critical periods exist in growth and development
   5. Hormonal changes can alter
      a. Physical stature and function
      b. Mental state and mood
      c. Oral status
   6. During growth and maturation, perceptions of self and self in relation to others change
   7. Health status generally progesses from acute illness to chronic illness
   8. Transition from one life stage to another is gradual and not necessarily based on chronologic age
   9. Biologic aging is not synonymous with chronologic age
   10. Signs of aging can appear at any age
B. U.S. health care system
   1. Current system is categorical, with many gaps in services
   2. Need to develop a continuum of services through the life stages to ensure
      a. Continuity of care
      b. Comprehensive philosophy of care
      c. System of planned change
   3. Services should stress
      a. Heterogeneity of people bearing the same label
      b. Individualized approach to care
   4. Dental needs and approaches to care can differ throughout the life cycle (Table 14-1)

Incidence/Prevalence of Special-Needs Patients

A. National statistics on incidence and prevalence figures are difficult to compile because of
   1. Unreliable reporting systems
   2. Variable definitions of conditions
   3. Differences between acute versus chronic conditions
   4. Overlap in data when dealing with multiple conditions
B. Estimated prevalence of selected handicapping conditions is shown in Table 14-2
C. Incidence, chronicity, and severity of health conditions increases with age
D. Table 14-3 identifies the most common chronic conditions in the elderly population

Table 14-1 Life span approach to dental care

Life stage	General care concerns	Usual oral concerns
Early childhood ↓	Teaching oral care skills Preventing early occurrence of caries or trauma (protecting developing teeth)	Oral infections Dental development
Childhood	Developing positive dental attitudes and behaviors	Caries Gingivitis
Adolescence ↓	Motivating toward self-responsibility for seeking and receiving care Controlling risk factors for disease	Caries Gingivitis Dental development
Young adult	Decreasing barriers and integrating dental care into daily schedule	Periodontal diseases
Midlife	Maintaining status and preventing deterioration	Periodontal diseases
Older adult ↓	Motivating to continue preventive care and accept new theories and techniques Decreasing barriers to care	Periodontal diseases Root caries Oral cancer
Elderly	Maintaining status and preventing deterioration	Periodontal diseases Root caries Oral cancer Fractures

Dental Hygienist's Role with Special-Needs Patients

A. Recognize physical, mental, medical, social and dental needs
B. Communicate with patients and caretakers in a positive, appropriate, nondiscriminatory manner
C. Communicate with other professionals and team members to facilitate planning, implementation, and coordination of care
D. Plan, implement, and evaluate community-based and office-based programs
E. Adapt dental hygiene procedures and treatment plans to meet patients' special needs, considering
   1. Barriers to care
   2. Resources
   3. Personal skills and abilities
F. Identify and eliminate potential barriers to care
G. Assess one's own attitudes, values, and commitment to provision of dental care to these patients.
H. Evaluate local, state, regional, and national trends for their potential impact on the provision of dental care
I. Advocate preventive dental programs, full use of dental auxiliaries, and development of a sound research base for use in dental health programs.

General Definitions

These tend to change frequently and often overlap
A. Labeling—process of classifying people for educational, medical, or financial reasons

Table 14-2 Prevalence of selected handicapping conditions

Estimated number	Condition
9 million	Mental illness
6.5 million	Mental retardation
6 million	Rheumatoid arthritis
4.5 million	Seizure disorders (including epilepsy)
1.7 million	Hearing loss (to the point of severe impairment)
1.4 million	Vision loss (to the point of severe impairment)
1.3 million	Emphysema
800,000	Total paralysis
700,000	Cerebral palsy
600,000	Diabetes
450,000	Multiple sclerosis
220,000	Muscular dystrophy
121,000	Cleft lip and/or palate

Modified from Robert Wood Johnson Foundation: Special report: dental care for handicapped Americans, Princeton, N.J., 1979, The Foundation.

Table 14-3 Leading chronic conditions in the elderly population

Noninstitutionalized	Nursing home residents
Arthritis	Arthritis
Hypertension	Heart disease
Hearing impairments	Mental illness
Heart disease	Paralysis

B. Barrier-free environment—facilities that are physically accessible to people with all types of disabilities
C. Normalization—making available patterns and conditions of everyday life that are as close as possible to the norms and patterns of the mainstream of society
D. Mainstreaming—integration of people with special needs into regular communities and services
E. Access to dental care—opportunity for each individual to enter into the dental care system and make use of all available services

Goals of Normalization for People with Special Needs

A. Ensure legal and civil rights
B. Guarantee appropriate education for continued learning
C. Increase or maintain social skills and problem-solving abilities
D. Increase employment options and decrease employer discrimination
E. Ensure comprehensive network of community resources

Potential Barriers to Dental Care

A. Accessibility
   1. Financial
      a. One fourth of the elderly population have an inadequate income level; percentages are higher for women, ethnic minorities, and single heads of households
      b. In 1977, 96% of the elderly's per capita dental expenditures were out-of-pocket; few third-party payment mechanisms exist for this group
      c. Between 65% and 85% of disabled people live near the poverty level
      d. More than 15 million handicapped adults are unable to be gainfully employed because of totally disabling conditions
      e. People working in sheltered workshops or training centers generally earn less than $2000 per year
      f. Medicaid coverage for dental care is extremely variable across states, sometimes not covering adult care or preventive services
      g. Medical expenses for many handicapped persons consume a major portion of their income
      h. Many special-needs patients on limited incomes cannot afford standard private practice fees for dental care

   2. Transportation/geography
      a. Over 50% of the handicapped and elderly population live in urban settings; the remainder live in small communities or farms
      b. Public transportation is often confusing and unaffordable, or nonexistent
      c. Patients with special needs often rely on others for transportation to dental appointments, thus increasing their dependence and making scheduling difficult
      d. Homebound, hospitalized, or institutionalized persons frequently cannot be transported for care in the community
   3. Physical facilities
      a. Minimum standards for accessibility must be met by dentists who receive monies (including Medicaid funds) from the U.S. Department of Health and Human Services or practice in newly constructed public buildings
      b. External barriers include parking lots and spaces, walkways, curbs, stairs, narrow doors and entryways, too-heavy or overpressurized doors, and small-print signs
      c. Internal barriers include narrow passageways or doors, cluttered rooms or hallways, loose rugs or heavy-shag carpets, abrupt changes in floor textures, noncontrasting colors, and bathrooms without grab-bars or other adaptations
B. Psychosocial concerns
   1. Over 50% of Americans express positive attitudes toward the elderly and people with disabilities, yet most really perceive them as different and inferior
   2. Society perceives disabilities, differences, and disease states before recognizing similarities
   3. Feelings of guilt, anxiety, apathy, inadequacy, embarrassment, depression, anger, and resentment about their special needs interfere with attempts to seek care
   4. Fear of or inability to comprehend dental procedures, antisocial or atypical behavior, or overdependency on dental providers interferes with provision of care
   5. Basic daily needs and activities are often overwhelming and can determine priorities for dental health care
   6. Perception of self-image and worth can affect treatment planning
C. Provider philosophy/provision of care
   1. Surveys indicate that about 20% of dentists are willing to treat handicapped persons

2. Reasons for not treating patients with special needs include
   a. Inadequate facilities and equipment
   b. Inadequate training (therefore, knowledge and skills)
   c. Not wanting to expose "normal" patients to "special" patients
   d. Inability to collect adequate fees
   e. Additional effort and time required
   f. Personal discomfort about perceived "differences" of special patients
D. Communication concerns
   1. Sensory impairments (hearing, visual) limit the ability to transmit and receive communications when scheduling or undergoing dental care or participating in dental health education
   2. Use of technical terminology, a foreign language, or inappropriate language levels may interfere with understanding
   3. Differences in communication styles (eye contact, physical proximity and contact, formal versus informal pronouns, cultural variations, use of nonverbal cues and verbal language) impair effective communication
   4. Use of condescending voice tones or language levels closes off communication lines
E. Medical concerns
   1. Situations compromising the provider or patient
      a. Inadequate sterilization procedures (control of disease transmission)
      b. Inadequate or inaccurate health histories
      c. Inadequate precautions for potential emergencies
      d. Inadequate knowledge of medical problems
   2. Types of treatment/conditions
      a. Medications
      b. Therapies that compromise dental status
      c. Conditions requiring premedication or alteration of treatment
      d. Conditions or situations that contraindicate treatment
      e. Terminal illness or the aging process may change treatment planning or the prognosis of treatment
      f. Medical problems or disabilities may necessitate provision of care in a setting other than the office
F. Mobility/stability concerns
   1. Impaired ambulation or use of a wheelchair may hinder access to care
   2. Uncontrolled or sudden movements may interfere with home care or treatment procedures

3. Uncontrolled or aggressive behavior may endanger the care providers and the patient
4. Spatial disorientation may interfere with patient relaxation in the dental chair or performance of oral care procedures

SPECIFIC CONDITIONS

See Chapters 6 and 7

Mental Retardation

A. Definition
   1. Subaverage intellectual functioning originating during the developmental period and associated with impairment in adaptive behavior
   2. Not the same as mental illness
   3. Label represents a highly heterogeneous group of people
B. Incidence—1% to 3% of the population, depending on criteria (2.3 to 6.7 million people)
C. Categories
   1. Mild (89%)
   2. Moderate (6%)
   3. Severe (3.5%)
   4. Profound (.5%)
D. Etiology—acquired (12%), inherited (13%), unknown (75%)
   1. Infections and intoxifications (rubella, meningitis, lead poisoning)
   2. Trauma or physical agents (child abuse)
   3. Disorders of metabolism or nutrition (phenylketonuria [PKU])
   4. Gross brain disease (atrophy or neoplasms)
   5. Chromosomal abnormalities (Down syndrome)
   6. Gestational disorders (Rh incompatibility, anoxia, prematurity)
   7. Environmental (lack of stimulation)
E. Signs/symptoms/clinical manifestations
   1. Variable, depending on the etiology
   2. Unusual difficulty in learning and applying what is learned to problems of daily living
   3. Skull or other craniofacial anomalies may exist
      a. Microcephaly—small cranium that restricts brain growth
      b. Hydrocephaly—expansion of the cranium from excessive accumulation of cerebrospinal fluid
      c. Malformation or asymmetry of growth
   4. General developmental delays
   5. Other possible manifestations include motor incoordination, visual and/or hearing disorders, specific learning disabilities, emotional disturbance, medical disabilities, and seizure disorder

F. Treatment
   1. Special education and vocational training
   2. Use of appropriate community resources for identified needs
G. Oral manifestations
   1. Most dental problems are not inherent to the disability but are related to extrinsic factors (e.g., neglect by caretakers or incoordination leading to poor oral hygiene)
   2. DMFS scores comparable to those of the general population, except decayed component is higher because of a lack of professional treatment
   3. Higher prevalence of periodontal conditions, probably related to poor oral hygiene and the lack of regular care
   4. Higher incidence of malocclusion and deviations in tooth eruption if associated with craniofacial syndromes or growth abnormalities
   5. Some instances of enamel dysplasia, more commonly seen in those with severe mental deficiencies resulting from severe prenatal or perinatal defects or insults
   6. Some instances of physical self-abuse if severely impaired

Down Syndrome

A. Definition/etiology
   1. Mental retardation disorder
   2. Associated with an anomaly of chromosome 21 (trisomy 21) in all or some body cells
B. Incidence—most common chromosomal abnormality (1700 newborns)
C. Signs/symptoms/clinical manifestations
   1. Mental retardation ranging from mild to profound
   2. Poor muscular development with hyperflexibility and hypotonia during childhood
   3. Short stature with delay in skeletal maturation
   4. Short neck and extremities with broad stubby fingers
   5. High incidence of congenital heart defects and hearing problems
   6. Abnormal craniofacial features
      a. Small brachycephalic skull
      b. Round flat facies
      c. Small nasomaxillary complex
      d. Ocular hypotelorism (eyes closer together)
      e. Epicanthal folds (Fig. 14-1)
      f. Strabismus (convergent eyes)
      g. Simian crease (single transverse palmar crease (Fig. 14-2)

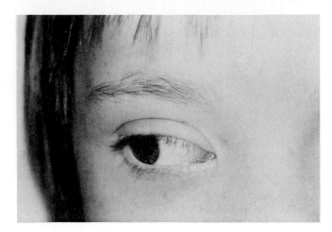

Fig. 14-1 Epicanthal fold, a characteristic of Down syndrome.

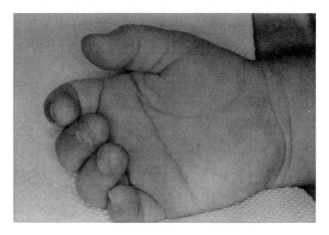

Fig. 14-2 Simean crease, one of the characteristics of Down syndrome.

D. Treatment
   1. No cure
   2. Prevention through amniocentesis
   3. Special education
E. Oral manifestations (Fig. 14-3)
   1. Relative mandibular prognathism as a result of the small nasomaxillary complex
   2. Dry skin and cracking of the lips
   3. Fissured tongue
   4. Hyperplasia of the adenoids and tonsils
   5. Altered salivary gland mechanism (decreased flow)
   6. Increased susceptibility to severe periodontal disease of early onset, especially in the anterior areas

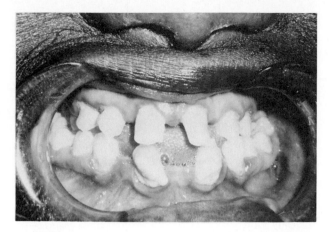

Fig. 14-3 Common oral conditions seen in Down syndrome.

7. Delayed eruption of teeth
8. Higher incidence of congenitally missing teeth
9. Small tooth crowns with short crown/root ratio
10. Enamel dysplasia
11. Malocclusion—anterior open bite or crossbite, posterior crossbite
12. Attrition

Autism

A. Definition
   1. Developmental disability with specific behavioral and communicative components
   2. Not the same as mental retardation or childhood schizophrenia, as previously thought
B. Incidence/prevalence
   1. Occurs in 5/10,000 births
   2. Four times more common in males
   3. Appears during first 3 years of life
   4. Approximately 60,000 autistic children in the United States
C. Etiology—different theories
   1. Psychogenic theories
      a. Result of adverse conditions in the child's psychologic environment
      b. Result of extreme negative feelings of parents toward child
   2. Genetic theories
   3. Biochemical theories (deficits in some)
   4. Neurophysiologic theories
D. Signs/symptoms/clinical manifestations
   1. Extreme aloneness, failure to develop eye contact, not cuddly as infants, failure to develop social relationships or perceive others' feelings
   2. Language disturbances—repetitious speech, pronoun reversals, lack of ability to use gestures; 50% never develop functional speech
   3. Comprehension problems, especially with verbal directions
   4. Obsessiveness about maintaining routines and sameness of the environment (resistance to change)
   5. Eating disturbances
   6. Constant movement and repetitious activity
   7. Intense attachments to objects
E. Treatment—variety of approaches tried with varying success
   1. Psychotherapy
   2. Behavior therapy
   3. Medications
   4. Special education
   5. Communication therapy
F. Oral manifestations—none directly associated with the syndrome

Specific Learning Disabilities and Minimal Brain Dysfunction

A. Definition
   1. Deficits in specific areas of learning that can cause problems in acquiring new skills
   2. Relates primarily to vision, hearing, language, and touch
B. Incidence/prevalence
   1. Not a distinct group
   2. Much controversy over diagnosis and treatment
   3. Occurs in 5% to 20% of the elementary school population
   4. More common in boys
C. Etiology
   1. Neurologic deficit
   2. Trauma
   3. Emotional factors
   4. Genetic or familial
   5. Cultural
D. Categories
   1. Areas of central nervous system (CNS) function affected
      a. Input—receiving, recognizing, and decoding messages (e.g., auditory or visual-perceptual problems)
      b. Organization—information storage, integration with other information, and prompt retrieval (e.g., short-term memory problem)
      c. Output—management of movement or utterances (e.g., hyperactivity, apraxia)

E. Signs/symptoms/clinical manifestations
 1. Hyperactivity or hypoactivity
 2. Irritability, impulsiveness, and need for immediate satisfaction
 3. Problems with concentration and memory
 4. Immaturity, clumsiness
 5. Lack of sense of direction, position, or time
 6. Speech and hearing problems
 7. Problems in reading, writing, or math
F. Treatment
 1. Remediation of weakness
 2. Compensation (creating new pathways)
 3. Exploitation of other areas (senses)
 4. Changing the environment
 5. Medications
G. Oral manifestations—none directly associated

Emotional Disturbance/Mental Illness

A. Definition
 1. By psychiatric diagnosis
 2. By psychologic tests
 3. By self-definition
 4. By cultural definition of maladjustment
B. Incidence/prevalence
 1. Of elementary children, 30% have at least mild, subclinical cases (10% need treatment)
 2. At some point in life 1/10 of all adults will need or benefit from some form of mental health intervention
C. Etiology—depends on the type of disturbance
 1. Familial
 2. Life stress (e.g., social, financial, marital)
 3. Depression
 4. Organic
D. Classifications (three common ones)
 1. Psychoneuroses—anxiety, depressive, obsessive, or conversion reactions
 2. Personality disorders—situational or adjustment reactions
 3. Psychoses—schizophrenia
E. Signs/symptoms/clinical manifestations (depend on the type of disorder)
 1. Inner tensions create anxiety, frustration, fears, and impulsive behavior
 2. Examples of behavior
  a. Translation of fears or anxieties into physical symptoms
  b. Regression to earlier forms of behavior
  c. Displays of hostility or aggression
  d. Withdrawal into fantasy (e.g., daydreams)
  e. Fear of failure and criticism
  f. Development of substitute fears, phobias, or compulsions

F. Treatment
 1. Stress management
 2. Psychotherapy
 3. Group therapy
 4. Medications
G. Oral manifestations
 1. None directly associated
 2. May see intraoral trauma resulting from unusual habits or aggressive behavior
 3. May have xerostomia as a side effect of medications

Alzheimer's Disease

A. Definition
 1. Progressive illness characterized by intellectual and cognitive disturbance, behavioral changes, and eventually a state of complete dependence
 2. Type of senile dementia
B. Incidence/prevalence
 1. Between 2% and 3% of the population
 2. Over age 65, 600,000 to 1.5 million are affected
 3. Accounts for the majority of cases of irreversible senile dementia
C. Etiology
 1. Unknown
 2. Postulated theories
  a. Viral agents causing selective cell death
  b. Excessive accumulation of toxic agents
  c. Genetic defect or disposition
  d. Age-related change in the immune system
D. Signs/symptoms/clinical manifestations
 1. Early
  a. Memory loss and inability to concentrate
  b. Anxiety, irritability, withdrawal, and petulance
  c. Abnormal sleep patterns
  d. Motor abnormalities, including exaggerated reflexes and gait disturbances
 2. Later
  a. Apathy, depression
  b. Disorientation and lack of judgment and understanding
  c. Incontinence
E. Treatment
 1. Medications—a variety are used, but none with significant success
 2. Maintenance of current abilities and reality orientation
 3. Provisions for ensuring safety
 4. Support for the family

F. Oral manifestations
1. None specific to the condition
2. Disease states usually are a result of neglect, the aging process, or any accompanying chronic illnesses

Epilepsy

See Chapter 18, section on seizures and convulsive disorders

A. Definition
1. Not a disease, but a term used to describe symptoms of recurrent or chronic brain dysfunction
2. Characterized by discrete, recurring behavioral manifestations that include disturbances of balance, sensation, behavior, perception, or consciousness
3. Should not be confused with one-time seizures that result from drug overdoses, brain tumors, or other problems
4. *Seizure* refers to an episode of cerebral dysfunction produced by abnormal, excessive neuronal discharge; not necessarily a recurring condition
5. *Convulsion* refers to a broad range of behavioral manifestations, including seizure activity
6. *Fit* is an outmoded synonym for *convulsion* or *seizure*
7. *Aura* refers to a specific sensation preceding a seizure, lasting from 1 to several seconds and manifested as
   a. Numbness, tingling
   b. Unusual smell
   c. Peculiar sound
   d. Feeling of nausea or fear
8. Status epilepticus
   a. Continuous convulsion lasting longer than 5 minutes
   b. May lead to death
   c. Constitutes a medical emergency
B. Incidence/prevalence
1. There are 1,000,000 cases in the United States
2. Incidence rate is 0.3% to 0.7% per year
3. Prevalence is highest in childhood
C. Etiology—prenatal, perinatal, postnatal, unknown (25% to 45%)
1. Prenatal
   a. Maternal infections
   b. Fetal growth abnormalities or prematurity
   c. Hormonal imbalances or Rh incompatibility
   d. Chromosomal disorders
   e. Toxicity or damage from drugs or radiation
   f. Genetic influences

2. Perinatal
   a. Delivery problems
   b. Anoxia
3. Postnatal
   a. Degenerative brain disease
   b. Injury
   c. Tumors
   d. Prolonged high fever
   e. Parasitic infections
   f. Toxic agents (including alcohol and drugs)
D. Types—can be classified by the site of the seizure origin in the brain, the etiology, or the type of seizure activity
E. Signs/symptoms/clinical manifestations
1. Generalized tonic-clonic (grand mal)
   a. May experience an aura
   b. Loss of consciousness
   c. Tonic movements (voluntary muscles experience continuous contractions)
   d. Clonic movements (intermittent muscular contraction and relaxation)
   e. Interruption of respiration and dilation of the pupils
   f. Loss of bladder or bowel control
   g. Seizure activity usually lasts 1 to 3 minutes
   h. Lethargy and disorientation follow the return of consciousness
   i. May occur any time during the day or only during sleep
2. Generalized absence (petit mal)
   a. Transient loss of consciousness
   b. May have minor motor movements of the eyes, head, or extremities
   c. Lasts 5 to 30 seconds
   d. Person may not be aware of having had a seizure
3. Complex partial (psychomotor)
   a. May be preceded by an aura
   b. Transient clouding of the consciousness
   c. Behavioral alterations
   d. Purposeless, repetitive, and stereotypic movements or actions
   e. Changes in affect or perception
   f. May become antisocial
   g. Person usually does not remember the incident
4. Mixed
F. Treatment
1. Drug therapy (70% of cases)
   a. Complete control is achieved in only about 5% of cases

b. One or more anticonvulsants (e.g., phenytoin [Dilantin], phenobarbital, primidone [Mysoline], phensuximide [Milontin], methsuximide [Celontin], trimethadione [Tridione], carbamazepine [Tegretol], acetazolamide [Diamox])

c. Common side effects
(1) Gingival overgrowth (phenytoin)
(2) Drowsiness and headaches
(3) Vision and gait disturbances
(4) Loss of appetite, nausea
(5) Blood dyscrasias

2. Surgery
3. Avoidance of precipitating factors (fatigue, stress, abnormal sensory stimuli, drugs, inadequate medication compliance)

G. Oral manifestations
1. Orofacial trauma—lips, tongue, buccal mucosa, teeth, facial or jaw bones
2. Gingival overgrowth from phenytoin (Fig. 14-4)
   a. More marked in anterior regions and buccal surfaces
   b. Does not occur in edentulous areas
   c. Correlated with poor oral hygiene
   d. Characteristically pale, pink, and fibrous
   e. Creates malpositioning of teeth and compromised esthetics
   f. Superimposed inflammation occurs from food retention or mouth breathing
   g. Can be alleviated through meticulous oral hygiene, surgery, or pressure appliances

Visual Impairment

A. Definition
1. Visual impairment—if after correction visual acuity in the best eye is no better than 20/200, or if central or peripheral vision impairment is present
2. Legally blind—visual acuity of less than 20/200 with correction

B. Incidence/prevalence
1. There are 450,000 legally blind persons in the United States
2. Of the legally blind, 50% are over age 60
3. Legally blind persons under age 20 make up 10% of the total
4. About 3% are totally blind
5. Half of the cases of blindness in the United States could have been prevented with proper diagnosis and treatment

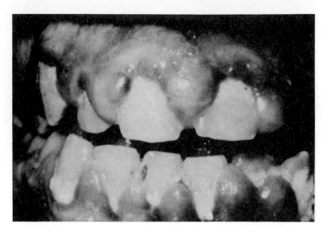

Fig. 14-4 Gingival overgrowth from phenytoin with superimposed inflammation.

C. Etiology—congenital, perinatal, postnatal
1. Trauma
2. Disease (infections, inflammation, toxicity)
3. Structural or developmental defects
4. Retrolental fibroplasia—high concentration of oxygen in the incubators of premature infants causes hemorrhage of retinal blood vessels, scarring, and retinal detachment
5. Macular degeneration (loss of central vision)
6. Retinal hemorrhages (e.g., complication of diabetes)
7. Glaucoma—failure of liquid in the eye to drain, resulting in increased pressure, pain, and destruction of the optic nerve
8. Cataracts—clouding and opacity of the lens blocks light perception (mainly associated with aging or congenital problems)

D. Signs/symptoms/clinical manifestations
1. Wears glasses or contact lenses
2. Awkward ambulation or bumping into objects
3. Eye pain
4. Constant tearing
5. Unusual squinting or blinking
6. Use of a guide dog or cane
7. Deliberate, slow actions
8. Attention to details and orderliness

E. Treatment
1. Cataracts—surgery, lens implants
2. Glaucoma—drugs or surgery
3. Laser treatment
4. Special education—auditory instruction and training in use of tactile senses (braille)
5. Prevention—use of safety glasses, regular checkups

Table 14-4 Hearing loss and probable effects

Classification	Loss (dB)	Hearing without amplification
Normal range	0-15	All speech sounds
Slight loss	15-25	Hears vowel sounds clearly; may miss unvoiced consonant sounds
Mild loss	25-40	Hears only louder-voiced speech sounds
Moderate loss	40-65	Misses most speech at normal conversational level
Severe loss	65-95	Misses all speech at normal conversational level
Profound loss	95+	Hears no speech or other sounds

From Lange, B.M., Entwistle, B.M., and Lipson, L.F.: Dental management of the handicapped: approaches for dental auxiliaries. Philadelphia, 1983, Lea & Febiger.

F. Oral manifestations
1. No particular dental problems
2. Gingivitis may be increased if oral hygiene habits are poor
3. Trauma to the orofacial area if the person experiences frequent accidents or falls

Hearing Impairment

A. Definition
1. Hearing impairment—defective, but functional hearing
2. Deaf—unable to understand speech, even with the use of an aid
3. Frequency—length of the sound wave (vibrations, or cycles, per second; human range is 16 to 30,000 cps)
4. Intensity—measured in decibels (human range is 1 to 100 dB)
B. Incidence/prevalence
1. There are 13,500,000 deaf and hearing-impaired persons in the United States; 51% of these are age 65 and over
2. Hearing losses are associated with a number of other handicapping conditions
   a. Cleft palate (90%)
   b. Cerebral palsy (20%)
   c. Down syndrome (70%)
C. Classifications—usually by severity of loss, as measured in decibel loss (Table 14-4)
D. Types
1. Conductive
   a. Injury or disease interferes with organs that conduct sound waves through the outer or middle ear
   b. Usually consistent over the entire range of sound
   c. Patient benefits most from the use of a hearing aid (sound conducted by bone)
   d. Speech is soft and low; patient hears own voice louder than that of others
2. Sensorineural
   a. Malfunction of organs that perceive sound (the inner ear, the auditory nerve, the auditory center in the brain)
   b. Most common cause is the process of aging
   c. Involves loss of sensitivity and acuity in one or more frequencies (usually higher frequencies and consonants)
   d. If individual wears a hearing aid, sound is conducted by air
   e. Speech is loud; person cannot hear own voice
E. Etiology
1. Prenatal or congenital
   a. Genetic defects
   b. Infections (rubella accounts for 20% of congenital types), influenza, and syphilis
   c. Blood incompatibilities
   d. Certain drugs (e.g., thalidomide, streptomycin)
   e. Unknown causes (10% to 20% of cases)
2. Acquired
   a. Infections (e.g., mumps, measles, poliomyelitis, chronic serous otitis media)
   b. Hereditary conditions
   c. Trauma
   d. Chronic use of certain drugs (e.g., aspirin, streptomycin)
   e. Lesions caused by trauma or disease
F. Signs/symptoms/clinical manifestations
1. May wear a unilateral or bilateral hearing aid
2. May lip-read or key in on other facial or nonverbal expressions

Table 14-5 Types of hearing aids

Type of aid	Characteristics	Indications for use
Body type hearing aid (monoaural or binaural)	Most powerful and durable, least cosmetic, broad frequency range	Used primarily for children and people with profound losses in whom power output is more important than cosmetics
Bone-conduction hearing aid	Used in body or eyeglass types; bone oscillator worn with a headband or as part of eyeglass bow	Used for people with a conductive loss that is not surgically correctable
Behind-the-ear aid	Most common; most esthetic; often good localization and isolation of signals	Can be used for the majority of hearing losses
Eyeglass aid	Cosmetic apeal; broad range of frequency responses	Usually for people who wear eyeglasses but object to the behind-the-ear type aid
CROS and BICROS aid	Microphone placed over worst ear; requires only slight amplification	Used for people with precipitous hearing loss
In-the-ear aid	Cosmetic, but much distortion and feedback	Used only for mild losses

From Lange, B.M., Entwistle, B.M., and Lipson, L.F.: Dental management of the handicapped: approaches for dental auxiliaries. Philadelphia, 1983, Lea & Febiger.

3. Speech may be characterized by aberrant modulations, pronunciations, or grammatical structures
4. May use sign language (American Sign Language) or finger spelling (American or manual alphabet)
5. May turn the head to one side if the loss is unilateral
6. Frequently asks people to repeat phrases
7. Person may not acknowledge having a loss

G. Treatment
  1. Depends on the patient's age at onset, and the type and cause of impairment
    a. Surgery
    b. Hearing aids (Table 14-5 lists types and indications for use)
    c. Education for development of communication skills
    d. Direct stimulation of the auditory nerve

H. Oral manifestations
  1. Not generally seen with hearing impairments unless associated with a syndrome (e.g., rubella syndrome)
  2. Prematurity or rubella may result in enamel dysplasia
  3. Bruxism may be evident

Cleft Lip or Palate

A. Definition—disturbances in embryologic formation resulting in incomplete closure of the lip and/or palatal area
B. Incidence/prevalence
  1. Occurs once in 1,750 live births

  2. One of the most common congenital malformations of the face and mouth

C. Classifications of cleft involvement
  1. Tip of the uvula
  2. Bifid uvula
  3. Soft palate (Fig. 14-5)
  4. Soft and hard palates (Fig. 14-6)
  5. Unilateral lip and palate
  6. Bilateral lip and palate

D. Etiology
  1. Most are genetic
  2. Other predisposing factors include maternal nutritional deficiencies or infectious diseases
  3. Cleft lip occurs during fetal weeks 4 through 7
  4. Cleft palate occurs during fetal weeks 8 through 12

E. Signs/symptoms/associated problems
  1. Oral-facial deformities
  2. Ear disease with resultant hearing loss
  3. Speech difficulties are a major handicap caused by
    a. Palatal insufficiency
    b. Missing or malpositioned teeth
    c. Hearing loss
  4. Feeding problems
  5. Predisposition to upper respiratory tract infections

F. Treatment
  1. Surgery—multiple operations at various developmental stages
  2. Speech therapy
  3. Insertion of an obturator or other appliance if needed for feeding or speech

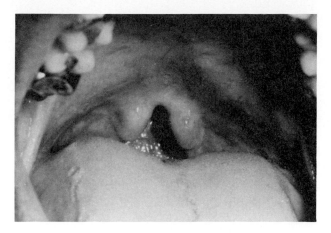

Fig. 14-5 Soft palate cleft.

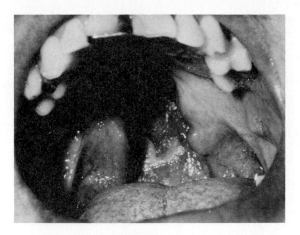

Fig. 14-6 Soft and hard palate cleft.

4. Antibiotics to prevent infections
5. Orthodontics
G. Oral manifestations
   1. High incidence of missing or maldeveloped teeth in the line of the cleft
   2. High incidence of malocclusion resulting from the structural defects
   3. Oral motor dysfunction
   4. Scar tissue from surgery

Cerebral Palsy

A. Definition—static, nonprogressive neuromuscular condition composed of a series of syndromes that result from damage to the brain
B. Incidence—3/1000 people in the United States, occurring more frequently in males
C. Etiology
   1. Prenatal (genetic or congenitally acquired; e.g., anoxia, infections, Rh incompatibility, metabolic disturbances)
   2. Natal—anoxia, hemorrhage
   3. Postnatal—trauma, infections, neoplasms, anoxia
D. Classification
   1. Motor disorders
      a. Spasticity (50% to 75%)—slight stimulus causes exaggerated muscle contraction
      b. Athetosis (15% to 25%)—muscles contract involuntarily
      c. Ataxia (10%)—muscles respond to a stimulus but cannot complete a contraction
      d. Hypotonia (<10%)—unable to respond to a volitional stimulus
      e. Rigidity (<10%)—increased initial muscle resistance; gives way with little force
      f. Mixed (5% to 10%)—two or more types appearing in the same person

   2. Limbs involved
      a. Monoplegic—one limb
      b. Hemiplegic—both limbs on the same side of the body
      c. Paraplegic—lower limbs
      d. Diplegic—major involvement of the lower limbs, minor involvement of the upper limbs
      e. Quadriplegic—all four limbs
      f. Triplegic—three limbs
E. Signs/symptoms/clinical manifestations (Fig. 14-7)
   1. Characterized by paralysis, weakness, muscle spasms, incoordination, or other aberrations of motor function, especially involving voluntary muscles
   2. Joint immobility and contractures increase with age
   3. Retained primitive reflexes (e.g., asymmetric or symmetric tonic neck reflex)
   4. Other associated conditions
      a. Speech/language disorders (60%)
      b. Hearing disorders (20%)
      c. Visual defects (40%)
      d. Mental retardation (40%)
      e. Seizures (40%)
   5. Wide range of limitation, from mild to totally dependent
F. Treatment
   1. Surgery for contractures
   2. Supportive therapies (physical therapy, occupational therapy, speech therapy)
   3. Adaptive equipment (braces, wheelchair, walkers, mouth sticks, voice synthesizer) (Fig. 14-8)
   4. Medications for seizures
   5. Special education

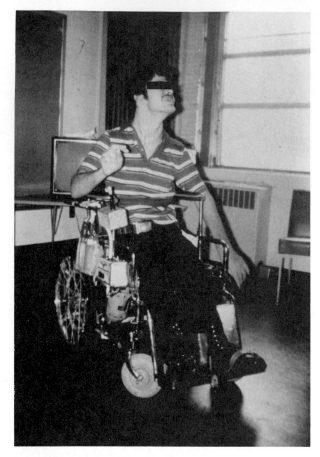

Fig. 14-7 Typical manifestations of cerebral palsy.

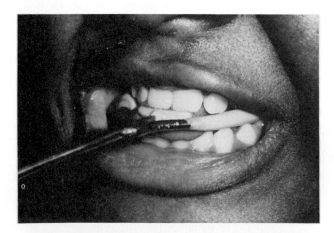

Fig. 14-8 Mouth stick used for typing or grasping.

G. Oral manifestations—marked variation among individuals
   1. Higher incidence of bruxism, dental caries, enamel dysplasia, malocclusion, and periodontal problems
   2. Phenytoin-induced gingival overgrowth if this drug is being given
   3. Oral motor dysfunction, (e.g., impaired swallowing), mouth breathing
   4. Trauma resulting from incoordination and frequent falls
   5. Attrition and possible joint disturbances from mouth sticks

Bell's Palsy

A. Definition—paralysis of facial muscles innervated by cranial nerve VII (facial nerve)
B. Incidence/prevalence—most common in adult years
C. Etiology
   1. Unknown
   2. Associated with bacterial and viral infections, trauma from oral extractions, or surgery on the parotid gland
D. Signs/symptoms/clinical manifestations
   1. Abrupt paralysis without preceding pain
   2. Occurs unilaterally
   3. Corner of the mouth droops, causing drooling
   4. Eyelids will not close; the lower eyelid droops; predisposes the eyes to infections
   5. Speech and chewing are difficult
   6. May have spontaneous remission in 2 to 8 weeks or permanent paralysis
E. Treatment
   1. Prednisone therapy
   2. Heat and massage to maintain circulation and muscle tone
   3. Eye drops or eye shield to prevent infections
   4. Surgery if needed
F. Oral manifestations—oral motor difficulties can cause food retention and the potential for increased caries or gingivitis

Myasthenia Gravis

A. Definition—immunologic neuromuscular disease characterized by variable weakness or fatigue of the striated, voluntary muscles
B. Incidence/prevalence
   1. Onset at any age
   2. If early onset, females affected more often
   3. If late onset, males affected more often
   4. No incidence figures available

C. Etiology—autoimmune mechanism causing a defect in nerve impulse transmission at the neuromuscular junction

D. Signs/symptoms/clinical manifestations
1. Affects muscles of the eyes (double vision), facial expression, mastication, and swallowing
2. Disturbs breathing and speech (weak, muffled voice)
3. Weakness may increase as the day progresses
4. Precipitated by
   a. Emotional excitement
   b. Surgical procedures
   c. Fatigue/loss of sleep
   d. Infections
   e. Alcoholic intake
5. Myasthenic crisis
   a. Patient nonresponsive to drugs
   b. Unable to clear secretions from the throat
   c. Impaired breathing
   d. Double vision

E. Treatment
1. Medications that block the action of cholinesterase at the myoneural junction (neostigmine [Prostigmin], pyridostigmine [Mestinon], ambenonium [Mytelase])
2. Radiation therapy or surgical removal of the thymus leads to partial remission
3. Corticosteroids or adrenocorticotropic hormone (ACTH)
4. Tracheostomy if needed during the crisis

F. Oral manifestations
1. Oral motor dysfunction
2. Retention of food increases susceptibility to dental caries and periodontal problems

Parkinson's Disease

A. Definition—progressive disorder of the central nervous system causing loss of postural reflexes, slowness of spontaneous movement, tremors, and muscle rigidity

B. Incidence/prevalence
1. Develops between ages 40 to 60
2. Over age 60, 1/100 persons affected
3. Higher incidence in men

C. Etiology
1. Cause unknown
2. Imbalance of dopamine and acetylcholine

D. Signs/symptoms/clinical manifestations
1. Mild, diffuse muscular pain
2. Tremors of the extremities, occurring mainly at rest

3. Shuffling, slow gait with the arms held to the side
4. Slurred, indistinct speech
5. Staring, masklike facial expression
6. Excessive salivation or dryness of mouth (side effects of medications)
7. Intellect not usually affected
8. Tremors in the lips, tongue, or neck; difficulty in swallowing
9. Feelings of stiffness and rigidity (particularly of the large joints)
10. Sensitivity to heat

E. Treatment
1. Medications (see Chapter 8)
   a. Levodopa to alleviate dopamine deficiency, tremors, and rigidity
   b. Side effects—orthostatic hypotension, dizziness
   c. Anticholinergic agents
   d. Antispasmodics
   e. Antihistamines
   f. Analgesics
   g. Sedatives
2. Physical and occupational therapy
3. Good nutrition
4. Surgery

F. Oral manifestations
1. Impaired oral motor functions may increase the incidence of dental caries or periodontal disease
2. Side effects of medications (dry mouth) may increase the incidence of dental caries

Arthritis

A. Definition
1. Term used to describe several disorders causing pain in the joints and connective tissue
2. Joint inflammation
3. *Polyarthritis* refers to involvement of many joints

B. Types (Table 14-6)
1. Osteoarthritis
2. Rheumatoid (adult type)
3. Rheumatoid (juvenile type)

C. Incidence/prevalence: common in all age groups (Table 14-6)

D. Etiology
1. Cause unknown
2. Theories (Table 14-6)

E. Signs/symptoms/clinical manifestations—affect various sites in different ways (Table 14-6)

Table 14-6 Characteristics of arthritis

	Osteoarthritis	Rheumatoid (adult type)	Rheumatoid (juvenile type)
Incidence/prevalence	12,000,000 in United States; onset at ages 50-70	5,000,000 in United States; onset at ages 20-40; affects females	250,000 in United States; occurs before age 16
Etiology	Unknown or from trauma, infection, or joint abnormality	Cause unknown; theories include autoimmunity, hereditary or psychosomatic factors, and infection	
Sites affected	Weight-bearing joints (hips, knees, vertebrae)	First affects fingers, hands, and knees; TMJ later	Involves many joints, especially fingers, knees, wrists, vertebrae, and TMJ
Signs/symptoms	Pain, aggravated by temperature changes; joint stiffness after inactivity; develops gradually; swelling rare; does not usually limit range of motion	Fatigue, loss of appetite, low-grade fever, migratory joint pain and swelling, stiffness after periods of inactivity, paresthesia, subcutaneous nodules, joint deformities, TMJ involvement, muscle atrophy near joints	Joint enlargement, stiffness, and pain; onset is acute with fever, rash, spleen and lymph node enlargement, tachycardia, and limited oral opening

F. Treatment
1. Primarily involves relief of pain and maintenance of function
2. Medications—aspirin, steroids, gold salts
3. Physical therapy and exercise to increase range of motion and prevent deformities
4. Application of heat or hydrotherapy
5. Surgery—joint replacement

G. Oral manifestations
1. Bruxism and occlusal imbalances
2. Temporomandibular joint (TMJ) pain and limited opening
3. Masking of inflammation by prolonged steroid therapy
4. Malocclusion occurs in the juvenile type
5. Delayed healing if long-term aspirin therapy is being given
6. Mucosal ulcerations or secondary oral infections (especially of gingiva) if gold salts are being given

Multiple Sclerosis

A. Definition—chronic degenerative disease of the central nervous system where
1. Myelin is destroyed through the formation of sclerotic tissue called plaque
2. Nerve impulses to the brain are disrupted or not transmitted
3. Scattered plaque accumulation causes widespread and varied symptoms with periods of exacerbation and remission

B. Incidence/prevalence
1. Affects 500,000 people in the United States
2. Varies geographically
3. More common in women
4. Onset occurs at any age, but usually between the ages of 20 to 45.

C. Etiology
1. Unknown
2. Possibly an autoimmune reaction or associated with viral infections

D. Signs/symptoms
1. Result from the location of lesions (Table 14-7)
2. Precipitating factors
   a. Infections
   b. Stress and emotional trauma
   c. Injury
   d. Heavy exercise and fatigue
   e. Pregnancy
3. Periods of remission
4. Death is usually the result of an infection
5. Fewer than 50% become nonambulatory

E. Treatment
1. No current cure
2. Physical and occupational therapy
3. Alternating periods of rest and exercise
4. Diet high in unsaturated fats
5. Medications
   a. Corticosteroids
   b. Hormones
   c. Muscle relaxants

Table 14-7 Symptoms associated with lesions in the central nervous system

Location of lesions	Possible symptoms
Spinal cord	Numbness
	Loss of sensitivity in appendages
	Sensitivity to heat
	Unsteady gait
	Loss of strength in the legs
	Impaired eye-hand coordination resulting in difficulty in fine motor movements
Brainstem	Blurred and/or double vision
	Difficulty in swallowing or chewing
	Diminished gag reflex
	Slurred speech
Cerebrum (lesions in the cerebrum usually occur in the latter stages of the disease process)	Disruptions in thinking
	Euphoria
	Depression
	Disruptions in behavior

From Lange, B.M., Entwistle, B.M., and Lipson, L.F.: Dental management of the handicapped: approaches for dental auxiliaries. Philadelphia, 1983, Lea & Febiger.

F. Oral manifestations
   1. None reported except as a result of poor oral hygiene or the side effects of drugs
      a. Ulcerations
      b. Xerostomia
      c. Gingival overgrowth (phenytoin given for pain)
   2. Facial pain

Muscular Dystrophies

A. Definition—group of progressive chronic diseases of the skeletal (striated) muscles characterized by the degeneration of muscle cells with replacement by fat or fibrous tissue
B. Incidence/prevalence
   1. Affects 150,000 to 200,000 people in the United States
   2. Most often affects children
C. Etiology—unknown, although thought to be biochemical in nature
D. Types (Table 14-8)
   1. Duchenne's
   2. Limb-girdle
   3. Fascioscapulohumeral
E. Signs/symptoms/clinical manifestations—varies by site and type (Table 14-8)
F. Treatment—goal is to maintain the person's activity and involvement
   1. Antimicrobial treatment
   2. Ventilation therapy, deep-breathing exercises
   3. Humidification and postural drainage for respiratory failure and infections
   4. Diuretics for cardiac problems

   5. Nutritional counseling if overweight
   6. Physical therapy involves muscle-stretching exercise and use of adaptive aids to
      a. Improve muscle strength
      b. Prevent and correct contractures
      c. Increase efficiency in the activities of daily living
   7. Speech therapy if needed
G. Oral manifestations
   1. Weakness in the masticatory muscles leads to decreased maxillary biting force
   2. Higher incidence of mouth breathing, open bite, and overexpansion of the maxilla
   3. In fascioscapulohumeral type, the lips appears thick because of involvement of the orbicularis oris muscle
   4. Increase in dental disease states if oral hygiene is neglected

Spinal Cord Injuries

A. Definition
   1. Fracture, dislocation, hyperextension, compression, or severance of components of the spinal column
   2. Occurs most often in the cervical and lumbar curves
   3. Cord damage can occur above or below the level of bone injury
B. Incidence/prevalence
   1. Affects 150,000 to 200,000 people in the United States
   2. About 10,000 new cases per year

Table 14-8 Types and characteristics of muscular dystrophies

	Duchenne's	Limb-girdle	Fascioscapulohumeral
Onset	Mainly affects boys; occurs before age 10	Occurs later (average age 20); affects both males and females	Males and females equally affected; usually occurs around puberty
Severity	Most severe and destructive form	Slower progression in most cases	Least destructive and progresses at slower rate; least common type
Etiology	Sex-linked recessive trait with high mutation rate	Autosomal recessive trait	Autosomal dominant trait
Sites affected	Pelvis, abdomen, hip, and spine affected first; spreads to trunk, extremities, and myocardium (cranial nerves *not* affected); osteoporosis also noted	Initial weakness in pelvic girdle, then in shoulder	Facial muscles affected first; weakness is asymmetric; progresses to shoulder girdle and upper arm
Limitations	Becomes confined to wheelchair and bed within a few years of diagnosis; may develop scoliosis, obesity, and cardiopulmonary problems; death usually occurs during adolescence	May be severely disabled by midlife, with decreased life span	May remain in state of indefinite remission, with some people living symptom-free, normal life span
Signs/symptoms	Clumsiness, frequent falls resulting from precarious balance, toe-walking, weakness of hips, lordosis, cramping of legs and abdomen, Gower's sign, enlargement of calves, decreased stamina	Begins as pain after exercise; then total muscle involvement	Masklike, wrinklefree, expressionless facial features; difficulty in closing eyes; muscles above elbow atrophy, below elbow are normal (Popeye effect); difficulty in raising arms

3. Seventy percent of patients are below the age of 40; only 15% are female

C. Etiology—acquired injury from accidents
 1. Automobile or motorcycle accidents cause 50% of injuries
 2. Occupational accidents cause 25% of injuries
 3. Sporting accidents cause 18% of injuries
 4. Falls, gunshot wounds, or other trauma cause 7% of injuries

D. Signs/symptoms/clinical manifestations
 1. Depend on the severity and level of injury
 2. Prognosis depends on
  a. First aid measures performed at the site of the accident
  b. Type and level of injury to the spinal cord
 3. *Paraplegia* refers to an injury below the cervical level that results in paralysis of the lower portion of the body

4. *Quadriplegia* refers to an injury occurring in the cervical region that results in paralysis of all four limbs and the trunk
 5. Most frequent cause of death is kidney stones or infection
 6. Functional limitations and specific manifestations depend on the level of the lesion (Tables 14-9 and 14-10)

E. Treatment
 1. Four phases of rehabilitation
  a. Physical—functional exercises to increase specific skills
  b. Equipment—development of adaptive equipment to allow for maximum independence
  c. Environment—implementation of structural and other changes in the home and work environment to accommodate the person's limitations

Table 14-9 Clinical manifestations of spinal cord injuries

Area affected	Clinical manifestations
Muscles (limb and trunk)	Innervation and perception to pain and touch disturbed; leads to 　Muscle atrophy 　Concerns for safety around varying temperatures 　Formation of decubitus ulcers (pressure sores) caused by breakdown of tissue from immobilization, bruises, or braces 　Decreased or absent self-care skills 　Spasticity and tremors 　Adaptive equipment required, especially for 　　Wrist stability 　　Pencil grasp 　　Arm movements
Respiration	Intercostal muscles may be paralyzed, resulting in need for diaphragmatic breathing or tracheostomy and total or partial dependence on a respirator
Bowel and bladder	Limited innervation, resulting in incontinence and encopresis, or retention Can lead to infections, particularly of kidneys Autonomic hyperreflexia can occur (medical emergency) 　Caused by sudden constriction of blood vessels 　Symptoms—rapid increase in blood pressure (e.g., 280/80), low pulse, pounding headache, skin blotching and sweating above site of injury, cold goosebumps below site of injury
Bones/joints	Contractures from spasticity and immobilization Heterotopic ossifications (bony accumulations) may develop around joints
Metabolism	Regulation of body temperature impaired
Social/emotional status	Problems associated with coping with a debilitating acquired injury May experience stages of shock, denial, anger, depression, mobilization, and coping

Table 14-10 Functional significance of lesion levels

Lesion level	Functional expectations for complete lesions
	CERVICAL LESIONS (C)
C4	Incapable of voluntary function in arms, trunk, or legs. Poor respiratory reserve. Totally dependent.
C5	Can stabilize and rotate neck; has rhontoids and deltoids, allowing some shoulder movement. Elbow flexion; biceps and brachiocardialis partially innervated.
C6	Can move shoulders well. Strong elbow flexion. Wrist muscles allow weak closure of hand; can use large-handled, lightweight objects. Can sit up in bed with help, and roll over. Still needs attendant.
C7	Patient can lift own body weight. Can use hands, which are weak and lack dexterity. Can eat independently, with some assistance. Most often confined to wheelchair.
	THORACIC LESIONS (T)
T1	Independent in bed, self-care (short of lifting weights). Lacks trunk stability, respiratory reserve, and trunk fixation of arm prime movers.
T6	Capable of heavy lifting (due to thoracic musculature). Increased respiratory reserve. Independent transfers, self-application of braces; doesn't need attendant.
T12	Can ambulate with crutches and braces.
	LUMBAR LESIONS (L)
L4	Patient is almost completely independent in all phases of self-care and ambulation, usually aided by crutches, canes, or prosthesis.

From Schubert, M.M., Snow, M., and Stiefel, D.J.: DECOD Series: Dental treatment of the spinal cord injured patient, Seattle, 1977, University of Washington.

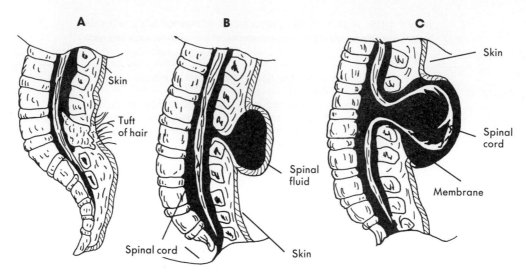

Fig. 14-9 Types of spina bifida. **A,** Spina bifida occulta. **B,** Meningocele. **C,** Myelomeningocele.

    d. Life—vocational training and reintegration into daily activities

2. Team approach required—physicians, nurse, occupational therapist, physical therapist, speech therapist, psychologist/counselor, vocational specialist, recreational therapist, dentist, dental hygienist, social worker

Spina Bifida

A. Definition
1. Congenital abnormality of the spinal column
2. Vertebrae fail to close completely around the spinal cord
B. Incidence/prevalence
1. Occurs in 2/1000 live births
2. A major cause of paraplegia in children
C. Etiology—specific cause unknown, but multiple factors, including genetic and environmental factors, are suspected
D. Types (Fig. 14-9)
1. Spinal bifida occulta
    a. Small defect in a vertebra, not involving the spinal cord
    b. Often undetected
2. Meningocele—bony defect that allows meninges and cerebrospinal fluid to form a sac protruding from the vertebral column
3. Myelomeningocele—severe defect where the spinal cord also protrudes into the sac
E. Signs/symptoms/clinical manifestations
1. Potential exposure of the nervous system to the external environment results in an increased chance for further damage from trauma or infection

2. Loss of motor function in the lower half of the body
    a. Differential involvement of muscle groups causes muscle imbalance, leading to spinal and limb deformities
    b. Loss of sensations of pain, touch, and temperature creates safety hazards and pressure sores
    c. Loss of bladder and bowel control
    d. Ambulation may be affected, creating a need for orthopedic devices or a wheelchair
3. Deformity of the brain
    a. Most have normal intelligence, but experience learning disabilities, especially visual-perceptual problems
    b. Some develop seizure disorders
    c. Sixty-five percent will develop hydrocephalus
       (1) Cerebrospinal fluid accumulates in the ventricles of the brain
       (2) Pressure expands the brain and skull
F. Treatment
1. Surgical correction of the defect
2. Insertion of ventriculoperitoneal or ventriculoatrial shunt if hydrocephalus is present (Fig. 14-10)
3. Orthopedic management through surgery, bracing, and physical therapy
4. Assisted urination or evacuation, catheterization
5. Medications to prevent or treat infections
6. Avoidance of decubitus ulcers
7. Weight control if fairly inactive
G. Oral manifestations—none directly associated

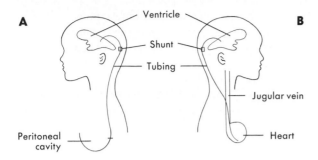

Fig. 14-10 Types of shunts for hydrocephalus. **A,** Ventriculoperitoneal shunt. **B,** Ventriculoatrial shunt.

Viral Hepatitis

See Chapter 7, section on infections of the gastrointestinal tract and Table 7-7

Acquired Immune Deficiency Syndrome

See Chapter 7, section on immunodeficiency

Sexually Transmitted Diseases

See Chapter 7, section on infections of the reproductive and urinary system

Tuberculosis

See Chapter 7, section on infections of the respiratory tract

A. Definition—infectious disease of bacterial origin that creates lesions in a number of organs, especially the lungs
B. Incidence
1. In cities over 500,000, the case rate is about 25.2/100,000 population
2. Rate drops to 10.6/100,000 in cities under 100,000
3. Varies significantly throughout the world
4. Is increasing in the United States as a result of recent immigrants
C. Etiology
1. Most cases caused by *Mycobacterium tuberculosis* (an aerobe)
2. Transmitted by infected, airborne droplets of mucus or saliva
D. Signs/symptoms/clinical manifestations
1. Often asymptomatic and diagnosed by a positive skin test (Mantoux test) or radiographic findings
2. Night fevers and sweating
3. Weight loss, anorexia

4. Specific symptoms depend on organs affected
   a. Pulmonary involvement—bloody sputum, dyspnea
   b. Localized lymphadenopathy
5. Common complications
   a. Pleuritis
   b. Meningitis
   c. Also affects pericardium, peritoneum, adrenal glands, kidney, and bone
E. Treatment
1. Prevention by BCG vaccine
2. Antituberculosis drugs—usually a combination
   a. Isoniazid
   b. Streptomycin
   c. Rifampin
F. Oral manifestations
1. Rare, but if they occur, they are deep, painless ulcers (usually with jagged undermined borders) on the dorsum of the tongue, palate, lips, mucosa, or gingiva
2. Usually caused by secondary spread from primary lung lesions
3. Biopsy required for definitive diagnosis

Cystic Fibrosis

A. Definition—inherited disorder of the exocrine glands
B. Incidence/prevalence
1. Occurs in 1/2000 live births in the United States
2. Between 2% and 5% of the population are carriers
3. Males and females equally affected
4. Most frequent cause of chronic lung disease in white children
C. Etiology—autosomal recessive disorder
D. Signs/symptoms/clinical manifestations—increased viscosity of mucus (obstructs the pancreatic ducts, leading to cyst formation, impaired metabolism, and progressive deterioration)
1. Accumulation of mucus in the lungs interferes with oxygen exchange
   a. Interferes especially with exhalation, causing a barrel-chested appearance
   b. Air sacs collapse, and infections occur, often leading to suppurative bronchitis, pneumonia, and obstructive emphysema
   c. Clubbing of fingers and toes
   d. Chronic cough
2. Sweat glands affected, leading to high levels of sodium in the sweat
3. Salivary glands also affected

4. Other findings and complications include a small gallbladder, cirrhosis of the liver, diabetes mellitus, and sterility in males
5. Linear growth and bone development delayed
6. Death usually occurs in early adulthood

E. Treatment
1. Antibiotics to eliminate lung infection (tetracycline used in the past)
2. Aerosol inhalants and postural drainage to maintain lungs as mucus free as possible
3. Dietary regimen
   a. Reduce total fat with increased calories and protein
   b. Powdered pancreatic enzyme supplements
   c. Regulate salt intake
4. General prevention of infections

F. Oral manifestations
1. Lower dental caries rate and plaque accumulation with increased calculus deposits; probably a result of alterations in saliva and long-term use of antibiotics
2. Enlargement of the salivary glands
3. Intrinsic staining of the teeth if tetracycline is administered during the formative years
4. Mouth breathing if sinuses are occluded

Bronchial Asthma

See Chapter 18, section on respiratory emergencies
A. Definition
1. Clinical state of hyperreactivity of the tracheobronchial tree characterized by recurrent paroxysms of dyspnea and wheezing
2. Results from bronchospasm, bronchial wall edema, and hypersecretion by mucous glands
3. Status asthmaticus—persistent exacerbation of asthma in spite of drug therapy (life threatening)

B. Incidence/prevalence
1. Nine million people in the United States; 2 to 3 million are children
2. Initial symptoms usually occur in the first 5 years of life
3. About 50% of affected children become asymptomatic before adulthood

C. Etiology—unknown, although precipitating factors and their effects are known
1. Extrinsic factors—dust, mold, pollen, animal dander, household sprays, smoke, wool, foods, air pollutants
2. Other factors—respiratory tract infections, aspirin and other anti-inflammatory drugs, exercise, emotional stress

D. Signs/symptoms/clinical manifestations
1. Wheezing, dyspnea, coughing, chest pain, sneezing, sputum production, fatigue
2. Expiratory phase of breathing is slower and more pronounced
3. Facial (sinus) pain, conjunctivitis, otitis media
4. More severe symptoms—syncope, respiratory failure, cyanosis

E. Treatment
1. Avoid precipitating factors
2. Immunotherapy (allergy shots)
3. Postural drainage (to loosen mucus)
4. Medications
   a. Bronchodilators such as aminophylline and theophylline
   b. Steroids
5. Exercise and physical fitness

F. Oral manifestations—no associated conditions except potential mouth breathing

Congenital Heart Disease

A. Definition
1. Anomalies of heart structure
2. Usually caused during the first 9 weeks in utero

B. Incidence/prevalence
1. Occurs in 0.5% of all live births (25,000 per year)

C. Etiology
1. Generally unknown
2. Genetic
3. Environmental
   a. Rubella infection (German measles) 2%
   b. Fetal hypoxia, endocarditis, or immunologic abnormalities
   c. Nutritional deficiencies (especially vitamin deficiencies)
   d. Drugs (e.g., thalidomide, alcohol)
   e. Radiation

D. Types of malformations
1. Cause initial left-to-right shunting of blood (e.g., atrial-septal defect, ventricular-septal defect, patent ductus arteriosus)
2. Initial right-to-left shunting (e.g., tetralogy of Fallot)—causes significant cyanosis
3. Malformations that obstruct blood flow (e.g., pulmonary stenosis)

E. Signs/symptoms/clinical manifestations
1. Dyspnea, fatigue, weakness (most common symptoms)
2. Cyanosis, dizziness, syncope, or ruddy color, leading to congestive heart failure
3. Clubbing of fingers or toes (Fig. 14-11)
4. Heart murmurs

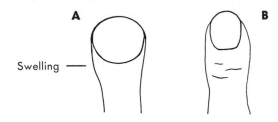

Fig. 14-11 A, Clubbing of finger observed in congenital heart disease. **B,** Normal finger.

5. Delayed growth and development
6. Complications—brain abscesses, bacterial endocarditis, congestive heart failure, acute pulmonary edema, bleeding problems
F. Treatment
   1. One fourth to one half of infants with these defects require treatment during the first year of life
   2. Surgery
   3. Medications
      a. Digitalis
      b. Anticoagulants
G. Oral manifestations
   1. None, except cyanosis or ruddy color of mucosa
   2. Developmental defects of teeth
   3. Slight hemorrhaging secondary to trauma if bleeding problems are present
   4. May have decreased ability to fight oral infections

Rheumatic Fever and Heart Disease

See Chapter 7, section on infections of the circulatory system and Appendix B
A. Definition
   1. Rheumatic fever—acute inflammatory condition occurring as a sequela to group A streptococcal infections
   2. Rheumatic heart disease—cardiac damage resulting from an acute attack of rheumatic fever
      a. Involves damage to the mitral or aortic valves
      b. Causes scarring and calcification
B. Incidence/prevalence
   1. Seventy-five percent of cases occur before age 20
   2. Accounts for 95% of all cases of childhood heart disease
   3. About 70% to 80% of those having rheumatic fever develop rheumatic heart disease
C. Etiology
   1. Group A streptococcal infections
   2. Autoimmune reaction to antibodies of group A streptococci
D. Signs/symptoms/clinical manifestations
   1. Low-grade fever
   2. Arthritis in the large joints of the knees and ankles for 2 to 3 weeks
   3. Carditis
   4. Subcutaneous nodules that are firm, painless, and colorless; last 1 to 2 weeks
   5. Chorea (involuntary and irregular muscle movements)
   6. Pink skin rash for 2 to 3 days
   7. Murmur
   8. Complications of rheumatic heart disease include dyspnea, angina pectoris, blood in sputum, and congestive heart failure
E. Treatment
   1. Rheumatic fever
      a. Penicillin G injection
      b. Codeine, aspirin, or steroids for arthritis
      c. Long-term antibiotic regimen
   2. Rheumatic heart disease
      a. No treatment if asymptomatic
      b. Surgery and placement of artificial valve if necessary
F. Oral manifestations—none

Cardiac Arrhythmias

A. Definition
   1. Irregular heartbeat manifested as abnormal pulse rates or rhythms
   2. Produces alterations in the normal sequence of contractions, leading to inadequate blood flow
   3. Produces aberrant electrical depolarization
   4. Adversely affects the ventricular rate
B. Types/etiology
   1. Bradycardia—slow heart rate
      a. May be unimportant in young people or athletes
      b. May cause syncope in elderly individuals
   2. Tachycardia—increased heart rate
      a. Normal response to exercise or fear
      b. Increased load on and oxygen consumption by the heart
   3. Atrial fibrillation—totally uncoordinated and ineffectual contractions
      a. Most common type
      b. Common causes—rheumatic or ischemic heart disease
      c. Impairs ventricular filling and rate
      d. Thrombi may form or heart failure can result

4. Ventricular fibrillation—irregular, uncoordinated, ineffective contractions of individual muscle bundles
   a. Results in heart failure and typically is fatal within a few minutes
   b. Most serious type and most common cause of death
   c. Can be a consequence of myocardial infarction or digitalis overdose
5. Heart block—defect in conducting mechanisms (usually sinoatrial node); impulses delayed or blocked (common causes include ischemic heart disease, rheumatic fever, and digitalis)
C. Signs/symptoms/clinical manifestations
   1. Abnormal pulse
   2. Palpitations
   3. Breathlessness or pallor
   4. Syncope
   5. Cyanosis
   6. Pain
   7. Cardiac failure
   8. May also be asymptomatic
D. Treatment
   1. Some require no treatment
   2. Digitalis or antiarrhythmic drugs
   3. Anticoagulants for atrial fibrillation
   4. Pacemaker
      a. Demand type—stimulates the heart only when the rhythm deviates from a predetermined norm
      b. Fixed rate type—rate is set independently of the natural heart rate
E. Oral manifestations—none

Hypertensive Disease

See Chapter 18, section on vital signs
A. Definition
   1. Hypertension—elevation in blood pressure greater than 140/90 mm Hg
   2. Hypertensive disease—sustained elevation of the diastolic blood pressure, creating an increased workload for the heart
B. Incidence/prevalence
   1. Hypertension affects 35 million people in the United States
   2. About 4% progress to a chronic disease state
   3. Most cases are primary hypertension
C. Etiology
   1. Most are of unknown cause
   2. Some are secondary to other conditions such as renal disease or endocrine disorders
   3. Predisposing factors include age, stress, smoking, weight gain, oral contraceptives, or excess salt in the diet

4. Chronic hypertension causes cardiac enlargement and eventually congestive heart failure
D. Signs/symptoms/clinical manifestations
   1. Early—occipital headache, dizziness, tingling of the extremities, vision changes, tinnitis, dyspnea
   2. Advanced—cardiac enlargement, ischemic heart disease, congestive heart failure, renal failure, stroke
E. Treatment (see Chapter 18, section on cardiac emergencies)
   1. Philosophies and therapies vary
   2. Life-style changes in terms of stress reduction, diet, and reduction of other risk factors
   3. Drug management with antihypertensives—usually a combination
      a. Diuretics
      b. Adrenergic-inhibiting agents
      c. Vasodilators
   4. Many side effects and precautions associated with drugs
F. Oral manifestations
   1. Generally no direct oral manifestations
   2. Facial palsy in those with chronic disease
   3. Oral lesions or xerostomia from drugs

Ischemic Heart Disease

A. Definition—coronary atherosclerotic heart disease that is symptomatic
B. Incidence/prevalence
   1. Affects 4.2 million people in the United States
   2. Leading cause of death after the age of 40 or 50
   3. Incidence and severity increase with age
C. Etiology
   1. Main cause is unknown
   2. Risk factors are the same as for hypertensive disease
   3. Accumulation of lipid plaque inside blood vessels impairs blood flow, and thus the oxygen supply to the heart
D. Signs/symptoms/clinical manifestations
   1. Angina pectoris—transient and reversible oxygen deficiency
      a. Pain—crushing or paroxysmal, usually less than 5 minutes; often mistaken for indigestion
      b. Sweating, anxiety, pallor, difficulty breathing
      c. Relieved by administration of nitroglycerine

2. Myocardial infarction—an infarct or necrosis caused by a sudden reduction or arrest of blood flow
   a. Pain in the sternum, radiating to the left arm; lasts longer than angina
   b. Not relieved by nitroglycerin
   c. Same other symptoms as angina, with nausea and vomiting, palpitations, and lowered blood pressure
   d. Often leads to sudden death from ventricular fibrillation
E. Treatment (see Chapter 18, section on cardiac emergencies)
   1. Same management as for hypertensive disease
   2. Drug therapy
      a. Nitroglycerin
      b. β-Adrenergic blockers
      c. Diuretics
      d. Coronary bypass operation if indicated
   3. Rest
F. Oral manifestations
   1. None directly associated
   2. Oral lesions or xerostomia may result as a side effect of drugs
   3. Pain may be radiated to the mandible

Congestive Heart Failure

A. Definition
   1. Represents a symptom complex that involves failure of one or both ventricles (usually the left ventricle)
   2. Imbalance between the demand placed on the heart and its ability to respond
B. Incidence/prevalence—most common cause of death in the United States
C. Etiology
   1. Underlying causes
      a. Heart valve damage
      b. Obstructive lung disease
      c. Damage to the walls of the heart muscle
   2. Precipitating causes that place an additional work demand on the heart
      a. Hypertensive crises
      b. Pulmonary embolism
      c. Arrhythmia
D. Signs/symptoms/clinical manifestations
   1. Dyspnea, irregular breathing pattern, coughing, weakness
   2. Swollen ankles late in the day, pitting edema
   3. Cyanosis, anxiety, fear
   4. Paleness, sweating, cold skin
E. Treatment (see Chapter 18, section on cardiac emergencies)
   1. Rest and limitation of activities
   2. Weight reduction (if necessary)

3. Dietary control (limit sodium intake)
4. Medications
   a. Diuretics
   b. Digitalis (increases the force of contractions)
F. Oral manifestations—none directly associated

Cerebrovascular Accident (Stroke)

A. Definition—sudden loss of brain function resulting from interference with the blood supply to a portion of the brain
B. Incidence/prevalence
   1. Initial strokes affect 74/1000 persons in the United States
   2. Third leading cause of death in the United States
   3. Blacks at greater risk than whites
   4. Males at greater risk than females
   5. Likelihood of having a stroke increases with age
C. Etiology
   1. Intracranial hemorrhage
   2. Blockage of vessels by thrombi or emboli (the most common cause)
   3. Vascular insufficiency
   4. Predisposing conditions
      a. Cerebral arteriosclerosis
      b. Dehydration
      c. Trauma
      d. Hypertension
      e. Diabetes
D. Signs/symptoms/clinical manifestations—depend on the area of the brain involved and the extent of damage (Table 14-11)
   1. Immediate
      a. Syncope, headache, chills, convulsions, nausea and vomiting
      b. Changes in the level of consciousness
      c. Transient paresthesias
      d. Mood swing
   2. Residual or chronic
      a. Paralysis—hemiparesis or localized
      b. Speech problems and aphasia (reduced capacity for the interpretation and formulation of language)
      c. Alterations in reflexes, especially the oral motor reflexes
      d. Functional disorders of the bladder or bowel
      e. Visual impairments
      f. Seizures
E. Treatment (see Chapter 18, section on cerebrovascular accident)
   1. Surgery
   2. Complete bed rest

Table 14-11 Functional limitations in stroke patients

Right hemiplegia (L-CVA)	Left hemiplegia (R-CVA)
Language problems Decreased *auditory* memory (cannot remember a long series of instructions) Vocabulary problems Slow, cautious, disorganized Anxious	Spatial-perceptual task difficulties—inability to judge distance, size, position, rate of movement, form and relation of parts to a whole Often thought to be unimpaired since able to speak and understand Visual field cuts; angles, etc., cannot be perceived Patient cannot use mirrors Patient cannot sequence tasks (such as toothbrushing) Decreased visual memory (loses place when reading) Cannot monitor self (keeps talking even though answered question already) May neglect left side Tendency to be impulsive and unaware of deficits. Spatial-perceptual difficulties are easy to miss

From Schubert, M.M., Snow, M., and Stiefel, D.J.: DECOD Series: Dental treatment of the stroke patient, Seattle, 1978, University of Washington.

3. Medications
    a. Anticoagulant therapy and vasodilators
    b. Antihypertensives
    c. Steroids
    d. Physical and occupational therapy
F. Oral manifestations
    1. Oral motor function
    2. Increased incidence of dental caries or periodontal disease because of oral motor problems or neglect

Sickle Cell Anemia

A. Definition
    1. Defect of hemoglobin that causes red blood cells to become sickle shaped
    2. Sickle cell trait—individual shows no symptoms unless experiencing abnormally low concentration of oxygen
    3. Sickle cell disease—progressively deteriorating and complex disease with multiple symptoms
B. Incidence/prevalence
    1. Found in blacks and other nonwhites; occurs in both sexes
    2. Sickle cell anemia found in 15% of this population; may die before age 40
    3. Sickle cell trait found in 9% of this population
    4. Babies do not show symptoms until age 6 months
C. Etiology
    1. Mutation in the globin gene of hemoglobin
    2. Sickle cell trait—individual has half normal hemoglobin and half sickle hemoglobin
    3. Sickle cell anemia—individual receives a sickle hemoglobin gene from both parents
    4. Sickled cells clog blood vessels

D. Signs/symptoms/clinical manifestations
    1. Infants
        a. Enlarged spleen, septicemia, and meningitis can develop
        b. Swelling of the feet and hands, pallor, tiredness, fever, pneumonia
    2. Preschoolers
        a. Severe pain crises affecting the extremities
        b. Strokes occur in 10% of those affected
    3. Adolescents
        a. Can develop gallstones, enlarged hearts, and lung infarctions
        b. Bones degenerate as a result of repeated sickling
        c. Delayed growth and late puberty
        d. Increased chance for stroke, impaired kidney and liver function, and arthritis
        e. Continued pain crisis
    4. Adulthood
        a. Hemorrhage or detached retina in the eye
        b. Pain crises—variable in each person
        c. Lung and kidney damage, gallstones
        d. Leg ulcers
    5. High altitude, chilling temperatures, stress, psychologic pressures, or infections can precipitate attacks
E. Treatment
    1. No cure
    2. Prevent complications
    3. Frequent transfusions (every 3 weeks) in some to prevent strokes
F. Oral manifestations
    1. Sore, painful, and red tongue
    2. Loss of taste sensation

3. Osteoporosis
4. Loss of trabecular pattern

Leukemias

A. Definition
1. Progressive malignant neoplasms characterized by an overproduction of abnormal leukocytes
2. Abnormal leukocytes displace hematopoietic tissue in the bone marrow, leading to decreased production of platelets, erythrocytes, and normal leukocytes
B. Classification
1. Chronicity
   a. Acute form—large numbers of immature nonspecific leukocytes are produced
   b. Chronic form—leukocytes are well differentiated and able to mature, but immunologic capacity is decreased
2. Type of white cell predominating
   a. Myeloid
   b. Lymphoid
   c. Monocytic
C. Incidence/prevalence
1. Acute type
   a. There are 3 to 4 cases per 100,000 persons in the United States
   b. Complete remission is gained by 85% to 90% using current treatment regimens
2. Chronic type—rare in children; 10 cases per 18,000 persons over age 75
3. Seventh leading cause of cancer death in adults; leading cause of cancer death in children
D. Etiology
1. Specific etiology unknown
2. Predisposing factors—genetic factors, ionizing radiation, other chemical agents
E. Signs/symptoms/clinical manifestations
1. Acute form appears suddenly and severely; chronic form is insidious
2. Fatigue, weakness, pallor
3. Ecchymoses of the skin and nosebleeds
4. Fever
5. Headache, nausea and vomiting
F. Treatment
1. Chemotherapy (alkylating agents)
2. Irradiation
3. Bone marrow transplant when indicated
G. Oral manifestations
1. Initial
   a. Leukemic infiltrate of the pulp and gingiva
      (1) Causes pain in teeth
      (2) Enlarged bluish-red, spongy, blunted papilla (Fig. 14-12)
      (3) Ulceration and necrosis

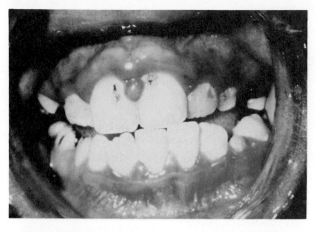

Fig. 14-12 Gingival enlargement in leukemia.

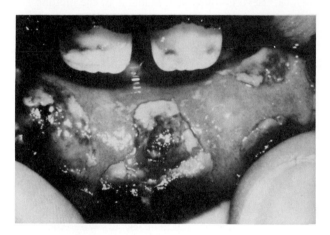

Fig. 14-13 Oral infections in leukemic patient.

   b. Mucositis, mucosal atrophy, and mucosal pallor
   c. Areas of spontaneous hemorrhage (intermittent oozing) and petechiae
   d. Loss of lamina dura, resorption of alveolar bone, cancellous bone destruction
2. Secondary
   a. Mucosal infections *(Candida, Pseudomonas)* and periapical infections (Fig. 14-13)
   b. Acute necrotizing ulcerative gingivitis (ANUG)
   c. Viral infections
   d. Osteomyelitis
3. Tertiary (treatment effects)
   a. Painful oral ulcerations
   b. Stomatitis
   c. Xerostomia and dental caries
   d. Jaw pain/Bell's palsy
   e. Secondary infections

Hemophilias

A. Definition—congenital disorder of the blood-clotting mechanism
B. Incidence/prevalence
   1. Occurs in 1/4000 males in the United States
   2. Majority have hemophilia A
   3. Ninety percent are under age 25
C. Classification
   1. Type
      a. Hemophilia A (factor VIII deficiency)
      b. Hemophilia B (factor IX deficiency)—Christmas Disease
      c. Von Willebrand's disease (lack of plasma—von Willebrand factor)
   2. Severity—level of clotting factor (normal level is 50% to 100%)
      a. Severe—have less than 1% of the clotting factor; may bleed spontaneously or from minor trauma
      b. Moderate—have 5% to 25% of the factor present; hemorrhage only with trauma
      c. Mild—have 25% to 50% of the factor present; bleed only after severe injuries and surgery
D. Etiology
   1. Hemophilia A and B
      a. Sex-linked recessive mode of inheritance (female carrier and manifested in males)
      b. High mutation rate
   2. Von Willebrand's disease—transmission by the dominant autosomal gene; occurs with equal frequency in both sexes
E. Signs/symptoms/clinical manifestations
   1. Bleeding and bruising from minor cuts or pressure
      a. Ecchymoses and hematomas
      b. Oozing
      c. Intramuscular bleeding causes pain
   2. Hemarthroses—bleeding into the soft tissues of the joints, leading to pain, swelling, and permanent joint contractures
   3. Renal function is impaired; exposure to hepatitis during transfusions
   4. Intracranial hemorrhages can cause seizures or other neurologic disorders
   5. Chronic complications include osteoarthritis, irregular growth, muscular atrophy, and tumor formation
   6. Inhibitor to antihemophilic factor can develop in hemophilia A, making the person resistant to replacement therapy
   7. Complications from bleeds include airway obstruction, intestinal obstruction, and compression of nerves and paralysis
F. Treatment
   1. Factor replacement therapy
      a. Fresh frozen plasma
      b. Cryoprecipitate (factor VIII and fibrinogen)
      c. Concentrates
   2. Amicar used for oral bleeds to help decrease bleeding
   3. Prevention of bleeds
   4. Joint replacement
   5. Physical therapy
G. Oral manifestations
   1. Ecchymoses, hematomas, and gingival oozing can be a problem (Fig. 14-14)
   2. Oral trauma is more evident and can be serious (Fig. 14-15)

Diabetes Mellitus

See Chapter 18, section on diabetes mellitus
A. Definition—hereditary disease of metabolism with
   1. Inadequate production and action of insulin from the pancreas
   2. Disorders in carbohydrate, protein, and fat metabolism
   3. Body cells unable to use glucose, leading to hyperglycemia
   4. "Brittle" diabetic patient has alternating extremes of hypoglycemia and hyperglycemia
B. Incidence/prevalence
   1. Diabetes mellitus affects 4.8 million people in the United States
   2. An additional 5.5 million have the potential for developing symptoms
   3. Both groups constitute 5% of the U.S. population
   4. Persons over age 45 constitute four fifths of patients
C. Types (Table 14-12)
   1. Type I, or insulin-dependent
   2. Type II, or noninsulin-dependent
D. Etiology
   1. Genetic disorder
   2. Destruction of the insulin-producing cells of the pancreas resulting from inflammation, cancer, or surgery
   3. Secondary to endocrine disorders (e.g., hyperthyroidism)
   4. Iatrogenic disease following the administration of steroids
E. Signs/symptoms/clinical manifestations
   1. Cardinal symptoms are those associated with hyperglycemia (Table 14-13)
   2. An overdose of insulin or inadequate glucose intake to balance the insulin intake can result in insulin shock (hypoglycemia) (Table 14-13)

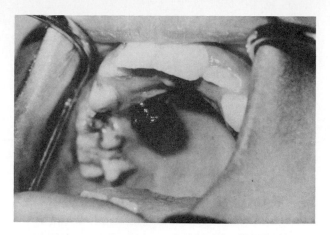

Fig. 14-14 Palatal bleed in hemophiliac patient.

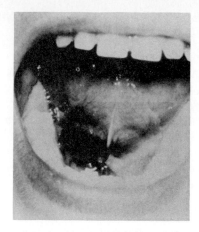

Fig. 14-15 Suction hematoma in hemophiliac patient.

Table 14-12   Comparison of type I and type II diabetes mellitus

Characteristic	Insulin-dependent diabetes mellitus	Noninsulin-dependent diabetes mellitus
Age of onset	Usually under 25 years; may appear later	Adulthood, particularly over 40 years; may appear at younger ages
Body weight	Normal or thin	High percent obese at the time of diagnosis
Rate of onset of clinical symptoms	Rapid	Slow
Severity	Severe	Mild
Diabetic emergency (ketoacidosis)	Common	Rare
Stability	Unstable	Stable
Insulin treatment required	Almost all	Less than 25%
Chronic manifestations	Uncommon before 20 years; prevalent and severe by age 30	Develop slowly with age

From Wilkins, E.M.: Clinical practice of the dental hygienist, ed. 5, Philadelphia, 1983, Lea & Febiger.

Table 14-13   Clinical manifestations of diabetes mellitus

Hyperglycemia	Hypoglycemia
Polydipsia	Early stage
Polyphagia	Diminished cerebral function
Polyuria	Changes in mood
Loss of weight	Decreased spontaneity
Fatigue	Hunger
Headache	Nausea
Blurred vision	More severe hypoglycemia
Nausea and vomiting	Sweating
Tachycardia	Tachycardia
Florid appearance	Piloerection
Hot and dry skin	Increased anxiety
Kussmaul respiration	Bizarre behavior patterns
Mental stupor	Belligerence
Loss of consciousness	Poor judgment
	Uncooperativeness
	Later severe stage
	Unconsciousness
	Seizure activity
	Hypotension
	Hypothermia

From Malamed, S.F.: Medical emergencies in the dental office, ed. 2, St. Louis, 1982, The C.V. Mosby Co.

3. Chronic complications include
   a. Atherosclerosis and other cardiovascular problems
   b. Renal failure
   c. Motor, sensory, and autonomic neuropathies
   d. Glaucoma and cataracts
   e. Associated with increased incidence of large babies, stillbirths, miscarriages, neonatal deaths, and congenital defects
F. Treatment—no known cure
   1. Management of acute symptoms
   2. Exercise and diet plan (food exchange system)
   3. Medications—insulin therapy (combination of short, intermediate, or long-acting insulin)
   4. Need to maintain a delicate balance between diet, exercise, and insulin
   5. Factors affecting the need for insulin
      a. Food intake
      b. Emotional events
      c. Exercise levels
      d. Infections
G. Oral manifestations (seen mainly in uncontrolled diabetics)
   1. Delayed wound healing and inability to manage oral infections (e.g., *Candida* infections)
   2. Decreased salivary flow may lead to increased caries
   3. Incidence of a rapidly progressing type of periodontal disease increases in type I diabetes

Thyroid Disease

A. Definition
   1. Hyperthyroidism (thyrotoxicosis)—excess of thyroid hormones in the bloodstream
   2. Graves' disease—toxic goiter
   3. Hypothyroidism—inadequate thyroid hormones in the bloodstream
      a. Cretinism—childhood onset (congenital)
      b. Myxedema—adult onset (acquired)
B. Incidence/prevalence
   1. Hyperthyroidism
      a. Disease is 7 times more common in women, especially being manifested during puberty, pregnancy, or menopause
      b. There are 3 cases per 10,000 adults per year
   2. Hypothyroidism
      a. Rare
      b. Myxedema is 5 times more common in females

C. Etiology
   1. Hyperthyroidism (Graves' disease)
      a. Etiology is unknown
      b. Autoimmune etiology or familial tendency is postulated
   2. Hypothyroidism
      a. Disease of the thyroid gland
      b. Myxedema may follow thyroid gland or pituitary gland failure resulting from irradiation, surgery, or excessive antithyroid drug therapy
D. Signs/symptoms/clinical manifestations—results of underproduction or overproduction of thyroid hormone (Table 14-14)
E. Treatment
   1. Hyperthyroidism
      a. Antithyroid drugs or iodine
      b. Surgery
   2. Hypothyroidism—daily thyroid supplement
F. Oral manifestations—primarily delayed or accelerated dental development (Table 14-14)

Chronic Alcoholism

A. Definition
   1. Chronic impairment in physical, mental, or social functioning caused by frequent ingestion (more than two drinks per day) of alcohol
   2. Can become dependent on its ingestion and also develop a tolerance to increasing amounts
B. Incidence/prevalence
   1. Heavy drinkers make up 7% to 10% of the U.S. population (two or more drinks per day)
   2. Majority are upper middle class
   3. Normal activities are maintained by 95%
   4. Eighty percent are heavy smokers
   5. One of every 12 adult drinkers has an alcohol dependency
C. Signs/symptoms/clinical manifestations
   1. Alcoholic breath
   2. Unexplained tremors
   3. Nausea and vomiting, gastrointestinal problems, ulcers
   4. Cutaneous lesions (redness, acne, spider angiomas)
   5. Edema of the eyelids and rest of the body
   6. Nutritional deficiencies (vitamin B, protein, calcium)

Table 14-14 Clinical features of thyroid disease

Hypothyroidism		Hyperthyroidism
Cretinism	Myxedema	
Dwarfism and obesity	Obesity	Weight loss
Coarse hair	Hair loss	Fine, friable hair
Eyes set apart	Puffy eyelids	Exopthalmus
	Muscle weakness	Tremors
	Dry cold skin	Warm, moist skin
	Decreased sweating	Increased sweating
	Cold intolerance	Heat intolerance
	Lethargy	Hyperactivity
	Bradycardia	Tachycardia
Delayed tooth eruption		Accelerated tooth eruption
Small jaws and malocclusion		Large jaws

Table 14-15 An overview of drug treatment modalities

Drug treatment may take the form of			
Supervisory-deterrent approaches	Medical-distributive approaches	Drug-free approaches	Crisis intervention approaches
Incarceration	Maintenance programs	Therapeutic communities	Hot lines
Criminal commitment	Detoxification programs	Self-help societies	Rap centers
Civil commitment	Antagonist programs		Free clinics
	Multimodality approaches		

From Duncan, D., and Gold, R.: Drugs and the whole person, New York, 1982, John Wiley & Sons, Inc. Reprinted by permission of John Wiley & Sons, Inc.

D. Long-term complications
   1. Hypertension and other types of heart disease
   2. Increased risk for various types of cancer
   3. Hepatitis, cirrhosis, and hypoglycemia
   4. Interference with the secretion of pancreatic enzymes
   5. Altered enzyme functioning and malabsorptive syndromes of the small intestine
   6. Irritation of the gastric mucosa leading to bleeding, inflammation, and ulceration
   7. Fetal alcohol syndrome (pregnant women)
   8. Impotence
E. Treatment
   1. Only about 10% of alcoholics receive treatment
   2. Table 14-15 provides an overview of drug treatment modalities for all types of drug dependence

   3. Some alcohol abuse programs involve use of disulfiram (Antabuse), which causes physical discomfort if alcohol is consumed
   4. Abstinence is an overriding goal
F. Oral manifestations—increased incidence of
   1. Caries caused by nausea and vomiting and neglected oral hygiene
   2. Periodontal disease caused by an impaired immune system and the effects on white blood cells
   3. Glossitis from nutritional deficiencies
   4. Leukoplakia and oral-pharyngeal cancer
   5. Swelling of the parotid glands leads to decreased salivation and increased caries incidence
   6. Trauma during inebriated states (accidents or fights)

Chronic Renal Failure

A. Definition
1. Progressive bilateral deterioration of renal function, resulting in uremia and eventually death
2. Uremia is the toxic condition produced by retention of urinary constituents in the blood

B. Incidence/prevalence
1. Affects 8 million people in the United States
2. Annually, 100,000 die (over 50% are over age 55)
3. Compromised life unless a successful transplant is performed (about 50% success rate)

C. Etiology
1. Infectious diseases (e.g., nephritis, viral and fungal infections)
2. Hypersensitivity states (e.g., glomerulonephritis)
3. Developmental defects of the kidneys
4. Circulatory disturbances (e.g., hypertension, hemorrhages)
5. Metabolic diseases (e.g., diabetes)

D. Signs/symptoms/clinical manifestations
1. Mental slowness or depression
2. Swelling and edema
3. Muscular hyperactivity
4. Hyperpigmentation of the skin (brownish yellow)
5. Anorexia and vomiting, diarrhea
6. Anemia
7. Possible functional defect in factor VIII protein, leading to hemorrhagic episodes
8. Hypertension, congestive heart failure
9. Complete natural history of the disease is displayed in the box on p. 561.

E. Treatment
1. Potassium regulation
2. Sodium regulation
3. Maintenance of water balance (depends on urine output, edema, and weight change)
4. Protein balance
5. Acid-base balance—correct acidosis with calcium carbonate (also give vitamin D)
6. Sedatives and hypnotics to manage neuromuscular complications
7. Dialysis when other methods alone are not effective
   a. Peritoneal—usually for acute renal failure
      (1) Injection of hypertonic solution into the peritoneal cavity
      (2) Draws out urea and other solutes
      (3) Less costly, easier to perform, but less effective than hemodialysis
      (4) More people using ambulatory type, where continuous dialysis is performed by the patient, with drainage into a bag
   b. Hemodialysis for chronic renal failure
      (1) Creation of an arteriovenous shunt (Fig. 14-16)
      (2) Blood runs from the artery to the dialysis machine, is filtered, and then returned to the vein
      (3) Heparin is added to prevent blood clotting
      (4) Patient is at risk for acquiring hepatitis from commercial blood products
   c. Kidney transplant—problems with graft rejections; use steroids, immunosuppressives, and antibiotics

F. Oral manifestations
1. Painful oral ulcerations and stomatitis from drugs
2. Candidiasis
3. Increased calculus deposits
4. Anemic mucosa
5. Oral petechia and hemorrhage
6. Ground-glass appearance of alveolar bone caused by leaching of calcium (uremic bone disease) (Fig. 14-17)
7. Bad taste and halitosis from urea in saliva
8. Enamel hypoplasia (Fig. 14-18)

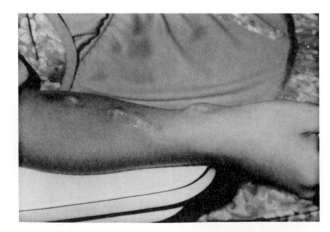

Fig. 14-16 Multiple access sites for arteriovenous shunts for hemodialysis.

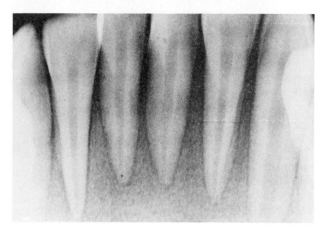

Fig. 14-17 Uremic bone disease in chronic renal failure.

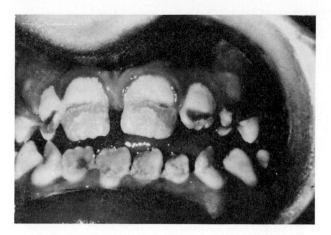

Fig. 14-18 Enamel hypoplasia associated with chronic renal failure.

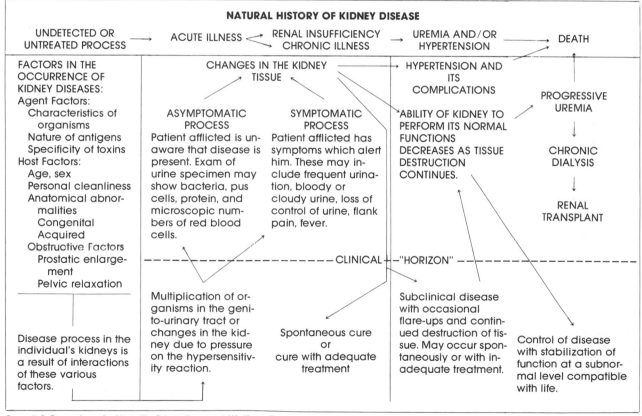

From U.S. Department of Health, Education and Welfare, Public Health Service: Kidney diseases—a guide for public health personnel, Washington, D.C., 1970.

DENTAL MANAGEMENT (Table 14-16) ▬▬▬▬▬

A. Personal and professional prerequisites
1. Interview in a sensitive manner to gather accurate data
2. Analyze and summarize data in oral or written format
3. Use problem-solving skills to develop alternative strategies to manage problems
4. Evaluate patient and professional goals and progress for appropriateness and effectiveness
5. Remain current in terms of new conditions, new methods of medical management, and advances in dental techniques
6. Apply new knowledge or techniques from other areas to dental management of special patients
7. Apply research principles and techniques to acquire clinical data that serve as the basis for treatment planning and preventive decision making

B. Office management issues
1. Stress a team concept with cooperation among members and coordination of information and activities
2. Identify and anticipate patient needs and problems before initiation of treatment; use of a previsit questionnaire is helpful (see box below)
3. Obtain informed consent for treatment from the patient or an appropriate representative before treatment
4. Explain office policies and procedures to the patient or guardian before or at the first appointment
5. Determine financial limitations that may affect treatment planning or payment procedures
   a. Determine additional resources available from other sources (e.g., community organizations)
   b. Attempt to provide flexible payment alternatives
6. If the patient is unable to receive care in the office because of physical limitations or geographic distance, care can be provided in a home or community setting using portable equipment
7. If office facilities are not physically accessible, make arrangements to
   a. Make them physically accessible
   b. Provide assistance to those who have difficulties
   c. Refer disabled patients to another practice that is accessible
8. Keep scheduling somewhat flexible to allow for transportation or other problems; block appointments are helpful when dealing with groups

Text continued on p. 575.

PREVISIT QUESTIONNAIRE FOR GATHERING DATA

Name _____ Phone _____

Address _____ Age _____

_____

Name/address of contact person (if different)

_____ Phone _____

_____

_____

Physician _____ Type _____ Phone _____

_____ Type _____ Phone _____

Medical problems/handicapping conditions _____

Potential barriers:

Transportation _____

Finances _____

Communication _____

Psychosocial _____

Medical _____

Mobility/stability _____

Other _____

Scheduling limitations _____

Other data _____

Table 14-16 Dental management considerations for special-needs patients

Condition	Medical issues	Barriers to care	Risk factors	Treatment considerations	Prevention/ education issues
Mental retardation	Syndrome? Associated medical conditions/other disabilities Treatment regimens	Limited financial resources Degree of reliance on others Limited mental ability	Oral motor dysfunction General incoordination Cariogenic foods/ reinforcers Self-abuse Resistant behavior	Gagging: radiographs, instrument placement, positioning Mental impairment: communication, cooperation, and stability in chair Limited finances: alternative treatment plans	"Tell, show, do" approach Simple language Frequent repetition and positive reinforcement Involve caretakers Frequent recall appointments Alternatives for food reinforcers
Down syndrome	Heart defects? (antibiotic premedication) Decreased resistance to infection	Same as for mental retardation	Same as for mental retardation	Same as for mental retardation plus: Small oral area: oral access for procedures Hearing disorders: communication	Same as for mental retardation plus: Stress oral hygiene and periodontal maintenance
Autism	No major problems	Behavior Degree of reliance on others	Eating disorders or fetishes Resistant behavior	Dependence on "routines": procedure sequencing Lack of useful language: communication Learning disabilities/ sensitivity to stimuli: communication distractions in the operatory	Combine verbal and nonverbal communication techniques and positive reinforcers Teach toothbrushing as a "motion" rather than a function Avoid metaphors and complex language structures
Learning disabilities/ minimal brain dysfunction	Medications and potential side effects	Depends on type of disability	Depends on disability Oral motor dysfunction General incoordination	Depends on disability Disorientation/ hyperactivity: stability in chair, length of appointments, physical contact	Tap skill areas Use combination of teaching approaches Maintain attention through eye contact and physical contact

Continued.

Table 14-16 Dental management considerations for special-needs patients — cont'd

Condition	Medical issues	Barriers to care	Risk factors	Treatment considerations	Prevention/ education issues
Emotional disturbance/ mental illness	Medications and potential side effects Psychologic causes of reported symptoms/ diseases, fears	Limited financial re- sources in some cases Emotional concerns, fears about dental care Disturbed thought processes	Depends on nature of disturbance Inadequate diet or strange food practices Phobias relating to oral care Self-abuse Side effects of medications	Anxiety, fear, aggression: stability in chair, cooperation, communication	Reality orientation techniques Possible dietary counseling Involve caretakers Positive reinforcement and repetition Decrease phobias and self-abuse Fluoride supplements if xerostomia from medications
Alzheimer's disease	Multiple medical problems Medications Reduced bowel and bladder control Fatigue from abnormal sleep patterns	Behavior Finances may be limited by disability and medical problems Wheelchair confinement Dependence on others	Oral motor dysfunction Depression or disorientation leading to oral neglect General motor dysfunction	Fluctuating moods and disorientation: length of appoint- ments, communication, cooperation Motor problems: oral access, radiographs, stability in chair Memory loss: data collection	Involve caretakers Involve patient when most lucid and positive Simple instructions and frequent repetition Positive reinforcement Frequent recall
Epilepsy	Medications and side effects Seizure information Degree of control Specific manifestations Presence of aura Frequency General management History of status epilepticus	Self-image problems Transportation if cannot drive	Side effects of medications Orofacial trauma during seizures	Seizure activity: treatment planning, appointment scheduling, stability in chair, communication Tissue overgrowth from phenytoin: treatment planning	Optimal oral hygiene and frequent recalls to decrease gingival overgrowth from phenytoin First-aid instructions for oral trauma Positive reinforcement and self-image building
Visual impairment	Degree of impairment? Sensitivity to light Treated versus untreated conditions	Partial or total dependence on others Attitudes and stereotypes about disability and toward guide dogs Limited income if not fully employed Locating dental providers Physical obstacles to or in office	No specific factors	Sight impairment: appointment scheduling, explanation of procedures, clinician position, communication, positioning of light, mobility into clinic, data collection, noise level Guide dog: placement in comfortable place in office (preferably not next to dental chair)	Watch tone of voice Comment on any changes in procedures Describe everything graphically Demonstrate procedures on finger, etc. Precede actions with verbal descriptions Teach toothbrushing in mouth Use audio aids or physical models for teaching

Condition					
Hearing impairment	Degree of impairment? Functioning of hearing aid	Partial or total dependence on others Limited income if not fully employed Locating dental providers	No specific factors	Hearing impairment: appointment scheduling, explanation of procedures, clinician position, communication, data collection, noise interference, use of aid during appointment	Determine appropriate communication techniques Provide paper and pencil if desired Involve translator if needed Watch facial expressions
Cleft lip or palate	Hearing impairment Upper respiratory tract infections Prosthetic appliances Medications	Fear of health care providers Self-image problems	Missing or malaligned teeth Oral motor dysfunction Feeding disorders	Cleft: clear communication, instrument positioning or fulcruming, suctioning and prevention of aspiration Fear: dental procedures, cooperation	Involve caretaker when appropriate Instruct in cleaning any prosthetic aids Nutritional counseling if needed
Cerebral palsy	Associated disorders Medications Other therapies Respiration impaired? Presence of primitive reflexes Degree of impairment	Communication Transportation if in wheelchair or cannot drive May have limited financial resources Dependence on others for care in many cases Mobility problems if in wheelchair Provider attitudes toward condition	Oral motor dysfunction General motor dysfunction Suboptimal fluoride intake possible Special diets	Primitive reflexes: patient or clinician position, stability, instrument positioning or fulcruming, oral access, suctioning and amount of water used, protection of airway, radiographs Use of wheelchair: transfers to dental chair, mobility in office, office accessibility	Involve caretakers as appropriate Be patient with slowness of responses and progress Use combination of communication methods Assess need for physical assistance or adaptive aids for home care Frequent recalls Fluoride supplements Nutritional counseling if needed
Bell's palsy	Therapies, especially prednisone Duration of condition	No specific barriers	Oral motor dysfunction	Lack of eye closure: protection of eyes (goggles) Oral motor dysfunction: protection of airway	Caution regarding effects of anesthesia Frequent rinsing or toothbrushing for food retention on affected side
Myasthenia gravis	Medications History of radiation therapy or surgery History of myasthenic crises	Communication	Oral motor dysfunction	Weakness increases during day: scheduling appointments Oral motor dysfunction/paralysis/impaired breathing, protection of airway, use of rubber dam, suctioning, chair position Weak voice: communication	Frequent recalls to prevent infection Frequent rinsing or toothbrushing for food retention

Continued.

Table 14-16 Dental management considerations for special-needs patients—cont'd

Condition	Medical issues	Barriers to care	Risk factors	Treatment considerations	Prevention/education issues
Parkinson's disease	Medications and side effects Rigidity of larger joints Sensitivity to heat	Mobility to and in office Communication Embarrassment about condition	Oral motor dysfunction Side effects of drugs Possible inadequate diet	Tremors: stability, instrumentation, radiographs Sensitivity to heat: temperature of operatory Muscular pain and joint rigidity: chair position, appointment length Slurred speech: communication	Frequent recalls Frequent rinsing and toothbrushing Adaptive equipment or assistance if needed Fluoride supplements Counseling re: side effects of medications
Arthritis	Medications Degree of impairment Joints affected Joint replacement (premedication may be needed)	Mobility to and in office Limited finances if disabled Weakness or fatigue decreases motivation to seek care	General motor impairment	Joint pain: chair position, appointment length Limited oral opening: positioning, instrumentation, radiographs	Adaptive equipment or assistance if needed Counseling re: side effects of medications
Multiple sclerosis	Medications and side effects Degree of facial pain Degree of impairment Sensitivity to heat	Mobility to and in office, especially if in wheelchair Depression or moodiness affects motivation Limited finances if on disability	Special diets Side effects of drugs Fine motor coordination problems Oral motor dysfunction	Weakness and numbness: wheelchair transfer, stability, appointment length Oral motor dysfunction: protection of airway Mood changes: communication, acceptance of treatment, cooperation Sensitivity to heat: room temperature Periods of exacerbation/remission: appointment scheduling	Adaptive equipment or assistance may be needed More frequent rinsing and brushing Assistance in dietary counseling Supplemental fluoride More frequent recalls to prevent infections
Muscular dystrophies	Medications Other therapies Type and degree of involvement Prognosis Check for obesity, scoliosis, or cardiopulmonary involvement	Depends on type Mobility to and in office, especially if in wheelchair Limited financial resources Weakness and possible decreased life span decreases motivation	Oral motor dysfunction General motor weakness and incoordination Dietary inadequacies Mouth breathing	Depends on type and degree of involvement Muscle weakness: stability in chair, wheelchair transfers, radiographs, instrumentation, appointment length Oral motor dysfunction: protection of airway, communication	Frequent recalls More frequent brushing and rinsing Fluoride supplements Adapted equipment or physical assistance for oral care

		Locating accessible office facilities		Incoordination: restorative treatment planning and possible emergency care Limited life span: treatment planning, motivation	
Spinal injuries	Depends on level of injury Medications Respiratory involvement Decubitus ulcers Incontinence/encopresis Contractures Heterotopic ossifications Body temperature regulation Potential for autonomic hyperreflexia Type of adaptive equipment	Mobility to and in office, especially if in wheel chair or on respirator Limited financial resources unless employed Psychosocial concerns/depression Locating accessible office facilities	Depends on level of injury Oral motor dysfunction Limited or total dependence on others Special diets	Psychologic state: communication, cooperation Spasticity, tremors: stability Paralysis: mobility, wheelchair transfers, stability in chair, length of appointment Impaired respiration/oral motor dysfunction: chair position, use of rubber dam, protection of airway, instrumentation	Adaptive equipment or physical assistance needed Fluoride supplementation Consider psychologic state
Spina bifida	Depends on type Similar to spinal injuries Shunt for hydrocephalus (antibiotic premedication) Seizure disorders	Depends on type and degree of impairment Similar to spinal injuries	Similar to spinal injuries, except oral motor dysfunction not apparent	Similar to spinal injuries, although psychologic state not as poor	Learning disabilities influence dental health education methods Fluoride supplementation
Viral hepatitis (see Chapter 7)	Type Degree of liver impairment Immunity versus active state versus carrier state Follow-up with physician if status unclear Good history Need for antigen or antibody test	Finding dentist if a chronic carrier	Potential for transmission of virus High-carbohydrate diet	Viral transmission: strict sterilization procedures, use of gloves and mask by clinician, no treatment if active state, use of aerosol-producing equipment	No specific concerns unless a chronic carrier Isolation of toothbrush from others if a carrier Counseling regarding transmission via saliva if type B or NANB Dietary counseling and fluoride supplements while on special diet
AIDS (see Chapter 7)	Systems involved Degree of impairment Consult with physician Kaposi's sarcoma Treatment regimens	Finding dentist who will treat Stigmas associated with disease Decreased motivation/depression Limited finances if unemployed	Oral infections	Viral transmission: same as for hepatitis Oral infections: treatment planning, transmission potential Kaposi's sarcoma: treatment planning Psychologic state: communication, motivation	Palliative care for oral infections Increased attention to oral hygiene

Continued.

Table 14-16 Dental management considerations for special-needs patients — cont'd

Condition	Medical issues	Barriers to care	Risk factors	Treatment considerations	Prevention/ education issues
Sexually transmitted diseases (gonorrhea, syphilis, genital herpes) (see Chapter 7)	Determine status: history of disease, active disease reported or observed, in high-risk group Treatment regimen and compliance Follow-up care Medication sensitivity Complications from long-standing untreated cases	Psychosocial stigma of diseases	Potential for disease transmission	Disease transmission: sterilization, use of mask and gloves by clinician Oral lesions: palliative care	Counseling regarding disease transmission concerns
Tuberculosis	Good history Treatment regimen (compliance and effectiveness) Appropriate follow-up care Instances of reinfection Organ systems affected	Stigma of condition	Potential for disease transmission	Disease transmission: same as for hepatitis	No specific recommendations except prevention of disease transmission
Cystic fibrosis	Degree of impairment, and prognosis Dietary changes Treatment regimens	Small stature may cause embarrassment Prognosis may decrease motivation Finances may be limited	Decreased resistance to infections	Mucus accumulations/ impaired breathing: chair position, appointment scheduling and length, coughing, protection of airway, use of rubber dam Fear of medical situations: cooperation Susceptibility to infections: appointment scheduling Tetracycline staining: esthetics, treatment planning	Fluoride supplements if dry mouth Frequent oral care due to mouth breathing Coordinate dietary suggestions with other professionals

Condition	Assessment	Barriers to care	Risk factors	Management	Preventive measures
Bronchial asthma	Type and severity of asthma Frequency and severity of attacks Precipitating factors Treatment regimens History of hospitalizations or status asthmaticus Instruct patient to bring inhalers if used	Fear of medical/dental environments	No specific risk factors	Anxiety: possible premedication or use of nitrous oxide Medications/precipitating factors: contraindications to prescribing or using certain drugs, appointment scheduling, medical emergency preparedness	Model relaxed, stress-free environment No specific preventive requirements
Congenital heart disease	Type and if repaired Extent of limitations Medications Prognosis Need for antibiotic premedication Physician consult	Financial constraints from medical bills Frequent illness Possibly debilitated state Overprotective attitude of parents	Decreased resistance to infections	Bleeding potential in some cases: treatment planning, need for lab tests, possible referral to specialist Heart condition: antibiotic premedication, stress management protocols, appointment length, chair position	Emphasize danger of intraoral infections in terms of aggravating heart condition Frequent recalls
Rheumatic fever and heart disease	Residual effects of rheumatic fever Physician consult regarding need for antibiotic premedication	No specific barriers	No specific risk factors	Heart defects: need for antibiotic premedication	Stress oral hygiene to prevent oral infections
Cardiac arrhythmias	Type and severity Symptoms Medications and side effects Presence of pacemaker and type	If pacemaker, avoidance of certain electric equipment	No specific risk factors	Pacemaker: avoidance of electromagnetic equipment Arrhythmia: stress management protocol, drug precautions, bleeding potential from medications	No specific preventive regimens

Continued.

Table 14-16 Dental management considerations for special-needs patients – cont'd

Condition	Medical issues	Barriers to care	Risk factors	Treatment considerations	Prevention/ education issues
Hypertensive disease	Vital sign monitoring Physician consult or referral Medications and side effects and other treatment regimens Cause: primary or secondary Predisposing or general risk factors Severity, symptoms Possibility of orthostatic hypotension	Anxiety about dental care	Side effects of medications	Hypertension: stress management protocols, chair position, treatment planning, monitoring vital signs, appointment scheduling, contraindications to treatment Medications: drug interactions, gag reflex, local anesthetics, bleeding potential	Counseling regarding reducing general risk factors Palliative care for oral infections from medications Fluoride supplements for xerostomia
Ischemic heart disease	Physician consult Angina or myocardial infarction episodes Hospitalizations Medications and side effects Surgery or pacemakers	Possible debilitated state Medical and other expenses Anxiety about dental treatment If pacemaker, avoidance of electromagnetic equipment	Side effects of medications Susceptibility to infections if debilitated	Heart condition: same considerations as for hypertensive disease and preparation for medical emergency, contraindications for treatment if uncontrolled or recent attack (within 6 months) Medications: same as for hypertensive disease Pacemaker: avoidance of electromagnetic equipment	Palliative care for side effects of medications Counseling regarding decreasing general risk factors Special oral hygiene instructions if hospitalized or bedridden Frequent recalls

Condition					
Congestive heart failure	Same as for severe ischemic or hypertensive heart disease				
Cerebrovascular accident (stroke)	Type of involvement, degree of limitation; Seizures?; Medications and side effects; Other therapies	Communication; Limited financial resources; Accessibility if need adaptive equipment or wheelchair; Partial or total dependence on others	Oral motor dysfunction; Side effects of medications; Impaired general motor coordination; Dietary inadequacies	Memory impairment, communication, data collection; Oral motor dysfunction/paralysis, instrumentation, jaw stability, radiographs, treatment planning; Impaired emotional control: cooperation, communication; General paralysis: mobility, possible wheelchair transfers, stability in chair	Use combination of teaching approaches; Reinforce and repeat instructions; Frequent recalls; Fluoride supplementation; Adaptive aids or supervision for oral care; Avoid sensory overload; Reorient patient to situations; Use one-step instructions; Dietary analysis/counseling
Sickle cell anemia	Precipitating factors for crises; Symptoms and severity; Associated conditions; Transfusions?; Lab tests needed?	Periods of pain; Debilitated condition at times; Fear of dental environment; Limited financial resources because of medical bills	Susceptibility to infections	Sickle cell crises: appointment scheduling, motivation, emergency care only; Susceptibility to infections: periodontal maintenance, physician consult for possible antibiotic premedication	Dietary counseling; Frequent recalls because of associated alveolar bone problems; Involvement of others in care

Continued.

Table 14-16 Dental management considerations for special-needs patients—cont'd

Condition	Medical issues	Barriers to care	Risk factors	Treatment considerations	Prevention/ education issues
Leukemias	Type Treatment regimens, frequency	Stages of acute disease versus remissions Fear of dental environment	Side effects of chemotherapy or radiation therapy Susceptibility to infections	Bleeding potential: preappointment lab tests, appointment scheduling, physician consult, surgical procedures Susceptibility to infections: periodontal maintenance, antibiotic premedication Acute versus remission stages: treatment planning, appointment scheduling Chemotherapy or radiation therapy: treatment planning	Palliative care for oral lesions Frequent recalls Fluoride program Involvement of others in care program
Hemophilias	Type and severity Frequency and location of bleeds Treatment regimens Joint replacements? Hepatitis? Seizures? Inhibitor status Lab tests needed?	Finding dentist who will treat Resources for emergency care	Potential for oral bleeds	Bleeding potential: preappointment lab tests, surgery, physician consult, factor replacement therapy, instrumentation, radiographs, use of rubber dam, suctioning, use of AMICAR Joint replacements: antibiotic premedication Hepatitis carrier: disease transmission procedures	Use of oral rinses and soft-bristled brush Counseling regarding first aid for oral trauma Frequent recalls

Diabetes mellitus	Type and severity Insulin regimens Dietary regimen Complications Hypertension and other heart conditions Frequency of episodes of hypoglycemia or hyperglycemia	Finding dentist who will treat if have chronic complications	Susceptibility to infections Decreased salivary flow in some	Insulin/sugar balance: potential for medical emergency, appointment scheduling, stress management protocol Susceptibility to infection: periodontal maintenance, possible antibiotic premedication, treatment planning Associated conditions (see management for each condition)	Frequent recalls Dietary analysis Fluoride program Need for immaculate plaque control
Thyroid disease	Type and cause Symptoms and severity Medications	No specific barriers	Abnormal dental development	Sensitivity to drugs: treatment planning, postoperative instructions, preparation for medical emergency Mental retardation in some (see management for mental retardation) Abnormal dental development: treatment planning Heat or cold intolerance: room temperature, length of appointment	Special hygiene instruction if mentally retarded Good oral hygiene to prevent infection

Continued.

Table 14-16 Dental management considerations for special-needs patients – cont'd

Condition	Medical issues	Barriers to care	Risk factors	Treatment considerations	Prevention/ education issues
Chronic alcoholism	Patient's perception of severity of problem Symptoms Treatment program Nutritional deficiencies Chronic complications Degree of liver impairment	Limited finances if not employed Potential for no-show appointments	Susceptibility to infection Nutritional deficiencies Nausea and vomiting Potential for oral trauma	Liver impairment and bleeding potential: preappointment lab testing, drug metabolism, instrumentation, treatment planning Inebriated states: emergency care, appointment scheduling, treatment planning, data collection Associated medical problems (see management for each problem)	Nutritional counseling Frequent recalls Fluoride programs Frequent soft tissue evaluation for oral cancer Counseling regarding first aid for oral trauma Firm approach regarding need for good oral hygiene Instill responsibility for oral care
Chronic renal failure	Symptoms and severity Hypertension Dialysis? Transplant? Special diets Need for antibiotic premedication	Finding dentist who will treat Debilitated condition at times Limited finances Fear of dental environment	Susceptibility to oral infection Dietary inadequacies	Hypertension and kidney failure: vital signs, drug interactions, drug metabolism Bleeding tendency: preappointment blood tests, instrumentation, physician consult AV shunt: antibiotic premedication Dialysis: appointment scheduling Transplants: premedication with steroids or antibiotics	Frequent recalls because of increased calculus Emphasis on good oral hygiene to prevent infection Palliative care for oral lesions Dietary counseling
Pregnancy	Trimester Side effects Nutritional status	Frequent sickness	Possible dietary inadequacies	Fetal sensitivity: avoidance of drugs, radiographs, elective dental procedures Pressure of fetus on mother: chair position, orthostatic hypotension (turn on left side to alleviate)	Prenatal counseling Good oral hygiene to decrease response to local irritants

C. Medical issues
1. Obtain a health history from the patient or caretaker, another professional, or agency records
2. Update the health history frequently
3. Be aware that many standard medical history forms will be inadequate for the multiple conditions and problems of some patients
4. Obtain specifics regarding medical treatment regimens or other therapies that may affect scheduling or treatment
5. Obtain names, addresses, and phone numbers for all the patient's physicians who might provide helpful data (e.g., generalist, cardiac specialist, endocrinologist)
6. Be particularly alert to the patient's physical status during the clinical appraisal
7. Monitor vital signs when appropriate
8. Record all medication information; update whenever it changes, which may be frequently
9. Note any indications or contraindications to treatment or premedication
10. Maintain records of all medical advice, prescriptions, or drugs given
11. If patients refuse to disclose medical information or follow recommended standard procedures for their own protection (e.g., antibiotic premedication), have them sign a statement to that effect for the records
12. Provide both written and verbal instructions for medication regimens or posttreatment suggestions
13. Develop an office policy for medical emergencies, differentiating between true emergencies and situations that just require common sense and appropriate responses (e.g., myocardial infarction versus a psychomotor seizure)

D. Treatment adaptations
1. Demonstrate understanding and acceptance of the conditions or problems to the patient and to significant others
2. Determine which special needs require provider adaptations versus patient adaptations
3. Demonstrate empathy, not sympathy
4. Discuss before treatment
   a. Behavioral expectations
   b. Overview of the entire treatment plan
   c. Procedures that will be performed at that appointment
   d. Approximate time required
   e. Communication techniques to be used during the appointment

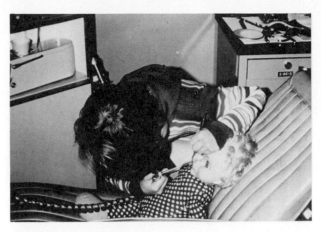

Fig. 14-19 Introducing child to dental treatment through role playing with doll.

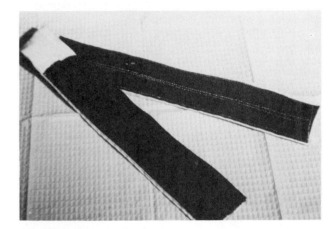

Fig. 14-20 Velcro strap used to provide patient stability in chair.

5. Introduce patients to the dental situation gradually, using desensitization, modeling, "show and tell," or other methods (Fig. 14-19)
6. Ensure patient comfort in the dental chair through frequent feedback, positioning, and supportive measures as needed (e.g., pillows)
7. Explain carefully the need for patient restraint for behavioral or stability purposes to ensure the patient's safety while in the chair; Velcro straps similar to seat belts are helpful for stability (Fig. 14-20)
8. Be aware that adaptations for specific procedures require problem solving and experimentation between the provider and patient; Fig. 14-21 shows various adaptations for procuring radiographs; Fig. 14-22 displays a variety of mouth props

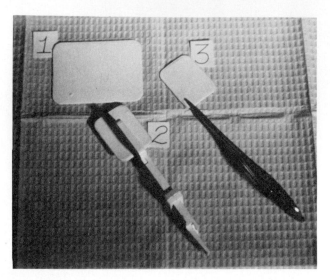

Fig. 14-21 Adaptations for procuring radiographs: *1*, occlusal size film; *2*, Snap-a-Ray, *3*, hemostat.

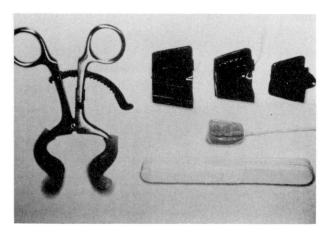

Fig. 14-22 Mouth props are useful for gaining intraoral access and jaw stability.

9. Discuss mechanisms for wheelchair transfers with each patient, since preferences and techniques vary
10. Protect the patient's airway through use of a rubber dam, adequate suctioning, and other means; this is of paramount importance because of the frequency of impaired oral reflexes
E. Preventive measures
  1. Identify risk factors for dental disease to plan preventive programs to
    a. Maximize positive health behaviors
    b. Eliminate risk factors
    c. Eliminate existing disease

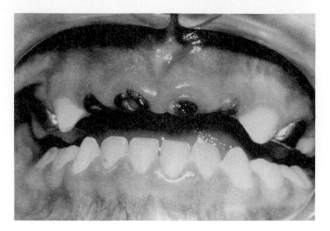

Fig. 14-23 Bottle mouth caries from prolonged bottle feeding.

  2. Common risk factors include
    a. Prolonged bottle feeding (Fig. 14-23)
    b. Inadequate diet
    c. Frequent snacking of cariogenic foods
    d. Suboptimal fluoride supplementation
    e. Oral motor dysfunction (e.g., hyperactive gag or impaired tongue control)
    f. General motor dysfunction interfering with oral hygiene care
    g. Crisis orientation to care
    h. Preoccupation with one's disability
  3. Develop individualized programs to reduce or eliminate the risk factors
  4. Consider the person's limitations when recommending home care procedures
    a. Problems with fluoride rinses or disclosing tablets if the patient has oral motor problems
    b. Problems performing the sequence of toothbrushing strokes if the patient has memory or general motor impairment
    c. Problems picking up and using a toothbrush and toothpaste if the patient has a spinal cord injury
  5. Schedule frequent recall appointments
  6. Coordinate preventive efforts in home, school, work place or dental office

SUGGESTED READINGS

American Dental Association: Prevention and control of dental disease through improved access to comprehensive care, Chicago, 1980, The Association.

Bond, A.W., and Mordarski, S.W.: Dental hygiene care of the special needs patient, Chicago, 1981, American Dental Hygiene Association.

Brown, J.P., and Schodel, D.R.: A review of controlled surveys of dental disease in handicapped persons, J. Dent. Child. **43**:17, 1976.

Burkhart, N.: Understanding and managing the autistic child in the dental office, Dent. Hyg. **58**:60, 1984.

Cooley, R.L., and Lubow, R.M.: AIDS: an occupational hazard? J. Am. Dent. Assoc. **107**:28, 1983.

Danforth, H.A., Snow, M., and Steifel, D.J.: Dental management of the cerebral palsied patient, Seattle, 1977, University of Washington.

Duncan, D., and Gold, R.: Drugs and the whole person, New York, 1982, John Wiley & Sons, Inc.

Engar, R.C., and Stiefel, D.J.: Dental treatment of the sensory impaired patient, Seattle, 1977, University of Washington.

Evans, B.E.: Dental care in hemophilia, New York, 1977, National Hemophilia Foundation.

Kokmen, E.: Dementia—Alzheimer type, Mayo Clini. Proc. **59**:35, 1984.

Lange, B.M., Entwistle, B.M., and Lipson, L.F.: Dental management of the handicapped: approaches for dental auxiliaries, Philadelphia, 1983, Lea & Febiger.

Little, J.W., and Falace, D.A.: Dental management of the medically compromised patient, ed. 2, St. Louis, 1984, The C.V. Mosby Co.

Malamed, S.F.: Handbook of medical emergencies in the dental office, ed. 2, St. Louis, 1982, The C.V. Mosby Co.

Nowak, A.J.: Dentistry for the handicapped patient, St. Louis, 1976, The C.V. Mosby Co.

Robert Wood Johnson Foundation: Special report: dental care for handicapped Americans, Princeton, 1979, The Foundation.

Schubert, M.M., Snow, M., and Stiefel, D.J.: Dental treatment of the spinal cord injured patient, Seattle, 1977, University of Washington.

Schubert, M.M., et al.: Dental treatment of the stroke patient, Seattle, 1978, University of Washington.

Scully, C., and Cawson, R.A.: Medical problems in dentistry, Boston, 1982, John Wright/PSG, Inc.

Segelman, A.E., and Doku, H.C.: Treatment of the oral complications of leukemia, J. Oral Surg. **35**:469, 1977.

Snow, M., Hale, J.M., and Stiefel, D.J.: Disabled dental patient—how many?, Seattle, 1978, University of Washington.

Snow, M.K., and Stiefel, D.J.: Dental treatment of the mentally retarded patient, Seattle, 1978, University of Washington.

Snyder, G.B., et al.: Your cleft lip and palate child, Evansville, Ind., Mead Johnson Lab.

Szymartis, D.S.: Dental considerations for treatment of the alcohol-consuming patient, J. Am. Dent. Assoc. **75**:592, 1977.

U.S. Department of Health, Education, and Welfare, Public Health Service: Kidney disease—a guide for public health personnel, Washington, D.C., 1970.

Wilkins, E.M.: Clinical practice of the dental hygienist, ed. 5, Philadelphia, 1983, Lea & Febiger.

Review Questions

1 Which of the following handicapping conditions is *not* generally associated with cerebral palsy?
1. Seizures
2. Visual defects
3. Hyperthyroidism
4. Hearing disorders
5. Speech disorders

2 The *most* optimal time to schedule a dental appointment for a patient on hemodialysis is
1. Immediately after dialysis
2. Dental treatment is contraindicated for patients on hemodialysis
3. 24 hours after dialysis
4. 4 hours after dialysis
5. Time is not a critical factor

3 All of the following groups are considered high risk for transmission of hepatitis virus, types B or NANB *except*
1. Hemodialysis patients
2. Hemophiliac patients with severe factor deficiency
3. Tuberculosis patients
4. Male homosexuals
5. Indochinese refuges

4 The *most* critical dental health problem for patients with Down syndrome is usually
1. The high dental caries rate
2. Malocclusion
3. Bruxism
4. The periodontal condition
5. Oral cancer

5 Premedication with antibiotics before dental treatment to prevent infectious endocarditis is recommended for patients with a history of *any* of the following conditions *except*
1. Myocardial infarction
2. Rheumatic heart disease
3. Prosthetic heart valves
4. Ventriculoatrial shunt for hydrocephalus
5. Pathologic heart murmur

6 Special dietary considerations are involved in *all* of the following conditions *except*
1. Diabetes
2. Chronic renal failure
3. Cystic fibrosis
4. Autism
5. Hypertension

7 Myasthenic crisis is a medical emergency because
1. The patient is unable to clear secretions from the throat, thus impairing breathing
2. The patient's muscles become rigid
3. Double vision impairs mobility
4. The patient cannot close the eyes
5. The patient can have a seizure

8 Initially, cystic fibrosis affects primarily the
1. Heart and lungs
2. Pancreas and exocrine glands
3. Liver and kidneys
4. Gallbladder and endocrine glands
5. Legs and arms

9 Status epilepticus
1. Is an outmoded synonym for a seizure
2. Refers to seizures that are preceded by auras
3. Refers to seizures that occur on a regular basis
4. Constitutes a medical emergency
5. Is the condition of an individual with epilepsy

10 ''Popeye'' arms are characteristic of
1. Duchenne's muscular dystrophy
2. Limb-girdle muscular dystrophy
3. Fascioscapulohumeral muscular dystrophy
4. Multiple sclerosis
5. Myasthenia gravis

11 Problems associated with cleft palate that can affect dental health or the receipt of dental care include *all* of the following *except*
1. Blood dyscrasias
2. Speech difficulties
3. Hearing loss
4. Feeding problems
5. Nasal problems

12 *All* of the following lesions of syphilis are contagious *except*
1. Gumma
2. Chancre
3. Mucous patch
4. Split papule
5. Granuloma

13 Special precautions to prevent disease transmission are required for patients with an uncertain history of all of the following *except*
1. Hepatitis B
2. Tuberculosis
3. AIDS
4. Alzheimer's disease
5. Syphilis

14 An 8-year-old boy runs into the office with his mother and proceeds to touch everything in sight. When you talk to him, he is constantly in motion and cannot concentrate on your questions. When you seat him in the dental chair and push the recline button, he exhibits a severe startle reflex. He cannot follow directions well and appears uncoordinated when brushing his teeth. This boy *most* probably is diagnosed as
1. Emotionally disturbed
2. Learning disabled/minimal brain dysfunction
3. Cerebral palsied
4. Epileptic
5. Leukemic

15 Dental development may be accelerated in patients with
1. Down syndrome
2. Hyperthyroidism
3. Hypothyroidism
4. Cretinism
5. Autism

16 Regulation of sodium intake is extremely important in *all* of the following conditions *except*
1. Hypertensive disease
2. Cystic fibrosis
3. Multiple sclerosis
4. Chronic renal failure
5. High blood pressure

17 Routine dental treatment is contraindicated in *all* of the following conditions *except*
1. Acute or recent myocardial infarction
2. Mild arrhythmias
3. Unstable angina
4. Congestive heart failure
5. Open heart surgery (within the past 3 months)

18 Xerostomia is a common oral manifestation accompanying *all* of the following conditions *except*
1. Leukemia
2. Radiation therapy
3. Mental retardation
4. Chronic alcoholism
5. Diuretic drug therapies

19 Use of aspirin is generally contraindicated in persons with *all* of the following conditions *except*
1. Arthritis
2. Leukemia
3. Hemophilia
4. Chronic alcoholism
5. Chronic renal failure

Situation: John, an adolescent boy with Down syndrome and mild mental retardation, arrives at the office for a new-patient examination. His health history reveals chronic congestion and a congenital heart defect. Oral examination reveals multiple carious lesions, early periodontitis, and oral motor dysfunction. Questions 20 and 21 refer to this situation.

20 What other health or physical problem is John *mostly likely* to have?
1. Bilateral cleft palate
2. Bronchial asthma
3. Hearing loss
4. Leukemia
5. Alzheimer's disease

21 Which of the following conditions are *atypical* of an adolescent with Down syndrome?
1. Early periodontitis
2. Multiple carious lesions
3. Congestion
4. Congenital heart defect
5. Epicanthal folds

Situation: Mr. Jones, a 35-year-old disc jockey, arrives alone with his seeing-eye dog at the dental office. His appointment is for a new-patient examination and oral hygiene instructions. Questions 22 and 23 refer to this situation.

22 When Mr. Jones *first* arrives, the dental hygienist or the receptionist should
1. Escort the dog outside
2. Hand Mr. Jones the health questionnaire and consent form
3. Describe the waiting room layout and office policies to Mr. Jones
4. Interview Mr. Jones in the waiting room regarding his medical and dental history
5. Question Mr. Jones about his blindness

23 The *most* appropriate educational strategy for providing Mr. Jones with oral hygiene instruction is
1. Physical guidance of the toothbrush intraorally, with verbal instructions
2. An audiotape
3. A videotape
4. Physical guidance and use of disclosing tablets for use at home
5. A mouth model

Situation: James, a 23-year-old, is confined to a wheelchair from a spinal cord injury at the C6 level, caused by a motorcycle accident 8 months ago. At the rehabilitation facility where he resides, he can move his shoulders and use his wrist muscles to some degree. He was formerly a high school athletic coach. Questions 24 to 27 refer to this situation.

24 James *most* likely will
1. Be depressed
2. Be ecstatic to see a dental hygienist
3. Refuse to see a dental hygienist
4. Get angry and throw a temper tantrum
5. Be enthusiastic

25 James' oral hygiene care will require
1. Total dependence on another person
2. Use of adaptive equipment
3. Use of a regular toothbrush that is angled at 90 degrees
4. No adaptations
5. Use of a mouth stick

26 Which of the following conditions represents a medical emergency for someone with a spinal injury?
1. Incontinence
2. Tremors
3. Heterotopic ossifications
4. Autonomic hyperreflexia
5. Muscle spasms

27 During an appointment in the dental office, this patient will *definitely* require
1. Transfer from a wheelchair to a dental chair
2. Diaphragmatic coughing
3. An upright chair position
4. That a rubber dam not be used
5. General anesthesia

Situation: Mrs. Clemens is a 45-year-old, regular dental patient. The dental hygienist notices that one corner of her mouth and one lower eyelid are drooping and that her speech is somewhat slurred. Mrs. Clemens noted a recent viral infection on her health history. Questions 28 and 29 refer to this situation.

28 Mrs. Clemens *most* likely is suffering from
1. Bell's palsy
2. Cerebral palsy
3. Alzheimer's disease
4. Parkinson's disease
5. None of the above

29 The *most* important precaution to take during dental treatment with Mrs. Clemens is
1. Adequate suctioning
2. Protection of the airway and eyes
3. Antibiotic coverage
4. Special sterilization procedures for the viral infection
5. Avoidance of quick movements

---

30 Oral lesions are *rare* in
1. Secondary syphilis
2. Tuberculosis
3. AIDS
4. Chronic alcoholism
5. Tertiary syphilis

31 Autonomic hyperreflexia is a condition that may occur in patients with
1. Emotional disturbance
2. Learning disabilities
3. Spinal cord injuries
4. Cardiac arrhythmias
5. Mental retardation

32 Treatment-related oral manifestations of leukemia include
1. Xerostomia and dental caries
2. Acute necrotizing ulcerative gingivitis (ANUG) and gingival enlargement
3. Osteomyelitis and tooth mobility
4. Enamel hypoplasia and staining
5. Mucous patches

33 The oral lesion associated with primary syphilis that is highly contagious is
1. Chancre
2. Gumma
3. Mucous patch
4. Split papule
5. Granuloma

34 Kaposi's sarcoma is associated with
1. Tuberculosis
2. AIDS
3. Leukemia
4. Chronic alcoholism
5. Down syndrome

35 Osteoarthritis affects primarily the
1. Weight-bearing joints (e.g., hips, knees) in children
2. Weight-bearing joints in adults
3. Small joints (e.g., fingers) in children
4. Small joints in adults
5. Large joints in children

36 Craniofacial features common to Down Syndrome include
1. Ocular hypertelerism
2. Small nasomaxillary complex
3. Elongated facial structure
4. Mandibular retrognathia
5. Simian crease

37 Which of the following conditions develops *most* often during childhood?
1. Bell's palsy
2. Parkinson's disease
3. Multiple sclerosis
4. Duchenne's muscular dystrophy
5. Alzheimer's disease

38 Secondary hypertension can result from *any* of the following *except*
1. Hyperthyroidism
2. Kidney disease
3. Oral contraceptives
4. Hyperactivity
5. Chronic renal failure

39 A person with a severe hearing loss (65 to 95 db loss)
1. Hears no speech or other sounds
2. Hears vowel sounds clearly, but not consonants
3. Misses all speech at normal conversational level
4. Hears only louder-voiced speech sounds
5. Hears only vowel sounds

40 Health professionals must be concerned about chronic carrier states in
1. Hepatitis A
2. Hepatitis B
3. Cystic fibrosis
4. Syphilis
5. Hypertensive disease

41 Inhaled and oral bronchodilators are used in cystic fibrosis to
1. Fight infection and slow the heart rate
2. Close airways and decrease the appetite
3. Open airways and help in removal of sputum
4. Fight infection and increase the appetite
5. Eliminate mucous secretions

42 Orofacial muscles are characteristically flaccid or rigid in *all* of the following conditions *except*
1. Parkinson's disease
2. Myasthenia gravis
3. Bell's palsy
4. Arthritis
5. Stroke

Answers and Rationales

1. (3) Hyperthyroidism does not generally accompany cerebral palsy.
   (1) Seizures occur in about 40% of cerebral-palsied persons.
   (2) Visual defects also occur in about 40% of cases of cerebral palsy.
   (4) Hearing disorders occur in 20% of cases of cerebral palsy.
   (5) Special disorders occur in 60% of cases of cerebral palsy.

2. (3) Twenty-four hours after dialysis is optimal, since the blood system is fairly clear, the patient is alert, and the anticoagulant is no longer a problem.
   (1) If anticoagulants are used, the potential for prolonged bleeding exists.
   (2) These patients can receive routine dental care as long as appropriate precautions are taken.
   (4) Bleeding problems from the anticoagulant still exist after 4 hours, and the patient is fatigued.
   (5) Time is a factor in this situation; see 3.

3. (3) Tuberculosis patients are not at any higher risk for acquiring or transmitting hepatitis virus.
   (1) Hemodialysis patients may acquire hepatitis virus from blood products used during dialysis.
   (2) Hemophiliac patients may acquire hepatitis virus during transfusions.
   (4) Male homosexuals are considered a high risk group for hepatitis transmission because of oral/anal transmission.
   (5) Indochinese refugees are considered a high-risk group for hepatitis transmission because of the environment from which they came.

4. (4) Periodontal conditions tend to be more severe and occur at an earlier age in patients with Down syndrome.
   (1) Epidemiologic data show a moderate to low caries rate.
   (2) Malocclusion is a problem, but not a critical problem.
   (3) Bruxism is also a problem, but not a critical one.
   (5) Oral cancer is not directly associated with Down syndrome.

For each question the correct answer and rationale are listed first. The other choices are presented in order with the reasons why they are not correct.

5. (1) Premedication to prevent infection is not a concern in myocardial infarction.
   (2) About 70% of patients with a history of rheumatic heart disease have residual heart damage, which requires premedication.
   (3) Bacteria can colonize in artificial heart valves, thus requiring premedication.
   (4) Bacteria can colonize in the artificial valves, causing heart damage.
   (5) Bacteria can colonize on heart valves and cause heart damage.

6. (4) No special dietary modifications are required in autism.
   (1) The balance between insulin and diet is important in diabetes.
   (2) Regulation of metabolites and nutrients is important in renal disease.
   (3) Dietary supplements are required in cystic fibrosis.
   (5) Restricted intake of sodium is important in hypertension.

7. (1) Impaired breathing is a medical emergency.
   (2) Muscular rigidity in this case does not constitute an emergency.
   (3) Impaired mobility is not an emergency.
   (4) Inability to close the eyes is not an emergency, but it can lead to eye damage from foreign particles.
   (5) Seizures do not generally occur with this condition.

8. (2) The original name for cystic fibrosis was coined because of the observed effects on the pancreas and exocrine glands
   (1) Cystic fibrosis affects the lungs, but not the heart.
   (3) The liver and kidneys are affected at later stages.
   (4) The gallbladder is affected, but not the endocrine glands.
   (5) Cystic fibrosis does not affect the arms and legs directly.

9. (4) Status epilepticus constitutes a medical emergency because respiration may be impaired.
   (1) The term *fit* is an outmoded synonym.
   (2) Any type of seizure may be preceded by an aura.
   (3) Status epilepticus refers to seizures lasting longer than 5 minutes.
   (5) This is an incorrect statement.

10. (3) Muscles above the elbow atrophy; below the elbow they are normal, resulting in the ''Popeye'' appearance.
    (1) Arms are not as affected as legs in Duchenne's muscular dystrophy.
    (2) Arms in limb-girdle muscular dystrophy do not show this characteristic.
    (4) Popeye arms are not a characteristic of multiple sclerosis.
    (5) Popeye arms are not a characteristic of myesthenia gravis.

11. (1) Blood dyscrasias are not generally associated with cleft palate.
    (2) Speech difficulties can influence communication in the dental office.
    (3) Hearing loss also interferes with communication.
    (4) Feeding problems can lead to retention of food or inappropriate diets, causing dental caries.
    (5) Breathing problems can influence communication, eating, and general comfort during dental care.

12. (1) Gummatous lesions occur in tertiary syphilis and do not contain viable organisms.
    (2) A chancre is the first lesion to occur at the site of inoculation and is highly contagious.
    (3) A mucous patch occurs in secondary syphilis and is highly contagious.
    (4) Split papules also occur in secondary syphilis and are contagious.
    (5) A granuloma is not a lesion of syphilis.

13. (4) There is no risk of disease transmission in Alzheimer's disease.
    (1) It is necessary to prevent transmission of hepatitis B virus via blood or saliva.
    (2) It is necessary to prevent transmission of tuberculosis by airborne droplets or sputum.
    (3) It is necessary to prevent transmission of the virus causing AIDS via saliva or other body fluids.
    (5) It is necessary to prevent transmission of *Treponema Paledum* via saliva or other body fluids.

14. (2) The constant activity, lack of impulse control, inattention, lack of coordination, and exaggerated reflexes are characteristics of those labeled as learning disabled or having minimal brain dysfunction.
    (1) People with the label ''emotional disturbance'' may exhibit some of these characteristics, but usually not all of them appear in one person.
    (3) The only characteristic of cerebral palsy is the heightened startle reflex.
    (4) The only characteristic of epilepsy is the periods of inattention
    (5) Individuals with leukemia present physiologic problems, not behavior problems.

15. (2) Premature eruption patterns may be observed in hyperthyroidism.
    (1) Dental development is delayed by Down syndrome.
    (3) Eruption patterns are delayed by hypothyroidism.
    (4) *Cretinism* is another name for hypothyroidism.
    (5) Eruption patterns are not affected by autism.

16. (3) There are no sodium restrictions in multiple sclerosis.
    (1) Reduction of sodium levels are recommended in hypertensive disease.
    (2) Loss of abnormal amounts of sodium through sweating interferes with the electrolyte balance, thus necessitating sodium supplements.
    (4) The sodium pump in the kidney is impaired, causing excess excretion of sodium.
    (5) High blood pressure is a hypertensive disease.

17. (2) Mild arrhythmias should present few problems during treatment.
    (1) Treatment should be delayed for 6 months on patients with acute or recent myocardial infarction.
    (3) Routine treatment should be postponed if the patient reports unstable angina.
    (4) Patients with congestive heart failure should not be treated until they are under good medical control.
    (5) Patients who have undergone open-heart surgery should not be treated until about 6 months postoperatively.
18. (3) Salivation is not affected in mental retardation.
    (1) Medications given for leukemia cause xerostomia.
    (2) Radiation therapy inactivates the parotid salivary glands.
    (4) Alcohol dehydrates the body, resulting in xerostomia.
    (5) Xerostomia is a common side effect in patients taking diuretics.
19. (1) Aspirin is generally prescribed for arthritis patients.
    (2) Aspirin increases the bleeding potential in leukemia.
    (3) Aspirin increases the bleeding potential in hemophilia.
    (4) Aspirin increases the bleeding potential in chronic alcoholism.
    (5) Aspirin increases the bleeding potential in chronic renal failure.
20. (3) Hearing loss occurs in about 70% of people with Down syndrome.
    (1) Bilateral cleft palate is not generally associated with Down syndrome, although there is a high occurrence of bifid uvula.
    (2) Bronchial asthma is not generally associated with Down syndrome.
    (4) Leukemia occurs in a small percentage of people with Down syndrome.
    (5) Alzheimer's disease is associated with Down syndrome but would not likely occur in early adolescence.
21. (2) A low caries incidence is generally seen in these patients.
    (1) Early developing peirodontal disease is common in adolescents with Down syndrome.
    (3) Congestion is common.
    (4) Congenital defects are also fairly common.
    (5) Epicanthal folds are typical of Down syndrome.
22. (3) Orienting him to the office will make him feel more comfortable.
    (1) The dog is a substitute for his vision and should remain in the office.
    (2) He will require an interview to complete all the forms.
    (4) An interview should be done in private, not in the waiting room.
    (5) Questions regarding Mr. Jones' visual impairment can wait until the health history is taken.

23. (1) Physical cues paired with verbal cues are best for people with visual impairments.
    (2) An audiotape may be confusing and does not provide feedback.
    (3) A videotape functions only as an audiotape and is inappropriate for peole with visual impairments.
    (4) Disclosing tablets are useless to the patient at home.
    (5) A mouth model might be helpful but could not be used alone.
24. (1) Depression is the most common psychologic reaction to disability.
    (2) His reaction to a stranger will probably be embarrassment and depression.
    (3) He may not feel he has a choice in seeing a dental hygienist.
    (4) He most likely will respond apathetically rather than becoming angry.
    (5) He is not likely to be enthusiastic because of his disability.
25. (2) The wrist muscles are weak, thus necessitating use of adaptive equipment for stability or grasping.
    (1) James still can use his arms to some degree.
    (3) He may require an adapted brush, but he will also require arm braces for stability.
    (4) He will require at least some type of adaptive equipment.
    (5) A mouthstick would be used by a quadraplegic.
26. (4) Autonomic hyperreflexia is a medical emergency that requires prompt action.
    (1) Incontinence is a problem, but not a medical emergency.
    (2) Tremors may interfere with treatment, but are not an emergency.
    (3) Heterotopic ossifications are a medical problem, not an emergency.
    (5) Muscle spasms may interfere with treatment, but are not an emergency.
27. (1) A C6 injury generally requires use of a wheelchair, and transference to the dental chair facilitates treatment.
    (2) Help with diaphragmatic coughing may not be needed.
    (3) A semireclined chair position is generally accepted.
    (4) Unless respiration is severely impaired or the patient has a phobia, a rubber dam is not contraindicated.
    (5) General anesthesia is not indicated.
28. (1) These symptoms and history are characteristic of Bell's palsy.
    (2) Cerebral palsy would affect more than just the facial muscles.
    (3) Alzheimer's disease involves more than unilateral paralysis.
    (4) Paralysis would be more diffuse and involves more of the body in Parkinson's disease.
    (5) Bell's palsy is the correct answer.

29. (2) Protection of the airway and eyes are important to prevent infections.
    (1) Swallowing may be impaired, but not significantly.
    (3) There is no indication for antibiotic coverage.
    (4) No special sterilization considerations are necessary.
    (5) Quick movements of the clinician or the patient would not be a problem for a patient with Bell's palsy.
30. (2) Tuberculosis lesions are uncommon in the mouth.
    (1) Mucous patches and split papules are common in secondary syphilis.
    (3) Oral infections and lesions are common in AIDs.
    (4) Oral lesions caused by increased susceptibility to infection are common in chronic alcoholics.
    (5) Gummatous lesions occur in tertiary syphilis.
31. (3) Autonomic hyperreflexia occurs usually when the bladder becomes too full and blood vessels suddenly constrict in patients with spinal injuries.
    (1) There is no association between autonomic hyperreflexia and emotional disturbance.
    (2) There is no association between the condition and learning disabilities.
    (4) There is no association between the condition and cardiac arrhythmias.
    (5) There is no association between the condition and mental retardation.
32. (1) Xerostomia and dental caries are related to chemotherapy treatments.
    (2) ANUG and gingival enlargement are caused by systemic factors.
    (3) Osteomyelitis and tooth mobility are caused by hyperplasia of the bone marrow.
    (4) Enamel hypoplasia and staining are related to the hyperbilirubinemia.
    (5) Mucous patches are oral manifestations of syphilis.
33. (1) The chancre occurs at the site of inoculation by *Treponema pallidum*.
    (2) Gummatous lesions are not contagious.
    (3) The mucous patch occurs in secondary syphilis.
    (4) Split papules also occur in the secondary stage.
    (5) Granulomas are not associated with syphilis.
34. (2) Kaposi's sarcoma occurs in the advanced stages of AIDS.
    (1) There is no known association between Kaposi's sarcoma and tuberculosis.
    (3) There is no direct association between Kaposi's sarcoma and leukemia.
    (4) There is no association between Kaposi's sarcoma and chronic alcoholism.
    (5) There is no association between Kaposi's sarcoma and Down syndrome.
35. (2) The weight-bearing joints in adults are most often affected in osteoarthritis.
    (1) Osteoarthritis usually does not affect children.
    (3) Children are not generally affected.
    (4) Large joints are affected more than small joints.
    (5) Osteoarthritis usually does not affect children.

36. (2) A small nasomaxillary complex is a basic characteristic of Down syndrome.
    (1) Ocular *hypo*telorism is common.
    (3) Round, flat facies are characteristic.
    (4) Relative mandibular prognathism is common.
    (5) Simian crease is characteristic but is not a craniofacial feature.
37. (4) Duchenne's muscular dystrophy generally develops around age 3.
    (1) Bell's palsy is most common in adult years.
    (2) Parkinson's disease develops between ages 40 and 60.
    (3) Multiple sclerosis usually occurs between ages 20 and 40.
    (5) Alzheimer's disease develops primarily in the elderly.
38. (4) Hyperactivity does not cause hypertension.
    (1) Excess hormone secretion increases peripheral resistance.
    (2) Renal artery obstruction or pyleonephritis can cause hypertension.
    (3) Hormones in oral contraceptives increase the peripheral resistance.
    (5) Hypertension can be a cause of chronic renal failure.
39. (3) A person with a severe hearing loss cannot hear most speech unless greatly amplified.
    (1) With a 65 to 90 dB loss, sounds can still be heard.
    (2) Vowels and consonants cannot be heard with a severe loss.
    (4) A person with a severe hearing loss cannot hear any language without amplification.
    (5) Vowels cannot be heard with a severe loss of hearing.
40. (2) Ten percent of individuals with hepatitis B are chronic carriers without symptoms.
    (1) There is no carrier state in hepatitis A.
    (3) Cystic fibrosis is not a viral condition.
    (4) Syphilis does not have a contagious chronic carrier state.
    (5) Hypertension is not a contagious disease.
41. (3) Opening the airway and removal of sputum are the main goals of treatment in cystic fibrosis.
    (1) Bronchodilators do not slow the heart rate.
    (2) The goal is to open the airway, not close it.
    (4) Antibiotics are used to fight infection, not bronchodilators.
    (5) Mucous secretions must be loosened and suctioned.
42. (4) The temporomandibular joint, not the facial muscles, is generally affected in arthritis.
    (1) Parkinson's disease is characterized by muscle rigidity and tremors.
    (2) Myasthenia gravis involves weakness of the facial muscles.
    (3) Bell's palsy is characterized by paralysis of the facial muscles.
    (5) A stroke can paralyze the facial musculature.

CHAPTER 15

Community Oral Health Planning and Practice

PAMELA ZARKOWSKI

Assessment, planning, implementation, and evaluation—the basic processes in dental hygiene practice—are used by the dental hygienist in community oral health practice. Community health extends the role of the dental hygienist from the traditional dental care setting to the community as a whole. In a sense, the community can be viewed as the patient/client and the dental care setting is the neighborhood health center, extended care facility, hospital, school, or other agency.

With increased emphasis on improving public access to dental care, the responsibilities of the dental hygienist to promote oral health in the community take on renewed importance. This chapter focuses on the knowledge and skills necessary for various roles in community oral health. Topics include basic concepts of epidemiology and trends in oral disease, assessment tools, dental health education strategies, basic statistical and research concepts, evaluation of dental literature, the provision and financing of dental care, and the need for, demand for, and utilization of dental services.

BASIC CONCEPTS

A. Health—state of complete physical, mental, and social well-being; not merely the absence of disease or infirmity
B. Public health—science and art of preventing disease, prolonging life, and promoting physical health and efficiency through organized community efforts
   1. Public health is concerned with the aggregate health of a group, a community, a state, a nation, or a group of nations
   2. Public health is people's health
C. Dental public health—science and art of preventing and controlling dental diseases and promoting dental health through organized community efforts; that form of dental practice that serves the community as a patient rather than the individual; concerned with the dental education of the public, with applied dental research, and with

the administration of group dental care programs, as well as the prevention and control of dental diseases on a community basis
D. Comparison of private versus community health (Table 15-1)
E. Criteria for a public health problem
   1. Disease or other threat is widespread
   2. Disease is one that can be prevented, alleviated, or cured
   3. Such knowledge is not being applied

EPIDEMIOLOGY

Basic Concepts

A. Epidemiology—study of health and disease in populations and how these states are influenced by the environment and ways of living; concerned with factors and conditions that determine the occurrence and distribution of health, disease, defects, disability, and deaths among individuals (Fig. 15-1)
B. Characteristics of epidemiology
   1. Groups rather than individuals are studied
   2. Disease is considered multifactorial
      a. Host
      b. Agent
      c. Environment
   3. Clinical trials versus epidemiologic surveys (Table 15-2)
C. Related concepts
   1. Epidemic—a disease of significantly greater prevalence than normal; more than the expected number of cases
   2. Endemic—continuing problem involving normal disease prevalence; the expected number of cases
   3. Pandemic—worldwide epidemic
   4. Mortality—death
   5. Morbidity—disease
   6. Rate—a proportion that uses a standardized denominator

Table 15-1 Comparison of private dental practice and community oral health practice

Private dental practice	Community dental practice
Assessment of patient's dental and medical history and oral health status	Survey of community dental status
Diagnosis of patient's oral health	Analysis of survey data to determine oral health needs
Treatment plan based on diagnosis and patient's needs and priorities	Program plan based on data analysis, priorities, and resources available
Treatment plan initiated; primary dentist may coordinate treatment with other providers (e.g., dental hygienists, specialists)	Program operation implemented; personnel will involve a varied group
Payment methods arranged between provider and patient	Financing takes place throughout process
Evaluation during treatment, at specific intervals, and/or on completion of treatment	Evaluation/appraisal is ongoing, conducted in terms of effectiveness, efficiency, appropriateness, and adequacy

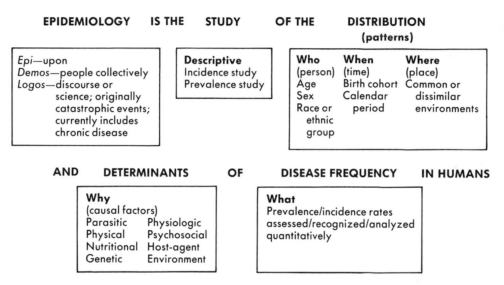

Fig. 15-1 Study of epidemiology.

D. Research concepts
  1. Research—"continual search for truth using the scientific method"[1]
  2. Sample—"a portion of the population that, if properly selected, can provide meaningful information about the entire population; a sample is examined when the researcher has neither the time, money, nor resources to study an entire population"[1]
  3. Random sample—"a sample composed of subjects who are chosen independently of each other, with equal opportunity for inclusion; increases external validity; controls intersubject differences"[1]
  4. Nonrandomized sample—"sample that is not randomly selected from a general population, therefore making generalizations to a larger population invalid; intact groups; threatens external validity"[1]
  5. Population—"that portion of the universe to which the researcher wants to generalize findings"[1]

Table 15-2 Comparison of clinical trials and epidemiologic surveys

	Clinical trial	Epidemiologic survey
Populations	Experimental and control groups are specially constituted as representative samples from from appropriate populations	Naturally occurring samples of target populations are usually studied
Sample size	Sample sizes are usually small, particularly when "treatments" are more complicated	Fairly large sample sizes are employed
Time frame	Trials are conducted over a period of time usually varying from 1 week to 6 months, depending on treatment involved, to compare treatment effects	Surveys are usually cross-sectional in design, using only one time period; longitudinal designs are used occasionally
Methods	While assessment methods may be indices, methods used should have acuity and clinical significance	Indices used for assessment establish a disease level of selected populations; these indices should be in general use to enable comparison of data for different populations
Data	Data generated from clinical trials should be applicable for specific hypothesis testing	Data generated from surveys are used to establish underlying etiologic factors and derive possible preventive methods, leading to development of hypotheses to be tested by controlled clinical trials

Science of Epidemiology

A. Uses of epidemiology
   1. Collecting data on normal biologic processes
   2. Determining the natural history of diseases
   3. Testing hypotheses for prevention and control of disease through special studies in populations
   4. Planning and evaluating health care services
B. Three classifications of epidemiologic research
   1. Descriptive research—"involves description, documentation, analysis, and interpretation of data to evaluate a current event or situation"[1]
      a. Incidence—"number of new cases of a specific disease within a defined population over a period of time"[1]
      b. Prevalence—"number of persons in a population affected by a condition at any one time"[1]
      c. Count—simplest sum of disease
   2. Analytical research—determines the cause of a disease, or if a causal relationship exists between a factor and a disease
      a. Prospective study (experimental study)— planning of the entire study is completed before data are collected and analyzed; population is followed through time to determine which members develop the disease; several hypotheses may be tested at one time
      b. Retrospective study (ex post facto study)— decision to carry out an investigation using observations or data that have been collected in the past; data may be incomplete or in a manner not appropriate for study
      c. Cross-sectional study—"study of subgroups of individuals in a specific and limited time frame to identify developmental changes in the overall group from the perspective of what is typical in each subgroup"[1]
      d. Longitudinal study—"investigation of the same group of individuals over an extended period of time to identify a change or development in that group))[1]
   3. Experimental research—used when the etiology of the disease is established and the researcher wishes to determine the effectiveness of altering some factor or factors
C. Distribution and determinants of disease
   1. Disease is multifactorial in nature
      a. Host factors
         (1) Immunity to disease/natural resistance
         (2) Heredity
         (3) Age, sex, race
      b. Agent factors
         (1) Biologic—microbiologic
         (2) Chemical—poisons, dosage levels
         (3) Physical—environmental exposure
      c. Environment factors
         (1) Physical—sunshine, rainfall
         (2) Biologic—animal hosts and vectors
         (3) Social—socioeconomic, education
   2. Interplay of these three factors is ongoing; to affect the disease, attack at the weakest link

Epidemiology of Oral Disease

A. Dental caries in the United States
 1. Statistics show that 25% to 80% of children between 1 and 5 years of age have suffered from dental caries
 2. Caries experience increases steadily with age
   a. DMF (decayed, missing, filled) values increase most significantly in youth and early adult years and more slowly in the later years of life
   b. Slowdown in caries attack may be influenced by such factors as the susceptible surfaces that have already been attacked, buildup of fluoride in the outer layers of enamel, and a change in dietary habits
   c. Root caries occurs in areas where gingival recession has occurred
 3. Females have higher DMF scores than males
   a. Higher scores do not indicate that females are more susceptible to caries than males
   b. Earlier eruption patterns allow teeth at risk to be in the oral environment for a longer period
   c. Females seek dental care more frequently than males; therefore, the treatment factor must be considered when evaluating DMF scores
 4. No inherent difference between blacks and whites
   a. Observed differences in caries between blacks and whites in the United States is related to socioeconomic and cultural differences, especially dietary practices and receipt of dental care
   b. Generally, the white population in the United States has better access to dental care than do blacks
 5. Environmental factors (e.g. diet) have a stronger influence than genetics
 6. Diet is the total oral intake of substances that provide nourishment and or calories; nutrition is the absorption of nutrients (see Chapter 9, section on nutritional counseling)
   a. Dietary factors, especially sugar, have an influence on dental caries prevalence
   b. Relationship exists between frequent consumption of fermentable carbohydrate and dental caries incidence
   c. Specific bacteria present in dental plaque ferment dietary carbohydrate to produce organic acids that demineralize tooth structure
   d. Plaque bacteria use carbohydrates to produce the sticky gel-like matrix of the plaque
   e. Fats and proteins have demonstrated noncariogenic effects
     (1) Fats may decrease caries activity by altering surface properties of enamel, reducing sugar solubilization, being toxic to oral bacteria, or simply by replacing dietary carbohydrates
     (2) Proteins may reduce caries posteruptively by a direct effect on plaque metabolism, replacement of dietary carbohydrates, or by increasing salivary urea levels

B. Periodontal disease
 1. Prevalence and severity of gingivitis increases with age, beginning at 5 years of age, reaching the highest point in puberty, and then gradually decreasing but remaining high throughout life
   a. Prevalence in children 6 to 11 years of age is approximately 38%
   b. Prevalence in adolescents 12 to 17 years of age is 62%
   c. Prevalence in young adults 18 to 24 years of age is 57%; prevalence of gingivitis decreases gradually with increasing age
   d. Recent study indicates a decrease in prevalence of gingivitis related to a decrease in oral hygiene scores and an increase in preventive services
 2. Precise method to determine the magnitude of periodontal disease does not exist, although data are available to allow a relatively accurate estimate of prevalence
   a. Of adults 18 to 79 years of age, 74% have some form of periodontal disease; approximately 25% have destructive periodontal disease
   b. Recent studies suggest a decrease in periodontal disease; 50% of the population have some form of periodontal disease, and 25% of the population have destructive periodontal disease
 3. Factors affecting the prevalence and severity of periodontal disease
   a. Prevalence and severity of periodontal disease increases directly with increasing age
     (1) When groups studied are equalized for sex, race, and oral hygiene, age appears to be an independent variable related to the increasing intensity of periodontal disease

(2) Some loss of attachment occurs with age, even with excellent oral hygiene
b. In general, males consistently have a higher prevalence and severity of periodontal disease than females
c. Blacks consistently appear to have more periodontal disease than whites; however, when oral hygiene status is taken into account, no difference exists
d. Periodontal disease is inversely related to increasing levels of education
e. Prevalence and severity of periodontal disease are higher in rural areas than in urban areas
f. There is a positive relationship between periodontal disease and the level of oral hygiene
(1) Statistically as well as clinically, plaque is a primary etiologic factor of periodontal disease
(2) Differences in periodontal disease levels between peoples of developed and developing countries are attributed to differences in oral hygiene levels
g. More study is necessary, but increased levels of prevalence and intensity of periodontal disease are found in areas of the world where generalized malnutrition is common
C. Oral cancer
1. Occurrence of oral cancer and site distribution within the mouth varies widely in different parts of the world (e.g., carcinoma of buccal mucosa as a result of chewing betel nuts in the Far East)
2. Oral cancer is two-and-a-half times more prevalent in males and there are twice as many deaths in males than in females; affects older men, heavy users of alcohol and tobacco, and individuals exposed to sunlight
3. Oral cancer is related to increasing age
D. Cleft lip and palate
1. Approximately 6000 children are born in United States each year with cleft lip and/or palate
2. Epidemiologic correlations indicate
a. Cleft lip and palate appear more frequently in plural births

b. More isolated cleft palates appear in girls
c. More facial clefts appear in boys
d. A relation exists between clefts and premature births
e. Infants with clefts are of lower birth weight than the general population of infants[3]
3. Clefts are associated with threatened spontaneous abortion during the first and second trimesters of pregnancy, influenza in the first trimester, and maternal drug consumption during the first trimester (e.g., opiates, penicillin, and salicylates)[3]
E. Malocclusion
1. Difficult to quantify because of varying cultural perceptions
2. Higher proportion of black females have severe malocclusion relative to black males; little difference is shown between white males and females

Indices in Dental Epidemiology

Indices aid in collection of data
A. Dental index—abbreviated measurement of the amount or condition of disease in a population; numerical scale with defined upper and lower limits designed to permit and facilitate comparison with other populations classified by the same criteria and methods
B. Attributes of a good index
1. Validity—measures what it is intended to measure
2. Reliability—measures consistently at different times; reproducibility, stability of measurement
3. Clear, simple, and objective
4. Sensitive to shifts in disease
5. Acceptable to the subjects involved[3]
C. Index may assess disease that is a reversible or irreversible condition or combination; therefore indices are classified as reversible or irreversible
1. Reversible index—measures conditions that can be reversed (e.g., gingivitis is reversible)
2. Irreversible index—measures cumulative conditions that cannot be reversed (e.g., dental caries)
D. Common dental indices used in oral health survey (Table 15-3)

Table 15-3 Common dental indices used in oral health surveys

Dental index	Procedure for use	Interpretation
DENTAL CARIES INDICES		
Decayed-Missing-Filled Teeth Index (DMFT): an irreversible index used to measure past and present caries experience of a population with permanent teeth. *D* indicates a carious tooth; *M* indicates a tooth missing because of caries; *F* indicates a filled tooth. The deft index, a variation of the DMFT, is used to measure observable caries experience in primary teeth. The *d* and *f* symbols are the same as in the DMFT. However, *e* indicates need for extraction, and missing teeth are not considered. A tooth that meets the criteria for both *d* and *f* is considered one decayed tooth. The deft does not take into account teeth that have been extracted or exfoliated because of past caries experiences.	Count and record the D, M, and F teeth in each member of the sample or population. Analyze the scores by using the following formulas: 1. $\text{DMFT count} = \dfrac{\text{Total DMFT}}{\text{Number of people examined}}$ (indicates number of teeth with a history of decay) $\text{deft count} = \dfrac{\text{Total deft}}{\text{Number of children examined}}$ (indicates observable caries experience) 2. $\text{FNM} = \dfrac{F}{\text{Total DMFT}}$ (indicates treatment received for decay [filling needs met]) 3. $\text{Percent of decayed teeth} = \dfrac{D}{\text{Total DMFT}}$ (indicates treatment required for decay) 4. $\text{Percent of missing teeth} = \dfrac{M}{\text{Total DMFT}}$ (indicates the number of teeth lost by decay) 5. $\text{Average D, M, or F per individual} = \dfrac{\text{D or M or F}}{\text{Number of people examined}}$	General guideline: total DMFT greater than or equal to an individual's age indicates high caries experience. DMFT rates are less indicative of caries experience in older age groups because of tooth loss from periodontal disease.
GINGIVITIS AND PERIODONTAL DISEASE INDICES		
Gingival Index (GI): a reversible index based on severity of inflammation and location. Can be used to determine prevalence and severity of gingivitis in epidemiologic surveys as well as individual dentition. GI often used in controlled clinical trial of preventive or therapeutic agents.	A score of 0 to 3 is assigned to four gingival scoring units: mesial, distal, buccal, and lingual surfaces of teeth. A blunt instrument, such as a periodontal probe, is used to assess bleeding potential. Totaling scores around each tooth yields GI score for area; divide by 4, score for tooth is determined. Totaling all scores and dividing by number of teeth examined provides GI score per person. Can be used on selected or all erupted teeth. Criteria include: 0 — Normal gingiva 1 — Mild inflammation: slight change in color; slight edema; no bleeding on probing 2 — Moderate inflammation: redness, edema, and glazing; bleeding on probing 3 — Severe inflammation: marked redness and edema, ulceration; tendency to spontaneous bleeding	0.1-1.0: Mild gingivitis 1.1-2.0: Moderate gingivitis 2.1-3.0: Severe gingivitis

Modified from Darby, M.L.: Community oral health: background, planning, and practice. In Petersen, S., editor: Comprehensive review of dental hygiene, ed. 4, St. Louis, 1980, The C.V. Mosby Co.
*For more detailed criteria of other factors see reference 2.

Continued.

Table 15-3 Common dental indices used in oral health surveys—cont'd

Dental index	Procedure for use	Interpretation
Periodontal Index (PI): a reversible index used to measure the periodontal condition of a population. Measures presence or absence of gingival inflammation and its severity, pocket formation, and masticatory function.	A score for each individual is obtained by arriving at a score for each tooth in the mouth, adding the scores, and dividing by the total number of teeth. The following scoring system is used: 0 — Negative: neither overt inflammation in the investing tissues nor loss of function due to destruction of supporting tissues. 1 — Mild gingivitis: an overt area of inflammation in the free gingivae, but this area does not circumscribe the tooth 2 — Gingivitis: inflammation completely circumscribes tooth, but there is no apparent break in epithelial attachment 4 — Not used in the field study 6 — Gingivitis with pocket formation: epithelial attachment has been broken and there is a pocket (not merely a deepened gingival crevice due to swelling in the free gingivae). No interference with normal masticatory function; the tooth is firm in its socket and has not drifted 8 — Advanced destruction with loss of masticatory function: tooth may be loose; may have drifted; may sound dull on percussion with a metallic instrument; may be depressible in its socket	0.0-0.2: Clinically normal 0.3-0.9: Gingivitis 0.7-1.9: Incipient destructive disease 1.5-5.0: Established destructive disease 3.8-8.0: Terminal states of disease
Periodontal Disease Index (PDI): used to measure the presence and severity of periodontal disease; measures reversible and irreversible disease. Used in epidemiologic surveys, longitudinal studies of periodontal disease, and clinical trials of therapeutic or preventive procedures. Gingival index of choice in longitudinal studies of periodontal disease.	Six teeth are examined: Nos. 3, 9, 12, 19, 25, and 28. PDI assesses gingivitis, gingival sulcus depth, calculus, plaque, occlusal and incisal attrition mobility, and lack of contact. Criteria used for evaluation of gingiva and gingival crevices are: 0 — Absence of inflammation 1 — Mild to moderate inflammatory gingival changes not extending all around tooth 2 — Mild to moderately severe gingivitis extending all around tooth 3 — Severe gingivitis, characterized by marked redness, tendency to bleed, and ulceration 4 — Gingival crevice in any of 4 measured areas (mesial, distal, buccal, lingual), extending apically to cementoenamel junction but not more than 3 mm 5 — Gingival crevice in any of 4 measured areas extending apically to cementoenamel junction (3-6 mm) 6 — Gingival crevice in any of 4 measured areas extending apically more than 6 mm from cementoenamel junction PDI score is obtained by totaling scores of the teeth and dividing by number of teeth examined.*	Sensitive index. Useful for measuring progress in periodontal patient.

Table 15-3 Common dental indices used in oral health surveys — cont'd

Dental index	Procedure for use	Interpretation
	ORAL HYGIENE INDICES	

Simplified Oral Hygiene Index (OHI-S): a reversible index used to measure oral hygiene status. Six teeth — the first fully erupted tooth distal to the second premolar in each quadrant (buccal surfaces on maxilla and lingual surfaces on mandible) and maxillary right and mandibular left central incisors (labial surface of each) — are assessed separately for debris and calculus. This assessment yields a DI-S score (debris index — simplified) and a CI-S score (calculus index — simplified).	Surfaces are examined for debris and scored using DI-S system:
	0 — No debris or stain present
	1 — Soft debris covering not more than one third of tooth surface being examined, or presence of extrinsic stains without debris regardless of surface area covered
	2 — Soft debris covering more than one third but not more than two thirds of exposed tooth surfaces
	3 — Soft debris covering more than two thirds of exposed tooth surface
	Surfaces are examined for calculus and scored using the CI-S system:
	0 — No calculus present
	1 — Supragingival calculus not more than one third of exposed tooth surface being examined
	2 — Supragingival calculus covering more than one third but not more than two thirds of exposed tooth surfaces, or presence of individual flecks of subgingival calculus around cervical portion of tooth
	3 — Supragingival calculus covering more than two thirds of exposed tooth surface, or a continuous heavy band of subgingival calculus around cervical portion of tooth
		OHI-S:
		  0.0-1.2: Good oral hygiene
		  1.3-3.0: Fair oral hygiene
		  3.1-6.0: Poor oral hygiene
		DI-S or CI-S:
		  0.0-0.6: Good oral hygiene
		  0.7-1.8: Fair oral hygiene
		  1.9-3.0: Poor oral hygiene

Plaque Index (PlI): used to assess extent of soft deposits; measures differences in thickness of debris at gingival margin used in conjunction with Gingival Index. Useful in longitudinal studies and clinical trials.	Four gingival scoring units: mesial, distal, buccal, lingual, are examined using mouth mirror, dental explorer, airdrying. PlI for area is obtained by totaling 4 plaque scores per tooth. If sum of PlI scores per tooth is divided by 4, PlI score for tooth is obtained. PlI score per person is obtained by adding PlI scores per tooth and dividing by number of teeth examined. May be obtained for a segment or group of teeth. 0 — No plaque in gingival area 1 — Film of plaque adhering to free gingival margin and adjacent area of tooth; plaque only noticed by running probe across tooth surface 2 — Moderate accumulation of soft deposits within gingival margin and/or on adjacent tooth surface can be seen by naked eye 3 — Abundance of soft matter within gingival pocket and/or gingival margin and adjacent tooth surface	

Continued.

Table 15-3 Common dental indices used in oral health surveys—cont'd

Dental index	Procedure for use	Interpretation
Patient Hygiene Performance (PHP): developed to assess individual's performance in removing debris after toothbrush instruction. Simple to use; can be performed quickly.	Teeth disclosed: Six teeth are evaluated: Nos. 3, 8, 14, 19, 24, and 30. Each tooth is divided into 5 areas: 3 longitudinal thirds, distal, middle, and mesial; the middle third is subdivided horizontally into incisal, middle, and gingival thirds. Score per person is obtained by totaling 5 subdivision scores per tooth surface and dividing by number of tooth surfaces examined.	

Index Selection

A. Index selection is determined by
   1. Type of condition to be assessed
   2. Age of the population to be studied
   3. Purpose of the research
B. Examiners should be calibrated or standardized in their use of index criteria
   1. Intrarater reliability—each individual examiner is scoring equivalently time and time again; "extent to which the same investigator remains consistent in scoring techniques when using a data collection instrument"[1]
   2. Interrater reliability—consistency exists between examiners; "degree to which different investigators can obtain the same results when using the data collection instrument on a population"[1]

Errors in Assessing Disease

A. Errors in sampling technique
   1. Incorrect sampling technique
   2. Use of nonrandom samples of the target population
   3. Nonparticipation of a segment of the target population
B. Errors in collecting and recording data
   1. Variation in assessment; lack of calibration; examiners are not collecting data in a consistent and accurate manner
   2. Observations are computed or recorded inaccurately

PREVENTING AND CONTROLLING ORAL DISEASES

Public Health Measures

A. Characteristics of a public health measure
   1. Not hazardous to life or function
   2. Effective in reducing or preventing the targeted disease
   3. Easily and efficiently implemented
   4. Potency maintained for a substantial time period
   5. Attainable regardless of socioeconomic status, education, or income
   6. Effective immediately on application
   7. Costs are inexpensive and within the means of the community
B. Examples of public health measures include vaccination programs and water purification

Measures for Preventing and Controlling Dental Caries

A. Water fluoridation
   1. Adjustment of the natural fluoride concentration to about 1 part of fluoride to 1 million parts of water (1 ppm)
   2. Most effective and efficient method of bringing the benefits of fluoride to a community
      a. Children reared in a fluoridated community show a 50% to 70% reduction in caries in their permanent dentition when compared to children in a nonfluoridated community
      b. Costs vary depending on the size of the community and the water system; for example, they range from 0.20 to $2.50 per person annually

3. Feeding machinery used for community fluoridation resembles machinery used for adding other materials
   a. Two types of machinery
      (1) Solution feeders—hand- or mechanically saturated solution of fluoride is fed into the main water supply at a carefully controlled rate
      (2) Dry feeder—solid material is fed into a dissolving tank at a measured rate by automatic machinery and the concentrated solution is carried to the main water supply in a sufficiently large amount of water
   b. Compounds used in fluoridation of water supplies include sodium silicafluoride (solid), sodium fluoride (solid) and fluosilicic acid (liquid)
4. Optimum fluoride levels range from 0.7 ppm to 1.2 ppm depending on the climate; the warmer the climate, the lesser the concentration because of increased water consumption; the colder the climate, the larger the concentration
5. Communities with excessive amounts of naturally occurring fluoride can use defluoridation equipment
6. Mottled enamel
   a. Chronic endemic form of hypoplasia of dental enamel caused by drinking water with a high fluoride content during the time of tooth formation; defective calcification of teeth giving a white chalky appearance, which gradually undergoes brown discoloration
   b. Occurs when water with a high fluoride content is ingested during the time of tooth development
7. Promotion of fluoride
   a. Two methods of implementation
      (1) Executive decision—a community leader introduces the idea of community water fluoridation through appropriate government channels and the idea is approved by the appropriate governing body
      (2) Referenda allowing members of the community to cast a vote for fluoridation of the water supply

   b. Public attitudes toward water fluoridation are both positive and negative
      (1) Recent increase in numbers of individuals opposed to water fluoridation; tactics used to oppose fluoridation include
         (a) Scare tactics that imply water fluoridation causes health hazards such as cancer, heart disease, and increased death rates
         (b) Suggestions that water fluoridation violates an individual's freedom of choice
         (c) Creation of an illusion of scientific controversy where none exists
      (2) Important for dental professionals to concentrate their efforts to obtain community support for fluoridation; tactics used to support water fluoridation include
         (a) Knowledge of medical and dental studies that provide the scientific foundation for fluoridation
         (b) Knowledge of the community (e.g., past efforts to either introduce water fluoridation or discontinue water fluoridation)
         (c) Work with all community leaders, community organizations, and members of the community having influence such as newspaper editors, or radio or television personalities
B. School water fluoridation
   1. Reduces dental caries among schoolchildren by about 40%
   2. School water is usually fluoridated at 4.5 times the optimum concentration recommended for the community in which the school is located
      a. Increased optimum amount is because children drink the water only when school is in session
      b. Uses same basic equipment and materials as used in community programs; monitored by an employee of the school system
   3. Major disadvantage is that children do not receive benefits until they begin school

Table 15-4 Daily dosage levels of supplemental fluoride recommended according to age and concentration of fluoride in water

	Concentration of fluoride in water (in ppm)*		
Age	0.3	0.3-0.7	0.7
0-2 years	0.25 mg	0.00 mg	0.00 mg
2-3 years	0.50 mg	0.25 mg	0.00 mg
3-13 years	1.00 mg	0.50 mg	0.00 mg

From Committee on Nutrition, American Academy of Pediatrics: Pediatrics **63:**150, 1979. Copyright American Academy of Pediatrics, 1979.
*2.2 mg sodium fluoride contains 1 mg fluoride.

C. Dietary fluoride supplements
1. Supplement forms include tablets, lozenges, drops, liquids, and fluoride-vitamin preparations
2. Tablets contain 1.0 mg of fluoride, although tablets for younger children are available with 0.5 or 0.25 mg (Table 15-4)
   a. Tablets contain neutral sodium fluoride (NaF) or acidulated phosphate fluoride (APF)
   b. Studies indicate that fluoride tablets taken daily result in a 50% to 80% reduction in caries
3. School-based programs use fluoride tablets
   a. Provides topical and systemic benefits
   b. Inexpensive and little time required
   c. Nondental personnel can supervise
4. Fluoridated salt brings the benefits of systemic fluoride to areas where piped water does not exist
   a. Studies indicate 250 ppm is a suitable concentration
   b. Reduction in caries parallels rates found in communities having water fluoridation
   c. Useful in developing countries
D. Topical application of fluorides (see Chapter 12, section on professionally administered topical fluoride treatments)
1. Professional application of topical fluorides is least cost-effective as a public health measure
2. Topical fluorides have an important role with patients in the private office setting
3. Materials used include sodium fluoride (NaF), stannous fluoride (SnF_2), and acidulated phosphate fluoride (APF)
   a. Reduction in caries
      (1) Reduction of 20% to 40% with a 2% NaF application

      (2) Reduction of 0 to 57% with an 8% to 10% SnF_2 application
      (3) Reduction of 25% to 67% with a 1.23% APF application
   b. Effects are primarily on smooth surfaces of teeth
E. Fluoride mouth rinses
1. Studies indicate a 20% to 50% reduction in caries
2. Sodium fluoride (NaF) and acidulated phosphate fluoride have been used in mouth rinses; sodium fluoride in a 0.2% concentration is used weekly or in a 0.05% concentration is used daily
   a. Sodium fluoride in 0.2% concentration on a weekly basis is suitable for school-based public programs
   b. Advantages of the school-based public programs include
      (1) Easy to learn
      (2) Inexpensive in time and resources
      (3) Nondental personnel can supervise
3. Daily rinsing appears to confer slightly greater benefits than weekly rinsing
4. Individual patients should rinse daily using a prescribed rinse from a dentist or mouth rinse available as an over-the-counter product
F. Pit and fissure sealants (see Chapter 12, section on dental sealants)
1. Studies indicate auxiliaries can apply sealants as successfully as dentists
2. Sealants have been successfully used in combination with fluorides
3. Cost-effectiveness of pit and fissure sealants is uncertain

Measures for Preventing and Controlling Periodontal Disease

A. No parallel to water fluoridation for the prevention of periodontal disease
B. Studies indicate that a thorough professional prophylaxis at 2 to 4-month intervals with daily self-care procedures by the patient will aid in maintaining periodontal health
C. Community activities should include
1. Public education to emphasize personal oral hygiene and regular dental visits
2. Education to convince dental professionals of the need for thorough prophylaxes for adult patients

Measures for Preventing and Controlling Other Dental Anomalies

A. Oral cancer
1. Primary prevention technique for cancer does not exist; avoiding risk factors such as alcohol and tobacco is recommended
2. Secondary prevention or control consists of early detection and treatment
3. Mass screening for oral cancer is costly; professionals should include oral cancer examinations as part of their prevention routines
4. Public education regarding signs and symptoms of oral cancer is important

B. Oral clefts
1. Primary prevention technique for cleft lip and palate does not exist
2. Multiple factors are involved with the occurrence of cleft palate; genetic counseling provides a valuable tool for identifying risk factors
3. Programs for treatment of the conditions are available through the state crippled children services
4. Dental professionals should be aware of the resources within the community

STEPS IN COMMUNITY PLANNING

General Considerations

A. Community groups vary
1. Planning principles can be applied to all groups
2. Principles are useful for all types of programs

B. Dental hygienist has potential for many roles in community health planning
1. Program planner or initiator
2. Consultant/resource person
3. Service provider
4. Director of a particular program/division
5. Researcher

Assessment

A. Definition—organized and systematic approach to identify a target group and define its oral health needs
1. Target group—group of individuals who are the focus of a particular dental health service or program
2. Health professional may identify the target group
3. Target group may contact health professionals

B. Data collection
1. Important to complete before planning
   a. Identify ongoing oral health programs or projects
   b. Assess oral health status and needs
   c. Develop a community profile of the area where the target population is located
2. Identify ongoing types of programs or projects
   a. Programs presently providing dental services
   b. Identify locations or facilities where dental health activities can occur
   c. Identify individuals, special equipment, facilities, and resources to meet the dental needs of the target population
3. Assess current dental status and needs
   a. Three methods for obtaining data to document dental status and needs
      (1) Identify and use an assessment method to obtain specific information related to the proposed project or program
      (2) Coordinate assessment with an agency or group seeking similar information about the identified target population
      (3) Research and collect data accumulated from records available from state or local health agencies, dental or medical programs, and public health or related agencies
   b. Assessment methods
      (1) Baseline data—data collected before program implementation; used for planning and evaluating a program
      (2) Used to identify the extent and severity of need and in determining objectives
      (3) Influenced by the type of information needed
      (4) Assessment methods can be used in combination with each other
      (5) Advantages and disadvantages of assessment methods (Table 15-5)
4. Types of assessment methods
   a. Four types of examinations and inspections as classified by the American Dental Association
      (1) Type 1—complete examination using a mouth mirror and explorer, adequate illumination, thorough radiographic survey, and when indicated, percussion, pulp vitality tests, transillumination, study models, and laboratory tests; because of the time, expense, and personnel required, seldom used in public health

Table 15-5 Data collection instruments and applications

Data collection methodology	Instrument	Indications	Advantages	Limitations
Direct observation of events, objects, people	Checklist, content analysis, evaluation forms, camera, tape recorder, videotape, thermometer, sphygmomanometer, rating and ranking scales	1. Used when subject recall may affect accuracy of data collection 2. Used to study behavior 3. Used to study psychomotor 4. Used in experimental research	1. Observations can be made as they occur in the "natural" setting 2. Observations can be made of behaviors that might not be reported by respondents	1. Time consuming 2. Difficulty in recording 3. Factors that may interfere with the situation 4. Difficulty in quantification of observations 5. Expensive 6. Observer-respondent interaction
Interview	Interview guide or interview schedule	1. Used for obtaining information on attitudes, beliefs, and opinions 2. Used in a survey 3. Used to gain information on past or present events	1. Flexibility 2. Questions can be clarified and explained 3. Complete data can be collected 4. Subjects do not have to read or write	1. Respondents may be inhibited to respond accurately and truthfully 2. Time consuming 3. Expensive 4. Interviewer may affect the responses
Asking questions	Questionnaire, opinionnaire	1. Used for obtaining information on attitudes, beliefs, and opinions 2. Used to gain information on past events 3. Used when impersonal interactions between researcher and respondent are required	1. Ease of administration 2. Relatively inexpensive 3. Standardization of instructions and questions 4. Economy of time 5. Data can be gathered over a wide geographical area	1. Misinterpretation of questions by respondents 2. Low return may bias results 3. Superficiality of responses 4. Incomplete data collection 5. Honesty of respondent
Survey	Questionnaire, interview, schedule, case study	1. Used for obtaining a broad range of information on the status quo 2. Used to study present conditions 3. Used in planning	1. Data can be gathered to reflect public opinion 2. Vast amount of data can be collected 3. Cross-sectional, generalized statistics can be obtained	1. Superficiality of responses 2. Control of extraneous variables is lacking
Epidemiological survey	Dental indices	1. Used to study disease patterns in a population 2. Used to evaluate the effectiveness of therapeutic or preventive treatments in a specific geographical area	1. Vast amount of data can be collected 2. Cross-sectional, generalized statistics can be obtained 3. Data are quantifiable	1. Difficulty in determining causation due to complexity of variables 2. Time consuming
Records, documents	Reports of legislative bodies and state or city officials, deeds, wills, appointment records, dental charts, report cards	1. Used to study posted events	1. Unbiased in terms of the investigator 2. Inexpensive 3. No subject-investigator interaction 4. Convenience and economy of time	1. Incomplete records 2. Accuracy of records may be unknown

From Darby, M.L., and Bowen, D.M.: Research methods for oral health professionals: an introduction, St. Louis, 1980, The C.V. Mosby Co.

(2) Type 2—limited examination using a mouth mirror, explorer, adequate illumination, and posterior bitewing radiographs (where indicated, periapical radiographs); useful where programs may include service to individuals; also helpful in surveys where time and money permit

(3) Type 3—inspection using a mouth mirror, explorer, and adequate illumination; most commonly used

(4) Type 4—screening with a tongue depressor and available illumination; identifies needs

b. Survey—common approach used to assess knowledge, oral health status, oral health behavior, values and attitudes

  (1) Can employ various techniques for data collection (e.g., questionnaire, interview, direct observation, indices, records, documents, etc.)

  (2) World Health Organization's suggested format for reporting survey results[4]

    (a) Statement of purpose of the survey (or assessment method)

    (b) Materials and methods

      [1] Description of the area and population surveyed

      [2] Types of information collected

      [3] Methods of collecting data

      [4] Sampling method

      [5] Examiner personnel and equipment

      [6] Statistical method and procedure

      [7] Cost analysis

      [8] Reliability and reproducibility

    (c) Results

    (d) Discussion and conclusions

    (e) Summary

C. Development of a community profile

  1. Community profile—provides information essential in planning a community health program; general areas for inclusion in the profile are

    a. Community overview

      (1) Number of individuals in the population

      (2) Population distribution by income, age, education, etc.

      (3) Geographic location and boundaries

      (4) Population setting (urban or rural)

      (5) Ethnic background, cultural heritages, languages

      (6) Diet, nutritional levels, nutrition programs

      (7) Amount, types, and influence of public services and utilities

      (8) Transportation schedules, routes, fares, reliability

      (9) Informed consent procedures

      (10) Distribution of public and private schools and religious organizations

      (11) Extent and type of fluoride therapies

    b. Community leadership and organization

      (1) Community leaders, liaisons, and councils and their attitudes toward oral health

      (2) Community power base for policy formulation

      (3) Governance structure (e.g., health council, city government, advisory board, school board, union)

      (4) Grassroots individuals with political influence

    c. Financing and funding of health services

      (1) Budget allocation procedures for dental health programs

      (2) Mechanism for requesting the necessary funding

      (3) Funding sources (e.g., federal, state, or local funding; individual or third party payment; private funds, grants, or endowments)

    d. Facilities, resources, and personpower

      (1) Location of space and facilities in the community or institution

      (2) Availability of equipment

      (3) Location of medical centers, clinics, and dental laboratories

      (4) Number of licensed practicing dentists, dental hygienists, dental assistants, medical personnel, or others with experience working with the target population

  2. Rationale for development of a community profile—to understand the environment in which the target population is located

  3. Size, location, and type of community dictates the type of information necessary for a community profile

D. Analysis of data

  1. Analysis includes organizing, tabulating, and interpreting data

  2. Data analysis can range from the simple to the complex

    a. Planner alone tabulates

    b. Statisticians and statistical tests are used

    c. Computers and other technology are used

3. Following analysis, needs and priorities can be identified
   a. Target group input is solicited
   b. Community representatives and/or advisory groups are consulted
      (1) Advisory groups provide an opportunity for dialogue and support
      (2) Members are determined by the unique characteristics of the project and can include consumers, political and financial leaders, and health and dental professionals

Program Planning

A. Definition—organized response to reduce or eliminate one or more problems; organized effort that includes the objective of reducing or eliminating one or more problems, performance of one or more activities, and utilization of resources
B. Elements of a program plan
   1. Identification of program goals and objectives
   2. Strategies and specific activities to meet objectives
      a. Sequence of activities
      b. Individuals responsible for each activity
   3. Resources required
      a. Location and facilities
      b. Equipment
      c. Personnel
   4. Timetables and deadlines
   5. Projected costs
   6. Program promotion
C. Goals and objectives
   1. For each need prioritized, a goal with related objectives needs to be determined
      a. Goal—broadly based statement of what changes will occur as a result of the program
      b. Objectives—specific statements that describe, in a measurable manner, the desired result of program activities
   2. Categories of goals and objectives
      a. Ultimate or long term
      b. Intermediate
      c. Short term or immediate (NOTE: Most activities may deal with immediate goals, but intermediate and long-term goals must be considered)
   3. Immediate objectives are stated in specific, measurable terms; factors considered
      a. What—identify the condition or situation to be attained
      b. Extent—scope and magnitude of situation or condition to be attained

c. Who—target group or portion of the community in which attainment is desired
d. Where—geographic area or physical boundaries of the program
e. When—time "at or by" which the desired situation or condition is to exist
D. Activities
   1. Program activities are the dynamic, energy-using procedures carried out by program objectives; programs might be preventive, educational, treatment oriented or research oriented
   2. To meet objectives, personnel, location, equipment, and costs are determined
E. Promotion
   1. Necessary for participation and success of a project
   2. Promotion techniques include an advisory committee, liaison groups, television and radio media, printed media, and special interest publications and programs
F. Implementation
   1. Process of putting plan into operation
   2. Monitoring plan for activities, personnel, equipment, and supplies
   3. Feedback mechanism from personnel and participants
   4. Ongoing evaluation mechanisms
G. Evaluation
   1. Key element—should take place at all stages
   2. Results of the program are measured against objectives developed during the early planning stages
   3. Assessment method may influence evaluation tool used (e.g., pretest versus posttest)

IMPLEMENTATION
Educational Strategies

A. Health education—provision of health information to people in such a way that they apply it in everyday living; a process with intellectual, psychologic, and social dimensions relating to activities that increase the abilities of people to make informed decisions affecting their personal, family, and community well-being; a process, based on scientific principles, that facilitates learning and behavioral change in both health personnel and consumers
B. Includes both formal and informal activities
   1. Formal activities include the deliberate provision of dental health education designed to elicit specific dental behavior (e.g., the curricula of elementary and secondary schools,

health professionals conducting in-service workshops and programs, health agencies providing education and service)
2. Informal activities include the acquisition of dental-related information that may lead to some specific dental behavior (e.g., interaction with colleagues, family, dental professionals and the dental environment)
C. Health education is an integral part of community activities and might involve
1. Allied health professionals
2. Elementary and secondary students
3. Educators
4. Special population groups
5. Adult groups
6. Institutionalized population
D. Health education topics are not limited to oral hygiene instruction; topics might include
1. Preventive measures such as fluorides, pit and fissure sealants, and others
2. Dental diseases such as periodontal disease, malocclusion, oral cancer, herpes simplex, and poor dental habits
   a. Assessment, prevention, and treatment
   b. Self-examination techniques
3. Dental safety and dental emergencies (e.g., what to do if a tooth is knocked out)
4. Roles of various dental and health professionals and their interrelationships
5. Care of teeth and prostheses
6. Careers in dentistry and dental hygiene
7. Becoming a discriminating dental consumer

Principles of Learning

See Chapter 12, section on disease control education, and Chapter 17, section on successful patient management
A. One learns by doing
B. Without a sufficient stage of readiness, learning is inefficient and may even be harmful
C. Without motivation, there can be no learning at all
D. Responses of the learner must be immediately reinforced
E. For maximum transfer of learning, responses should be learned in the way they are going to be used
F. Individuals' responses will vary according to how they perceive the situation
G. All persons perform to the best of their ability based on their physical ability, their background of learning, and the present forces acting on them; individuals must be motivated to learn; individuals possess some basic physical needs and some personal or social needs—desire for recognition, security, response, and new experiences; wants,

needs, and motives of the learner should be identified
H. Learners progress in any area of learning only as far as they need to progress to achieve their purposes
I. Learning proceeds much more rapidly and is retained much longer when what is learned possesses meaning, organization, and structure
J. Individuals are more apt to become involved whole-heartedly if they have participated in the selection and planning of the project

Principles of Teaching

A. Identify learner needs and audience level
B. Establish objectives
C. Design learning experiences and methodology based on objectives
D. Plan evaluation

Instruction versus Instructional Objectives

A. Instruction is based on a combination of
1. Instructional objectives
2. Learning experiences based on the objectives
3. Evaluation of learning
B. Instructional objectives are important to successful instruction and learning
C. Components of a good objective include
1. Performance—an objective always says what a learner is expected to be able to do, using a verb that denotes an observable behavior (e.g., "the patient will *demonstrate* the Bass toothbrushing technique")
2. Conditions—an objective always describes the important conditions (if any) under which the performance is to occur (e.g., *"given a soft-bristled toothbrush,* the patient will demonstrate the Bass toothbrushing technique")
3. Criterion—wherever possible, an objective describes the criterion of acceptable performance by describing how well the learner must perform in order to be considered acceptable (e.g., "given a soft-bristled toothbrush, the patient will demonstrate the Bass toothbrushing technique and remove *all plaque detected by a disclosing agent"*)

Lesson Plan Development

A. Lesson plan—organization of topics and learning experiences so that they relate to a central theme or problem; lesson plan should include an organized plan with objectives, activities, materials, and evaluation techniques
B. Objective—provides educators with an organized approach in presenting specific topics and ideas in order to achieve stated objectives

C. Rationale—to provide a basic foundation on which teaching and learning can be assessed, planned, implemented, and evaluated

Methods of Teaching Instructional Units

A. Lecture—informative talk, prepared beforehand and given before an audience or group
1. Purposes
   a. Introduce new topics
   b. Summarize facts and ideas
   c. Review concepts
   d. Convey information to large numbers of individuals
2. Advantages
   a. Preparation takes place before presentation
   b. Allows for organization
3. Disadvantages
   a. No active participation by the learner
   b. Poor presentation technique may present a barrier to learning
B. Lecture-demonstration—informative talk that presents information supplemented by a demonstration to reinforce learning
1. Purposes
   a. Introduce information
   b. Demonstrate skills or techniques to supplement information
2. Advantages
   a. Sets forth information in a complete format
   b. Allows for concentration of attention and economical use of time
   c. Useful for reinforcing material
3. Disadvantages
   a. Difficult for large groups to see a demonstration
   b. Requires careful preparation for success
C. Discussion—group activity in which the student and teacher define a problem and seek a solution
1. Purposes
   a. Allows interaction among participants
   b. Can include the use of questions by the leader to stimulate interaction
   c. Provides two-way communication between the group leader and members
2. Advantages
   a. Encourages members to contribute personally to the discussion
   b. Stimulates participants to problem solve
   c. Participant learns to work within a group setting and accept the group's opinion
3. Disadvantages
   a. Individuals with strong personalities can influence a group

b. A poor group leader may contribute to the failure of the discussion
c. Nothing is achieved because discussion goes in many directions without coming to a decision

EVALUATION AND RESEARCH
Statistics in Dental Literature
Basic Concepts

A. Population—entire group or whole unit to which results of an investigation can be inferred
1. Target population—"all members of a specific group who possess a clearly defined set of characteristics"[1]
2. Sample—"portion of the population, that if properly selected, can provide meaningful information about the entire population; a sample is examined when the researcher has neither the time money nor resources to study an entire population"[1]
B. Sampling techniques
1. Random sample—"sample composed of subjects who are chosen independently of each other, with equal opportunity for inclusion; increases external validity; controls intersubject difference"[1]
2. Stratified sample—"method of sampling used to represent subgroups proportionately in the sample when they are known to exist in the population"[1]
3. Systematic sample—"sample achieved by drawing every n^{th} subject from a list or file of the total population; considered to be random if the list or file is in random order"[1]
4. Convenience sample with random assignment—used when access to the total population is not feasible; potential members are numbered consecutively, and a table of random numbers is used for experimental and control group assignments[1]
   a. Experimental group—"sample group in a study that is exposed to the experimental variable under study; a group who receives the independent variable"[1]
   b. Control group—"sample group in an experiment that does not receive the experimental treatment (independent variable) but rather receives a placebo treatment or no treatment at all"[1]
C. Sample size
1. Large sample, if selected properly
   a. Accurately represents the defined population
   b. Increases the precision and accuracy of collected data

c. Reduces the standard error of the sample mean
2. Small sample
   a. May be necessary depending on the purpose of the research
   b. When inappropriate for the type of research, may lead to inaccurate conclusions
D. Definitions
   1. Research—"continual search for truth using the scientific method"[1]
   2. Scientific method—"methodology used in any type of research involving procedures which increase the likelihood that information gathered will be relevant, reliable, and unbiased; steps of the method include
      a. Identification and statement of the problem
      b. Formulation of a hypothesis
      c. Collection, organization, and analysis of data
      d. Formulation of conclusions
      e. Verification, rejection, or modification of the hypothesis by the list of its consequences in a specific situation"[1]
   3. Statistic—"numerical characteristic of a sample derived from the data collected; a characteristic of a sample, identified symbolically with Arabic letters ($\overline{X}$, sd)"[1]
   4. Parameter—"characteristic of a population; indicated symbolically by Greek letters (μ, σ)"[1]
   5. Variable—"state, condition, concept, construct, or event whose value is free to vary, e.g., height, dental caries"[1]
      a. Independent variable—"condition of the experiment that is manipulated or controlled by the investigator; the experimental variable; the experimental treatment"[1]
      b. Dependent variable—"measure thought to change as a result of the presence, absence or manipulation of the independent variable"[1]
      c. Extraneous variables—"uncontrolled variables that are not related to the purpose of the study but may influence the dependent variable and therefore influence the outcome of the study"[1]

Data

A. Data—numbers collected from measurements or counts
   1. Continuous data—numerical data capable of any degree along a continuum; measurements made from values (e.g., time or temperature)
   2. Discrete data—numerical variables or data that are counted only in terms of whole numbers (e.g., set, number of patients examined)
B. Scales of measurement—used to measure variables
   1. Nominal scale—observations fitted into classes or categories (e.g., Republicans/Democrats; male/female; good oral hygiene/poor oral hygiene)
   2. Ordinal scale—ranking of characteristic in some empirical order (e.g., ranking students according to grades received; student with highest score is assigned rank of one, second best, rank of two, and so on)
   3. Interval scale—measurement scale characterized by equal intervals along the scale; has no absolute zero (e.g., a Fahrenheit thermometer)
   4. Ratio scale—measurement scale characterized by the presence of an absolute zero (e.g., age, weight, and height)

Statistics[1]

A. Statistics—science that describes, summarizes, analyzes, and interprets numerical data for the purpose of making an inference about a population
B. Descriptive statistics—that branch of statistics used to numerically describe and summarize data collected; no attempt is made to generalize research findings beyond the immediate sample
   1. Measures of central tendency—used to describe what is typical in the sample group based on the data gathered
      a. Mean—sum of the values, divided by the number of items
         (1) Incorporates the value of each score
         (2) Affected by extreme scores
         (3) Interval or ratio statistic
      b. Median—point of a distribution with 50% of the scores falling above it and 50% of the scores falling below it; arrange scores of distribution in ascending order of magnitude and locate the midpoint
         (1) When the total number of scores is odd, the median is the middle score
         (2) When the total number of scores is even, take two middle scores, sum them, and divide by 2
         (3) Median can be a decimal
         (4) Not affected by extreme scores
         (5) Ordinal statistic
      c. Mode—determined by observing the most frequently occurring score in a distribution
         (1) Distribution may be unimodal, bimodal, multimodal, or have no mode
         (2) Nominal statistic

2. Measures of dispersion—used to describe variability of scores in a distribution
   a. Range—the spread between the highest and lowest scores in a distribution
      (1) Ordinal statistic
      (2) Easily determined
      (3) Somewhat unreliable because it is determined by only two scores of the distribution
   b. Variance—sum of the squared deviations from the mean divided by N; square root of the variance yields the standard deviation
   c. Standard deviation—used to analyze descriptively the spread of scores in a distribution; the positive square root of the variance
      (1) The greater the dispersion of scores from the means of the distribution, the greater will be the standard deviation and variance
      (2) Small standard deviation indicates that the distribution of scores is clustered around the mean; large standard deviation indicates that scores are widely dispersed around the mean
C. Correlation—statistical measure for determining the strength of the linear relationship between two variables
   1. Correlational technique is based on the number of variables to be correlated, the nature of the variables to be correlated, the nature of the variable (discrete or continuous), and the scale of measurement (nominal, ordinal, interval, and ratio)
   2. Procedures yield a measure called a correlation coefficient, ranging from −1.0 to +1.0; the sign indicates the direction of the correlation, whereas the number indicates the strength of the correlation
   3. Types of correlations
      a. Positive correlation—value of one variable increases as the value of the second variable also increases; perfect positive correlation is a +1.0
      b. Negative correlation—inverse relationship between two variables; perfect negative correlation is a −1.0

D. Inferential statistics—that branch of statistics used to infer research findings from the sample to the general population from which the sample was taken; used to generalize results to a larger population of interest
   1. Parametric statistics—inferential statistical procedures in which the following assumptions are made about population parameters
      a. Data are intervally or ratio scaled
      b. Population from which the data are taken is normally distributed
      c. Sample is large and randomized
      d. Variables measured are continuous
   2. Nonparametric statistics—inferential statistical procedures in which there are fewer assumptions about the population parameters
      a. Data are nominally or ordinally scaled
      b. Population from which the sample is drawn is distribution free
      c. Sample small
      d. Variables are discrete

Statistical Decision Making

A. Types of hypotheses
   1. Hypothesis—proposition, condition, or principle that predicts or indicates a relationship among or behavior of variables under certain conditions
   2. Null hypothesis (Ho)—hypothesis that assumes that there are no statistically significant differences between the population groups; hypothesis being tested
   3. Research hypothesis or positive hyposthesis is stated in terms that express the opinion or prediction of the researcher
   4. Failing to accept the null hypothesis means accepting the alternate
B. Type I and type II errors
   1. Type I error (alpha)—based on statistical results, the researcher rejects the null hypothesis and concludes that a statistically significant difference exists when in fact, no true difference is present; rejecting a null hypothesis that is true
   2. Type II error (beta)—Researcher concludes that no statistically significance difference exists and accepts the null hypothesis when in fact a significant difference does exist; accepting a null hypothesis that is false
   3. Relationship between two types of testing errors (Fig. 15-2)

		Null hypothesis is	
		Accepted	Not accepted
Null hypothesis is actually	True	No error	Type I error $(p = \alpha)$
	Not true	Type II error $(p = \beta)$	No error

Fig. 15-2 Type I and type II errors.

C. Statistical significance—"according to the odds established by the alpha level, the obtained result is less likely to be a chance occurrence and more likely the result of the independent variable; does not necessarily mean that data are important, valid, or meaningful"[1]
  1. Statistical decision making—tool used by the researcher to aid in the interpretation of findings
  2. Statistical decision making is not the sole means by which research findings are interpreted and applied
  3. Clinical significance—practical implications of research that may or may not be inherent in research results; findings may have statistical significance without having clinical significance
D. Probability level—"researcher's odds for determining the operation of chance factors in producing the obtained research result; cut-off point for failing to reject or rejecting the null hypothesis; also known as significance level, alpha value, and P-value"[1]
  1. P-value—"probability of observing a value of the test statistic equal to or more extreme than its table value"[1]
    a. "Small P-values indicating rare chance occurrences lead to the rejection of the null hypothesis and the assertion of a statistically significant result"[1]
    b. "Large P-values indicate that chance occurrences were likely to have accounted for the result and therefore the null hypothesis should be retained"[1]
  2. Maximum P-values typically used on the table of values of the test statistic are 0.10, 0.05, 0.01, and 0.0001
    a. If probability is less than 0.05 (P < 0.05) two sets of data are reported as significantly different

  b. Factor of more than 0.05 (P > 0.05) indicates data are not significantly different
  c. Test statistic used depends on the size of the sample, the number of samples, the type of data, and other factors
E. Inferential statistical techniques—parametrics
  1. *t*-Test for independent samples—inferential statistical analysis of choice for determining if a statistically significant difference exists between two sample groups drawn independently from a population and when only one or two independent variables are tested
    a. Designed for normally distributed, randomly selected data
    b. Data are interval or ratio scaled
    c. Used when sample groups have fewer than 30 observations
  2. *t*-Test for dependent samples—inferential statistic for determining if a statistically significant difference exists between two samples that are related and when only one independent variable is tested; also known as *t*-test for correlated samples
    a. Formula for the test takes into account the fact that two groups are related
    b. More sensitive than the *t*-test for independent samples because groups are paired, eliminating a possible source of variance
  3. Analysis of variance (ANOVA)—inferential statistic used to analyze the effects of two or more independent variables simultaneously within the same research design and to determine interactions among the variables in multiple sample groups
    a. Samples should be randomly and independently selected from normal populations with equal variances
    b. Data must be at least interval or ratio scaled

    c. *F* ratio—value that results when ANOVA computed
      (1) Ratio of the variance between the group means over the variance within the groups; determines if the observed differences among the sample means is significant
      (2) Determines if the observed difference among the sample means is large enough to reject the null hypothesis
F. Inferential statistical techniques—nonparametrics
  1. Chi square test (χ^2)—statistical test for determining if a statistically significant differences exists between observed frequencies and expected frequencies; used to analyze discrete, nominally scaled data; has two applications
    a. Used in the single-sample situation to determine whether or not a significant difference exists between the observed number of cases within designated categories and the expected number of cases within designated categories and the expected number predicted in the null hypothesis
    b. Chi square test of the independence of categorical variables is used with two or more samples; allows the testing of hypotheses regarding the interrelationship between and among categorical variables
  2. Chi square analysis used primarily to analyze questionnaire data that are discrete and nominally scaled

Evaluating Dental Literature

A. Professional responsibility includes keeping current with new developments
B. Reviewing dental literature is important for the dental hygiene professional
  1. Necessary to study dental literature before and during planning for community programs
  2. Dental literature will provide impetus and support for various types of community activities
C. Reviewing dental literature is a valuable source of continuing education for a professional

Criteria for Reviewing Dental Literature

A. Overall description of the article
  1. Title concise and descriptive
  2. Author's affiliations and credentials are noted
    a. Researcher has a satisfactory reputation for well-conducted research
    b. Researcher is not affiliated with a commercial firm

  3. Article found in a reputable journal
    a. Journal has an editorial review board
    b. Journal is affiliated with a professional group or specialty group
    c. Journal is not a "popular" magazine, sponsored by a cause, or published by a commercial firm
  4. Data published indicates current knowledge and is not outdated by more recent research
B. Author has qualifications to write the article
  1. Author's current or past position supports expertise in a particular area
  2. There is evidence of finances and facilities to support the research
C. References are available for articles
  1. References are comprehensive, accurate, and recent
  2. Given the topic, there is an appropriate number of current references
D. Research problem is clearly, accurately, and completely described
  1. Purposes of the study are clearly stated
  2. There is a thorough review of the literature
  3. Important terms and concepts are defined adequately
  4. Hypotheses or objectives are adequate and clearly stated; hypotheses or objectives follow directly from the statement
E. Experimental or descriptive research requires a different evaluation
  1. Characteristics of the population sampled are described
  2. Sampling techniques are described and adequate
  3. There is no bias in selection or assignment of objects or persons in the sample
  4. Research design is described; there is control indicated for variables that might influence the results
  5. Tests and instruments used give reasonable measures of the factors under study
    a. Test and instruments used are valid and reliable
    b. Conditions in which measurements are made are completely described
  6. All factors needed to test the hypotheses or achieve the objectives are included in the analysis
    a. Statistical tests are described
    b. Hypotheses are tested through statistical analysis
  7. Findings are presented in a clear manner
    a. Statistical tables are clear and easy to understand

b. Data are presented in a straightforward manner

c. Tables highlighting information within article are presented accurately and are easy to evaluate

8. Discussion highlights significant issues that are the result of the research
   a. Author may speculate on the significance of the findings
   b. Strengths and weaknesses of the study are stated
   c. Results should be related to the current literature

9. Conclusions are supported by the findings

PROVIDING DENTAL CARE
Dental Delivery System

A. Definition—resolution of explicit dental needs through the delivery or provision of dental services by means of organized and sometimes interdependent activities

B. Dental delivery system is complex
   1. Structure of the system is related to the manner in which patients and providers get together for the provision of health care services
   2. Financing arrangements
   3. Supply of provider personnel

Diverse Modes of Providing Dental Care in the United States

A. Private sector
   1. Solo practice—dental practice in which there is a single proprietorship by a dentist who may employ dental hygienists, dental assistants, and staff
      a. Advantages
         (1) Provider and patient flexibility in terms of the availability of services
         (2) Inherent economic incentive to be efficient because of the investment involved
         (3) Provider can accept or refuse patients
         (4) Provider determines policies and staffing
      b. Disadvantages
         (1) Total responsibility for care of patients lies with one practitioner; may limit times absent from the office
         (2) Limits types of care available to patients

2. Group practice—dental practice in which dentists, sometimes in association with the members of other health professions, agree formally among themselves on certain arrangements to provide efficient dental services; practice formally organized to provide dental care through the services of three or more dentists using office space, equipment, and/or personnel jointly; generally treats patients on a fee-for-service basis; prepaid programs in limited numbers
   a. Advantages
      (1) Dentists in group practices enjoy higher levels of income than their solo colleagues
      (2) Provides for improved personal freedom because colleagues can substitute when a dentist is absent
      (3) Quality may improve because of built-in peer review
      (4) Fringe benefits are possible because of the numbers employed within the practice
      (5) Potential exists for a variety of specialties to be represented within the practice; more varieties of services can be provided for patients
   b. Disadvantages
      (1) Personality conflicts may occur, affecting the practice
      (2) Loss of individuality; identity belongs to the group, not the individual practitioner

3. Closed panel—prepayment plan in which patients eligible for dental services in a public or private program can receive services only at specified facilities from a limited number of dentists
   a. Professional groups have expressed concern about closed-panel groups because patients are denied freedom of choice of dentists
   b. Another argument against the closed panel is related to the quality of care provided, although charges of poor quality cannot be substantiated

4. Open panel—prepayment plan in which patients eligible for dental services can receive care from any licensed dentist they choose; any licensed dentist may participate; dentist may accept or refuse any patient
   a. Prepaid group practice is a group practice that provides dental services on a prepaid basis
   b. Prepaid group practices are generally regarded as open panels

5. Health maintenance organization (HMO)—legal entity that provides a prescribed range of health services to each individual who has enrolled in the organization in return for a prepaid, fixed, and uniform payment; uses prepaid capitation system
   a. Includes five elements
      (1) Managing organization
      (2) Delivery system
      (3) Enrolled population
      (4) Benefit package
      (5) System of financing and prepayment
   b. Only a small proportion of HMOs offer dental services
   c. Qualifies for federal funds if certain statutory conditions are met
   d. Reduces cost of care to the consumer because of emphasis on ambulatory care reducing unnecessary hospitalization
6. Dental department in a hospital
   a. Dental care is provided for special situations, such as patients requiring general anesthesia or other hospital resources
   b. Routine care for patients with special needs such as patients with cleft palate repair, trauma to the head and neck region, or specific disease or disability
   c. Routine care for the indigent
7. Retail dental clinics—dental clinics located in department store or shopping mall settings; dental clinic franchises
   a. Department stores view the dental clinics as an extra service for their customers similar to pharmacies or optical departments
   b. Most dental practice acts require ownership by a dentist
   c. If state laws allow ownership by nondentists, department stores can own their own clinics and hire dental personnel as salaried employees
   d. Purported to increase access to dental care because of location, hours, flexible appointment scheduling, and marketing techniques
B. Public sector
1. Community health centers—federally funded group practices, primarily medical with a dental component; located in areas to provide services to communities where dental and medical practitioners are not found in adequate numbers
   a. Similar to a well-developed group practice with different financing arrangements
   b. Provide primary medical and dental care; referral services and ease of access for members of the community
   c. Centers include neighborhood health centers, family health centers, and rural initiative centers
2. U.S. Public Health Service (USPHS)—component of the Department of Health and Human Services
   a. Major responsibilities of the U.S. Public Health Service include health research and the promotion of health through public health efforts
   b. Responsible for dental care provided to American Indians, federal prisoners, Coast Guard personnel, coast and geodetic survey personnel, Merchant Marine personnel, merchant seamen, and individuals suffering from Hansen's disease
   c. States, counties, and cities have established programs aimed at providing care for indigent populations eligible to receive public welfare

FINANCING DENTAL CARE
Mechanisms of Payment

A. Fee for service—two-party arrangement in which a fee scale is developed for a service; charge or payment for performed services[3]
   1. Most American dental patients pay for their care using fee for service
   2. Culturally acceptable method of payment
   3. Only system under which some forms of dental treatment are available
B. Postpayment or budget payment plans—mechanisms whereby the patient borrows money from a bank to pay dental fees; patient repays the loan with interest to the bank in budgeted amounts[3]
   1. Initially proposed to bring benefits of routine dental care to a large segment of the population
   2. Studies indicate budget plans are used by middle-income rather than low-income individuals
   3. Credit card payment is currently more popular and achieves a similar purpose by allowing postpayment
C. Private third-party prepayment plans
   1. Definition—third-party payment for dental services is payment for services by some agency other than the beneficiary of those services (e.g., insurance company, employer)[3]
      a. Dentist and patient are the first and second parties; administrator of the finances is the third party

b. Third party may collect premiums, assume financial risk, pay claims, and provide administrative services

c. Third party also known as the carrier, insurer, underwriter, or administrative service

d. Purchaser of plan can be an organized private group such as a union or employer

2. Prepayment allows the spread of the financial burden of dental care over a group because prepayment plans apply to groups of people (e.g., unions, all state employees, etc.)

3. Reimbursement for prepayment plans is done by the usual, customary, and reasonable (UCR) fee

a. Usual fee—fee usually charged by a dentist to private patients

b. Customary fee—customary because it is in the range of the fee charged by dentists with similar training within a specific geographic area

c. Reasonable fee—considered reasonable if it meets the above two criteria or if it is justifiable considering special circumstances[3]

4. Types of prepayment plans

a. Dental service corporations—legally constituted nonprofit organizations incorporated on a state-by-state basis and sponsored by a constituent dental society (e.g., Delta Dental Plans)

b. Health service corporations—offer limited dental coverage as part of their hospital/surgical/medical policies (e.g., Blue Cross/Blue Shield)

c. Commercial insurance plans—operate for profit

(1) Have no obligation to dental health of the community

(2) Organize levels of reimbursement differently; do not use usual, customary, and reasonable fees; develop a fee for particular services, based on reported experience of fees in the area, and dentists are paid at that rate

(3) Can be selective about groups to which they offer insurance

(4) Compete with dental service corporations because, through promotion and marketing, they can provide attractive total health package plans to potential purchasers

d. Prepaid group practice—can have a variety of financing arrangements

(1) Income can be divided equally

(2) Income can be divided among practitioners in the practice according to different criteria such as specialty or number of patients

(3) In some group practices all dentists are salaried

e. Health maintenance organizations (HMOs)—capitation-based, prepaid practices that must meet certain statutory requirements to be eligible to receive federal subsidies

f. Capitation plan—system in which a dentist or group of dentists agree to participate in a panel and accept a predetermined level of reimbursement for services provided

(1) Receives the predetermined sum on a monthly or yearly basis

(2) Fee is paid whether the patients use the care or not

Public Financing of Care

A. Social Security amendments as of 1965 amended the Social Security Act of 1935 and introduced a plan to remove barriers for obtaining health care

1. Title XVIII Medicare—insurance program from trust funds to pay medical bills for insured people

a. All people over 65 are eligible; no income limitations

b. Federal program

c. Dental segment is limited

2. Title XIX Medicaid—assistance program; money from federal, state, and local taxes pays bills for eligible people

a. Certain groups of needy and low-income people are eligible, including the aged, blind, disabled, and members of families with dependent children

b. Federal and state governments form a partnership in financing care; varies from state to state

c. Dental care not mandatory except for persons under 21 years of age

d. Extremely complex program

B. Veteran's Administration (VA) provides some dental care through its hospital system

C. Treatment for children with cleft lip and palate is funded by state and federal money

D. Federal government provides financing for dental treatment of children in Headstart, the preschool child development program

NEED FOR, DEMAND FOR, AND UTILIZATION OF DENTAL SERVICES

Definitions

A. Need—normative, usually professional judgment as to the amount and kind of health or medical care services required by an individual having certain characteristics to attain or maintain some standard level of health
B. Demand—volume and type of health care services that an individual desires to consume at some level of price
   1. Effective demand—desire for care and ability to obtain care
   2. Potential demand—desire for care and inability to obtain care
C. Utilization—proportion of the population that uses dental services over a period of time; volume and type of services actually consumed

Health Behavior and Utilization

A. Health belief model (see Chapter 12, section on health belief model)
   1. Individuals must feel susceptible to the disease
   2. Individuals must feel that the disease is potentially serious in its effects on them
   3. Individuals must feel that a course of action that will prevent or alleviate the disease is available to them
B. Utilization patterns for dental care
   1. Shift in dental services used has been reported (e.g., there has been an increase in examinations; extractions and dentures show a slight decline)
   2. Age, gender, and race—young and old demonstrate the least dental care utilization rates; females have more dental visits than males; nonwhites have a lower number of dental visits than whites
   3. Higher education and income levels mean higher dental care utilization rates
   4. Utilization of dental care is lower in rural farm and nonfarm communities than in urban areas; overall, individuals in rural areas are showing a substantially greater increase in utilization than city dwellers

5. Dental insurance shows no significant impact on dental care utilization
   a. Effect of dental insurance coverage varies with socioeconomic class of insured population
   b. Groups who voluntarily purchased dental insurance have the highest dental care utilization rates
   c. Marketing and enrollment characteristics of the plan affect dental care utilization
   d. Insurance coverage affects utilization with an increase in utilization initially, followed by a decline in utilization rates

Barriers to Dental Care

A. Noncost barriers
   1. Patients do not see a need for dental care
   2. Pain is associated with dental care
   3. Access to care is difficult or impossible
   4. Patient's time is more valuable than interest in obtaining care
   5. Dental personnel are not viewed favorably
B. Cost-related barriers
   1. Fees are considered too high
   2. Insurance coverage is limited or not available
C. Social and psychologic barriers
   1. Dental care and appearance of teeth are not valued
   2. Prior experience has been unpleasant
   3. Emotional factors such as fear of dental care

Current Status

A. Approximately 50% of the population seek care annually
   1. Need to reach other 50% and make them aware of available dental care services
   2. Caries rates are declining
B. Must be a change in philosophy on the part of dental personnel
   1. Identify those individuals currently not seeking care (e.g., special population groups, low income individuals)
   2. Increase access to care (e.g., vary office hours; offer care in nontraditional settings)
   3. Continue to educate the public; emphasis on periodontal disease as well as caries

DENTAL PERSONNEL

A. Types—dentist, dental assistant, dental hygienist, expanded-function dental auxiliary, dental laboratory technician, denturist, dental therapist

B. Patterns of dental school enrollment
  1. Between 1975 and 1981 the number of applicants to U.S. dental schools has decreased 10% per year
  2. Factors affecting the decline include but are not limited to the financial conditions of the dental care market, the cost of education, and demographic changes
  3. Dental school enrollments will continue to decline, but the total number of practicing dentists will continue to increase because more new graduates will enter the profession than those who will retire or leave dentistry

C. Distribution of dentists
  1. Traditionally measured in a population/dentist ratio
  2. Population/dentist ratio not always accurate because of location, population involved, community need, and demand for dental services
  3. Uneven distribution of dentists exists for various reasons
    a. Dentists have freedom to choose their practice location
    b. Location of dental schools provides an abundant number in some areas, too few in other areas
    c. Popular areas are those with a high demand for services
    d. Rural areas have a lower demand for care
    e. Restrictions in movements from state to state because of licensing requirements

D. Trends in distribution of dentists
  1. Dentists will continue to locate in areas of demand and economic opportunity
  2. Dental profession has recognized a need to develop programs to help in resolving maldistribution problems

E. Supply of auxiliary personnel
  1. Currently 202 accredited dental hygiene programs, 291 for dental assisting, and 56 for dental laboratory technology
  2. Supply and employment of auxiliary personnel fluctuates because of changes in market conditions
  3. Dental hygienists as a profession are seeking alternative avenues to help dentistry meet unmet dental needs

REFERENCES

1. Darby, M.L., and Bowen, D.M.: Research methods for oral health professionals: an introduction, St. Louis, 1980, The C.V. Mosby Co.
2. Ramfjord, S.P.: Indices for prevalence and incidence of periodontal disease, J. Periodontol. **30:**51, 1959.
3. Strifter, D.F., Young, W.O., and Burt, B.A.: Dentistry, dental practice, and the community, Philadelphia, 1983, W.B. Saunders Co.
4. World Health Organization: Oral health surveys—basic methods, Geneva, 1971, World Health Organization.

SUGGESTED READINGS

Carranza, F.A., Jr.: Glickman's clinical periodontology, Philadelphia, 1984, W.B. Saunders Co.
Chilton, N.W., and Miller, M.F.: Paper presented at International Conference on Research in the biology of periodontal disease, June 12-15, 1977, Chicago, Ill.
Committee on Nutrition, American Academy of Pediatrics: Daily dosage levels of supplemental fluoride, Pediatrics **63:** 150, 1979.
Darby, M.L.: Community oral health planning and practice. In Peterson, S., editor: Comprehensive review of dental hygiene, ed. 4, St. Louis, 1980, The C.V. Mosby Co.
Greene, J.C., and Vermillion, J.R.: The simplified oral hygiene index: a method for classifying oral hygiene status. J. Am. Dent. Assoc. **68:**7, 1964.
Gruebbel, A.O.: A measurement of dental caries prevalence and treatment service for deciduous teeth, J. Dent. Res. **23:** 163, 1944.
Jong, A.: Dental public health and community dentistry, St. Louis, 1981, The C.V. Mosby Co.
Klein, H., Palmer, C.E., and Knutson, J.W.: Studies on dental caries. I. Dental status and dental needs of elementary school children, Public Health Rep. **57:**751, 1938.
Kostiw, U., Stephenson, M., and Zarkowski, P.: The dental health consultant in the community, Chicago, 1982, American Dental Hygienists' Association.
Löe, H.: The gingival index, the plaque, and the retention index systems, J. Periodontol. **38:**610, 1967.
Podshadley, A.G., and Haley, J.V.: A method for evaluating oral hygiene performance, Public Health Rep. **83:**259, 1968.
Russell, A.C.: A system of classification and scoring for prevalence surveys of periodontal disease, J. Dent. Res. **35:**250, 1956.
Silness, J., and Löe, H.: Periodontal disease in pregnancy. II. Correlation between oral hygiene and periodontal condition, Acta. Odont. Scand. **22:**112, 1964.

Review Questions

Situation: A dental hygienist conducted an in-service workshop on dental health and related topics for teachers in an elementary school system. Questions 1 and 2 refer to this situation.

1 This *best* describes which kind of a community program?
1. Educational
2. Preventive
3. Treatment
4. Therapeutic
5. Review

2 One important aspect of the in-service workshop is the development of dental health plans. A lesson plan should be
1. Organized and related to a central theme
2. Written in vague terms to allow creativity
3. Logical and meaningful
4. Unnecessary for a dental health unit
5. 1 and 3

3 A 10-year study on the use of a fluoride mouth rinse and subsequent reduction in dental caries in an elementary school population demonstrates which use of epidemiology?
1. Collecting data for normal biologic processes
2. Study of the natural history of diseases
3. Testing hypotheses for prevention and control of disease with population studies
4. Planning and evaluating health care services
5. 1 and 2

4 The type of study used in the 10-year fluoride mouth rinse study can also be described as a (an)
1. Case history study
2. Cross-sectional study
3. Count study
4. Experimental study
5. Retrospective study

Situation: A random sample of cigarettes indicated the following nicotine levels: 13.1, 11.8, 17.6, 17.4, 21.2, and 14.3 milligrams. Questions 5 and 6 refer to this situation.

5 The mean for the sample is
1. 9.4
2. 14.9
3. 15.9
4. 17.9
5. 15.4

6 The median nicotine content in the sample is
1. 15.8
2. 16.3
3. 17.2
4. 9.4
5. 31.7

7 In reviewing a research article, the reader noted that the author presented the following information in the methods and materials section of the paper
(a) Research problems and design are clearly stated
(b) Tests and instruments used are reasonable
(c) Important terms and concepts are defined
(d) Examiners are calibrated
Information omitted but that should appear in this section of the paper is
1. Author's credentials
2. Conclusions
3. Population characteristics and sampling techniques
4. An abstract
5. a, b, and c

8 A type of private third-party prepayment plan that is a nonprofit organization incorporated on a state-by-state basis and sponsored by a constituent dental society is a (an)
1. Health Maintenance Organization (HMO)
2. Department store clinic
3. Health service corporation
4. Dental service corporation
5. Prepaid group practice

9 Health education occurs formally and informally. An example of formal health education is
1. A health education brochure
2. An advertisement for toothpaste
3. An in-service program for nurses' aides
4. Answering a patient's questions about fees
5. A billboard advocating good oral health

10 Ranking students from the individual with the highest grade-point average to the lowest is an example of a (an)
1. Ordinal scale
2. Nominal scale
3. Interval scale
4. Ratio scale
5. Count

11 To reinforce the skills necessary for toothbrushing, it is important to have the learner
1. Describe the technique
2. Read about the technique
3. Watch the dental hygienist brush
4. Use a disclosing agent for evaluation
5. Practice the toothbrushing

12 A random sample suggests that
1. A person in a control group will not be a member of the experimental group
2. Any member of a group to be studied has an equal opportunity to be included in the study
3. Every n^{th} name on a list is selected
4. Subjects are volunteers

13 Use of type A toothpaste and type B toothpaste will show no difference in caries reduction. This statement is an example of a (an)
1. Alternative hypothesis
2. Null hypothesis
3. Rejected hypothesis
4. Type I error
5. Type II error

14 In a nonfluoridated community which preventive dental health program would have the maximum cost benefit for the control of caries in elementary school children?
1. A dental health education program
2. A fluoride mouth rinse program
3. A restorative care program
4. A parent-teacher education program
5. A pit and fissure sealant program

15 The purpose of Title XIX of the Social Security Amendments of 1965 was to
1. Develop an insurance program from trust funds to pay medical bills
2. Provide medical payments for veterans
3. Develop Headstart programs
4. Develop an assistance program for eligible individuals
5. 2 and 3

16 In writing a behavioral objective, it is important to include what the learner is expected to do. Which of the following is the *best* learner performance term?
1. To believe
2. To know
3. To demonstrate
4. To understand
5. To feel

17 Which of the following has been a factor in the declining enrollment in dental schools?
1. Dental schools have increased the number of auxiliary programs
2. There are less qualified dental faculty; therefore class size has decreased
3. Tuition costs and the job market have discouraged applicants
4. Dental disease is decreasing
5. Dental schools make it difficult to get accepted

18 One method to decrease variation in assessing and recording observations when conducting a study is to
1. Use a more sensitive index instead of the simple ones
2. Have examiners evaluate common subjects, compare results, and come to agreement
3. Have examiners take more time in scoring subjects
4. Increase the number of examiners
5. Rotate the number of examiners

19 In statistical analysis, a P-value of 0.001 indicates that the group studied is
1. Significantly different
2. Barely insignificant
3. Very insignificant
4. Very highly insignificant
5. Data are the same—no significance

20 To evaluate the statistical significance of the difference between two means, one uses a _____, whereas to evaluate the expected values versus the observed values of two or more samples of data, one uses a _____ . Which combination makes the statement correct?
1. Chi square test, t-test
2. Chi square test, f test
3. t-test, chi square test
4. t-test, f test
5. Correlation coefficient, chi square test

21 Epidemiologic studies of dental caries suggest that
(a) Males have higher DMF (decayed, missing, filled) scores than females
(b) A relationship exists between dental caries and the level of oral hygiene
(c) Caries experience increases steadily with age
(d) Females have higher DMF scores than males
(e) There is no inherent difference between blacks and whites
1. a, c, and e
2. b, c, d, and e
3. a, b, c, and e
4. c, d, and e
5. b, c, and d

22 In comparing epidemiologic surveys with clinical trials, epidemiologic surveys are characterized by
(a) Small samples
(b) Cross-sectional or longitudinal approaches
(c) The fact that data gathered often is used to establish etiologic factors
(d) The use of dental indices
(e) The use of experimental and control groups
1. a, b, c, and d
2. b, c, d, and e
3. b, c, and d
4. b and d
5. d and e

23 In developing a community profile, the information gathered
(a) Provides an overview of all aspects of the community
(b) Is limited to geographic boundaries, population size, and demographic data
(c) Is useful when working with large or small communities
(d) Is only necessary for large dental health programs
(e) Is a crucial step in the planning process for many reasons
1. a, b, c, and e
2. a, b, d, and e
3. a, c, and e
4. a, b, and c
5. a only

24 The following plaque scores were recorded for a group of senior citizens participating in a plaque control study: 2, 2.5, 3, 3, 3, 2. The mean score for the group was computed and recorded as 2.5. Because the scores are clustered around the mean, statistical analysis would *most* likely indicate a
1. Large standard deviation
2. Large variance
3. Small standard deviation
4. Small range
5. 1 and 2

25 The following National Board Dental Hygiene Examination scores were recorded for six dental hygienists living in the same dormitory: 83, 85, 79, 92, 98, 84. What is the range of scores?
1. 86.8
2. 84.5
3. 19
4. 18
5. 88.5

26 A local restaurant was the focus of a botulism outbreak. The state epidemiologist *most* likely used which format to determine the cause of the disease?
1. Retrospective study
2. Prospective study
3. Cross-sectional
4. Case-control
5. Longitudinal

27 A dental hygienist surveyed a group of nurses concerning their understanding of dental health and oral hygiene procedures using a written questionnaire. Following compilation and evaluation of the answers, the dental hygienist planned the in-service program for the nurses. The activities parallel which of the following private practice activities?
1. History taking and diagnosis
2. Diagnosis and treatment planning
3. History taking, diagnosis, and treatment planning
4. History taking, diagnosis, and treatment
5. History taking, treatment planning, implementation, and evaluation

28 A dental hygienist records the amount of caries detected by the dentist on 100 patients since their last prophylaxis appointments 1 year ago. Of the 100 patients observed, there are 20 new carious lesions requiring treatment. This type of quantification of disease is known as
1. A score
2. A count
3. An assessment
4. Incidence
5. Prevalence

29 In the def index, the *d* indicates
1. All decayed teeth indicated for filling by amalgam
2. All decayed primary teeth
3. All decayed primary anterior teeth indicated for filling
4. All decayed primary canines and molars indicated for filling
5. None of the above

30 The dental index *most* age-specific is
1. OHI-S
2. PI
3. DMF
4. def
5. None of the above

31 The Periodontal Index would be *most* useful in
1. Screening a group of individuals to determine which of them needs periodontal surgery
2. Determining the relative severity of periodontal disease in three adult population groups
3. Determining a treatment plan for one patient in a private practice setting
4. Determining the amount of gingivitis in a group of patients
5. 3 and 4 only

32 The ideal epidemiologic study of periodontal disease or dental caries is one in which
1. All possible factors are recorded in detail
2. Elaborate mechanisms are used to evaluate all aspects of the disease
3. Simple indices and calibrated examiners are used
4. Only 500 to 1000 people are studied
5. All of the above

33 Which of the following is a disadvantage of the DMF index?
1. It is time consuming
2. It is a sum of dissimilar items
3. It is difficult to determine true caries using the criteria provided in the index
4. It measures cumulative experience and is not necessarily indicative of current caries activity
5. It is expensive to apply

34 The PHP index is designed to
1. Evaluate plaque and calculus on specific tooth surfaces
2. Score plaque on specific tooth surfaces
3. Score plaque and gingivitis
4. Score plaque, calculus, and gingivitis
5. 1 and 3 only

35 An individual recognizes a dental need, has a desire to correct it, and an ablity to obtain care. This *best* describes
1. The dental care market
2. Effective demand
3. Potential demand
4. Dental need
5. Potential need

36 Which of the following is *not* considered a host factor for dental caries?
1. Age
2. Bacteria
3. Immunity
4. Race
5. Sex

37 The group of people *most* likely to use dental services would be
1. College-educated, high-income females
2. College-educated, high-income males
3. Nonwhite males and females
4. Older, low-income males
5. Older, low-income females

38 The statistic useful in determining need for dental care in an adult population is
1. D/DMFT
2. DMFT
3. DFMS
4. D/OHI
5. F/DMFT

39 A dental public health program in a metropolitan area *most* likely would
1. Provide care only for the indigent
2. Provide preventive treatment for everyone
3. Provide treatment for the indigent population and preventive treatment for everyone
4. Prevent and improve all people's dental health
5. Provide restorative care for individuals with third-party coverage

40 A state health department plans to conduct a study of 100 factory workers who have died within the last 10 years. All have been employees of the same factory. The evaluation will include the study of health records and death certificates on the 100 employees. This *best* describes a (an)
1. Incidence study
2. Prevalence study
3. Cross-sectional study
4. Longitudinal study
5. Retrospective study

41 A mean PlI score of 2.8 for a population of schoolchildren indicates that the examiners *most* likely found within the study group
1. An abundance of soft deposits
2. A moderate accumulation of soft deposits
3. A slight film of plaque detected by running the probe along tooth surfaces
4. No plaque
5. Difficult to determine

42 Providing evening and weekend hours in a dental office for care is an example of
1. Educating the public about their dental needs
2. Improving patient accessibility
3. Decreasing patient accessibility
4. Identifying those currently not seeking care
5. 1 and 4

43 Criteria used to evaluate an author of a scientific article include
1. Number of pages of articles published previously
2. Quantity of degrees and titles listed after the name
3. Current or past position of the author to support expertise in a particular area
4. Evidence of facilities to support research
5. 1, 2, 3, and 4

44 The variable controlled or manipulated in a study is a (an)
1. Population parameter
2. Dependent variable
3. Independent variable
4. Variable
5. Discrete number

45 Another name for population characteristic is a (an)
1. Dependent variable
2. Parameter
3. Datum
4. Variable
5. Independent variable

46 An important advantage in using a large sample is that it
1. Makes record keeping complicated
2. Increases precision and accuracy of data
3. Costs less
4. More likely represents the defined population
5. 2 and 4

47 Two thirds of all dental hygienists interviewed smoked some brand of cigarettes. The statement could be classified as a
1. Statistic
2. Descriptive statistic
3. Inferential statistic
4. Range
5. Median

48 The number of children born annually in the United States with cleft lip or palate is
1. Less than 500
2. 1000
3. 4000
4. 6000
5. 9000

49 Donations in dollars were received for a dental health clinic and were recorded as follows: 2, 3, 4, 5, 6, 6, 6, 7, 7, 8. the mode for the contributions is
1. 12
2. 6
3. 6 and 7
4. 54
5. Cannot be determined

50 The *least* expensive type of examination to quickly ascertain dental needs is a
1. Type 1 complete examination
2. Type 2 limited examination
3. Type 3 inspection
4. Type 4 screening
5. Combination of types 3 and 4

51 A medically compromised patient requiring special resources would receive the *best* dental care in a
1. Community clinic
2. Solo practice
3. Health Maintenance Organization (HMO)
4. Dental department in a hospital
5. Group practice

52 Community health centers are characterized by
1. Solo practitioners in the facility
2. Usually being located in an area with a high dentist-to-population ratio
3. Providing primary medical and dental care
4. 1, 2, and 3
5. 2 and 3

53 A type of prepayment practice plan in which patients can receive services only at specific facilities from a limited number of dentists *best* describes a (an)
1. Closed panel
2. Open panel
3. Public health clinic
4. Solo practice with referrals
5. Group practice

54 One of the advantages of a prepayment dental plan is
1. The patient pays directly out-of-pocket immediately following the service
2. The interest on the amount not paid is minimal
3. Groups of people can spread the financial burden
4. It is a traditional and acceptable method of payment
5. Dentists charge lower fees

Answers and Rationales

1. (1) The program increases the knowledge of the teachers.
   (2) A preventive program would use a known preventive agent or procedure
   (3) Treatment programs provide dental services (e.g., restorative care).
   (4) A therapeutic program is concerned with the treatment and cure of diseases.
   (5) Given the population group, a review program does not apply.

2. (5) The lesson plan should be organized, logical, and written in an organized manner.
   (1) A lesson plan should also be logical and meaningful.
   (2) A vague lesson plan is not a useful teaching tool.
   (3) A lesson plan should also be organized and relate to a central theme.
   (4) To allow a dental health unit to run smoothly, lesson plans are useful.

3. (3) The study demonstrates evaluating the effects of a particular preventive caries agent using a field trial or population study.
   (1) Such a study includes collecting data to describe biologic processes such as growth patterns.
   (2) Study of the natural history of diseases includes observations about the progress and effects of particular diseases.
   (4) Planning and evaluating health care include evaluating the availability, utilization, and productivity of health care services, while this study demonstrates prevention and control of disease using a population study.
   (5) This answer is not appropriate.

4. (4) An experimental study alters or manipulates a particular variable and observes results.
   (1) A case history study evaluates from effect to cause.
   (2) A cross-sectional study evaluates a segment of the population at one particular time.
   (3) A count study counts or assesses a particular aspect.
   (5) A retrospective study uses data already collected.

5. (3) $\dfrac{13.1 + 11.8 + 17.6 + 17.4 + 21.2 + 14.3}{6} = 15.9$
   (1) 9.4 is too low.
   (2) 14.9 is too low.
   (4) 17.9 is too high.
   (5) 15.4 is not exactly correct.

6. (1) To determine a median, arrange the values in order of magnitude and then find the arithmetic mean of the two middle values—15.8.
   (2) 16.3 is too high.
   (3) 17.2 is too high.
   (4) 9.4 is the range.
   (5) 31.7 is the sum of the two middle values.

7. (3) Materials and methods includes sampling techniques and steps taken to eliminate biases.
   (1) The author's credentials appear after the title or at the end of the paper.
   (2) The conclusion is in another section of the paper.
   (4) The abstract and introduction come before the methods and materials section.
   (5) This information (a, b, c) was included.

8. (4) A dental service corporation is a legally constituted nonprofit organization, incorporated on a state-by-state basis.
   (1) An HMO is capitation based and must meet certain statutory requirements.
   (2) Department store clinics were developed to make a profit and allow accessibility to consumers.
   (3) A health service corporation offers limited dental coverage.
   (5) *Prepaid* implies that payment is made before service.

9. (3) An in-service program requires assessing, planning, implementing, and evaluating in an organized manner.
   (1) Brochures represent a passive kind of learning.
   (2) An advertisement for toothpaste would emphasize a particular product, with health education given a minor emphasis.
   (4) Answering questions is an example of an informal interaction.
   (5) Use of a billboard is not a controlled situation, but more a visual stimulus.

10. (1) Ranking of characteristics in some empirical order is an ordinal scale.
    (2) Observations fitted into classes or categories would be a nominal scale.
    (3) An interval scale is used to measure a variable characterized by equal intervals.
    (4) A ratio scale is used to measure a variable characterized by the presence of an absolute zero.
    (5) The count is the sum of certain characteristics or variables.

11. (5) Individuals learn by doing.
    (1) Verbal description does not mean the skill is learned.
    (2) Reading may provide knowledge but not skill.
    (3) The patient is not reinforcing the skill.
    (4) A disclosing agent is useful for evaluating, but is not part of learning the actual skill.

12. (2) A random sample is composed of subjects who are chosen independently with an equal opportunity for inclusion.
    (1) Research design suggests a person will not be a member of the control and experimental group.
    (3) Systematic sampling occurs by selecting every n^{th} subject from a list or file of the total population.
    (4) This is a method of acquiring participants, not a random sample.

For each question the correct answer and rationale are listed first. The other choices are presented in order with the reasons why they are not correct.

13. (2) Stated negatively, there is no difference.
    (1) The alternative hypothesis states that there is a difference.
    (3) This is not a rejected hypothesis.
    (4) In a type I error the null hypothesis is true and not accepted.
    (5) In a type II error the null hypothesis is not true and is accepted.
14. (2) The cost of a fluoride mouth rinse program is low; there is approximately a 35% reduction in caries; such a program can use nondental personnel.
    (1) An increase in health education does not result in caries reduction.
    (3) Restorative care is expensive.
    (4) Education of parents and teachers is not related to a preventive program for children.
    (5) A pit and fissure sealant program requires professional application, and this increases cost.
15. (4) Medicaid is an assistance program where money from federal, state, and local taxes pays medical bills for individuals who meet certain requirements.
    (1) Medicare, Title XVIII, is an insurance program available to individuals 65 and older.
    (2) This is a separate program.
    (3) This is part of a different program.
    (5) This is an inappropriate combination.
16. (3) To demonstrate, which implies the learner must perform an activity.
    (1) This does not make clear what the learner must do.
    (2) This indicates knowledge.
    (4) This indicates comprehension.
    (5) This indicates a value.
17. (3) Tuition costs and the dental care market have discouraged applicants.
    (1) Dental schools have not increased numbers; some programs have been discontinued.
    (2) Qualified faculty exist; some schools are consolidating faculty or implementing hiring freezes.
    (4) Dental caries rates are decreasing, but periodontal disease is increasing.
    (5) Dental schools are fair in their application requirements.
18. (2) Calibrating examiners by examination of a few subjects and comparison of results reduce variation in assessing and recording.
    (1) Simple criteria will be sensitive.
    (3) Increased time will not necessarily decrease variation. The objective is to use a quick-scoring instrument.
    (4) Increasing the number of examiners will increase variation.
    (5) Rotating examiners will increase chances of less agreement.

19. (1) Probability of less than 0.05 indicates two sets of data are significantly different.
    (2) Probability of greater than 0.05 indicates data are not significantly different.
    (3) Very insignificant probability would require a greater score than 0.05.
    (4) Very highly insignificant probability would require a much greater score than 0.05.
    (5) The value of P indicates the significance level.
20. (3) The t-test determines the significance of the statistical difference between two means; the chi square test determines if there is a statistical difference between expected values and observed values.
    (1) These are in incorrect order.
    (2) The f test is used to compare variances of two samples of data.
    (4) Both these tests are used for normally distributed, randomly selected, measured data.
    (5) The correlation coefficient determines the strength of the linear relationship between two variables.
21. (4) Caries rates increase with age; females have higher scores; and studies indicate, with all other factors equal, that there is no difference between blacks and whites.
    (1) Females have higher DMF scores than males.
    (2) A relationship exists between oral hygiene and periodontal disease.
    (3) This is an inappropriate combination.
    (5) This is an inappropriate combination.
22. (3) Surveys are cross-sectional; data generated establish underlying etiologic factors, and derive possible preventive methods. Indices are used so that data can be compared with different populations.
    (1) A small sample is used in a clinical trial; a large sample is used in an epidemiologic survey.
    (2) Experimental and control groups are used in a clinical trial; an epidemiologic survey uses naturally occurring samples.
    (4) This excludes using data for determining etiologic factors.
    (5) This is not an appropriate combination.
23. (3) The overview includes leadership, finance, funding, geographic boundaries, demographics, and other related material. The overview is an important process in planning programs for all types of communities.
    (1) An overview is not limited to boundaries, size, etc.
    (2) An overview is important for small groups as well as large communities.
    (4) Limiting information may influence the success of the program.
    (5) Providing an overview is not the only reason for developing a community profile.

24. (3) A small standard deviation indicates the distribution of scores is clustered around the mean.
    (1) The greater the dispersion of scores from the mean, the greater the standard deviation.
    (2) The greater the dispersion of scores from the mean, the greater the variance.
    (4) Range would not require statistical analysis.
    (5) This is incorrect.
25. (3) 98 − 79 = 19, the range of scores.
    (1) The mean score is 86.8
    (2) Mode is 84.5
    (4) 18 is a miscalculation of range.
    (5) The average of the highest and lowest scores is 88.5
26. (4) Looking backward from effect to cause is a case-control format.
    (1) Using observations collected previously is a restrospective study.
    (2) Population studied through time is a prospective study.
    (3) A sample evaluated at one time is a cross-sectional format.
    (5) A sample studied on two or more occasions over a period of time is a longitudinal format.
27. (3) History taking parallels surveying; diagnosis parallels analyzing survey data; treatment planning parallels program planning.
    (1) This does not include treatment planning.
    (2) History taking is not included.
    (4) Treatment is not parallel in the situation given.
    (5) Treatment initiation and evaluation are not included in the situation given.
28. (4) *Incidence* refers to the number of new cases of a disease within a given time period.
    (1) A score is not an evaluation comparing two things.
    (2) A count is only a sum of disease.
    (3) Assessment is a general term for initial evaluation.
    (5) Prevalence refers to the number of persons in a population affected by a condition at one time.
29. (2) "*d*" indicates decayed.
    (1) *d* does not indicate that an amalgam filling is required.
    (3) *d* does not signify anterior teeth only.
    (4) *d* does not indicate canines and molars only.
    (5) This is incorrect, since the correct answer is 2.
30. (4) The def is only used with groups who have primary dentitions.
    (1) The OHI-S scores debris and calculus and can be used with all age groups.
    (2) This index can be used with adolescent to older adult groups.
    (3) This index can be used with all groups who have permanent dentitions.
    (5) The correct answer is 4.

31. (2) This index is useful for screening large groups and determining the prevalence of periodontal disease.
    (1) The index is based on signs of periodontitis from gingivitis to severe disease. It is not detailed enough to determine the need for surgery.
    (3) The index is not useful for one patient. Other assessment tools can be used.
    (4) The index is not specific for gingivitis.
    (5) The correct answer is 2.
32. (3) An index is useful for studying large numbers of people to acquire information on trends and occurrence of disease. Calibration of examiners using the index increases the reliability of the study.
    (1) An epidemiologic study does not allow all details to be recorded.
    (2) Elaborate mechanisms are costly and time consuming.
    (4) Sample sizes vary according to the purpose of research; larger sample sizes are ideal.
    (5) The correct answer is 3.
33. (4) The DMF measures lifetime caries experience only.
    (1) The index has three criteria that can be used in little time.
    (2) All criteria are related to experience with dental disease.
    (3) Each tooth is rated for decay.
    (5) The DMF index is not expensive to apply.
34. (2) The PHP evaluates plaque on six teeth using a disclosing agent, light, air, and mouth mirror.
    (1) The OHI index scores plaque and debris on specific teeth.
    (3) This is not the objective of the index.
    (4) These assessments are made with other indices.
    (5) This is not indicative of the PHP.
35. (2) Effective demand is a desire for care and the ability to obtain care.
    (1) *Dental care market* is a general term for the need for and demand for dental services.
    (3) Potential demand is a desire for care and the inability to obtain care.
    (4) Dental need is the professional judgment as to the amount of service required.
    (5) Potential need is another term for possible dental needs.
36. (2) Bacteria is an agent factor rather than a host factor.
    (1) Caries experience increases with age.
    (3) Immunity to disease means that a natural resistance may exist.
    (4) There is no inherent difference between blacks and whites.
    (5) Gender is a host factor.
37. (1) Higher education and income levels are positively related to higher dental care utilization rates. Females have more dental visits than males.
    (2) Females seek dental care more frequently than males.
    (3) Nonwhites have a lower number of dental visits.
    (4) Older citizens have lower dental care utilization rates.
    (5) Lower income groups have lower dental care utilization rates.

38. (1) D/DMFT provides the percentage of dental decay in relation to total DMFT score.
    (2) DMFT provides cumulative dental experience.
    (3) DFMS is the cumulative dental experience using a finer measurement.
    (4) D/OHI cannot be computed: they are two different indexes.
    (5) F/DMFT provides the percentage of treatment in relation to the DMFT score.

39. (4) A dental public health program prevents and controls dental disease and promotes dental health through organized community efforts for all people.
    (1) Dental public health programs are concerned about all citizens' health.
    (2) The program would provide preventive and other dental services.
    (3) Dental public health activities are not limited to certain services for particular population groups.
    (5) Programs vary in the kinds of patients that receive services. Payment methods vary from fee-for-service to insurance reimbursement.

40. (5) A retrospective study uses observations or data that have been collected in the past. Data may be incomplete or inappropriate.
    (1) An incidence study describes the number of new cases of a disease within a given time period.
    (2) The number of persons in a population affected by a condition at any one time describes a prevalence study.
    (3) A cross section of a population evaluated is called a cross-sectional study.
    (4) The same sample of people studied on two or more occasions describes a longitudinal study.

41. (1) An abundance of soft deposits receives a score of 3. The high mean score indicates the study group displayed an abundance of soft deposits.
    (2) A moderate accumulation of soft deposits receives a score of 2.
    (3) A slight film of plaque detected by a probe receives a score of 1.
    (4) No plaque receives a score of 0.
    (5) Examiners were able to determine this because of the high mean score.

42. (2) Nontraditional hours provide increased opportunities for treatment.
    (1) Public education requires a major effort on the part of professional and consumer groups.
    (3) Improved availability will not decrease accessibility.
    (4) Survey methods are necessary to identify those not seeking care.
    (5) This is an inappropriate selection.

43. (3) The author's credentials and location should support his or her expertise and ability to successfully complete research.
    (1) The length of the article is not a reflection of the author's skills.
    (2) The number of degrees does not always reflect the quality of skill.
    (4) Evidence of facilities to support research does not always reflect the quality of skill.
    (5) This is not an appropriate combination.

44. (3) An independent variable is controlled or manipulated.
    (1) Characteristics of a population are a population parameter.
    (2) An uncontrolled characteristic is a dependent variable.
    (4) A value that can vary from subject to subject is a variable.
    (5) A number that cannot be subdivided meaningfully is a discrete number.

45. (2) A parameter is a characteristic of a population.
    (1) A dependent variable is an uncontrolled characteristic in a study.
    (3) A datum is qualitative and quantitative information gathered.
    (4) A variable is a characteristic whose value can vary from subject to subject.
    (5) An independent variable is a controlled or manipulated characteristic study.

46. (4) A larger sample more likely will represent the defined population and increase the accuracy of the data collected.
    (1) Complicated record keeping may be a disadvantage because of the personnel and storage involved.
    (2) A large sample does not always indicate more precision or accurate data.
    (3) Depending on the type of study, larger samples mean increased cost.
    (5) This is not an appropriate combination.

47. (2) A descriptive statistic summarizes data collected and no attempt is made to generalize research findings beyond the immediate sample.
    (1) *Statistic* is a general term for the science that describes, summarizes, analyzes, and interprets numerical data to make an inference about a population.
    (3) Research findings that generalize from a sample to the general population of interest are inferential statistics.
    (4) Range is obtained by subtracting the lowest score from the highest scores.
    (5) This cannot be inferred from the statement given.

48. (4) There are 6000 cases of cleft lip or palate reported annually in the United States.
    (1) Less than 500 is an incorrect number of reported cases.
    (2) One thousand is an incorrect number of reported cases.
    (3) Four thousand is an incorrect number of reported cases.
    (5) Nine thousand is an incorrect number of reported cases.

49. (2) 6 is the donation that occurs with most frequency and is the mode.
    (1) 12 is the sum of the two middle values.
    (3) 6 occurs more frequently than 7.
    (4) 54 is the sum of all donations.
    (5) This is not true; the mode can be determined.
50. (4) Type 4, screening with a tongue depressor and available illumination, is the least expensive.
    (1) Type I uses a mouth mirror, explorer, radiographs, and other assessment tests.
    (2) Type 2 uses a mouth mirror, explorer, and posterior bitewings.
    (3) Type 3 uses a mouth mirror and explorer.
    (5) Types 3 and 4 are similar types of screening.
51. (4) An individual would have medical personnel and expertise available in a dental department in a hospital.
    (1) A community clinic may not be able to cope with a medically compromised patient.
    (2) An individual practitioner may not be able to provide all the treatment services necessary.
    (3) An HMO emphasizes ambulatory care to minimize hospitalization.
    (5) A dental group practice does not always have resources available for medically compromised patients.

52. (3) Community health centers provide medical and dental care and easy access for community members.
    (1) Community health centers are similar to a well-developed group practice, rather than a solo practice.
    (2) Community health centers are located in areas where dental and medical practitioners are not found in adequate numbers.
    (4) This is an incorrect grouping.
    (5) This is an incorrect grouping.
53. (1) In a closed-panel plan, patients are limited to particular facilities and practitioners.
    (2) Any licensed dentist can participate and the patient has a choice of all licensed dentists in an open-panel plan.
    (3) A public health clinic provides services for all individuals and is not a prepayment plan.
    (4) Solo practice involves one practitioner.
    (5) Dentists provide dental services and accept prepayment and postpayment in a group practice.
54. (3) A prepayment plan applies to groups, such as unions, and allows the spread of the financial burden.
    (1) *Fee-for-service* indicates the patient pays immediately following service.
    (2) Interest must be paid on loans taken from banks for budget payment plans.
    (4) Fee-for-service is a culturally acceptable and traditional method.
    (5) Dentists should charge the same fees to both insured and noninsured patients.

CHAPTER 16

Concepts and Practice of Four-handed, Six-handed, and TEAM Dentistry

HAZEL O. TORRES

Flexibility of roles and the stimulus of performing multiple services are possible within the various modalities of current dental practices. The dental hygienist who obtains proficiency in functioning in the practice of four-handed, six-handed, and TEAM (training in expanded auxiliary management) dentistry finds the role of the dental hygienist more diversified, stimulating, and rewarding. The challenge of participating with the other members of the dental team provides a stimulus and creates an atmosphere wherein dental procedures may be performed with less fatigue for the individuals. This chapter prepares the dental hygienist by providing the knowledge base necessary to work successfully in various modes of dental care delivery. Topics include principles of four-handed, six-handed, and TEAM dentistry, instrument grasp and oral evacuation techniques, and basic functions performed in TEAM dentistry.

HISTORICAL BACKGROUND

A. Since 1948 the concept and practice of four-handed dentistry has been researched by the Department of Health and Human Services, Division of Dentistry, Public Health Service, Human Resources Administration, Bethesda, Md., and by other dental researchers
B. Training of dental personnel in the concepts and practice of four-handed dentistry was introduced into curricula and clinical experiences in dental schools throughout the United States; full implementation of training of students in this area occurred in 60 dental schools from 1960 into the early 1970s; instruction in the full utilization of the chairside assistant (four-handed dentistry) was incorporated into what was titled the Dental Auxiliary Utilization (DAU) Program; since that time the DAU concept has become widely accepted also in the private-practice sector of dentistry; implementation of training in DAU,

including utilization of all auxiliaries, was made possible through federal grants to the dental schools
C. TEAM dentistry concept (an acronym for *training in expanded auxiliary management*), in which the services of the dental hygienist, chairside assistant, and dental laboratory technician are fully used, was initiated in dental schools in the 1970s; four-handed, six-handed, and/or TEAM dentistry models of practice have been adopted and emulated by dental graduates as they have established their own dental practices

BASIC CONCEPTS

A. Concept of four-handed (as well as six-handed) dentistry includes several characteristics
   1. Availability of modern dental equipment (i.e., dental chair, stools, lighting, and mobile cabinets
   2. Multiple treatment areas
   3. Positioning of the dental chair to accommodate the patient, operator, and chairside assistant
   4. Establishing and maintaining patient rapport with effective communication
   5. Utilization of the dental assistant at the chairside by
      a. Standardizing basic instrument trays for all dental procedures
      b. Adopting a system of passing and receiving dental instruments and materials
      c. Preparing and delivering dental materials
      d. Rinsing and evacuating fluids from the oral cavity
   6. Systematized appointment control

B. In four-handed dentistry the dental team is made up of an operator (dentist) and a chairside assistant; operator could also be the dental hygienist and/or the expanded-function dental auxiliary (dental hygienist or assistant with additional training in particular procedures); chairside assistant would assist the operator in the traditional role

PRINCIPLES AND DEFINITIONS

A. Four-handed dentistry—principles and practice of four-handed dentistry include the full use of the services of a trained chairside assistant; operator and assistant assume a seated position near the head of the patient, with the assistant's hands readily accessible to assist the operator during the delivery of dental procedures
B. Six-handed dentistry—six-handed dental delivery system entails the full utilization of a second individual, a coordinating assistant, who is capable of chairside assisting and/or providing supportive assistance to the operator and chairside assistant; six-handed model of dental delivery lends itself to provide assistance for the performance of more complicated dental procedures in an efficient and effective manner
C. TEAM dentistry—TEAM (training in expanded auxiliary management) relates to the full use of services of all individual members of the dental team; operator coordinates activities with TEAM members: dental hygienist, chairside assistant, and dental laboratory technician
   1. With each auxiliary trained to a specific competence level, performance of nontraditional services may be delegated to each one
   2. Dental operator (dentist) coordinates dental treatment procedures and delegates the performance of specific services to the member of the team educationally qualified with clinical skills to perform the function; limiting factor is compliance with the dental practice act of a particular state
   3. Services that may be delegated vary with the state dental practice act; might include
     a. Dental radiographic surveys
     b. Construction of custom trays
     c. Oral clinical examinations
     d. Obtaining of preliminary and final impressions
     e. Fabricating and seating of temporary coverages
     f. Root planing, deep scaling, and gingival curettage

ESSENTIALS FOR THE PRACTICE OF FOUR-HANDED DENTISTRY
Organization of Dental Procedures

To achieve full implementation of four-handed dentistry, the operator determines the sequence in which the dental procedures are performed and the essentials needed to provide the specific dental treatment
A. Sequence of a given procedure
   1. Preliminary examination and preparation of diagnostic aids; aids may include radiographs, study casts, and laboratory reports on tests requested by the dentist
   2. Examination of patient records of prior and scheduled treatment
   3. Updating of the medical and dental history of the patient
B. Preset trays for dental procedures
   1. Instrumentation—includes the basic instrument setup (i.e., two mouth mirrors, explorer, cotton (college) pliers, cotton rolls and pellets, high-velocity evacuator, handpieces, burs, and stones, along with additional instrumentation that relates to specific procedures
   2. Examples
     a. Amalgam restoration—matrices and retainer, wedge, amalgam carrier, condensers, and carvers
     b. Composite restoration—etching solution, composite, base and catalyst, separator, plastic instrument, finishing disks and stones, and lubricant
     c. Prophylaxis—right-angle handpiece, disclosing material, rubber cup, mounted polishing brush, polishing abrasive, floss, tape, and oral cavity rinse
     d. Preliminary impression—perforated or rim-lock impression tray, alginate material, water graduate and measure for alginate, 4-inch rubber bowl (flexible), and broad-tip rigid spatula

Use of Time and Motion in Performing Dental Procedures

A. Time and motion
   1. Dentistry has borrowed the concept of "time and motion" from industry to increase the efficiency of dental practice
   2. For several years dental researchers studied the applicability of time and motion and analyses of the motions needed to perform dentistry effectively

3. Application of time-and-motion principles coincided with the implementation of four-handed dentistry; essential motions performed by the dental operator and the chairside assistant were recorded; formal classifications of hand, arm, and body movements were determined

B. Classifications of motions (movements of hand, arm, and body)[1]

1. Essential motions in four-handed dentistry (from a seated position)
   a. Class I motions—involving fingers-only movements
   b. Class II motions—involving movements of the fingers and wrist
   c. Class III motions—involving movements of the fingers, wrist, and elbow
   d. Class IV motions—involving movements of the entire arm from the shoulder
   e. Class V motions—involving movements of the arm and twisting of the body

2. Examples of classification of motions (one goal of four-handed dentistry is to have the dental team use class I to III motions to avoid fatigue as much as possible)
   a. Class I motion—dental hygienist maintains a fulcrum when scaling the patient's teeth during a prophylaxis
   b. Class II motion—dental hygienist maintains a fulcrum and rotates the wrist slightly to reach the lingual or facial surface of the root during the scaling procedure
   c. Class III motion—dental hygienst performs the clinical examination of the lymph nodes and the temporomandibular joint on each side of the patient's head

d. Class IV motion—dental hygienist or assistant dispenses, mixes, and loads alginate in the impression tray and places the impression tray in the patient's oral cavity; in this instance both arms are used simultaneously; fingers are used to flex the cheeks away from the tray during insertion into the oral cavity

e. Class V motion—dental hygienist uses the extended hand and arm motion to adjust the ultrasonic scaler or the compressed air for the right-angle handpiece; another example is the assistant turning from the patient (swiveling the stool and twisting the body at the waist) to spot weld a custom matrix on the electric welder placed on the cabinet near the dental chair, or to turn on the amalgamator for triturating amalgam

Position of the Dental Team

A. Seated position
1. Four-handed dentistry uses the seated position of the dental team (operator and chairside assistant)
2. Dynamics of dental procedures are performed around the focal area, the oral cavity of the patient
3. Team remains in a seated position throughout the performance of a given procedure

B. Clock configuration (Fig. 16-1)
1. Oral cavity of the patient becomes the center of an imaginary clock used to describe the focus of activity as dentistry is performed
2. Clock configuration is imaginary; however, if a clock were laid over the patient, the center would be the patient's oral cavity and the 12 o'clock position would be at the patient's forehead

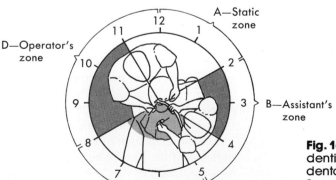

A—Static zone
D—Operator's zone
B—Assistant's zone
C—Transfer zone

Fig. 16-1 Clock configuration zones for four-handed dentistry. (From Torres, H.O., and Ehrlich, A.: Modern dental assisting, ed. 3, Philadelphia, 1985, W.B. Saunders Co.)

3. With the center of the clock as the focal point, the clock is divided into four sections, or *operating zones,* defined as the dynamic areas used by the operator and assistant to accomplish the performance of dental procedures; these basic four-handed dentistry positions would be reversed if the operator were left handed; in that instance the assistant would be on the right side of the patient, with the operator on the left side of the chair
   a. Static zone (11 o'clock to 2 o'clock area)—area for the placement of mobile equipment or a mobile cart to hold the preset instrument tray; static zone is at the knees of the seated chairside assistant and at the left side of the operator
   b. Assistant's zone (2 o'clock to 4 o'clock area)—area at the left side of the patient between the 2 o'clock to 4 o'clock area; assistant and dental procedure will dictate exactly where within the 2 o'clock to 4 o'clock area the assistant will be seated
   c. Transfer zone (4 o'clock to 8 o'clock area)—space over the lap of the patient, between the assistant's left arm and the operator's right arm; this area may be used for positioning heavy tubing or the handpiece attachment, and for passing the tubing or large instruments such as dental forceps and loaded impression trays
   d. Operator's zone (8 o'clock to 11 o'clock area)—area reserved for the operator for the performance of all dental procedures; usually the operator (dental hygienist or dentist) will be seated from the 9 o'clock to 11 o'clock position to deliver treatment; 8 o'clock position may be used for sharing information with or making inquiries of the patient before or after treatment
C. Positions of individual dental team members
   1. Operator's position (9 o'clock to 12 o'clock)
      a. Exact position of the operator will vary during performance of the various dental procedures; access to a particular tooth or area of the quadrant within the oral cavity may dictate a slight modification of the positions for specific treatment
      b. Positioning of the dental chair and the patient must be accomplished *before* final positioning of the operator
         (1) Dental chair is lowered and positioned with the back upright for safe admission of the patient

(2) Chair back is reclined until the patient's head is slightly lower than the feet or parallel with the knees
         (3) Patient's head is positioned up to the top of the chair (headrest); patient's arms are supported at the side by the arms of the dental chair
      c. Operator moves into position with his or her legs under the head of the dental chair; objective is to place the head of the patient on the dental chair in the lap of the operator
      d. Operator functions from the 9 o'clock to 12 o'clock position for access to the mandibular area, anterior of the oral cavity, and facial surfaces of the maxillary teeth (Fig. 16-2)
      e. Operator functions from the 11 o'clock or 12 o'clock position for preparation or treatment of the teeth of the maxillary arch, the palatal area, or the posterior or anterior (lingual surfaces) of the dentition; indirect vision principle (use of a mouth mirror to view the work area) is applied for visibility of the maxillary lingual or occlusal area; 12 o'clock position is obtained frequently to polish the lingual surfaces of the maxillary teeth during an oral prophylaxis
   2. Chairside assistant's position (2 o'clock or 3 o'clock)
      a. Chairside assistant's position at 2 o'clock or 3 o'clock remains more static; operator moves from the 9 o'clock position to the 12 o'clock position to obtain visibility and to accommodate the procedure
      b. Assistant determines exactly which position is best for assisting with most procedures; a move to a second position will be the exception
      c. Assistant is seated with the feet supported on the platform part of the stool; assistant's stool is adjustable to provide
         (1) Support to the middle back
         (2) Flat platform to support the feet
         (3) Seat parallel to the floor
         (4) Adjustable ring to support the assistant at the waist
         (5) Optional—a rod support on the assistant's stool (this is not advised, since the circulation of the feet may be affected if the feet are hung over the rod for any length of time)

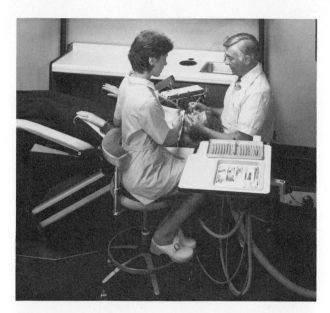

Fig. 16-2 Four-handed dentistry (side delivery), operator at 12 o'clock position. (Courtesy A-dec, Inc. © Copyright 1982.)

d. Position of the assistant 4 inches above the height of the operator
   (1) Provides access to the oral cavity without blocking the operator's view
   (2) Provides visibility of the field of operation
   (3) Enables the beam of the operating light to shine on the patient's oral cavity without creating a shadow
   (4) Allows space to place the high-velocity evacuator, and mouth mirror or index finger to retract tissues
   (5) Enables the thighs to be parallel with the left side of the chair and the patient's upper arms
   (6) Enables the knees of the assistant to be parallel with the patient's shoulders or neck
   (7) Provides space for the mobile cart to cover the assistant's knees, with the instrument tray at the assistant's lap
3. Position of the instrument tray
   a. Position of the mobile cart and instrument tray for four-handed dentistry is usually at the 1 o'clock to 2 o'clock position
   b. If the operator is at the left side of the dental chair, the assistant's position, mobile cart, and instrument tray are at the 11 o'clock to 12 o'clock position

c. If the operator is at the 12 o'clock position, the mobile cart and instrument tray are moved to the 2 o'clock position
d. Mobile cart and instrument tray are placed over the knees of the assistant
e. Small amounts of material may be placed on the instrument tray or placed on a secondary tray to be moved into place as the preparation or preliminary treatment of a tooth is completed; examples of materials and trays include
   (1) Trays and material for topical application of fluorides
   (2) Local anesthesia instrumentation
   (3) Instrumentation for placement of a temporary coverage
f. Dental materials in large containers (e.g., alginate impression material, accessories, and impression trays) may be placed on the cabinet adjacent to the chairside assistant; these materials are placed chairside on the mobile cart when needed
g. Amalgamator or pulp vitalometer is placed on the cabinet adjacent to the chairside assistant and near an electrical outlet; these heavier pieces of equipment are placed in this manner for safety and for accessibility when needed

Instrument Delivery

A. Front delivery—over-the-patient delivery system provides accessibility to accomplish dental procedures by placing the instrument tray, handpieces, and power controls over the chest or lap of the patient (Fig. 16-3)
   1. Front delivery is not totally conducive to the four-handed dentistry concept, since the operator reaches for and returns the handpieces, air-water syringe, and instruments that may be placed in the midpatient position
   2. In this practice the function of the dental assistant is limited; in addition, there is the possibility of instruments and materials dropping on the patient's lap or chest
B. Rear delivery—accomplishes performance of dental procedures by placing a mobile dental unit or instrument cart directly in back of the patient's head and at a right angle to the dental chair; instrument tray and supplemental materials are placed on top of the dental unit or mobile cart (Fig. 16-4)

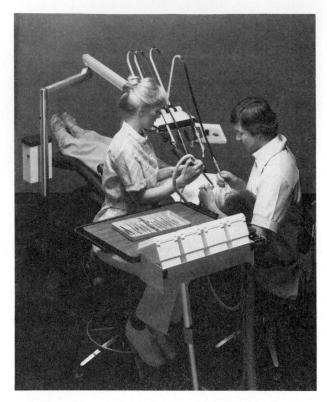

Fig. 16-3 Four-handed dentistry (front delivery), operator at 11 o'clock position. (Courtesy A-dec, Inc. © Copyright 1982.)

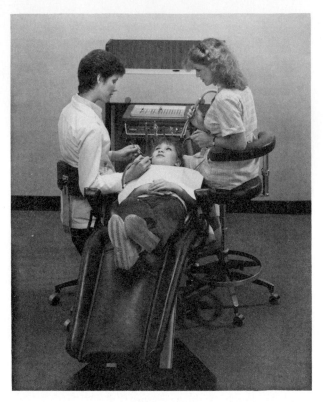

Fig. 16-4 Four-handed dentistry (rear delivery), operator at 9 o'clock position. (Courtesy A-dec, Inc. © Copyright 1982.)

1. Mobile dental unit contains high- and low-speed handpiece capability, the compressed air-water-spray syringe, and the high-velocity evacuator
2. Unless an additional mobile cart is placed alongside of the chairside assistant, space may be limited for the instrument tray; also there is limited flat surface space for mixing dental materials unless a second mobile cart is used

ESSENTIALS FOR THE PRACTICE OF SIX-HANDED DENTISTRY

Organization of Dental Procedures

Same as in four-handed dentistry

Use of Time and Motion in Performing Dental Procedures

Same as in four-handed dentistry

Position of the Dental Team

Same as in four-handed dentistry

Instrument Delivery

Same as in four-handed dentistry

Role of the Individual Team Member

A. Operator
  1. Operator performs the dental procedure or delegates the performance of the particular function to the chairside assistant or coordinating assistant; operator is the dentist or dental hygienist, with the chairside assistant and coordinating assistant providing support services
  2. Examples of functions performed in six-handed dentistry
     a. Preparation and placement of impression material
     b. Preparation and placement of cavity preparation liners and bases
     c. Preparation, placement, and finishing of restorative materials
     d. Administration of nitrous oxide and oxygen (N_2O and O_2) as analgesia before deep scaling and curettage

B. Chairside assistant
1. Chairside assistant functions in the traditional role, providing the second pair of hands in supporting the function of the operator
2. Assistant retracts tissues, directs the high-velocity evacuator, and passes and receives instruments and materials
C. Coordinating assistant
1. Coordinating assistant functions as a support to aid the operator and chairside assistant in their performance of dental procedures
2. Tasks that may be performed by the coordinating assistant
   a. Dispensing and preparing additional dental materials as needed (e.g., triturating amalgam during multiple restorations)
   b. Mixing the elastomer, polysulfide, polyether, and silicone rubber base tray impression material and loading the material into the tray; chairside assistant prepares the syringe mix and passes the loaded syringe to the operator, who places it in the tooth preparation
   c. Exposing and processing dental radiographic surveys as prescribed by the dentist

Examples of Six-handed Dentistry in the Performance of Dental Procedures

A. To prepare multiple amalgam preparations for restoring teeth in a quadrant, the coordinating assistant prepares supplemental mixes of amalgam that are triturated as needed, and loads the carriers with amalgam and passes them to the chairside assistant; chairside assistant receives the loaded amalgam carrier, places the amalgam in the prepared tooth, and passes and receives condensors and carvers to and from the operator, who condenses and carves the amalgam
B. During the extraction of a mandibular impacted tooth, the coordinating assistant supports the mandible; operator may use a chisel and mallet to fracture the decayed or impacted crown while the chairside assistant directs the surgical vacuum tip to remove tooth fragments and fluids from the oral cavity
C. During a medical emergency the coordinating assistant provides the emergency kit and/or oxygen, prepares the syringe with medication as requested by the dentist, and calls for an emergency squad (paramedics) or the patient's physician as directed; if cardiopulmonary resuscitation (CPR) or basic first aid is indicated, the chairside assistant or coordinating assistant provides support as one rescuer while the operator provides support as the second rescuer

APPLICATION OF THE PRINCIPLES OF FOUR-HANDED DENTISTRY ▬▬▬▬

Maintaining the Safety and Comfort of the Patient

A. Patient is placed in the subsupine position with the head at the center top of the back of the dental chair
B. Patient is draped to protect clothing from accidental spills of material
C. Patient is advised to wear protective glasses throughout the dental procedure; this protects the eyes from accidental injury from objects dropped or bits of material or tooth fragments loosened from the teeth; keeping the eyes closed also prevents the glare of the operating light from irritating the eyes

Maintaining a Comfortable Seated Position for the Dental Team

Assumes a right-handed operator
A. Operator is seated at the right side of the patient at the 9 o'clock position for mandibular teeth and at the 11 o'clock position for maxillary teeth
1. Operator uses the direct-vision approach on the mandibular arch and indirect vision (image in the mouth mirror) for the maxillary arch
2. Operator is seated with the feet flat on the floor with one foot (right) near the rheostat (power control for handpieces); operator's back is straight and placed against the back of the stool; seat of the stool is positioned approximately 13 to 15 inches (average, 14 inches) from the floor; operator's thighs are parallel to the floor; with proper back support and the feet flat on the floor, the operator is able to lean forward slightly and maintain balance
3. Operator's arms and hands encircle the face of the patient; operator's arms are parallel to the side; access to the patient's oral cavity is possible without the operator raising the arms
4. Operator's shoulders remain erect and parallel with the floor; with a slight lowering of the head, the field of operation is readily visible
NOTE: As mentioned, the patient's head (head of the dental chair) is placed on the lap of the operator; with a slight turn, depression, or tilt of the patient's head, the operator is able to view all quadrants of the patient's oral cavity
B. Chairside assistant is seated at the 2 o'clock to 3 o'clock position at the left side of the patient
1. Assistant is seated approximately 4 inches higher than the operator to maintain a line of vision of the field of operation and to keep out of the operator's line of vision

2. Assistant's stool is placed parallel with the upper left side of the dental chair
3. Assistant's left thigh is parallel to the patient's left upper arm and shoulders
4. Assistant's knees may extend beyond the head of the dental chair and the patient
5. Back of the stool supports the assistant's back at the lower lumbar area; optional—a padded bar may extend from the back of the chair to encircle the waist of the assistant
6. Assistant's feet are placed flat on the platform at the base of the stool
7. Assistant's position accommodates a class IV or V motion to reach objects placed on the cabinet near the assistant's side of the dental chair
8. Mobile cart with instrument tray is placed over the knees of the assistant

Establishing and Maintaining Accessibility and Visibility of the Field of Operation

A. Establishing and maintaining accessibility and visibility of the field of operation is essential and constant
B. As the patient is directed to move his or her head on the headrest, visibility must be maintained
   1. Operator and chairside assistant modify their positions to keep the field of operation clearly visible
   2. Patient is directed to keep his or her mouth open and tongue away from the area to be operated

Establishing and Maintaining a Fulcrum

A. Operator
   1. Operator obtains a fulcrum with the little and fourth fingers, right hand, on the quadrant near the area to be treated
   2. With the right hand maintaining the fulcrum, the handpiece or instrument is directed toward the tooth under preparation or treatment
   3. Operator stabilizes the mouth mirror with the left hand, retracting the cheek or tongue depending on the area of the oral cavity under treatment
B. Chairside assistant
   1. Assistant adjusts the operating light, focusing it on the area of the oral cavity to be treated
   2. Assistant positions the tip of the high-velocity evacuator following the operator's placement of the mouth mirror and handpiece; high-velocity evacuator is placed with the slanted lumen (opening) toward the distal aspect of the oral cavity if a posterior tooth is being treated, or along the gingiva of a tooth being prepared in the anterior area of the oral cavity

   a. Right quadrant—evacuator is placed across the oral cavity toward the lingual surface of the maxillary and mandibular teeth; assistant places the evacuator tip and retracts or depresses the tongue
   b. Left quadrant—retracting the cheek, the assistant places the evacuator tip on the facial surface for the maxillary and mandibular teeth; using the mouth mirror, the operator retracts the tongue away from the quadrant
3. Chairside assistant retracts the cheek and tongue using the index finger, mouth mirror, and high-velocity evacuator; air-water syringe is directed toward the oral cavity with the left hand; water rinse is directed onto the tooth preparation, into the floor of the oral cavity, at the cul-de-sac, in a trough formed by stretching the lower lip sightly
4. Chairside assistant avoids directing the water onto a flat tooth surface or on the tongue to prevent splashing the face or clothes of the patient and team

INSTRUMENT GRASPS

Basic Concepts

A. Various instrument grasps are applied to safely *pass, use,* and *receive* a dental instrument, forceps, handpiece, or accessory instrument for placing a medicament (e.g., a cotton roll or cotton pallet) (Fig. 16-5)
B. Instrument grasps used in four- and six-handed dentistry are the result of time-and-motion studies identifying the necessary movement and the space needed to supply the instrument or material at the chairside
C. Assistant picks up an instrument by the nib or the end opposite the end to be used (double-ended instrument); index finger and thumb of the left hand are used to grasp the instrument from the instrument tray; when grasped, the instrument is moved into position near the *area of exchange*
D. Area of exchange is near the chin of the patient; operator uses a prearranged signal at the time of exchange; chairside assistant grasps the used instrument and places the next instrument into the hand of the operator
E. Operator maintains a fulcrum during the exchange (e.g., retains the fulcrum and rotates the hand and instrument slightly away from the oral cavity and in position to receive or exchange the instrument)

Types

A. Pen grasp (Fig. 16-6)
   1. Similar to holding a pencil or pen for writing
   2. Necessitates a fulcrum near the tooth or area to be treated to stabilize the instrument and avoid slippage and injury to the tooth
   3. Fourth finger and little finger of the right hand are used to establish the fulcrum; on receipt, the instrument is stabilized with the index finger, thumb, and third finger
B. Inverted or modified pen grasp (Fig. 16-7)
   1. For the inverted or modified pen grasp, the index, third finger and thumb support the instrument in a manner similar to that of the pen grasp.
   2. A slight clockwise rotation of the wrist turns the hand slightly to the side (e.g., using a gold or finishing knife on its side in the process of trimming excess restorative material from the facial surface of an anterior tooth)
C. Palm grasp (Fig. 16-8)
   1. Instrument handle is grasped and held in the palm of the hand as all fingers and the thumb surround the instrument

2. Provides strength and support to the instrument
3. Used for anterior maxillary dental forceps for extracting teeth or for rubber dam clamp forceps
D. Palm-thumb grasp (Fig. 16-9)
   1. All four fingers encompass the bulbous handle of the instrument, such as a root or third molar elevator
   2. Thumb or index finger is used to stabilize the instrument tip (provide leverage) when pressure is brought to bear during its use
   3. Usually reserved for instruments that require a push or thrust action
E. Modified palm-thumb grasp (Fig. 16-10)
   1. During the performance of some procedures, two fingers may grasp and surround the instrument while the other two fingers are pressed against it
   2. Movement of the instrument may be more flexible than the palm-thumb grasp action

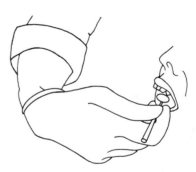

Fig. 16-7 Modified pen grasp (inverted pen grasp). (Modified from Torres, H.O., and Ehrlich, A.: Modern dental assisting, ed. 3, Philadelphia, 1985, W.B. Saunders Co.)

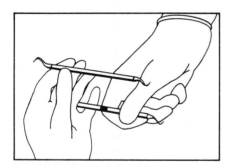

Fig. 16-5 Position for passing and receiving instruments. (Modified from Torres, H.O., and Ehrlich, A.: Modern dental assisting, ed. 3, Philadelphia, 1985, W.B. Saunders Co.)

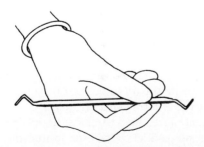

Fig. 16-6 Pen grasp of instrument in position of use. (Modified from Torres, H.O., and Ehrlich, A.: Modern dental assisting, ed. 3, Philadelphia, 1985, W.B. Saunders Co.)

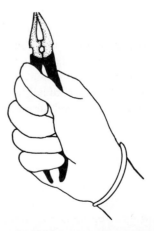

Fig. 16-8 Palm grasp of forceps. (Modified from Torres, H.O., and Ehrlich, A.: Modern dental assisting, ed. 3, Philadelphia, 1985, W.B. Saunders Co.)

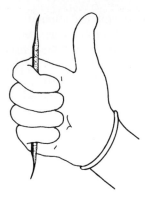

Fig. 16-9 Palm-thumb grasp of instrument. (Modified from Torres, H.O., and Ehrlich, A.: Modern dental assisting, ed. 3, Philadelphia, 1985, W.B. Saunders Co.)

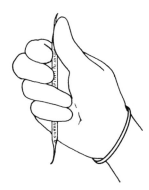

Fig. 16-10 Modified palm-thumb grasp. (Modified from Torres, H.O., and Ehrlich, A.: Modern dental assisting, ed. 3, Philadelphia, 1985, W.B. Saunders Co.)

Passing and Receiving Accessories of the Dental Unit

A. Background setting
   1. Accessories and mobile dental unit are in place in back of the patient, between the operator and chairside assistant
   2. Electrical power to the dental unit is turned on
   3. Syringe with compressed air and warm water is available
B. Right-angle handpiece for a prophylaxis
   1. Assistant extends the tubing and coupling for the handpiece away from the mobile dental unit; tubing is locked in the extended position; straight handpiece is coupled to the tubing
   2. Assistant picks up the sterile low-speed right-angle handpiece and attaches it to the straight handpiece
   3. Rubber cup accessory is placed on the right-angle handpiece

   4. Assistant adjusts the power control at the dental unit to select a low speed of the right-angle handpiece for the polishing procedure
   5. Aspirating tip of the high-velocity evacuator is placed adjacent to the handpiece in each quadrant

Passing and Receiving Instruments Simultaneously

A. On a signal from the dental hygienist the last scaling instrument is received, by the chairside assistant, in the little and fourth fingers of the left hand
B. Instrument is placed on the instrument tray
C. With the index finger and thumb, the handpiece is placed in the operator's right hand as the operator maintains a fulcrum
   1. At a signal from the operator the assistant retracts the tongue, directs the air-water-spray syringe, and rinses the teeth and quadrant being polished
   2. When the last teeth are polished, at a signal from the operator the assistant retrieves the right-angle handpiece using the little and fourth fingers
   3. Using the thumb and index finger, the assistant passes dental floss to the operator, who flosses the patient's teeth to remove polishing debris from the interproximal spaces
   4. Assistant receives the used floss in the palm of the left hand and, using the water control of the syringe, rinses the patient's oral cavity
   5. Assistant directs the high-velocity evacuator and removes all excess fluid and debris from the oral cavity
   6. Optional—patient is provided a small cup with antiseptic mouth rinse; high-velocity evacuator is used to remove the rinse from the patient's oral cavity

Picking Up, Passing, and Receiving Individual Instruments

A. Operator maintains a fulcrum at the area of exchange and keeps fingers open to receive the instrument
B. Assistant picks up the dental instrument near the end opposite the tip to be used from a preset tray and carries it to the area of exchange
C. Assistant places the instrument in the operator's right hand parallel to the used instrument
D. Assistant, using the extended little and fourth fingers, grasps the used instrument and tucks it into the closed fingers

E. Assistant extends the index finger and thumb, placing the new instrument into the hand of the operator with the working end near the oral cavity

F. With a slight pivot of the fulcrum, the operator places the instrument in position for use

G. Assistant moves the left hand and arm to return the used instrument to its original position on the instrument tray

H. Assistant picks up the high-velocity evacuator with the right hand; at a signal from the operator, the assistant places the evacuator tip (lumen slanted toward the distal aspect) and vacuums the oral cavity

I. Holding a mouth mirror in the left hand, the assistant retracts the tongue or tissue away from the field of operation

J. As the operator completes the procedure, the assistant lays the mouth mirror and high-velocity evacuator tubing on the instrument tray

K. Placing both hands in the area of exchange simultaneously, the assistant grasps the instrument and mouth mirror from the operator

Manipulating, Passing, and Receiving Dental Materials

A. Mobile cart is positioned over the assistant's knees

B. Assistant dispenses and mixes the dental material on the instrument tray or on the mobile cart

C. Example procedure is for the application of topical fluoride
1. Picking up the maxillary tray partially filled with topical fluoride gel, the assistant passes it to the operator (dental hygienist)
2. Dental hygienist places the fluoride tray over the patient's maxillary teeth
3. Picking up the high-velocity evacuator, the assistant vacuums the excess saliva from the patient's oral cavity
4. Turning to the instrument tray, the assistant lays the high-velocity evacuator on the tray, picks up the mandibular tray partially filled with fluoride gel, and passes it into the operator's right hand
5. Operator receives the tray and places it over the patient's mandibular teeth
6. If one tray is seated, the assistant places a salvia ejector in the oral cavity
7. With both arches covered with a tray, the patient is advised to close his or her mouth, thus eliminating some of the flow of saliva
8. Assistant turns to the instrument tray and cleans the receptacle of gel, discards soiled tissues and cotton rolls or squares, and places used instruments on the tray

ORAL EVACUATION
Basic Concepts

A. Patient is in a supine position for the four-handed (or six-handed) dentistry mode of treatment delivery

B. Control of oral fluids and debris is indicated

C. High-velocity evacuation system
1. High-velocity tubing attached to the dental unit or to a central vacuum system is used
2. Amount of vacuum is controlled on the dental unit or handle of the vacuum tubing attachment
3. Sterile, contoured plastic tip is attached to the end of the vacuum tubing on the dental unit or wall central vacuum
4. Extension tip
   a. Extension tip is approximately 8×10 inches long and contoured slighty in a V formation, with a slanted lumen at each end
   b. Tip is reversible and adjustable to adapt to various positions by swiveling the plastic extension tip in the coupling attachment
   c. High-velocity evacuation tip is held by friction only
5. The two openings (lumens) at extreme ends of the tip are adaptable to the
   a. Posterior positions in the quadrants
   b. Anterior positions of the oral cavity
   c. Facial or lingual surfaces of the teeth depending on the area of the oral cavity being treated
6. Tip is placed with the assistant at the patient's left side (for a left-handed operator the assistant is at the right side of the patient)

Positions for Placement of the High-Velocity Evacuator

A. Oral evacuation system is used for two basic purposes
1. Removing debris and fluids
2. Retracting tissues or the tongue, lips, and cheeks

B. High-velocity evacuator tubing and tip are held in two general positions by the chairside assistant
1. Modification pen grasp (wand grasp)— extension tip is held with a modified pen grasp with the hand placed at the junction of the extension tip at the vacuum coupling of the tubing
2. Thumb-to-nose grasp
   a. Tubing is placed slightly under the right arm next to the right side of the assistant's body
   b. The four fingers of the right hand grasp the extension tip and vacuum tubing on top, at the location of the coupling

c. Right thumb is placed and stabilized on the underside of the metal end of the vacuum tubing

d. Thumb is positioned toward the assistant's face

e. Optional—if the operator is left handed, the oral evacuation tip is held in the right hand, simulating the same basic position

C. Positions for placement of the evacuator

1. Operator places the mouth mirror and handpiece *first* before placement of the oral evacuator tip by the assistant

2. Evacuator tip is placed from the left side of the dental chair and the patient

3. Goal is to place the oral evacuator tip and/or mouth mirror and to maintain a clear line of vision for the operator and assistant; tip aids in retracting the cheek

  a. Maxillary right quadrant posterior

    (1) Occlusal and lingual surfaces— evacuator tip is placed at the gingival mucosa at the palatal surface and near the tooth under treatment

    (2) Facial surfaces—evacuator tip is placed across the palate from the left to the right and near the occlusal surface of the tooth or teeth being treated

  b. Maxillary left quadrant—evacuator tip is placed at the facial surface in back of the tooth under preparation

  c. Mandibular right quadrant posteriors

    (1) Lingual surfaces—using the mouth mirror, the assistant retracts the tongue toward the left of the oral cavity

    (2) Oral evacuator tip is placed intermittently into the floor of the oral cavity to remove the fluids and debris

    (3) Facial surfaces—operator retracts the right cheek and places the handpiece with the bur or polishing cup at the tooth's facial surface

    (4) Assistant intermittently vacuums the arch and the floor of the oral cavity as the fluids and debris accumulate

    (5) Evacuator tip is placed from the left across the oral cavity over the tongue and near the occlusal surfaces of the teeth under preparation

  d. Maxillary anterior teeth

    (1) Lingual surfaces—operator may approach from the 12 o'clock position

      (a) Operator places the mouth mirror into the anterior area of the palate for indirect vision of the lingual tooth surfaces

      (b) Assistant intermittently places the evacuator tip into the anterior floor of the oral cavity

    (2) Facial surfaces—operator retracts the patient's lip and approaches the teeth from the front or right side of the patient

    (3) Assistant places the evacuator tip at the midline with the lumen placed at the lingual surface and incisal edge of the teeth

  e. Mandibular left quadrant

    (1) Lingual surfaces—operator retracts the tongue with a mouth mirror

      (a) Handpiece is placed near the tooth

      (b) As fluids and debris accumulate, the evacuator tip is placed in the floor of the oral cavity

    (2) Facial surfaces—operator places the handpiece in position near the tooth

      (a) Evacuator tip is placed distal to the tooth being treated; lumen is pointed distally

      (b) Left cheek is retracted by the application of the evacuator tip

  f. Mandibular anterior teeth

    (1) Lingual surfaces—operator may approach the tooth from the 12 o'clock position

      (a) Operator places a mouth mirror in the anterior area of the floor of the oral cavity (indirect vision) and retracts the tongue

      (b) Assistant intermittently swabs the anterior floor of the oral cavity with the evacuator tip

      (c) To accomplish evacuation of the floor of the oral cavity, the operator momentarily moves the handpiece and mouth mirror away from the immediate field of operation

    (2) Facial surfaces—seated at the 9 o'clock position, the operator retracts the lip and approaches the teeth to be treated from the front

      (a) Using a sweeping action with the evacuator tip, the assistant intermittently vacuums the area

(b) Optional—assistant flexes the lower lip slightly, creating a trough; fluids and debris are collected in the trough; evacuator tip is used for evacuation

Retraction of Tissues Using High-Velocity Evacuation

A. Adaptive placement of the high-velocity evacuator will effect retraction of the tongue and cheeks out of the line of vision and field of operation
   1. Tongue—retraction of the tongue is accomplished with the evacuator tip placed against the lingual mucosa of the maxillary right quadrant
   2. Evacuator tip is placed to lay on the tongue across the anterior floor of the oral cavity
   3. Lips—evacuator tip may be used to retract the lower lip away from the teeth to provide accessibility to the facial surfaces of the lower anterior teeth
   4. Cotton roll may be placed under the evacuator tip to avoid traumatizing the tissues
B. Retraction of the cheeks using a mouth mirror
   1. Side of the oral evacuator tip is laid against the left commissure of the lips
   2. With firm but gentle pressure the cheek is retracted away from the operator's line of vision
   3. To avoid traumatizing the lips or cheeks, a cotton roll may be placed under the evacuator tip
   4. Position of the evacuator tip is maintained until the procedure is completed
   5. If the cheek is released for some reason, the procedure is repeated to obtain retraction of the cheek
C. Retraction of the tongue and cheeks using the fingers
   1. Tongue may be retracted by grasping it with a gauze sponge square and placing it to the side or extending it upward and out of the oral cavity; used to achieve a thorough examination of each surface of the tongue and of the floor of the mouth
   2. Cheeks may be retracted by hooking the index finger into the commissures of the lips; this is indicated during brief procedures or during procedures on the teeth that are more posterior in the quadrant
   3. Optional—for traditional retraction of the tongue or cheeks, the operator and assistant use mouth mirrors

4. Commercial plastic and metal cheek retractors are also available for retracting the cheeks
5. Caution is advised to avoid injury to the soft tissues of the oral cavity

Isolation of Segments of the Oral Cavity

Segments of the oral cavity are isolated by strategic placement of cotton rolls
A. Cotton rolls are placed
   1. Under the lips (maxillary and mandibular) next to the mucosa
   2. In the facial areas of the cheeks
   3. In the floor of the oral cavity, anteriorly under the tongue and posteriorly on the top of the tongue near the facial or occlusal areas of the teeth
B. Automaton is a mechanical C-shaped clamp device that extends into the oral cavity and under the chin to stabilize cotton rolls and maintain the tongue in position

Use of the Triple Syringe

A. Triple syringe is an accessory of the mobile dental unit
   1. Capable of spraying warm water, compressed warm air, or a warm water mist into the oral cavity
   2. Controls are placed at the back of the syringe and easily changed by a simple touch of the finger or thumb
B. Passing and receiving the syringe
   1. Assistant picks up the syringe, holds it in the left hand with the index finger and thumb, and extends and locks the tubing away from the dental unit
   2. Assistant selects the control of the syringe and, holding it in a gunlike position, directs the spray toward the oral cavity; water spray is directed under the tongue and at an angle into the quadrants of the oral cavity
   3. Caution is advised to avoid directing the water onto a hard flat surface, which will result in splattering water on the patient, operator, and assistant
   4. To pass the syringe to the operator, the assistant places the syringe nozzle into the index finger and thumb of the left hand and moves it into position near the area of exchange
   5. Following the used instrument retrieval, the assistant extends the index finger and thumb and passes the syringe into the operator's right hand

6. To retrieve the syringe after use, the assistant extends the little and fourth fingers of the left hand to grasp the syringe
7. Syringe exchange is completed
C. Evacuating the field of operation—evacuation is accomplished as described previously
D. Drying the field of operation
1. Cotton rolls and cotton pellets are used to dry moist areas of the oral cavity that are under treatment
2. Warm air is selected on the triple syringe
3. Soft blasts of warm air from the syringe are directed toward the area (tooth) under treatment; syringe is moved back and forth to avoid overheating and overdrying the tooth, particularly exposed dentin
4. Caution—dessication, extreme dryness from overdrying tissues of the tooth, causes injury to exposed dentin and possible injury to the pulp of the tooth

Placement of the Saliva Ejector-Retractor

A. Device known as an ejector-retractor is designed to retract the tongue and eject fluids from the oral cavity during periods when material (e.g., cements) may be setting
B. Tongue is gently positioned away from the field of operation
C. Ejector-retractor is placed on the salivia ejector tubing attachment of the mobile dental unit
D. Control for the saliva ejector-retractor is turned on after the ejector-retractor is placed in position in the oral cavity

MAINTAINING SAFETY THROUGHOUT THE PERFORMANCE OF DENTAL PROCEDURES

A. Through effective communication the operator and assistant function as a team, conveying a feeling of confidence to the patient
B. Chairside assistant must be particularly alert at all times to prevent injury or trauma to tissues of the oral cavity during
1. Evacuation
2. Placement of materials
3. Exchange of instruments
C. General condition or physical appearance of the patient is observed by the assistant throughout the dental procedure
D. Assistant checks for signs of fatigue or pallor, indicating illness of the patient
E. Assistant quietly alerts the operator if the condition of the patient changes during the dental procedure

F. To ensure the comfort of the patient, the operator concentrates on performing the dental procedure as quickly as possible
G. For the management of emergencies that may arise, see Chapter 18

TEAM DENTISTRY
Basic Concepts

A. Training in expanded auxiliary management (TEAM) stimulates the practice of dentistry, fully using the contribution of each member of the dental team; individual team member is qualified through special training (licensed in some states) to perform more complicated services (reversible procedures) for the patient
B. Individual team member (other than the dentist) is referred to as an expanded-function auxiliary; however, the full concept of TEAM dentistry utilizes expanded-function dental auxiliaries in traditional and in expanded roles
C. TEAM concept includes the dentist trained in the utilization of personnel (e.g., the chairside assistant [expanded and traditional functions], the dental hygienist [expanded and traditional functions], and the dental laboratory technician [expanded and traditional functions])

Roles of the Members of the Dental Team – Examples

A. Dentist performs the operative, surgical procedure and, as the coordinator, delegates the performance of particular functions to the professional staff
B. Dental hygienist might be delegated responsibility for prevention, nutritional counseling, charting of pocket depths, administration of local anesthesia, deep root scaling and curettage, dental radiographic surveys, placement and removal of sutures following the laying of a flap in periodontal survey by the dentist, and placement and removal of periodontal surgical packs
C. Chairside assistant might perform traditional chairside functions—rinsing and evacuating fluids from the oral cavity; passing and retrieving instruments; dispensing, mixing, and placing intermediate-type dental materials (e.g., cavity varnish, bases, liners, and intermediary restorative materials); and constructing and placing temporary coverages such as custom acrylic, aluminum, or stainless steel temporary crowns
D. Expanded-function dental auxiliary (EFDA [assistant] or EFDH [dental hygienist]) might perform acid etching of enamel for bonding of brackets and/or placement of pit and fissure sealants

E. Coordinating assistant maintains the flow of patients in and out of the multiple treatment areas; prepares sterile instrument trays; exposes, processes, and mounts radiographs; prepares the treatment area for the next patient; assists with medical emergencies; and assists with multiple impressions and restorations by preparing the dental materials for the chairside assistant, dental hygienist, or dentist

F. Dental laboratory technician receives the impressions and prepares study and working casts, temporary coverages (acrylic crowns and bridges), permanent crowns and bridges, and partial and full dentures

Basic Functions Performed

Basic Concepts

A. Concept of efficient TEAM dentistry is modeled on the delegation of a function by the operator (dentist) to the most logical qualified staff member

B. TEAM dentistry typifies the full implementation of time and motion to effect a more efficient delivery system for a dental practice and to delegate a function to individually qualified personnel without stopping or halting productivity

Administration of Topical and Local Anesthesia

A. Assistant places the topical anesthetic at the site of injection

B. Dentist or dental hygienist administers block infiltration of a local anesthetic solution

Rubber Dam Placement and Removal

A. Chairside or coordinating assistant or expanded-function auxiliary (dental hygienist or assistant) prepares, places, and removes the rubber dam isolating the tooth (or teeth) to be prepared

B. Individual team member selects the clamp and frame, prepares the rubber dam, and places it on the tooth as the need arises

Application of Medicaments for a Prepared Tooth—Example of TEAM Concepts

A. Prepared tooth is rinsed and dried with the warm air syringe

B. Cavity varnish
 1. Thin layer of cavity varnish (Copal) is spread throughout the floor and walls of the cavity preparation
 2. Operator indicates if a second application is needed

C. Cavity liner
 1. Calcium hydroxide (Ca_2OH) is mixed; with a small ball-type applicator a layer of calcium hydroxide is placed gently over the nearly exposed pulpal area of the preparation; cavity liner is used to form a protective layer of insulation between the pulpal tissue and the restoration; calcium hydroxide encourages the formation of secondary dentin
 2. Assistant mixes the calcium hydroxide paste and, holding the mixing pad in the right hand near the area of exchange, hands the applicator to the operator with the left hand
 3. Operator applies a thin layer of calcium hydroxide on the floor of the cavity preparation near the area of the pulp; applicator is retrieved by the assistant with the little and fourth fingers of the left hand

D. Cement base application
 1. Zinc phosphate cement is spatulated on a cool, dry glass slab to a puttylike consistency
 2. With a small spoon excavator, smooth condenser, or small plastic-type instrument, base material is distributed evenly and gently tamped into the floor (base), over the dentin of the cavity preparation
 3. If there is an excess of base that is to be removed, an inverted cone or round bur is placed in a contraangle handpiece, or a spoon excavator is used to remove the excess

E. Topical fluoride application (varies with the type of fluoride used; see Chapter 12, section on professionally administered topical fluoride treatments)

Obtaining Alginate Impressions for Study Casts

A. Alginate impression provides a negative of the patient's dental arch and the dentition

B. Alginate impressions for study casts must meet the following minimum criteria
 1. Registration of the retromolar areas, tuberosities, palatal area, alveolar ridges, dentition, attached frena of the dental arches, and free and attached gingivae
 2. Accurate representation of the morphology of the erupted dentition
 3. Adequate space within the tray to allow for material beyond the facial and incisal/occlusal surfaces of the teeth within the impression of the individual arch

C. Instrumentation and selection of the impression trays
   1. Instrumentation—flexible rubber bowl, stiff beaver-tail laboratory spatula, water, alginate powder, and measuring graduates (measurers with gradations)
   2. Selection of trays
      a. Maxillary tray—extends beyond the posterior tooth in the dentition or the area of the tuberosities; must be adequate space to provide a minimum of 2 mm of material around the margin and throughout the tray; tray extends beyond the postdam area of the palate
      b. Mandibular tray—extends beyond the most posterior tooth in the arch and beyond the retromolar area; tray seats over the mandibular teeth and avoids injury to the muscle attachments at the lingual floor of the oral cavity
D. Preparation of alginate impression material
   1. Scoops of alginate powder are measured— average of 2 scoops for mandibular area; average of 3 scoops for maxillary area
   2. Water is measured—one line on water graduate for each scoop of powder; water should be a maximum of 68° F (20° C); too hot, it accelerates the set of alginate; too cold, it retards the set of alginate
   3. Powder is placed in the bowl; water is then added
   4. Alginate powder and water are incorporated and spatulated a maximum of 60 seconds to obtain a creamy consistency; if creamy consistency can be reached more quickly, no harm is done to the material
E. Loading of the impression tray (assumes a right-handed operator)
   1. Mandibular arch
      a. With the spatula in the right hand and the bowl in the left hand, the material is scooped up with the spatula; with the tray in the left hand, the spatula is scraped on the lingual margin of the tray
      b. Alginate is loaded into the tray from the lingual approach with one major motion
      c. Tip of the spatula is placed vertically into the alginate mass to break air bubbles as the material is loaded into the tray
      d. Surface of the alginate is smoothed by placing wetted fingers over the occlusal surface of the material in the tray

   2. Maxillary arch
      a. Spatula loaded with alginate is scraped over the posterior (postdam area) margin of the tray
      b. Alginate is loaded forward to avoid bubbles; surface is smoothed with wetted fingers
      c. Bulk of the alginate material is loaded into the anterior of the tray to avoid extrusion of the material onto the soft palate as the impression tray is seated
F. Receipt and seating of the loaded impression tray
   1. Mandibular arch.
      a. Assistant hands the loaded tray to the operation (dental hygienist)
      b. Operator turns the tray sidewise, flexes the right cheek, and slips the tray into the oral cavity
         (1) Tray is straightened and centered over the alveolar ridge; operator uses both index fingers and thumbs to seat the tray on the mandiular arch
         (2) Index fingers of the operator's hands flex the cheeks outward
         (3) Patient is advised to lift the tongue upward; patient's tongue is then relaxed in the floor of the oral cavity
         (4) Alginate impression material is permitted to set (setting time depends on the type of alginate used)
   2. Maxillary arch
      a. Assistant hands the loaded tray to the operator (dental hygienist)
      b. Operator turns the tray sidewise and slips it into the oral cavity
         (1) With the upper lips and cheeks flexed, the maxillary tray is straightened and seated upward onto the maxillary teeth and palate
         (2) Lips relax over the tray
         (3) Operator places the index finger onto the palatal area of the tray and with a thrust *upward* seats the tray on the palate
G. Removal of the impression tray from the dental arch
   1. Cheeks are flexed away from the tray in the mandibular arch
      a. Mandibular tray is grasped by the handle
      b. Tray is snapped off the arch without injury to the maxillary teeth; operator's fingers serve as a cushion between the arches
      c. Impression is examined to determine that it represents the mandibular arch

2. Cheeks are flexed away from the tray in the maxillary arch
   a. Maxillary tray handle is grasped firmly and tray is pulled straight down
   b. Fingers of the left hand are placed between the arches to protect the teeth of the mandibular arch
   c. If suction prevents removal of the maxillary tray, the air syringe is handed to the operator, who blows compressed air into the posterior side of the tray to break the seal; this action can also be applied to each side and the anterior area of the impression tray to break the suction seal without damage to the impression
H. Storage of the alginate impression before pouring
   1. If the impression is rinsed and cannot be poured immediately, it may be stored in
      a. A damp cloth or paper towel until poured
      b. A 2% potassium sulfate solution
   2. Maximum storage time for the alginate impression should not exceed 20 minutes
I. Alginate impressions are checked for excess material beyond the periphery of the trays, particularly the postdam area of the maxillary impression
   1. Excess impression material is trimmed away using a laboratory knife
   2. Alginate impressions are poured in dental stone or plaster

FOUR-HANDED, SIX-HANDED, AND TEAM DENTISTRY IN THE DENTAL SPECIALTIES

A. Four-handed, six-handed, and TEAM concepts and principles are applicable to the dental specialties
B. Cited are examples of procedures that may be delegated to educationally qualified and clinically competent dental hygienists; services will vary from state to state according to state laws
   1. Pedodontics
      a. Impressions for study casts, space maintainers, and occlusal guards
      b. Complete clinical oral examination
      c. Application of topical fluorides
      d. Selection, sizing, and placement of temporary stainless steel crowns
      e. Placement of liners and bases in a prepared tooth
      f. Application of acid etching and pit and fissure sealants
      g. Exposure of radiographs
   2. Orthodontics
      a. Impressions for study casts
      b. Prophylaxis procedures
      c. Acid etching for direct bonding of brackets
      d. Selection and sizing of orthodontic bands
      e. Placement and removal of ligature ties
      f. Instructing the patient in the placement and removal of headgear
   3. Endodontics
      a. Pulp vitality testing
      b. Placement and removal of a rubber dam
      c. Irrigation and drying of the open root canal
      d. Temporization of the coronal area of the tooth under treatment or for root canal therapy
   4. Periodontics
      a. Temporary stabilization of teeth
      b. Scaling and root planing
      c. Prophylaxis
      d. Administration of local anesthesia
      e. Gingival curettage
      f. Placement and removal of periodontal surgical dressings
      g. Placement and removal of sutures
      h. Dental disease control instructions
      i. Postsurgical instructions and follow-up
   5. Oral surgery
      a. Administration of nitrous oxide and oxygen (N_2O and O_2) for analgesia before administration of general anesthesia administered by the oral surgeon
      b. Removal of sutures
      c. Assistance with medical emergencies
      d. Assistance with surgery
      e. Irrigation of dry sockets and placement of palliative medicaments
      f. Exposure of radiographs
   6. Crown and bridge prosthetics
      a. Cord retraction of the gingiva
      b. Obtaining of impressions for cast restorations
      c. Formulation of indirect patterns for endodontic posts and core castings

REFERENCE

1. Robinson, G.E., et al.: Four-handed dentistry manual, ed. 2, Birmingham, 1971, University of Alabama School of Dentistry.

SUGGESTED READINGS ▬▬▬▬▬▬

Anderson, P.C., and Burkard, M.R.: The dental assistant, ed. 4, Albany, N.Y., 1982, Delmar Publishers, Inc.

Building and maintaining a successful dental practice, Chicago, 1983, Marketing Services Department, American Dental Association.

Castano, F.A., and Alden, B.A.: Handbook of clinical dental auxiliary practice, ed. 2, Philadelphia, 1980, J.B. Lippincott Co.

Chasteen, J.E.: Four-handed dentistry in clinical practice, St. Louis, 1978, The C.V. Mosby Co.

Chasteen, J.E.: Essentials of clinical dental assisting, ed. 3, St. Louis, 1984, The C.V. Mosby Co.

Comptroller General Report to the Congress of the United States: Increased use of expanded function dental auxiliaries would benefit consumers, dentists and taxpayers, Springfield, Va., March 1980, USAO, HRD 8-9-51, U.S. Department of Commerce.

Conference on training dental students to use chairside assistants, Bethesda, Md., April 1968, Division of Dental Health, U.S. Department of Health, Education, and Welfare.

Description and documentation of the private practice dental delivery system, Reading, Mass., 1981, DHHS Publication No. (HRA) 81-11, U.S. Department of Health and Human Services, Public Health Service, Human Resources Administration, Division of Dentistry, prepared by Systematics, Inc.

Froelich, R.E., Bishop, F.M., and Dworkin, S.F.: Communication in the dental office: a programmed manual for the dental profession, St. Louis, 1976, The C.V. Mosby Co.

Spohn, E.E., Halwowski, W.A., and Berry, T.G.: Operative dentistry procedures for the dental auxiliaries, St. Louis, 1981, The C.V. Mosby Co.

Steele, F.: Dimensions of dental hygiene, ed. 3, Philadelphia, 1982, Lea & Febiger.

Torres, H.O., and Ehrlich, A.: Modern dental assisting, ed. 3, Philadelphia, 1985, W.B. Saunders Co.

Wilkins, E.M.: Clinical practice of the dental hygienist, ed. 5, Philadelphia, 1983, Lee & Febiger.

Workshop on future requirements of dental manpower and the training and utilization of auxiliary personnel, Detroit, Jan. 1962.

Review Questions

1 Which of the following describes the practice of four-handed dentistry?
1. Early research in dentistry
2. Utilization of the chairside assistant
3. Utilization of the dental hygienist
4. Utilization of the dental laboratory technician
5. Its role in TEAM dentistry

2 Which of the following individuals assists the operator, functioning as a component in four-handed dentistry?
1. Dental hygienist
2. Chairside assistant
3. Dentist
4. Coordinating assistant
5. Dental laboratory technician

3 Which of the following pieces of dental equipment lends itself to the practice of four-handed (or six-handed) dentistry?
1. Upright dental chair
2. Mobile dental unit
3. Fixed dental cabinet
4. Wall-mounted x-ray unit
5. Portable lead shield

4 Which of the following functions are performed by the chairside assistant in the practice of four-handed dentistry?
1. Sterilize dental instruments
2. Pick up, pass, and receive instruments
3. Prepare the tooth for a restoration
4. Place, condense, and carve amalgam
5. Check the occlusion of the amalgam restoration

Situation: The patient enters the operatory and is requested to be seated in the contoured dental chair. Using the four-handed dentistry mode of delivery, the dental team proceeds to prepare and treat the patient for an intermediary temporary restoration of a maxillary molar. Questions 5 to 8 refer to this situation.

5 Which of the following would be essential to the four-handed dentistry mode of delivery?
1. The chair is in an upright position
2. The instrument tray is placed on a fixed cabinet
3. The patient is seated at an 80-degree angle
4. The patient is placed in a supine position
5. The operator is standing at the patient's right

6 For mixing and placing the intermediary restoration, which type of dental cement is selected?
1. Calcium hydroxide
2. Zinc phosphate
3. Glass ionomer
4. Alginic acid
5. Zinc oxide–eugenol

7 Which of the following are the instruments the assistant passes to the operator to place the mix for a temporary restoration?
1. Explorer, smooth condenser, and contraangle handpiece
2. Spoon excavator, smooth condenser, and explorer
3. Plastic instrument, smooth condenser, and explorer
4. Contraangle handpiece, mouth mirror, and explorer
5. Serrated condenser, smooth condenser, and explorer

8 Which of the following describes the patient's head position for placing the temporary restoration on a maxillary molar?
1. Head straight and forward on the headrest
2. Head steady on the headrest area and turned slightly to the right
3. Head steady on the headrest area and turned slightly to the left
4. Head turned to the left, chin down
5. Head turned to the right, chin up

9 Which of the following may be excluded from the TEAM practice in direct patient treatment?
1. Dentist
2. Dental hygienist
3. Chairside assistant
4. Secretarial manager
5. Dental laboratory technician

10 One nonessential of four- and six-handed dentistry practices is
1. Diagnostic aids
2. Updated medical/dental records
3. Preset instrument trays
4. Third-party fee for service
5. Mobile equipment

11 Which of the following is an inappropriate form of motion when using four-handed dentistry during dental treatment?
1. Rising from the stool and obtaining a medicament from a fixed cabinet
2. Use of fingers and thumb to pick up and pass dental instruments
3. From a seated position, turning to a spot welder on the cabinet
4. Holding vacuum tubing to the side (under the arm) and directing the tip in a thumb-to-nose position
5. Directing the high-velocity evacuator tip in a wand position

12 What classification of motion is used to adjust the controls on the dental unit for the ultrasonic scaler or compressed air?
1. Class I motion
2. Class II motion
3. Class III motion
4. Class IV motion
5. Class V motion

13 Maintaining a fulcrum when using a curette for deep scaling during a prophylaxis uses what class of motion?
1. Class I
2. Class II
3. Class III
4. Class IV
5. Class V

14 Which of the following relates to the patient's position in the clock configuration for four- and six-handed dentistry?
1. The forehead is the center of the clock
2. The oral cavity is the center of the clock
3. The chin is the center of the clock
4. The head is the static zone
5. The head is the area of exchange

15 Which of the following would be placed first in the patient's oral cavity?
1. Mouth mirror by the operator to retract the tissues, tongue, or cheek
2. Contraangle handpiece to establish a fulcrum
3. Index finger of the assistant
4. High-velocity evacuator
5. Mouth mirror by the assistant

16 Which of the following identifies the seated position of the dental operator in TEAM dentistry?
1. Head tilted upward and forward
2. Upper body leaning forward at the hips
3. Knees higher than the hips
4. Feet flat on the floor
5. Elbows higher than the hands

17 When working with a right-handed operator, the assistant passes the handpiece or air-water syringe to the operator, using the left hand
1. Index and third fingers
2. Fourth and third fingers
3. Thumb and index finger
4. Fourth and little fingers
5. Index finger only

18 Which of the following instrument grasps is used to pass carvers and condensers for an amalgam restoration?
1. Inverted pen grasp
2. Modified pen grasp
3. Palm grasp
4. Palm-thumb grasp
5. Pen grasp

19 In TEAM dentistry the expanded-function dental auxiliary (dental hygienist) is delegated functions that are
1. Irreversible
2. Reversible
3. Traditional
4. Surgical
5. Reparative

20 To prepare an adequate quantity and distribution of impression material in the maxillary tray, the alginate is loaded from the
1. Side of the tray
2. Posterior
3. Postdam area
4. Anterior of the tray
5. Cuspid area

21 Which of the following procedures is considered an expanded responsibility for the dental hygienist in periodontics?
1. Deep scaling
2. Root planing
3. Obtaining impressions for study casts
4. Suturing tissue of a surgical flap
5. Removing sutures of surgical flap

22 To seat the impression tray on the maxillary arch, the tray is turned with the handle vertical to the anterior teeth, and the
1. Handle is pressed upward
2. Sides of tray are pressed upward
3. Postdam area of the tray is tilted
4. Index finger is pressed on the palatal area
5. Thumb is pressed on the anterior of the tray

23 If a medical emergency occurs during an operative procedure, which of the following personnel in six-handed dentistry would probably contact the paramedics?
1. Dentist
2. Chairside assistant
3. Dental hygienist
4. Dental laboratory technician
5. Coordinating assistant

24 The six-handed dentistry mode of dental practice uses the coordinating assistant for
1. Passing and receiving instruments
2. Preparing and passing the anesthetic syringe
3. Rinsing and vacuuming the patient's oral cavity
4. Dispensing, mixing, and loading impression material in the tray
5. Dispensing, mixing, and loading impression material in the syringe

25 In a full-crown preparation, which of the following is the accepted method of placing medicated cord to retract the gingiva?
1. Poking it into the gingival crevice
2. Laying it clockwise at the circumference of the cervix
3. Placing it at the mesial and distal aspects of the gingiva
4. Placing it at the facial and lingual aspects of the cervix
5. Placing it on the gingival crest at the cervix

26 During a comprehensive clinical examination to determine tooth vitality the dental hygienist uses a
1. Radiographic survey
2. Vitalometer on suspected teeth
3. Periodontal probe
4. Fiberoptic light
5. Precussion technique

27 Which of the following materials would be used to place a cavity liner over an exposed area of the pulp?
1. Copal varnish
2. Zinc oxide–eugenol
3. Calcium hydroxide
4. Light-cured composite
5. Zinc phosphate cement

28 What area of the clock configuration represents the chairside assistant's zone?
1. 2 o'clock to 4 o'clock
2. 4 o'clock to 8 o'clock
3. 8 o'clock to 11 o'clock
4. 8 o'clock to 12 o'clock
5. 12 o'clock to 2 o'clock

29 Functioning at the chairside, the operator and chairside assistant refer to the dynamic area of exchange as the patient's
1. Chest
2. Lap
3. Chin
4. Oral cavity
5. Middle of the face

30 Which of the following is positioned by the chairside assistant to retract the cheek or tongue before placement of the handpiece by the operator?
1. Mouth mirror
2. Handpiece
3. Saliva ejector
4. Explorer
5. High-velocity evacuator tip

31 Considering the clock configuration (in four-handed dentistry), the delivery of instruments and materials from in back of the patient's head is referred to as
1. Side delivery
2. Rear delivery
3. Front delivery
4. The static zone
5. The dynamic zone

32 In four-handed dentistry it is essential that a fulcrum be used by the operator to stabilize the
1. Explorer
2. Mouth mirror
3. Handpiece
4. Impression tray
5. Holder with articulating paper

33 Following placement of a Ferrier (No. 212) rubber dam clamp, the jaws of the clamp rest
1. On the enamel of the crown
2. At 3 mm below the cementoenamel junction
3. On the margin of the rubber dam
4. Below the rubber dam at the cementoenamel junction
5. Above the inverted dam at the cementoenamel junction

34 When placing a Ferrier (No. 212) rubber dam clamp for a class V restoration, for visibility of the tooth during preparation, the gingiva
1. Remains in its normal position
2. Is retracted a minimum of 0.25 mm
3. Is retracted a minimum of 0.75 mm
4. Is retracted a maximum of 0.75 mm
5. Is retracted a maximum of 1 mm

35 To avoid contamination of an instrument when grasping it for passing to the operator, the assistant picks it up
1. Near the nib of the instrument
2. At the point
3. At the end opposite the one to be used
4. At the center of the handle
5. At the end to be used

36 During oral evacuation of the posterior oral cavity using the high-volume evacuator, the tip is placed with the lumen (opening)
1. Directed toward the operator
2. Near the tooth under preparation
3. Near the tooth under preparation and toward the posterior
4. Directed toward the anterior
5. Directed toward the tooth under preparation toward the anterior

37 In four-handed dentistry the side of the high-velocity evacuator tip may be used to
1. Dry the oral cavity
2. Retract the cheek
3. Hold the tongue
4. Retract the gingiva
5. Retract the lips

38 To change a bur or mandrel in the high-speed handpiece, the operator positions the handpiece for the assistant at the
1. Back of the patient's head
2. Oral cavity
3. Area of exchange at the chin of the patient
4. Area of exchange, maintaining a fulcrum
5. Side of the patient's face

39 In preparing the anesthetic syringe, passing of the syringe to the operator is accomplished at the area of exchange
1. On the chest of the patient
2. At the oral cavity
3. At the rear of the patient's head
4. Near the patient's chin
5. Over the instrument tray

40 The pad with a mix of sedative dressing is held by the assistant at the area of exchange at the
1. Oral cavity
2. Chest of the patient
3. Cheeks of the patient
4. Upper half of the face
5. Chin of the patient

41 To enable the operator to place a sedative dressing at the base of a deep cavity preparation in a tooth, the instrument passed is a (an)
1. Wedelstaedt chisel
2. Cotton pliers
3. Spoon excavator
4. Plasic-type instrument
5. Angle former

42 When assisting a right-handed operator who is using a mouth mirror and a handpiece, what hand will the assistant use to receive and pass the air-water syringe and the explorer?
1. The mouth mirror is received in the assistant's left hand; the explorer is passed
2. The handpiece is received in the assistant's left hand; the air-water syringe is passed
3. The handpiece is received in the assistant's right hand; the explorer is passed
4. The air-water syringe and explorer are passed simultaneously
5. The operator retains the handpiece in the left hand and receives the explorer from the assistant's right hand.

43 Seated at the 9 o'clock position, the operator uses the inverted or modified pen grasp to
1. Examine the cingulum of a maxillary anterior tooth
2. Hold the high-speed handpiece for preparation of tooth No. 19
3. Use an enamel chisel
4. Condense amalgam for a restoration in a mandibular molar
5. Extract a maxillary premolar

44 When using the high-velocity evacuator tip during restorative dentistry or oral surgery, the dental team avoids injuring the soft tissues of the oral cavity with the suction tip, particularly the
1. Free gingiva
2. Tongue
3. Buccal mucosae
4. Floor of the oral cavity
5. Soft palate

45 Functioning within the TEAM concept, a dental prosthesis is prepared for the patient by the
1. Dental hygienist under a prescription
2. Dentist under written specifications
3. Expanded-function dental auxiliary under a prescription
4. Dental laboratory technician under a prescription
5. Coordinating assistant under a prescription

46 Of the five specialty dental practices, six-handed dentistry most readily lends itself to
1. Prosthodontics
2. Pedodontics
3. Orthodontics
4. Oral surgery
5. Periodontics

47 According to the dental practice act of some jurisdictions, the clinical examination of the patient's oral cavity may be delegated to a (an)
1. Expanded-function dental auxiliary
2. Dental laboratory technician
3. Dental hygienist
4. Chairside assistant
5. Coordinating assistant

48 The individual of the dental staff responsible for patient accounts receivable, receipt of payment, and scheduling of appointments is the
1. Chairside assistant
2. Administrative assistant
3. Coordinating assistant
4. Dental laboratory technician
5. Dental hygienist

49 In some jurisdictions the administration of nitrous oxide and oxygen (N_2O and O_2) for conscious sedation may be delegated legally to which of the following if special training has been received?
1. Dentist
2. Dental hygienist
3. Chairside assistant
4. Coordinating assistant
5. Expanded-function dental auxiliary

50 The dental material frequently used for a cavity liner is known generically as
1. Calcium hydroxide
2. Zinc oxide–eugenol
3. Zinc phosphate cement
4. Copal varnish
5. Reversible colloids

51 Thirty-five to forty percent of phosphoric acid is used for etching enamel before direct bonding of brackets in orthodontics and also in
1. Insulating bases
2. A cavity sealer
3. Pit and fissure sealants
4. Zinc phosphate cement base
5. Zinc oxide–eugenol insulation

52 Criteria for an acceptable alginate impression of the maxillary dentulous arch includes the representation of the teeth, a lack of bubbles (voids) or distorted tissues, the alveolus, and the palatal and
1. Retromolar area
2. Mylohyoid ridge
3. Genial tubercles
4. Frenum
5. Oblique ridge

53 If an alginate impression is to be poured later, it should be stored in a
1. Damp cloth or paper towel
2. 2% potassium sulfate solution
3. Humidor
4. Safe place at the back of the bench
5. 2% saline solution

54 A cement that forms a bond between the dentin and enamel and is favorable for luting a cast restoration is
1. Ortho-ethoxybenzoic acid (EBA)
2. Calcium hydroxide
3. Zinc phosphate
4. Polycarboxylate (polyacrylate)
5. Zinc oxide–eugenol

55 In cosmetic dentistry, specifically the acid etching of enamel procedure, the enamel surface is etched with phosphoric acid and the
1. Facial surface is covered with composite resin
2. Entire crown is covered with composite resin
3. Surface is prepared for a full crown
4. Surface is prepared for retention of a composite veneer
5. Temporary coverage (custom) is placed

Answers and Rationales

1. (2) The chairside assistant gives the operator support by providing extra hands during the performance of dental procedures.
   (1) Early research determined the ground rules for appreciation of four-handed dentistry.
   (3) The dental hygienist may become the operator in the performance of some dental procedures.
   (4) The dental laboratory technician works in the laboratory from a written prescription from the dentist.
   (5) Four-handed dentistry is the basis for TEAM dentistry and the delegation of expanded functions for auxiliaries.

2. (2) The four-handed dentistry team is composed of the dentist as the operator and usually a chairside assistant.
   (1) The dental hygienist may function as the operator.
   (3) The dentist is the operator.
   (4) The coordinating assistant serves as a backup person (in six-handed dentistry).
   (5) The dental laboratory technician fabricates prostheses from laboratory prescriptions provided by the dentist.

3. (2) The mobile dental unit adapts readily to the practice of four-handed (or six-handed) dentistry because it can be moved from one position to another.
   (1) The upright dental chair is rigid; the back cannot accommodate positioning the patient in a supine position.
   (3) Fixed dental cabinets are immobile (attached to the wall).
   (4) The wall-mounted x-ray unit is used for radiographic surveys.
   (5) The portable lead shield, part of the operatory equipment, is adaptive to use during radiation exposures in radiographic technique.

4. (2) In four-handed dentistry the chairside assistant is solely responsible for maintaining order on the instrument tray—picking up, passing, and receiving used dental instruments.
   (1) Sterile dental instruments are prepared by the coordinating assistant in the sterilization area.
   (3) The dentist prepares the tooth.
   (4) The assistant places, and the dentist condenses and carves the amalgam.
   (5) The dentist places articulating paper and checks the occlusion in four-handed dentistry.

5. (4) The patient is in a supine position for the performance of dental procedures using four-handed dentistry. This is basic positioning for a dental procedure.
   (1) The chair must be in a reclined position.
   (2) The instrument tray is placed on a mobile cabinet.
   (3) The patient is in a supine position with the feet slightly higher than the head.
   (5) The operator is seated at the right of the patient.

6. (5) Zinc oxide–eugenol cements are selected for temporary restorations for their palliative effect on the pulpal tissues and exposed dentin.
   (1) Calcium hydroxide is used for a cavity liner placed over the nearly exposed or exposed pulpal area. It has very low crushing strength and would crush during mastication.
   (2) Zinc phosphate is used more frequently as a base or for cementing cast restorations.
   (3) Glass ionomer cement is used to cement permanent restorations.
   (4) Alginic acid is a component of alginate powder, an irreversible impression material.

7. (2) The spoon excavator is used to carry the material to the tooth, the smooth condenser to pack it, and the explorer to remove excess at the cavity margin.
   (1) The explorer is unable to place mix; the contraangle hand-piece is not needed in most cases.
   (3) The plastic instrument is used for carrying mix.
   (4) The contraangle handpiece, mouth mirror, and explorer are an incomplete setup; the contraangle hand-pice is used for tooth preparation.
   (5) Mix would stick to the serrations of a serrated condenser

8. (5) For ease of placement of a temporary restoration, the chin is slightly elevated and the head is turned to the right toward the operator.
   (1) It is difficult to retract tissues and see the tooth preparation with the head straight and forward.
   (2) The head turned slightly to the right is somewhat helpful.
   (3) The head turned to the left causes difficulty in reviewing the tooth.
   (4) The head turned to the left and the chin down prevents viewing of the oral cavity.

9. (4) The secretarial manager manages the appointment scheduling and business aspect of a practice and is not directly involved with patient treatment.
   (1) The dentist is the operator.
   (2) The dental hygienist provides preventive therapy.
   (3) The chairside assistant assists at chairside.
   (5) The dental laboratory technician fabricates prostheses from impressions.

For each question the correct answer and rationale are listed first. The other choices are presented in order with the reason why they are not correct.

10. (4) Third-party fee for service has no direct effect on the practice of dentistry.
    (1) Diagnostic aids help the dentist prepare the diagnosis.
    (2) Updated records determine the immediate need for treatment.
    (3) Preset trays aid in efficiency.
    (5) Mobile equipment is essential to efficient delivery of treatment.

11. (1) The dental team remains seated throughout the performance of a procedure.
    (2) Use of fingers and thumb constitutes a class I motion.
    (3) Turning at the waist constitutes a class V motion.
    (4) Using the fingers, wrist, and elbow constitutes a class IV motion.
    (5) Using the fingers and wrist constitutes a class II motion.

12. (4) Class IV motion extends the hand and arm from the shoulder to reach the controls on the dental unit.
    (1) Class I motion is finger motion only.
    (2) Class II motion is finger and wrist motion.
    (3) Class III motion is finger, wrist, and elbow motion.
    (5) Class V motion involves moving the arm and twisting the body.

13. (1) Maintaining a fulcrum to scale calculus from the teeth uses the fourth and little fingers (class I motion).
    (2) Class II motion includes rotating the wrist.
    (3) Class III motion involves movements of the fingers, wrist, and elbow.
    (4) Class IV motion involves movements of the arm from the shoulder.
    (5) Class V motion involves movements of the arm and twisting the body at the waist.

14. (2) The oral cavity is the dynamic center of the clock in four- and six-handed dentistry.
    (1) The forehead is too high.
    (3) The chin is too low.
    (4) The static zone is the area from 11 o'clock to 2 o'clock.
    (5) The area of exchange is near the chin.

15. (1) The operator first retracts the tissues, tongue, or cheek.
    (2) A fulcrum (with handpiece) is established after retraction of the tissues.
    (3) The assistant uses the index finger to retract tissue as needed.
    (4) The high-velocity evacuator is placed after the operator places the instruments or handpiece out of the line of vision.
    (5) The mouth mirror is used by the assistant to retract the tongue or cheeks at the left side of the oral cavity *after* the operator has completed placement.

16. (4) Both feet are placed flat on the floor with one foot free to touch the rheostat.
    (1) The head is tilted slightly downward; the neck is straight.
    (2) The upper body is with the back against the back of the stool.
    (3) The knees are level with the hips; the thighs are parallel with the floor.
    (5) The elbows are close to the body; the hands are slightly elevated to encircle the patient's oral cavity.

17. (3) Holding the handpiece or syringe from the base, the assistant passes it to the operator in line of use, with the thumb and index finger.
    (1) The index and third finger would not provide control.
    (2) The fourth and third fingers aid in receiving instruments.
    (4) The fourth and little fingers receive instruments.
    (5) The index finger only is used to retract the cheek.

18. (5) The pen grasp is used for this purpose, because the instruments are used in a manner similar to that of writing with a pencil or pen.
    (1) The inverted pen grasp uses a clockwise rotation of the wrist.
    (2) The modified pen grasp is the same as the inverted pen grasp.
    (3) The palm grasp is for bulbous-handled instruments, such as pliers and forceps.
    (4) The palm-thumb grasp is similar to the palm grasp, except two fingers grasp and two fingers press against the instrument.

19. (2) Reversible functions (procedures) are delegated because they may be redone by the operator if incorrect or injury to the patient would result.
    (1) Irreversible functions are permanent.
    (3) Traditional functions are those that are recognized as being within the role of the dental hygienist.
    (4) A surgical function would be the cutting of hard and soft tissues.
    (5) A reparative function would be repair following the performance of a surgical function or perhaps the placement of a dressing or a base in a prepared tooth.

20. (3) Loading the perforated or rim-lock tray from the postdam area places the bulk of the material forward into the anterior area.
    (1) The side of the tray is difficult to load.
    (2) The posterior is near the postdam area.
    (4) The anterior of the tray is contoured and thus difficult to load.
    (5) It is difficult to load the bulk of the material in the cuspid area.

21. (4) Suturing tissue of a surgical flap laid by the periodontist by a dental hygienist is an expanded responsibility.
    (1) Deep scaling and curettage is a traditional function for a dental hygienist.
    (2) Root planing is a traditional function for a dental hygienist.
    (3) Making impressions for study casts is a traditional function for a dental hygienist and dental assistant.
    (5) Removing sutures is often delegated to the dental hygienist.

22. (4) The index finger presses on the palatal area, which aids in seating the tray and distributing material evenly throughout the arch.
    (1) The handle goes up as the tray is seated.
    (2) The sides of the tray go up as the tray is seated.
    (3) Tilting the postdam area distorts the impression.
    (5) Pressing on the anterior of the tray is ineffective.

23. (5) The coordinating assistant usually is in the area near the dental team and is therefore the logical person to contact the paramedics.
    (1) The dentist provides immediate first aid.
    (2) The chairside assistant provides support to the dentist.
    (3) The dental hygienist is treating a patient in the adjacent operatory.
    (4) The dental laboratory technician is working in the dental laboratory away from the stricken patient.

24. (4) The coordinating assistant dispenses, mixes, and loads the impression material into the impression tray and then hands the tray to the chairside assistant.
    (1) The chairside assistant passes and receives instruments.
    (2) The chairside assisant prepares and passes the anesthetic syringe.
    (3) The chairside assistants rinses and vacuums the patient's oral cavity.
    (5) The chairside assistant prepares the syringe with impression material.

25. (2) The chemically treated cord is laid at the distal aspect and then around the facial, mesial, and lingual aspects of the tooth with the cord extending slightly at the overlap to effect easy removal.
    (1) Poking the gingiva could cause trauma.
    (3) The mesial and distal aspects are one half of the gingiva to be retracted.
    (4) The facial and lingual aspects are one half of the gingiva to be retracted.
    (5) The gingiva should be displaced slightly as cord is placed into the sulcus.

26. (2) The vitalometer reading of a suspected tooth could be compared with the response of a normal tooth.
    (1) A radiographic survey is diagnosed by the dentist.
    (3) A periodontal probe is used to measure pocket depth.
    (4) A fiberoptic light is used as a reflector and with a handpiece to illuminate the operating field.
    (5) Percussion technique means tapping the tooth with the handle of an instrument to determine sensitivity.

27. (3) Calcium hydroxide is the mildest ingredient that can be placed over a pulpal exposure; if the area is free of contamination, the pulp may regenerate to heal itself.
    (1) Copal varnish is used to seal the exposed dentinal tubules.
    (2) Zinc oxide–eugenol is a palliative substance that may be placed over the calcium hydroxide.
    (4) A light-cured composite is a restorative material.
    (5) Zinc phosphate cement is used as a base over zinc oxide–eugenol and as a cementing medium for cast restorations.

28. (1) The 2 o'clock to 4 o'clock area at the left side of the patient is the area for the chairside assistant.
    (2) The 4 o'clock to 8 o'clock area is the transfer zone.
    (3) The 8 o'clock to 11 o'clock area is the operator's zone.
    (4) Optional—the 12 o'clock area is the operator's zone for indirect vision of the lingual aspect of the maxillary and mandibular anteriors.
    (5) The 12 o'clock to 2 o'clock area is the static zone for mobile equipment.

29. (3) The patient's chin is the dynamic area where instruments and materials are passed and received.
    (1) The chest is too low for exchange.
    (2) The lap is too far from the oral cavity.
    (4) The operator's hand in the fulcrum position at the oral cavity pivots toward the chin to receive and pass instruments.
    (5) The chance of injury to the patient by accidentally dropping an instrument is imminent.

30. (5) The high-velocity evacuator tip is positioned by the chairside assistant to retract the cheek or tongue before placement of the handpiece by the operator.
    (1) The mouth mirror could be positioned to retract the cheek or tongue after the assistant has placed the evacuator tip.
    (2) The operator positions the handpiece following placement of the high-velocity evacuator.
    (3) The saliva ejector would be appropriate if the operator were operating without a chairside assistant and not practicing four-handed dentistry.
    (4) The explorer is used briefly to examine the tooth before and intermittently during the preparation. It is not held in the mouth during the preparation.

31. (2) In rear delivery, a mobile dental unit or instrument cart placed perpendicular to the patient's head holds the instruments and materials for the assistant to pick up, pass, and receive from the operator.
    (1) In side delivery, the assistant passes instruments and materials from the instrument tray on the mobile cart placed in the traditional position.
    (3) In front delivery, the mobile instrument cart is at the upper left side of the patient. The assistant passes and receives the instruments and materials at the chin of the patient.
    (4) The static zone is the 12 o'clock to 2 o'clock area that may be used to position the mobile cart or dental unit.
    (5) The dynamic zone is at the chin of the patient and is also referred to as the area of exchange.

32. (3) A fulcrum (point of stabilization of an instrument using the fourth and fifth fingers) placed on teeth adjacent to the tooth being prepared is used to control the position and maneuverability of the handpiece.
    (1) The explorer is used with or without a fulcrum by placing the fine wirelike tip into the fissures and pits of tooth enamel to detect caries.
    (2) A mouth mirror is used without a fulcrum. It is used briefly for viewing (straight and indirect vision) the teeth and a preparation or restoration.
    (4) An impression tray does not require a fulcrum; it is loaded with material placed into the oral cavity and seated onto the teeth and dental arch.
    (5) A holder with articulating paper is held like a wand; it is used to place the articulating paper over the occlusal surfaces of the mandibular teeth. The patient is requested to occlude on the paper to enable the operator to detect high points on the restoration.

33. (5) Placing the jaws of the clamp just above the inverted dam at the cementoenamel junction would stabilize the dam and prevent leakage of moisture.
    (1) Placing the clamp on the tooth enamel could diminish stabilization and cause the clamp to slip off the tooth.
    (2) To avoid injury to the cementum, the clamp should not be placed far down on the cementum.
    (3) Placing the clamp on the margin of the rubber dam would prevent inversion of the dam.
    (4) The jaws of the rubber dam clamp placed at the cementoenamel junction just below the inverted rubber dam would not assure retraction or freedom from moisture.

34. (5) The operator may carefully retract the gingiva 1 mm from the proposed margin of the preparation.
    (1) Gingiva would be in the way of instruments and burs and could be injured.
    (2) Retraction of 0.25 mm is not sufficient clearance of the area for the operator.
    (3) Retraction of 0.5 mm is the minimum amount of retraction.
    (4) Retraction of 0.75 mm may be sufficient in some cases depending on the location of the class V caries.

35. (3) The instrument for passing and receiving is grasped at the end opposite the one to be used.
    (1) Grasping at the nib of the instrument will contaminate it.
    (2) Grasping at the point will contaminate the instrument.
    (4) Grasping at the center of the handle will make it difficult to pass the instrument.
    (5) Grasping at the end to be used will contaminate the instrument.

36. (3) The tip (lumen) of the high-velocity evacuator is placed near the posterior tooth being prepared and directed to the posterior of the oral cavity to be out of the line of vision of the operator.
    (1) The tip must be placed near the tooth being prepared to evacuate the debris.
    (2) The tip must be near the tooth under preparation and directed toward the posterior to keep out of the operator's line of vision.
    (4) If a posterior tooth is being prepared, the tip is directed to the posterior of the arch.
    (5) To direct the lumen toward the anterior when preparing a posterior tooth would block the line of vision of the operator.

37. (2) The side of the high-velocity evacuator tip is placed to retract the patient's cheek and/or tongue before placement of the handpiece by the operator.
    (1) The high-velocity evacuator is used to remove excess fluids and debris and is not designed to dry the oral cavity.
    (3) The high-velocity evacuator may be used to displace the tongue to the side of the floor of the mouth, as when the mandibular posteriors are under preparation; however, the tongue tissue would be injured by the suction of the tip if the tongue were held by the high-velocity evacuator.
    (4) The high-velocity evacuator does not retract gingiva or other soft tissues; to do so would cause trauma.
    (5) The *side* of the tip extension of the high-velocity evacuator may be laid against the lip for partial retraction. The suction of the high-velocity evacuator tip would injure the soft tissue if the tip were held intentionally for a period of time.

38. (3) For safety, the handpiece is held at the upper chest (chin) of the patient during removal and insertion of burs, stones, and mandrels.
    (1) Changing burs at the back of the patient's head creates an extra motion for the operator and the assistant.
    (2) Exchanging burs, mandrels, and stones in the handpiece at the oral cavity might result in injury to the patient if the accessory were dropped or if the handpiece slipped when the accessory was forced into the clutch or sleeve of the handpiece.
    (4) Maintaining a fulcrum is appropriate for the exchange of instruments only.
    (5) Changing burs, stones, and mandrels in the handpiece at the side of the patient's face is acceptable if it is done away from the dynamic area of treatment.

39. (4) The area of exchange is at the patient's chin to prevent dropping instruments or material and causing injury to the patient.
    (1) The chest of the patient is too low, requiring extra motions for the operator and the assistant.
    (2) Passing the syringe at the oral cavity could produce an injury if it were dropped; also, the patient is able to see the syringe at that location.
    (3) The rear of the patient's head is used only if the patient is extremely tense or, in the case of small children, to prevent unnecessary fear.
    (5) Passing the syringe over the instrument tray would cause an awkward motion for the operator, resulting in an unnatural position.

40. (5) The chin of the patient is the safe area to pass or receive instruments or materials.
    (1) The oral cavity does not provide maneuverability for instruments, pads, and materials.
    (2) The chest of the patient is too low for effective passing of material, since it might drop from the carrying instrument. In addition, the operator must make an additional motion to pick up the material.
    (3) The upper part of the face could incur possible injury to the eyes or cheeks of the patient if something were accidently dropped.
    (4) The cheeks might be injured if the material or an instrument were dropped.

41. (3) A small excavator is used to carry and to place a slight depth of sedative dressing over the pulpal area of a deep preparation.
    (1) A Wedelstaedt chisel is used to remove undermined enamel in the preparation of the tooth.
    (2) Cotton pliers are used to hold cotton pellets moistened with cavity varnish, not a thick or semithick sedative dressing.
    (4) A plastic-type instrument is used to place a bulk of malleable plastic-type material into a cavity preparation (e.g., a composite restorative material in an anterior tooth).
    (5) An angle former is used to finish the retention or marginal area of a cavity preparation.

42. (2) The handpiece is received by the dental assistant with the fourth and fifth fingers of the left hand; the air-water syringe is passed into the operator's right hand in the position of use.
    (1) In this instance the mouth mirror would be held in the operator's left hand and the assistant would receive it in the right hand.
    (3) The assistant's right hand would be receiving the mouth mirror, not the handpiece, because the handpiece is in the operator's right hand.
    (4) It is acceptable to pass the air-water syringe and explorer at the same time if the two hands of the operator pass both instruments simultaneously; this was not stated, however.
    (5) The handpiece would be in the operator's right hand, since he is right handed.

43. (1) Seated at the 9 o'clock position, the operator examines the lingual surface of a maxillary anterior tooth by rotating the wrist and inserting the mouth mirror into the oral cavity from the side.
    (2) The pen grasp and fulcrum are used to stabilize the handpiece for preparation of tooth No. 19 (first mandibular molar, left quadrant).
    (3) The enamel chisel would be used with a palm-thumb grasp.
    (4) The pen grasp is used to condense amalgam on the occlusal of the mandibular teeth.
    (5) A palm grasp is used to direct and to stabilize a forceps used to extract a tooth.

44. (5) The soft palate is avoided at all times when placing the high-velocity evacuator tip. To touch the soft palate would stimulate a violent choking and gagging reflex, causing extreme discomfort to the patient.
    (1) The free gingiva is very short in length and would not be affected by the high-velocity evacuator.
    (2) The high-velocity evacuator tip is laid on its side over the tongue to avoid injury to soft tissues.
    (3) The buccal mucosae (cheeks) are retracted by placing the side of the tube extension against the cheek; if suction occurs, the tube is twisted to break free of the tissue.
    (4) The tube extension of the high-velocity evacuator is laid across the floor of the oral cavity. A quick fluorish of the vacuum tip will remove the saliva and debris without injury to the soft tissues.

45. (4) The dental laboratory technician is qualified through training to receive a prescription (work order) specifying requirements for a prosthesis. The technician is legally authorized to construct the prosthesis for the dentist.
    (1) The dental hygienist is educationally qualified to perform other dental procedures (not fabricating a prosthesis), particularly in the preventive area of dentistry.
    (2) The dentist could construct the dental prosthesis; however, it is a time-consuming effort and his or her services are needed for direct patient care. Delegation of the fabrication of a prosthesis to the dental laboratory technician is legal in all states.
    (3) The expanded-function dental auxiliary is effective in the area of supportive restorative procedures and construction of diagnostic aids, not in fabricating a prosthesis. Fabrication of custom trays and custom temporary coverage of teeth may be delegated to the extended-function dental auxiliary, however.
    (5) The coordinating dental assistant provides supportive assistance to the dental team, (e.g., exposing film for radiographic surveys, obtaining preliminary impressions, etc.).

46. (3) Orthodontics lends itself readily to using six-handed dentistry, particularly during the direct bonding of brackets, cementing of bands, taking of alginate impressions, etc.

    (1) Prosthodontics would use six-handed dentistry during the taking of multiple impressions.

    (2) Pedodontics would use six-handed dentistry during the taking of impressions and administration of sedation analgesia (nitrous oxide and oxygen).

    (4) Oral surgery would be closest to orthodontics in using six-handed dentistry—during surgery with a patient under general anesthesia (e.g., maintaining a free airway, evacuation of the oral cavity, monitoring the patient's vital signs and intravenous medication etc.)

    (5) Periodontics would be the least likely to adapt to six-handed dentistry. Periodontics does however, use the services of the dental hygienist.

47. (1) According to the individual state dental practice act (board of dental examiners, rules and regulations interpreting and implementing the dental practice act), the expanded-function dental auxiliary may be trained to perform the clinical examination of a patient's oral cavity, usually under the general supervision of a dentist.

    (2) The dental laboratory technician is qualified to construct casts, custom trays, temporary appliances, and prostheses. The technician works by prescription (work order) from the dentist to the laboratory and does not work directly with the patient.

    (3) The dental hygienist may assume the role of the expanded-function dental auxiliary with special training in the expanded function to be delegated: the oral examination.

    (4) The chairside assistant too may be trained in the role of the expanded-function dental auxiliary if the particular state dental practice act and the rules and regulations stipulate the delegation.

    (5) The coordinating assistant is responsible for the supportive services (e.g., radiographic surveys, primary impressions, and assisting in medical emergencies as needed by the dental team and patient).

48. (2) The administrative assistant is the office manager, responsible for all records, payroll, payments on accounts by patients, purchasing for the office, and accounts payable.

    (1) The chairside assistant is assigned responsibility primarily to the dental operatory, the patient, and to assisting the dentist.

    (3) The coordinating assistant assists as a backup for the chairside assistant and is responsible for sterilization of instruments, tray setups, equipment for preparing the operatory, receiving and dismissing the patients, etc.

    (4) The dental laboratory technician works in the dental laboratory on cases that are prescribed in the various work orders. Most states demand that each patient's case be accompanied by a work order (prescription).

    (5) The dental hygienist performs preventive treatment for patients and may through additional training administer local anesthesia, nitrous oxide and oxygen as analgesia sedation, etc.

49. (2) The dental hygienist may legally be delegated the administration of the analgesia (nitrous oxide and oxygen) in a state that permits it if the dental hygienist has had special training.

    (1) The dentist is legally qualified to administer the analgesia following special training in the chemistry and reaction of the nitrous oxide and oxygen used for conscious sedation.

    (3) The chairside assistant is trained to assist with the administration of nitrous oxide and oxygen under the direct supervision of the dentist. The chairside assistant is not permitted to administer the gases.

    (4) The coordinating assistant is limited to assisting with the administration of nitrous oxide and oxygen as a sedation, assisting the dentist, under direct supervision.

    (5) The expanded-function dental auxiliary may have the function of administering analgesia included in the training program if it is allowed by the particular state where the expanded-function dental auxiliary is employed.

50. (1) Calcium hydroxide (Ca_2OH) is a mild-acting cavity liner that encourages the formation of dentinal cells by forming a protective layer between the pulp and the restorative material.

    (2) Zinc oxide–eugenol is effective as a sedative base material.

    (3) Zinc phosphate cement is effective as an insulating base; however, it should not be used on a near pulpal exposure or an exposure.

    (4) Copal varnish (sealer) is an effective sealer of dentinal tubules that have been exposed during the preparation of the cavity.

    (5) Reversile colloids, commonly referred to as hydrocolloids, are fine impression materials that must be processed in airtight containers in a water bath.

51. (3) Pit and fissure sealants are placed on enamel surfaces that have been etched with phosphoric acid, rinsed thoroughly, and dried.

    (1) An insulating base is placed on the dry floor of the preparation to insulate the pulp of the tooth from thermal changes.

    (2) A cavity sealer (varnish) is used to seal the tubules and the cavity margins of a freshly prepared tooth before placement of a restoration.

    (4) Zinc phosphate cement base is placed in the base of the cavity preparation and serves as insulation of the pulp from a metallic restoration.

    (5) Zinc oxide–eugenol base is insulative and palliative to the pulp of the tooth. It is not used with the acid-etching procedure.

52. (4) Representation of the frenum (frena) of the maxillary arch within the maxillary impression is essential to produce an exact reproduction of the arch when the cast is poured. The postdam area must also be represented.
    (1) The retromolar area is a landmark posterior to the third molars in the mandibular arch.
    (2) The mylohyoid ridge is a landmark relating to muscle attachments on the lingual or mesial surface of the mandible.
    (3) The genial tubercles are landmarks relating to muscle attachments at the lingual midline area near the inferior border of the mandible.
    (5) The oblique ridges are landmarks on the facial surface of the mandible caused by muscle attachments.

53. (2) A 2% solution of potassium sulfate prevents the alginate impression from dehydrating and prevents inhibition if stored in the solution for a brief period (10 to 15 minutes).
    (1) A damp cloth or paper towel is used as the second choice if the potassium sulfate solution is not available. Storage of a fresh impression in a moist towel should be for a very brief period only.
    (3) A humidor provides 100% humidity and is used to prevent shrinkage of the stone that has just been poured into an impression.
    (4) A safe place is a fair substitute, but the answer needs to be more specific, such as the 2% potassium sulfate solution.
    (5) A 2% saline solution does not serve as a neutral solution; in fact, the saline would possibly draw water from the impression if left for any length of time.

54. (4) Polycarboxylate (polyacrylate) cement forms a favorable bond with the enamel and the dentin.
    (1) EBA permanent cementation is added to eugenol and increases the strength of the mix; however it is not as favored as polycarboxylate.
    (2) Calcium hydroxide, used as a cavity liner, has very low crushing strength and is not effective as a cementing medium.
    (3) Zinc phosphate cement is used as an insulative base or as a temporary restoration.
    (5) Zinc oxide–eugenol, used as an insulative base, has low crushing strength and is not effective as a cementing medium.

55. (4) After the enamel surface (usually the facial surface) is etched, rinsed, and dried, the facial surface is prepared with a slight mechanical retention to help retain the composite.
    (1) To cover the etched enamel surface with composite veneer would probably not be sufficient to retain the veneer.
    (2) Covering the enire crown in cosmetic dentistry is effective; however, it is a more radical mode of treatment, when veneer is usually sufficient.
    (3) Preparing a full crown would be a radical mode of treatment.
    (5) Temporary coverage usually entails preparing a custom-made temporary crown and is not included in the category of cosmetic dentistry.

CHAPTER 17

Practice Management and Career
Development Strategies

SANDRA KRAMER

Achieving and maintaining a successful position as a valued health care provider requires not only knowledge and skill in one's profession, but also a basic understanding of business management and career development strategies. This chapter is designed to bridge the gap between the educational preparation of the dental hygienist and the reality of the working world. Topics reviewed in this chapter include practice building and management, marketing skills and strategies, employment situations, compensation, job performance, communication techniques, résumé preparation, interviewing, job search strategies and job selection considerations, employment retention and mobility, and personal financial planning. Intentional involvement of the dental hygienist in these concepts should contribute to increased effectiveness as a team member and greater personal career satisfaction.

THE DENTAL HYGIENIST AS A MEMBER
OF THE DENTAL TEAM

The Team Concept

A. Definition—combined actions with interdependence of the entire dental office staff to promote the unit and efficiency of the group rather than individual interests; "team spirit" is affected by each member
B. Team members
  1. Dentists
  2. Dental hygienists
  3. Dental assistants
  4. Receptionists
  5. Office managers
  6. Dental laboratory technicians
  7. Bookkeepers
  8. Patients

C. Goals
  1. High-quality dental care
  2. Decentralized management, with each person accepting responsibility and participating in decision making
  3. Work simplification
  4. Increased efficiency
  5. Reduction in work time
  6. Increased practice profitability
  7. Office harmony and comradery within an enjoyable and supportive environment
  8. Job satisfaction for all individuals with achievement of self-esteem and self-actualization
  9. Professional growth for each individual
D. Characteristics of an effective work team[9]
  1. Group atmosphere is informal, comfortable, relaxed, and supportive, producing a feeling of belonging
  2. Flexibility exists to accommodate for change
  3. People talk to one another, mostly about the job to be done
  4. Job tasks, roles, and functions are well understood and accepted by the staff, with recognition of the special contributions of each individual
  5. Staff members respect and value one another
  6. Staff members maturely listen to one another and are unafraid to express ideas and opinions; attempts are made to resolve differences, and personnel can accept unresolvable disagreement
  7. There is fusion of ideas, energy, and individual expertise
  8. Most decisions are reached by consensus, with individuals realizing the importance of a total and united team effort for ultimate benefit to all

9. Criticism is frequent, honest, and relatively comfortable
10. People express their feelings
11. Innovation and change are accepted and are frequent
12. When action is taken, clear assignments are made and accepted; action is immediate
13. Goals are periodically reevaluated, with adjustments made as needed
14. Leader of the group does not dominate; leadership may shift from person to person

E. Team elements
   1. Interpersonal
      a. Open and frequent communications throughout each day maintain fluid patient and procedural activities
      b. Regular staff meetings
         (1) Purposes
             (a) Review goals
             (b) Evaluate progress
             (c) Share updated information
             (d) Air grievances
             (e) Problem solve and reach agreement on solutions
         (2) Design
             (a) State the purpose of the meeting
             (b) Prepare and distribute the agenda in advance
             (c) Consider agenda items and suggestions from all staff members
             (d) Share discussions among all members; no single person dominates the meeting
             (e) Reach decisions by consensus
             (f) Stay on track; do not stray off of the agenda
             (g) End on a positive, team-building note
      c. Includes quality human relations between all office personnel, patients, and members of the professional community
   2. Organizational
      a. Practice philosophy, goals, and objectives are determined by the team and written to direct daily activities
      b. Policy and procedures manuals systematize the practice and clearly familiarize personnel with responsibilities
      c. Staff meetings include organizational and administrative evaluation and control

F. Team building
   1. Definition—synergistic process of developing group goals with motivation and commitment

2. Technique
   a. Participation of all members
   b. Dissemination of information
   c. Sharing of ideas
   d. Formulation of goals, objectives, and priorities
   e. Critique of plans and anticipation of obstacles
   f. Modification of goals and objectives
   g. Activation of plans
   h. Evaluation of plans
   i. Revisions as needed

Successful Patient Management

A. Attitudes toward patients
   1. Patient is the most important person in the practice, the purpose for work and for the existence of the dental practice
   2. Patient is a member of the "team" and must be included in all decisions about his or her oral care
   3. Each individual is approached as a whole person, including medical, psychologic, and emotional aspects
   4. A variety of value systems exist, which are different; intrinsic worth of each individual person is appreciated
   5. Patient's personal resources are acknowledged[12]
      a. Level of self-esteem
      b. Experiential background and previous history
      c. Intelligence
      d. Motivation
      e. Values
      f. Socioeconomic level

B. Communications[12]
   1. People communicate to satisfy needs
      a. Need to survive—physiologic
      b. Need for safety and comfort—physical and psychologic security
      c. Interpersonal needs—social needs for acceptance, love, and recognition
      d. Intrapersonal needs—self-esteem and self-actualization
   2. Clear and accurate communication between members of the dental team and patients is critical to successful patient management
      a. Effective communication requires skills in both sending and receiving messages
         (1) Verbal
         (2) Nonverbal
         (3) Written

b. Dental appointments often cause increased stress and anxiety partly by
  (1) Dental discomfort, pain, or problems
  (2) Treatments and procedures
  (3) Exclusive behavior of personnel
  (4) Unfamiliar environment
  (5) Fear of the unknown or outcome
3. All communications and behaviors have meaning and result from inner thoughts or feelings
4. Maintain an open, accepting environment by being understanding, permissive, nonjudgmental, and honest
5. Recognize the patient as an individual person
  a. Call the patient by name
  b. Refer to others in the office by name
  c. Be courteous to the patient and others who may accompany the patient
  d. Respect the patient's personal privacy
  e. Support the patient's dignity
  f. Maintain confidentiality
6. Eliminate barriers created by the dental office whenever possible
  a. Be flexible in carrying out routines and policies
  b. Explain procedures before beginning
  c. Avoid the use of dental jargon that excludes the patient
  d. Encourage patient participation in discussions and decision making
7. Identify the patient's needs and determine priorities for care
  a. Educate the patient about the findings
  b. Help the patient understand the nature of the findings and accept needed care and consequences
  c. Gain patient input to establish priorities together
  d. Be nonjudgmental and nonpunitive in your response and behavior; do not "lecture" the patient
C. Establishment of a teaching-learning environment[12] (see Chapter 12, section on stages in commitment to a new behavior, and Chapter 15, section on implementation)
  1. Definitions
    a. Teaching—communication designed to produce learning
    b. Learning—activity by which knowledge, attitudes, and skills are acquired, resulting in behavior change
  2. Goals of learning
    a. Acquiring knowledge—cognitive
    b. Developing attitudes—effective
    c. Developing psychomotor skills—conative

3. Principles of the teaching-learning process
  a. Learning occurs best when there is a perceived need or readiness to learn
    (1) Identify the patient's motivational readiness
    (2) Identify the patient's experiential readiness
    (3) Determine the patient's level of adaptation
    (4) Consider the patient's level of human needs
    (5) Recognize the signs of learning readiness
      (a) Awareness—patient develops awareness of the oral health problem
      (b) Interest—patient asks direct questions
      (c) Desire—patient seeks information
      (d) Action—patient's dental disease condition allows the dental personnel to intervene through teaching
    (6) Once the need has been recognized by the patient and readiness has been determined, develop a plan and teach
  b. Method of presentation of material influences the patient's ability to learn
    (1) Keep information organized, accurate, and brief
    (2) Institute appropriate teaching methods
      (a) Concepts are best taught with discussions and visual aids
      (b) Attitudes are best taught by exploration of feelings, discussion, and an atmosphere of acceptance
      (c) Skills are best taught by illustrations, models, demonstration, return demonstration, feedback, and practice
    (3) Encourage patients to ask questions and answer them directly
    (4) Provide opportunities for evaluation
  c. Learning is easier when new material is related to what the learner already knows
    (1) Find out what the patient knows about the situation or problem
    (2) Reinforce the knowledge base, then relate new information to similar, previous experiences
    (3) Teach at the patient's level of understanding, based on the foundation of the present knowledge
    (4) Avoid the use of technical jargon

d. Learning is purposeful—short-term and long-term goals identify desired behavior
   (1) Set goals with the patient
   (2) Criteria of goals
       (a) Specific—state exactly what is to be accomplished
       (b) Measurable—set a minimum acceptable level of performance
       (c) Realistic—must be reasonably achievable
e. Learning is an active process and takes place within the learner
   (1) Use a teaching approach that actively involves the learner
   (2) Provide opportunities for the patient to practice new skills
   (3) Encourage self-directed activities
f. Every individual has capabilities and strengths that can help him or her to learn
   (1) Identify the patient's personal resources
   (2) Build on identified strengths
   (3) Use personal resources
   (4) Try to adapt recommended behavior changes to the patient's life-style
g. Overall health, outside stresses, and energy will affect the patient's ability to learn and perform
h. Learning does not always advance straight ahead—expect plateaus and remissions with a resulting change in needs
   (1) Accept the patient's feelings regarding lack of progress
   (2) Identify progress that has been made
   (3) Be patient; do not cause additional stress to the patient
   (4) Try alternative approaches for achieving goals
   (5) Identify short-term goals with which the patient can agree
   (6) Alter long-term goals if necessary
4. Motivation
   a. Definition—progress of stimulting a person to assimlate certain concepts or behavior
   b. Principles related to dental hygiene approaches
      (1) Each patient deserves to be cared for as a whole being, as a complex product of life's experiences—be accepting and respectful
      (2) Learning is best when information coincides with the patient's own attitudes and value system

(3) A motivated learner assimilates new information more rapidly than a nonmotivated learner
(4) Intrinsic motivation (stimulated from within the learner) is preferable to extrinsic motivation (stimulated from outside the learner)
    (a) Identify factors that are essential for the patient to have a meaningful achievement
    (b) Satisfaction with learning progress promotes additional learning; therefore design teaching to assist the patient in attaining a feeling of meaningful achievement
    (c) Encourage the patient to participate and be self-directed
(5) Information is learned more readily when it is relevant and meaningful to the patient
    (a) Help the patient interpret why the information is important and how new information will be useful
    (b) Relate information by building on the patient's foundation of knowledge, experience, attitudes, and feelings
(6) Learning motivated by success or rewards is preferable to learning by failure or punishment
    (a) Help the patient set realistic goals, focusing on abilities and strengths
    (b) Select learning tasks in which the patient is likely to succeed
    (c) Help the patient master or feel successful at each stage of instruction before going on to the next
    (d) Accept errors as part of the learning process
    (e) Teach tolerance for failure by recalling previous successes
(7) Planned reinforcement is essential for learning
    (a) Identify factors that are stimulants or incentives
    (b) Provide visible reinforcements
    (c) Use repetition as a form of reinforcement (repeated activities become habitual)
        [1] Provide opportunity for the patient to practice old and new skills
        [2] Review information previously taught

(8) Evaluation of performance aids in
learning
   (a) Purpose
      [1] Measure and interpret results
         compared with goals set
      [2] Reinforce correct behavior
      [3] Help the learner realize how to
         change incorrect behavior
      [4] Help the teacher determine
         adequacy of teaching
   (b) Teacher and learner observe and
      evaluate together in relation to the
      desired behavior
   (c) Reasons for a good or poor
      evaluation require explanation
   (d) Criticism and value judgments must
      relate to the performance, not the
      individual
D. Case presentations
   1. Definition—process of presenting examination
      data to the patient along with treatment options
      and recommendations to reach agreement on the
      treatment plan
   2. Elements
      a. Information—share the findings of the
         examination with the patient; use charts,
         radiographs, photographs, and study models
         to give clear and complete explanation
      b. Education—explain the significance of the
         findings to the patient in terms of short- and
         long-range consequences; ask questions that
         bring the patient into the discussion so you
         can determine his or her interest
      c. Options—present alternative methods of
         treatment including benefits, time, risk, and
         cost for each
      d. Choice—based on the patient's
         understanding of data presented, desires,
         and perceived needs
      e. Agreement—patient and professional concur
         on a course to follow and who will be
         responsible for what
   3. Case presentations for dental hygiene therapy
      a. Dental hygienist may be responsible for data
         collection and presentation of findings and
         records to the dentist for agreement on
         treatment options; dental hygienist then
         presents the findings and alternatives to the
         patient

      b. Dentist may perform data collection and
         case presentation and then present the dental
         hygienist with a prescription for the total
         dental hygiene therapy plan as agreed on by
         the patient; in this case the dental hygienist
         should review the plan with the patient
         before beginning treatment procedures
E. Failure to communicate
   1. Dental hygienists play an important role in the
      continuity of care and must report observations
      to the supervising dentist, especially alterations
      in dental health progress
   2. Failure or delay in communicating important
      patient findings is considered unethical and can
      result in a malpractice lawsuit against the dental
      hygienist
   3. Documenation of data without provision of
      verbal information can also lead to liability;
      although dental hygienists are not legally
      allowed to diagnose or plan treatments, the
      courts believe dental hygienists possess the skill
      necessary to recognize dental disease and make
      discriminating professional judgments (see
      Chapter 19, section on legal relationships in
      dental hygiene practice)
F. Patient noncompliance[3]
   1. Definition—lack of patient cooperation with
      recommended dental care
   2. Examples
      a. Routine tardy arrival for scheduled
         appointments
      b. Failure to keep appointments
      c. Unwillingness to have necessary diagnostic
         tests, such as radiographs
      d. Unwillingness to accept recommended
         specific procedures or the treatment plan
      e. Unwillingness to accept referrals to
         specialists
      f. Failure to use medications as instructed
      g. Failure to follow the oral hygiene regimen
   3. Significance
      a. Results in compromised dental care
      b. If there is a lawsuit, the decision outcome
         or amount of settlement may be altered
         based on negligence
   4. Managing noncompliance
      a. Recognize it when it happens
      b. Document any instances in the patient's
         records
         (1) Note your explanation of recommended
            care
         (2) Note observation that instructions are
            not being followed

(3) Note the patient's disinclination to follow instructions and the reason
(4) Note your discussion of consequences of not following instructions
G. Patient correspondence
1. Written communications from the dental hygienist to the patient might include
a. Follow-up to review what was discussed during the appointment
b. Reinforcement to encourage new skills and behavior
c. Reminder of the need to schedule an appointment
d. Personal congratulations, well wishes, or sympathy note
e. Thank-you notes
2. Value
a. Establishes the dental hygienist as an individual within the dental practice
b. Promotes the practice in general

The Dental Hygienist as a Team Member

A. Dental hygienist's role
1. Contributes knowledge, skills, and experience to the dental office team
2. Establishes a mutually cooperative relationship with co-workers to support one another and gain individual daily satisfaction
3. Develops office friendships
4. Establishes and maintains professional behavior with genuine interest in quality patient care and the success of the dental practice
B. Dental hygienist's clinical contributions to the practice
1. Data collection
a. Medical health history
b. Dental health history
c. Nutritional/dietary history
d. Vital signs—body temperature, blood pressure, pulse, and respiration
e. Extraoral examination
f. Intraoral examination
g. Periodontal examination
h. Dental examination—restorations, caries, defects, wear, etc.
i. Occlusal examination
j. Myofunctional examination
k. Plaque and calculus examination
l. Radiographic survey
m. Impressions for study models
n. Exfoliative cytology
o. Photography

2. Data organization
a. Charting and record keeping for all of the preceding
b. Legal evidence
3. Prioritization of treatments
a. Sequencing of services
b. Case presentation to the dentist and/or the patient
4. Dental hygiene therapy (services vary according to state practice acts)
a. Plaque control instruction
b. Dietary/nutritional counseling
c. Pain control
(1) Topical anesthesia
(2) Local anesthesia
(3) Nitrous oxide and oxygen analgesia
d. Scaling and root planing
e. Soft tissue curettage
f. Coronal polishing
g. Instrument sharpening
h. Overhanging restoration removal
i. Amalgam restoration carving and polishing
j. Fluoride therapy
k. Occlusal pit and fissure sealants
l. Desensitization of exposed root surfaces
m. Temporary restoration placement and removal
n. Periodontal dressing placement and removal
o. Suture removal
p. Removable appliance care
q. Cardiopulmonary resuscitation
5. Case evaluation
a. Repeated data collection
b. Comparison of data to assess treatment results
c. Recommendation for further care or maintenance interval
C. Integral contributions of the dental hygienist[7]
1. Assumes responsibility for services rendered with a respectable level of competence
2. Provides release time for the dentist—performs all procedures legal for dental hygienists, thereby freeing the dentist's time for highest-level services
3. Markets dental services—reports dental needs to patients or dental work that will be needed in the future if restorations deteriorate or the patient wishes to change existing dental conditions (see section on marketing dentistry—practice promotion)
4. Professional associate of the dentist—participates in case evaluation and treatment planning for dental hygiene therapy

5. Practice builder—communicates with patients as a professional relations specialist, interpreter, confidante, practice ambassador, and friend
6. Public relations promoter—speaks highly of dentistry in general when away from the dental office
7. Dental disease prevention specialist—educates patients to assume responsibility and care for their own dental health

Practice Administration

A. Definition—organization and management of a professional practice; effective practice management benefits patients and staff members alike by serving more people with increased efficiency, saving time and money, reducing pressure and tension, and increasing personal satisfaction
B. Personnel management
   1. Policy manual
      a. Purpose—outlines practice principles
      b. Content
         (1) Practice philosophy
            (a) General attitudes and goals
            (b) Specific objectives
            (c) Issues regarding the success of the practice, standards of patient care, and satisfaction for all
         (2) Team approach/personnel involvement
         (3) Specific standards of patient care for quality assurance and education
         (4) Personnel policies
         (5) Employment regulations
         (6) Work arrangements
         (7) Guidelines of professional ethics and conduct
         (8) Referrals to specialists
         (9) Office charts, forms, and documentation guidelines
         (10) Appointment administration/fees and financing
         (11) Office safety and emergencies
         (12) Service to the community
   2. Procedures manual
      a. Purpose
         (1) Assigns responsibility and describes routines
         (2) Provides a job description for each position in the office (clearly defining all aspects of performance), outlines expectations, and serves as a guideline for performance review
      b. Contents
         (1) Job titles
         (2) Job summaries—key elements of positions; examples include
            (a) Updating of medical histories
            (b) Oral examinations
            (c) Exposing and processing of radiographs
            (d) Oral hygiene instruction
            (e) Scaling, root planing, and coronal polishing
            (f) Application of fluorides
            (g) Adjunctive services
            (h) Record keeping and documentation
            (i) Scheduling of appointments
         (3) Duties—examples
            (a) Daily routines
               [1] Opening the office
               [2] Greeting patients
               [3] Communicating with the dentist and support staff
               [4] Preparing tray setups
               [5] Sterilizing instruments
               [6] Sanitizing the operatory
               [7] Closing the office
            (b) Operatory maintenance
               [1] Decor for comfort, beauty, and personalization
               [2] Overall organization and cleanliness
               [3] Regular maintenance of the dental equipment
               [4] Care of dental instruments
               [5] Restocking of supplies/ inventory control
               [6] Light housekeeping
               [7] Special tasks
         (4) Qualifications—requirements for job applicants
   3. See sections on the team concept and dentist– dental hygienist relationship
C. Patient management
   1. See section on successful patient management
   2. Scheduling of patients[13]—time management is critical to the success of the practice and to quality patient care
      a. Appointment control—appointment book
         (1) Clearly block out time for staff meetings, lunch hours, days off, holidays, vacations, time away from the office for professional meetings, etc., as far in advance as possible

(2) Appointment book management systems
    (a) Unlimited future booking—appointments are scheduled as far in advance as is necessary to accommodate all patients; requires careful advance planning for time away from the office
    (b) Restricted appointment booking—limits appointments to a specified time period, such as 1 to 3 months; patients who are not scheduled during this time are placed on a call list and are telephoned when appointments become available
    (c) Waiting list is maintained of patients who need appointments and are available on short notice to fill cancellations

(3) Scheduling time allotments
    (a) Specific amount of time is designated for each appointment based on the needs of each patient
    (b) Usual dental hygiene appointments run from 45 minutes to 1 hour
    (c) Additional time may be scheduled for new patients, patients with difficult periodontal conditions, management problems, etc.
    (d) Less time may be scheduled for children or patients with partial dentitions

(4) Appointment book entries (write in pencil)
    (a) Patient's name
    (b) Daytime telephone number—identify if it is a work *(w)* or home *(h)* number
    (c) Service/type of appointment—*R,* recall; *NP,* new patient; *Q,* quadrant root planing and curettage
    (d) Length of appointment time/number of time units
    (e) Special instructions—''premedicate,'' ''local anesthesia,'' ''dentist appointment follows''

b. ''Recall'' health maintenance systems
(1) Purposes
    (a) Organizes and maintains dental checkups and periodontal maintenance therapy on a regular schedule according to patient needs
    (b) Ensures maximum number of patients receive periodic dental care

(2) Types
    (a) Advance scheduling—definite future reservation is made, requiring that the appointment book be available 6 to 12 month in advance; patients are reminded by a postcard and/or telephone call approximately 2 weeks before the actual date
    (b) Reminder card—notifies the patient by mail that it is time for the health maintenance checkup and requests the patient to phone the office to schedule an appointment; assigns responsibility to the patient to set up the appointment, and the office maintains cross-reference of who is due
    (c) Telephone reminder—patient is contacted by phone, and a definite appointment is scheduled
    (d) Combination—all systems are available within the office with flexibility of choice based on patient preference

(3) Recall references
    (a) Triplicate appointment card—one copy is given to the patient, the second one is filed with the patient's chart, and the third one becomes a postcard reminder to be mailed before the appointment; can schedule a definite appointment or note it is time for the patient to call the office to schedule an appointment
    (b) Tickler file—monthly grouping of patients' cards needing appointments; each contains a record of previous appointments, what is needed now, and how to best contact and schedule the patient
    (c) Alphabetical file—by patient name; card lists previous appointments and what is needed next
    (d) Cross-references combine duplicates of the above

c. Patient ''reclamation''
(1) Definition—periodic purging of all files to harvest ''fugitive'' patients to either complete unfinished therapy or return after an extended absence from dental care

(2) Systems
  (a) Send a card or note stating the date of the last appointment and what needs to be done
  (b) Telephone the patient to discuss dental needs and learn patient preferences
3. Payment arrangements
  a. Payment at the time of service is usual and customary for dental practices
  b. Some offices offer a small discount (5%) for payment on the day of service to encourage immediate payment
  c. For dental care more extensive than routine dental hygiene services, arrangements may be made to extend payments over 30 to 60 days
  d. Some offices assess a finance charge for accounts delinquent over 30 days
  e. Patients covered by insurance benefits may pay for services themselves and be reimbursed by the insurance carrier, or the office may bill and collect from the insurance company first and then bill the patient for the balance.
  f. For financial arrangements, options should be available to accommodate different patient preferences
D. Office management
  1. Operatory and equipment maintenance
    a. Written guidelines outline required procedures with recommended intervals for best results
    b. Each staff member is assigned appropriate areas of responsibility
  2. Supply and inventory control
    a. Aids office efficiency to maintain an adequate stock and avoid accumulation or waste from excess items
    b. Consists of itemized lists of supplies and materials used in the office
      (1) Storage location
      (2) Purchase information
        (a) Item
        (b) Cost
        (c) Supplier
        (d) Quantity
        (e) Frequency
        (f) Date ordered and when received
      (3) Minimum stock for reorder

c. May group items and assign inventory control to different staff members
  (1) Receptionist—administrative supplies
  (2) Dental assistant—general dental supplies
  (3) Dental hygienist—oral hygiene supplies
E. Records management
  1. Value/purposes
    a. Permanent documents provide a "written memory" of what transpired
    b. Organization of data collection—should be brief, neat, complete, accurate, and easy to read
    c. Evaluation aids for diagnosis
    d. Management aids for decision making and treatment planning
    e. Educational aids for patient information and instruction
    f. Protection of the patient regarding general health and discovery of dental diseases
    g. Behavior modification tools to establish the patient's goal orientation
    h. Enhancement of patient confidence in professionals and the practice
    i. Communication devices to enhance professionals' mutual case comprehension
    j. "Roadmap" for instrumentation guide
    k. Regulation of care to identify conditions beyond normal limits or variations from previous conditions
    l. "Trend analysis" of data for long-term evaluation and decision making
    m. Guidance for consistent-quality therapy
    n. Integration for correlation of tissue conditions, oral hygiene, treatment, and responses
    o. Third-party justification and satisfaction
    p. Accountability for demonstration of responsible care
    q. Legal protection to present documentary evidence for defense if necessary
  2. Elements
    a. Written patient records
      (1) Patient registration form with administrative information
      (2) Health history, including nutritional information
      (3) Dental history
      (4) Dental and periodontal charts
      (5) Treatment records of initial examination findings, diagnosis, and treatment plan

(6) Treatment records of procedures performed—include who, when, what, where, why, how, and what is needed next

(7) Consent forms to authorize treatment or decline recommended care such as radiographs, premedication, or fluoride therapy

b. Nonwritten records

(1) Photographs
(2) Radiographs
(3) Models
(4) Cephalometric tracings

Marketing Dentistry[9]

A. Definition—planning and management of dental services that benefit patients at a profit to the dental practice
B. Purpose—to obtain and maintain the desired share of the patient population market
C. Strategy
   1. Identify target market—groups with similar needs
   2. Develop a complete marketing plan to meet and satisfy the desires and needs of the target group
      a. Prices/fees
      b. Location/convenience
      c. Promotion
      d. Services
   3. Incorporate systems for changes with a step-by-step plan to build the practice
   4. All staff members participate in the marketing effort
D. Personnel/groups for marketing relations
   1. Oral health professionals—dentists, dental hygienists, dental assistants, office managers, receptionists, and dental laboratory technicians
   2. Business consultants to dental practice— bookkeepers, accountants, and lawyers
   3. Practice management consultants
   4. Physicians
   5. Allied health professionals
   6. Dental suppliers
   7. Prominent community and business members
   8. General public
   9. Patient population
E. Goals
   1. Goal setting
      a. Identify desired situations for the future to guide and direct behavior
      b. Involve staff members in discussions
      c. Establish step-by-step objectives
      d. Review and redefine goals on a regular basis

2. Types
   a. Practice organizational goals
   b. Procedural goals for staff members
   c. Personal goals
F. Practice promotion—all staff members project the desired image for professionals and gain public exposure for the practice
   1. Write articles for local newspapers on prevention, dental service updates, dental emergencies, evaluation of over-the-counter dental products, etc.
   2. Get a feature article about the practice in the local newspaper
   3. Participate in broadcast media (local radio and television) programing with special interest information, talk shows, community service announcements, etc.
   4. Participate in civic, religious, and fraternal group activities (provide opportunities to meet many people at once)
   5. Use business contacts within the community patient population—distribute your business to many
   6. Sponsor community projects
   7. Participate in community cultural and recreational events
   8. Become a public speaker
   9. Teach health information and cardiopulmonary resuscitation workshops to consumers and other professionals
   10. Become a student—attend local classes and workshops of interest to you
   11. Meet and cooperate with neighboring health professionals; provide business cards and referral slips
   12. Volunteer professional services and demonstrations
   13. Perform dental screenings in schools, health fairs, community and athletic programs, civic groups, and at special events
   14. Actively participate in your professional association
   15. Participate creatively in the community
   16. Use advertising—telephone book, newspaper, radio, and other community media
   17. Use mass direct mail—sending dental health education materials, practice brochures, or a newsletter to the patient population or the community at large

G. Patient satisfaction considerations
1. Offer a wide spectrum of dental services
   a. Prevention
   b. Maintenance
   c. Restoration
   d. Counseling
   e. Reconstruction
2. Provide quality care
3. Provide personalized care—recognize each patient as an individual, listen to each one, be responsive, and develop special relationships
4. Be a consumer advocate—stay abreast of consumer trends
5. Educate patients about dentistry, using common language
6. Include alternatives in treatment planning, explain all the options, and make recommendations; differentiate between what is necessary and what is ideal
7. Maintain fair and reasonable fees
8. Consistently offer dependable care and caring
9. Extend office hours to include early morning, evening, and weekend appointments
10. Appeal to all age ranges—children through senior citizens
11. Offer current treatment modalities
12. Allow patients to take responsibility for their own dental health
13. Run an efficient practice—minimize waiting time
14. Promote positive psychologic attitudes by all staff members
15. Maintain warm, respectful interpersonal relations between staff members and patients
16. Establish a pleasant, comfortable, attractive office decor
17. Offer a variety of financial arrangements
18. Process insurance forms expediently
19. Be prepared for and incorporate changes in the practice as needed
20. Develop and fully utilize auxiliaries
21. Provide strong technical expertise
22. Develop rapport with specialty practices for referrals, coordination of patient care, and close follow-through
23. Choose a convenient access location with easy parking
24. Provide "give-aways"—toothbrushes and other oral hygiene aids, health education brochures, toys or balloons for children, flowers, etc.
25. Exchange written correspondence with patients—outlines of treatment plans and copies of letters to other professionals concerning the patient's needs and care
26. Send patients personalized thank-you notes, congratulatory notes, special occasion notes, or get-well wishes
27. Maintain positive, satisfactory telephone contacts
28. Use follow-up telephone calls after complex treatments and to check on anxious patients
29. Keep patients informed by providing written treatment plans and briefly explaining procedures before beginning work
30. Quote fees for the treatment plan and make fair financial arrangements
31. Schedule time realistically
32. Maintain an effective "recall" dental health maintenance program to continue dental care on a routine schedule
33. Develop a practice brochure introducing staff members, the range of services, office hours, financial arrangements, etc.
34. Make accommodations for emergency patients

H. Recognition—express appreciation for staff cooperation daily, note patient support and patronage, and recognize referral sources with thank-you notes

I. Evaluation of marketing effectiveness
1. Internal analysis
   a. Compare gross revenues of the practice—daily, weekly, monthly, and annually
   b. Count patients—maintained and new
   c. Perform an overall financial analysis of the practice
      (1) Budget
      (2) Balance sheet of accounts receivable and accounts payable
      (3) Productivity per hour, day, week, month, and year
   d. Interview all staff members
2. External analysis
   a. Survey patients by interviews or questionnaires—Are they satisfied? Recommendations for changes?
   b. Survey other community and referral sources—can any further services be offered?

DENTIST–DENTAL HYGIENIST RELATIONSHIP

Employment

A. State dental practice act regulates the dental hygienist's performance of duties under general, indirect, or direct supervision of a licensed dentist and within specified physical settings; each state establishes its own legal guidelines

B. Financial arrangements between the dentist and dental hygienist are solely the concern of those two individuals and are separate from and not controlled by the state dental practice act

C. Employment arrangements
1. Employer-employee—dental hygienist as an employee, works within the office structure of a dentist
   a. All financial concerns of operating the practice are the responsibility of the dentist, the employer
   b. Employer pays the employee on an hourly wage, salary, or commission basis, withholding federal, state, and Social Security taxes from the employee's paycheck
   c. Dental hygienist's employer may also be an independent management firm, health maintenance organization, or state, county, or private agency employing individuals for dental offices or other specific work settings
2. Independent contractor—Internal Revenue Service (IRS) classification of a contractual arrangement between the dentist and self-employed dental hygienist
   a. Dental hygienist provides services to the patients of the dentist, adhering to the dentist's supervision and settings regulated by the state dental practice act
   b. Financial arrangements for operating the dental hygiene portion of the practice are contracted between the dentist and dental hygienist
   c. No taxes are withheld by the dentist from the dental hygienist's paycheck; dental hygienist pays self-employment (Social Security) tax and files estimated income tax payments
   d. IRS sets rules that establish qualifying criteria for independent contractors; it is illegal for a dentist-employer to arbitrarily "assign" the status of "independent contractor" to a dental hygienist–employee
   e. Independent contractor may hire employees and function as an employer

3. Independent dental hygiene practice—currently illegal but in the conceptual form might include
   a. Dental hygienist providing services to the public in a separate dental hygiene facility without a dentist's supervision
   b. Dental hygienist would assume all financial responsibility for the practice, would be self-employed, and would function as an employer to the employees of the facility

D. Terms of employment
1. Permanent—employee service with the employer is secure and of unlimited duration
2. Temporary—employee service is known to be of limited duration
3. Probationary—service trial period, usually 1 to 3 months, when employee and employer can evaluate one another and working together; employee may resign or be dismissed immediately for any reason
4. Full time—employee works solely in one office the customary number of hours that the facility functions, normally 30 to 40 hours per week
5. Part time—employee works less than the full hours of the facility's operation, usually less than 30 hours per week
6. Job sharing—two or more people share one full-time job by the day, week, month, or year; time can be split in any fashion agreeable to the job sharers and the employer; salary and benefits are shared proportionally with the time worked
7. Regular hours—coincide with normal office hours
8. Staggered hours—established working hours that fit the life-schedule of the employee, hours vary from routine office hours but are stable daily for that employee
9. "Flex" time—employee arrives and leaves work whenever he or she chooses; can change daily

E. Employment rights
1. Non-Discrimination Act, Title VII of the Civil Rights Act of 1964—establishes equal employement opportunity for all during the hiring process and throughout the course of employment; requires fairness and impartiality with regard to race, color, religious belief, gender, national origin, and age

2. Pregnancy Discrimination Act, 1979 amendment to Title VII of the Civil Rights Act of 1964—prohibits discrimination on the basis of pregnancy, childbirth, or related medical conditions; protects women from being fired or refused a job or promotion because of pregnancy; provides that, following maternity leave, the job will be returned with no loss in seniority or fringe benefits
3. Working conditions—each state sets minimum standards for working conditions, including
   a. Hours and days of work
   b. Minimum wage and reports for pay
   c. Employee records
   d. Uniforms and equipment
   e. Meal periods and eating area
   f. Rest periods and rest facilities
   g. Environmental temperature
4. Occupational Safety and Health Standards Board (OSHA)—sets minimum federal requirements for industrial safety
5. Employee Retirement Income Security Act of 1974 (ERISA)
   a. Purpose
      (1) Ensures that benefit plan participants know to what they are entitled
      (2) Guarantees that participants receive benefits, even if the business fails
   b. Elements
      (1) Required communications from corporation to employee with a summary of the corporate plan and updates, summary of annual reports, and announcement of plan modifications
      (2) On employee request, the corporation must provide a complete annual report, complete description of the document plan, and full vesting statements of total benefits accrued, nonforfeitable pension benefits, and the earliest date benefits become nonforfeitable

Compensation

A. Methods of remuneration
1. Fixed salary—guaranteed fixed wage for hourly, daily, weekly, or monthly employment
2. Salary plus commission—base salary plus an additional percentage of fees charged for dental hygiene services
3. Commission with guaranteed minimum salary— pays a percentage of fees charged for dental hygiene services, with an assured minimum wage per day regardless of daily gross production

4. Commission—earnings based on a percentage of fees charges for dental hygiene services
5. Independent contractor—sets and collects all fees and pays overhead costs, with profit fluctuation based on production, collection, and expenses
6. Overtime—usually for hourly wage earners; pays time-and-a-half for all time in excess of the contracted hours per week
7. Compensatory time off ("comp" time)—given for hours worked in excess of the established work week; used in place of overtime pay
8. Profit-sharing bonus—work incentive awarded to employees when profit goals are set and achieved for a specified period; may be calculated monthly, quarterly, or annually
9. Fringe benefits—required and optional services paid by the employer in addition to regular wages (see section on fringe benefits)

B. Negotiating a starting salary
1. Considerations
   a. It is your right to be paid what you are worth
   b. Before interviewing, determine a definite starting salary range that is acceptable to you
   c. Be prepared to discuss salary, including fringe benefits, with facts and a prepared strategy
   d. Think of the employer as the buyer and yourself as the seller; the commodity is your service: personal skills and technical expertise
   e. Unless you participate in negotiating, your salary is often less than it should be; dental practices often expect employees to accept satisfaction of service instead of a reasonable salary
   f. First salary offer from the employer is one of the most negotiable points of a new job; do not be too intimidated to make a counteroffer; first offer is usually not final, and employers expect negotiation
   g. You have the power to say no to an unacceptable offer
2. Determining factors
   a. Current education, skill level, experience
   b. Office fees, services rendered, daily production
   c. Responsibility for patient care and disease recognition
   d. Supply and demand

3. Need to get agreements in writings
   a. Initial probationary period may carry a reduced salary; establish a date for the salary to increase and what the increase will be
   b. Establish intervals for regular salary discussions with expected wage increases
C. Salary increases
   1. Usually sporadic and highly subjective for dental hygienists
   2. Based on one or more of the following
      a. Responsibility
      b. Seniority
      c. Merit
      d. Production
      e. Cost of living
      f. Educational advancement
      g. Supply and demand
   3. Negotiating a raise
      a. Set a definite appointment for the discussion
      b. Be prepared with all the reasons why you deserve a raise, emphasizing your value to the practice, not that you need more money
         (1) List your accomplishments
         (2) Use specific examples
         (3) Present facts and figures
         (4) Be direct and brief
         (5) Show how you have exceeded expectations
      c. Present the specific dollar-figure increase you are seeking with clear justification
D. Payroll
   1. Each payroll period includes a written compensation statement identifying gross earnings and itemizing deductions to reach the net amount of the paycheck
   2. Required and voluntary deductions are made from the gross compensation to arrive at the net paycheck
      a. Required employee deductions
         (1) Federal income tax withheld, based on declared exemptions
         (2) State income tax withheld, based on declared exemptions
         (3) Federal Insurance Contributions Act (FICA, Social Security), percentage set by the federal government
         (4) State disability insurance (limited to certain states)
         (5) City income tax (limited to certain cities)
      b. Optional employee deductions
         (1) Voluntary contribution to a retirement account
         (2) Professional expenses paid by the employee
         (3) Credit union savings account automatic deposit
   3. Employer payroll expenses
      a. Social Security matching funds
      b. Workers' compensation
      c. Federal Unemployment Tax Act
      d. Disability insurance (required by some states)
      e. Pension and profit-sharing plans
      f. Fringe benefits
      g. Bookkeeping and accounting fees

Fringe Benefits[2]

A. Definition—paid services in addition to direct pay
   1. Standard part of compensation programs in all sectors of the American economy—private, government, and nonprofit
   2. Some are legally required; others are optional
   3. Desirable because of the tax advantage of receiving services and benefits from the employer rather than paying for them with posttax paycheck dollars
B. Legally required benefits
   1. Social Security—Federal Old Age Survivors' Disability and Hospital Insurance Program includes
      a. Old age benefits—at age 65, provides a tax-free annual family benefit; amount is based on average yearly earnings while working
      b. Survivors' benefits—in case of the employee's death, survivors (including dependent children) may receive a monthly family income
      c. Disability benefits—for some medically caused total disabilities at any age; provides a tax-free monthly income
      d. Hospital insurance—after age 65, covers basic hospitalization, some related care, and, at a modest cost to the retiree, supplemental insurance (Medicare) for doctor bills and other medical services
   2. Workers compensation—protects the employee from medical expenses and loss of income in the event of injury on the job or job-related disability
      a. Financed entirely by employers via state payroll taxes; rate varies according to job-risk category
      b. Covers all medical expenses
      c. Income benefits vary according to salary level

3. Disability insurance—required in some states to provide benefits for nonoccupational accidents or illnesses
   a. Financing usually combines employer and employee contributions
   b. Disability must be medically certified
   c. Income benefits vary according to salary level
4. Unemployment insurance—provides benefits to individuals involuntarily unemployed
   a. Financed entirely by employers through state and federal unemployment taxes; rate varies based on the employer's past use record
   b. Weekly tax-free payments are made to those eligible
   c. Income benefits vary according to prior earnings
C. Optional fringe benefits (''perks'')—depend on office policy; may vary within the office from employee to employee; flexible program allows employer and employees to design a benefits package with services selected to best suit each individual's needs and life-style
   1. Paid absences
      a. Sick leave—salary paid during occasional short-term illnesses; usually sick-leave benefits are allowed to accumulate if not used, or unused days are paid at the end of the year as a bonus
      b. Holidays—salary paid for usual, nationally observed holidays
      c. Vacation—salary paid for vacation time off; schedule may vary according to the length of service with the employer; may be able to accumulate unused vacation time; for part-time employees vacation days are prorated (divided proportionally with the work schedule)
      d. Educational leave—salary paid for time off to attend educational programs that are work related; may have an annual specified maximum limit; may be given leave without pay
      e. Professional activities—salary paid for time off to attend professional meetings that are work or career related; may have an annual specified maximum limit; may be given leave without pay
      f. Emergency personal leave—paid time off for unexpected events such as a family illness, death, or funeral; jury duty, legal depositions, or court witness appearances; or extreme weather conditions
      g. Maternity leave—time off, usually without pay, but with the guarantee of job protection on return from the leave; reasonable time limits usually apply
      h. Extended or sabbatical leave—usually leave without pay for a few weeks to several months for the purpose of travel, education, family, or personal needs; job is held during the absence with an agreed-on time of return
   2. Insurance benefits
      a. Health insurance—program protects the insured from major medical costs; coverage may be
         (1) Fee-for-service plan where the individual selects the health care provider and submits a bill for payment to the private insurance carrier; usually has a deductible, pays a percentage of costs, excludes some types of care, and has a lifetime dollar value limit on claims per individual
         (2) Health maintenance organization for comprehensive health care services
         (3) Prepaid service plans such as Blue Cross and Blue Shield for service contracts to specific health care providers
         (4) Self-insured plans, which reimburse employees directly for medical expenses without third-party involvement
      b. Dental insurance—program protects the insured from usual dental expenses; types include
         (1) Schedule plans with specific dollar limits for each dental procedure, usually without a deductible
         (2) Comprehensive plans that reimburse on a ''reasonable and customary'' basis, with the insurance carrier paying a percentage of the actual charges
      c. Vision insurance—program covers the expenses of eye examinations, eye care, and prescription corrective lenses
      d. Liability (malpractice) insurance—protects the insured against liability for
         (1) Injuries arising out of professional services rendered, including errors, negligence, or omissions
         (2) Injuries from acts or omissions while participating as a member of a professional organization or committee
         (3) Personal injury against claims of slander, libel, defamation of character, false arrest, etc.

(4) Legal fees and court costs paid whether or not the insured is found liable

e. Long-term permanent disability insurance—in the event of severe and/or permanent disability, coverage provides a percentage of the basic wage; usually includes

   (1) "Elimination" or waiting period before the policy starts paying benefits, usually 30 days or longer

   (2) Benefit period may be a specified number of years, for the length of the disability, until regular retirement benefits begin, or for a lifetime

   (3) Partial benefits may be available if the insured is able to return to work on a limited basis

f. Life insurance—provides assistance to building a financial estate for surviving family; basic types include

   (1) Term insurance—considered "pure death protection," covering a specific, temporary period; renewal costs increase as the insured ages

   (2) Whole life insurance—called "straight," "permanent," or "cash value"; more expensive initially, with costs leveling and the policy building a cash value; may pay dividends or provide borrowing equity

g. Pension plans (see section on retirement)

3. Professional expenses—employer makes direct payment or reimburses for

a. Professional license renewal

b. Uniform allowance—for purchase and/or maintenance of office attire

c. Professional education assistance—tuition reimbursement and related expenses, such as books, supplies, equipment, and travel expenses, usually with a specified annual limit; may also include salary for time away from home; educational loan program may provide short- or long-term repayment program or "loan forgiveness" (considered paid) if the employee stays with the employer for an agreed-on period of time

d. Professional activities—reimbursement or payment for registration fees and related travel expenses for participation at meetings related to the field of dental hygiene; usually with a specified annual limit

e. Professional journals and texts—subscriptions and purchase

f. Paid parking, transportation, and/or automobile expenses related to commuting to work

g. Expense account—reimbursement for purchase of items for the office, instruments, forms, equipment, etc.

4. Other benefits

a. Child care and baby-sitting expenses

b. Personal legal services

c. Personal financial counseling

d. Notary service

e. Staff functions—meals, parties, and other special events

Employment Agreement/Letter of Intent

A. Definition—written contract describing the terms of employment agreed on by the dental hygienist (employee) and dentist (employer)

B. Functions

1. Clarifies specific details of employment issues for both parties

2. Establishes a stable working relationship

3. May or may not be legally binding

4. Provides psychologic security for both parties

C. Contents

1. Terms of agreement

a. Names of the parties—dental hygienist (employee) and dentist (employer)

b. Job title

c. Date the contract takes effect (employment commencement) and date the contract expires

d. Option of contract renewal

2. Settings and terms of employment

a. Address of dental office(s) and name of supervising dentist(s)

b. Agreement of both parties to adhere to the rules and regulations of the state dental practice act

c. Statement of equipment, supplies, and instruments to be provided by the dentist

d. Work arrangement of days of the week or days per month agreed on

e. Work load by hours and scheduling of appointments

f. Overtime to be paid by "comp" time or financial compensation

g. Payment for time not worked, such as holidays, vacation, sick leave, etc.

3. Job description

a. Specific services to be performed

b. Other characteristic duties and responsibilities of the position

c. Opportunities for growth and promotion

4. Compensation
   a. Method—hourly, daily salary, commission, or combination
   b. Starting remuneration or method of calculation
   c. Payroll schedule
   d. Increases in remuneration
      (1) Dates of review
      (2) Basis for increase
   e. Fringe benefits—listed individually
      (1) Requirements of initial qualification
      (2) Vesting increments
      (3) Accrual techniques
5. Probationary period
   a. Terms and date of probation
   b. Agreement for mutual evaluation at the conclusion of probation
   c. Employment termination options for each party
6. Performance evaluation
   a. Dates for review
   b. Method of evaluation
   c. Criteria for performance success
7. Termination procedures
   a. Advance notice—required length of time
   b. Statement of cause
   c. Employee replacement procedures
8. Signatures of each party with the date
9. Witness signatures (optional)

Job Performance

A. Employment issues affecting job performance[1]
   1. Factors positively influencing dental hygiene employment conditions
      a. Attitudes (self-image) of dental hygienists
      b. Attitudes of dentists
      c. State dental practice acts
      d. Consumer/patient awareness and education
      e. Demand for dental hygiene services
      f. Role of the dental hygienist as a practice builder
      g. Role of the dental hygienist as a dental disease prevention specialist
   2. Factors negatively influencing dental hygiene employment conditions
      a. Attitudes (self-image) of dental hygienists
      b. Attitudes of dentists
      c. Dentists' lack of knowledge of full capabilities of dental hygienists
      d. State dental practice acts
      e. Lack of consumer/patient awareness and education
      f. Lack of demand for dental hygiene services
      g. Maldistribution and/or overpopulation of dental hygienists
      h. Inflation and/or economic recession
      i. Economic exploitation of dental hygienists
      j. Unfair, financially discriminatory employment practices
      k. Poor practice management by dentists
      l. Lack of business knowledge by dentists
      m. Lack of business knowledge by dental hygienists
      n. Pressure to practice illegally
      o. Overall lack of recognition of the dental hygienist as a professional making valuable contributions as a team member to the dental practice
B. Job expectations—employer and employee must plan the job together and discuss and agree on minimum performance expectations and results concerning
   1. What is done on the job (basic work functions)
   2. The manner in which it is accomplished (standards of performance)
   3. Why it is done (importance of function)
   4. Skills necessary to perform the job
   5. Goals and limits for achieving expectations
C. Job satisfaction—employment fulfillment is largely dependent on the employee to assert self in using skills and assuming maximum job responsibility leading to professional growth; as one gains competence and respect, job satisfaction follows
D. Performance evaluation
   1. Definition—communication tool based on the agreed-on performance plan; measures work progress and provides constructive feedback; includes criticism and compliments regarding specific elements of employment actions and behavior; should be separate from the salary review
   2. Value
      a. Provides a progress report, recognizes and supports desired behavior, develops strengths, pinpoints weaknesses, and gives specific direction for change; can give a psychologic boost and rekindle employee interest
      b. Can assist in determining a salary increase
      c. Can be used as a legal tool for dismissal
   3. Frequency
      a. At the completion of the probationary period if the job is new—1 to 3 months after employment commencement
      b. Once or twice a year for continuing employment

4. Technique
   a. Completion of the office "performance review form" by both the employer and the employee
   b. Meeting of the employer and employee to share, compare, and discuss results of the review form; appraisal should
      (1) Measure progress toward the goal of task and behavior performances
      (2) Compare actual results with the agreed-on plan, citing specific incidents
      (3) Praise accomplishments when performance meets or exceeds stated standards
      (4) When differences occur, determine the cause, then consider alternatives to facilitate reaching desired outcomes
      (5) If corrective action is indicated, state the specific plan with measurable results and gain agreement of both parties
      (6) Modify performance standards if indicated and agreed on by both parties
      (7) Enhance communications between the employer and employee, giving an opportunity for "coaching" to achieve performance goals, rather than merely "judging" performance
   c. Format
      (1) Direct statement of behavioral objectives in terms of quality and quantity; standards to achieve a satisfactory performance level
      (2) Clear, self-explanatory statements to facilitate both the employer's evaluation of the employee and the employee's self-evaluation
      (3) Written document directs the interview and allows for reexamination of all information following the interview
   d. Content areas—address all areas of the job description
      (1) Participation with the practice and staff as a team member
      (2) Knowledge of the dental hygiene field
      (3) Treatment procedures and clinical skills
      (4) Practice routine with patients
      (5) Communication skills with the staff and patients
      (6) Dependability to the office and work schedule
      (7) Responsibility for the operatory, equipment, and supplies
      (8) Work habits
      (9) Initiative, leadership, and problem-solving skills

   e. Daily verbal feedback—critical to successful performance
      (1) Praise good behavior and tell the feelings produced
      (2) Observe discrepancies, describing specific incidents and the feelings produced
E. Changing performance[2]
   1. Planning
      a. Describe the performance discrepancy as specifically as possible, listing
         (1) Desired standard of performance
         (2) Present level of performance
         (3) Analysis of performance discrepancy—why is it not satisfactory?
         (4) Definition of what needs to be done differently and how it should be properly performed
      b. Gain mutual agreement on the desired change; be sure each party is clear
      c. Divide changes into small successive steps to progressively implement the ultimate desired result
   2. Evaluation
      a. Ask for immediate feedback and reinforcement for the new, desired performance
      b. Monitor progress, gaining reinforcement often at first, then gradually less often
      c. Steadily follow the guidelines for change
      d. Be specific in acknowledging how performance is changing
   3. Incorporation
      a. Strive for high-quality performance
      b. Be fair and honest in efforts to change performance
      c. Consistently include the desired performance as soon as possible to achieve self-responsibility
F. Job termination
   1. Dismissal
      a. Clearly understand the grounds for dismissal
         (1) Ask for the true, complete picture
         (2) Ask for clarification of vague statements
         (3) Remember that it is the work performance that is unacceptable, not the person
      b. Clarify the severance arrangements
         (1) Date of termination
         (2) Severance pay
         (3) Benefits accrued and due to the employee
      c. Behave professionally and with dignity

d. Acknowledge your feelings and mourn the loss
e. Put the terminated job into perspective and enter the job market
   (1) Inventory your career goals
   (2) Update your résumé
   (3) Begin the interviewing process
   (4) Move confidently on to the next career stage
2. Resignation
   a. Notify your employer of your intentions as soon as possible
   b. Do not tell co-workers before notifying your employer
   c. Clearly state your grounds for resigning or state that it is time for career advancement
   d. Clarify the severance arrangements
      (1) Date of termination
      (2) Benefits accrued and due to the employee
      (3) Whether or not the employee plans to find and train a successor
   e. Tie up loose ends
   f. Depart with dignity and behave professionally
G. Changing jobs
   1. Consider the risk of a job change when there is lack of employment satisfaction or growth stagnation on one job
   2. New job should offer new duties, more responsibility, opportunity for professional growth, and/or increased compensation
   3. Goal is to find a job that offers the best opportunities and become a permanent employee
   4. See section on career mobility

Dentist–Dental Hygienist Communications

A. Overall relationship should be based on adult, professional interdependence
   1. Each respects and recognizes the other's level of competence
   2. Dental hygienist begins a new job with immediate professional behavior, demonstrating knowledge, skills, judgment, and caring
   3. Dental hygienist expresses ideas, opinions, and feelings and encourage reciprocal sharing from the dentist
   4. Each assumes responsibility for the treatment rendered and quality patient care
B. Dental hygienists role is that of self-responsibility
   1. State your standards and priorities for all office functions

2. Set limits on what you can effectively and competently accomplish
3. When you need information or assistance, ask the dentist for input or guidance
4. Welcome criticism from mistakes to enhance your learning and growth
5. Be cooperative, diplomatic, and friendly
6. Use an assertive communication style to enhance your office effectiveness
7. Model the behavior you want to receive
C. Disagreement
   1. Conflicts are to be expected, and confrontation should not be avoided
   2. Take the risk to discuss problems assertively and unemotionally
      a. Identify conflict as soon as you recognize it
      b. Discuss issues privately, with diplomacy and tact
      c. Describe the issue first, factually and accurately, then note your feelings
      d. Be ready, and present a solution for the disagreement
      e. Strive for a ''win-win'' solution for both parties
   3. Ability to deal effectively with conflict increases the dental hygienist's value to the dental practice and wins respect from others

PROFESSIONAL MANAGEMENT ▬▬▬▬
Seeking Employment

A. Résumé
   1. Purpose
      a. Inventories professional qualifications and assets
      b. Is an introduction; creates a first impression
      c. Generates an interview
      d. Can eliminate purposeless interviews
      e. After an interview the résumé becomes a visible reminder of the applicant to the potential employer
   2. Types
      a. Blanket—general résumé for all jobs in the related field
      b. Specific—designed with one particular job in mind
   3. Styles
      a. Descriptive/traditional—lists education, experience, and qualifications in chronologic order; biographic
      b. Functional—states effective accomplishments that support a specific job position; reflects ability

4. Contents
   a. Personal identification
      (1) Name
      (2) Address
      (3) Telephone number
   b. Job objective
      (1) Statement of the exact job being sought
      (2) May include a brief philosophic statement and professional goals
   c. Professional education applicable to the job objective
      (1) Postgraduate degree
      (2) College degree
      (3) Associate degree
      (4) Dental hygiene licensure with license number and special certificates
   d. Professional experience
      (1) New graduates—list special skills and interests from school or jobs in related fields as appropriate
      (2) Midcareer professionals—divide experiences into categories such as private practice, teaching, administrative, research, community health, etc.
   e. Professional data—optional
      (1) Professional affiliations
      (2) Community/professional services
      (3) Continuing education courses related to the position sought
      (4) Professional projects
   f. References—optional
      (1) "Available on request" or
      (2) List two sources who speak well of you; include their names, positions, addresses, and telephone numbers
      (3) Notify listed references that they may be contacted
   g. Eliminate unnecessary personal information, such as gender, age, race or color, religion, marital status, children, height, weight, hobbies, etc.
5. Format
   a. Brief—one page
   b. Neat, accurate, typed letter-perfect with correct spelling and grammar
   c. Organized with functional headings to introduce each category
   d. Spaces and wide margins used for easy readability
   e. Original or high-quality photocopy on medium-weight white or ivory bond paper; no carbon copies

B. Cover letter
   1. Purpose
      a. Introduces the applicant and the résumé
      b. Highlights important qualifications
   2. Content
      a. Introduce yourself courteously and professionally
      b. Tell how you heard of the job or why you like this office
      c. Emphasize your qualifications to fit this job
         (1) Demonstrate your understanding of the employer's needs
         (2) Indicate your skills that specifically fit this job
         (3) Demonstrate your interest
      d. Do not repeat yourself in the résumé
      e. State your availability for an interview and your intention to contact the office to schedule an interview
   3. Format
      a. Brief and simple—one or two paragraphs
      b. Original, indiviudally typed
      c. Neat, accurate, typed letter-perfect on bond paper with correct spelling and grammer
   4. Address the letter to the person of authority, using this person's name and title
   5. Sign the cover letter
   6. Enclose your résumé
C. Interviews[8,15]
   1. Types
      a. Information—about the job market and where to look in the field; can use to gather job descriptions
      b. Job search—regarding a specific job being sought
   2. Purpose—mutual opportunity of reciprocal information and impressions to evaluate for congruent job objectives
      a. Interviewer appraises the candidate's
         (1) Résumé
         (2) Work qualifications
         (3) Professional philosophy
         (4) Behavior
         (5) Appearance
      b. Candidate appraises the interviewer and employment situation with regard to
         (1) Job description and responsibility
         (2) Staff members
         (3) Practice philosophy
         (4) Office environment
         (5) Working conditions
         (6) Opportunity for job satisfaction, professional growth, challenge, and responsibility

c. Fact finding for both parties
d. Initiation of a relationship between the two parties
3. Styles
   a. Directed
      (1) Follows a specific pattern
      (2) Highly structured format with a checklist of questions
      (3) Usually impersonal and dominated by the inteviewer
      (4) Little opportunity for the candidate to initiate questions
   b. Open
      (1) Loosely structured format
      (2) Broad, general questions
      (3) Allows for interaction between the interviewer and candidate
   c. Combination
      (1) Includes both direct and open questions
      (2) Opportunity for sufficient information exchange while both parties get the necessary facts
   d. Group interview
      (1) Several candidates and one or more interviewer
      (2) May begin as or become nondirective, allowing the candidates to conduct the process, while the interviewer does not participate
      (3) Expect one candidate to emerge from the others
   e. Board interview
      (1) One candidate and several interviewers
      (2) Each interviewer asks questions in his or her special interest area
4. Obtaining an interview
   a. Screening—identify potential acceptable positions; eliminate unacceptable positions
      (1) Telephone the office
      (2) Ask basic questions about the position
      (3) Listen for the office "tone"
   b. Make an interview appointment
      (1) Set the date, time, and location
      (2) Get directions to the office
      (3) Ask what is expected to be the length of the interview
      (4) Ask who will be the interviewer
5. Preparation
   a. Develop self-knowledge—know who you are and what you have to offer
      (1) Job qualifications, skill strengths, and weaknesses
      (2) Employment expectations

(3) Professional philosophy
(4) Short- and long-range career goals
(5) Personal attributes and philosophy
   b. Research the position—limit yourself to job descriptions that meet your goals and suit your practice philosophy
      (1) Learn the reputation of the practice, dentist, and employees
      (2) Talk to current or previous employees or other dentists
   c. Role-play a mock interview
      (1) Write possible questions that you may be asked
      (2) Present your answers out loud
      (3) Write your questions about the position
      (4) Present your questions out loud
      (5) Ask for a critique from a colleague
      (6) Repeat—continuing until you feel, act, and sound informed and professional
   d. Imagine the interviewer—plan your approach
      (1) Interviewer's position in the office
      (2) Interviewer's area of expertise, attitudes, and expectations
      (3) Knowledge of job position and dental hygiene skills and services
      (4) Personality, disposition, and honesty
      (5) Communication skills
      (6) Practice philosophy
6. Preliminary interview
   a. Introductions
      (1) Initial contact, first impressions
      (2) Establish rapport
   b. Presentation of the candidate's qualifications
      (1) Résumé reviewed
      (2) Professional philosophy shared
      (3) Specific strengths of education and experience stressed
   c. Presentation of the position
      (1) Job description of specific procedures and the work load
      (2) Dental hygienist's general responsibilities, participation with the practice team, and opportunity for professional growth
      (3) Description of the office atmosphere and work environment
      (4) Philosophy and goals of practice
      (5) Compensation

d. Compatibility established between the candidate and position
   (1) Candidate's skills and strengths linked with the job description and needs of the practice
   (2) Plans made to accommodate for weaknesses in the match
e. Conclusion
   (1) Summary of findings
   (2) Possible job offer
   (3) Plans for a follow-up interview
7. Selection interview/second interview
   a. Opportunity for a second look at each other
   b. Opportunity for office observation—details and work situation
   c. Opportunity for additional questions between the candidate and employer
   d. Discussion of details
      (1) Job description and office procedures
      (2) Office policies
      (3) Work schedule
      (4) Compensation—starting package and raises
   e. Job offer
      (1) Starting date
      (2) Probationary period
      (3) Discussion of an employment agreement or letter of intent
8. Candidate selection criteria
   a. Interviewer's subjective feelings about the candidate, the human factor of simply liking another person
   b. Overall characteristics of appearance, body language, human relations skills, and verbal communication skills
   c. Strength of the candidate's qualifications, performance record, achievements, and success potential
   d. Recommendations from references
   e. Candidate's attitude—interest, ability, and willingness to do the job
   f. Candidate's personality—pleasantness, poise, enthusiasm, intelligence, judgment, maturity, self-confidence, and motivation
9. Strategies
   a. Initiate discussion of personally and professionally important issues if they are not covered by the interviewer
   b. If the exact job desired does not exist, design it and then promote it to the employer

10. Recommendations for successful interviews
    a. Be prompt for a good first impression
    b. Attire makes the second impression
       (1) Appearance must be professional—present a serious image
       (2) Look conservative—wear simple, tasteful attire with soft, blended colors
       (3) Avoid distractors such as heavy makeup, elaborate hairstyles, strong or lingering scents, extensive jewelry, and frilly, gaudy, sexy, cute, or overdone dressing
       (4) Be neat, clean, fresh, and perfect from head to toe
       (5) Dress as though you represent the dentist with whom you are interviewing
    c. Verbal communications
       (1) Address the interviewer by name
       (2) Wait for the interviewer to begin the questioning first; follow the interviewer's lead
       (3) Listen carefully to each question and answer the actual question asked
       (4) Respond to questions with concise answers
       (5) Reply to questions with information that demonstrates your knowledge and skills and will establish credibility and trust
       (6) Say "I don't know" when you do not know the answer to a question
       (7) Be diplomatic and tactful—avoid complaining or negatively judging past experiences, jobs, employers, colleagues, schools, or teachers
       (8) State your questions to the interviewer succinctly
       (9) Use good grammer and pronunciation; avoid slang and minimize jargon
    d. Nonverbal communications and body language
       (1) Display your dental hygiene smile
       (2) Maintain good posture
       (3) Shake hands firmly on meeting the interviewer
       (4) Be seated at the direction of the interviewer
       (5) Use eye contact throughout the interview
       (6) Assume an open, calm body position
       (7) Pay attention, demonstrate interest, show eagerness, and take notes if you like

(8) Be human; act as natural as possible

(9) Do not smoke, chew gum, chew nails, bite lips, wiggle feet, or display other nervous habits

e. Attitude

(1) Interview the interviewer on a parity basis

(2) Believe in yourself

(3) Heed your own feelings

(4) Be positive and enthusiastic

(5) Be courteous, sincere, and genuine

(6) Be consistent

D. Job search strategies

1. Preparation—focus on yourself

a. Clarify your career goals

(1) Practice philosophy and values

(2) Work objectives related to goals

(3) Compensation needs

b. Identify all your professional skills and personal strengths necessary to achieve your goals

c. Imagine the ideal job situation, and seek or create one that fits this fantasy as closely as possible

d. Know your full value to a dental practice

2. Investigate the job market

a. Research local trends

(1) Job opportunities and growth potential

(2) Job descriptions

(3) Work loads and job sharing

(4) Compensation packages

(5) Job turnovers and layoffs

b. "Shop around" and interview for information

(1) Learn all the options and make comparisons

(2) Do not underrate your abilities or undercut a wage

(3) Choose the best opportunity for you

3. Job sources

a. Friends, colleagues, and other professional contacts—word-of-mouth

b. Verbal or printed announcements at meetings and conferences

c. Dental hygiene association component employment placement services

d. Dental society employment placement services

e. Private health care providers' employment placement agencies

f. Public or county health departments

g. Dental hygiene school job announcement bulletin boards

h. Dental hygiene and dental association newsletters and journal job announcements

i. Bulletin board job announcements in large office buildings

j. Contact

(1) People at offices near where you would like to work

(2) People mentioned in association newsletters

(3) Association leaders, authors, speakers, and educators

k. Canvas

(1) Local dental association membership directories

(2) Alumni association membership directories

(3) Telephone book yellow pages with listings of dentists located near you

l. Dental supply houses or supply salespersons

m. Newspaper classified advertisements

E. Job selection considerations[15]

1. Purpose—candidate compares career needs and desires with what the practice offers

2. Factors

a. Overall practice ambience and atmosphere

b. Practice philosophy, goals, and values

c. Personnel harmony

d. Interactions with patients

e. Quality of care provided

f. General job description

(1) Specific duties of the job

(2) Variety of services

g. General work conditions

(1) Work load, scheduling, and hours

(2) Equipment, instruments, and supplies

h. Overall role of the dental hygienist— respect and responsibility

i. Compensation package

(1) Salary

(2) Fringe benefits

(3) Schedule for increases

j. Opportunity for professional growth

k. Job security

(1) Assured patient load

(2) Employee turnover rate

l. Location of the office, commute, and parking

m. Solo or group practice

n. Well-established or new, growing practice

3. Choose the job that offers the most for you

Career Development

A. Professional stationery and business cards
  1. Purpose
    a. Establish professional identity
    b. Demonstrate personal style
  2. Uses
    a. Exchange of cards at professional introductions
      (1) Job interviews
      (2) Dental professional meetings, conferences, and educational programs
      (3) Nondental professional associations, agencies, and professional contacts
    b. Professional correspondence
    c. Practice promotion
  3. Styles
    a. Engraved business cards
    b. Engraved or printed stationery
    c. Printed memo pads
  4. Design
    a. Name and degrees
    b. Title
      (1) Registered dental hygienist (R.D.H.)
      (2) Expanded certificate(s)
      (3) Other identifying information such as "dental health specialist" or "oral disease prevention educator"
    c. Home or office address and telephone number
    d. For an office card, may include the dentist's name, such as "in the office of _____, D.D.S."
    e. Select a quality of paper and a design that represent your professional image and abilities
    f. May need more than one card design to represent different affiliations
B. Employment retention
  1. Career planning
    a. Definitions
      (1) Career—course or progress of a person's life related to some noteworthy activity or pursuit; total of one's lifework in a chosen field
      (2) Occupation—one's regular or principal business or line of work
      (3) Job—position of employment to gain a livelihood
    b. Career elements
      (1) Continual education to expand knowledge and skills in the field
      (2) Maturation of professional and technical skills

      (3) Responsible contributions for directing the success of patient care or other work objectives and creating a positive work environment
      (4) Participation in the growth of the profession through research, education, politics, organizational leadership, and/or public awareness
      (5) Personal gratification gained through involvement
    c. Goals—short-term objectives that support long-range goals for career development and professional achievement
      (1) Record goals to continually guide direction and contribute to commitment
      (2) Revise goals for growth, advancement, or change
  2. Starting a new job—quickly establish, then maintain, your "professional personality"
    a. Fill your work role with intelligent, responsible behavior
    b. Use time productively
    c. Demonstrate standards for quality care
    d. Establish a communications style for verbal and written interactions
    e. Mutually with your employer, define performance standards, then meet and surpass your employer's expectations for your performance
    f. Demonstrate your substance
    g. Be consistent
    h. Initially be investigative to learn about this new position and others in the office
    i. Gain respect and build a loyalty base
  3. Continuing education—keep current with research developments, new trends in dentistry, and the state of the art of dental hygiene through
    a. Didactic meetings
    b. Clinical workshops
    c. Study groups
    d. Journals, literature, and new and revised texts
    e. Discussions with colleagues
  4. Postlicentiate degrees—expand your knowledge and gain additional skills for job retention or career mobility
    a. Bachelor of science or arts
    b. Master of science or arts
    c. Doctoral degree

C. Stress and burnout
  1. Definitions
     a. Stress—strain or tension from compulsive pressures; usually diminishes one's resistance
     b. Burnout—combination of physical, emotional, and behavioral changes in an individual as a response to high-intensity or long-duration stress; adaptive capabilities are exceeded
  2. Relationship to dental hygiene[4]
     a. "Giving" role of health care providers
     b. Intense interpersonal relations with patients and staff members
     c. Monotonous job tasks
     d. Lack of appreciation (reduced self-esteem)
     e. Being taken for granted (reduced self-worth)
     f. Lack of accomplishment of personal and/or professional goals
     g. Lack of change
  3. Strategies for reducing stress and burnout
     a. Identify when you are experiencing burnout
     b. Identify the causes of stress
        (1) Analyze your feelings to achieve self-awareness of internal issues
        (2) Evaluate your environment and work situation to make external changes
     c. Reprioritize your goals or reevaluate your methods to accomplish reconfirmed goals
     d. Attempt to make changes at work to reduce stress—delegate duties, be creative, or try something new
     e. Modify your behavior to better enjoy the life process
        (1) Take classes to learn assertiveness training, success strategies, communication skills, or time management techniques
        (2) Take good care of your body; get regular sleep, adhere to a physical fitness program, and follow sound nutrition guidelines
        (3) Enjoy recreation
        (4) Try techniques for mind and body relaxation, such as catnaps, slow, deep breathing, stretching, conscious relaxation, meditation, biofeedback, visualization, guided imagery, yoga, or prayer
        (5) Try body relaxation experiences of message, hot tubs, or saunas
        (6) Try new behavior

D. Assertive behavior[2,14]
  1. Value—assertive behavior enables one to negotiate mutually satisfactory solutions in a variety of situations with employers, co-workers, patients, and colleagues
  2. Definitions
     a. Assertive behavior—communicating honestly and openly in a manner that equalizes the parties involved to gain reasonable results; it is personally satisfying and socially effective
     b. Passive behavior—submission to others' wants and needs; timidity, usually because of a lack of confidence, fear, or low self-esteem; may lead to frustration and depression
     c. Aggressive behavior—attacking, harsh, and demanding; often blaming and hurtful to the other party; aimed at domination and humiliation
  3. Self-concept—assertive behavior is dependent on self-confidence; self-concept can be enhanced by repeated positive thoughts, statements, and images; believe in your right to be treated honestly, with respect, and as a professional
  4. Verbal communications
     a. Express your thoughts and feelings directly and honestly
     b. Use a positive approach in comments you make about yourself without hurting others
     c. Take responsibility for your rights
  5. Speech patterns[14]
     a. Tone and pitch of voice can be intimidating or reassuring; can show weakness or strength
     b. Rate of speaking can be paced to include or exclude others; can demonstrate confidence or nervousness
  6. Body language[14]—up to two thirds of overall communication is done without speaking; nonverbal messages speak loudly; body language can say something completely opposite from the words being spoken, confusing the listener; nonverbal messages can undermine or support the actual words spoken
     a. Gestures—use of the hands can emphasize or distract
     b. Eye contact—sets the stage for assertive communication; establishes trust and confidence
     c. Facial expression—influences credibility of what is said

d. Habitual mannerisms—can be distracting

e. Laughter—if inappropriate, will subvert communication; may show nervousness or insincerity

f. Posture—stance demonstrates self-image while sitting, standing, and walking

g. Body movements—can demonstrate discomfort and insincerity or sincerity and interest

7. Implementing assertive behavior—begin with small steps in assertiveness skills[2]

a. Identify successful assertive behavior you are already using

b. Watch others who are successfully assertive

c. Plan your new assertiveness; imagine, then write, an assertive script

(1) Describe the exact thing you want to change; be objective and specific

(2) Express what you think and how you feel about the specific situation

(3) Specify the exact change you desire; work on one thing at a time; request must be reasonable and within the power of the other person to meet

(4) Consequences in the form of rewards and penalties for each party should be spelled out; emphasize the positive consequences; negative consequences must be realistic and believable, not idle threats

d. Practice assertive behavior in front of a mirror, then with a friend

e. Initiate assertive behavior in your speech, eye contact, appearance, body language, and actions

Career Mobility

A. Definitions[11]

1. Allied health personnel—supporting, complementing, and supplementing the professional functions of dentists in the delivery of health care to patients

2. Vertical career ladder—moving up the technical ladder from dental assistant to dental hygienist to dentist to dentist in a specialty practice; entry may occur at any of the first three levels

3. Lateral career mobility—combines existing knowledge, skills, and licensure with additional study to qualify for employment in related fields (see *D* on employment opportunity alternatives to traditional dental hygiene practice)

B. Job changes

1. Periodically review your employment situation, job status, technical skill level, and knowledge

a. Are you satisfied?

b. Are you still experiencing professional growth?

2. Compare your present situation with your stated career goals

a. Are you accomplishing objectives?

b. Is it time to move on?

3. Decide if it is time for a job change

a. Expand your present employment situation

b. Switch to a new office in a similar work position

c. Change to a job that is an alternative to traditional clinical practice with new duties and responsibilities, part time or full time

4. Enhance success at career mobility

a. Make professional contacts throughout your career

b. Investigate all possible career options

c. Plan changes carefully with a clear, thorough idea of what you want to do

d. Be creative—look for opportunities; redesign your present job or design a new one and sell it to your employer, part time or full time.

e. Be willing to take risks

C. Networks of professional connections

1. Networking—sharing and extending professional contacts to establish friendships and business relationships; exchanging knowledge and information; advising and developing a professional and moral support system for achievement of goals

2. Value—professional networks can keep those involved informed of professional developments and apprised of job opportunities, assist in making job changes, and create synergism for participants

3. Participants

a. Professional colleagues

b. Business and professional acquaintances

c. College classmates and faculty

d. Present and former co-workers

e. Friends and relatives

4. Types

a. General—all the contacts made during one's professional career

b. Specific—organized group of professionals meeting on a regular basis to promote growth and development of one another

D. Employment opportunity alternatives to traditional dental hygiene practice—part-time and full-time jobs for dental hygienists are available or may be created in (and are not limited to) the following areas
  1. Private dental practices
    (a) Clinical supervision
    (b) Administration
    (c) Practice management
  2. Dental hygiene schools
    (a) Education—didactic and clinical
    (b) Administration
    (c) Research
  3. Public schools
    (a) Dental inspection and disease prevention programs for students and teachers
    (b) Nutritional counseling
    (c) Sports dentistry
    (d) Curriculum development
  4. Community dental health projects
    (a) Prenatal care
    (b) Parents' and children's groups
    (c) Senior citizens' groups
    (d) Research
  5. Consulting and education
    (a) Practice management
    (b) Designing and teaching continuing education workshops for health professionals
  6. Continuing education business—own and operate
  7. Sports dentistry—mouth protection, education, and planning
    (a) Park and recreation departments
    (b) Youth teams
    (c) Schools
  8. Public and private institutions
    (a) Hospitals
    (b) Nursing and convalescent homes
    (c) Residential care facilities
    (d) Homes for the elderly
    (e) Hospices
  9. Myofunctional therapy
  10. Dental products industry
    (a) Retail representative
    (b) Manufacturer's (wholesale) representative
    (c) Product marketing
    (d) Sales management
    (e) Product research and design
    (f) Product manufacturing
    (g) Professional relations representative
    (h) Dental products supply house representative
  11. Insurance industry
    (a) Clinician
    (b) Dental claims examiner
    (c) Marketing and underwriting
    (d) Professional relations
  12. Government service
    (a) Armed forces
    (b) Veteran's Administration
    (c) Public Health Service
    (d) Indian Health Service
    (e) State agencies
  13. Health professionals recruiting and placement agency
    (a) Own and operate
    (b) Associate as personnel consultant
  14. Scientific research
  15. Professional organizations (constituent or American Dental Hygienists' Association [ADHA])
    (a) Administration
    (b) Management
  16. Professional media
    (a) Technical or scientific writing and publishing
    (b) Educational video production
  17. Foreign country dental hygiene

PERSONAL BUSINESS INTERESTS
Financial Planning

A. Definition—setting financial goals for the future, taking steps to achieve maximal money management
B. Steps
  1. Evaluate your present financial situation by computing your net worth: the difference between assets (amounts owned) and liabilities (amount owed); include real property, life insurance, stocks, bonds, retirement accounts, household and personal property, and bank accounts; calculate your net worth annually to check progress in reaching your financial goal, then review and update your plan
  2. Set goals for the future, stating specific objectives for short-term accomplishments and long-range goals; plan to spread investments over the years
    a. Set long-range goals, including the desired income at retirement
    b. State other objectives, including income now and in 5 years, then 10 years, etc.; specify investments such as residential property, securities, retirement accounts, education of children, travel, etc.

c. Plan a budget as an effective money management tool; anticipate basic needs and expenses, allocate funds, analyze spending habits, control impulsive buying, and live within income limits; plan for some fun and recreation as well as for emergency expenses; regularly monitor actual expenses as compared with the budget to see if you are on the right track or need to compensate for unexpected bills

d. Keep records—complete and accurate accounting assists with taxes, expense accounts, and forecasting the financial future

e. Establish a credit rating in your own name to facilitate getting loans, a mortgage, or other credit and to function with independence financially; check your credit profile from time to time for accuracy

f. Use credit effectively—for major purchases, spread payments over a long period and pay reasonable finance charges; avoid unnecessary debts, finance charges, and penalties for late payments

g. Pay yourself first—with interest, dividends, and appreciation; begin with small, guaranteed investments; make your money work for you by investigating interest-bearing checking accounts, savings accounts, money market accounts, mutual funds, bonds, certificates of deposit, Treasury bills, etc.; establish a reserve fund for emergencies

h. Purchasing a home is an important major investment, usually the largest single investment of a lifetime; provide your own housing and eliminate paying rent to someone else; financially valuable because it offers safety and security, provides financial leverage as collateral, gains appreciation, and offers a tax advantage

i. Diversify other investments—spread and reduce risks, obtain the highest possible return, and gain income-producing securities

j. Protect yourself with disability insurance to safeguard your earning power

k. Plan a retirement fund

3. Goals for investments
   a. Produce income
   b. Provide a tax advantage
   c. Hedge inflation
   d. Show capital growth/appreciation in value
   e. Furnish safety and security
   f. Have liquidity conversion potential
   g. Be maintained management free or with minimal expenses

4. Professional assistance for financial planning
   a. Make personal investigations through research, reading, classes, talking with others, studying market indicators, and/or participation in investment clubs
   b. Design a carefully planned strategy to achieve financial goals, using the expertise of specialists for help with laws, regulations, intricacies, and refinements
      (1) Banker
      (2) Real estate broker
      (3) Stock broker
      (4) Insurance broker
      (5) Investment advisor
      (6) Accountant
      (7) Lawyer

5. Types of investments—consider how much risk you are willing and able to assume, consider both short- and long-term investments, evaluate income needs now and in the future
   a. Tangibles (hard assets)
      (1) Real estate
      (2) Gold, silver, coins, and gems
      (3) Antiques, art, stamps, rare books, etc.
   b. Intangibles (paper with a guarantee, securities, or liquid assets)
      (1) Banks, savings and loans, or thrifts
         (a) Interest-bearing checking accounts
         (b) Savings accounts
         (c) Money market certificates
         (d) Certificates of deposit
      (2) Government securities
         (a) U.S. Treasury bills
         (b) U.S. Treasury notes and bonds
         (c) U.S. saving bonds
         (d) Federal agency lending programs
         (e) Short-term tax-exempt notes
         (f) Municipal bonds for estates, counties, and municipalities
      (3) Investment firms
         (a) Money market funds
         (b) Stocks
         (c) Corporate bonds
         (d) Mutual funds
         (e) Tax-deferred annuities
         (f) Commodities/financial futures
         (g) Limited partnerships
         (h) Tax shelters
         (i) Trust deeds
         (j) Foreign currency

6. Estate planning
   a. Definition—provides for intentional disposition of possessions and assets on one's death to organize family resources and provide for their future
   b. Value
      (1) Requires careful financial planning and management during one's lifetime
      (2) Intentionally creates, defines, and retains assets of the estate
      (3) Provides for disability
      (4) Plans and provides for retirement
      (5) Can spread family income and ensure prudent money management during one's lifetime
      (6) Trusts can be established to reduce administrative and management costs and protect assets
      (7) Minimizes or avoids taxes imposed on estates and inheritances
      (8) Guarantees financially secure property will be disposed of as one desires
   c. Includes
      (1) Titles of properties
      (2) Insurance
      (3) Pension plans
      (4) Investments
      (5) Management plan
      (6) Disposition of property

Taxes[6]

A. Tax system
   1. Taxes are the largest single item in the budget of the average American; it is worth the additional time and money to be certain one is getting all the possible tax breaks available
   2. One's "tax bracket" is the combined federal and state percentage of taxes paid on the total dollars earned
   3. U.S. tax system is a "marginal progressive" style; it is advantageous to maximize tax deductions to reduce tax liabilities to the lowest tax bracket possible; further, one's tax bracket will help determine the best types of investments for one's financial situation
B. Tax considerations for professionals—in addition to the tax savings available to all tax payers, professionals are entitled to special tax adjustments, deductions, and credits if these expenses are employment related
   1. Record keeping and substantiation requirements
      a. Calendar of professional activities
      b. Explanation of the professional event, including the date, activity, how it is related and helpful to the job, the sponsor, location, cost, and transportation required
      c. Expense record
      d. Proof of all expenses, such as receipts, cancelled checks, or credit card vouchers
      e. Overall complete, accurate, and permanent
      f. Retain federal records for at least 3 years after filing; check for individual state requirements
      g. Keep copies of federal and state income tax returns forever
   2. Professional activities
      a. Meetings of professional organizations
      b. Staff meetings
      c. Educational programs related to the profession
      d. Study groups
      e. Employment-seeking expenses for a job change within the same profession
   3. Professional expenses are deductible only to the extent that the professional is not reimbursed and can establish his or her right to deduct them
C. Travel and transportation expenses
   1. Definitions
      a. Travel—ordinary and necessary expenses incurred while away from home (overnight) for the purpose of a professional or job-related activity; deduct as "Employee Business Expense," IRS Form 2106, as an adjustment to income; these include
         (1) Fares for airplane, train, bus, etc.
         (2) Meals and lodging
         (3) Automobile expenses
         (4) Related necessary expenses such as telephone calls and laundry
      b. Transportation—actual cost of transportation to professional activities not away from home (not overnight); allowable only as an itemized deduction, Schedule A, IRS Form 1040; permits commuting between two jobs on the same day; does not permit basic commuting from home to job and back; these include
         (1) Actual automobile expenses
         (2) Bus and cab fares
         (3) Bridge tolls and parking fees
   2. Methods of computation
      a. Mileage rate method—multiply the total number of miles driven by the rate allowed by the IRS; instructions for Form 2106 state the rate for each tax year

b. Actual expenses method—compute the ratio of business mileage to total mileage; multiply the ratio times the cost of actual operating expenses (gasoline, oil, repairs, maintenance, licenses, insurance, depreciation or lease payments, loan interest, etc.)

c. Both options require keeping an odometer dairy at the beginning and end of each trip; nonprofessional portions are to be excluded from total

3. Calculation of deductible travel

a. If the trip is entirely for professional activities, all expenses are deductible

b. If the trip is primarily professional, with a small portion for personal travel, travel expenses to and from the destination, as well as direct professional expenses, are deductible

c. If the trip is primarily for pleasure, none of the travel expense is deductible, but direct professional expenses at the destination are deductible

4. Travel outside the United States

a. If the trip is entirely professional, all expenses may be deducted

b. If the trip is a combination of professional activities and pleasure, expenses must be divided, with no deduction for the personal portion

c. Limit is two foreign conventions or trips per tax year

d. Substantiation requires a written statement, signed by the attendee, showing the total number of days spent at the convention, the number of hours devoted each day to scheduled professional activities, and an actual program of scheduled activities; a written statement of an officer of the convention is attached with other required statements to the federal tax return

D. Miscellaneous professional expenses—may be deducted only if deductions are itemized; Schedule A, Form 1040

1. Professional education expenses

a. Deducted as ordinary and necessary if they meet express requirements of the employer or the law for retaining professional status and/or licensure; or to maintain or improve skills required in performing the duties of the present profession, including education that leads to a degree

b. If new educational requirements are placed on the present profession, necessary education expenses to meet these stipulations are deductible

c. Expenses for training in a new profession may not be deducted

d. Include tuition, fees for correspondence courses, books, supplies, travel, and transportation costs

e. Proof of attendance may be required

2. Professional uniform expenses

a. Purchase and upkeep costs of work clothes can be deducted if they are specifically required as a condition of employment and are not suitable for general or everyday wear; must be recognizable as a "uniform"

b. Upkeep includes laundering, dry cleaning, repairs, and alterations

c. Uniform items include dresses, pants and tops, laboratory coats and jackets, clinic shoes, caps, white or support hoisery, protective clothing (such as safety eyeglasses, masks, and gloves), and name tags and pins

3. Other miscellaneous professional expenses

a. Dues to professional organizations

b. Employment-seeking expenses, including agency fees, résumé typing and printing, telephone calls, postage, travel, and transportation expenses

c. Liability (malpractice) insurance premiums

d. Instruments, professional equipment, and supplies

e. Medical examinations required by the employer

f. Subscriptions to professional and trade journals

g. Professional legal expenses

h. Professional license renewal

i. Telephone toll and long-distance calls for professional reasons

E. Retirement accounts

1. Individual Retirement Arrangements (IRAs) are allowed for any person with earned income, regardless of participation in another qualified retirement plan

2. Amount contributed to the IRA is subtracted from the gross income, regardless of whether itemized deductions are made

3. Allowable contributions and interest earned are not taxable during working years

4. One may not borrow from the IRA before the specified age (59½) without being taxed and penalized
5. See section on retirement

F. Child and dependent care
1. Expenses allowed for children under age 15 or disabled dependents while one is at work or looking for work
2. Credit available is a maximum of 30%, related to the tax payer's adjusted gross income

G. Tax audits
1. Tax returns are reviewed by agents and computers for errors and omissions, deductions that are beyond the norm relative to a given profession, and other variables
2. Letter of notification indicates specific categories for audit
3. All elements of proof are presented for acceptance of deductions
4. Although all auditors rely on the same reference sources, each may interpret the law slightly differently
5. Repetitive audits for the same items are not allowed for 2 years following a clear audit; if an audit finds additional tax liability, the audit can be repeated on that item until the audit is clear; one can be audited every year for a different issue
6. IRS auditors are responsible to both the taxpayer and the government and are charged to be fair
7. Legitimate deductions should not be eliminated to avoid an audit

Retirement

A. Focus on goals
1. Life-style, home location, and living conditions
2. Activities, travel, recreation, hobbies, and business involvement
3. Consider your projected living costs and the income required to accommodate your retirement plans; note possible illness or disability
4. Consider your projected income from Social Security, retirement funds, and whole life insurance policies in addition to other investments
5. Write out a plan and review it periodically

B. Tax-deferred retirement accounts
1. Purpose
a. Establish a retirement account
b. Taxes on amounts deposited and interest earned are deferred until withdrawal
c. Reduce the annual adjusted gross income to reduce the income tax debt
2. Types
a. Corporate—may establish a pension plan at the principal's discretion
(1) Requirements—rules set by the corporation
(a) Minimum number of hours per year
(b) Minimum age of employee
(c) May establish a waiting period before the employee can participate in the plan (usually 1 to 3 years)
(d) Vesting schedule options—grants the employee full ownership of monies contributed in his or her name by the corporation
(e) When and if requirements are met, the employee must be included in the plan
(2) Contributions
(a) Maximum allowable is 25% of the annual salary to a maximum of $25,000
(b) Employer contributions (percentage) equal employee contributions
(c) Monies are held in a single corporate account
(d) Lump-sum or regular deposits may be made during the year
(e) Contributions are allowed until April 15 of the following year or the end of the fiscal year
(f) All amounts deposited by the employer are deductible by the employer as a business expense
(3) Termination—employee who leaves employment where there is a retirement plan may take the fund (amount vested) and "roll it over" into an IRA

b. Keogh plan
(1) Requirements
  (a) Dentist must be self-employed and have a Keogh plan for self
  (b) Employee needs
    [1] Minimum of 3 years continuous employment
    [2] Minimum of 1000 hours per year
    [3] Vesting of 100% is immediate when the above requirements are met
(2) Contributions
  (a) Maximum allowable is 15% of the annual earned income to a maximum of $7500
  (b) Employer contributions (percentage) equal employee contributions
  (c) Separate account for each plan participant
  (d) Lump-sum or regular deposits may be made during the year
  (e) Contributions allowed until April 15 of the following year or the end of the fiscal year
  (f) All amounts deposited by the employer are deductible by the employer as a business expense
(3) Termination—employee who leaves employment where there is a Keogh plan may take the fund and "roll it over" into an IRA
c. Individual Retirement Arrangement (IRA)
(1) Requirements
  (a) Allowable for anyone with earned income regardless of inclusion in another retirement account
  (b) Spouse may have a separate account, even if no income
(2) Contributions
  (a) Maximum allowable is up to 100% of earned income to a maximum of $2000
  (b) For a married couple filing a joint tax return when only one partner earns income, a separate spousal IRA may be established for the nonworking spouse; maximum allowable to both accounts is $2500

  (c) Lump-sum or regular deposits may be made throughout the year
  (d) Contributions are allowed until April 15 of the following year or extended filing of taxes
  (e) All amounts deposited are tax deductible as adjustments to income
3. Termination and withdrawal for all retirement accounts
  a. All accounts may be terminated at any time
  b. Funds must be left on deposit until minimum age 59½, or funds will be taxed and assessed a penalty fee
  c. Withdrawal begins after retirement, age 59½, or disablement
  d. Withdrawal must begin at age 70½, and contributions may continue
4. Mechanisms
  a. Savings account
  b. Mutual funds
  c. Retirement bonds
  d. Retirement annuities
  e. Trust accounts

Wills[10]

A. Definition—written, legal arrangement for distribution of assets when death occurs
B. Value
  1. Ensures disposal of belongings as one chooses and lets others know of these wishes
  2. Requires that one think about the consequences of one's death and decide what one wants and plan for proper distribution
  3. Protects beneficiaries' rights to receive assets without dispute
  4. Safeguards and ties up all loose ends of financial affairs
  5. Provides for financial and guardian care of minor children
  6. Minimizes expenses of transfers and unnecessary fees
  7. Ensures minimum delay in distributing the estate
  8. Covers payment of debts of the decedent
  9. Provides for tax planning
C. Contents
  1. Identifies beneficiaries
  2. Identifies all aspects of financial affairs
  3. Divides assets
  4. Codicil can give away special items

D. Wills are best prepared in consultation with a lawyer to ensure validity and best interests overall

E. Executor duties
   1. Carries out provisions of the will
   2. Directs financial concerns of the state following death
   3. Gathers and preserves property
   4. Collects income due
   5. Pays bills and taxes
   6. Identifies and distributes all remaining assets
   7. Provides record keeping to the court

F. Probate—legal process alerting the community of the death, then attending to financial distribution of the estate

REFERENCES

1. American Dental Hygienists' Association: Current employment conditions for practice, Annual Report, 1979-1980.
2. Bower, S.A., and Bower, G.H.: Asserting yourself, Reading, Mass., 1976, Addison-Wesley Publishing Co., Inc.
3. The Dentists' Insurance Company: Patient non-compliance, TDIC Newsletter **3**:3, 1982.
4. Dreyer, R.: Is burnout inevitable? Career Dir. Dent. Hyg. **10**(11):1, 1983.
5. Jensen, J.: How to design your agency's employee benefits program, Grantsmanship Center News, p. 41, Sept.-Oct. 1979.
6. Kramer, S.: Tax guide for allied health professionals, Oakland, Calif., 1981, Professional Press.
7. Lampner, J.: Effective career management for hygienists, Los Altos, Calif., 1977, Lange Medical Publications.
8. Medley, H.A.: Sweaty palms: the neglected art of being interviewed, Belmont, Calif., 1978, Wadsworth Publishing Co.
9. Milone, C.L., Blair, W.C., and Littlefield, J.E.: Marketing for the dental practice, Philadelphia, 1982, W.B. Saunders Co.
10. Porter, S.: Sylvia Porter's new money book, New York, 1979, Doubleday & Co., Inc.
11. Resurreccion, R.L., and Wilson, S.: A perspective on career mobility in the dental hygiene profession, J. S.C. Dent. Hyg. Assoc., fall 1980.
12. Saxton, D.F., et al.: Mosby's comprehensive review of nursing, ed. 11, St. Louis, 1984, The C.V. Mosby Co.
13. Schwarzrock, S., and Jensen, J.: Effective dental assisting, ed. 6, Dubuque, Iowa, 1982, Wm. C. Brown Group.
14. Schwimmer, L.D.: How to ask for a raise without getting fired, New York, 1980, Harper & Row, Publishers, Inc.
15. Woodall, I.R.: Leadership, management, and role delineation, St. Louis, 1977, The C.V. Mosby Company.

SUGGESTED READINGS

Anders, D.M.: Dental team finds success by passing the ball, Dent. Economics **71**:72, 1981.

Biggs, J.: Staff evaluation and control, Quintessence Int., p. 1978.

Blanchard, K., and Johnson, S.: The one minute manager, New York, 1982, William Morrow & Co., Inc.

Catalyst staff: making the most of your first job, New York, 1981, Ballantine/Del Rey/Fawcett Books.

Council, J.D., and Plachy, R.J.: Performance appraisal is not enough, J. Nurs. Admin. **10**(10):20, 1980.

Grates, A.: 21 steps to a better job, New York, 1983, Monarch Press.

Irish, R.K.: Go hire yourself an employer, ed. 2, New York, 1978, Anchor Press.

Malmin, O.: Viewpoint: misdiagnosis-misdirection, Dent. Economics **72**:29, 1982.

Muchmore, P.: Dental marketing: from research to service, Dent. Economics **73**:34, 1983.

Pattison, G., and Pattison, A.: Periodontal instrumentation, Reston, Va., 1979, Reston Publishing Co., Inc.

Peters, T.J., and Waterman, R.H.: In search of excellence, New York, 1982, Harper & Row, Publishers, Inc.

Peterson, S.: Comprehensive review for dental hygienists, ed. 4, St. Louis, 1980, The C.V. Mosby Co.

Rogers, M., and Joyce, N.: Women and money, New York, 1978, McGraw-Hill Book Co.

Saleebey, W.M.: Study skills for success, San Pablo, Calif., 1981, Learning Resource Institute.

Stratton, D.J.: Coping with success, Leadership, Dec. 1980.

Weinstein, B.: 20 ways to be more creative in your job, New York, 1983, Simon & Schuster, Inc.

Wilkins, E.: Clinical practice of the dental hygienist, ed. 5, Philadelphia, 1983, Lea & Febiger.

Review Questions

1 The concept of practice management is related to
1. Laws governing dental practices
2. Written forms and documents of dental practices
3. Organization of the processes and personnel of dental practices
4. Economics of dental practices
5. Investments

2 The "team concept" in dentistry discourages
1. Decentralized management
2. Work simplification
3. Individual professional growth
4. Independent decision making
5. Group practice

3 Which of the following would *inhibit* an effective work team?
1. A relaxed and informal work atmosphere
2. Accommodation for change
3. Frequent, honest criticism
4. Emotions controlled and withheld
5. Job satisfaction

4 Regular staff meetings to discuss goals, evaluate progress, and solve problems demonstrate
1. Interpersonal team building
2. Organizational team building
3. Public relations promotion
4. Psychologic relations building
5. Marketing principles

5 An objective method for data collection includes
1. Direct observation of the patient
2. Questioning the patient
3. Requesting previous dental records
4. Clinical periodontal probing
5. Self-reporting

6 The determining factor in a revised case presentation for dental hygiene therapy is the
1. Correctness of the original hypothesis
2. Method of providing care
3. Availability of time
4. Effectiveness of implementation
5. Availability of supplies

7 Which of the following *best* defines the term *dental hygiene therapy?* Dental hygiene therapy is the
1. Activities a dental hygienist employs to identify patient needs
2. Process the dental hygienist uses to determine dental hygiene goals
3. Steps the dental hygienist employs in planning and giving dental hygiene care
4. Implementation of dental hygiene care by the hygienist
5. Evaluation of dental hygiene care by the dentist

8 To begin dental hygiene therapy, the dental hygienist must first
1. State the patient's dental hygiene needs
2. Identify goals for dental hygiene care
3. Obtain information about the patient
4. Evaluate the effectiveness of dental hygiene care
5. Evaluate the effectiveness of dental care

9 The effectiveness of dental hygienist–patient communication is validated by
1. Office staff meetings
2. Dental health assessments
3. Patient feedback
4. The patient's oral hygiene adaptations
5. The dentist's feedback

10 The goals of dental hygiene therapy teaching are
1. Acquiring knowledge—cognitive
2. Developing attitudes—affective
3. Developing psychomotor skills—conative
4. A combination of the above
5. None of the above

11 The learning process in dental hygiene education ends with
1. Dissemination of educational information and materials
2. Demonstration of oral hygiene aids and techniques
3. Patient feedback of information and techniques
4. Evaluation of patient understanding and techniques
5. Patient participation

12 What is the *greatest value* in getting to know each patient personally?
1. The patient will want to return to the office for further care
2. The dental hygienist can assess the patient's learning capabilities and strengths to enhance patient education
3. The patient will want to refer others to the dental practice
4. Establishment of community participation by the practitioner
5. Establishment of personal friendships

13 What term denotes a patient's lack of cooperation?
1 Noncompliance
2. Collusion
3. Noncomprehension
4. Denial
5. Noncommunicative

14 As a dental office team member, the dental hygienist
1. Contributes knowledge, clinical skills, and intangible attributes to the practice
2. Concentrates on rendering quality dental hygiene therapy
3. Actively participates in staff meetings
4. Develops office friendships
5. Follows the directives of the dentist

15 Which of the following is *most important* in positive dental office team relations?
  1. Well-defined responsibilities
  2. High salaries
  3. Open, honest communication between team members
  4. Regularly scheduled staff meetings
  5. Regularly scheduled vacations

16 A patient is *most* likely to judge the success of a dental practice by the
  1. Number of patients in the reception room
  2. Interpersonal relations between staff with one another and with patients
  3. Physical office environment
  4. Demonstrated professional competence of the practitioners
  5. Personality of the dentist

17 Employee questions regarding practice standards and principles should be directed to the
  1. Procedures manual
  2. Policy manual
  3. Employee handbook
  4. State dental practice act
  5. American Dental Hygienists' Association

18 Which of the following guidelines would *not* appear in the office policy manual?
  1. Operatory maintenance
  2. Office safety and emergencies
  3. Practice philosophy, values, and goals
  4. Referrals to specialists
  5. Vacation times

19 The *least* time-consuming method of recall is
  1. Advance scheduling
  2. Telephone
  3. Letter or postcard
  4. Cross-reference
  5. All methods are time consuming

20 Recall cards are part of which management system?
  1. Personnel
  2. Patient
  3. Records
  4. Office
  5. All systems use recall cards

21 At an initial interview you meet with the dentist, office manager, and staff dental hygienists. This type of interview is termed
  1. Individual
  2. Group
  3. Board
  4. Open
  5. Team

22 Your first step in preparing for the interview is
  1. Screening the office by telephone
  2. Developing self-knowledge of career goals
  3. Role playing the interview
  4. Researching the office
  5. Writing the resumé

23 The overall goal of the interview is to
  1. Introduce the candidate to the potential employer
  2. Present the available position to the candidate
  3. Present the candidate's qualifications to the potential employer
  4. Establish whether or not there is compatability between the candidate and the office
  5. Negotiate salary

24 A discussion of fringe benefits would *not* include which of the following insurances
  1. Workers' compensation
  2. Medical
  3. Liability
  4. Disability
  5. Life

25 You might accept a job offer before finalization of the
  1. Salary establishment
  2. Outline of fringe benefits
  3. Projected work schedule
  4. Written employment agreement
  5. Outline of the job description

26 The interviewer's selection of a candidate primarily is based on the
  1. Interviewer's subjective feelings about the candidate
  2. Strength of the candidate's qualifications
  3. Candidate's salary request
  4. Candidate's projected work schedule
  5. Candidate's résumé

27 A good candidate interviewing strategy is to
  1. Be polite and allow the interviewer to lead all discussion
  2. Lead the interview to be certain all of your issues are covered
  3. Share the lead in discussion with the interviewer to cover interests of both parties
  4. Ask as many questions as possible to demonstrate your interest in the job, but do not overexpose yourself
  5. Demonstrate your knowledge of the dental literature

28 The most important job selection consideration is
  1. The practice philosophy, values, and goals
  2. Personnel harmony
  3. The quality of dental care provided
  4. The candidate's personal values priority
  5. The annual salary

29 Patient *reclamation* refers to
  1. Contacting patients who have transferred to other practices
  2. Scheduling multiple appointments for dental hygiene therapy
  3. Contacting patients who have unfinished therapy or extended absences from the office
  4. Scheduling appointments to upgrade existing restorations
  5. Attracting patients who have never received dental care

30 Which of the following can be *most* effective for marketing relations?
1. Dentists
2. Dental auxiliaries
3. Dental suppliers
4. Patients
5. Other health professionals

31 *Marketing dentistry* is defined as
1. Advertising the practice
2. Managing services to benefit patients and profit the practice
3. Community participation by all staff members
4. Identifying target patient populations
5. Retail dentistry

32 The dental hygienist can *best* participate in marketing the dental practice by
1. Maintaining warm, respectful relations with patients and staff members
2. Processing insurance forms expediently
3. Providing ''give-away'' oral hygiene devices
4. Exchanging written correspondence with patients
5. Attending a marketing course

33 The final step in dental marketing is
1. Advertising
2. Profits to the practice
3. Recognition of all participants
4. Evaluation of the program
5. Implementation of the program

34 A dental hygienist providing services directly to the public is the definition for an
1. Employee service arrangement
2. Employer service arrangement
3. Independent contractor
4. Independent practitioner
5. Entrepreneur

35 Employment service known to be limited in duration is termed
1. Probationary
2. Temporary
3. Trial
4. Part time
5. Tenure

36 Which of the following protects employees against unfair discrimination?
1. Occupational Safety and Health Standards Board
2. State dental practice act
3. Code of ethics
4. Title VII of the Civil Rights Act
5. Equal Rights Amendment (ERA)

37 In negotiating a starting salary, a dental hygienist who makes a counteroffer
1. Demonstrates his or her intention to be paid what he or she is worth
2. Surprises the prospective employer
3. May lose the job offer
4. Starts off on the wrong foot with the new employer
5. May appear too assertive

38 In negotiating a salary increase, the *best* approach is to
1. Request an automatic annual cost-of-living raise to avoid further uncomfortable discussions
2. Demand your right to a raise proportional to each fee increase
3. Explain your personal need for more money
4. Present your value to the practice
5. Submit an update resume

39 Which of the following is *not* an employer payroll expense?
1. Federal income tax
2. Social Security matching funds
3. Federal unemployment tax
4. Workers' compensation
5. Federal Insurance Contributions Act (FICA) matching funds

40 Old age benefits, survivors' benefits, disability benefits, and hospital insurance are all included in which of the following?
1. Workers' compensation
2. Federal unemployment
3. Social Security
4. State disability insurance
5. State taxes

41 An employer's direct payment for professional expense
1. Is taxed twice
2. Is considered a fringe benefit and should be included in calculating the employee's compensation package
3. Is separate from the compensation package
4. Is illegal
5. Is a component of salary

42 The primary purpose of an employment agreement is
1. To legally bind the employer to promises made during the job interview
2. To describe and clarify the terms of employment for the dental hygienist and the dentist
3. To guarantee continuous employment to the dental hygienist
4. To eliminate the need for future negotiations
5. To guarantee an employee for the employer

43 Who is *primarily* responsible for employment issues affecting the dental hygienist's job performance?
1. The dentist
2. The dental hygienist
3. The combination of the dentist and dental hygienist
4. The patient
5. The dental office manager

44 During a performance evaluation, the dental hygienist should *least* expect
1. Recognition of strengths and an outline of weaknesses of performance
2. To participate in self-evaluation
3. A monthly progress report
4. Specific corrective action requested
5. Feedback about performance

45 When achieving its greatest expanse of opportunity, the practice of dental hygiene can be defined as
1. A job
2. Employment
3. An occupation
4. A career
5. A science

46 One common reason dental hygienists often suffer from stress and burnout is related to
1. Expression of self-esteem
2. Expression of self-worth
3. The "giving role" of health practitioners
4. Job tasks
5. Low salaries

47 The first step in reducing stress and burnout is
1. Reprioritization of goals
2. Behavior modification
3. Finding a new job
4. Identifying that you are experiencing stress and burnout
5. Asking for a raise in salary

48 Communicating honestly and openly to equalize both parties in an interaction describes which type of behavior?
1. Passive behavior
2. Nonassertive behavior
3. Assertive behavior
4. Aggressive behavior
5. Nonverbal behavior

49 Your behavior is *most* determined by
1. Your self-concept
2. Others' behavior toward you
3. Your mood at the given moment
4. Your body language
5. Your parents

50 The dental hygienist's personal business management would *not* include which of the following?
1. Financial planning
2. Tax planning
3. Will preparation
4. Employment agreements
5. Investment planning

Answers and Rationales

1. (3) Practice management includes overall elements of the entire operation of a dental practice.
   (1) Laws governing dental practices are only a portion of practice management.
   (2) Written forms and documents are only a portion of practice management.
   (4) Economics are only a portion of practice management.
   (5) Investments are only a portion of practice management.
2. (4) The "team concept" requires participative decision making.
   (1) Decentralized management results in shared responsibility.
   (2) Work simplification allows for ease of shared responsibility.
   (3) Individual professional growth results in job satisfaction.
   (5) Group practice encourages the "team concept."
3. (4) Expression of feelings is the key to successful team relations.
   (1) A relaxed and informal work atmosphere produces a feeling of belonging.
   (2) Flexibility is necessary to all teams.
   (3) Frequent, honest criticism provides comfortable guidance for change.
   (5) An effective work team creates job satisfaction.
4. (1) Interpersonal team building keeps communications open.
   (2) Organizational team building represents policy and procedures.
   (3) Public relations promotion relates to outside connections.
   (4) Staff meetings are not intended to be therapy sessions.
   (5) Staff meetings are not intended to discuss marketing principles.
5. (4) Periodontal probing measures specific information, which is objective.
   (1) Direct observation without precise measurement is subjective.
   (2) Verbal history is subjective.
   (3) Previous records may be sketchy and incomplete.
   (5) Self-reporting is subjective.

For each question the correct answer and rationale are listed first. The other choices are presented in order with the reasons why they are not correct.

6. (4) When a plan does not produce the desired outcome, the plan should be changed.
   (1) Patient response is the determinant, not the dental hygienist's hypothesis.
   (2) Various methods may have the same outcome; effectiveness is most important.
   (3) Time is not relevant in the revision of therapy.
   (5) Availability of supplies is not relevant in the revision of therapy.

7. (3) Dental hygiene therapy is more than cleaning teeth; it is the step-by-step process that scientifically provides for patient needs.
   (1) Dental hygiene therapy goes beyond needs identification.
   (2) Goal establishment is only one aspect of dental hygiene therapy.
   (4) Implementation is only one aspect of dental hygiene therapy.
   (5) Evaluation is only one aspect of dental hygiene therapy.

8. (3) The initial step in any process using problem solving is the collection of data.
   (1) Dental hygiene needs can only be determined after assessment.
   (2) Goals are set after dental hygiene needs are established.
   (4) Evaluation is the last phase of the process.
   (5) Evaluation is the last phase of the process.

9. (3) Feedback allows the patient to ask questions and express feelings and allows the dental hygienist to assess the patient's understanding.
   (1) Staff meetings are subject to all members' evaluations of patient status.
   (2) Dental health assessment does not necessarily include dental hygienist–patient relationships.
   (4) Dental hygienist–patient communication should be evaluated by the patient's verbal and behavioral responses.
   (5) The dentist's feedback does not relate to the dental hygienist–patient communication.

10. (4) The teaching-learning environment includes the combination of cognitive, affective, and conative changes.
    (1) Cognitive change is only one aspect of the teaching-learning process.
    (2) Affective change is only one aspect of the teaching-learning process.
    (3) Conative change is only one aspect of the teaching-learning process.
    (5) The correct answer is 4.

11. (4) Evaluation is the last phase of the teaching-learning process.
    (1) Information dissemination is the first step in teaching.
    (2) Demonstration precedes evaluation in the teaching-learning process
    (3) Feedback precedes evaluation in teaching.
    (5) Patient participation is not the final phase in the learning process.

12. (2) The goal of dental hygiene therapy is to provide the best possible care for each patient, with care designed to reach each individual.
    (1) Future care is not the goal of the present appointment.
    (3) Practice enhancement is not the goal of the present appointment.
    (4) Community outreach is not the goal of the present appointment.
    (5) Establishing personal friendships is not the goal of the present appointment.

13. (1) Noncompliance is lack of patient agreement or cooperation with recommended dental care.
    (2) Collusion is secret agreement with wrongful purpose.
    (3) Noncomprehension is lack of understanding.
    (4) Denial is a declaration that a statement is untrue.
    (5) Noncommunicative is a lack of conversation or exchange of talk, ideas, etc.

14. (1) The dental hygienist's membership on the team requires all-encompassing participation with the entire practice.
    (2) Quality care is only one aspect of the team concept.
    (3) Staff meeting attendance is only one aspect of the team concept.
    (4) Office friendships are only one aspect of the team concept.
    (5) Following the dentist's directives is only one aspect of the team concept.

15. (3) Communications facilitate all aspects of office functioning.
    (1) Defined responsibilities may actually limit team building and cooperation.
    (2) Financial arrangements may have a minor influence on interpersonal relations.
    (4) Staff meetings may facilitate open communications.
    (5) Vacations away from the office may have a minor influence on interpersonal relations.

16. (2) Human behavior toward others will most greatly influence patients; likeability influences perceived success.
    (1) Waiting for other patients may be frustrating.
    (3) The office atmsphere often reflects the decorating tastes of individuals, not success.
    (4) Professional competence is difficult for patients to assess.
    (5) The personality of the dentist is difficult for patients to equate with success of the practice.

17. (2) The policy manual outlines practice principles, values, and goals.
    (1) A procedures manual describes routines.
    (3) The employee handbook outlines personnel data.
    (4) State dental practice acts are state laws governing the practice of dentistry.
    (5) The American Dental Hygienists' Association does not regulate the policies of the private-practice office.

18. (1) Operatory maintenance is described in the procedures manual.
    (2) Office safety and emergencies are described in the policy manual.
    (3) The practice philosophy is described in the policy manual.
    (4) Referrals are outlined in the policy manual.
    (5) Vacation benefits are outlined in the policy manual.
19. (1) Advance scheduling fills the appointment book quickly.
    (2) Telephoning may require several attempts to reach patients.
    (3) Correspondence requires patients to respond at their will.
    (4) Cross-reference requires double the time to ensure correct booking.
    (5) The benefits of advance scheduling offset the small amount of time required.
20. (2) Patient management includes all phases of patient care.
    (1) Personnel management relates to staff members.
    (3) Records management is the treatment of records and nonwritten elements.
    (4) Office management relates to supplies and equipment.
    (5) All management systems do not use recall cards.
21. (3) During a board interview, one candidate meets with several interviewers.
    (1) An individual interview is one in which one candidate meets with one interviewer.
    (2) Group interviews are conducted with several candidates at the same time.
    (4) An open interview describes a technique used during an interview.
    (5) A team interview is not a recognized type of interview.
22. (2) Self-knowledge is the basis for all successful job searches.
    (1) Telephone screening follows self-evaluation.
    (3) Role playing follows contacting the office.
    (4) Researching the office follows telephone screening.
    (5) Writing the résumé precedes the interview process.
23. (4) Compatibility determines a reason to continue the interviewing process.
    (1) Introduction only begin the interviewing process.
    (2) Presentation of the position is only half of the consideration.
    (3) The candidate's qualifications are only half of the consideration.
    (5) Negotiating the salary is only a portion of the process.
24. (1) Workers' compensation is legally required for all employees.
    (2) Medical insurance is an optional fringe benefit.
    (3) Liability insurance is an optional fringe benefit.
    (4) Disability insurance is an optional fringe benefit, except in a few states.
    (5) Life insurance is an optional fringe benefit.

25. (4) The written agreement can follow the interview.
    (1) The salary should be established before job acceptance.
    (2) Fringe benefits should be established before job acceptance.
    (3) The work schedule should be agreed on before job acceptance.
    (5) The job description should be agreed on before job acceptance.
26. (1) Personal feelings and liking another individual are key reasons for choosing a candidate.
    (2) General qualifications are secondary to subjective feelings.
    (3) A salary request is negotiable.
    (4) The work schedule can be changed later.
    (5) The candidate's résumé is secondary to subjective feelings.
27. (3) Equalizing the "give/get" ratio by shared discussion is a good interviewing strategy.
    (1) Allowing the interviewer to totally lead puts the candidate in a passive role.
    (2) Dominating the interview puts the candidate in an aggressive role.
    (4) Covering up real personality and expectations misleads the interviewer.
    (5) A demonstration of knowledge of the dental literature will not necessarily impress the interviewer.
28. (4) Job selection criteria are subjective and require self-knowledge.
    (1) Practice philosophy may be most important to some people, but not to all.
    (2) Personnel harmony may be most important to some people, but not to all.
    (3) The quality of dental care provided may be most important to some people, but not to all.
    (5) Annual salary may be most important to some people, but not to all.
29. (3) *Reclamation* refers to contacting patients of record.
    (1) Transferred patients are under current treatment
    (2) Scheduling is for patients already under care.
    (4) Upgrading restorations is unrelated to contacting patients in need of care.
    (5) *Reclamation* does not refer to patients who have never received dental care.
30. (4) Patients can directly refer others to the practice.
    (1) Dentists usually make direct referrals only to specialists.
    (2) Dental auxiliaries make fewer direct referrals than patients.
    (3) Dental suppliers make few referrals.
    (5) Other health professionals make few referrals.
31. (2) By definition, *marketing* includes the entire process of services to patients and profits to the practice.
    (1) Advertising may be one marketing technique.
    (3) Community activities may be one marketing technique.
    (4) Targeting populations is a preliminary marketing step.
    (5) Retail dentistry may be one marketing technique.

32. (1) Demonstration of good human relations skills will win more approval for a practice than any other quality.
    (2) Expediency is a small factor in marketing.
    (3) "Give-aways" are a small factor in marketing.
    (4) Only a few patients warrant correspondence.
    (5) Attending a marketing course is a small factor in marketing.

33. (4) Evaluation is the final step in the marketing process.
    (1) Advertising is one technique used in marketing.
    (2) Profits are evaluated.
    (3) Recognition precedes evaluation.
    (5) Implementation precedes evaluation.

34. (4) An independent practitioner would directly offer services to patients, without the dentist employer or supervision.
    (1) An employee dental hygienist works for the dentist.
    (2) Employer service arrangement is currently unknown.
    (3) An independent contractor uses a contractual agreement beween the dentist and dental hygienist.
    (5) An entrepreneur does not relate to a service arrangement.

35. (2) *Temporary,* by definition, is known to be of limited duration.
    (1) *Probationary* refers to a service trial period.
    (3) *Trial* refers to a probationary period.
    (4) *Part time* refers to working less than the full facility hours.
    (5) *Tenure* does not refer to a dental employment service.

36. (4) Title VII of the Civil Rights Act is the Non-discrimination Act.
    (1) The Occupational Safety and Health Board sets industrial standards.
    (2) State dental practice acts are state laws governing the practice of dentistry.
    (3) A Code of ethics is optional.
    (5) ERA does not exist.

37. (1) A dental hygienist making a counteroffer of salary demonstrates seriousness about self and the job and is showing assertive behavior.
    (2) Employers expect to negotiate starting salaries.
    (3) If making a counteroffer of salary causes loss of the job, the job may not have been the right job for that dental hygienist.
    (4) The first offer of salary is the most negotiable.
    (5) A counteroffer can be made without appearing too assertive.

38. (4) Presenting one's full value to the practice is the most relevant to deserving a salary increase.
    (1) An automatic cost-of-living increase may be less than one deserves.
    (2) Demanding an increase presents an irrelevant emotional and aggressive attitude and may result in loss of the job.
    (3) Personal need for more money is irrelevant.
    (5) An updated resume would be ineffectual in receiving an increase in salary

39. (1) Federal income tax is an employee expense.
    (2) Social Security funds are matched by the employer.
    (3) Federal unemployment tax is an employer expense.
    (4) Workers compensation is an employer expense.
    (5) FICA matching funds would be an employer expense.

40. (3) All of the benefits listed are part of the Social Security benefits package.
    (1) Workers' compensation is for on-the-job injury only.
    (2) Federal unemployment is for the involuntarily unemployed.
    (4) State disability is for nonoccupational accidents.
    (5) State taxes help pay for the benefits package.

41. (2) All fringe benefits combine with salary to total the compensation package.
    (1) Benefits are taxed once.
    (3) Benefits are a part of the total compensation package.
    (4) Benefits are legal and common business practice.
    (5) A benefit is not a component of salary.

42. (2) Employment agreements include all factors discussed during the interview.
    (1) An employment agreement may or may not be legally binding.
    (3) An agreement does not necessarily guarantee continuous employment.
    (4) An agreement should open future negotiations on a regular basis.
    (5) An agreement does not guarantee that the employee will stay.

43. (3) The dental hygienist and dentist must share the responsibility for job performance together.
    (1) The dentist is not solely responsible for employment issues.
    (2) The dental hygienist is not solely responsible for employment issues.
    (4) The patient is a minor participant in job satisfaction but does play a role.
    (5) The dental office manager could play a minor role in the dental hygienist's performance as it relates to inter-office relationships.

44. (3) Monthly progress reports are too frequent and unrealistic.
    (1) Performance strengths and weaknesses are important to evaluations.
    (2) Self-evaluation is half the process of performance evaluation.
    (4) Corrective action requested must be stated specifically to be effective.
    (5) Feedback about performance is important to evaluations.

45. (4) A carrer is a noteworthy activity in one's lifetime.
    (1) A job is employment to gain a livelihood.
    (2) Employment is a job to gain a livelihood.
    (3) An occupation is a line of work.
    (5) A science is a branch of knowledge.

46. (3) Health practitioners experience intense interpersonal relations, which can lead to stress and burnout.
    (1) Self-esteem may be suppressed, but this does not necessarily cause stress.
    (2) Self-worth may be suppressed, but this does not necessarily cause stress.
    (4) Job tasks are often monotonous, but are not necessarily stressful.
    (5) Low salaries may cause unfulfillment but not necessarily stress.

47. (4) One must identify the signs and symptoms of stress and burnout before corrective actions can be taken.
    (1) Goals are reprioritized after the cause is identified.
    (2) Behavior is modified after the cause is identified.
    (3) A new job will not cure the problem unless it is first identified.
    (5) Asking for a raise in salary may produce more stress if it is denied.

48. (3) Assertive behavior is effective and useful for both parties; it is an open and honest expression of one's feelings.
    (1) Passive behavior is submission to the other.
    (2) Nonassertive behavior is submission to the other.
    (4) Aggressive behavior is attacking and harsh, and denies another's rights.
    (5) Nonverbal communication is not an open and interactive behavior.

49. (1) Self-confidence determines assertive behavior.
    (2) Behavior of others may influence one's self-confidence.
    (3) Moods are a reflection of self-confidence.
    (4) Body language is an example of nonverbal communication.
    (5) Parents may influence one's behavior and self-confidence.

50. (4) Employment agreements are part of the professional business management of the dentist–dental hyginist relationship.
    (1) Financial planning is part of personal business.
    (2) Tax planning is part of personal business.
    (3) Will preparation is part of personal business.
    (5) Investment planning is part of personal business.

CHAPTER 18

Medical Emergencies

MARCIA K. BRAND

Dental hygienists must prepare to manage any medical emergency that might occur in the dental setting. Careful observation and questioning before the dental appointment enables the dental hygienist to identify, prepare, and care for the patient who experiences a medical complication. A working knowledge of the principles of first aid, cardiopulmonary resuscitation, and basic life support is essential. Equally important is the ability to measure and record vital signs, recognize signs and symptoms of medical disorders, and prevent further complications through appropriate intervention.

This chapter reviews the basic principles of measuring vital signs and preventing and managing medical emergencies. Periodic review of this knowledge and practice of these skills are necessary to maintain competence in this critical area.

GENERAL CONSIDERATIONS

A. Medical emergency
1. Dental patient experiencing an unforeseen medical difficulty or problem, or a combination of problems, is said to present a medical emergency
2. These complications make it necessary for the dentist or dental hygienist to take immediate action to alleviate the situation and prevent further injury
B. Dental hygienist's legal responsibility
1. Dental hygienist has a legal duty to provide patient care that meets standards for quality; these standards generally are determined on a state-by-state basis; accepted standards of care include training in medical emergency management and cardiopulmonary resuscitation
2. Dental hygienist who is not prepared to manage a medical emergency that occurs in the dental operatory, according to the standard of care for that state, may be held liable for damages
3. Dental hygienist has a responsibility to maintain complete records that describe the onset and management of a medical emergency in the dental setting; complete records include a description of the emergency, the patient's vital signs, drugs administered and dosages, emergency procedures performed, and the patient's responses to treatment; these records should be made at the time of treatment, for they document the incident and protect the dental staff in the event that any legal complications arise as a result of the emergency

C. Preventing medical emergencies
1. Thorough medical history reveals conditions that predispose a patient to medical complications; medical history is taken at the first appointment and updated at each subsequent appointment
2. Information obtained from the medical history is used to modify the patient's treatment plan and reduce the likelihood that the patient will experience a medical complication in the dental treatment setting
3. If more information regarding the patient's medical status is needed, the dentist or dental hygienist should consult the patient's physician
4. Taking and recording the patient's vital signs (generally, blood pressure, pulse, respiration rate) provides the dental hygienist with information regarding the patient's medical status
5. Medical complications may result from the patient's response to stress and anxiety in the dental environment; careful appointment planning, stress reduction measures, or premedication may reduce the likelihood that a patient will experience a stress-induced medical emergency

D. Preparing for medical emergencies
1. Every dental treatment setting should maintain an emergency kit; materials and drugs should be kept current, the kit should be accessible to all treatment rooms, and personnel should be familiar with its contents; equipment essential for emergency management includes a positive-pressure oxygen delivery system, clear

face mask, self-inflating resuscitation bag (ambu bag), oral airway tubes, and blood pressure measurement device

2. Each member of the dental staff should maintain current certification in basic cardiac life support and receive training in the recognition and management of common medical emergencies

3. Some states may require dental hygienists to have certification in cardiopulmonary resuscitation (CPR) to be eligible for licensure

4. Each member of the dental staff should have specific responsibilities in the event that a patient experiences a medical emergency

5. Staff drills in emergency procedures should be conducted regularly; arrangements should be made to familiarize new staff members with these procedures

VITAL SIGNS

Basic Concepts

A. Vital signs are the numerical values given to blood pressure, body temperature, pulse rate, respiration rate, and body height and weight

B. Patient's vital signs, along with the information gained from the medical history, are necessary to determine the patient's ability to safely and comfortably undergo dental treatment

C. Any value that is not within normal limits should be brought to the attention of the dentist, the patient, and the patient's physician, as indicated

D. Vital sign values should be recorded in the patient's chart at each visit; for most dental visits, blood pressure, pulse rate, and respiration rate are routine; body temperature should be recorded if infection is suspected; height and weight should be measured and recorded as indicated

E. Dental hygienist should explain the purpose of and method for measuring vital signs to the patient before initiating these procedures

Blood Pressure

A. Definition—force exerted by the blood on the walls of the blood vessels during the contraction and relaxation of the heart

1. Systolic pressure—force exerted during ventricular contraction (heartbeat); the highest pressure in the cardiac cycle

2. Diastolic pressure—resting pressure; occurs during ventricular relaxation (heart rest) and is the lowest pressure of the cardiac cycle

3. Pulse pressure—value obtained when the diastolic pressure is subtracted from the systolic pressure

4. Hypertension—sustained, abnormally high blood pressure

5. Hypotension—sustained, abnormally low blood pressure

B. Factors that affect blood pressure values

1. Blood pressure is the result of three variables—force of the heart's contraction, resistance of the peripheral blood vessels, and volume of blood in the circulatory system

2. Blood pressure may increase with age as a result of a decreased elasticity of the blood vessel walls

3. Blood pressure increases in response to exercise, stress, eating, and medications (such as stimulants)

C. Normal values for adults and children

1. Patient's blood pressure should be measured at the initial visit; routine measurements thereafter are necessary to determine a normal range, or nonemergency value, for the patient

2. Blood pressure is recorded as millimeters of mercury, with the systolic pressure over the diastolic pressure

$$\frac{\text{(Systolic mm Hg)}}{\text{(Diastolic mm Hg)}}$$

3. Normal systolic values for adults range from 100 to 140 mm Hg

4. Normal diastolic values for adults range from 60 to 90 mm Hg

5. Value of 140 to 160 mm Hg (systolic) over greater than 90 to 95 mm Hg (diastolic) should be rechecked for accuracy

6. Elevated readings should be reported to the dentist, the patient, and the patient's physician

7. Normal blood pressure values for children range from about 65 to 140/40 to 70 mm Hg; after age 7, systolic pressure rises about 2 mm Hg per year until age 16; diastolic pressure rises about 1 mm Hg

8. At age 16, blood pressure values average about 110/70 mm Hg

D. Measuring blood pressure

1. Equipment

a. Mercury manometer is the most frequently used instrument for measuring blood pressure

b. Sphygmomanometer is the device used to measure blood pressure; it has an inflatable cuff, a central bulb, and a pressure gauge; cuffs come in different sizes

c. Width of the cuff should be 20% greater than the diameter of the upper arm

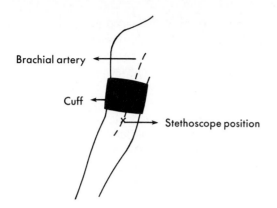

Fig. 18-1 Stethoscope position for blood pressure measurements.

d. Stethoscope is used to listen to the sounds of the blood as it passes through the brachial artery (Fig. 18-1)

2. Technique—palpatory-auscultatory method

a. Patient is seated in an upright position, with the arm bared at chest level, palm up; right arm is usually used

b. Cuff is placed snugly around the upper arm so that it is 1 inch above the antecubital fossa; bladder is over the brachial artery

c. Radial artery is palpated, and cuff is inflated until the radial pulse disappears; cuff is then inflated an additional 30 mm Hg

d. Cuff is deflated at a rate of 2 to 3 mm Hg/sec until the radial pulse returns; this value is the palpatory systolic pressure

e. Diaphragm of the stethoscope is placed over the brachial artery; stethoscope earpieces are directed forward

f. Cuff is inflated again to a level 30 mm Hg above the palpatory systolic pressure

g. Cuff is deflated at a rate of 2 to 3 mm Hg/sec

h. Sounds heard through the stethoscope are called Korotkoff sounds; they are produced by the brachial artery; their intensity decreases as the pressure in the cuff decreases

i. First sound heard through the stethescope is the systolic blood pressure

j. Last sound heard is the diastolic blood pressure

k. Blood pressure is recorded as a fraction, systolic/diastolic; measurement should be recorded as measured on the right or left arm

Body Temperature

A. Basic concepts

1. Body temperature should be measured orally in the dental setting

2. Body temperature of greater than 99.5° F is considered to be elevated; elevated temperature suggests the presence of infection, disease, or other pathologic condition

3. Patient with an elevated temperature should see the dentist or physician for further evaluation

B. Factors that affect body temperature

1. Body temperature is elevated by smoking, exercise, and eating and drinking hot foods and beverages; body temperature is decreased by starvation or shock

2. Body temperature is lowest in the morning and highest in the late afternoon or early evening

C. Normal values

1. Normal oral temperature for an adult is between 96.0° to 99.5° F (35.5° to 37.5° C)

2. Value greater than 101° F may indicate an active disease process; values greater than 99.5° indicate a fever

D. Measuring body temperature

1. Several different types of thermometers exist; most common are the oral, rectal, and external thermometers; most thermometers employ a mercury column, although electric and chemical thermometers are also available

2. Oral thermometers are contraindicated for small children and unconscious or unstable patients

E. Technique for measuring body temperature with a mercury-column thermometer

1. Thermometer should be shaken until the mercury level is below the mark indicating 96° F

2. If the patient has been eating, smoking, or drinking, the temperature should not be measured for 15 minutes

3. Thermometer bulb is placed under the patient's tongue

4. Thermometer should be in the patient's mouth for 2 minutes

5. Temperature measurements are given at 0.2, or 2 tenths, of a degree; highest reading is recorded

Pulse

A. Basic concepts

1. Pulse is the force of the blood through an artery created by the heart's contraction; each contraction creates a wave of blood that can be felt by gently pressing a superficial artery against underlying tissue

2. Pulse is evaluated according to three criteria: rate, rhythm, and quality
3. Pulse rate is measured as the number of heartbeats per minute

B. Factors that affect the pulse rate
1. Pulse rate increases in response to exercise, certain drugs, anxiety or emotional distress, heat and cold, eating, heart disease, and smoking
2. Pulse rate is decreased by sleep, drugs, fasting, and disease

C. Normal resting heart rate
1. Adult—ranges from 60 to 90 beats/min
2. Infant—ranges from 130 to 160 beats/min
3. Children—ranges from 100 to 130 beats/min; older children generally have pulse rates of between 80 and 100 beats/min

D. Determining the pulse rate
1. Sites—pulse may be felt at several superficial arteries (Fig. 18-2)
   a. Brachial pulse—located on the medial aspect of the antecubital fossa of the elbow
   b. Radial pulse—located on the lateral aspect of the wrist (thumb side) on the ventral surface
   c. Carotid pulse—located in the neck groove, just anterior to the sternocleidomastoid muscle
   d. Femoral pulse—located on the medial aspect of the thigh
2. In nonemergency situations the brachial or radial pulse is monitored; in emergency situations the carotid pulse, indicating that blood is flowing to the brain, is monitored

E. Technique for palpating the radial pulse
1. First three fingers are used to locate the radial pulse on the thumb side of the wrist
2. Number of beats in 1 minute is counted and recorded; some practitioners prefer to count the number of beats for 30 seconds and multiply by 2 to obtain the pulse rate
3. Number of beats, as well as any irregularities in quality (weak, strong, steady) and regularity, is recorded

Respiration Rate

A. Basic concepts
1. Respiration is the body's inspiration and exhalation of air
2. Respiration rate is the frequency of the body's respiration
3. Qualities to examine include depth, rhythm, quality, breathing sounds, and patient position during respiration
4. Respiration rate should be evaluated while the patient is unaware of being observed

B. Factors that affect respiration
1. Respiration rate is increased by exercise, pain, drugs, smoking, anxiety and distress, disease, severe bleeding, and shock
2. Respiration rate is decreased by drugs, sleep, and severe disease
3. Normal range for adults is between 12 and 20 respirations/min
4. Normal respiration rate for children is approximately 20 respirations/min

C. Evaluating respiration
1. After the pulse rate has been determined, the dental hygienist continues to hold the patient's wrist for 60 seconds; during this time, the number of times that the chest rises and falls is counted
2. Number of respirations per minute is recorded, along with any observed variations in the depth (shallow, deep), rhythm (regularity), quality (labored, easy), sounds (rales, wheezes) and patient positioning (sitting, leaning)

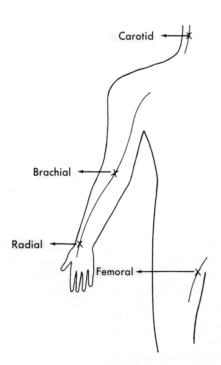

Carotid

Brachial

Radial

Femoral

Fig. 18-2 Location of pulse points.

BASIC CARDIAC LIFE SUPPORT ▪▪▪▪▪▪▪▪
Definition

A. Basic cardiac life support (BCLS) maintains an individual's heart (cardiac or circulatory) and lung (pulmonary or respiratory) functions through cardiopulmonary resuscitation (CPR)

B. BCLS minimizes damage from insufficient or impaired respiratory and circulatory function, prevents collapse through intervention, or supports the patient's respiratory and circulatory systems during arrest

C. CPR requires three basic skills: maintaining an open airway, providing ventilation by rescue breathing, and providing circulation by cardiac compression; these skills are acquired through certification courses taught according to the criteria established by the American Heart Association or American Red Cross

D. Certification requires testing in the knowledge and skills of basic cardiac life support and may be required for dental hygiene licensure in some states

Basic Concepts

A. Basic concepts of medical emergency care and basic life support can be remembered as the "ABCDs" of emergency management, where

A Airway—establishing a clear air passage
B Breathing—providing respiration through rescue breathing
C Circulation—providing circulation and cardiac support through external cardiac compressions
D Definitive treatment—providing therapy (such as drugs) and accessing the community's emergency medical system

B. Emergency medical system (EMS) is a community-wide, coordinated system of providing care for individuals who are injured or experience a sudden illness; includes paramedical rescue personnel and transportation to hospitals or emergency care facilities

C. Cardiac arrest is a sudden unexpected cessation of breathing and circulation

D. Respiratory arrest is a sudden cessation of breathing

E. Biologic death, defined as brain death, occurs within 4 to 6 minutes after cardiac arrest, unless life support measures are initiated; biologic death results from permanent, cellular damage to the brain caused by an inadequate supply of oxygenated blood

F. Clinical death occurs when the heart stops beating; will progress to biologic death unless CPR is initiated within 4 to 6 minutes; CPR might reverse clinical death or maintain a patient in clinical, rather than biologic, death until definitive therapy can be initiated

Performing CPR
Single-Rescuer CPR

The steps for performing single-rescuer CPR follow; however, it is important to remember that advances in scientific knowledge and clinical research result in frequent changes in these techniques; periodic review and recertification in CPR is necessary to remain up to date

A. Determining consciousness
 1. Look around any individual who appears to be unconscious to see if the cause, such as drugs or electric shock, can be determined
 2. Determine the person's level of consciousness by gently shaking the person's shoulder and asking, "Are you okay?" several times; this should take 4 to 10 seconds; an unresponsive individual may be unconscious
 3. Summon help if the person does not respond to attempts at arousal
 4. Carefully turn the person to a supine position, if necessary, by rolling the body as a unit; kneel beside the head and shoulder

B. Opening the airway
 1. Place one hand on the person's forehead and the other under the neck; lift the head back until the lower jaw moves forward and the tongue lifts away from the back of the throat, opening the airway
 2. Hyperextending the head might cause further injury to a person who has a neck or spine injury; it is helpful to remove loose dentures (Fig. 18-3)

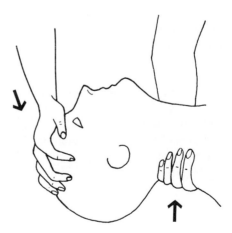

Fig. 18-3 Head tilt to open airway.

C. Determining breathlessness
   1. Kneel next to the person's shoulders and place your ear next to the person's mouth and nose, looking toward the person's chest; watch the chest to see if it rises and falls, and listen and feel for the exchange of air
   2. If the person is breathing, monitor the vital signs until help arrives
   3. If the person is not breathing, begin rescue breathing immediately
   4. Checking for breathlessness should take 3 to 5 seconds
D. Performing rescue breathing for an adult
   1. Kneel near the person's shoulder
   2. Pinch the nostrils shut with the thumb and index finger
   3. Take a deep breath and place your mouth tightly over the person's mouth to create a seal
   4. Exhale into the person's lungs and repeat three more times in rapid succession; turn your head aside for fresh air between ventilations
   5. If there is a pulse, deliver one breath every 5 seconds
   6. Monitor the person's vital signs until help arrives
E. Performing rescue breathing for a child—make these modifications
   1. Use less force or volume when inflating the child's lungs
   2. Seal the child's mouth and nose with your mouth, if possible
   3. Inflate the lungs approximately once every 4 seconds
   4. For an infant, make tiny "puffs" rather than full ventilations
   5. For an infant, breathe once every 3 seconds, or 20 times/min
F. Performing cardiac compressions
   1. Determine the absence or presence of the pulse by checking the carotid pulse; take 7 to 10 seconds to make this determination, since the heart may be beating faintly or slowly
   2. If there is no pulse, begin cardiac compressions immediately
   3. Cardiac compressions achieve artificial circulation by squeezing the heart between the sternum (breast bone) and spine; with alternate squeezing and releasing of the heart between these structures, the heart is forced to empty and refill as though it is contracting

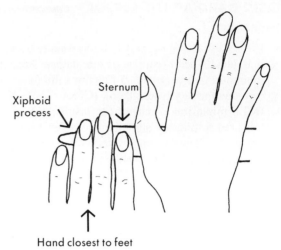

Fig. 18-4 Locating hand position for performing cardiac compressions.

   4. To perform external cardiac compressions, locate the sternum and the xiphoid process; place the third finger of the hand closest to the patient's feet on the xiphoid process, and place the middle and index fingers on the sternum
   5. Place the heel of the other hand (closest to the head) next to the index finger, on the lower half of the sternum (Fig. 18-4); without moving this hand, place the other hand (closest to the feet) on top
   6. Use both hands to alternately depress the sternum 1½ to 2 inches, then fully release the pressure on the sternum
   7. Compressions, when performed by a single rescuer, are completed at a rate of 80/min; to achieve this rate, count "one-and-two-and . . ." until 15 compressions are performed
   8. After every fifteenth compression, administer two breaths, for a 15:2 cycle; patient's lungs should not deflate between breaths
   9. Check the pulse after four cycles to see if it has returned; if not, continue performing CPR; if the pulse has returned, continue rescue breathing
   10. Never interrupt the performance of CPR for more than 5 seconds
   11. Evaluate the effectiveness of the CPR by assessing the patient's color and the responsiveness of the pupils to light
   12. To perform cardiac compressions for a child, depress the midsternum about 1 to 1½ inches, using the heel of one hand

13. To perform cardiac compressions for an infant, use two or three fingers to depress the midsternum one half to three fourths of an inch. When performing CPR for an infant, administer a single ventilation after every fifth compression, for a ratio of 5 compressions to 1 ventilation and a rate of 100 to 120 compressions/min

Two-Rescuer CPR

Two-rescuer CPR is more effective than single-rescuer CPR, since one individual performs ventilations while the other performs compressions; there is no need to interrupt cardiac compressions for ventilations as there is with single-rescuer CPR

A. Rescuers kneel on opposite sides of the patient: one at the patient's shoulders to perform ventilations, the other at the patient's chest to perform compressions
B. Rescuer performing compressions administers five compressions; on the fifth upstroke, the rescuer performing rescue breathing inflates the patient's lungs; in this manner the rescuer administering ventilations does not have to oppose the force of the compressions
C. Count for two-rescuer CPR is "one–one thousand, two–one thousand . . ." until the count of five is completed; this achieves a rate of 60 compressions/min, with a ratio of 5 compressions to 1 ventilation
D. Rescuers may switch positions, since CPR can be very tiring; cycle should not be interrupted for more than 5 seconds during the switch
E. Rescuer performing the ventilations should monitor the pulse, pupil response, and color of the patient's skin to assess the effectiveness of the CPR

Duration of CPR

A. CPR may be discontinued when the patient revives, the rescuer(s) are too exhausted to continue, another qualified individual takes over its performance, or an individual who is legally qualified pronounces the patient dead
B. Continue CPR until the patient is entered into the emergency medical system; if rescue workers, such as paramedics, arrive, continue CPR until they are prepared to take over and provide advanced cardiac life support measures

MANAGEMENT OF AN OBSTRUCTED AIRWAY

A. Basic concepts
1. Obstructed airway occurs when a foreign object or material suddenly prevents an individual from exchange of air
2. Foreign body obstruction of the upper cavity usually occurs while an individual is eating, but may occur when an individual becomes unconscious, permitting the tongue to fall back into the pharynx and block air exchange; obstructed airway may also result from the aspiration of vomitus or blood, as well as dental materials
3. Airway may be partially or completely obstructed; individual with a partial airway obstruction will be able to cough or talk; individual with a partial obstruction should be supported in efforts to dislodge the block, but no attempt should be made to remove it
4. Obstructed airway may be prevented by cutting food into smaller pieces, limiting alcohol intake with meals, and keeping small objects out of the reach of infants and small children
B. Recognizing an obstructed airway in a conscious person
1. Someone experiencing an obstructed airway may be coughing weakly, making high-pitched noises (crowing), or becoming cyanotic (blue in color)
2. Person may be unable to speak or cough
3. Person may clutch at the neck
C. Treating an obstructed airway in a conscious person
1. Determine if the person has a complete airway obstruction by asking the person to speak; if the person can speak, do not interfere with his or her own attempts to dislodge the foreign object
2. If the person cannot speak, deliver four back blows; these are sharp blows delivered between the shoulder blades with the heel of the hand; support the individual's chest at the sternum with the other hand*

---

*The American Heart Association and American Red Cross, on the recommendation of Dr. Henry Heimlich, are currently considering revising this standard.

3. If the back blows do not dislodge the obstruction, deliver four abdominal thrusts; these are quick, upward motions into the abdomen, delivered from behind the individual; place the thumb side of the fist between the xiphoid and navel, support the fist with the other hand, and make four quick, upward motions

4. If an individual is obese or pregnant, deliver the thrusts to the center of the sternum; stand behind the person, place your arms under the armpits, encircling the chest, and make four rapid compressions of the sternum

5. Continue these two measures (back blows and abdominal thrusts) until the obstruction is dislodged or the person becomes unconscious

D. Treating an obstructed airway in an unconscious person (prone position)

1. Determine unconsciousness, call for help, open the airway, establish breathlessness, and attempt to ventilate (standard procedure for managing an unconscious person)

2. If attempts to ventilate are unsuccessful, reposition the head and try to ventilate again
   a. Most common reason for failure to achieve a ventilation is improper positioning of the patient's head
   b. Repositioning the head to establish an open airway will usually allow the rescuer to achieve an adequate ventilation

3. If repositioning the head does not permit ventilation, deliver four back blows by kneeling next to the patient, rolling the patient against the thigh, and administering four sharp blows between the shoulder blades with the heel of the hand*

4. Next deliver four abdominal thrusts; place the person in a supine position, straddle or kneel next to the person, and deliver four upward thrusts with the heel of one hand between the navel and sternum

5. To deliver abdominal thrusts for an obese person or pregnant woman, use the same hand position as for CPR and compress the sternum forcefully four times

6. Clear the person's mouth of any dislodged material by turning the person's head to one side and sweeping out any debris with the fingers

---

*The American Heart Association and American Red Cross, on the recommendation of Dr. Henry Heimlich, are currently considering revising this standard.

7. Attempt to ventilate again; if attempts to ventilate are unsuccessful, repeat the sequence of four back blows, four abdominal thrusts, and clearing the mouth

8. If the obstruction is removed, continue with the procedure for an unconscious victim

ADMINISTRATION OF OXYGEN

A. Basic concepts
1. Purpose
   a. Oxygen is essential for most chemical reactions in the body, whereas carbon dioxide is the major waste product of these reactions
   b. Circulatory and respiratory systems transport these gases
   c. During a medical emergency the body's increased need for oxygen or diminished ability to obtain or use oxygen may require administration of higher concentrations of oxygen than exist in regular air
   d. System for delivering this oxygen to a patient is essential in the management of emergency situations
2. Indications for oxygen administration include syncope, cardiac problems, and respiratory difficulties (with the exception of hyperventilation)

B. Equipment—portable oxygen unit consists of an oxygen tank (an E cylinder is recommended), tubing, a self-inflating resuscitation bag (ambu bag), and a clear mask that covers the face and nose

C. Technique for administering oxygen to an unconscious patient
1. Place the patient in a supine position and open the airway
2. Start the oxygen flow from the cylinder, and adjust the rate so that the flow inflates the positive-pressure bag
3. Secure the mask over the patient's face to cover the nose and mouth
4. Compress the positive pressure bag once every 3 to 5 seconds to inflate the patient's lungs
5. Observe for chest movement and exhalation
6. If the patient is breathing but breaths appear to be weak or shallow, time the administration of ventilations to support the patient's respirations

D. Technique for administering oxygen to a conscious patient
1. Place the patient in a supine position, or encourage the patient to assume a comfortable position

2. Disconnect the positive-pressure apparatus (ambu bag)
3. Start the oxygen flow from the cylinder, and adjust the rate so that the reservoir bag fills at a rate of approximately 7 to 12 L/min
4. Place the clear mask over the patient's face to cover the nose and mouth
5. Allow the patient to breathe at his or her own rate
6. Do not permit the reservoir bag to deflate; monitor the patient's breathing and vital signs

UNCONSCIOUSNESS

A. Unconsciousness is inability to respond to stimuli, make purposeful movements, or gain awareness of events taking place
B. Levels of unconsciousness range from syncope (transient, simple fainting) to coma (prolonged, deep unconsciousness)
C. Etiology
   1. Unconsciousness may result when there is a diminished blood supply to the brain (inadequate cerebral circulation), the quality of the blood flowing to the brain is altered (because of metabolic changes), there is a central nervous system disorder, or there is an emotional disturbance
   2. Most common cause of unconsciousness in the dental setting is psychic factors, such as fear and anxiety; treatment for this type of unconsciousness is aimed at increasing the amount of oxygenated blood received by the brain
D. Preventing loss of consciousness
   1. To reduce the likelihood that a patient will become unconscious in the dental setting, the dental hygienist should perform a thorough medical history, evaluate the patient's vital signs, and determine if the patient is stressed or anxious about dental care
   2. Patients who are anxious about receiving dental care may require premedication or increased measures to ensure pain control
E. Managing unconsciousness
   1. If a patient becomes unconscious in the dental setting, the dental hygienist should initiate the procedures established for BCLS; also, if the patient is in the dental chair, the back of the chair may be lowered to increase blood flow to the patient's brain
   2. Procedures for emergency management should be initiated immediately, according to the preestablished plan

MANAGING OTHER MEDICAL EMERGENCIES

Syncope

A. Syncope is a sudden, transient loss of consciousness
B. Etiology
   1. Syncope is caused by decreased cerebral function resulting from impaired circulation or altered metabolism
   2. Syncope may result from psychogenic factors, such as anxiety and fear, or from nonpsychogenic factors, such as hunger, heat, or a sudden change in position
C. Preventing syncope
   1. Reducing the likelihood that the patient will experience syncope in the dental setting may be accomplished by completing a thorough medical history to determine a previous history of this occurrence
   2. Anxiety reduction through premedication, good patient rapport, and stress reduction may reduce the chances that an anxious patient will experience syncope
   3. Patients who "feel faint" may be aided by reclining the dental chair to the Trendelenberg position (head lower than legs)
D. Signs and symptoms—syncope occurs in three stages: presyncope, syncope, and postsyncope; each stage has its signs and symptoms
   1. Signs and symptoms of presyncope include the patient's subjective feelings of malaise, warmth, or nausea; dental hygienist may observe pallor, sweating, and a rapid pulse
   2. Signs and symptoms of syncope include dilated pupils, irregular or shallow breathing, a slow pulse, lowered blood pressure, and unconsciousness (of less than 5 minutes' duration)
   3. Postsyncope signs and symptoms include the patient's subjective feelings of confusion, nausea, and weakness; objective signs and symptoms include pallor, weakness, sweating, and a return to normal blood pressure and pulse rate
E. Managing syncope
   1. If it appears that the patient may faint, place him or her in a supine position, with the head lower than the legs if possible, and discontinue dental treatment; these actions may prevent syncope

2. If syncope occurs, follow these procedures
   a. Open the airway
   b. Determine if the patient is breathing; if the patient is not breathing, initiate BCLS procedures
   c. If the patient is breathing, loosen tight clothing and monitor the blood pressure, pulse, and respiration rate
   d. Keep the patient warm
   e. Administer oxygen if possible
   f. Administer a respiratory stimulant, such as an ammonia capsule, if available; gently pass the crushed capsule under the patient's nose
   g. Patient who has experienced syncope will generally return to consciousness within 5 minutes; when the patient regains consciousness, reassure the patient that he or she will be fine, and keep the patient in the supine position; it is advisable to discontinue dental treatment and make arrangements for the patient to be escorted home
   h. If it is likely that the patient became unconscious from causes other than simple fainting, medical follow-up may be necessary

Shock

A. Shock results from diminished blood volume or increased peripheral vascularity
B. Etiology and pathophysiology—there are five commonly accepted categories, or causes, of shock
   1. Hypovolemic shock—caused by inadequate blood volume
   2. Anaphylactic shock—caused by an acute allergic reaction
   3. Septic shock—caused by prolonged metabolic disease
   4. Cardiogenic shock—caused by heart failure
   5. Neurogenic shock—caused by psychologic or neurologic disorder
C. Signs and symptoms
   1. Patient may complain of thirst or restlessness
   2. Blood pressure may drop, pulse rate may increase, and skin may be pale and clammy; patient may, in severe cases, go into a coma

D. Treatment
   1. Although it is unlikely that a patient will experience shock in the dental setting, anaphylactic shock may occur as a result of administration of a local anesthetic, or hypovolemic shock (caused by decreased blood volume) may occur if an individual is seriously injured in an accident
   2. If a patient exhibits signs and symptoms of shock, place him or her in a supine position
   3. Provide reassurance
   4. Keep the patient warm
   5. Monitor the vital signs
   6. Maintain an open airway
   7. Administer oxygen
   8. Enter the patient into the emergency medical system for definitive therapeutic care

Respiratory Emergencies

See Chapter 14, section on bronchial asthma
A. Respiratory emergencies occur when an individual's ability to inhale or exhale and use oxygen or exchange carbon dioxide is impaired; patients are usually conscious during the early stages of a respiratory emergency, so effective patient management by the dental hygienist is critical in these situations
B. Preventing respiratory emergencies
   1. Thorough medical history may identify an individual who is more likely to experience a respiratory difficulty in the dental setting
   2. Patient's treatment plan may be modified to reduce stress and decrease the likelihood that the patient will experience an anxiety-induced respiratory difficulty in the dental setting
C. Chronic obstructive pulmonary disease
   1. Several respiratory diseases fall into the category of chronic obstructive pulmonary disease (COPD); they result from an obstruction of airflow into and out of the lungs; COPD includes asthma, bronchitis, and emphysema; of these, only asthma causes a true "emergency" situation
   2. Asthma results from an obstruction of the bronchioles caused by stress, infection, or allergy; acute episodes are usually self-limiting although the condition of status asthmaticus is a life-threatening, persistent attack of asthma
      a. Asthma attacks may be prevented by identifying the patient at risk through a thorough medical history and reducing stress during the dental appointment

b. Signs and symptoms of asthma include the patient's subjective feelings of anxiety, fatigue, weakness, and dypsnea (shortness of breath); dental hygienist may observe dypsnea, wheezing, and cyanosis
c. Treatment for an asthma attack
  (1) Encourage the patient to assume a position that facilitates breathing
  (2) If the patient has medication available, assist him or her in its administration; many asthmatics carry bronchodilators or medication
  (3) Administer oxygen
  (4) Seek the assistance of the dentist or physician if indicated
D. Hyperventilation is characterized by rapid breathing and is often brought about by pain, anxiety, or drugs; rapid breathing causes an excessive elimination of carbon dioxide, which results in respiratory alkalosis
  1. Signs and symptoms of hyperventilation include the patient's subjective report of tingling, giddiness, light-headedness, dizziness, and heart palpitations; dental hygienist may observe rapid respirations and a rapid pulse
  2. To assist the hyperventilating patient, the dental hygienist should reassure the patient that he or she will be all right, loosen tight clothing, and encourage the patient to breathe slowly and deeply
  3. It may be helpful to have the patient breathe into a small paper bag to decrease the oxygen intake; do not administer oxygen

Cardiac Emergencies

See Chapter 14, sections on congenital heart disease, rheumatic fever and heart disease, cardiac arrhythmias, hypertensive disease, ischemic heart disease, and congestive heart failure
A. Cardiac emergencies result from many causes; most require immediate, definitive medical treatment
  1. Sudden, unexpected cessation of cardiac activity is called cardiac arrest; it will lead to sudden death unless the heart's function can be maintained by CPR until it can be started again (management of cardiac arrest and sudden death is described in the section on basic cardiac life support)
  2. Cardiac arrest may be caused by accidents (such as electric shock or drowning) as well as by heart disease, which is the focus of this review

B. Etiology and pathophysiology—heart disease and cardiac emergencies may result from changes in the blood's composition (such as leukemia or anemia), the heart's function (such as arrhythmia or angina pectoris), blood vessels (such as arteriosclerosis), and blood volume (from shock or hemorrhage)
C. Preventing cardiac emergencies in the dental setting is accomplished through identification of patients at risk by a thorough medical history, evaluation by a physician when the past history or present signs and symptoms indicate the need for consultation, stress reduction measures, and premedication as indicated
D. Cardiovascular diseases
  1. Hypertension—term used to describe elevated blood pressure; although hypertension is not in itself an "emergency" it may indicate an impending circulatory or cardiac emergency
    a. Etiology and pathophysiology
      (1) In primary hypertension, the etiology is unknown, but contributing factors include smoking, heredity, race, age, diet, and obesity
      (2) Secondary hypertension results from an underlying condition, such as kidney disease
    b. Signs and symptoms
      (1) Patient may complain of headaches, dizziness, and breathing difficulties
      (2) Clinically, the patient will exhibit an elevated blood pressure
    c. Patient who exhibits hypertension should be referred to a physician for evaluation
  2. Angina pectoris
    a. Angina pectoris is a transient (temporary) ischemia (lack of oxygenated blood) of the myocardium (heart muscle) usually caused by coronary artery disease; generally manifested by chest pain
    b. Signs and symptoms
      (1) Patients experiencing angina usually complain of chest pain on exertion, weakness, and shortness of breath; pain may be described as crushing, and it may be felt in the left shoulder and mandible, as well as in the chest
      (2) Dental hygienist may observe that the patient is experiencing labored breathing; patient may be sweaty or pale

c. Treating the patient with angina
   (1) If the patient begins to experience chest pain or shortness of breath, discontinue dental treatment and alert the dentist and staff
   (2) Administer the patient's prescription of nitroglycerin, if available, or have the dentist administer this medication from the office emergency drug kit
   (3) Administer oxygen
   (4) Monitor the patient and vital signs; if the patient responds, encourage him or her to rest; discontinue oral health services for that appointment
   (5) If the patient does not respond, and if a second administration of nitroglycerin does not provide relief, assume that the patient is having a myocardial infarction and alert the emergency medical system immediately

3. Myocardial infarction
   a. Myocardial infarction is a diminished or interrupted supply of oxygenated blood to the heart that causes death (necrosis) of part of the heart muscle, resulting in impaired heart function and diminished cardiac output; if a large area of the heart is affected, the heart may be unable to function and stop beating
   b. Signs and symptoms
      (1) Patient may complain of sudden, severe, crushing chest pain that radiates to the arms, neck, or back; there may be nausea and vomiting, as well as overwhelming fear and anxiety
      (2) Dental hygienist may observe that the patient has decreased blood pressure, weakness, and cold and clammy skin
   c. Treatment
      (1) If myocardial infarction is suspected, immediately stop treatment, alert the dentist, and seek medical assistance through the emergency medical system
      (2) Administer the patient's nitroglycerin or other medication; if this does not relieve the pain within 3 minutes, suspect impending cardiac arrest
      (3) Monitor the patient's vital signs
      (4) Administer oxygen
      (5) Begin BCLS and CPR if indicated
      (6) Continue these measures until definitive treatment is available

4. Congestive heart failure
   a. Congestive heart failure results when the heart is unable to meet the demands placed on it by the body; factors that precipitate these increased demands include hypertension and heart damage from rheumatic heart disease or ischemia
      (1) If the right side of the heart is failing, there will be an impairment of systemic circulation
      (2) If the left side of the heart is in failure, there will be diminished respiratory capacity
   b. Signs and symptoms
      (1) May differ, depending on whether the patient is experiencing right- or left-sided fatigue
      (2) Patient may complain of weakness and fatigue, cold hands and feet, cough, or swelling
      (3) Dental hygienist may observe edema, cyanosis or pallor, shortness of breath, a rapid heart rate, and prominent jugular veins
   c. Treatment
      (1) Patient with congestive heart failure will probably be under a physician's care for this condition; consult the patient's physician before initiating dental treatment
      (2) If the patient experiences a crisis in the dental setting, discontinue treatment
      (3) Seat the patient upright or encourage the patient to assume a comfortable position
      (4) Administer oxygen
      (5) Monitor vital signs
      (6) Obtain medical assistance for the patient

5. Sudden death (from cardiac arrest)
   a. Sudden death is clinical death that occurs within 24 hours of the onset of symptoms; is usually attributable to cardiovascular disease, an obstructed airway, anaphylaxis, drug overdose, pulmonary embolism, or accident
   b. Etiology of cardiac arrest
      (1) Cardiac arrest results from cardiovascular collapse caused by ventricular fibrillation or cardiac standstill
      (2) Respiratory arrest (cessation of breathing) will result in cardiac arrest if not treated within 2 minutes

c. Signs and symptoms of sudden death from cardiac arrest are unconsciousness, absence of a pulse or blood pressure, absence of respirations, and fixed, dilated pupils

d. Treatment is BCLS, including CPR, until definitive therapy can be administered

Allergic Reactions

A. Allergic reactions describe a wide range of the body's physiologic responses caused by hypersensitivity to an allergin

B. Etiology and pathophysiology

1. Allergic responses may be evoked by many substances, including drugs, pollens, foods and chemicals

2. When the body contacts these substances, there is an inappropriate response of the body's immune system caused by an antigen-antibody reaction

C. Preventing allergic reactions

1. Thorough medical history should reveal a previous history of allergic reaction to dental therapeutics, or drugs and materials used in the dental setting

2. Patient who previously has experienced a reaction should be asked to describe the type of reaction and its severity

3. Patient with a suspected allergy should be referred to a physician for testing and confirmation

D. Types

1. Delayed allergic reactions

a. Delayed allergic reactions are characterized by skin or respiratory signs and symptoms; skin reactions include erythema, urticaria (hives), and angioedema (swelling of the orofacial structures); respiratory reactions include respiratory distress, wheezing, dypsnea, and angioedema of the larynx

b. Treatment

(1) Delayed reactions may be mild and necessitate no treatment

(2) If the reaction is more severe, the dentist may administer antihistamines or epinephrine; if the patient has difficulty breathing, it may be necessary to support respiration through the administration of oxygen

(3) If the reaction persists, the patient should be accompanied to a physician

2. Immediate reaction or anaphylaxis

a. Immediate allergic reactions are characterized by urticaria, nausea, angioedema, and respiratory distress; reaction may progress to cardiovascular collapse; patient may have a very rapid, weak pulse, heart palpitations, and may become cyanotic

b. Treatment

(1) Immediate allergic reaction or anaphylaxis poses a life-threatening situation requiring definitive treatment; patient must be entered into the emergency medical system immediately

(2) Place the patient in a supine position

(3) Administer oxygen

(4) Monitor vital signs

(5) Dentist or physician may administer epinephrine

(6) Initiate basic cardiac life support if necessary

Drug-related Emergencies and Poisoning

Basic Concepts

A. Drug-related emergencies include allergic response, overdose, psychogenic response (syncope or hyperventilation), and idiosyncratic reaction

B. Thorough medical history should reveal the patient's drug allergies and previous adverse reactions; these agents and materials and drugs containing these materials must be avoided during dental treatment

C. Dental hygienist should be prepared to manage reactions to administration of a local anesthetic or fluoride

Specific Reactions

A. Local anesthesia reactions may be the result of psychogenic or allergic response or toxic overdose

1. Psychogenic response is usually manifested as syncope or hyperventilation; generally the result of fear of the injection rather than the local anesthesia; these reactions (syncope and hyperventilation) should be managed according to the criteria described in related sections of this chapter

2. Allergic reactions occur more frequently with amide-type anesthetics (procaine, benzocaine), are relatively rare, and should be managed by the criteria established under the section on allergic reactions in this chapter

3. Toxic overdoses of local anesthetic agents are usually the result of an intravascular injection of the local anesthetic, rather than the administration of too much of the agent
    a. Patient who experiences a toxic overdose may be anxious and confused; may have a rapid pulse and respirations, followed by shock, respiratory arrest, and cardiovascular collapse
    b. Toxic overdose is managed by discontinuing the injection, entering the patient into the emergency medical system, and treating the patient for syncope; BCLS may be necessary if the patient experiences respiratory or cardiac arrest
B. Fluoride poisoning by ingestion may be acute (caused by a single large administration of an agent) or chronic (caused by long-term ingestion)
    1. Acute toxic reactions to fluoride in adults are rare, although fatal fluoride poisoning may be caused by accidental ingestion of large quantities of fluorides, such as those contained in insecticides with sodium fluoride; ingestion of 15 to 30 mg of fluoride per kilogram of body weight may cause death in adults
    2. Some dental products contain enough fluoride to be hazardous, especially to children; one ounce of topical fluoride gel or one 8-ounce tube of fluoridated tooth paste could be life threatening to a small child
    3. Child who ingests a toxic dose of fluoride will complain of nausea and abdominal pain; symptoms may include excessive salivation, vomiting, and diarrhea; convulsions, hypotension, profuse sweating, and a mucoid discharge from the mouth and nose may also be present.
    4. Acute fluoride poisoning is treated by
        a. Inducing emesis
        b. Administering milk
        c. Entering the patient into the emergency medical system or transporting the person to a hospital for definitive treatment

Bleeding and Hemorrhage

A. Patient may experience a bleeding problem in the dental treatment setting because of a dental procedure, accident, or spontaneous bleeding (such as a nosebleed)
B. Patients taking certain types of medications may be more susceptible to bleeding problems; such patients may be identified by a thorough medical history

C. Modifications in the patient's medication regimen may be necessary to reduce the likelihood that the patient will experience a bleeding problem as the result of dental treatment; patient's physician must be consulted before any modifications are suggested
D. Bleeding may be arterial or venous; arterial bleeding is usually more red in color and "spurts" with the contraction of the heart; venous bleeding is darker in color and "oozes"
E. Treatment of hemorrhage usually can be managed by direct pressure on the bleeding area; use clean gauze to apply pressure
    1. If bleeding is from a dental extraction or surgery site, pack the area with gauze and have the patient close until bleeding stops
    2. For nosebleed, apply cold compresses to the nose and apply pressure to the bleeding side; it may also help reduce bleeding if the nostril is gently packed with gauze
    3. If bleeding is severe, watch for signs of shock and enter the patient into the emergency medical system

Cerebrovascular Accident (Stroke)

A. Pathophysiology and etiology
    1. Cerebrovascular accident (CVA), or stroke, results when the supply of oxygen to the brain cells is disrupted by ischemia, infarction, or hemorrhage of the cerebral blood vessels
    2. Factors that make persons more susceptible to cerebrovascular accident include smoking, high blood pressure, and diabetes
B. Prevention
    1. Persons may decrease the likelihood that they will experience a CVA by reducing their risk factors, such as controlling hypertension or eliminating the cigarette-smoking habit
    2. Thorough medical history might identify an individual at risk for a CVA
C. Signs and symptoms
    1. Conscious person who is experiencing a stroke may exhibit temporary or transient symptoms, including dizziness, weakness on one side, difficulty in speaking, and increased blood pressure; pulse may be described as "bounding" when palpated at the brachial or radial pulse point
    2. More serious signs and symptoms that may occur include paralysis, convulsions, nausea, dyspnea, and severe headache
    3. Unconscious CVA victim may have an elevated blood pressure and a bounding pulse

D. Treatment
  1. Conscious patient
    a. If the signs and symptoms of a CVA persist for 2 to 10 minutes, stop treatment, alert the staff, and enter the patient into the emergency medical system
    b. Assist the patient to assume a comfortable position
    c. Monitor the patient's vital signs
    d. If the patient experiences difficulty breathing, administer oxygen
    e. Continue to support the patient's breathing and monitor vital signs until medical assistance arrives
  2. Unconscious patient
    a. Alert the staff and enter the patient into the emergency medical system
    b. Place the patient in a supine position
    c. Monitor vital signs
    d. Administer oxygen
    e. Initiate BCLS if necessary, and support the patient until medical assistance arrives

Seizures and Convulsive Disorders

See Chapter 14, section on epilepsy
A. Seizures and convulsive disorders are the result of changes in brain function
  1. Seizures are characterized by alterations in consciousness, motor function, and sensory perceptions; usually have a rapid onset and brief duration
  2. Convulsions are involuntary contractions of the voluntary muscles
  3. Epilepsy is a condition characterized by recurrent seizures and convulsions
B. Etiology and pathophysiology
  1. Seizures and convulsions result from a disturbance of the brain's electrical activity
  2. Disruptions may include tumors, congenital abnormalities, injuries, drugs, and idiopathic causes
C. Preventing seizures
  1. Thorough medical history should identify an individual with a history of seizures or convulsive disorders
  2. If a patient has a previous history of seizures, determine if medications have been prescribed to control the seizures and if the patient has taken the required medication before that appointment
  3. Short appointments, scheduled early in the day, may reduce the likelihood that a susceptible patient will experience a seizure in the dental setting

D. Types of seizures
  1. Generalized or grand mal seizures are the most common type
    a. Person who is about to have a grand mal seizure may experience an "aura," characterized by numbness, changes in the senses of sight, smell, and taste, and hallucinations
    b. Seizure will progress to loss of consciousness and involuntary clonic and tonic muscle contractions
    c. Affected individual may make the characteristic "epileptic cry" caused by forcible exhalation
    d. After the seizure, respiration will return, the person may perspire, and the muscles will relax
    e. Affected individual may experience headache, muscle ache, and drowsiness
  2. Generalized absence or petit mal seizures usually occur in children
    a. Person experiencing a petit mal seizure will experience sudden, momentary loss of consciousness
    b. Person may not be aware of having experienced an attack; may twitch, but usually will not fall
  3. Psychomotor seizures are characterized by purposeless movements and trancelike confusion that may last from several minutes to several hours; person's speech and consciousness may be impaired
E. Treatment for generalized absence or psychomotor seizures is generally not indicated; to care for a patient who experiences a grand mal seizure in the dental setting, the dental hygienist should
  1. Lower the dental chair and clear the area
  2. Establish an airway
  3. Loosen tight clothing
  4. Make no attempts to restrain the patient or place any objects in the mouth
  5. Monitor vital signs
  6. After the seizure, permit the patient to rest
  7. Arrange for the patient to be assisted when leaving the dental office

Diabetes Mellitus

See Chapter 14, section on diabetes mellitus
A. Diabetes is characterized by elevated levels of blood glucose, resulting from an impaired ability to produce or use the hormone insulin

B. Patients with diabetes mellitus will exhibit a number of clinical manifestations of the disease and have an increased susceptibility to infection and diseases of the blood vessels

C. Etiology and pathophysiology
1. Insulin is normally produced by β-cells of the pancreas
2. Cells of the body need insulin to take in glucose, and the liver uses insulin to store glucose as glycogen
3. If glucose and glycogen are unavailable to the body as energy sources, the body must break down other materials for "fuel"
4. Dental setting emergencies related to diabetes may occur as the result of two different situations
   a. Patient has too much insulin, resulting in hypoglycemia (low blood sugar)
   b. Patient has inadequate insulin, resulting in hyperglycemia (high blood sugar)

D. Types
1. Type I, or insulin-dependent, diabetes mellitus usually occurs in childhood and is more likely to precipitate a diabetic emergency
2. Type II, or noninsulin-dependent, diabetes mellitus usually occurs in adulthood and rarely results in an emergency situation

E. Preventing diabetic emergencies
1. Thorough medical history is essential to prevent diabetic emergencies in the dental office; factors to be determined during the medical history include the type and severity of diabetes, medications, and their frequency, duration, and dosage; medical consultation may be necessary
2. Patient whose diabetes is not under control should postpone dental treatment except for emergency procedures
3. Dental hygienist should establish that the patient's medications have been taken according to prescription and that the patient has eaten meals according to schedule on the day of the appointment
4. Efforts should be made to minimize the patient's stress and anxiety
5. Appointments should be scheduled to ensure that the patient is rested and that the patient's meal and medication schedule is not interrupted; unless a patient is taking long-acting insulin, appointments should be scheduled 1½ to 3 hours after insulin administration

F. Diabetic emergency—insulin reaction (hypoglycemia or hyperinsulinism)
1. Insulin reaction occurs when there is too much insulin available, with the result that the patient's blood glucose is abnormally low; this reaction may occur when the patient takes medication and omits a meal, or engages in excessive exercise
2. Signs and symptoms of insulin reaction may occur suddenly and include hunger, headache, pale moist skin, and feelings of dizziness and weakness; patient undergoing an insulin reaction will not be thirsty and will have a normal breath odor
3. Treatment for insulin reaction includes the administration of sugar in the form of orange juice, cola, or sugar water; this will usually bring about a rapid recovery; if the patient becomes unconscious, seek assistance through the emergency medical system

G. Diabetic emergency/diabetic coma (hyperglycemia, hypoinsulinism ketoacidosis)
1. Diabetic coma occurs when there is insufficient insulin available, with the result that some cells cannot metabolize blood glucose
2. Signs and symptoms of impending diabetic coma in a conscious patient include the "classic" signs of polydipsia (excessive thirst), polyuria (excessive urination), polyphagia (excessive hunger), nausea, dry, flushed skin, and a "fruity" breath odor, followed by unconsciousness
3. Treatment for a patient experiencing symptoms of diabetic coma include discontinuance of dental care, entry into the emergency medical system; and patient support through BCLS if necessary
4. If the dental hygienist has doubts regarding the etiology of a diabetic-related problem, it is advisable to administer a small amount of sugar; since hyperinsulinism is more common than diabetic coma, the administration of sugar will probably improve the patient's condition

Acute Adrenal Insufficiency, or Adrenal Crisis

A. Acute adrenal insufficiency (adrenal crisis) occurs when the adrenal gland produces insufficient amounts of cortisol, a glucosteroid that enables the body to respond to stress

B. Dental treatment may induce considerable stress for some patients, causing this serious complication

C. Adrenal crisis is a life-threatening situation, and patients experiencing adrenal insufficiency may go into cardiac arrest or shock

D. Etiology and pathophysiology—adrenal gland is unable to produce enough cortisol to enable the body to respond to a stressful situation

E. Signs and symptoms
   1. Patient undergoing acute adrenal insufficiency may experience confusion, weakness, and abdominal pain
   2. Pulse may be rapid and weak; patient may develop hypotension, followed by unconsciousness

F. Treatment
   1. Alert the staff and enter the patient into the emergency medical system
   2. Discontinue dental treatment
   3. Place the patient in a supine position
   4. Monitor vital signs
   5. Administer oxygen
   6. Dentist or physician may administer glucocorticosteroid
   7. If the patient becomes unconscious, BCLS may be necessary until definitive treatment is available

Foreign Body in the Eye

A. Having a foreign body in the eye may happen to the dental hygienist, as well as the patient, in the dental environment

B. Safety glasses should be worn by both the dental hygienist and the patient to prevent splatter of agents or materials during dental hygiene care

C. Foreign material in the eye will usually cause tearing, pain, and blinking

D. Procedure for removing a solid particle from the eye
   1. While the patient looks down, pull the upper eyelid down over the lower lid
   2. If the particle is not removed, turn the lower eyelid down and examine it for irritants
   3. If the solid particle is visible and cannot be removed by tearing, remove it with a moistened cotton-tip applicator
   4. After the particle is removed, irrigate the eye with an eye cup or with gently running water
   5. If the particle cannot be easily removed, refer the person to a physician for prompt treatment; it may be necessary to cover the eye with sterile gauze and adhesive tape to prevent the patient from further damaging the eye by rubbing

E. Procedure for removing a caustic solution from the eye
   1. If a chemical solution is splashed in the eyes, irrigate them with gently running water for 15 minutes
   2. Refer the person to a physician for medical assistance if damage to the eye is suspected

MANAGING DENTAL EMERGENCIES
Dislocated Jaw

A. Dislocated jaw, or mandible, may occur as the result of trauma or forced movement

B. Patient with a dislocated jaw cannot return the mandible to a normal position because the head of the condyle is anterior to the articular eminence

C. Patient with a dislocated mandible may experience considerable pain and anxiety

D. To return the mandible to its normal position, the dental hygienist should wrap both thumbs in a cloth or towel to protect them and place the thumbs directly on the occlusal surfaces of the mandibular teeth; fingers should be placed under the patient's mandible at the curve; to move the mandible back into place, press down and back with the thumbs and pull up and forward with the fingers; mandible should slip into place

Avulsed Tooth

A. Avulsed tooth is a tooth that is forcibly removed from the mouth by trauma

B. Such a tooth should be handled only by the crown

C. Tooth should be reimplanted into the socket immediately after being rinsed with water if possible

D. If the tooth cannot be placed into the socket, the patient should transport the tooth to the dental setting for emergency treatment by holding it under the tongue

E. Less preferred transport medium is milk; as a last resort, distilled water may be used

F. Patient should receive immediate emergency treatment in the dental setting

Aspirated Materials

A. Dental materials and instruments may be easily aspirated during dental care because of the patient's position, diminished responses caused by drugs, and diminished "oral awareness" caused by local anesthesia

B. Prevent aspiration of materials through the use of a rubber dam; patients with conditions that predispose them to coughing (COPD) or who may be poor management cases (such as the developmentally disabled) merit careful attention

C. If a patient is reclining in the dental chair and aspirates an object into the oropharyngeal area, lower the back of the chair, using gravity to assist the patient's efforts to dislodge the object

D. If an object is aspirated into the trachea, begin BCLS maneuvers for management of an obstructed airway

E. If an object that has been swallowed cannot be located, the patient must be escorted to seek further medical evaluation

Broken Dental Hygiene Instruments

A. Instrument breakage can be minimized by careful sharpening and frequent inspection

B. If an instrument breaks, stop the procedure immediately and isolate the area where the tip is believed to be located

C. Inform the patient of the situation

D. Dry the area and examine it for the tip; if the tip is believed to be in a sulcus or periodontal pocket, use gentle instrumentation to explore the area; take care to avoid pushing the broken tip further into the sulcus

E. If the tip cannot be located, inform the dentist of the situation and use radiographs and transillumination to locate the broken piece

F. Follow-up by a dentist or physician may be necessary

SUGGESTED READINGS

American Heart Association: Manual for instructors of basic cardiac life support, Dallas, 1978, The Association.

Burke, S.R.: Human anatomy and physiology for the health sciences, New York, 1980, John Wiley & Sons, Inc.

Blair, D.M., and Cantrell, J.R.: Symposium on medical emergencies in the dental office, Dent. Clin. North Am. **26**(1), 1982.

Kutscher, A.H., et al.: Pharmacology for the dental hygienist, Philadelphia, 1982, Lea & Febiger.

Malamed, S.F.: Handbook of medical emergencies in the dental office, ed. 2, St. Louis, 1982, The C.V. Mosby Co.

McCarthy, F.M.: Medical emergencies in dentistry, Philadelphia, 1982, W.B. Saunders Co.

Monrotus, S.C.: Practical pharmacology for the dental hygienist, Philadelphia, 1980, W.B. Saunders Co.

Requa, B.S., and Holroyd, S.V.: Applied pharmacology for the dental hygienist, St. Louis, 1982, The C.V. Mosby Co.

Whitford, G.M.: Fluorides: metabolism, mechanism of action and safety, Dent. Hyg. **57**(5):16, 1983.

Wilkins, E.W.: Clinical practice of the dental hygienist, ed. 5, Philadelphia, 1983, Lea & Febiger.

Woodall, I.R., et al.: Comprehensive dental hygiene care, ed. 2, St. Louis, 1985, The C.V. Mosby Co.

Review Questions

1 If a young man came into the office for dental hygiene services, the dental hygienist would probably treat him that day *unless* he were to present which of the following vital signs?
1. A respiration rate of 15 breaths/min
2. A temperature of 99° F
3. A blood pressure of 140/110
4. A pulse rate of 70 beats/min
5. A respiration rate of 12 breaths/min

2 The state in which one is completely unaware of one's surroundings and is unable to make any meaningful or purposeful movements is called
1. Local anesthesia
2. Sedation
3. Unconsciousness
4. Coma
5. Syncope

Situation: A 52-year-old man with known diabetes, which is apparently well under control, arrives for a 9 AM appointment for a mandibular third molar extraction. He was advised by a friend not to eat before having oral surgery. The patient is given 1.8 ml injection of 2% lidocaine containing 1:100,000 epinephrine to block the inferior alveolar nerve. About 5 minutes after the injection, he has the following symptoms: sweating, pallor, hunger, trembling, headache, dizziness, and weakness. The pulse rate is 105, and the blood pressure is 140/90. The patient's symptoms do not improve after he is placed in a supine position. Questions 3 and 4 refer to this situation.

3 The most probable diagnosis of the patient's condition is
1. Epinephrine reaction
2. Anaphylaxis
3. Anesthetic toxicity
4. Insulin shock
5. Diabetic coma

4 Which of the following is the best treatment for this patient?
1. Have the dentist or physician administer an antihistamine
2. Administer sugar in a liquid form
3. Administer the patient's insulin as prescribed
4. Administer oxygen
5. Do nothing; this situation is self-limiting

5 A condition characterized by high blood pressure is
1. Hyperthyroidism
2. Hypotension
3. Hyperthermia
4. Hypertension
5. Hypothermia

6 The dental hygienist's responsibility for medical emergency management is described by which of the following statements?
1. The dental hygienist cannot be held legally responsible for patient care in an emergency situation because of the Good Samaritan Act
2. The dental hygienist is expected to meet an accepted standard of care in the management of an office emergency situation
3. The dental hygienist cannot be held responsible for remaining up to date in medical emergency management
4. The dentist is responsible for documenting any medical emergencies that arise in the dental office
5. The dental hygienist is expected to know CPR

Situation: A 51-year-old woman arrived 10 minutes late for a 6-month dental hygiene recall appointment. She was immediately escorted to the operatory, and the hygienist began scaling. After 10 minutes, the patient complained of nausea, dizziness, and a very warm sensation. The dental hygienist stopped treatment and placed the patient in a position so that her head was lower than her legs. The patient began to feel better, and the dental hygienist continued scaling. Questions 7 and 8 refer to this situation.

7 Which of the following might have prevented this medical complication?
(a) Premedicating the patient to reduce anxiety associated with dental treatment
(b) Reviewing the patient's medical and dental histories before treatment
(c) Consulting with the patient's physician
(d) Administering oxygen
(e) Taking and recording the patient's vital signs
1. a, b, and c
2. b, c, and e
3. b, c, d, and e
4. d and e
5. e only

8 The patient in this situation probably experienced
1. Syncope
2. Acute adrenal insufficiency
3. Hyperventilation
4. An insulin reaction
5. Angina

9 The patient's respiration rate should be monitored
1. For a period of 2 minutes
2. After the patient has completed the written medical history
3. After the pulse has been taken and while the patient is unaware that the respiration rate is being observed
4. Periodically during the initial appointment as a method of assessing the patient's anxiety
5. Only in an emergency situation

10 The vital signs are numerical values given to blood pressure, pulse rate, body temperature, respiration rate, body height, and weight. For most dental visits, which of these signs should be recorded?
1. Blood pressure, pulse rate, height, and weight
2. Blood pressure, body temperature, and weight
3. Blood pressure, pulse rate, and respiration rate
4. Pulse rate and respiration rate
5. None; vital signs are taken only in an emergency

11 In which of the following medical complications would you expect the patient to exhibit a lowered blood pressure?
(a) Shock
(b) Syncope
(c) Anaphylaxis
(d) Hyperventilation
(e) Congestive heart failure
1. a only
2. a and b
3. a, b, and c
4. b, c, and d
5. d only

12 Once cardiac arrest occurs, the brain cells generally begin to die within
1. 1 to 2 minutes
2. 4 to 6 minutes
3. 3 to 5 minutes
4. 6 to 8 minutes
5. 8 to 10 minutes

13 Frequent urination, thirst, and a dry mouth are symptoms of
1. Hypertension
2. Angina pectoris
3. Kidney disease
4. Diabetes mellitus
5. Impending myocardial infarction

14 In shock the patient's blood pressure shows a
1. Marked drop
2. Marked rise
3. Rise
4. Normal reading
5. Drop, followed by a rapid rise in blood pressure

15 Myocardial infarction results from
1. Heart valve damage
2. Occlusion of coronary arteries
3. Infective endocarditis
4. Adrenal gland disorder
5. Thrombocytopenia

16 The range for the normal adult pulse rate is
1. 40 to 60 beats/min
2. 60 to 90 beats/min
3. 90 to 130 beats/min
4. 130 to 150 beats/min
5. 150 to 170 beats/min

17 When should vital signs be recorded in the patient's chart?
(a) At every dental appointment
(b) Once every year
(c) When medical complications are suspected
(d) To document the patient's physical status and responses to treatment during an emergency situation
1. a only
2. b and c
3. c and d
4. a, c, and d
5. d only

18 Which of the following blood pressure readings is considered to be elevated for an adult patient?
1. 120/80
2. 140/80
3. 120/90
4. 140/90
5. 150/95

19 In a dental office emergency situation the best site for determining the patient's pulse rate is the
1. Femoral artery
2. Temporal artery
3. Jugular vein
4. Radial artery
5. Carotid artery

20 Permanent cellular damage to the brain caused by an inadequate supply of oxygenated blood results in
1. Shock
2. Respiratory arrest
3. Cardiac arrest
4. Biologic death
5. Clinical death

21 What type of shock is caused by an acute allergic reaction?
1. Hypovolemic
2. Anaphylactic
3. Septic
4. Cardiogenic
5. Neurogenic

22 The most common cause of unconsciousness in the dental office is
1. Allergic reaction to a local anesthetic
2. Diabetes-related crisis
3. Poor patient positioning
4. Fear and anxiety
5. Shock

Situation: The patient for whom you are providing care has related a history of swollen ankles that have improved following treatment with digoxin, 0.25 mg a day. While lying in a horizontal position in the dental chair, your patient becomes progressively short of breath. The pulse is 104 and regular, Questions 23 to 28 refer to this situation.

23 Which of the following conditions is the most likely cause of the patient's problem?
1. Congestive heart failure
2. Myocardial infarction
3. Anaphylaxis
4. Cerebrovascular accident (CVA)
5. Anxiety

24 On placing the patient in an upright position, you note that the patient's breathing improves. The patient develops chest pains and collapses. Which of the following should be used to determine if the patient has stopped breathing?
1. Palpate the patient's femoral pulse in the groin area
2. Palpate the patient's carotid pulse using the index and middle fingers
3. Tap the patient on the shoulder, shake, and shout
4. Evaluate the size of the patient's pupils
5. Look at the patient's chest, listen, and feel for air from the mouth and nose

25 Effective performance of chest compressions during CPR includes all of the following *except*
1. Compressing the chest over the xiphoid process at the tip of the sternum
2. Interlocking the fingers so that they remain off the patient's chest during compressions
3. Keeping the heel of the hand in light contact with the chest wall during the relaxation phase of chest compression
4. Using smooth, regular, uninterrupted movements to compress the chest
5. Depressing the chest 1½ to 2 inches during chest compressions

26 Which of the following is the proper ratio of breaths to compressions when performing one-rescuer CPR for an adult?
1. 5 compressions to 1 breath
2. 7 compressions to 1 breath
3. 10 compressions to 2 breaths
4. 12 compressions to 2 breaths
5. 15 compressions to 2 breaths

27 As you are giving CPR, you find that the pulse begins again, but the patient does not begin breathing. What should you do?
1. Continue to administer CPR until breathing begins
2. Continue giving compressions without mouth-to-mouth breathing
3. Continue giving breaths without chest compressions
4. Wait for the patient to begin breathing on his own
5. Deliver four back blows and four abdominal thrusts

28 You continue to provide rescue breathing for this patient. How often should you deliver a ventilation?
1. Once every second
2. Once every 5 seconds
3. Once every 15 seconds
4. On every fifth heart beat
5. On every fifteenth heart beat

---

29 Which of the following positions are effective for performing external cardiac compressions?
(a) Having the patient in a seated position
(b) Placing the patient in a horizontal position
(c) Placing the patient with the head lower than the heart
(d) Placing the patient with the head higher than the heart
1. a only
2. a and b
3. b and c
4. b, c, and d
5. a, b, c, and d

Situation: Your patient complains that his right hand is numb and that the polishing agent you are using tastes peculiar. He makes a sharp crying sound, becomes unconscious, and makes convulsive motions. Questions 30 to 32 refer to this situation.

30 All of the following statements are true *except*
1. The patient experienced an ''aura'' before the seizure
2. The patient experienced a petit mal seizure
3. The patient experienced a grand mal seizure
4. The patient experienced a disruption of the electrical function of the brain
5. The patient's condition is probably self-limiting

31 To assist your patient in this situation, you should
1. Have the dentist administer diazepam (Valium)
2. Place a tongue blade wrapped in gauze between the patient's teeth to prevent him from biting his tongue
3. Place him in an upright position
4. Lower the chair and clear the area
5. Restrain him

32 When the seizure is over, you should
1. Seek medical assistance immediately
2. Administer the patient's anticonvulsant medications
3. Permit the patient to rest
4. Use an ammonia capsule to arouse the patient
5. Dismiss the patient immediately

---

33 All of the following statements are true except
1. The normal range for oral temperatures for adults is 96.0° to 99.5° F
2. The normal range for pulse rate for adults is 60 to 90 beats/min
3. The normal range for respiration rates for adults is 12 to 20 respirations/min
4. The normal respiration rate for a child is approximately 20 respirations/min
5. The normal pulse rate for an infant is 80 to 100 beats/min

34 Respiratory distress frequently may be alleviated by the administration of oxygen. This may be true of all of the following except
1. Hyperventilation
2. Bronchitis
3. Congestive heart failure
4. Asthma
5. Emphysema

Situation: Your patient needs impressions for the fabrication of study models. After the impressions are made, he washes his hands and face with hand soap and water, while you wrap and store the impression trays. On your return, you begin scaling the patient's teeth. He complains that his face is ''itchy,'' and you notice that his hands and face are reddened and that there appear to be hives on his hands. Questions 35 and 36 refer to this situation.

35 The patient has probably experienced
1. A mild, delayed allergic reaction
2. A severe delayed allergic reaction
3. An immediate allergic reaction
4. A skin reaction
5. A mild case of anaphylaxis

36 Treatment for immediate or delayed allergic reactions may include all of the following *except*
1. Administration of oxygen
2. Administration of antihistamines
3. Administration of epinephrine
4. Administration of amphetamines
5. Administration of diphenhydramine (Benadryl)

---

37 Which of the following medical complications present a truly life-threatening situation?
(a) Myocardial infarction
(b) High blood pressure
(c) Acute adrenal insufficiency
(d) Anaphylaxis
(e) Delayed allergic reactions
1. a and d
2. a, b, c, and d
3. a, c, and d
4. a only
5. d only

Situation: A parent calls you on the dental office phone certain that her 3-year-old son has ingested the contents of a bottle of fluoride mouth rinse. Questions 38 and 39 refer to this situation.

38 What symptoms might the child exhibit if he has ingested a toxic dose of fluoride?
1. Nausea, excessive salivation, vomiting, profuse sweating, and mucoid discharge from mouth
2. Nausea, dry, pale skin, hypertension, and xerostomia
3. Abdominal pain, xerostomia, and diarrhea
4. Nausea and caustic burns on the mouth and throat
5. Sloughing oral mucosa, caustic burns around the mouth, and abdominal pain

39 What would you tell the mother to do in this situation?
1. Bring the child into the office
2. Induce vomiting, administer milk, and take the child to the hospital for evaluation or definitive care
3. Disregard the situation; fluoride is essentially nontoxic
4. Do not induce vomiting; do administer milk
5. Take the child immediately to the emergency room

---

40 If a dental material is aspirated into the oropharyngeal area, the dental hygienist should
1. Lower the back of the chair to assist the patient's efforts to dislodge the object
2. Try to remove the object with a pair of college pliers
3. Immediately administer four back blows
4. Perform an abdominal thrust
5. Seat the patient upright

Answers and Rationales

1. (3) This value, 140/110, exceeds the range of normal for an adult.
   (1) Fifteen breaths per minute is within the normal range.
   (2) A temperature of 99° F is within the normal range.
   (4) A pulse of 70 is within the normal range.
   (5) Twelve breaths per minute is within the normal range.
2. (3) The stem gives the definition of the term *unconsciousness*.
   (1) Local anesthesia does not bring about unconsciousness.
   (2) Sedation does not bring about unconsciousness, but rather an altered response.
   (4) A coma is very profound unconsciousness from which an individual cannot be aroused.
   (5) Syncope is a transient state during which an individual may become unconscious.
3. (4) The symptoms describe insulin shock; the patient's choice to skip breakfast also suggests that he is experiencing an insulin reaction.
   (1) Reactions to the epinephrine in local anesthesia are rare.
   (2) The symptoms of anaphylaxis differ from those of insulin shock.
   (3) The patient only received one injection; it was not administered into a major blood vessel.
   (5) Diabetic coma has a slow onset and different symptoms.
4. (2) This patient is probably experiencing insulin shock; administering sugar may relieve his hypoglycemia.
   (1) An allergic reaction warranting the use of an antihistamine is unlikely.
   (3) The patient probably has too much insulin at this time.
   (4) Although oxygen may become necessary, it is not immediately indicated.
   (5) This situation could be self-limiting, but probably will be alleviated by the administration of sugar.
5. (4) *Hypertension* is defined as an abnormally high elevation of blood pressure.
   (1) This is excessive activity of the thyroid gland.
   (2) This is abnormally low blood pressure.
   (3) This is an abnormal rise of body temperature without the presence of infection.
   (5) This is subnormal body temperature.

For each question the correct answer and rationale are listed first. The other choices are presented in order with the reasons why they are not correct.

6. (2) Minimum standards may vary from state to state; accepted standards usually include training in CPR and managing common medical emergencies.
   (1) The dental hygienist is legally responsible for managing emergency situations within the dental hygiene scope of practice.
   (3) The dental hygienist is expected to remain up to date in emergency care.
   (4) The dental hygienist should assist in the documentation of the management of emergency situations that arise in the dental office.
   (5) The minimum standard of care includes training in CPR; however, this alone does not prepare the dental hygienist to manage an emergency.

7. (2) Reviewing the patient's histories might reveal past or recent medical complications necessitating treatment plan modification, the need for a consultation with a physician, or stress reduction measures. Taking the patient's vital signs might have revealed a diminished capacity to undergo dental treatment.
   (1) Premedication for anxiety is probably unwarranted in this situation.
   (3) The administration of oxygen is appropriate treatment, but an unwarranted preventive measure.
   (4) See 3.
   (5) Correct, but reviewing the histories and consulting the physician are also correct.

8. (1) Syncope is a transient loss of consciousness, frequently from psychogenic causes.
   (2) Adrenal insufficiency is a life-threatening situation, characterized by confusion, weakness, abdominal pain, and hypotension.
   (3) Hyperventilation may be induced by anxiety, but is characterized by rapid breathing.
   (4) An insulin reaction is caused by the administration of insulin without adequate food intake; signs and symptoms include hunger and weakness.
   (5) Angina is characterized by chest pain.

9. (3) This prevents the patient from changing the respiration rate because he or she is aware of observation.
   (1) One minute of observation is adequate to determine the patient's respiration rate.
   (2) It would be difficult to observe the respiration rate from any distance.
   (4) The respiration rate should be determined over a 1-minute period.
   (5) The respiration rate should be observed in a nonemergency situation to establish a baseline of normal values for the patient.

10. (3) Blood pressure, pulse rate, and respiration rate provide critical information regarding the patient's ability to withstand dental procedures and form a baseline for comparison should an emergency occur.
    (1) Height and weight are usually not recorded.
    (2) Temperature is generally not recorded unless infection is suspected; weight is usually not recorded.
    (4) Temperature is not recorded unless infection is suspected.
    (5) Vital signs are necessary in nonemergency situations for the reasons given in 3.

11. (3) Shock, syncope, and anaphylaxis all may be characterized by a decreased blood pressure value.
    (1) Correct, but b and c are also characterized by falling blood pressure.
    (2) Correct, but c is also characterized by a falling blood pressure value.
    (4) Hyperventilation is not characterized by a falling blood pressure; congestive heart failure may be characterized by an increase in blood pressure.
    (5) See 4.

12. (2) The brain cells begin to undergo irreparable damage caused by a lack of oxygen with 4 to 6 minutes after cardiac arrest.
    (1) Brain cells begin to die with 4 to 6 minutes.
    (3) Brain cells begin to die with 4 to 6 minutes.
    (4) Brain cells begin to die with 4 to 6 minutes.
    (5) Brain cells begin to die with 4 to 6 minutes.

13. (4) These symptoms, as well as hunger and susceptibility to infection, are indicative of diabetes.
    (1) Symptoms of hypertension may be absent or include headache or dizziness.
    (2) Symptoms of angina include chest pain.
    (3) Frequent urination could indicate a kidney dysfunction; however, thirst and a dry mouth may not.
    (5) Symptoms of myocardial infarction include chest pain and anxiety.

14. (1) Shock is brought on by a marked drop in blood pressure from a decreased blood supply or increased peripheral vascularity.
    (2) Blood pressure drops as a patient experiences shock.
    (3) Blood pressure drops as a patient experiences shock.
    (4) Blood pressure drops as a patient experiences shock.
    (5) Blood pressure drops as a patient experiences shock.

15. (2) Myocardial infarction is a result of reduced or occluded coronary blood flow.
    (1) Heart valve damage is a result of a congenital defect or rheumatic fever.
    (3) Infective endocarditis is a result of bacterial invasion of a defective heart valve.
    (4) Adrenal gland disorder is a possible cause of secondary hypertension.
    (5) Thrombocytopenia results in an increase in the number of white blood cells.

16. (2) The normal range for an adult pulse rate is from 60 to 90 beats/min.
    (1) The 40 to 60 range is too low.
    (3) The 90 to 130 range is too high.
    (4) The 130 to 150 range is too high.
    (5) The 150 to 170 range is too high.

17. (4) Vital signs should be recorded before each dental appointment to assess the patient's ability to undergo dental treatment.
    (1) This is not the only correct answer.
    (2) Vital signs should be evaluated at each appointment, as well as when medical complications are expected.
    (3) Both answers are correct; however, selection a is also correct.
    (5) This is not the only correct answer.

18. (5) Systolic values greater than 140 mm Hg and diastolic values greater than 90 mm Hg are considered to be elevated.
    (1) This value is within the normal range for adults (systolic = 100 to 140 mm Hg; diastolic = 60 to 90 mm Hg).
    (2) The value 140/80 is within the normal adult range.
    (3) The value 120/90 is within the normal adult range.
    (4) The value 140/90 is within the normal adult range.
19. (5) The carotid artery carries blood to the brain. The brain must receive oxygenated blood, or it will begin to undergo irreparable damage within 4 to 6 minutes.
    (1) The femoral artery does not indicate blood flow to the brain.
    (2) The temporal artery does not indicate blood flow to the brain.
    (3) Veins are not used to determine the presence or absence of a pulse.
    (4) The radial artery does not indicate blood flow to the brain.
20. (4) Biologic death occurs when the brain does not receive an adequate supply of oxygenated blood; irreparable cellular damage occurs within 4 to 6 minutes.
    (1) Shock may cause biologic death; shock is caused by diminished blood volume or increased peripheral vascularity.
    (2) This occurs when the patient is not breathing; if untreated, it will lead to biologic death.
    (3) This occurs when the patient's heart is not beating; if untreated, it will lead to biologic death.
    (5) This occurs within the 4 to 6 minutes between the time when a patient's breathing and heartbeat cease and the onset of biologic death.
21. (2) Anaphylactic shock results from an acute allergic reaction.
    (1) Hypovolemic shock results from inadequate blood volume.
    (3) Septic shock results from prolonged metabolic disease.
    (4) Cardiogenic shock results from heart failure.
    (5) Neurogenic shock is caused by a neurologic disorder.
22. (4) Fear and anxiety may cause a patient to experience syncope, which is the most common cause of unconsciousness.
    (1) Allergic reactions to local anesthetic agents are rare.
    (2) A diabetes-related crisis is uncommon in the dental office and may be prevented by completing a thorough medical history and patient questioning.
    (3) Patients may become light-headed or experience syncope from postural hypotension if they sit or stand too rapidly; this is not a common occurrence and results from the change, not the position.
    (5) Shock is uncommon in the dental office.

23. (1) Edema and shortness of breath are symptoms of congestive heart failure. Digoxin is commonly prescribed for this condition.
    (2) Myocardial infarction is characterized by crushing chest pain.
    (3) Anaphylaxis is characterized by a rapid onset, urticaria, angioedema, and respiratory distress, followed by cardiovascular collapse.
    (4) A CVA is characterized by dizziness, difficulty speaking, and impaired function.
    (5) Edema is not a symptom of anxiety.
24. (5) Observing the patient's chest, listening, and feeling for air from the mouth and nose is the correct procedure for determining if the patient is breathing.
    (1) Palpating the patient's femoral pulse in the groin area assesses the presence of a pulse but does not determine if the patient is breathing.
    (2) Determining the patient's pulse does not determine if the patient is breathing.
    (3) Shaking the patient determines consciousness, not breathing.
    (4) The size of the pupils helps to assess the amount of oxygenated blood the brain is receiving but does not determine if the patient is breathing.
25. (1) The xiphoid process must be avoided, since it may be fractured during the compressions and puncture the lungs and surrounding soft tissue.
    (2) This is correct performance of cardiac compressions.
    (3) This is correct performance of cardiac compressions.
    (4) This is correct performance of cardiac compressions.
    (5) This is correct performance of cardiac compressions.
26. (5) A 15:2 ratio of compressions to ventilations is correct for performing single-rescuer CPR.
    (1) A 5:1 ratio is correct for performing two-rescuer CPR.
    (2) A 7:1 ratio is incorrect.
    (3) A 10:2 ratio is incorrect.
    (4) A 12:2 ratio is incorrect.
27. (3) Provide rescue breathing until the patient begins to breathe on his own or definitive therapy is initiated by trained personnel.
    (1) Compressions are unnecessary; the patient's heart is beating.
    (2) Mouth-to-mouth breathing is essential, since the patient is not breathing on his own.
    (4) The patient's brain must continue to receive oxygenated blood; the rescuer cannot wait for the patient to breathe on his own.
    (5) This is unnecessary; the patient is not experiencing an obstructed airway.
28. (2) An adult normally breathes 12 times/min; therefore, you would deliver a ventilation once every 5 seconds.
    (1) Once every second is too fast a rate.
    (3) Once every 15 seconds is too slow a rate.
    (4) The pulse rate does not determine the frequency of ventilations.
    (5) The pulse rate does not determine the frequency of ventilations.

29. (3) CPR is most effective when the patient is in a horizontal position, or when the head is lower than the heart.
    (1) CPR cannot be performed effectively when the patient's head is higher than the heart (seated position), since the blood must be forced up to the patient's brain against gravity.
    (2) Having the patient in a seated position is incorrect.
    (4) Placing the patient's head higher than the heart is incorrect.
    (5) See 2 and 4.
30. (2) Petit mal seizures are brief and are not characterized by clonic and tonic muscle contractions.
    (1) An aura may precede a grand mal seizure and is characterized by changes in sensory perception.
    (3) The symptoms are consistent with those of a grand mal seizure.
    (4) Seizures result from disturbances in the brain's electrical activity.
    (5) Seizures are generally self-limiting and require no definitive treatment.
31. (4) The best course of action is to protect the patient from falling or striking any objects until the seizure is over.
    (1) Administering diazepam is unnecessary, since the seizure is probably self-limiting and the patient requires no medications.
    (2) No objects should be placed in the patient's mouth.
    (3) The patient should be kept supine and low to prevent injury by falling.
    (5) The patient should not be restrained.
32. (3) The patient may be tired and need to rest.
    (1) Additional medical care or definitive treatment is usually not indicated.
    (2) Additional medical care or definitive treatment is usually not indicated.
    (4) The patient will probably not require this measure.
    (5) The patient should be encouraged to rest.
33. (5) The normal pulse rate for an infant is 130 to 160 beats/min, not 80 to 100.
    (1) Normal oral temperatures for adults range between 96.0° and 99.5° F.
    (2) The normal adult pulse rate is 60 to 90 beats/min.
    (3) The normal adult respiration rate is 12 to 20 respirations/min.
    (4) The normal respiration rate for a child is 20 respirations/min.
34. (1) The patient who has hyperventilated is in respiratory alkalosis caused by excessive elimination of carbon dioxide; administering oxygen will not alleviate the situation.
    (2) Bronchitis may be alleviated by the administration of oxygen.
    (3) Congestive heart failure may be alleviated by the administration of oxygen.
    (4) Asthma may be alleviated by the administration of oxygen.
    (5) Emphysema may be alleviated by the administration of oxygen.

35. (1) Mild delayed allergic reactions are characterized by respiratory and skin reactions to agents.
    (2) This was a mild reaction; a more severe reaction might be characterized by angioedema and respiratory distress.
    (3) This is a more severe reaction that develops immediately and may progress to cardiovascular collapse.
    (4) True, but this is not the response that best describes the patient's condition.
    (5) This is a more severe reaction that develops immediately and may progress to cardiovascular collapse.
36. (4) Amphetamines are stimulants and are not indicated for the treatment of allergic reactions.
    (1) Oxygen may be necessary to support the patient's respiration.
    (2) Antihistamines are used to treat allergic reactions.
    (3) Epinephrine may be used to treat severe allergic reactions.
    (5) Diphenhydramine is an antihistamine and may be used to treat allergic reactions.
37. (3) Myocardial infarction, acute adrenal insufficiency, and anaphylaxis pose a serious threat to the individual's life.
    (1) Acute adrenal insufficiency is also correct.
    (2) High blood pressure may cause a cardiovascular accident or cardiovascular collapse; however, it is more a symptom than a life-threatening situation itself.
    (4) Selections c and d also pose life-threatening situations.
    (5) Selections a and c also pose life-threatening situations.
38. (1) These are symptoms of fluoride poisoning.
    (2) Fluoride poisoning is not known to cause dry skin or xerostomia; it may cause hypotension and excessive salivation.
    (3) Fluoride poisoning does not cause xerostomia.
    (4) Caustic burns are not usually seen with fluoride poisoning.
    (5) Sloughing and burned oral tissues are not usually seen with fluoride poisoning.
39. (2) This is considered to be the best out-of-hospital treatment for fluoride poisoning.
    (1) The child may require immediate or definitive treatment unavailable in the dental office.
    (3) Fluoride can be toxic; this dose could be toxic for a 3-year-old child.
    (4) Vomiting should be induced.
    (5) Out-of-hospital treatment should be attempted first; the child should then be taken to the emergency room.
40. (1) Lowering the back of the chair will use "gravity" to assist the patient in efforts to remove the obstruction.
    (2) The use of college pliers may force the object further ino the patient's oropharyngeal area.
    (3) The patient should be assisted with efforts to cough up the obstruction.
    (4) The patient should be assisted in efforts to cough up the obstruction.
    (5) Seating the patient upright may make it more difficult for the patient to dislodge the obstruction.

CHAPTER 19

Historical, Professional, Ethical, and Legal Issues

LINDSAY L. RETTIE

Although the formal recognition and training of dental hygienists began at the beginning of the twentieth century, dental practitioners were discussing the value of preventive care and the need for preventive specialists more than 50 years before dental hygiene's inception. The modern dental hygienist needs to be aware of the beginning of his or her profession, as well as its development, to appreciate the responsibilities of the present and the opportunities of the future.

For professional growth, dental hygienists must contribute to their professional organization. Each dental hygienist has a professional obligation to become a part of that organization, and in return the American Dental Hygienists' Association stands ready to support all dental hygienists as it works to ensure the future of the profession. A knowledge of the history of the profession and a working understanding of the structure and purpose of the professional association are essential.

As health care providers, dental hygienists are confronted with ethical questions. Decisions regarding the health and welfare of others lead to moral dilemmas. To meet the demands of caring for others, dental hygienists must be prepared with scientific knowledge, professional skill, and sound moral judgment. The study of ethical theory and principles helps the dental hygienist to appreciate the moral perspective and leads to ethical decision making.

Finally, some acquaintance with the law and the U.S. legal system is essential for all health care providers today. The greatest defense against malpractice is an understanding of the legal rights and duties of providers and consumers alike. A brief overview of the legal system and relevant legal issues serves to alert the dental hygienist to the benefits and liabilities of becoming a professional in the 80s.

This chapter reviews the history of the idea and practice of dental hygiene, describes the structure and function of the American Dental Hygienists' Association and its constituent and component organizations, reviews the principles and theories of ethics to set standards and provide a frame of reference for future ethical decision making, and provides a synopsis of the U.S. legal system and its relationship to the health professional. Taken together, the four topics addressed make the dental hygienist aware of the rights, privileges, and responsibilities of the profession.

HISTORY OF THE DENTAL HYGIENE PROFESSION IN THE UNITED STATES

Establishment of a New Profession in Dentistry — 1844 to 1924

A. Recognition of the importance of preventive measures in oral health
  1. 1844—editorial discussing the value of oral hygiene measures appeared in *The American Journal of Dental Science*
  2. 1865—Henry S. Chase emphasized the importance of diet for good dental health
  3. 1870—Andrew McLain published a paper entitled ''Prophylaxis or Prevention of Dental Decay,'' which discussed the principles of mouth hygiene and diet
  4. 1879—George A. Mills published a paper that advocated clean mouths in children and described the use of the explorer
  5. 1884—Meyer L. Rhein
    a. Urged dentists to teach their patients to use a toothbrush and waxed floss
    b. Designed a toothbrush for this purpose
    c. Recommended the establishment of oral health programs in the public schools
  6. 1890—Charles B. Atkinson defined dental prophylaxis
  7. 1894—David D. Smith initiated the first recorded preventive practice
  8. 1896—x-rays first used in the detection of dental disease
  9. 1897—Robert R. Andrews suggested mandatory oral examinations of all schoolchildren
  10. 1901—David D. Smith differentiated between home care and professional dental prophylaxis

B. Identification of a new subspecialty in dentistry
   1. 1902—Cyrus M. Wright
      a. Proposed a subspecialty in dentistry to carry out the tedious work of dental prophylaxis
      b. Specifically recommended women for this subspecialty
   2. 1902—Thaddeus P. Hyatt
      a. Advocated educating the public in oral hygiene techniques
      b. Proposed that the tasks related to oral prophylaxis and patient education become the responsibility of a new dental specialty
   3. 1903—Meyer L. Rhein
      a. Advocated the training of women to perform dental prophylaxes
      b. Named this subspecialty "dental nurse"
      c. Suggested licensure for the new subspecialty
   4. 1903—F.W. Low proposed a new profession of "odontocure" to be practiced by women in the private homes of clients
   5. 1906—Alfred Civilion Fones
      a. Became a recognized instructor in the technique of oral prophylaxis
      b. Taught his assistant, Irene Newman, to perform oral prophylaxes
      c. Became known as the "father" of dental hygiene '
   6. 1907—Connecticut dental law was amended to
      a. Limit the duties of unlicensed assistants in dental offices
      b. Allow the cleaning of teeth by trained assistants under supervision
C. Concern for children's dental health
   1. 1887—Alabama Dental Association resolved that preventive dental education should be
      a. Routinely conducted in all public schools
      b. Provided by experienced dental health lecturers
   2. 1914—Bridgeport School Dental Health Plan provided a program of dental health education and preventive services in the public schools, based on the premise that
      a. Dental decay was the most prevalent defect found in schoolchildren
      b. Prevention, not restoration, was the way to control dental disease
   3. Dental dispensaries founded to take care of the dental needs of children
      a. 1910—Forsyth Dental Infirmary (Boston, Mass.)
      b. 1910—Rochester Dental Clinic (Rochester, N.Y.)
      c. 1929—Guggenheim Foundation Clinic (New York City)

D. Early dental hygiene programs—1910 to 1925
   1. 1910—Ohio College of Dental Surgery
      a. Started a 1-year course to train dental nurses
      b. Discontinued it in 1914 because of opposition from local dentists
   2. 1913—Dr. A.C. Fones
      a. Started a training program to supply the Bridgeport School Dental Health Plan with trained dental health personnel
      b. Named the new profession "dental hygiene" because he wanted to stress prevention, not illness
   3. 1914—Colorado College of Dental Surgery initiated a dental nurse program that became a dental hygiene program in 1920
   4. 1916 to 1925—10 new dental hygiene programs were started
      a. 1916—Columbia University took over the dental hygiene program that had been started by Hunter College during that year
      b. 1916—Rochester Dental Dispensary initiated a dental hygiene program
      c. 1916—Forsyth Dental Infirmary started a training program for dental hygienists
      d. 1918—University of California Dental School began a 1-year program for dental hygienists; changed to a 2-year program in 1924
      e. 1920 to 1925—dental hygiene training programs started at the University of Minnesota, University of Michigan, Temple University, University of Pennsylvania, Northwestern University, and Marquette University
E. Dental hygiene licensure, the first 10 years—1915 to 1925
   1. 1915—Connecticut dental statute first outlined the scope of practice of dental hygiene
   2. 1915—Connecticut Board of Dental Examiners presented the first dental hygiene license to Irene Newman, the first person trained by Dr. Fones and a graduate of his first class
   3. 1915—Massachusetts dental law was amended to include the duties of dental hygienists
   4. 1916—New York enacted legislation defining dental hygiene practice
   5. 1916—American Dental Association recognized and endorsed licensure for dental hygienists
   6. 1922—American Dental Association adopted a model dental hygiene practice act to be used by the remaining states
   7. 1917 to 1924—legislation to allow the practice of dental hygiene was adopted in an additional 20 states, as well as in Hawaii and the District of Columbia

Establishment of the American Dental Hygienists' Association

A. State associations
1. 1914—Connecticut Dental Hygienists' Association
   a. Established by a group of graduates from Dr. Fones' program
   b. Irene Newman elected as the first president
2. 1920—there were four state associations: California, Connecticut, Massachusetts, and New York
B. Organization of a national association
1. 1922—organizational meeting held at the annual meeting of the American Dental Association
2. 1923—first annual meeting of the American Dental Hygienists' Association
   a. Held in Cleveland, Ohio
   b. Forty-six dental hygienists representing 11 states attended
   c. Winifred A. Hart elected the first President of the American Dental Hygienists' Association
3. 1925—second national meeting, at which the Constitution and Bylaws of the American Dental Hygienists' Association were adopted
4. 1926—first code of ethics specifying the responsibilities of members was drafted
   a. Adopted as the Principles of Ethics in 1931
   b. Principles of Ethics revised in 1953, 1969, and 1974
5. 1927—*The Journal of the American Dental Hygienists' Association*
   a. Recognized as the official publication of the American Dental Hygienists' Association
   b. Published monthly beginning with its January 1927 issue
   c. Changed to quarterly publication in the mid-1930s
   d. Title changed to *Dental Hygiene* in 1972, and monthly publication resumed in 1975
6. 1927—American Dental Hygienists' Association was incorporated as a nonprofit organization
7. 1927—first continuing education course was offered to dental hygienists by the University of Buffalo
8. 1928—American Dental Hygienists' Association
   a. Accepted its first official seal
   b. Revised the Constitution and Bylaws to meet requirements of incorporation
9. 1935—membership in the American Dental Hygienists' Association reached approximately 1000
10. 1938—establishment of the Junior American Dental Hygienists' Association, later renamed the Student American Dental Hygienists' Association

Events Influencing the Development of Dental Hygiene—1918 to 1944

A. National attention on public health
1. 1918—North Carolina established the first dental division of a state department of health
2. 1921—Children's Bureau established, which provided
   a. Health care for mothers and children
   b. Jobs for dental hygienists in state health departments
3. 1930—White House Conference produced a Children's Charter that promoted preventive programs for children; conference led to
   a. Children's Fund of Michigan dental program
   b. W.K. Kellogg Foundation's support of pedodontic clinics
   c. Children's National Dental Health Week
B. 1932—American Dental Association established the Committee on Dental Hygiene to
1. Survey the curricula of all existing dental hygiene programs
2. Determine the number of graduate dental hygienists
3. Determine the number of practicing dental hygienists
4. Review requirements of state departments of education
5. Review state dental practice acts
C. 1935—Social Security Act enacted
1. Title V provided for
   a. Maternal and child health services
   b. Preventive services as a part of the health plan
2. Title VI provided for
   a. Public health services
   b. Training of health professionals
D. 1937—American Dental Association established the Council on Dental Education to oversee educational programs in dentistry and dental hygiene
E. 1941 to 1944
1. World War II
   a. American Dental Hygienists' Association annual sessions discontinued during the war years (1942 to 1945)

b. Dental hygienists served as civil service employees

c. Requests from the American Dental Hygienists' Association to commission dental hygienists in the armed forces were denied

2. National Dental Hygiene Association established by black dental hygienists

Era of Dental Research—1943 to 1953

A. 1943 to 1949—dental research on fluoride
1. Indicated the effectiveness of fluoride in reducing tooth decay
2. Established the need for fluoride rinse programs for preschool children and schoolchildren
3. Involved dental hygienists in
   a. Advocating and educating the public regarding water fluoridation
   b. Topical fluoride demonstration projects
   c. Conducting dental screenings
   d. Public health and school fluoride programs
B. 1946 to 1953—dental care delivery research
1. U.S. Public Health Service initiated projects to determine the effectiveness of the expanded use of auxiliaries in the delivery of dental care to schoolchildren
2. Forsyth Dental Clinic
   a. Initiated a 5-year research project to evaluate the feasibility of dental hygienists restoring primary teeth
   b. Terminated the project in its third year because of the opposition of local dentists
C. 1948—National Institute of Dental Research
1. Established by the National Dental Research Act
2. Involved dental hygienists in water fluoridation, topical application of fluoride, and oral cancer research

Growth of the Profession During the 1940s and 1950s

A. 1947—American Dental Association Council on Dental Education
1. Required all dental hygiene programs to be no less than 2 years in length
2. Surveyed colleges and universities to determine the transferability of dental hygiene courses
3. Proposed a standard curriculum for all programs
4. Conducted a curriculum survey of all dental hygiene programs; additional curriculum surveys conducted in 1951, 1958, and 1964

B. 1948—American Dental Hygienists' Association established the
1. Position of Executive Secretary
2. Central office in Washington, D.C.
C. 1951—Texas became the last state in the continental United States to grant dental hygiene licensure
D. 1951—American Dental Association Council on Dental Education
1. Recommended that dental hygienists receive training in expanded duties
2. Began accrediting dental hygiene programs
E. 1953 to 1954—Alaska and Puerto Rico granted dental hygiene licensure, making it possible to be licensed in the 48 states plus Alaska, the District of Columbia, Hawaii, and Puerto Rico
F. 1957 to 1958—American Dental Hygienists' Association
1. Established the Educational Trust Fund (ETF)
2. Reaffirmed that membership would not be denied because of race, creed, or color
3. Requested that all constituents comply with the American Dental Hygienists' Association's membership policy
4. Moved the central office to Chicago
5. Instituted the Dental Hygiene Aptitude Test
   a. As a measure of predicting academic success in dental hygiene
   b. As an admission criterion, adopted by most dental hygiene programs from 1958 to 1964

National Interest in the Delivery of Health Care in the 1950s and 1960s

A. 1952—President's Commission on the Health Needs of the Nation
1. Studied
   a. Availability of health care
   b. Personnel in the health professions
2. Recommended
   a. Delegation of duties to auxiliary personnel
   b. That dental care be considered part of comprehensive health care
   c. Fluoridation of all public water supplies
   d. Support for research
B. 1953—establishment of the Department of Health, Education, and Welfare (DHEW) indicated the nation's interest in the general welfare; dental hygienists became involved in programs funded by the DHEW
C. 1953 to 1957—dental hygiene labor study conducted by the U.S. Public Health Service revealed
1. Thirty-four dental hygiene programs in existence

2. Approximately 15,000 graduate dental hygienists
D. 1963 to 1968—federally supported programs included
  1. Vocational Education Act of 1963, which
    a. Contributed to the growth of dental hygiene programs
    b. Introduced dental hygiene programs in technical schools and community colleges
  2. Health Professions Educational Assistance Amendments of 1965 provided
    a. Funds to educational programs that increased the number of students accepted
    b. Funds for the renovation of training facilities
    c. Start-up funds for new programs in the health professions
    d. Loans and scholarships for health professionals in training
  3. Allied Health Professions Personnel Training Act of 1966 provided
    a. Capitation grants to dental hygiene programs
    b. Funds for improvement or initiation of new programs
  4. National Advisory Commission on Health Manpower of 1967 identified the need for additional allied health professionals
  5. Health Manpower Act of 1968 provided funds for
    a. Basic education of health professionals
    b. Advanced training of health professionals
    c. Special projects
  6. National Institute of Health Research Training Grants in Dental Health of 1968 provided grant funds to dental and dental hygiene faculty for research, teaching, and related activities

Expansion of Dental Hygiene in the 1960s and 1970s

A. 1960 to 1965—graduate programs in dental hygiene initiated at Columbia University, the University of Michigan, and Iowa State University provided advanced training in
  1. Education and administration for dental hygiene educators
  2. Principles of public health for dental hygienists
B. 1961—American Dental Hygienists' Association adopted proportional representation in the House of Delegates
  1. Allowing each constituent to have 1 delegate for up to 100 members
  2. Plus 1 delegate for each additional 100 members

C. 1962—National Board Dental Hygiene Examinations
  1. Developed by the Committee on Dental Hygiene National Boards of the American Dental Hygienists' Association
  2. Administered by the American Dental Association's Council on National Board Dental Examiners
  3. Recognized by 25 states immediately; ultimately recognized by all 50 states and Puerto Rico
  4. Open to graduates of all accredited dental hygiene programs; however, those graduating before 1955 had to pass the examination by 1965 to use it as a criterion for licensure
D. 1964 to 1970—acceptance of men for
  1. Dental hygiene licensure in all states except Alabama, Indiana, Louisiana, Mississippi, Nebraska, Rhode Island, and Utah
  2. Membership in the American Dental Hygienists' Association and its constituents
E. 1965—survey of dental practice indicated
  1. Employed dental hygienists numbered 15,400
  2. Decline in public health positions for dental hygienists
  3. Most dental hygienists were employed in private practices
F. 1965—Dental Hygiene Educators Conference
  1. Identified the responsibilities of dental hygienists
  2. Identified the competence students must achieve
  3. Established a network of dental hygiene educators
G. 1965—American Dental Hygienists' Association produced the recruitment film *Bright Future*
H. 1967—American Dental Hygienists' Association studied the need for and design of associate, baccalaureate, and master's level dental hygiene programs
I. 1969—American Dental Hygienists' Association established a Washington office to
  1. Monitor legislation of interest to the profession
  2. Provide information to lawmakers
  3. Represent the views of the association
J. 1970—American Dental Hygienists' Association
  1. Sponsored the First International Symposium on Dental Hygiene, held in Italy
  2. Produced the first *Curriculum Essentials* for dental hygiene programs
K. 1970—Community Oral Health Managers instituted by the U.S. Army resulted in
  1. Commissioning of baccalaureate-trained dental hygienists as officers
  2. Preventive oral health programs for military personnel and dependents

L. 1970—training in expanded auxiliary management (TEAM) demonstration projects were established to determine the feasibility of teaching registered dental hygienists to perform nontraditional duties under the supervision of a dentist
1. Registered dental hygienists were taught to
   a. Administer anesthesia
   b. Cut hard and soft tissue
   c. Place restorative materials
2. Studies conducted at the Forsyth Dental Clinic, the University of Pennsylvania, the University of Iowa, and Howard University
3. Studies indicated that graduate dental hygienists could be trained to perform expanded functions successfully
4. Several projects were stopped because of the objections of local dentists

M. 1971—dental hygienists became involved in dental auxiliary utilization (DAU); demonstration projects in North Carolina, Iowa, Alabama, Kentucky, Florida, Maryland, Missouri, and Ohio

N. 1972—*The Journal of the American Dental Hygienists' Association* adopted the title *Dental Hygiene;* changed from quarterly to monthly publication in 1975

O. 1973—Commission on Accreditation of Dental and Dental Auxiliary Programs
1. Established by the American Dental Association
2. Two members on the commission represent dental hygiene

P. 1976—American Dental Hygienists' Association publication *Educational Directions* for dental auxiliaries became the second official publication of the American Dental Hygienists' Association

Q. 1976—Linda Krol, R.D.H., became the first dental hygienist to own and manage a practice in dental hygiene

R. 1977—Alabama, the last state to allow preceptorship, amended its practice act to require formal training

S. 1978—denturists won permission of the respective legislatures to practice in Arizona, Maine, and Oregon

T. 1978—American Dental Hygienists' Association
1. Established District XIII and added the Virgin Islands as a constituent
2. Changed the name of the Educational Trust Fund (ETF) to the American Dental Hygienists' Association Foundation
3. Established the Hygienists' Political Action Committee (HY-PAC)

U. 1979—California amended its dental practice act to allow registered dental hygienists to practice in their own offices by referral/general supervision

V. 1979—American Dental Hygienists' Association created the Dental Hygiene Commission for Assurance of Competency to
1. Define competence in dental hygiene
2. Study methods currently used to ensure competence

W. 1979—ended two decades of rapid expansion in dental hygiene education and practice, resulting in
1. Two hundred and one dental hygiene programs in operation, the majority in community colleges and technical institutes
2. Dental hygiene programs in 50 states and Puerto Rico
3. Estimated number of licensed dental hygienists reaching 73,500
4. Some expanded functions for dental hygienists legalized by 47 states

Issues for the 1980s

A. 1980—*Horizons,* the newsletter of the American Dental Hygienists' Association
1. Distributed bimonthly to all members of the American Dental Hygienists' Association
2. Funded by Johnson & Johnson

B. 1980—state activities
1. After a decade of lobbying, 33 states had dental hygienist representation on boards of dental examiners
2. Sunset review process continued in 23 states whereby programs, agencies, and regulatory boards are reviewed to determine duplication of effort in preparation for possible elimination
3. Continuing education became mandatory for recertification in 12 states

C. 1980—Federal Trade Commission proposed nullification of state restrictions requiring dental hygienists to work under the supervision of a dentist because this constitutes restraint of trade

D. 1981—American Dental Hygienists' Association
1. Began meeting twice a year
   a. House of Delegates meeting held for the first time in June
   b. Scientific session held in the fall of each year
2. Established the council structure, incorporating standing committees into six councils
3. Membership reached over 22,000

E. 1981—*RDH* magazine for dental hygienists first published to address the professional, financial, legal, and personal needs of dental hygienists

F. 1981—Consumer-Patient Radiation Health and Safety Act of 1981 proposed common standards for all health care providers using ionizing radiation

G. 1982—American Dental Hygienists' Association produced the film *Dental Hygienist: Your Preventive Professional*

H. 1982—Federal Trade Commission's authority to control state-regulated health professions was challenged by the American Medical Association and the American Dental Association

I. 1983—International Liasion Committee (ILC) for dental hygiene
   1. Held the Ninth International Symposium on Dental Hygiene in Philadelphia
   2. Drafted a constitution and bylaws

J. 1983—Dental Hygiene Aptitude Test (DHAT) was discontinued because it no longer was recognized as the best predictor of success in dental hygiene; SAT and ACT scores used as reliable predictors

K. 1984—American Dental Hygienists' Association established a Universal Registry for Continuing Education

L. 1984—Florida and Washington dental hygienists lobbied for separate dental hygiene boards of examiners

M. 1984—Congress reaffirmed the Federal Trade Commission's authority over the health professions; this was recognized as a political victory by the American Dental Hygienists' Association

N. 1984—Washington and Colorado adopted amendments to permit dental hygienists to work without supervision of a dentist in limited alternate practice settings

O. 1985—state dental hygiene associations, with the assistance of the American Dental Hygienists' Association, focused on issues of regulation and access to care

AMERICAN DENTAL HYGIENISTS' ASSOCIATION

Purpose of the Organization

A. Constitution, Bylaws, Principles of Ethics, and Policy Manual were written, adopted, and may be amended by the House of Delegates
   1. Constitution of the American Dental Hygienists' Association describes
      a. Mission and goals of the organization
      b. Composition of its membership
      c. Organizational structure
      d. Governing units
      e. Officers
      f. Meeting schedule
   2. Bylaws are the rules that govern the association

3. Principles of Ethics outline the moral obligations of each member to the profession and the public
4. Policy Manual describes the association's position on issues confronting the dental hygiene profession

B. Purpose and mission of the American Dental Hygienists' Association as stated in the Policy Manual
   1. Purpose of the association is to
      a. Improve the health of the public
      b. Advance the art and science of dental hygiene
      c. Maintain the highest standards of dental hygiene education and practice
      d. Represent and protect the interest of the dental hygiene profession
      e. Improve the professional competence of the dental hygienist
      f. Foster research in oral health
      g. Provide professional communications
      h. Publish a scientific journal (i.e., *Dental Hygiene*)
   2. Mission of the American Dental Hygienists' Association is to
      a. Improve the public's total health by increasing
         (1) Awareness of quality care
         (2) Access to quality oral health care
      b. Position the dental hygienist as *the* preventive oral health professional

C. Goals of the American Dental Hygienists' Association as stated in the American Dental Hygienists' Association Policy Manual are to
   1. Increase the quality of care provided by the dental hygienist
   2. Increase the number of people who use the services of a dental hygienist
   3. Reduce obstacles to the public's access to alternate practice settings
   4. Increase the membership of the American Dental Hygienists' Association to represent the majority of licensed dental hygienists
   5. Improve the quality of work life for dental hygienists

D. American Dental Hygienists' Association subscribes to the following Principles of Ethics, which state the moral obligations of the membership to
   1. Provide oral health care using the highest levels of professional knowledge, judgment, and ability

2. Serve all patients without discrimination
3. Hold professional relationships in confidence
4. Use every opportunity to increase public understanding of oral health practices
5. Generate public confidence in members of the dental health professions
6. Cooperate with all health professions in meeting the health needs of the public
7. Recognize and uphold the laws and regulations governing this profession
8. Participate responsibly in the professional association and uphold its purposes
9. Maintain professional competence through continuing education
10. Exchange professional knowledge with other health professions
11. Represent dental hygiene with high standards of personal conduct

Structure of the American Dental Hygienists' Association

A. Governance of the American Dental Hygienists' Association
   1. National level
      a. House of Delegates
         (1) Attends to matters of policy
         (2) Approves the budget of the association
         (3) Establishes councils and standing committees
         (4) Is presided over by the Speaker of the House
      b. Board of Trustees
         (1) Attends to administrative matters
         (2) Appoints and directs
            (a) Executive Director
            (b) Editorial Director
         (3) Hires administrative staff
         (4) Is presided over by the President
   2. District level—13 districts
      a. Established by the House of Delegates
      b. Incorporates a number of constituents
      c. Represented by a district trustee who sits on the Board of Trustees and is elected by delegates from the incorporated constituents
   3. Constituent level—53 constituents or state associations
      a. Chartered by the Board of Trustees; each state, commonwealth, federal district, territory, or possession of the United States is eligible to become a constituent of the American Dental Hygienists' Association
      b. Incorporates a number of components

c. Represented by delegates who sit in the House of Delegates of the American Dental Hygienists' Association
   4. Component level—approximately 260 components or local associations
      a. Established by constituent houses of delegates
      b. Not limited to a specific geographic area or designated number
      c. Represented by delegates who sit in the house of delegates of the constituent (state)
B. Representation in the American Dental Hygienists' Association
   1. Classification and privileges of members of the American Dental Hygienists' Association; membership in the American Dental Hygienists' Association requires simultaneous membership in the constituent (state) and component (local) associations
      a. Voting members shall have the right to vote, hold office, and such other privileges as the House of Delegates may determine
         (1) Active member—any dental hygienist who
            (a) Graduates from an accredited dental hygiene program or is licensed under the provision of a "grandfather" clause
            (b) Is licensed to practice dental hygiene in the United States or its territories
            (c) Agrees to adhere to the Bylaws and Principles of Ethics of the American Dental Hygienists' Association
            (d) Agrees to hold membership in constituent and component organizations if they exist
         (2) Life member—any active member who
            (a) Has made outstanding contributions to dental hygiene
            (b) Is nominated by the Board of Trustees
            (c) Is elected by the House of Delegates or
            (d) Served as President of the American Dental Hygienists' Association
         (3) Retired member—any active member who has
            (a) Reached the age of 62 or has retired from the practice of dental hygiene because of disability

(b) Been an active member for at least one of the following
[1] Twenty-five years
[2] Twenty consecutive years
[3] Continuously from the date of eligibility

b. Nonvoting members shall have such privileges as the House of Delegates shall determine, but shall not have the right to vote or hold office
(1) Associate member—any dental hygienist who
(a) Is practicing outside the United States under a current license or certificate
(b) Holds membership in the association of that country
(c) Agrees to adhere to the Bylaws and Principles of Ethics of the American Dental Hygienists' Association
(2) Student member—any full-time student who is
(a) Enrolled in one of the following programs of study
[1] Accredited dental hygiene program
[2] Baccalaureate or graduate degree program that is complementary to a career in dental hygiene
(b) Recommended by the director or a duly appointed representative of an institution
(3) Honorary member—any individual who
(a) Is not a dental hygienist
(b) Has made outstanding contributions to dental hygiene or dental health
(c) Has been nominated by the Board of Trustees
(d) Has been elected by the House of Delegates
(4) Allied member—any individual who
(a) Supports the purposes and mission of the association
(b) Is not otherwise qualified for any other class of membership
(5) Corporate member—any corporation, institution, or organization that supports the mission of the American Dental Hygienists' Association

2. Officers of the American Dental Hygienists' Association
a. Elected officers
(1) Officers assuming a 1-year term as the result of a previous election by the House of Delegates
(a) President
(b) Immediate Past President
(2) Officers elected by the House of Delegates for 1 year
(a) President-Elect
(b) First Vice-President
(c) Second Vice-President
(3) Officers elected by the House of Delegates for 2 years
(a) Treasurer
(b) Speaker of the House
(4) District trustees are elected
(a) By the delegates of the constituents of their respective districts
(b) From among the voting delegates of the respective district
(c) To represent the district on the Board of Trustees
(d) For a 2-year term
b. Appointed officers who serve under the direction of the Board of Trustees
(1) Executive Director
(2) Editorial Director

3. House of Delegates, legislative body of the American Dental Hygienists' Association
a. Is presided over by the Speaker of the House
b. Consists of
(1) Voting members who represent each constituent based on the proportional formula
(a) One delegate for up to 100 members plus
(b) One delegate for each additional 100 members
(2) Nonvoting members
(a) Elected officers of the association
(b) Appointed officers of the association
(c) One student delegate from each district

4. Board of Trustees, administrative body of the American Dental Hygienists' Association
   a. Is presided over by the President
   b. Consists of
      (1) Voting members
         (a) President
         (b) President-Elect
         (c) First Vice-President
         (d) Second Vice-President
         (e) Treasurer
         (f) Immediate Past President
         (g) District trustees (13)
      (2) Nonvoting or exofficio members without vote
         (a) Executive Director
         (b) Editorial Director
C. American Dental Hygienists' Association policies
   1. Meetings shall be at least twice a year
      a. June meeting shall consist of
         (1) House of Delegates meeting
         (2) Board of Trustees semiannual meeting
      b. Fall meeting shall be
         (1) In conjunction with the American Dental Association annual meeting
         (2) Scientific session for the American Dental Hygienists' Association
         (3) Board of Trustees semiannual meeting
   2. Councils of the American Dental Hygienists' Association
      a. Include
         (1) Council on Administration (composed of elected officers plus two trustees)
         (2) Council on Dental Hygiene Practice
         (3) Council on Consumer and Government Relations
         (4) Council on Educational Services and Research
         (5) Council on Member Services
         (6) Council on House of Delegates Administration
      b. Are established by the House of Delegates
      c. Have members and chairs appointed by the President with the approval of the Board of Trustees

3. Districts, constituents, and components of the American Dental Hygienists' Association
   a. There are 13 districts, each represented by a district trustee
   b. There are 53 constituent associations, representing each of the 50 states plus the District of Columbia, Puerto Rico, and the Virgin Islands
   c. Components represent the local organizational divisions within each state and are not restricted to a specific number, membership, or geographic area
4. Policy Manual of the American Dental Hygienists' Association specifies the association's position on
   a. American Dental Hygienists' Association's mission and goals
   b. Ethics
   c. Licensure
   d. Education
   e. Continuing education
   f. Practice
   g. Public health
   h. Research
5. Official publications of the American Dental Hygienists' Association
   a. *Dental Hygiene*—journal of the American Dental Hygienists' Association; published monthly
   b. *Horizons*—American Dental Hygienists' Association Newsletter; published bimonthly
   c. *Legislative Bulletin*—published every 6 weeks; provides news regarding legislative activities
   d. *Educational Directions*—aimed at dental hygiene educators; published quarterly

PROFESSIONALISM IN DENTAL HYGIENE
Defining a Profession

A. Characteristics of a profession
   1. Special education or preparation
   2. Identifiable membership
   3. Dedicated to service
   4. Promotion of knowledge in the field (e.g., research)
B. Standards for a profession
   1. Codes of ethics
      a. Ancient codes
         (1) Code of Hammurabi—2100 BC
            (a) First code of ethical standards for business

(b) Guaranteed justice for all
(c) Invoked ''an eye for an eye'' and ''a tooth for a tooth''
(2) Hippocratic Oath—400 BC
    (a) Stated, ''Above all, do no harm''
    (b) Protected the rights of the patient
    (c) Admonished physicians to keep the confidence of patients
    (d) Placed the needs of the patient above those of society
    (e) Placed an obligation on physicians to teach the next generation of physicians
(3) Oath of Maimonides—thirteenth century; admonished physicians
    (a) To do good
    (b) To be sympathetic
    (c) Not to be greedy
  b. Common elements of codes
    (1) Self-imposed
    (2) Set rules governing behavior
    (3) Serve to protect the public
    (4) Strive to enhance the profession
  c. Patient's Bill of Rights
    (1) Focuses on the needs of the patient
    (2) Encourages informed choice by the patient
    (3) Guarantees quality care to the patient
2. Credentials, type of credentials
  a. Licensure—state regulation of professionals
    (1) Granted by a state agency or board
    (2) Limits practice to
      (a) Duties prescribed by law in the state practice act or
      (b) Duties delineated by rules and regulations
    (3) Authorizes practice by professionals meeting specified qualifications
  b. Registration—qualified professionals listed in a directory or file
  c. Certification—state or national recognition
    (1) Recognition by a nongovernmental agency (e.g., a professional association)
    (2) Identification of professionals who have met specified qualifications
3. Accountability—professionals are expected to demonstrate
  a. Competence in skill and knowledge
  b. Adherence to standards in delivering services
  c. Dedication to the best interests of the patient or client
  d. Integrity in professional activities

Ethical Issues in Dental Hygiene

A. Definitions
  1. Ethics
    a. Study of moral conduct
    b. Establishes principles that
      (1) Serve as a guide for conduct and thought
      (2) Are based on theory
  2. Morals
    a. Standards of conduct and thought
    b. Based on ethical principles
    c. Measure conduct against standards
  3. Mores
    a. Customs of a group
    b. Standards for behavior
    c. Change with time
  4. Values
    a. Beliefs and attitudes
    b. Motivate behavior
    c. Dynamic; may change with time and circumstances
B. Values
  1. Types
    a. Intrinsic—attitudes or beliefs related to the maintenance of life (e.g., valuing health care)
    b. Extrinsic—attitudes or beliefs related to alternatives not essential to life (e.g., valuing a specific health care provider or agency)
    c. Instrumental—attitudes or beliefs related to a process (e.g., valuing a healthy life-style)
    d. Terminal—attitudes or beliefs related to an outcome or product (e.g., valuing health)
  2. Criteria for adopting values—values are
    a. Freely chosen
    b. Chosen from alternatives
    c. Chosen after consideration
    d. Prized and cherished
    e. Publicly held
    f. Action oriented
    g. Integrated into one's life-style
  3. Values clarification
    a. Outcome of an activity that
      (1) Leads to an understanding of personal thoughts and actions
      (2) Does not dictate rules, behavior, or thought
      (3) Does not impose or judge the values held by others

b. Process involves the individual in
   (1) Choosing or identifying his or her own values
   (2) Prizing and affirming his or her own values
   (3) Acting on his or her values
4. Hierarchy of values—some values are more important than others in motivating action and are therefore considered higher on the scale of values
5. Values dissonance
   a. Occurs when
      (1) Personally held values are not congruent with
         (a) Those held by the profession
         (b) Those held by others (colleagues, family, clients, supervisors)
      (2) Values come in conflict (e.g., when the value to respect the life-style of others conflicts with the value to improve the oral hygiene of the patient)
   b. May result in a change in values
6. Value judgment—evaluation of the beliefs and behavior of others based on the values held by self
7. Origin of values
   a. Personal values are influenced and instilled by
      (1) Home and family
      (2) Peers and colleagues
      (3) Professional expectation
      (4) Custom and national mores
      (5) Events and circumstances of life
   b. Values accepted by a group are influenced by
      (1) Leaders
      (2) Members
      (3) Time, events, and circumstances
C. Moral reasoning
   1. Characterized by
      a. Cognitive judgment
      b. Independence from prevailing norms, mores, or customs
      c. Philosophic thought rather than behavior
   2. Moral development theory of L. Kohlberg
      a. Assumes that moral development is
         (1) Cognitive—based on thinking and influenced by experience
         (2) Sequential—one stage builds on the previous one
         (3) Hierarchical—each stage is better than the previous one
         (4) Universal—applicable to all persons and cultures

b. Catagorizes moral reasoning into three levels divided into six stages
   (1) Preconventional level—children and adolescents reason at this level
      (a) Stage 1—punishment and obedience orientation; response to punishment or reward
      (b) Stage 2—instrumental relativist orientation; personal interest is paramount, or "I'll scratch your back if you scratch mine"
   (2) Conventional level—most adults reach this level of reasoning
      (a) Stage 3—interpersonal concordance of "good boy–nice girl" orientation; in search of praise
      (b) Stage 4—law-and-order orientation; self-respect through social order and obedience
   (3) Postconventional level—few adults reach this level of reasoning
      (a) Stage 5—social-contract legalistic orientation; upholding those societal standards that are seen as fair
      (b) Stage 6—universal ethical-principle orientation; guided by principles, not rules and laws
D. Ethical theories—are unchanging, do not change with custom
   1. Criteria that identify an ethical theory; ethical theories
      a. Are systematic approaches to knowledge relevant to ethical thought and action
      b. Make up principles and rules
      c. Assist in decision making
   2. Two major ethical theories
      a. Utilitarianism—focuses on consequences; best possible outcome for the greatest number of people; also known as the "greatest happiness" theory; if one thinks as a utilitarian, one might believe that "the ends justify the means"
         (1) Act utilitarians concentrate on the outcome of a single act under specific circumstances (e.g., tell the patient whatever is necessary to achieve a positive outcome)
         (2) Rule utilitarians concentrate on the outcome of types of acts (e.g., in general, tell patients the truth as long as it will not result in harm)

b. Deontology—focuses on ethical principles rather than the consequence of actions; if one thinks as a deontologist, one might say, "It's the principle of the thing"
  (1) Act deontologists consider the ethical principles involved in an action in light of the circumstances (e.g., do not lie, but you may avoid telling the truth if the whole truth is harmful)
  (2) Rule deontologists concentrate on principles and rules in general as they apply to types of actions (e.g., always tell the whole truth)
3. Ethical principles governing health care
  a. Autonomy—health professional should
    (1) Include the patient in the decision regarding treatment
    (2) Fully inform the patient
    (3) Obtain informed consent for treatment
    (4) Respect the patient as an individual
    (5) Protect the confidentiality of the patient
  b. Nonmaleficence—health professional should
    (1) Above all, do no harm
    (2) Prevent harm or the risk of harm
    (3) Consider the risks as well as the benefits of treatment alternatives
    (4) Present the alternative of minimal or no treatment if this is feasible
  c. Beneficence—health professional should
    (1) Promote well-being or benefit
    (2) Consider whose well-being is being benefited (the patient, the family, society, or the health professional)
    (3) Consider the costs as well as the benefits of treatment
    (4) Resist being paternalistic whereby the patient's autonomy is violated when treatment is dictated; paternalism occurs when the health professional insists on the treatment that he or she believes is best for the patient
  d. Veracity—health professional should
    (1) Be truthful
    (2) Keep promises
    (3) Refrain from deception
    (4) Report known violations of the standard of care by colleagues to the proper authority
  e. Justice—health professional should consider treatment in terms of fairness
    (1) Noncomparative justice—patient's claims are not in competition with the claims of others or society

    (2) Comparative justice—patient's claims are in competition with others (e.g., should one individual have the right to drink nonfluoridated water, or should the water system be fluoridated for the good of the community?)
    (3) Distributive justice or allocation of scarce resources (e.g., who should receive treatment when all cannot be treated?); services may be allocated on the basis of
      (a) Equity—all persons receive equal treatment
      (b) Need—treatment allocated on the basis of need
      (c) Effort—treatment allocated to those who have earned it
      (d) Contribution—treatment allocated to those who are making a contribution to society or
      (e) Merit—treatment allocated to those who are worthy
E. Ethical decision making—what is an ethical dilemma, and how should decisions be made?
  1. Ethical dilemmas
    a. Involve two or more opposing ethical principles that are equally important (e.g., telling the whole truth when doing so will cause harm)
    b. Concern several alternative actions (e.g., lying to spare pain, or telling the truth and causing pain)
    c. Choice of action must be made from several unsatisfactory alternatives (e.g., lying violates the patient's autonomy and his or her right to be informed, but telling the truth may hurt the patient's chances of recovery)
  2. Decisions should be made based on
    a. Ethical theory (e.g., deontologic or utiliarian)
    b. Ethical principles and rules (e.g., autonomy, beneficence, etc.)
    c. Relevant facts
    d. Selection from alternatives
F. Ethical issues and public policy
  1. Distributive justice—fair allocation of resources involved
    a. Macroallocation of resources based on the needs of the public (e.g., water fluoridation)
    b. Microallocation of resources based on the needs of the individual (e.g., fluoride treatment)

2. Health policy questions
   a. Should public tax dollars support
      (1) Financial assistance and care of the needy or elderly?
      (2) Financial aid for victims of
         (a) Chronic diseases?
         (b) Acute and devastating diseases?
      (3) Research and experimentation?
         (a) Who should decide what research should be done?
         (b) Who should support research?
   b. What proportion of the national budget should be spent on health care?
   c. For whom is health care beneficial?
      (1) Public
      (2) Individual
      (3) Health care practitioner
   d. Who should decide about treatment?
      (1) Patient
      (2) Practitioner
      (3) Third-party payer (Blue Cross/Blue Shield or Medicare)
      (4) Legislature or Congress

LEGAL RELATIONSHIPS IN DENTAL HYGIENE PRACTICE

Basis of Law in the United States

A. Jurisprudence—defined as
   1. Philosophy of law
   2. Concerns the principles of positive law and legal relations
B. Sources of American law—based on English common law
   1. Statutes (statutory law)
      a. Federal statutes or legislation—U.S. Constitution stipulates that all powers not given to the federal government are reserved to the states; these include the authority to
         (1) Police the health and welfare of its citizens (police powers)
         (2) Empower elected or appointed agencies or boards to regulate the practice of the professions
      b. State statutes or legislation—practice acts and rules and regulations governing the practice of selected professions
   2. Judicial decisions (common law)
      a. Unwritten, based on custom
      b. Made by judges or based on previous decisions under the principle of *stare decisis*

C. U.S. legal system is based on adversarial relations
   1. No legal action can be initiated between parties or between an agency and an individual without an adversarial relationship or one party injuring the other
   2. Constitutionality of a law cannot be tested before its enactment
D. Types of law
   1. Criminal law—offense against society punishable by imprisonment or fine (e.g., a person who practices dentistry or dental hygiene without a license is committing an offense against society)
      a. Felonies—more serious offenses against individuals or society
      b. Misdemeanors—less serious crimes
   2. Civil law—concerned with the legal rights and duties of private persons (e.g., the relationship between a dental health professional and a patient is governed by civil law)
      a. Contract—conditions of agreement between parties (e.g., once the treatment plan has been presented and the patient has agreed to the fee, a contract is in effect)
      b. Property—wills, copyrights, deeds, etc.
      c. Tort—civil wrong or injury committed by one individual against another
         (1) Intentional torts—also may be considered crimes against society and as such fall under both criminal and civil law
            (a) Murder—unlawful killing with premeditated malice
            (b) Manslaughter—unlawful killing without malice
            (c) Assault—violent physical or verbal attack
            (d) Battery—beating or use of force
            (e) False imprisonment—confining without cause
            (f) Defamation of character
               [1] Libel—written defamation
               [2] Slander—oral defamation
            (g) Fraud—deception or misrepresentation with the intention of taking something of value

(2) Unintentional torts—negligence (also called malpractice)
  (a) Occurs when four conditions exist
    [1] Duty was owed
    [2] Duty was breached
    [3] Damages or injury resulted
    [4] Breach of duty was the direct cause of the injury (proximate cause)
  (b) May result from omission or commission of acts
E. Legal doctrines
  1. Doctrine of Personal Liability—holds every person liable for his or her own negligent conduct even though others also may be negligent
  2. Doctrine of the Reasonably Prudent Man—holds a professional responsible for maintaining the standard of care that is considered reasonable or customary by his or her peers in his or her community
  3. Doctrine of *Respondeat Superior*—holds an employer liable for the negligent acts of his or her employees that occur while they are carrying out their duties in the general course of employment
  4. Doctrine of the Borrowed Servant—holds the supervising physician or dentist liable for the negligent acts of those who are working under his or her supervision, even if he or she is not the employer
  5. Doctrine of Corporate Negligence—holds a hospital or health care agency liable for negligent acts of its employees or professional staff
  6. Doctrine of *Res Ipsa Loquitur* (the thing speaks for itself)—shifts the burden of proof from the plaintiff to the defendant because
    a. That type of injury normally does not occur unless there was negligence (e.g., an infection occurred as the result of unsterile instruments)
    b. Injury was caused by something completely under the control of the defendant (e.g., the instrument slipped)
    c. Injury was not caused by any voluntary action of the plaintiff (e.g., the patient did not contribute to the injury)
  7. Doctrine of Foreseeability—holds an individual liable for negligent acts or natural consequences that could or should have been foreseen

8. Doctrine of *Res Judicata*—holds that once the matter has been decided in court, the case cannot be retried
9. Doctrine of *Stare Decisis*—requires judges to adhere to the precedents of prior decisions; this results in common law or judge-made law
10. Doctrine of *Res Gestae*—admits pertinent statements made by others (third parties) at the time of the accident as admissible evidence, thereby making an exception to the hearsay rule, which normally excludes statements not made in court
11. Doctrine of Comparative Negligence—compares the negligence of the plaintiff and that of the defendant to determine degrees of failure to exercise due care

Legal Relationships

A. Professional duties
  1. Standard of care or due care—professional's duty to
    a. Possess the skill and knowledge expected
    b. Exercise the skill and knowledge standard in the community
  2. Duty to refer to a specialist, when indicated, who possesses and exercises the standard of care
  3. Duty to render treatment only extends to patients already accepted for treatment (e.g., a health professional is not required by law to accept any new patient)
  4. Duty to continue or complete treatment started within a reasonable time or to arrange alternative sources of treatment for patients already accepted for treatment
  5. Duty to obtain informed consent from responsible parties (may be a parent or guardian) before treatment; informed consent must be based on
    a. Adequate maturity of the patient or guardian
    b. Complete information presented to the patient regarding the risks, cost, and benefits of the proposed treatment
B. Malpractice—professional negligence
  1. Criteria for malpractice
    a. Health professional owed a duty to the client; relationship between the client and health care provider established a duty
    b. Duty was breached by the health care provider (failure to exercise due care)
    c. Client sustained injury or damage
    d. Injury or damage was the direct result of the breach of duty

2. Common grounds for malpractice
   a. Poor results when success was guaranteed (e.g., the health professional may have indicated that the results of treatment would be perfect or near perfect)
   b. Failure to exercise proper technique in
      (1) Sterilization
      (2) Radiographs
   c. Failure to adequately inform the patient regarding treatment procedures, outcomes, and risks
   d. Failure to obtain permission
      (1) Technical assault—touching or treating without consent (e.g., the health professional treats a child without the parent's consent)
      (2) Invasion of privacy—divulging private information without consent (e.g., the health professional discusses the case in public using the client's name)
3. Defense against malpractice
   a. Exercise due care, using reasonable skill and care
   b. Keep accurate and complete records of each case
   c. Contributory negligence by the patient relieves the health professional of liability
   d. Statute of limitations limits the length of time in which a suit may be brought
      (1) For adults this is usually 2 years after the injury or damage has been recognized or discovered
      (2) For children this is a reasonable period of time after the child reaches the age of majority
   e. Question of proximate cause; if there are possible intervening causes or contributory negligence, these may relieve the health professional from liability
4. Types of damages or redress
   a. Nominal damages—monetary compensation for the loss
   b. Compensatory damages—actual costs to cover repair or treatment plus general damages to cover pain and suffering
   c. Punitive damages—additional monetary compensation to punish the defendant, usually awarded in cases where the professional acted with recklessness or indifference

C. Dental health professionals in court—dental hygienist may be required to appear in court as a witness, as an expert witness, as a defendant, or as a plaintiff
   1. Expert witness
      a. May testify for either the defendant or the plaintiff
      b. Should testify as to the standard of care in the community
      c. Should not advocate or give opinion regarding the guilt or innocence of the defendant
   2. Witness may be required to repeat what he or she saw or heard at the time of an incident
      a. Report accurately what occurred
      b. Should not participate in a "conspiracy of silence"
   3. Defendant is best served by
      a. Telling the truth
      b. Having accurate and complete records of the case
      c. Remaining silent on some points—most states allow "privileged communications" to remain confidential
   4. Plaintiff is best served by
      a. Accurate records
      b. Timely action
      c. Knowledge of facts
      d. Familiarity with legal rights
D. Contractual relationships
   1. Contract—promissory agreement between two or more parties that creates, modifies, or destroys a legal relationship; nature of the relationship between the patient and health professional becomes contractual when the treatment plan and fee for service are agreed on
   2. Elements of a contract
      a. Mutual assent
      b. Promises or consideration
      c. Two or more parties
      d. Must be a lawful act and not against public policy
   3. Breach of contract is the unjustified failure to perform the terms of a contract as agreed on
   4. Classification of contracts—all are legally binding
      a. Expressed
         (1) Are those where the terms are expressly agreed on
         (2) May be oral or written

b. Implied
   (1) Are those without specific terms, or the terms of the agreement are "understood"
   (2) May be oral or written
c. Oral contracts are those verbally agreed on
d. Written contracts are those with the terms in writing
E. Practice arrangements
   1. Partnership—association of two or more persons for the purpose of conducting business
      a. Partners share equally in the profits, expenses, and debts
      b. Partners share equally in liability, one for the other
      c. Partners share equally in liability for acts of employees
      d. Partnership agreement may be verbal or written
      e. Partnerships are dissolved on the loss of any partner
   2. Corporation—single persons or associations of two or more persons for the purpose of conducting business
      a. Members are employees of the corporation
      b. Members are protected from the negligence of the others; only the member involved in the negligence and the corporation are liable
      c. Members of the corporation are not liable for the acts of other employees of the corporation
      d. Articles of incorporation must be written and filed with the state
      e. Corporation continues even if a member is lost
      f. Corporation is subject to regulation by the state
   3. Independent contractors
      a. Are expected to achieve the specified result (e.g., a dental prophylaxis)
      b. Independently make judgments and perform techniques to achieve the specified result
      c. Receive a fee for service rather than a salary
      d. Are not employees per se; receive no benefits or salary from the supervising physician or dentist

Legislation Governing the Practice of Dental Hygiene

A. Dental practice acts, including rules and regulations
   1. Are enacted into law by state legislatures
   2. Regulate the dental health professional's relationship with the state
   3. Provide for a board of dental examiners empowered to regulate the pracice of dentistry and dental hygiene within the state
   4. Set criteria for licensure and the renewal thereof
      a. Educational requirements
      b. Competence examination and procedures thereof
   5. Set grounds for revocation of a license
   6. Specify duties permitted by the respective professions
      a. Duties permitted may be listed; these are called list regulations
      b. Duties permitted may be left open to interpretation by the supervising professional; these are called open regulations
   7. Specify supervision requirements—supervision of dental hygienists may be
      a. General—supervising dentist prescribes the treatment but does not immediately oversee the treatment
      b. Indirect—similar to general
      c. Direct—supervising dentist prescribes and directs the treatment by on-site supervision
B. Boards of dental examiners
   1. Are appointed or elected officials who are
      a. Dentists
      b. Dental hygienist representatives in most states
      c. Consumer representatives in a few states
   2. Regulate application for licensure
   3. Implement mechanisms for measuring competence of prospective registrants (e.g., licensing examinations or "boards")
   4. Implement mechanisms for investigating complaints made against practitioners
   5. Are empowered to grant and revoke licenses
   6. Draft laws pertaining to dentistry and dental hygiene, which must be enacted by state legislatures
   7. Design the rules and regulations pertaining to the practice of dentistry and dental hygiene that augment the practice acts

C. Boards of dental hygiene examiners
  1. The State of Washington regulates dental hygiene practice through a board of dental hygiene examiners
    a. Serves the same function as a board of dental examiners
    b. Is composed of dental hygienists
  2. The State of Florida is reviewing a proposal by the Florida Dental Hygienists' Association to institute a board of dental hygiene examiners

SUGGESTED READINGS

American Dental Hygienists' Association: Grassroots, Dent. Hyg. **53**(1):14, 1979.

American Dental Hygienists' Association: Association policy manual, Chicago, 1983, The Association.

American Dental Hygienists' Association: Bylaws—principles of ethics, Chicago, 1984, The Association.

Beauchamp, T.L., and Childress, J.F.: Principles of biomedical ethics, New York, 1979, Oxford University Press.

Fales, M.J.: History of dental hygiene education in the United States, 1913-1975, unpublished dissertation, Ann Arbor, 1975, University of Michigan.

Helmelt, M.D., and Mackert, M.E.: Dynamics of law in nursing and health care, Reston, Va., 1978, Reston Publishing Co., Inc.

Mayuga, P.W.: Linda Krol—independent contractor, Dent. Hyg. **53**(4):169, 1979.

Motley, N.E.: Ethics, jurisprudence and history for the dental hygienist, ed. 3, Philadelphia, 1983, Lea & Febiger.

Purtilo, R.B.: The American Physical Therapy Association Code of Ethics: its historical foundations, Phys. Ther. **57**(9):1001, 1977.

Rest, J.R.: Development in judging moral issues, Minneapolis, 1979, University of Minnesota Press.

Sarner, H.: Dental jurisprudence, Tampa, Fla., 1963, W.F. Poe Associates, Inc.

Steele, S.M., and Harmon, V.M.: Values clarification in nursing, New York, 1979, Appleton-Century-Crofts.

Woodall, I.R.: Legal, ethical, and management aspects of the dental care system, ed. 2, St. Louis, 1983, The C.V. Mosby Co.

Review Questions

1 The members of the dental profession who first suggested the need for a new specialty in dentistry devoted to prevention intended to develop a group of professionals who would
  1. Go on to dental school
  2. Become dentists eventually
  3. Become independent practitioners
  4. Improve the dental health of schoolchildren
  5. Perform services the dentists did not have the expertise to perform

2 The "father" of dental hygiene is considered to be
  1. Dr. A.C. Fones
  2. Dr. T.P. Hyatt
  3. Dr. G.A. Mills
  4. Dr. M.L. Rhein
  5. Dr. D.D. Smith

3 The "father" of dental hygiene really wanted to call practitioners in the new dental specialty
  1. Dental aides
  2. Odontocurists
  3. Dental nurses
  4. Dental hygienists
  5. Subspecialty dentists

4 The first state to license dental hygienists was
  1. Ohio
  2. New York
  3. California
  4. Connecticut
  5. Massachusetts

5 Irene Newman was all of the following *except*
  1. Dr. A.C. Fones' assistant
  2. President of the Connecticut Dental Hygienists' Association
  3. The first president of the American Dental Hygienists' Association
  4. The first licensed dental hygienist in the United States
  5. A member of the first dental hygiene class conducted in Bridgeport, Conn.

6 The American Dental Hygienists' Association held its first meeting in
  1. 1913
  2. 1923
  3. 1935
  4. 1941
  5. 1943

7 During World War II dental hygienists working for the armed forces were given the status of
  1. Volunteers
  2. Commissioned officers
  3. Private practitioners
  4. Civil service employees
  5. Noncommissioned officers

8 The Forsyth research project to evaluate the feasibility of dental hygienists performing restorative procedures was terminated because of
1. Lack of funding
2. Lack of interest
3. Opposition of local dentists
4. Opposition of the federal government
5. Opposition of the citizens of Massachusetts

9 The first central office of the American Dental Hygienists' Association was established in 1948 in
1. New York City
2. Washington, D.C.
3. Cleveland, Ohio
4. Chicago, Ill.
5. Boston, Mass.

10 The last state within the continental United States to grant dental hygiene licensure was
1. Texas
2. Maine
3. Oregon
4. Virginia
5. New York

11 Until 1964 one group was excluded from dental hygiene licensure in most states, and from membership in the American Dental Hygienists' Association. This group was made up of
1. Men
2. Blacks
3. Women
4. Native Americans
5. Foreign-trained dental hygienists

12 The office that monitors legislation of interest for the American Dental Hygienists' Association is the
1. Chicago office
2. Central office
3. New York Office
4. Washington office
5. Bridgeport office

13 The American Dental Hygienists' Association sponsored the First International Symposium on Dental Hygiene in 1970 in
1. Italy
2. France
3. England
4. The United States
5. Australia

14 The Commission on Accreditation of Dental and Dental Auxiliary Programs was established in 1973 by the
1. American Dental Association
2. Council on Allied Health Education
3. American Dental Hygienists' Association
4. Council on Medical and Dental Education
5. American Association of Dental Schools

15 The last state to allow preceptor training in lieu of formal training was
1. Texas
2. Oregon
3. Alabama
4. Kentucky
5. Massachusetts

16 HY-PAC was initiated in 1978 and stands for
1. Hygiene Policy Advisory Committee
2. Hygiene Planning Alliance Commission
3. Hygiene Pilot Articulation Committee
4. Hygienists' Political Action Committee
5. Hygiene Program Accreditation Committee

17 The first state to amend its dental practice act to allow registered dental hygienists to practice in their own offices by referral was
1. Maine
2. Oregon
3. New York
4. California
5. North Carolina

18 By 1979 there were 201 programs in operation; most of these are in
1. Universities
2. Proprietary schools
3. Academic health centers
4. Senior colleges and institutions
5. Community colleges and technical institutions

19 The federal agency that proposed nullification of state restrictions that require dental hygienists to work under the supervision of a dentist was the
1. Federal Trade Commission
2. Council of State Governors
3. National Institutes of Health
4. Department of Health and Human Services
5. Department of Health, Education, and Welfare

20 The official journal of the American Dental Hygienists' Association is called
1. *Directions*
2. *The Bulletin*
3. *Dental Hygiene*
4. *Dental Hygiene Science*
5. *The Journal of the American Dental Hygienists' Association*

21 The document that describes the mission and goals of the American Dental Hygienists' Association is the
1. Bylaws
2. Charter
3. Constitution
4. Practice Act
5. Principles of Ethics

22 The detailed rules for governing the American Dental Hygienists' Association are found in the
1. Bylaws
2. Charter
3. Practice act
4. Constitution
5. Principles of Ethics

23 The mission of the American Dental Hygienists' Association includes the following *except*
1. To improve the public's total health
2. To increase the awareness of quality care
3. To increase access to quality oral health care
4. To position the dental hygienist in alternative practice settings
5. To position the dental hygienist as *the* preventive oral health professional

24 The Principles of Ethics outline the moral obligations of
1. The House of Delegates only
2. The officers of the association only
3. The members of boards of dental examiners
4. Each individual member of the American Dental Hygienists' Association
5. The American Dental Hygienists' Association as an organization

25 The policy-making body of the American Dental Hygienists' Association is the
1. Central office
2. Executive board
3. Board of Trustees
4. Washington office
5. House of Delegates

26 There are two major functional governing bodies of the American Dental Hygienists' Association; one is responsible for policy, and the other for administration. They are the
1. Districts and the components
2. Constituents and the components
3. State and local associations
4. Constituents and the Council of Presidents
5. House of Delegates and the Board of Trustees

27 The Board of Trustees of the American Dental Hygienists' Association
1. Is self-perpetuating
2. Appoints the President
3. Is the legislative body of the association
4. Is presided over by the Speaker of the House
5. Is the administrative body of the association

28 The House of Delegates of the American Dental Hygienists' Association
1. Hires the staff
2. Reports to the Executive Director
3. Is the legislative body of the association
4. Is the administrative body of the association
5. Conducts the business affairs of the association

29 The House of Delegates of the American Dental Hygienists' Association has the responsibility for all of the following *except*
1. The election of the President
2. Setting the policies of the association
3. Approving the budget of the association
4. The election of the Speaker of the House
5. The administrative affairs of the association

30 In order to be a member of the American Dental Hygienists' Association, a dental hygienist must hold membership at each level, with the *exception* of the
1. Local level
2. District level
3. National level
4. Component level
5. Constituent level

31 An individual, not a dental hygienist, who has gained recognition for contributions to the art and science of dental hygiene may become a (an)
1. Allied member of the American Dental Hygienists' Association
2. Active member of the American Dental Hygienists' Association
3. Associate member of the American Dental Hygienists' Association
4. Honorary member of the American Dental Hygienists' Association
5. Retired member of the American Dental Hygienists' Association

32 The President of the American Dental Hygienists' Association presides over the Board of Trustees and is
1. Elected by the district trustees
2. Elected by the House of Delegates
3. Elected by the general membership
4. Appointed by the Board of Trustees
5. Appointed by the Executive Director

33 The Speaker of the House is elected by the House of Delegates and presides over the
1. District meetings
2. House of Delegates
3. Component meetings
4. Council of Presidents
5. International Liasion Council

34 Members of the American Dental Hygienists' Association have influence over its policies through
1. The Washington lobbyist
2. Trustee representation on the Board of Trustees
3. A direct or referendum vote on each issue or policy
4. Delegate representation in the House of Delegates
5. The state president, who sits on the Council of Presidents

35 The Executive Director is responsible for the day-to-day administrative operation of the American Dental Hygienists' Association and is
1. Appointed by the President
2. Elected by the membership
3. Elected by the House of Delegates
4. Appointed by the Board of Trustees
5. Appointed by the Council of Presidents

36 Members of the American Dental Hygienists' Association have representation on the Board of Trustees through the district trustee, who is
1. Elected by local vote
2. Appointed by the President
3. Elected by the membership
4. Appointed by the Executive Director
5. Elected by delegates from the constituents

37 The appointed officials of the American Dental Hygienists' Association are the
1. District trustees
2. First Vice-President and Second Vice-President
3. President and President-Elect
4. Secretary and Treasurer
5. Executive Director and Editorial Director

38 The study of moral conduct based on theory is known as
1. Mores
2. Ethics
3. Morals
4. Values
5. Value clarification

39 Valuing a healthy life-style is an example of attitudes or beliefs that represent
1. Value judgment
2. Terminal values
3. Intrinsic values
4. Extrinsic values
5. Instrumental values

40 When personally held values are not congruent with those held by the profession or peers, this may result in
1. Value judgment
2. Terminal values
3. Values dissonance
4. A hierarchy of values
5. Values clarification

41 Moral reasoning is characterized by
1. Mores
2. Feelings
3. Behavior
4. Cognitive judgment
5. Beliefs and attitudes

42 In Kohlberg's hierarchy of moral development the final, or postconventional, level is reached by
1. No adults
2. All adults
3. Few adults
4. All adolescents
5. All adolescents and adults

43 In Kohlberg's hierarchy of moral development, stage 4, the law-and-order orientation, is found in the
1. Conventional level
2. Preconventional level
3. Postconventional level
4. Preconventional and conventional levels
5. Conventional and postconventional levels

44 If you say, "The ends justify the means," you are thinking as a
1. Theorist
2. Legalist
3. Utilitarian
4. Kohlbergian
5. Deontologist

45 If you say, "It's the principle of the thing," you are thinking as a
1. Theorist
2. Legalist
3. Utilitarian
4. Kohlbergian
5. Deontologist

46 A person who concentrates on principles and rules in general as they apply to types or classes of actions is a (an)
1. Legalist
2. Act utilitarian
3. Act deontologist
4. Rule utilitarian
5. Rule deontologist

47 The person who focuses on the outcome of a single act under specific circumstances is a (an)
1. Legalist
2. Act utilitarian
3. Rule utilitarian
4. Act deontologist
5. Rule deontologist

48 The principle that states, "Above all, do no harm" is the principle of
1. Justice
2. Autonomy
3. Veracity
4. Beneficence
5. Nonmaleficence

49 The ethical principle that requires health professionals to fully inform their patients and protect the confidentiality of the patients is the principle of
1. Justice
2. Autonomy
3. Veracity
4. Beneficence
5. Nonmaleficence

50 When resources are scarce and treatment is allocated only to those who have earned it, this is an example of distributive justice based on
1. Need
2. Merit
3. Equity
4. Effort
5. Contribution

51 Suppose a dental hygienist performs treatment that is not within the legal limits of dental hygiene. Although the patient is not injured by the treatment, this can be considered
1. A civil wrong
2. A federal crime
3. A criminal wrong
4. Both a civil and a criminal wrong
5. Neither a civil nor a criminal wrong

52 Statutory law includes all *except* which of the following
1. State legislation
2. Dental practice acts
3. The U.S. Constitution
4. Previous court decisions
5. Amendments to the U.S. Constitution

53 Common law is all *except* which of the following
1. Unwritten
2. Statutory
3. Made by judges
4. Based on custom
5. Based on previous court decisions

54 A dental professional may be criminally liable if the tort he or she commits is
1. Accidental
2. Intentional
3. Contributory
4. Unintentional
5. Caused by negligence

55 The legal area covered by the term *tort* usually applies to
1. Property
2. Civil offenses
3. Practice agreements
4. Contract agreements
5. Dental practice acts

56 The act that directly results in an injury, and without which the injury would not have occurred, is known in law as
1. *Res Gestae*
2. *Stare Decisis*
3. Proximate cause
4. Breach of contract
5. *Respondeat Superior*

57 Intentionally defaming someone in writing is known as
1. Libel
2. Fraud
3. Assault
4. Slander
5. Battery

58 The dental health professional's relationships with individual patients are governed by
1. Civil law
2. Common law
3. Federal law
4. Criminal law
5. Military law

59 Suppose a dental hygienist, without the employer's knowledge, uses the office after hours to render preventive services to a friend and the treatment results in injury to the friend. Who would be held liable?
1. The employer
2. All three parties
3. The dental hygienist
4. The employer and the hygienist
5. The friend under contributory negligence

60 The application of the Doctrine of *Res Ipsa Loquitur* places a burden of proof on
1. The court
2. The plaintiff
3. The defendant
4. The expert witness
5. Both the plaintiff and the defendant

61 Suppose a dental hygienist is employed by and working for Dr. A, who pays her salary and benefits. She is loaned to Dr. B for a day while Dr. B's hygienist is sick. While working in Dr. B's office, the hygienist cuts a patient's tongue. In addition to the hygienist, who would be liable?
1. Dr. A
2. Dr. B
3. Both Dr. A and Dr. B
4. Neither Dr. A nor Dr. B
5. The dental hygienist alone

62 The name given to the principle that states that a case, once tried, cannot be retried for the same offense is
1. *Res Gestae*
2. *Res Judicata*
3. *Stare Decisis*
4. *Res Ipsa Loquitur*
5. Statute of limitations

63 The use of unsterilized instruments renders a dental professional liable for malpractice
1. Under all circumstances
2. If the patient contributes to the negligence
3. If the assistant testifies that the instruments were unsterile
4. If the patient is injured as a result of the unsterilized instruments
5. If the patient sees the dental professional drop the instrument on the floor

64 A physician or dentist is responsible for the negligent acts of his or her assistant
1. At all times
2. In the general course of employment
3. When in the presence of patients
4. Only when carrying out specific instructions
5. When the assistant acts on his or her own initiative

65 A dental professional may legally discontinue treatment
1. By moving out of town
2. Under no circumstances
3. By refusing to give further appointments
4. By refunding any money collected for the treatment
5. By referring the patient to another qualified practitioner

66 The most important question in a malpractice suit is whether the practitioner
1. Was experienced
2. Had an assistant
3. Exercised due care
4. Had advanced training
5. Had been in practice for 2 years

67 All *except* which of the following must occur in a case of negligence?
1. The duty is breached
2. A procedure is omitted
3. The breach of duty caused the injury
4. There is injury to the patient
5. There is a duty owed by the practitioner to the patient

68 In a case of proven contributory negligence the
1. Court becomes liable
2. Parents become liable
3. Patient becomes liable
4. Health professional remains liable
5. Health professional is relieved of liability

69 The statute of limitations for bringing a malpractice suit against a practitioner because of a negligent act committed against an adult is usually
1. 1 year
2. 2 years
3. 6 years
4. 10 years
5. 12 years

70 A civil complaint may be made by a patient against a dental health professional who performs unauthorized treatment. Such touching without consent is known as
1. Fraud
2. Slander
3. Battery
4. Technical assault
5. Breach of contract

71 In law, an acceptable defense against malpractice is
1. Good faith
2. High ethics
3. Reasonable skill and care
4. The practitioner's education
5. The practitioner's reputation

72 In considering the liability of a dental professional for technical assault, which of the following is *most* relevant?
1. There was no charge for the service
2. The treatment performed was exploratory
3. The patient benefited from the treatment
4. The patient had not consented to the treatment
5. The dental professional was well trained and skillful

73 Expressed contracts differ from implied contracts in that expressed contracts
1. Are always written
2. Have specified terms
3. Are not legally binding
4. Are general understandings
5. Are in effect for only 1 year

74 If a patient is injured because of the negligence of one of two partners
1. Both partners are liable
2. Neither partner is liable
3. Only the partner who caused the injury is liable
4. Everyone, including employees of the partnership, is liable
5. No one is liable, because proximate cause cannot be established

75 Dental practice acts regulate the dental health professional's relationship with the
1. State
2. Consumer
3. Professional association
4. Internal Revenue Service (IRS)
5. Federal Trade Commission (FTC)

76 Dental and dental hygiene practice acts are enacted by the
1. Local courts
2. Federal courts
3. State legislatures
4. American Dental Association
5. State boards of dental examiners

Answers and Rationales

1. (4) Improvement of the dental health of schoolchildren was of major concern to the dental community and the public alike during the latter part of the nineteenth century.
   (1) Going on to dental school was not intended for the subspecialty.
   (2) Becoming dentists was not expected; in fact, women were suggested because it was thought that they would not wish to overstep the bounds of dental hygiene.
   (3) Becoming independent practitioners was not the suggestion of most proponents of the new specialty.
   (5) Dentists had the skill to provide the service but did not wish to take the time.
2. (1) Dr. A.C. Fones is known as the "father" of dental hygiene because he named the profession "dental hygiene" and started the first successful training program.
   (2) Dr. T.P. Hyatt proposed a new dental specialty.
   (3) Dr. G.A. Mills described the use of the explorer.
   (4) Dr. M.L. Rhein advocated preventive home care and school programs.
   (5) Dr. D.D. Smith had the first preventive practice.
3. (4) "Dental hygienists" was the name given to the new professionals by Dr. Fones because he wanted to stress health, not disease.
   (1) "Dental aide" indicates assistant, not specialist.
   (2) "Odontocurists" was the name suggested by F.W. Low.
   (3) "Dental nurses" was the name suggested by M.L. Rhein.
   (5) "Subspecialty dentists" was a description used by C.M. Wright.
4. (4) Connecticut was the first state to license dental hygienists.
   (1) Ohio was the location of the first meeting of the American Dental Hygienists' Association.
   (2) New York was the third state to license dental hygienists.
   (3) California was one of the early states, but not the first.
   (5) Massachusetts was the second state to license dental hygienists.

For each question the correct answer and rationale are listed first. The other choices are presented in order with the reasons why they are not correct.

5. (3) The first president of the American Dental Hygienists' Association was Winifred A. Hart.
   (1) Irene Newman was Dr. A.C. Fones' assistant.
   (2) Irene Newman was the first president of Connecticut Dental Hygienists' Association.
   (4) Irene Newman was the first licensed dental hygienist in the United States.
   (5) Irene Newman was a member of the first dental hygiene class conducted by Dr. Fones.
6. (2) The first meeting of the American Dental Hygienists' Association was held in 1923.
   (1) The year the first class was accepted to Dr. Fones' program was 1913.
   (3) The year that the Social Security Act was signed into law was 1935.
   (4) World War II began in 1941.
   (5) Fluoride research began in 1943.
7. (4) Dental hygienists served as civil service employees during World War II.
   (1) Some dental hygienists may have been volunteers, but most were employed by the civil service.
   (2) The American Dental Hygienists' Association requested commissioned officer status for dental hygienists to make them comparable to nurses with similar training; this request was denied.
   (3) Dental hygienists were not private practitioners during World War II.
   (5) Dental hygienists did not generally serve as noncommissioned officers during World War II.
8. (3) The opposition of local dentists caused the Forsyth research project to be discontinued.
   (1) The project was not discontinued because of a lack of funds.
   (2) The project was not discontinued because of a lack of interest.
   (4) The project was not discontinued because of opposition by the federal government.
   (5) The project had the support of the citizens of Massachusetts.
9. (2) Washington, D.C., was the site of the first central office of the American Dental Hygienists' Association
   (1) It was not New York.
   (3) Cleveland was the site of the first American Dental Hygienists' Association meeting.
   (4) Chicago is the current site of the central office.
   (5) Boston was the site of the Forsyth research project.
10. (1) Texas was the last state within the continental United States to license dental hygienists in 1951.
    (2) Maine licensed dental hygienists in 1917.
    (3) Oregon licensed dental hygienists in 1949.
    (4) Virginia licensed dental hygienists in 1950.
    (5) New York licensed dental hygienists in 1916.

11. (1) Men were excluded from dental hygiene licensure until 1964 in most states.
    (2) Black women were not excluded from licensure.
    (3) Women (as opposed to men) were eligible for licensure.
    (4) Native American women were not excluded from licensure.
    (5) Foreign-trained dental hygienists as a group were not denied licensure.

12. (4) Washington, D.C., is the site of the office that monitors legislation.
    (1) Legislation is not the primary focus of the Chicago office.
    (2) The central office is located in Chicago.
    (3) There has never been an American Dental Hygienists' Association office in New York.
    (5) There has never been an American Dental Hygienists' Association office in Bridgeport, Conn.

13. (1) Italy was the site of the First International Symposium on Dental Hygiene in 1970.
    (2) France has not been a site for a symposium.
    (3) England was the site of a later conference.
    (4) The United States was the site of the Ninth International Symposium on Dental Hygiene.
    (5) Australia was not the site of the first symposium.

14. (1) The American Dental Association established the Commission on Accreditation of Dental and Dental Auxiliary Programs.
    (2) It was not established by the Council on Allied Health Education.
    (3) The American Dental Hygienists' Association has representation on the commission but is not its sponsor.
    (4) There is no "Council on Medical and Dental Education."
    (5) The American Association of Dental Schools did not establish the commission.

15. (3) Alabama was the last state to allow preceptor training.
    (1) Texas did not allow preceptor training.
    (2) Oregon did not allow preceptor training.
    (4) Kentucky did not allow preceptor training.
    (5) Massachusetts did not allow preceptor training.

16. (4) HY-PAC stands for Hygienists' Political Action Committee.
    (1) The "Hygiene Policy Advisory Committee" does not exist.
    (2) The "Hygiene Planning Alliance Commission" does not exist.
    (3) The "Hygiene Pilot Articulation Committee" does not exist.
    (5) The "Hygiene Program Accreditation Committee" does not exist.

17. (4) California was the first state to allow dental hygienists to practice in their own offices.
    (1) In Maine, denturists may practice independently.
    (2) In Oregon, denturists may practice independently.
    (3) New York does not allow dental hygienists to operate their own offices.
    (5) North Carolina has litigation pending that may result in dental hygienists being allowed to own their own offices.

18. (5) Most of the dental hygiene programs are located in community colleges and technical schools.
    (1) Universities are not the site of most dental hygiene programs.
    (2) Proprietary schools are not the site of most dental hygiene programs.
    (3) Academic health centers are not the site of most dental hygiene programs.
    (4) Senior colleges are not the site of most dental hygiene programs.

19. (1) The Federal Trade Commission was the agency that proposed nullification of state restrictions regarding supervision of dental hygienists by dentists.
    (2) The Council of State Governors has produced a report recommending less supervision of licensed professionals.
    (3) The National Institutes of Health have not made any recommendations regarding supervision.
    (4) The Department of Health and Human Services has not made any recommendations regarding supervision.
    (5) The Department of Health, Education, and Welfare did not make any recommendations regarding supervision.

20. (3) *Dental Hygiene* has been the official title of the journal of the American Dental Hygienists' Association since 1972.
    (1) *Directions* is not the title of the journal of the American Dental Hygienists' Association, but *Educational Directions* is a publication of the American Dental Hygienists' Association aimed at dental hygiene educators.
    (2) *The Bulletin* is not the title of the journal of the American Dental Hygienists' Association, but the *Legislative Bulletin* is a publication of the American Dental Hygienists' Association that reviews legislative issues relevant to dental hygienists.
    (4) *Dental Hygiene Science* is not the name of a publication.
    (5) *The Journal of the American Dental Hygienists' Association* was the official title from 1927 to 1972.

21. (3) The Constitution of the American Dental Hygienists' Association describes the mission and goals of the association.
    (1) The Bylaws are the rules that govern the American Dental Hygienists' Association.
    (2) A charter applies to constituent associations that receive a charter from the Board of Trustees.
    (4) A practice act refers to state law governing the practice of each dental professional.
    (5) The Principles of Ethics govern the moral conduct of the members.

22. (1) The Bylaws of the American Dental Hygienists' Association are the rules that govern the association.
    (2) A charter applies to constituent associations that receive a charter from the Board of Trustees.
    (3) A practice act refers to state law.
    (4) The Constitution describes the mission and goals.
    (5) The Principles of Ethics govern the moral conduct of the members.

23. (4) To position dental hygienists in alternative practice settings is not one of the stated missions of the American Dental Hygienists' Association.
    (1) To improve the public's total health is part of the mission statement.
    (2) To increase the awareness of quality care is part of the mission statement.
    (3) To increase access to quality oral health care is part of the mission statement.
    (5) To position the dental hygienist as the preventive oral health professional is part of the mission statement.

24. (4) The Principles of Ethics outline the moral obligations of each individual member of the American Dental Hygienists' Association.
    (1) The House of Delegates is governed by the Principles of Ethics in the same way that each member of the American Dental Hygienists' Association is governed.
    (2) The officers of the association are not the only members governed by the Principles of Ethics.
    (3) The members of boards of dental examiners are not affected by the Principles of Ethics of the American Dental Hygienists' Association unless they are dental hygienists.
    (5) The Principles of Ethics pertain to individual members, not the organization per se.

25. (5) The House of Delegates is the policy-making body of the American Dental Hygienists' Association.
    (1) The central office assists in the administration of the organization.
    (2) The executive board is the entire Board of Trustees; the former Executive Committee is now known as the Council on Administration.
    (3) The Board of Trustees is the administrative body of the association.
    (4) The Washington office is responsible for legislative representation for the association.

26. (5) The House of Delegates and the Board of Trustees are the two major functional bodies of the American Dental Hygienists' Association.
    (1) The districts and the components are regional and state bodies of the American Dental Hygienists' Association.
    (2) The constituents and the components are state and local organizations.
    (3) The state and local associations are also known as the constituent and component associations, respectively.
    (4) The constituents are the state organizations, and there is no "Council of Presidents."

27. (5) The administrative body of the association is the Board of Trustees.
    (1) The Board of Trustees is not self-perpetuating.
    (2) The President is elected by the House of Delegates.
    (3) The legislative body of the association is the House of Delegates.
    (4) The Speaker of the House presides over the House of Delegates, whereas the President presides over the Board of Trustees.

28. (3) The legislative body of the association is the House of Delegates.
    (1) The staff is hired by the Board of Trustees.
    (2) The Executive Director reports to the Board of Trustees.
    (4) The administrative body is the Board of Trustees.
    (5) The Board of Trustees and the Executive Director conduct the business of the association.

29. (5) The administrative affairs of the association are not the responsibility of the House of Delegates.
    (1) The President is elected by the House of Delegates.
    (2) The policies of the association are set by the House of Delegates.
    (3) The House of Delegates approves the budget; the Board of Trustees prepares the budget.
    (4) The House of Delegates elects and is presided over by the Speaker of the House.

30. (2) The district level does have individual members but does have a district trustee elected by delegates representing the constituents within the district.
    (1) The local level is the same as the component level; components are subdivisions of state associations.
    (3) To be a member of the American Dental Hygienists' Association, a dental hygienist must hold membership at the national level.
    (4) The component level is the local level, and a dental hygienist who wishes to be a member of the American Dental Hygienists' Association must also be a member of this organization if one exists.
    (5) The constituent level is the state level, and a dental hygienist who wishes to be a member of the American Dental Hygienists' Association must also be a member of this organization.

31. (4) An honorary member of the association is one who has gained recognition for contributions to the art and science of dental hygiene but who is not a dental hygienist.
    (1) An allied member is any individual who supports the purposes and mission of the association.
    (2) An active member must be a licensed, graduate dental hygienist.
    (3) An associate member must be a dental hygienist who is practicing outside of the United States.
    (5) A retired member is a dental hygienist who had been an active member of the American Dental Hygienists' Association before retirement.

32. (2) The House of Delegates elects the President.
    (1) The district trustees are not involved with the election of the President.
    (3) The general membership does not vote per se; delegates representing the membership of each constituent sit in the House of Delegates, which elects the President.
    (4) The Board of Trustees is presided over by the President, but it does not elect the President.
    (5) The Executive Director is appointed by the Board of Trustees and does not have the power to appoint the President.

33. (2) The House of Delegates is presided over by the Speaker of the House.
    (1) District meetings are presided over by the district trustee
    (3) Component meetings are presided over by each president of the components, respectively.
    (4) The "Council of Presidents" does not exist.
    (5) The International Liaison Council does not have a direct relationship with the Speaker of the House of the American Dental Hygienists' Association.

34. (4) Delegate representation in the House of Delegates allows the membership of the American Dental Hygienists' Association to have influence over the policies of the association.
    (1) The Washington lobbyist provides the association with a way to have some influence over legislative matters at the national level.
    (2) Trustee representation on the Board of Trustees allows influence over the administrative decisions but not over the policies of the association.
    (3) Direct or referendum votes do not exist in the American Dental Hygienists' Association.
    (5) The state president has influence over the affairs of the constituent organization only, not over the American Dental Hygienists' Association; there is no "Council of Presidents."

35. (4) The Executive Director is appointed by the Board of Trustees.
    (1) The President appoints council members and chairpersons but does not appoint the Executive Director.
    (2) The membership per se does not vote on national matters.
    (3) The House of Delegates elects the President and other elected officers, but the Executive Director is not an elected officer.
    (5) There is no "Council of Presidents."

36. (5) The district trustee is elected by delegates from the constituents.
    (1) There is no local vote on issues of the American Dental Hygienists' Association.
    (2) The President appoints council members and chairpersons but not the trustees.
    (3) The membership of the American Dental Hygienists' Association votes on component officers and issues but not directly for the trustee.
    (4) The Executive Director does not make appointments.

37. (5) The Executive Director and the Editorial Director are the appointed officials of the American Dental Hygienists' Association.
    (1) The district trustees are elected by and from among the delegates of the respective districts.
    (2) The First Vice-President and Second Vice-President are elected by the House of Delegates.
    (3) The President assumes the presidency as a result of an earlier election by the House of Delegates; the President-Elect is elected by the House of Delegates.
    (4) The Secretary and Treasurer are elected by the House of Delegates.

38. (2) Ethics is the study of moral conduct based on theory.
    (1) Mores are the customs of a group.
    (3) Morals are standards of conduct based on ethical principles.
    (4) Values are beliefs and attitudes that motivate behavior.
    (5) Value clarification is an activity that leads to an understanding of personal thoughts and actions.

39. (5) Valuing a healthy life-style is an example of attitudes or beliefs that represent instrumental values (values related to a process).
    (1) Value judgment is the evaluation of the beliefs and behavior of others based on the values held by self.
    (2) Terminal values are attitudes or beliefs related to an outcome or product.
    (3) Intrinsic values are attitudes or beliefs related to the maintenance of life.
    (4) Extrinsic values are attitudes or beliefs related to alternatives not essential to life.

40. (3) Values dissonance occurs when personally held values are not congruent with those held by the profession or peers.
    (1) Value judgment occurs when one evaluates the thoughts or behavior of others based on personally held values.
    (2) Terminal values are attitudes or beliefs related to an outcome or product.
    (4) Hierarchy of values occurs when some values hold more importance than others in motivating action.
    (5) Values clarification occurs as the result of an activity that leads to an understanding of personal thought or actions.

41. (4) Cognitive judgment is a characteristic of moral reasoning and is based on thinking and experience.
    (1) Mores are customs of a group.
    (2) Feelings are unreasoned opinion or belief.
    (3) Behavior is a manner of conducting oneself.
    (5) Beliefs and attitudes constitute values and may not be based on reason or knowledge.

42. (3) Few adults reach the postconventional level of Kohlberg's hierarchy of moral development.
    (1) Not correct; some adults do reach the postconventional level. As the name implies, postconventional is beyond conventional.
    (2) Not correct; only a few adults reach this level.
    (4) Not correct; adolescents very rarely reach this level.
    (5) Not correct; few adults and very, very few adolescents reach this level.

43. (1) The conventional level contains stage 3 and stage 4. Stage 3 is the interpersonal concordance or "good boy–nice girl" stage, and stage 4 is the law-and-order stage.
    (2) The preconventional level contains stage 1 and stage 2. Stage 1 is the punishment and obedience orientation, and stage 2 is the instrument relativist orientation.
    (3) The postconventional level contains stage 5 and stage 6. Stage 5 is the social-contract legalistic orientation, and stage 6 is the universal ethical principle orientation.

(4) Not correct; stage 4 appears only in the conventional level.

(5) Not correct; stage 4 appears only in the conventional level.

44. (3) A utilitarian may say, "The ends justify the means" because he or she focuses on outcomes or consequences of actions.

    (1) Theorists produce and study theories; they are not particularly likely to say, "The ends justify the means."

    (2) Legalists view things from the legal standpoint; they are not likely to say, "The ends justify the means."

    (4) Kohlbergians are the followers of the theories of Kohlberg; they are not likely to say, "The ends justify the means."

    (5) Deontologists focus on principles, not consequences; they would say, "It's the principle of the thing" rather than "The ends justify the means."

45. (5) A deontologist focuses on principles, not consequences of actions. He or she may say, "It's the principle of the thing."

    (1) Theorists produce and study theories; they are not particularly likely to say, "It's the principle of the thing."

    (2) Legalists view things from the legal standpoint; they are not particularly likely to say, "It's the principle of the thing."

    (3) Utilitarians focus on the consequences of actions; they would say, "The ends justify the means" rather than "It's the principle of the thing."

    (4) Kohlbergians are the followers of the theories of Kohlberg; they are not particularly likely to say, "It's the principle of the thing."

46. (5) A rule deontologist concentrates on principles and rules in general as they apply to types or classes of actions.

    (1) Legalists concentrate on things from the legal standpoint.

    (2) Act utilitarians concentrate on the outcome of a single act.

    (3) Rule utilitarians concentrate on the outcome of types of acts.

    (4) Act deontologists consider the ethical principles involved in an action in light of the circumstances.

47. (2) An act utilitarian focuses on the outcome of a single act under specific circumstances.

    (1) Legalists focus on the legal point of view.

    (3) Rule utilitarians focus on the outcome of types of acts.

    (4) Act deontologists focus on the ethical principles involved in an action in light of the circumstances.

    (5) Rule deontologists focus on ethical principles and rules in general as they apply to types of actions.

48. (5) The principle of nonmaleficence states, "Above all, do no harm."

    (1) The principle of justice requires fairness.

    (2) The principle of autonomy requires respect for the rights of the patient.

    (3) The principle of veracity requires truthfulness.

    (4) The principle of beneficence requires the promotion of well-being.

49. (2) The principle of autonomy requires health professionals to fully inform their patients and protect their confidentiality.

    (1) The principle of justice requires fairness.

    (3) The principle of veracity requires truthfulness.

    (4) The principle of beneficence requires the promotion of well-being.

    (5) The principle of nonmaleficence states, "Above all, do no harm."

50. (4) Distributive justice based on effort would result in the allocation of treatment only to those who have earned it.

    (1) Allocation of treatment based on need would result in all who are in need receiving treatment.

    (2) Allocation of treatment based on merit would result in only those who are considered worthy receiving treatment.

    (3) Allocation of treatment based on equity would result in each person having an equal share in or an equal chance of receiving treatment.

    (5) Allocation of treatment based on contribution would result in only those who have contributed to society receiving treatment.

51. (3) A criminal wrong occurs when a dental hygienist performs dental treatment that is not within the legal limits of dental hygiene, even if the patient is not harmed.

    (1) A civil wrong occurs when the dental hygienist is negligent and harms a patient.

    (2) A federal crime is not involved in this case, because the law that delineates the limits of practice of dental hygiene is a state law.

    (4) Both a civil and a criminal wrong is not correct, since the patient was not injured in this case.

    (5) Not correct; practicing dentistry without a dental license is a criminal wrong.

52. (4) Previous court decisions do not constitute statutory law.

    (1) Statutory law is written law and includes state legislation.

    (2) Dental practice acts are statutory laws.

    (3) The U.S. Constitution is statutory.

    (5) Amendments to the U.S. Constitution are statutory.

53. (2) Statutory law is written and therefore is not common law.

    (1) Common law is unwritten.

    (3) Common law is made by judges.

    (4) Common law is based on custom.

    (5) Common law is based on previous court decisions.

54. (2) An intentional tort may be considered a crime.

    (1) An accidental tort constitutes a civil wrong, not a crime.

    (3) A contributory tort may or may not be considered a civil wrong, but it does not constitute a crime.

    (4) An unintentional tort constitutes a civil wrong, not a crime.

    (5) A tort resulting from negligence is a civil wrong, not a crime.

55. (2) Civil offenses are the legal area usually applicable when using the term *tort*.
    (1) The term *tort* is not used in relation to a property issue.
    (3) The term *tort* is not used in relation to practice agreements.
    (4) The term *tort* is not used in relation to contract agreements.
    (5) The term *tort* is not used in relation to dental practice acts.
56. (3) *Proximate cause* is the legal term used to describe an act that directly results in an injury.
    (1) *Res Gestae* admits pertinent statements made by third parties as admissible evidence.
    (2) *Stare Decisis* requires judges to adhere to the precedents of prior decisions.
    (4) Breach of contract occurs when one party fails to comply with the terms of the contractual agreement.
    (5) *Respondeat Superior* holds an employer liable for the negligent acts of his or her employees.
57. (1) *Libel* is the term used when one is guilty of intentionally defaming someone in writing.
    (2) *Fraud* is the term used in deception or misrepresentation with intent to take something of value from someone.
    (3) *Assault* is the term used for violent physical or verbal attack.
    (4) *Slander* is the term used for intentional verbal defamation of someone's character.
    (5) *Battery* is the term used for beating or use of force.
58. (1) Civil law governs the relationship between dental health professionals and patients.
    (2) Common law pertains to unwritten or judge-made law.
    (3) Federal law pertains to statutes promulgated by the federal government.
    (4) Criminal law pertains to acts against society.
    (5) Military law governs the actions of military personnel.
59. (3) The dental hygienist would be liable because he or she presumably did not use due care, which resulted in injury to the friend.
    (1) The employer would not be liable, since he or she did not know that the office was being used.
    (2) All three parties would not be liable, because the employer and the friend would not be liable.
    (4) Not correct; the employer was not aware of the incident; therefore the hygienist alone would be liable.
    (5) The friend would not be liable even though there was contributory negligence, because a person cannot hold himself or herself liable.
60. (3) *Res Ispa Loquitur* (the thing speaks for itself) places the burden of proof on the defendant.
    (1) The court must decide the matter of facts but does not bear the burden of proof.
    (2) The plaintiff normally bears the burden of proof, but when "the thing speaks for itself," the burden of proof is shifted to the defendant.

(4) The expert witness has the responsibility of testifying to the standard of care but does not bear the burden of proof.
(5) The defendant alone bears the burden of proof in this case.
61. (3) Both Dr. A and Dr. B would be liable in addition to the dental hygienist: Dr. A as a result of being the employer (the Doctrine of *Respondent Superior* applies) and Dr. B under the Doctrine of the Borrowed Servant.
    (1) Dr. A alone would not be liable, because Dr. B also would be liable.
    (2) Dr. B alone would not be liable, because Dr. A also would be liable.
    (4) Not correct; both Dr. A and Dr. B would be liable.
    (5) Not correct; both Dr. A and Dr. B would be liable in addition to the dental hygienist.
62. (2) *Res Judicata* states that a case once tried cannot be retried for the same offense.
    (1) *Res Gestae* admits pertinent statements made by third parties at the time of the accident as admissible in court.
    (3) *Stare Decisis* requires judges to adhere to the precedents of prior decisions.
    (4) *Res Ipsa Loquitur* shifts the burden of proof from the plaintiff to the defendant.
    (5) Statute of limitations is the limit placed on the length of time in which a suit may be initiated.
63. (4) If the patient is injured as a result of the use of the unsterilized instruments, the dental professional becomes liable for malpractice.
    (1) Not correct; injury must occur in order for malpractice to exist.
    (2) Not correct; the patient would not contribute to the use of unsterilized instruments.
    (3) Not correct; without injury there would be no case.
    (5) Not correct; injury must occur for a malpractice suit to be initiated.
64. (2) A physician or dentist is responsible for the negligent acts of his or her assistant in the general course of employment under the Doctrine of *Respondent Superior*.
    (1) A physician or dentist is not responsible for the negligent acts of his or her assistant at all times.
    (3) The presence of patients has no bearing on the responsibility.
    (4) The responsibility of the physician or dentist is not limited to when the assistant is carrying out specific instructions.
    (5) The physician or dentist is not responsible for the negligent acts of his or her assistant when the assistant acts on his or her own initiative.

65. (5) Referring the patient to another qualified practitioner is the only way that a dental professional may legally discontinue treatment.
    (1) Moving out of town does not relieve the professional from responsibility unless he or she refers the patient to another professional.
    (2) Not correct; the practitioner may legally refer a patient to another professional.
    (3) Refusing to give further appointments is not legal unless some other arrangement can be made for the treatment, or the patient has been so uncooperative as to have caused the practitioner to be unable to treat the case (contributory negligence).
    (4) Refunding any money collected for unfinished treatment does not relieve the professional from responsibility, but this should be done when a patient is referred to another qualified professional.

66. (3) The exercise of due care is the most important question in a malpractice suit.
    (1) The practitioner's experience is not as pertinent as due care.
    (2) Having an assistant is not relevant.
    (4) Having advanced training is not as pertinent as due care.
    (5) Having been in practice for 2 years is not relevant.

67. (2) A procedure being omitted is the only condition that is *not* necessary for negligence to occur.
    (1) A duty must be breached for there to be negligence.
    (3) The breach of duty must cause an injury for there to be negligence.
    (4) There must be injury to the patient for there to be negligence.
    (5) There must be a duty owed by the practitioner to the patient for there to be negligence.

68. (5) The health professional is relieved of liability in the case of proven contributory negligence.
    (1) The court never becomes liable.
    (2) The parents normally do not become liable.
    (3) The patient cannot assume liability, since one cannot bring charges against oneself.
    (4) The health professional does not remain liable.

69. (2) The statute of limitations for an adult to bring a malpractice suit is 2 years in most states.
    (1) The usual statute of limitations is not 1 year.
    (3) The usual statute of limitations is not 6 years.
    (4) The usual statute of limitations is not 10 years.
    (5) The usual statute of limitations is not 12 years.

70. (4) Technical assault is the civil complaint made by a patient against a dental health professional who performs unauthorized treatment.
    (1) Fraud is the criminal charge in the case of deception or misrepresentation with intent to take something of value from someone.
    (2) Slander is the criminal charge in the case of intentional verbal defamation of someone's character.
    (3) Battery is the criminal charge in the case of beating or ue of force.
    (5) Breach of contract is the civil complaint made when one party fails to comply with the terms of a contractual agreement.

71. (3) Reasonable skill and care is an acceptable defense against malpractice.
    (1) Good faith cannot prevent malpractice.
    (2) High ethics does not guarantee protection from malpractice.
    (4) The practitioner's education does not guarantee protection from malpractice.
    (5) The practitioner's reputation does not guarantee protection from malpractice.

72. (4) The fact that the patient had not consented to the treatment is the most relevant fact in a case of technical assault.
    (1) The fact that there was no charge for the service is not relevant.
    (2) The fact that treatment was exploratory is not relevant.
    (3) The fact that the patient benefited from the treatment is not relevant.
    (5) The fact that the dental professional was well trained and skillful is not relevant.

73. (2) Expressed contracts have specified terms.
    (1) Expressed contracts may be written or oral.
    (3) Expressed contracts are legally binding.
    (4) Expressed contracts are not general understandings but have specific terms, unlike implied contracts, which have understandings rather than specific terms.
    (5) There are no standard limits as to the length of time an expressed or an implied contract may be in effect; the contract itself usually specifies the length of time it will be in effect.

74. (1) Both partners are liable in a case where a patient is injured by one of two partners.
    (2) Not correct; both partners are liable.
    (3) Not correct; this would be true in a corporation but not in a partnership.
    (4) Not correct; only the two partners are liable.
    (5) Not correct; proximate cause has been established, and one of the partners was negligent.

75. (1) The dental health professional's relationship with the state is regulated by the dental practice act.
    (2) The relationship between the dental health professional and the consumer is regulated by contract.
    (3) The relationship between the professional and the professional association is regulated by the terms of membership, the constitution, and the bylaws of the association.
    (4) The relationship between the professional and the IRS is regulated by federal tax laws.
    (5) The relationship between the professional and the FTC is regulated by the antitrust laws.

76. (3) State legislatures enact dental and dental hygiene practice acts.
    (1) Local courts uphold, but do not enact, dental and dental hygiene practice acts.
    (2) The federal courts have no relationship to the practice acts.
    (4) The American Dental Association may influence the state boards of dental examiners but does not enact the dental practice acts.
    (5) State boards of dentistry draft the practice acts, which are enacted by the state legislatures.

Medical Terminology

PREFIXES

a, ab-, abs- From; away; departing from the normal
ad- Addition to; toward; nearness
amb-, ambi- Both; ambidextrous, having the ability to work effectively with either hand
amphi- On both sides
ampho- Both
an- Negative; without or not
ana- Upper, away from
andro- Signifying man
ant-, anti- Against
ante-, antero- Front; before
bili- Pertaining to bile
brady- Slow
brom-, bromo- A stench
broncho- Relating to the bronchi
cac- Bad
cardi-, cardio- Relating to the heart
cata- Down or downward
cervico- Relating to the neck
circa- About
circum- Around
co- With or together
con- Together with
contra- Opposite; against
demi- Half
di- Twice
dia- Through
dialy- To separate
en- In
end-, endo-, ento- Inward; within
ep-, epi- On; in addition to
ex- Out; away from
exo- Without; outside of
extra- Outside of; in addition to
fibro- Relating to fibers
gaster-, gastr-, gastro- Pertaining to the stomach
hemi- Half
hemo- Relating to the blood
hepat-, hepatico-, hepato- Pertaining to the liver
heter-, hetero- Meaning other; relationship to another
homeo- Denoting likeness or resemblance
homo- Denoting sameness
hyal-, hyalo- Transparent
hyper- Above; excessive; beyond
hypo- Below; less than
ideo- Pertaining to mental images

idio- Denoting relationship to one's self or to something separate and distinct
in- Not; in; inside; within; also intensive action
infra- Below
inter- In the midst; between
intra- Within
intro- In or into
iso- Equal or alike
juxta- Of close proximity
karyo- Relating to a cell's nucleus
kypho- Humped
laryngo- Pertaining to the larynx
medi- Middle
myelo- Pertaining to the spinal cord or bone marrow
oari-, oaric- Pertaining to the ovary
omni- All
per- Through; by means of
peri- Around; about
post- Behind or after
postero- Relating to the posterior
pre- Before
pro- Before, in front of
pseudo- False
re- Back; again (contrary)
retro- Backward
semi- Half
steato- Fatty
sub- Under; near
syn- Joined together
trans- Across; over
un- Not; reversal

SUFFIXES

-able, -ible, -ble The power to be
-ad Toward; in the direction of
-aemia, -emia Pertaining to blood
-age Put in motion; to do
-agra Denoting a seizure; severe pain
-algia Denoting pain
-ase Forms the name of an enzyme
-blast Designates a cell or a structure
-cele Denoting a swelling
-centesis Denoting a puncture
-ectomy A cutting out
-esthesia Denoting sensation
-facient That which makes or causes
-gene, -genesis, -genetic, -genic Denoting production; origin

-*gog*, -*gogue* To make flow
-*gram* A tracing; a mark
-*graph* A writing; a record
-*iasis* Denoting a condition or pathologic state
-*id* Denoting shape or resemblance
-*ite* Of the nature of
-*itis* Denoting inflammation
-*logia* Denoting discourse, science, or study of
-*oid* Denoting form or resemblance
-*oma* Denoting a tumor
-*osis* Denoting any morbid process
-*ostomosis*, -*ostomy*, -*stomy* Denoting an outlet; to furnish
    with an opening or mouth
-*plasty* Denoting molding or shaping
-*rhagia* Denoting a discharge; usually a bleeding
-*rhaphy* Meaning suturing or stitching
-*rhea* Meaning a flow or discharge
-*scopy* Generally an instrument for viewing
-*tomy* Denoting a cutting operation
-*trophy* Denoting a relationship to nourishment

COMBINING FORMS

aer-, *aero-* Denoting air or gas
alge-, *algesi-*, *algo-* Relating to pain
allo- Other; differing from the normal
anomalo- Denoting irregularity
arthro- Relating to a joint or joints
brevi- Short
celio- Denoting the abdomen
centro- Center
cheil-, *cheilo-* Denoting the lip
chol-, *chole-*, *cholo-* Relating to bile
chondr-, *chondri-* Relating to cartilage
chrom-, *chromo-* Relating to color
cole-, *coleo-* Denoting a sheath
colp-, *colpo-* Relating to the vagina
cranio- Relating to the cranium of the skull
crymo-, *cryo-* Denoting cold
crypt- To hide; a pit
cyano- Dark blue
cyclo- Pertaining to a cycle
cysto- Relating to a sac or cyst
cyto- Denoting a cell
dacryo- Pertaining to the lacrimal glands
dactylo- Relating to digits
dent-, *dento-* Relating to teeth
derma-, *dermat-* Relating to the skin
desmo- Relating to a bond or ligament
dextro- Right
diplo- Double; twofold
dorsi-, *dorso-* Referring to the back
duodeno- Relating to the duodenum
electro- Relating to electricity
encephalo- Denoting the brain
entero- Relating to the intestines
episio- Relating to the vulva
eso- Inward
esthesio- Relating to feeling or sensation

facio- Relating to the face
gangli-, *ganglio-* Relating to a ganglion
geno- Relating to reproduction
gero-, *geronto-* Denoting old age
giganto- Huge
gingivo- Relating to the gingiva or gum
gloss-, *glosso-* Relating to the tongue
gluco- Denoting sweetness
glyco- Relating to sugar
gnath-, *gnatho-* Denoting the jaw
gon- Denoting a seed
grapho- Denoting writing
hapt-, *hapte-*, *hapto-* Relating to touch or a seizure
helo- Relating to a nail or a callus
hist-, *histio-*, *histo-*, Relating to tissue
holo- Relating to the whole
hydr-, *hydro-* Denoting water
hygro- Denoting moisture
hyl-, *hyle-*, *hylo-* Denoting matter or material
ileo-, *ilio-* Relating to the ileum
ipsi- Meaning self
irido- Relating to a colored circle
iso- Equal
jejuno- Referring to the jejunum
kerato- Relating to the cornea
kino- Denoting movement
labio- Pertaining to the lips
lacto- Relating to milk
laparo- Pertaining to the loin or flank
latero- Pertaining to the side
leido-, *leio-* Smooth
leuk-, *leuko-* Denoting deficiency of color
lip-, *lipo-* Pertaining to fat
litho- Denoting a calculus
macr-, *macro-* Large; long
mast-, *mastro-* Relating to the breast
meg-, *mega-* Great; large
meli- Sweet
meningo- Denoting membranes; covering the brain and
    spinal cord
micr-, *micro-* Small in size or extent
mono- One
morpho- Relating to form
multi- Many
my-, *myo-* Relating to muscle
myc- *mycet-* Denoting a fungus
myringo- Denoting tympani or the eardrum
myx-, *myxo-* Pertaining to mucus
narco- Denoting stupor
naso- Relating to the nose
necro- Denoting death
neo- New
nephr-, *nephro-* Denoting the kidney
normo- Normal or usual
oculo- Denoting the eye
odyno- Denoting pain
oleo- Denoting oil
onco- Denoting a swelling or mass

onyco- Relating to the nails
oo- Denoting an egg
opisth-, opistho- Backward
ophthal-, ophthalmo- Pertaining to the eye
optico- Relating to the eye or vision
orchi-, orcho- Relating to the testes
oro- Relating to the mouth
ortho- Straight; right
oscillo- Denoting oscillation
osteo- Relating to the bones
ot-, oto- Denoting the ear
ovario- Denoting the ovary
ovi-, ovo- Denoting an egg
palato- Denoting the palate
patho- Denoting disease
pedia-, pedo- Denoting a child
perineo- A combining form for the region between the anus and scrotum or the vulva
phago- Denoting a relationship to eating
pharyngo- Pertaining to the pharynx
phleb-, phlebo- Denoting the veins
phon-, phono- Denoting sound
phot-, photo- Relating to light
phren- Relating to the mind
picr-, picro- Bitter
pilo- Denoting hair
plasmo- Relating to plasma or the substance of a cell
pneuma-, pneumono-, pneumoto- Denoting air or gas
pod-, podo- Meaning foot
poly- Many
proct-, procto- Denoting the anus and rectum
psych-, psycho- Relating to the mind
ptyalo- Denoting saliva
pubio-, pubo- Denoting the pubic region
pulmo- Denoting the lung
pupillo- Denoting the pupil
pyel-, pyelo- Denoting the pelvis
pyloro- Relating to the pylorus
py-, pyo- Denoting pus
recto- Denoting the rectum
rhin-, rhino- Denoting the nose
rrhagia- Denoting abnormal discharge
salpingo- Denoting a tube, specifically the fallopian tube
schizo- Split
sclero- Denoting hardness
scoto- Relating to darkness
sero- Pertaining to serum
sialo- Relating to saliva or the salivary glands
sidero- Denoting iron
sinistro- Left
somato- Denoting the body
somni- Denoting sleep
spasmo- Denoting a spasm
spermato-, spermo- Denoting sperm
sphero- Denoting a sphere; round
sphygmo- Denoting a pulse

splen-, spleno- Denoting the spleen
staphyl-, staphylo- Resembling a bunch of grapes
steno- Narrow; short
sterco- Denoting feces
steth-, stetho- Relating to the chest
stomato- Denoting the mouth
sym-, syn- With; along
tacho-, tachy- Swift
tarso- Relating to the flat of the foot
terato- Denoting a marvel, prodigy, or monster
thoraco- Relating to the chest
thrombo- Denoting a clot of blood
toxico-, toxo- Denoting poison
tracheo- Denoting the trachea
trichi-, tricho- Denoting hair
ur-, uro-, urono- Relating to urine
varico- Denoting a twisting or swelling
vaso- Denoting a vessel
veno- Denoting a vein
ventri-, ventro- Denoting the abdomen
vertebro- Relating to the vertebra
vesico- Denoting the bladder
viscero- Denoting the organs of the body
vivi- Denoting alive
xantho- Denoting yellow
xero- Denoting dryness

TERMINOLOGY FREQUENTLY USED TO DESIGNATE BODY PARTS OR ORGANS

anus Anal, ano
arm Brachial, brachio-
blood Hem, hemat-
chest Thoracic, thorax
ear Auricle, oto-
eye Ocular, oculo-, ophthalmo-
foot Pedal, ped-, -pod
gallbladder Chole, chol-
head Cephalic, cephalo-
heart Cardium, cardiac, cardio
intestines Cecum, colon, duodenum, ileum, jejunum
kidney Renal, nephric, nephro-
lip Cheil-
liver Hepatic, hepato-
lungs Pulmonary, pulmonic, pneumo
mouth Oral, os, stoma, stomat-
muscle Myo-
neck Cervix, cervical, cervico-
penis Penile
rectum Rectal
skin Derma, integumentum
stomach Gastric, gastro-
testicle Orchio-, orchi-, orchido-
urinary bladder Cysti-, cysto-
uterus Hystero, metra
vagina Vulvo, vaginal

Prevention of Bacterial Endocarditis:

A Committee Report of the

American Heart Association

COUNCIL ON DENTAL THERAPEUTICS

Recommendations for the prevention of bacterial endocarditis are revised periodically to use current scientific information for the improvement of patient care. This latest revision was done, as were past revisions, by the Committee on Rheumatic Fever and Infective Endocarditis of the American Heart Association in consultation with the Council on Dental Therapeutics of the American Dental Association through its representative on the committee. The Council on Dental Therapeutics has reviewed and approved those sections pertinent to dentistry. The full text of the revision appears in the December 1984 issue of *Circulation*. The report from the Council on Dental Therapeutics that follows is abridged to include only those parts related to dental practice.

Dental treatment, surgical procedures, or instrumentation involving mucosal surfaces or contaminated tissue may cause transient bacteremia. Blood-borne bacteria may lodge on damaged or abnormal heart valves or on endocardium near congenital anatomic defects and result in bacterial endocarditis or endarteritis. However, it is impossible to predict which patients will develop this infection or which procedures will be responsible. Therefore, prophylactic antibiotics are recommended for patients at risk who are undergoing those procedures most likely to cause bacteremia. It is important that such

antibiotics be initiated shortly before, not several days before, a procedure. Certain patients, for example, those with prosthetic heart valves and surgically constructed systemic-pulmonary shunts or conduits, are at higher risk of endocarditis than others (Table B-1). Likewise, certain dental procedures (for example, extractions) are much more likely to initiate significant bacteremia than are others (Table B-2). Although the importance of such factors is difficult to quantitate, they have been considered in developing these recommendations.

Because there are no controlled clinical trials, the choice of antibiotic regimens for prevention of endocarditis in humans must be based on indirect information. The present recommendations are based on a review of available data, including in vitro studies, clinical experience, experimental animal model data, and assessment of both the bacteria most likely to produce bacteremia from a given site and those most likely to result in endocarditis. The substantial morbidity and mortality in patients who have infective endocarditis and the paucity of controlled clinical studies emphasize the need for continuing research into the epidemiology, pathogenesis, prevention, and therapy of endocarditis.

Antibiotic regimens used to prevent recurrences of acute rheumatic fever are inadequate for the prevention of bacterial endocarditis. Appropriate additional antibiotics should be prescribed at times of procedures associated with risk of development of endocarditis.

Warning

The committee recognizes that it is not possible to make recommendations for all possible clinical situations. Practitioners must exercise their clinical judgment in determining the duration and choice of antibiotic when special circumstances apply. Furthermore, because endocarditis may occur despite antibiotic prophylaxis, physicians and dentists should maintain a high index of suspicion regarding any unusual clinical events after dental or surgical procedures.

From J. Am. Dent. Assoc. **110**:98, 1985. Copyright by the American Dental Association. Reprinted by permission. This report was prepared by the Committee on Rheumatic Fever and Infective Endocarditis, American Heart Association, in consultation with the Council on Dental Therapeutics, American Dental Association. Committee members include Stanford T. Schulman, M.D., chairman; Don P. Amren, M.D.; Alan L. Bisno, M.D.; Adnan S. Dajani, M.D.; David T. Durack, M.D., D. Phil.; Michael A. Gerber, M.D.; Edward L. Kaplan, M.D.; H. Dean Millard, D.D.S., M.S.; W. Eugene Sanders, M.D.; Richard H. Schwartz, M.D.; and Chatrchai Watanakunakorn, M.D. The foreword was prepared by Dr. H. Dean Millard, dental member to the committee. Address requests for reprints to the Council on Dental Therapeutics, American Dental Association, 211 E. Chicago Ave., Chicago, 60611. The American Heart Association is located at 7320 Greenville Ave., Dallas, 75211. For a copy of the full report, address requests to the American Heart Association, Report No. 71-005-c.

Table B-1   Cardiac conditions*

Endocarditis prophylaxis recommended
  Prosthetic cardiac valves (including biosynthetic valves)
  Most congenital cardiac malformations
  Surgically constructed systemic-pulmonary shunts
  Rheumatic and other acquired valvular dysfunctions
  Idiopathic hypertrophic subaortic stenosis
  Previous history of bacterial endocarditis
  Mitral valve prolapse with insufficiency†
Endocarditis prophylaxis not recommended
  Isolated secundum atrial septal defect
  Secundum atrial septal defect repaired without a patch 6 or more months earlier
  Patent ductus arteriosus ligated and divided 6 or more months earlier
  Postoperative coronary artery bypass graft surgery

*This table lists common conditions but is not meant to be all-inclusive.
†Definitive data to provide guidance in management of patients with mitral valve prolapse are particularly limited. It is clear that in general such patients are at low risk of development of endocarditis, but the risk-benefit ratio of prophylaxis in mitral valve prolapse is uncertain.

Patients Receiving Anticoagulants

Intramuscular injections are contraindicated in patients receiving heparin. Therefore, regimens employing intramuscular antibiotics should not be used. Intravenous or oral regimens should be substituted. Anticoagulation with warfarin sodium (Coumadin) is a relative contraindication to intramuscular injections. The risk of hematoma formation is lower than with heparin, and with careful technique intramuscular injections can be given if necessary. However, oral or intravenous regimens are more appropriate in patients receiving warfarin sodium.

Dental Procedures and Upper Respiratory Tract Surgical Procedures

Patients at risk for bacterial endocarditis should maintain the best possible oral health to reduce potential sources of bacterial seeding because poor dental hygiene or periodontal or periapical infections may induce bacteremia even in the absence of dental procedures. Edentulous patients may develop bacteremia from ulcers caused by ill-fitting dentures. Antibiotic prophylaxis is recommended with all dental procedures (including routine professional cleaning) likely to cause gingival bleeding. Because the spontaneous shedding of primary teeth or simple adjustment of orthodontic appliances do not present a significant risk of endocarditis, antibiotics are not necessary. Similarly, endotracheal intubation is not an indication for antibiotic prophylaxis unless associated with another procedure for which prophylaxis is recommended.

Because alpha-hemolytic (viridans) streptococci are most commonly implicated in endocarditis after dental procedures, prophylaxis should be specifically directed against these organisms. Certain upper respiratory tract procedures (for example, tonsillectomy, adenoidectomy, or bronchoscopy—especially with a rigid bronchoscope—and surgical procedures including biopsy involving respiratory mucosa) may also cause bacteremia with organisms having similar antibiotic susceptibilities to those producing bacteremia after dental procedures. Therefore, the same regimens are recommended. Endocarditis has not been reported in association with insertion of tympanostomy tubes. However, studies to define the risk of bacteremia with this procedure are not available.

Table B-3 contains suggested regimens for prophylaxis for dental procedures, and for surgical procedures and instrumentation of the upper respiratory tract. In those patients at particularly high risk for endocarditis (for example, those with prosthetic heart valves or surgically constructed systemic-pulmonary shunts), the committee favors the use of parenteral prophylactic antibiotics.

Table B-2   Procedures for which endocarditis prophylaxis is indicated

All dental procedures likely to induce gingival bleeding (not simple adjustment of orthodontic appliances or shedding of primary teeth)
Tonsillectomy or adenoidectomy (or both)
Surgical procedures or biopsy involving respiratory mucosa
Bronchoscopy, especially with a rigid bronchoscope*
Incision and drainage of infected tissue

*The risk with flexible bronchoscopy is low, but the necessity for prophylaxis is not yet defined.

Prophylaxis Recommendations for Dental Procedures and Surgery of Upper Respiratory Tract

1. Standard Regimen

ORAL PENICILLIN. For adults and children over 60 lb (27 kg): penicillin V 2 g 1 hour before the procedure and then 1 g 6 hours later. For children less than 60 lb: 1 g 1 hour before the procedure and then 500 mg 6 hours later.

For patients unable to take oral antibiotics before a procedure, 2 million units of aqueous penicillin G (50,000 units/kg for children) intravenously (IV) or intramuscularly (IM) 30 to 60 minutes before the procedure and 1 million units (25,000 units/kg for children) 6 hours later may be substituted. (Children's antibiotic dosages should not exceed the maximum adult doses.)

2. For Patients with Prosthetic Valves and Others with Highest Risk of Endocarditis

PARENTERAL AMPICILLIN AND GENTAMICIN. Ampicillin 1 to 2 g (50 mg/kg for children) plus gentamicin 1.5 mg/kg for children) both IM or IV one-half hour before the procedure, followed by 1 g oral penicillin V (500 mg for children under 60 lb) 6 hours later. Alternatively, the parenteral regimen should be repeated once 8 hours later. (Children's antibiotic dosages should not exceed the maximum adult dosages.)

Table B-3 Summary of recommended antibiotic regimens for dental/respiratory tract procedures

STANDARD REGIMEN	
For dental procedures that cause gingival bleeding, and oral/respiratory tract surgery	Penicillin V 2 g orally 1 hour before, then 1 g 6 hours later. For patients unable to take oral medications, 2 million units of aqueous penicillin G intravenously or intramuscularly 30-60 minutes before a procedure and 1 million units 6 hours later may be substituted
SPECIAL REGIMENS	
Parenteral regimen for use when maximal protection desired (for example, for patients with prosthetic valves)	Ampicillin 1-2 g intramuscularly or intravenously, plus gentamicin 1.5 mg/kg intramuscularly or intravenously, one-half hour before procedure, followed by 1 g oral penicillin V 6 hours later. Alternatively, the parenteral regimen may be repeated once 8 hours later
Oral regimen for penicillin-allergic patients	Erythromycin 1 g orally 1 hour before, then 500 mg 6 hours later
Parenteral regimen for penicillin-allergic patients	Vancomycin 1 g intravenously slowly over 1 hour, starting 1 hour before. No repeat dose is necessary

NOTE: Pediatric doses: Ampicillin 50 mg/kg per dose; erythromycin 20 mg/kg for first dose, then 10 mg/kg; gentamicin 2.0 mg/kg per dose; penicillin V full adult dose if greater than 60 lb (27 kg), one-half adult dose if less than 60 lb (27 kg); aqueous penicillin G 50,000 units/kg (25,000 units/kg for follow-up); vancomycin 20 mg/kg per dose. The intervals between doses are the same as for adults. Total doses should not exceed adult doses.

3. Standard Regimen for Patients Allergic to Penicillin

ORAL ERYTHROMYCIN. Erythromycin 1 g (20 mg/kg for children) 1 hour before the procedure and then 500 mg (10 mg/kg for children) 6 hours later. (Children's antibiotic dosages should not exceed the maximum adult dosages.)

For patients unable to tolerate oral erythromycin, changing to a different erythromycin preparation may be beneficial. For those who cannot tolerate either penicillin or erythromycin, an oral cephalosporin (1 g 1 hour before the procedure plus 500 mg 6 hours later) may be useful, but data are lacking to allow specific recommendation of this regimen. Tetracyclines cannot be recommended for this purpose.

4. Regimen for High-Risk Patients Allergic to Penicillin

IV VANCOMYCIN. Vancomycin 1 g (20 mg/kg for children) IV slowly over 1 hour starting 1 hour before the procedure. (Children's antibiotic dosages should not exceed the maximum adult dosages.) Because of the long half-life of vancomycin, a repeat dose should not be necessary.

NOTES: In unusual circumstances or in the case of delayed healing, it may be necessary to provide additional doses of antibotics even though bacteremia rarely persists longer than 15 minutes after the procedure. Penicillin V is the preferred form of oral penicillin because it is relatively resistant to gastric acid.

For those patients taking an oral penicillin for secondary prevention of rheumatic fever or for other purposes, viridans streptococci that are relatively resistant to penicilln may be present in the mouth. In such cases, the physician or dentist should select erythromycin or one of the parenteral regimens.

Some patients with a prosthetic heart valve in whom a high level of oral health is being maintained may be offered oral antibiotic prophylaxis for routine dental procedures. Parenteral antibiotics are recommended, however, for patients with prosthetic valves who require extensive dental procedures, especially extractions, or oral or gingival surgical procedures.

Cardiac Surgery

Patients undergoing open-heart surgery—especially with placement of prosthetic heart valves or prosthetic intravascular or intracardiac materials—are at risk for bacterial endocarditis. Because the morbidity and mortality of endocarditis in such patients are high, maximal preventive efforts including prophylactic antibiotics are recommended.

Endocarditis associated with open heart surgery is most often caused by *Staphylococcus aureus,* coagulase-negative staphylococci, or diphtheroids. Streptococci, gram-negative bacteria, and fungi are less common. No single antibiotic regimen is effective against all these organisms. Furthermore, prolonged use of broad-spectrum antibiotics may predispose to superinfection with unusual or resistant microorganisms.

Therefore, prophylaxis at the time of cardiac surgery should be directed primarily against staphylococci and should be of short duration. Penicillinase-resistant penicillins or "first-generation" cephalosporins are most often selected, although the choice of antibiotics should be influenced by each hospital's antibiotic susceptibility data. For example, high prevalence of infection by methicillin-resistant staphylococci in a particular institution should prompt consideration of vancomycin for preoperative prophylaxis. Prophylaxis should be started immediately before the operative procedure and continued for no more than 2 days after surgery to minimize emergence of resistant microorganisms. The effects of cardiopulmonary bypass and compromised postoperative renal function on serum antibiotic levels should be considered, and doses timed appropriately before and during the procedure.

Careful preoperative dental evaluation is recommended so that required dental treatment can be completed at least several weeks before cardiac surgery whenever possible. Such measures may decrease the incidence of late postoperative endocarditis.

Status after Cardiac Surgery

The same precautions should be observed in the years after open heart surgery that have been outlined for the unoperated patient undergoing dental procedures. The risk of endocarditis appears to continue indefinitely and is particularly significant in patients with prosthetic heart valves, in whom the mortality from endocarditis is considerable. Patients with an isolated secundum atrial septal defect repaired without a prosthetic patch and those who have had ligation and division of a patent ductus arteriosus are not at increased risk of developing endocarditis after a 6-month healing period after surgery. There is no evidence that patients who have undergone coronary artery bypass graft surgery are at risk to develop endocarditis unless another cardiac defect is present. Therefore antibiotics to protect against endocarditis are not needed for these individuals.

Other Indications for Antibiotic Prophylaxis to Prevent Endocarditis

In susceptible patients, prophylaxis to prevent endocarditis is also indicated for surgical procedures on any infected or contaminated tissues, including incision and drainage of abscesses. In these circumstances, regimens should be individualized but in most instances should include antibiotics effective against *S. aureus*.

Antibiotic prophylaxis for the foregoing surgical and dental procedures should also be given to patients with a documented previous episode of bacterial endocarditis, even in the absence of clinically detectable heart disease.

Patients with indwelling transvenous cardiac pacemakers appear to present a low risk of endocarditis: when such cases occur they are predominantly caused by staphylococci. However, dentists and physicians may choose to use prophylactic antibiotics when dental and surgical procedures are performed in these patients. The same recommendations apply to renal dialysis patients with arteriovenous shunt appliances. Endocarditis prophylaxis also deserves consideration in patients with ventriculo-atrial shunts for hydrocephalus, because there are documented cases of bacterial endocarditis in these patients.

Prophylactic antibiotics are not required in diagnostic cardiac catheterization and angiography because with adequate aseptic techniques the occurrence of endocarditis after these procedures is extremely low.

SELECTED REFERENCES

Bisno, A.L., ed. Treatment of infective endocarditis, New York, Grune & Stratton, 1981.

Kaplan, E.L., and Taranta, A.V., eds. Infective endocarditis. American Heart Association Monograph No. 52, Dallas, AHA, 1977.

Rahimtoola, S.H., ed. Infective endocarditis. New York, Grune & Stratton, 1977.

Kaye, D., ed. Infective endocarditis. Baltimore, University Park Press, 1976.

Freedman, L.R. Infective endocarditis and other intravascular infections. New York, Plenum Publishing Corp., 1982.

Kaplan, E.L., and Shulman, S.T. Infective endocarditis. In Adams, F.H., and Emmanouilides, G.C., eds. Moss' heart disease in infants, children, and adolescents, ed 3. Baltimore, Williams & Wilkins Co, 1983.

Gersony, W.M. Infective endocarditis. In Behrman, R.E., and Vaughn, V.C., eds. Nelson's textbook of pediatrics, ed 12. Philadelphia, W.B. Saunders Co., 1983.

Durack, D.T. Infective and noninfective endocarditis. In Hurst, J.W., ed. The heart, ed 5. Hightstown, N.J., McGraw-Hill Book Co., 1981.

Durack, D.T. Prophylaxis of infective endocarditis. In Mandell, G.L., Douglas, R.G., Jr., and Bennett, J.E., eds. Principles and practice of infectious diseases, ed 2. New York, John Wiley & Sons, Inc., 1984.

Index

COMPREHENSIVE DENTAL HYGIENE CARE

New 2nd Edition! By Irene R. Woodall, R.D.H., M.A., Ph.D.; Bonnie R. Dafoe, R.D.H., B.S.; Nancy Stutsman Young, R.D.H., M.Ed.; Leslie Weed-Fonner, R.D.H., M.Ed., M.S.W.; and Samuel L. Yankell, Ph.D., F.D.H.

". . . (It) reads easily, is concise and interesting, and progresses logically from basic dental hygiene skills to skills of a more advanced level . . . the authors are well qualified to write this book . . . Comprehensive Dental Hygiene Care is exciting, new and very worthwhile." (Dental Hygiene, review of the last edition)

- focuses on patient-centered care
- emphasizes methods of including the patient in the decision-making process and instructing him/her in self-care
- presents technical procedures step-by-step — including instrumentation
- integrates theory and practice
- includes a new chapter on instrument sharpening

1985. 732 pages, 694 illustrations. (Book Code: 5700-8) $37.95.

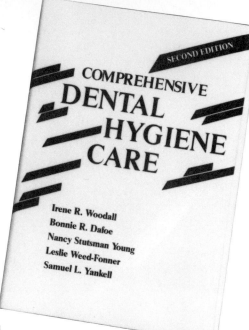

COMPREHENSIVE DENTAL HYGIENE CARE
SECOND EDITION

Irene R. Woodall
Bonnie R. Dafoe
Nancy Stutsman Young
Leslie Weed-Fonner
Samuel L. Yankell

OUTLINE OF CONTENTS

Please contact your Mosby representative or medical book distributor. You can also call Mosby at 800-345-8500, ext. 15. Canadian customers call 416-298-1588. Prices differ outside the U.S. and are subject to change. In the U.S., mail this coupon to: Linda Anderson, The C.V. Mosby Company, 11830 Westline Industrial Dr., St. Louis, MO 63146. 30-day approval good in U.S., Canada, and U.S. Possessions only. In U.S., add applicable sales tax. Canadian customers, please mail to: The C.V. Mosby Company, Ltd., 5240 Finch Ave. East, Scarborough, Ontario M1S 4P2. OUTSIDE the U.S. and Canada, all orders must be prepaid. A pro forma invoice will be sent. **ALL PRICES SUBJECT TO CHANGE WITHOUT NOTICE.**

MOSBY
TIMES MIRROR

AMS489-005